Rehabilitation Techniques

for Sports Medicine and Athletic Training

SIXTH EDITION

Rehabilitation Techniques
for Sports Medicine and Athletic Training

SIXTH EDITION

Editor

William E. Prentice, PhD, PT, ATC, FNATA
Professor, Coordinator of the Sports Medicine Program
Department of Exercise and Sport Medicine
University of North Carolina at Chapel Hill
Chapel Hill, North Carolina

Laboratory Manual Prepared By
Thomas W. Kaminski, PhD, ATC, FNATA, FACSM
Professor, Director of Athletic Training Education
University of Delaware
Newark, Delaware

PowerPoint Presentations Prepared By
Jason Scibek, PhD, LAT, ATC
Duquesne University
Pittsburgh, Pennsylvania

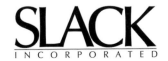

SLACK
INCORPORATED

www.Healio.com/books

ISBN: 978-1-61711-931-6

Instructors: *Rehabilitation Techniques for Sports Medicine and Athletic Training, Sixth Edition Laboratory Manual* is also available from SLACK Incorporated. Don't miss this important companion to *Rehabilitation Techniques for Sports Medicine and Athletic Training, Sixth Edition*. To obtain the Laboratory Manual, please visit http://www.efacultylounge.com.

The procedures and practices described in this publication should be implemented in a manner consistent with the professional standards set for the circumstances that apply in each specific situation. Every effort has been made to confirm the accuracy of the information presented and to correctly relate generally accepted practices. The authors, editors, and publisher cannot accept responsibility for errors or exclusions or for the outcome of the material presented herein. There is no expressed or implied warranty of this book or information imparted by it. Care has been taken to ensure that drug selection and dosages are in accordance with currently accepted/recommended practice. Off-label uses of drugs may be discussed. Due to continuing research, changes in government policy and regulations, and various effects of drug reactions and interactions, it is recommended that the reader carefully review all materials and literature provided for each drug, especially those that are new or not frequently used. Some drugs or devices in this publication have clearance for use in a restricted research setting by the Food and Drug and Administration or FDA. Each professional should determine the FDA status of any drug or device prior to use in their practice.

Any review or mention of specific companies or products is not intended as an endorsement by the author or publisher.

SLACK Incorporated uses a review process to evaluate submitted material. Prior to publication, educators or clinicians provide important feedback on the content that we publish. We welcome feedback on this work.

Published by: SLACK Incorporated
                      6900 Grove Road
                      Thorofare, NJ 08086 USA
                      Telephone: 856-848-1000
                      Fax: 856-848-6091
                      www.Healio.com/books

Contact SLACK Incorporated for more information about other books in this field or about the availability of our books from distributors outside the United States.

Library of Congress Cataloging-in-Publication Data

Rehabilitation techniques for sports medicine and athletic training / [edited by] William E. Prentice. -- Sixth edition.
    p. ; cm.
Includes index.
ISBN 978-1-61711-931-6 (alk. paper)
I. Prentice, William E., editor.
[DNLM: 1. Athletic Injuries--rehabilitation. 2. Physical Therapy Modalities. QT 261]
RD97
617.1'027--dc23
                            2014042486

For permission to reprint material in another publication, contact SLACK Incorporated. Authorization to photocopy items for internal, personal, or academic use is granted by SLACK Incorporated provided that the appropriate fee is paid directly to Copyright Clearance Center. Prior to photocopying items, please contact the Copyright Clearance Center at 222 Rosewood Drive, Danvers, MA 01923 USA; phone: 978-750-8400; website: www.copyright.com; email: info@copyright.com

Printed in the United States of America.

Last digit is print number: 10   9   8   7   6   5   4   3   2   1

DEDICATION

This book is dedicated to my family—Tena, Brian, and Zachary—who make an effort such as this worthwhile. They keep me grounded and help me to maintain the focus in both my personal life and my professional life.

CONTENTS

ACKNOWLEDGMENTS

The preparation of the manuscript for a textbook is a long-term and extremely demanding effort that requires input and cooperation on the part of many individuals. I would like to personally thank each of the contributing authors. They were asked to contribute to this text because I have tremendous respect for them both personally and professionally. These individuals have distinguished themselves as educators and clinicians dedicated to the field of athletic training. I am exceedingly grateful for their input. Brien Cummings, my Acquisitions Editor, has provided tremendous support throughout the transition to my new publisher. He has been persistent and diligent in the completion of this text. As always, Gary O'Brien, my long time developmental editor, has been instrumental in organizing and embedding hundreds of instructional videos into the eBook version of this text. None of my projects would be possible without his invaluable input.

— Bill Prentice

ABOUT THE EDITOR

William E. Prentice, PhD, PT, ATC, FNATA is recognized as an author, educator, and clinician. He received both BS and MS degrees from the University of Delaware, a PhD degree in sports medicine and applied physiology from the University of Virginia, and BSPT degree in physical therapy from the University of North Carolina. He is a Professor in the Department of Exercise and Sport Science, and has served as the Program Director of the NATA Accredited Post-Professional Athletic Training Education Program at the University of North Carolina at Chapel Hill since 1980. He started his career as an Assistant Athletic Trainer at Temple University prior to beginning his PhD at Virginia. He also served for 10 years as the Director of Sports Medicine Education for the Healthsouth Corporation.

Dr. Prentice is the author of 49 editions of nine different textbooks most notably *Principles of Athletic Training, Essentials of Athletic Injury Management, Athletic Training: An Introduction to Professional Practice, Therapeutic Modalities in Sports Medicine and Athletic Training, Rehabilitation Techniques in Sports Medicine and Athletic Training, Therapeutic Modalities for Physical Therapists, Musculoskeletal Intervention: Techniques for Therapeutic Exercise,* and *Get Fit, StayFit.* He has published more than 100 journal articles and abstracts, and has made more than 220 lectures and presentations. Prentice served as the athletic trainer for the Women's Soccer Program at the University of North Carolina for 26 years since 1980 and during that period the team won 17 NCAA and 1 AIAW National Championships.

Dr. Prentice has been the recipient of numerous awards from the NATA, including most notably the Sayers "Bud" Miller Distinguished Athletic Training Educator Award in 1999; the Educational Multimedia Committee Videotape Production Award in 1997; and the Most Distinguished Athletic Trainer Award in 1999. In 2004, Dr. Prentice was inducted into the National Athletic Trainers Association's Hall of Fame. In 2006, the NATA established the William E. Prentice Scholarship that is presented annually in his name. In 2008, Dr. Prentice was selected in the inaugural class as an NATA Fellow. In 2012, Dr. Prentice was inducted into the Mid-Atlantic Athletic Trainer's Association Hall of Fame. In 2014, Dr. Prentice received the Dr. Ernst Jokl Sports Medicine Award from the United States Sports Academy.

CONTRIBUTING AUTHORS

Jolene L. Bennett, MA, PT, OCS, ATC, CertMDT
(Chapter 5)
Clinical Specialist for Orthopedics and Sports
  Medicine
Spectrum Health Rehabilitation and Sports
  Medicine
Visser Family YMCA
Adjunct Faculty
Clinical Doctorate of Physical Therapy
Grand Valley State University
Grandville, Michigan

Troy Blackburn, PhD, ATC (Chapter 6)
Associate Professor
Department of Exercise and Sport Science
University of North Carolina
Chapel Hill, North Carolina

Michelle C. Boling, PhD, LAT, ATC (Chapter 21)
Associate Professor
Department of Athletic Training and
  Physical Therapy
University of North Florida
Jacksonville, Florida

Michael Clark, DPT, MS, PT, PES, CES (Chapter 5)
Chairman, Founder and CEO
Fusionetics
Alpharetta, GA

Bernard DePalma, MEd, PT, ATC (Chapter 20)
Head Athletic Trainer
Cornell University
Ithaca, New York

Joe Gieck, EdD, PT, ATC (Chapter 4)
Professor Emeritus, Sports Medicine
University of Virginia
Charlottesville, Virginia

Kevin Guskiewicz, PhD, ATC, FNATA, FACSM
(Chapter 7)
Senior Associate Dean, College of Arts and
  Sciences
Professor, Department of Exercise and
  Sport Science
University of North Carolina
Chapel Hill, North Carolina

Doug Halverson, MA, ATC, CSCS (Chapter 20)
Staff Athletic Trainer
Campus Health Service
Division of Sports Medicine
University of North Carolina
Chapel Hill, North Carolina

Elizabeth G. Hedgpeth, EdD (Chapter 4)
Lecturer, Sport Psychology
Department of Exercise and Sport Science
University of North Carolina
Chapel Hill, North Carolina

Christopher J. Hirth, MSPT, PT, ATC (Chapter 22)
Rehabilitation Coordinator
Campus Health Service
Division of Sports Medicine
University of North Carolina
Chapel Hill, North Carolina

Barbara J. Hoogenboom, EdD, PT, SCS, ATC
(Chapters 5 and 15)
Professor
Physical Therapy Program
Grand Valley State University
Grand Rapids, Michigan

Daniel N. Hooker, PhD, PT, ATC (Chapter 24)
Athletic Trainer/ Physical Therapist
Campus Health Service
Division of Sports Medicine
University of North Carolina
Chapel Hill, North Carolina

Stuart L. (Skip) Hunter, PT, ATC (Chapter 23)
Owner, Clemson Sports Medicine
Clemson, South Carolina

Scott Lephart, PhD, ATC (Chapter 6)
Dean
College of Health Sciences
University of Kentucky
Lexington, Kentucky

Nancy E. Lomax, PT (Chapter 15)
Staff Physical Therapist
Spectrum Health Rehabilitation and Sports
  Medicine Services
Visser Family YMCA
Grandville, Michigan

Michael McGee, EdD, LAT, ATC (Chapter 16)
Chair, School of Health, Exercise and
  Sport Science
Program Director of Athletic Training
Director and Head Athletic Trainer
Program Coordinator of Community Health
Hickory, North Carolina

Joseph B. Myers, PhD, ATC (Chapter 17)
Professor
Department of Exercise and Sport Science
University of North Carolina
Chapel Hill, North Carolina

Darin A. Padua, PhD, ATC (Chapters 3 and 21)
Professor
Chair, Department of Exercise and Sport Science
University of North Carolina
Chapel Hill, North Carolina

Terri Jo Rucinski, MA, PT, ATC (Chapter 17)
Staff Physical Therapist/Athletic Trainer
Campus Health Service
Division of Sports Medicine
University of North Carolina
Chapel Hill, North Carolina

Anne Marie Schneider, OTR/L, CHT (Chapter 19)
Certified Hand Therapist/Office Manager
Proaxis Therapy
Carrboro/Durham, North Carolina

Rob Schneider, PT, MS, LAT, ATC (Chapter 17)
Co-owner Balanced Physical Therapy
Carrboro/Durham, North Carolina

Patrick Sells, DA, CES (Chapter 10)
Associate Professor
School of Physical Therapy
Belmont University
Nashville, Tennessee

Steven R. Tippett, PhD, PT, SCS, ATC (Chapter 11)
Professor and Department Chair
Department of Physical Therapy and Health
  Science
Bradley University
Peoria, Illinois

C. Buz Swanik, PhD, ATC (Chapter 6)
Associate Professor
College of Health Sciences
University of Delaware
Newark, Delaware

*Michael L. Voight, DHSc, PT, SCS, OCS, ATC,
  CSCS, FAPTA (Chapter 11)*
Professor
School of Physical Therapy
Belmont University
Nashville, Tennessee

Steven M. Zinder, PhD, ATC (Chapter 23)
Assistant Professor
Department of Orthopedics and Sports Medicine
University of South Florida
Tampa, FL

Pete Zulia, PT, SCS, ATC (Chapter 18)
Co-founding Partner
Oxford Physical Therapy Centers
Oxford, Ohio

PREFACE

Historically the authors of *Rehabilitation Techniques for Sports Medicine and Athletic Training* have tried diligently to stay on the cutting edge of the athletic training profession with regard not only to presenting a comprehensive and ever expanding body of knowledge, but also with the latest techniques of delivering educational content to students. As will become readily apparent, this latest sixth edition reflects what is perhaps the most exciting and revolutionary revision in the 27 year history of this text. This text is now being published by SLACK Incorporated in Thorofare, NJ. Most evident in this edition, is the addition of four-color images and illustrations throughout the text, which markedly enhances the student's ability to learn visually. In addition to the hard copy of this text, the editor has created an eBook version of this text that will facilitate direct access to nearly 700 instructional videos from within the body of the text that clearly demonstrate specific clinical techniques, rehabilitative exercises, and manual therapy skills that are used by experienced athletic trainers.

ORGANIZATION

This sixth edition is divided into four sections. Section I discusses the basics of the rehabilitation process. It begins by discussing the important considerations in designing a rehabilitation program for the injured patient and providing a basic overview of the rehabilitation process (Chapter 1). It is essential for the athletic trainer to understand the importance of the healing process and how it should dictate the course of rehabilitation (Chapter 2). The evaluation process is critical in first determining the exact nature of an existing injury and then designing a rehabilitation program based on the findings of that evaluation (Chapter 3). It is also essential to be aware of the psychological aspects of rehabilitation with which the injured patient must deal (Chapter 4).

Section II deals with achieving the goals of rehabilitation. The chapters address primary goals of any sports medicine rehabilitation program: establishing core stability (Chapter 5), reestablishing neuromuscular control (Chapter 6), regaining postural stability and balance (Chapter 7), restoring range of motion and improving flexibility (Chapter 8), regaining muscular strength, endurance, and power (Chapter 9), and maintaining cardiorespiratory fitness during rehabilitation (Chapter 10). Athletic trainers have many rehabilitation "tools" with which they can choose to treat an injured athlete. How they choose to use these tools is often a matter of personal preference.

Section III discusses in detail how these tools can be best incorporated into a rehabilitation program to achieve the goals identified in the first section. The chapters in Section III focus on primary tools of rehabilitation: plyometric exercise (Chapter 11), open vs closed kinetic chain exercise (Chapter 12), joint mobilization and traction techniques (Chapter 13), proprioceptive neuromuscular facilitation techniques (Chapter 14), aquatic therapy (Chapter 15), and functional progressions and functional testing (Chapter 16).

Section IV of this text goes into great detail on specific rehabilitation techniques that are used in treating a variety of injuries. Specific rehabilitation techniques are included for the shoulder (Chapter 17), the elbow (Chapter 18), the wrist, hand, and fingers (Chapter 19), the groin, hip, and thigh (Chapter 20), the knee (Chapter 21), the lower leg (Chapter 22), the ankle and foot (Chapter 23), and the spine (Chapter 24). Each chapter begins with a discussion of the pertinent functional anatomy and biomechanics of that region. An extensive series of photographs illustrating a wide variety of rehabilitative exercises is presented in each chapter. The last portion of each chapter involves in-depth discussion of the pathomechanics, injury mechanism, rehabilitation concerns, rehabilitation progressions, and finally, criteria for return to activity for specific injuries.

The updated sixth edition of *Rehabilitation Techniques for Sports Medicine and Athletic Training* offers a comprehensive reference guide emphasizing the most current techniques of sport injury rehabilitation for the athletic trainer overseeing programs of rehabilitation.

COMPREHENSIVE COVERAGE OF EVIDENCE-BASED MATERIAL

Growth of the athletic training profession, dictates the necessity for expanding our research efforts to identify new and more effective methods and techniques for dealing with sport-related injury. Any athletic trainer charged with the responsibility of supervising a rehabilitation program knows that the most currently accepted and up-to-date rehabilitation protocols tend to change rapidly. A sincere effort has been made by the contributing authors to present the most recent information on the various aspects of injury rehabilitation currently available in the literature. Additionally, this manuscript has been critically reviewed by selected athletic trainers who are well-respected clinicians, educators, and researchers in this field to further ensure that the material presented is accurate and current.

PERTINENT TO THE ATHLETIC TRAINER

Many texts are currently available on the subject of rehabilitation of injury in various patient populations. As in the past, the sixth edition of this text concentrates exclusively on the application of rehabilitation techniques in a sport-related setting for a unique sports medicine emphasis.

PEDAGOGICAL AIDS

The teaching aids provided in this text to assist the student include the following:

- *Objectives:* These goals are listed at the beginning of each chapter to introduce students to the points that will be emphasized.

- *Figures and Tables:* The number of new photos and tables included throughout the text has been significantly increased and are now in four-color in an effort to provide as much visual and graphic demonstration of specific rehabilitation techniques and exercises as possible.

- *Clinical Decision-Making Exercises:* About 150 clinical decision-making exercises are found throughout the text to challenge the student to integrate and apply the information presented in this text to clinical cases that typically occur in an athletic training setting. Solutions for each exercise are presented at the end of each chapter.

- *Rehabilitation Plans:* Rehabilitation Plans can be found in each chapter in Section IV as examples of case studies that help apply the thought process an athletic trainer should use in developing and implementing a rehabilitation program.

- *Summary:* Each chapter has a summary list that reinforces the major points presented.

- *References:* A comprehensive list of up-to-date references is presented at the end of each chapter to guide the reader to additional information about the chapter content.

- *Glossary:* A glossary of terms is provided for quick reference.

ANCILLARIES

A Laboratory Manual accompanies the sixth edition of *Rehabilitation Techniques for Sports Medicine and Athletic Training*. It has been prepared by Dr. Tom Kaminski of the University of Delaware to provide hands-on directed learning experiences for students using the text. It includes practical laboratory exercises designed to enhance student understanding. The Laboratory Manual is available for download at www.efacultylounge.com

INTRODUCTION

This sixth edition of *Rehabilitation Techniques for Sports Medicine and Athletic Training* is for the professional student of athletic training who is interested in gaining more in-depth exposure to the theory and practical application of rehabilitation techniques used in a sports medicine environment. The purpose of this text is to provide the athletic trainer with a comprehensive guide to the design, implementation, and supervision of rehabilitation programs for sport-related injuries. It is intended for use in courses in athletic training that deal with practical application of theory in a clinical setting. The contributing authors have collectively attempted to combine their expertise and knowledge to produce a text that encompasses all aspects of sports medicine rehabilitation.

SECTION I

The Basis of Injury Rehabilitation

CHAPTER 1

Essential Considerations in Designing a Rehabilitation Program for the Injured Patient

William E. Prentice, PhD, PT, ATC, FNATA

After completing this chapter, the athletic training student should be able to do the following:

- Describe the relationships among the members of the rehabilitation team: the athletic trainers, team physicians, coaches, strength and conditioning specialists, athlete, and athlete's family.

- Express the philosophy of the rehabilitative process in a sports medicine environment.

- Realize the importance of understanding the healing process, the biomechanics, and the psychological aspects of a rehabilitation program.

- Arrange the individual short-term and long-term goals of a rehabilitation program.

- Discuss the components that should be included in a well-designed rehabilitation program.

- Propose the criteria and the decision-making process for determining when the injured patient may return to full activity.

One of the primary goals of every sports medicine professional is to create a playing environment that is as safe as it can possibly be. Regardless of that effort, the nature of participation in sport and physical activity dictates that injuries will eventually occur. Fortunately, few of the injuries that occur in an athletic setting are life-threatening. The majority of the injuries are not serious and lend themselves to rapid rehabilitation. When injuries do occur, the focus of the athletic trainer shifts from

Prentice WE, ed.
Rehabilitation Techniques for Sports Medicine and Athletic Training (pp 3-21).
© 2015 SLACK Incorporated.

injury prevention to injury treatment and reha-bilitation. In a sports medicine setting, the ath-letic trainer generally assumes primary respon-sibility for the design, implementation, and supervision of the rehabilitation program for the injured athlete. The athletic trainer respon-sible for overseeing an exercise rehabilitation program must have as complete an understand-ing of the injury as possible, including knowl-edge of how the injury was sustained, the major anatomical structures affected, the degree or grade of trauma, and the stage or phase of the injury's healing.[3,18]

THE REHABILITATION TEAM

Providing a comprehensive rehabilitation program for an injured patient in an athletic environment requires a group effort to be most effective. The rehabilitation process requires communication among a number of individu-als, each of whom must perform specific func-tions relative to caring for the injured athlete. Under ideal conditions, an interprofessional team that includes the athletic trainer (and the athletic training students), the athlete, the phy-sician, nurses, physical therapists, the coaches, the strength and conditioning specialist, and the injured athlete's family will communicate freely and function as a team. This group is intimately involved with the rehabilitative process, beginning with patient assessment, treatment selection, and implementation, and ending with functional exercises and return to activity. The athletic trainer directs the post-acute phase of the rehabilitation, and it is essential that the patient understand that this part of the recovery is just as crucial as surgical technique to the return of normal joint func-tion and the subsequent return to full activity. All decisions made by the physician, the athletic trainer, and the coaches that dictate the course of rehabilitation ultimately affect the injured patient.

> ### Clinical Decision-Making Exercise 1-1
> A team physician has diagnosed a swimmer with thoracic outlet syndrome. The athletic trainer is developing a rehabilitation plan for this patient. What considerations must be taken into account?

Of all the members of the rehabilitation team charged with providing health care, per-haps none is more intimately involved than the athletic trainer. The athletic trainer is the one individual who deals directly with the patient throughout the entire period of rehabilitation, from the time of the initial injury until the complete, unrestricted return to activity. The athletic trainer is most directly responsible for all phases of health care in an athletic envi-ronment, including preventing injuries from occurring, providing initial first aid and injury management, evaluating and diagnosing inju-ries, and designing and supervising a timely and effective program of rehabilitation that can facilitate the safe and expeditious return to activity.

In 2010 the Board of Certification (BOC) completed the latest role delineation study, which defines the profession of athletic train-ing. This study was designed to examine the primary tasks performed by the entry-level athletic trainer and the knowledge and skills required to perform each task. The panel deter-mined that the roles of the practicing athletic trainer could be divided into five major areas or performance domains: injury/illness preven-tion and wellness protection, clinical evaluation and diagnosis, immediate and emergency care, treatment and rehabilitation, and organiza-tional and professional health and well-being.

An athletic trainer must work closely with and under the supervision of the team physi-cian with respect to designing rehabilitation and reconditioning protocols that make use of appropriate therapeutic exercise, rehabilita-tive equipment, manual therapy techniques, or therapeutic modalities. The athletic trainer should then assume the responsibility of over-seeing the rehabilitative process, ultimately returning the patient to full activity.

Certainly, the athletic trainer has an obliga-tion to the patient to understand the nature of the injury, the function of the structures damaged, and the different tools available to safely rehabilitate that patient. Additionally, the athletic trainer must understand the treatment philosophy of the patient's physician and be careful in applying different treatment regimens because what may be a safe but outdated technique in the opinion of one physician may be the treatment of choice to another. The successful athletic trainer must demonstrate flexibility in his or her approach to rehabilitation by incorporating techniques that are evidence-based and effective, but somewhat variable from one patient to another, as well as from one physician to another.

Communication is crucial to prevent misunderstandings and a subsequent loss of rapport with either the patient or the physician. The patient must always be informed and made aware of the why, how, and when factors that collectively dictate the course of an injury rehabilitation program.

Any personal relationship takes some time to grow and develop. The relationship between the coach and the athletic trainer is no different. The athletic trainer must demonstrate to the coach his or her capability to correctly manage an injury and guide the course of a rehabilitation program. It will take some time for the coach to develop trust and confidence in the athletic trainer. The coach must understand that what the athletic trainer wants is exactly the same as what the coach wants—to get an injured patient healthy and back to practice as quickly and safely as possible.

This is not to say, however, that the coaches should not be involved with the decision-making process. For example, when a patient is rehabilitating an injury, there may be drills or technical instruction sessions that the individual can participate in without exacerbating the injury. Thus the coaches, athletic trainer, and team physician should be able to negotiate what that individual can and cannot do safely in the course of a practice.

Athletes are frequently caught in the middle between coaches who tell them to do one thing and medical staff who tell them something else. The athletic trainer must respect the job that the coach has to do and should do whatever can be done to support the coach. Close communication between the coach and the athletic trainer is essential so that everyone is on the same page.

Clinical Decision-Making Exercise 1-2

A gymnast has just had an anterior cruciate ligament (ACL) reconstruction. The orthopedist has prescribed some active range of motion (AROM) exercises to start the rehabilitation process. The patient is progressing very quickly and wants to increase the intensity of her activity. What should the athletic trainer do to address the patient's request?

When rehabilitating an injured patient, particularly in a secondary school or middle school setting, the athletic trainer, the coach, and the physician must take the time to explain and inform the patient's parents about the course of the injury rehabilitation process. With a patient of secondary school age, the parents' decisions regarding health care must be of primary consideration. In certain situations, particularly at the secondary school and middle school levels, many parents will insist that their child be seen by their family physician rather than by the individual who may be designated as the team physician. This creates a situation in which the athletic trainer must work and communicate with many different "team physicians." The opinion of the family physician must be respected even if that individual has little or no experience with injuries related to sports.

It should be clear that the physician working in cooperation with the athletic trainer assumes the responsibility of making the final decisions relative to the course of rehabilitation for the patient from the time of injury until full return to activity. The coaches must defer to and should support the decisions of the medical staff in any matter regarding the course of the rehabilitative process.

THE PHILOSOPHY OF SPORTS MEDICINE REHABILITATION

The approach to rehabilitation is considerably different in a sports medicine environment than in most other rehabilitation settings.[4] The competitive nature of athletics necessitates an aggressive approach to rehabilitation. Because the competitive season in most sports is relatively short, the patient does not have the luxury of being able to sit around and do nothing until the injury heals. The goal is to return to activity as soon as is safely possible. Consequently, the athletic trainer tends to play games with the healing process, never really allowing enough time for an injury to completely heal. The athletic trainer who is supervising the rehabilitation program usually performs a "balancing act"—walking along a thin line between not pushing the patient hard enough or fast enough and being overly aggressive. In either case, a mistake in judgment on the part of the athletic trainer can hinder return to activity.

Understanding the Healing Process

Decisions as to when and how to alter or progress a rehabilitation program should be based primarily on the process of injury healing. The athletic trainer must possess a sound understanding of both the sequence and the time frames for the various phases of healing, realizing that certain physiological events must occur during each of the phases. Anything that is done during a rehabilitation program that interferes with this healing process will likely increase the length of time required for rehabilitation and slow return to full activity. The healing process must have an opportunity to accomplish what it is supposed to. At best the athletic trainer can only try to create an environment that is conducive to the healing process. Little can be done to speed up the process physiologically, but many things can impede healing (see Chapter 2).

Exercise Intensity

The SAID Principle (an acronym for Specific Adaptation to Imposed Demand) states that when an injured structure is subjected to stresses and overloads of varying intensities, it will gradually adapt over time to whatever demands are placed upon it.[17] During the rehabilitation process, the stresses of reconditioning exercises must not be so great as to exacerbate the injury before the injured structure has had a chance to adapt specifically to the increased demands. Engaging in exercise that is too intense or too prolonged can be detrimental to the progress of rehabilitation. Indications that the intensity of the exercises being incorporated into the rehabilitation program exceed the limits of the healing process include an increase in the amount of swelling, an increase in pain, a loss or a plateau in strength, a loss or a plateau in ROM, or an increase in the laxity of a healing ligament.[24] If an exercise or activity causes any of these signs, the athletic trainer must back off and become less aggressive in the rehabilitation program.

Clinical Decision-Making Exercise 1-3

A baseball player recently underwent surgery to repair a superior labrum anterior and posterior (SLAP) lesion and torn rotator cuff. He wants to know why he can't start throwing right away. What is your reason for why he must progress slowly?

In most injury situations, early exercise rehabilitation involves submaximal exercise performed in short bouts that are repeated several times daily. Exercise intensity must be commensurate with healing. As recovery increases, the intensity of exercise also increases, with the exercise performed less often.[2] Finally, the patient returns to a conditioning mode of exercise, which often includes high-intensity exercise three to four times per week.

Understanding the Psychological Aspects of Rehabilitation

The psychological aspects of how an individual deals with an injury are a critical yet often neglected factor in the rehabilitation process. Injury and illness produce a wide range of emotional reactions; therefore the athletic trainer needs to develop an understanding of the psyche of each patient.[9] Individuals vary in terms of pain threshold, cooperation and compliance, competitiveness, denial of disability, depression, intrinsic and extrinsic motivation, anger, fear, guilt, and the ability to adjust to injury. Besides dealing with the mental aspect of the injury, sports psychology can also be used to improve total athletic performance through the use of visualization, self-hypnosis, and relaxation techniques (see Chapter 4).

Understanding the Pathomechanics of Injury

When a joint or other anatomic structure is damaged by injury, normal biomechanical function is compromised. Adaptive changes occur that alter the manner in which various forces collectively act upon that joint to produce motion. Thus the biomechanics of joint motion are changed as a result of that injury.[15]

It is critical that the athletic trainer supervising a rehabilitation program has a solid foundation in biomechanics and functional human anatomy to be effective in designing a rehabilitation program. An athletic trainer who does not understand the biomechanics of normal motion will find it very difficult to identify existing adaptive or compensatory changes in motion and then to know what must be done in a rehabilitation program to correct the pathomechanics.

Understanding the Concept of the Kinetic Chain

The athletic trainer must understand the concept of the kinetic chain and must realize that the entire body is a kinetic chain that operates as an integrated functional unit.[12] The kinetic chain is composed of not only the muscular system including muscles, tendons, and fascia, but also the articular system and neural system. Each of these systems functions simultaneously with the others to allow for structural and functional efficiency. The central nervous system sorts the cumulative information from these three systems and allows for neuromuscular control. If any system within the kinetic chain is not working efficiently, the other systems are forced to adapt and compensate; this

can lead to tissue overload, decreased performance, and predictable patterns of injury.[6]

The functional integration of the systems allows for optimal neuromuscular efficiency during functional activities. In reality, movements in everyday life require dynamic postural control through multiple planes of motion and at different speeds of motion. Optimal functioning of all contributing components of the kinetic chain results in appropriate length-tension relationships, optimal force-couple relationships, precise arthrokinematics, and optimal neuromuscular control. Efficiency and longevity of the kinetic chain requires optimal integration of each system.[6]

Injury to the kinetic chain rarely involves only one structure. Since the kinetic chain functions as an integrated unit, dysfunction in one system leads to compensations and adaptations in other systems. The myofascial, neuromuscular, and articular systems all play a significant role in the functional pathology of the kinetic chain. Rehabilitation should focus on functional movements that integrate all components necessary to achieve optimal movement performance. Concepts of muscle imbalances, myofascial adhesions, altered arthrokinematics, and abnormal neuromuscular control need to be addressed by the athletic trainer when developing a comprehensive rehabilitation program.[6]

Understanding the Concept of Integrated Functional Movement

To develop a comprehensive rehabilitation program, the athletic trainer must not only fully understand the concept of the functional kinetic chain but also, most importantly, the definition of function. Function is integrated, multiplanar movement that requires acceleration, deceleration, and stabilization.[6,22] Functional kinetic chain rehabilitation is a comprehensive approach that strives to improve all components necessary to allow a patient to return to a high level of function. The athletic trainer must understand that the kinetic chain operates as an integrated functional unit.[12] Functional kinetic chain rehabilitation must therefore address each link in the kinetic chain and strive to develop functional strength and neuromuscular efficiency. Functional strength is the ability of the neuromuscular system to reduce force, produce force, and dynamically stabilize the kinetic chain during functional movements in a smooth and coordinated fashion.[6] Neuromuscular efficiency is the ability of the central nervous system (CNS) to allow agonists, antagonists, synergists, stabilizers, and neutralizers to work efficiently and interdependently during dynamic kinetic chain activities.[6]

Traditionally, rehabilitation has focused on isolated absolute strength gains, in isolated muscles, using single planes of motion. However, all functional activities are naturally multiplanar and require a blend of acceleration, deceleration, and dynamic stabilization.[22] Movement may appear to be one plane dominant, but the other planes need to be dynamically stabilized to allow for optimal neuromuscular efficiency.[6] Understanding that functional movements require a highly complex, integrated system allows the athletic trainer to make a paradigm shift. The paradigm shift focuses on training the entire kinetic chain using all planes of movement and establishing high levels of functional strength and neuromuscular efficiency.[6,22] The paradigm shift dictates that we train to allow force reduction, force production, and dynamic stabilization to occur efficiently during all kinetic chain activities.[6,22]

Using the Tools of Rehabilitation

Athletic trainers have many tools at their disposal—such as manual therapy techniques, therapeutic modalities, aquatic therapy, and the use of physician-prescribed medications—that can individually or collectively facilitate the rehabilitative process. How different athletic trainers choose to use those tools is often a matter of individual preference and experience.

Additionally, patients differ in their individual responses to various treatment techniques. Thus the athletic trainer should avoid "cookbook" rehabilitation protocols that can be followed like a recipe. In fact, use of rehabilitation "recipes" should be strongly discouraged. Instead, the athletic trainer must develop a broad theoretical knowledge base from which specific techniques or tools of rehabilitation can be selected and practically applied to each individual case.

Using Therapeutic Modalities in Rehabilitation

Athletic trainers use a wide variety of therapeutic techniques in the treatment and rehabilitation of sport-related injuries.[20] One of the more important aspects of a thorough treatment regimen is the use of therapeutic modalities. At one time or another, virtually all athletic trainers make use of some type of therapeutic modality. This might involve a relatively simple technique, such as using an ice pack as a first aid treatment for an acute injury, or more complex techniques such as the stimulation of nerve and muscle tissue by electrical currents. There is no question that therapeutic modalities are useful tools in injury rehabilitation. When used appropriately, these modalities can greatly enhance the patient's chances for a safe and rapid return to full activity. The athletic trainer must have knowledge of the scientific basis of the various modalities and their physiological effects on a specific injury. When applied to practical experience, this theoretical basis can produce an extremely effective clinical method.

A comprehensive rehabilitation program should focus on achieving specific short-term and long-term objectives. Modalities, though important, are by no means the single most critical factor in accomplishing these objectives. Therapeutic exercise that forces the injured anatomic structure to perform its normal function is the key to successful rehabilitation. However, therapeutic modalities certainly play an important role and are extremely useful as adjuncts to therapeutic exercise.[20]

It must be emphasized that the use of therapeutic modalities in any treatment program is an inexact science. There is no way to "cookbook" a treatment plan that involves the use of therapeutic modalities. Athletic trainers should make every effort to understand the basis for using each different type of modality and then make their own decisions as to which will be most effective in a given clinical situation.

Despite the fact that therapeutic modalities are commonly used by athletic trainers as an integral tool in the rehabilitation process, they will not be discussed further in this text. (The reader is referred to *Therapeutic Modalities in Rehabilitation, Fourth Edition*, for detailed information relative to the use of specific modalities in rehabilitation.)

Using Medications to Facilitate Healing

Prescription and over-the-counter medications can effectively aid the healing process during a rehabilitation program. An athletic trainer supervising a program of rehabilitation must have some knowledge of the potential effects of certain types of drugs on performance during the rehabilitation program. Patients might be expected to respond to medication just as anyone else would, but the patient's situation is not normal. Intense physical activity requires that special consideration be given to the effects of certain types of medication. On occasion, the athletic trainer, working with guidance from the team physician, must make decisions regarding the appropriate use of medications based on knowledge of the indications for use and the possible side effects in patients who are involved in rehabilitation programs.

Those medications commonly used to aid the healing process are discussed in detail in Chapter 2.

Therapeutic Exercise vs Conditioning Exercise

Exercise is an essential factor in fitness conditioning, injury prevention, and injury rehabilitation. To compete successfully at a high level, the patient must be fit. A patient who is not fit is more likely to sustain an injury. Coaches and athletic trainers both recognize that improper conditioning is one of the major causes of sport injuries. It is essential that the patient engage in training and conditioning exercises that minimize the possibility of injury while maximizing performance.[5]

The basic principles of training and conditioning exercises also apply to techniques of therapeutic, rehabilitative, or reconditioning exercises that are specifically concerned with restoring normal body function following injury. The term therapeutic exercise is perhaps most widely used to indicate exercises that are used in a rehabilitation program.[16]

ESTABLISHING SHORT- AND LONG-TERM GOALS IN A REHABILITATION PROGRAM

Designing an effective rehabilitation program is relatively simple if the athletic trainer routinely integrates several basic components. These basic components can also be considered the short-term goals of a rehabilitation program. They should include (1) providing correct immediate first aid and management following injury to limit or control swelling; (2) reducing or minimizing pain; (3) establishing core stability; (4) reestablishing neuromuscular control; (5) improving postural stability and balance; (6) restoring full ROM; (7) restoring or increasing muscular strength, endurance, and power; (8) maintaining cardiorespiratory fitness; and (9) incorporating appropriate functional progressions. The long-term goal is almost invariably to return the injured patient to practice or competition as quickly and safely as possible.

Establishing reasonable, attainable goals and integrating specific exercises or activities to address these goals is the easy part of overseeing a rehabilitation program. The difficult part comes in knowing exactly when and how to progress, change, or alter the rehabilitation program to most effectively accomplish both long- and short-term goals.

> ### Clinical Decision-Making Exercise 1-4
> A volleyball player has a second-degree ankle sprain. X-rays reveal no fracture. The athletic trainer wants to begin rehabilitation right away so the patient may be able to play again before the season is over. What are the short- and long-term goals for this patient?

Athletes tend to be goal-oriented individuals. Thus, the athletic trainer should design a goal-oriented rehabilitation program in which the patient can have a series of progressive "successes" in achieving attainable short-term goals throughout the rehabilitation process. Injured athletes are almost always most concerned to know precisely how long they will be out and when exactly they can return to full activity. The athletic trainer should not make the mistake of giving an injured patient an exact time frame or date. Instead, the patient should be given a series of sequenced challenges, involving increasing skill and ability, that must be met before progressing to the next level in his or her rehabilitation program. It is critical that the patient be actively involved in planning the process of rehabilitating his or her injury.[19]

The Importance of Controlling Swelling

The process of rehabilitation begins immediately after injury. Thus, in addition to understanding exactly how the injury occurred, the athletic trainer must be competent in providing correct and appropriate initial care. Initial first aid and management techniques are perhaps the most critical part of any rehabilitation program. The manner in which the injury is initially managed unquestionably has a significant impact on the course of the rehabilitative process.[20]

The one problem all injuries have in common is swelling. Swelling can be caused by any number of factors, including bleeding, production of synovial fluid, an accumulation of inflammatory by-products, edema, or a combination of several factors. No matter which mechanism is involved, swelling produces an increased pressure in the injured area, and increased pressure causes pain.[10] Swelling can also cause neuromuscular inhibition, which results in weak muscle contraction. Swelling is most likely during the first 72 hours after an injury. Once swelling has occurred, the healing process is significantly retarded. The injured area cannot return to normal until all the swelling is gone. Therefore everything that is done in first aid management of any of these conditions should be directed toward controlling the swelling.[20] If the swelling can be controlled initially in the acute stage of injury, the time required for rehabilitation is likely to be significantly reduced.

To control and significantly limit the amount of swelling, the PRICE principle—Protection, Restricted activity, Ice, Compression, and Elevation—should be applied (Figure 1-1). Each

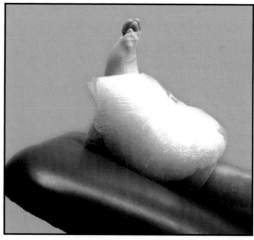

Figure 1-1. The PRICE technique should be used immediately following injury to limit swelling.

factor plays a critical role in limiting swelling, and all of these elements should be used simultaneously.

Protection

The injured area should be protected from additional injury by applying appropriate splints, braces, pads, or other immobilization devices. If the injury involves the lower extremity, it is recommended that the patient go non-weight-bearing on crutches at least until the acute inflammatory response has subsided.

Restricted Activity (Rest)

The period of restricted activity following any type of injury is absolutely critical in any treatment program. Once an anatomical structure is injured, it immediately begins the healing process. In an injured structure that is not rested and is subjected to unnecessary external stress and strains, the healing process never really gets a chance to begin. Consequently, the injury does not get well, and the time required for rehabilitation is markedly increased. This is not to minimize the importance of early mobility. Controlled mobility has been shown to be superior to immobilization for scar formation, revascularization, muscle regeneration, and reorientation of muscle fibers and tensile properties.[8] The amount of time necessary for resting varies with the severity of the injury, but most minor injuries should rest for about 24 to 48 hours before an active rehabilitation program is begun.

It must be emphasized that rest does not mean that the patient does nothing. The term rest applies only to the injured body part. During this period, the patient should continue to work on cardiovascular fitness and strengthening and flexibility exercises for the other parts of the body not affected by the injury.[25]

Ice

The use of cold is the initial treatment of choice for virtually all conditions involving injuries to the musculoskeletal system.[20] It is most commonly used immediately after injury to decrease pain and promote local vasoconstriction, thus controlling hemorrhage and edema. Cold applied to an acute injury will lower metabolism in the injured area, and thus the tissue demands for oxygen, thus reducing hypoxia. This benefit extends to uninjured tissue, preventing injury-related tissue death from spreading to adjacent normal cellular structures. It is also used in the acute phase of inflammatory conditions, such as bursitis, tenosynovitis, and tendinitis, in which heat can cause additional pain and swelling. Cold is also used to reduce the reflex muscle guarding and spastic conditions that accompany pain. Its analgesic effect is probably one of its greatest benefits. One explanation of the analgesic effect is that cold decreases the velocity of nerve conduction, although it does not entirely eliminate it. Cold can also bombard cutaneous sensory nerve receptor areas with so many cold impulses that pain impulses are lost. With ice treatments, the patient reports an uncomfortable sensation of cold, followed by burning, an aching sensation, and finally complete numbness.[1,20]

Because of the low thermal conductivity of underlying subcutaneous fat tissues, applications of cold for short periods are ineffective in cooling deeper tissues. For this reason longer treatments of 20 to 30 minutes are recommended. Cold treatments are generally believed to be more effective in reaching deeper tissues than most forms of heat. Cold applied to the skin is capable of significantly lowering the temperature of tissues at a considerable depth. The extent of this lowered tissue temperature depends on the type of cold applied to the skin, the duration of its application, the thickness of the subcutaneous fat, and the region of the body to which it is applied. Ice should be applied to the injured area until the signs and symptoms of inflammation have disappeared and there is little or no chance that swelling will be increased by using some form of heat. Ice should be used for at least 72 hours after an acute injury.[20]

Compression

Compression is likely the single most important technique for controlling initial swelling. The purpose of compression is to mechanically reduce the amount of space available for swelling by applying pressure around an injured area. The best way of applying pressure is to use an elastic wrap, such as an Ace bandage, to apply firm but even pressure around the injury.

Because of the pressure build-up in the tissues, having a compression wrap in place for a long time can become painful. However, the wrap must be kept in place despite significant pain because it is so important in the control of swelling. The compression wrap should be left in place continuously for at least 72 hours after an acute injury. In many overuse problems, such as tendinitis, tenosynovitis, and particularly bursitis, which involve ongoing inflammation, the compression wrap should be worn until the swelling is almost entirely gone.

Elevation

The fifth factor that assists in controlling swelling is elevation. The injured part, particularly an extremity, should be elevated to eliminate the effects of gravity on blood pooling in the extremities. Elevation assists venous and lymphatic drainage of blood and other fluids from the injured area back to the central circulatory system. The greater the degree of elevation, the more effective the reduction in swelling. For example, in an ankle sprain, the leg should be placed in such a position that the ankle is virtually straight up in the air. The injured part should be elevated as much as possible during the first 72 hours.

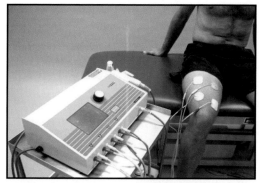

Figure 1-2. Several modalities, including electrical stimulating currents, may be used to modulate pain.

The appropriate technique for initial management of the acute injuries discussed in this chapter, regardless of where they occur, would be the following:

1. Apply a compression wrap directly over the injury. Wrapping should be from distal to proximal. Tension should be firm and consistent. Wetting the elastic wrap to facilitate the passage of cold from ice packs might be helpful.

2. Surround the injured area entirely with ice bags, and secure them in place. Ice bags should be left on for 45 minutes initially and then 1 hour off and 30 minutes on as much as possible over the next 24 hours. During the following 48-hour period, ice should be applied as often as possible.

3. The injured part should be elevated as much as possible during the initial 72-hour period after injury. Keeping the injured part elevated while sleeping is particularly important.

4. Allow the injured part to rest for about 24 hours after the injury.

Controlling Pain

When an injury occurs, the athletic trainer must realize that the patient will experience some degree of pain. The extent of the pain will be determined in part by the severity of the injury, by the patient's individual response to and perception of pain, and by the circumstances in which the injury occurred. The patient's pain is real. The athletic trainer can effectively modulate acute pain by using the PRICE technique immediately after injury.[21] A physician can also make use of various medications to help ease pain.

Persistent pain can make strengthening or flexibility exercises more difficult, thus interfering with the rehabilitation process. The athletic trainer should routinely address pain during each individual treatment session. Making use of appropriate therapeutic modalities—including various techniques of cryotherapy, thermotherapy, and electrical stimulating currents—will help modulate pain throughout the rehabilitation process[20] (Figure 1-2). To a great extent, pain will dictate the rate of progression. With initial injury, pain is intense and tends to decrease and eventually subside altogether as healing progresses. Any exacerbation of either pain, swelling, or other clinical symptoms during or following a particular exercise or activity indicates that the load is too great for the level of tissue repair or remodeling.

Establishing Core Stability

Core stability is absolutely essential to every aspect of the rehabilitation process (Figure 1-3). The core is considered to be the lumbo-pelvic-hip complex, which functions to dynamically stabilize the entire kinetic chain during functional movements. Without proximal or core stability, the distal movers cannot function optimally to efficiently use their strength and power. Chapter 5 will discuss the concept of core stabilization in great detail.[6,13]

Reestablishing Neuromuscular Control

Reestablishing neuromuscular control should be of prime concern to the athletic trainer in all rehabilitation programs[26] (see Chapter 6). The ability to sense the position of

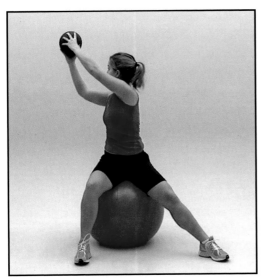

Figure 1-3. Core stability forms the basis for all aspects of a rehabilitation program.

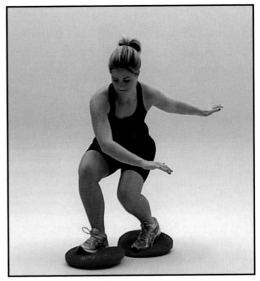

Figure 1-4. Reestablishing neuromuscular control and balance is critical to regaining functional performance capabilities.

a joint in space is mediated by mechanoreceptors found in both muscles and joints, in addition to cutaneous, visual, and vestibular input. Neuromuscular control relies on the central nervous system to interpret and integrate proprioceptive and kinesthetic information and then to control individual muscles and joints to produce coordinated movement.[24]

Following injury and subsequent rest and immobilization, the central nervous system "forgets" how to put together information coming from muscle and joint mechanoreceptors, and from cutaneous, visual, and vestibular input. Regaining neuromuscular control means regaining the ability to follow some previously established sensory pattern.[26] Neuromuscular control is the mind's attempt to teach the body conscious control of a specific movement. Successful repetition of a patterned movement makes its performance progressively less difficult, thus requiring less concentration, until the movement becomes automatic. This requires many repetitions of the same movement, progressing step-by-step from simple to more complex movements. Strengthening exercises, particularly those that tend to be more functional, such as closed kinetic chain exercises, are essential for reestablishing neuromuscular control.[26] Addressing neuromuscular control is

critical throughout the recovery process, but it is perhaps most critical during the early stages of rehabilitation to avoid reinjury.[26]

Restoring Postural Control and Stability (Balance)

Postural stability involves the complex integration of muscular forces, neurological sensory information received from the mechanoreceptors, and biomechanical information.[11] The ability to maintain postural stability and balance is essential to acquiring or reacquiring complex motor skills.[24] Patients who show a decreased sense of balance or a lack of postural stability following injury might lack sufficient proprioceptive and kinesthetic information and/or might have muscular weakness, either of which can limit the ability to generate an effective correction response when there is not equilibrium. A rehabilitation program must include functional exercises that incorporate balance and proprioceptive training that prepares the patient for return to activity (Figure 1-4). Failure to address balance problems can predispose the patient to reinjury (see Chapter 7).

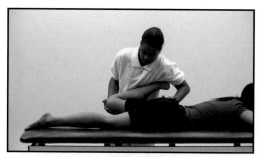

Figure 1-5. Stretching techniques are used with tight musculotendinous structures to improve physiological ROM.

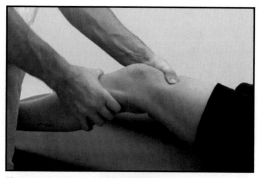

Figure 1-6. Joint mobilization techniques are used with tight ligamentous or capsular structures to improve accessory motion.

Restoring Range of Motion

Following injury to a joint, there will always be some associated loss of motion. That loss of movement can usually be attributed to a number of pathological factors, including resistance of the musculotendinous unit (ie, muscle, tendon, fascia) to stretch; contracture of connective tissue (ie, ligaments, joint capsule); or some combination of the two. Muscle imbalances, postural imbalance, neural tension, and joint dysfunction can also lead to a loss in ROM.

It is critical for the athletic trainer to closely evaluate the injured joint to determine whether motion is limited due to physiological movement constraints involving musculotendinous units or due to limitation in accessory motion (joint arthrokinematics) involving the joint capsule and ligaments. If physiological movement is restricted, the patient should engage in stretching activities designed to improve flexibility (Figure 1-5) (see Chapters 8 and 14). Stretching exercises should be used whenever there is musculotendinous resistance to stretch. If accessory motion is limited due to some restriction of the joint capsule or the ligaments, the athletic trainer should incorporate joint mobilization and traction techniques into the treatment program (Figure 1-6) (see Chapter 14). Mobilization techniques should be used whenever there are tight articular structures.[16] Traditionally, rehabilitation programs tend to concentrate more on passive physiological movements without paying much attention to accessory motions.

Restoring Muscular Strength, Endurance, and Power

Muscular strength, endurance and power are among the most essential factors in restoring the function of a body part to preinjury status. Isometric, progressive resistive (isotonic), isokinetic, and plyometric exercises can benefit rehabilitation. A major goal in performing strengthening exercises is to work through a full pain-free ROM.

Most strength-training programs involve single-plane force production using either free weights or exercise machines. A functional rehabilitative strengthening program should involve exercises in all three planes of motion, concentrating on a combination of concentric, eccentric, and isometric exercises designed both to increase strength through a full multiplanar ROM and to improve core stabilization and neuromuscular control.[6]

Isometric Exercise

Isometric exercises are commonly performed in the early phase of rehabilitation when a joint is immobilized for a time. They are useful when using resistance training though a full ROM might make the injury worse. Isometrics increase static strength and assist in decreasing the amount of atrophy. Isometrics also can lessen swelling by causing a muscle pumping action to remove fluid and edema (see Chapter 9).

Progressive Resistive Exercise

Progressive resistive exercise (PRE) is the most commonly used strengthening technique

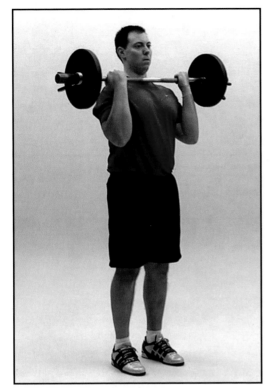

Figure 1-7. Progressive resistive exercise using isotonic contractions is the most widely used rehabilitative strengthening technique.

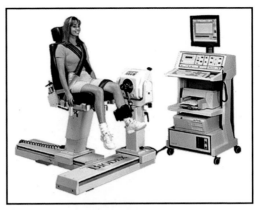

Figure 1-8. Isokinetic exercise is most often used in the later stages of rehabilitation. (Reproduced with permission from Biodex Medical Systems)

in a rehabilitation program. PRE may be done using free weights, exercise machines, or rubber tubing (Figure 1-7). Progressive resistive exercise uses isotonic contractions in which force is generated while the muscle is changing in length. Isotonic contractions may be either concentric or eccentric. In a rehabilitation program the athletic trainer should incorporate both eccentric and concentric strengthening exercises. Traditionally, progressive resistive exercise has concentrated primarily on the concentric component and has to some extent minimized the importance of the eccentric component (see Chapter 9).

Isokinetic Exercise

Isokinetic exercise is occasionally used in the rehabilitative process. It is most often incorporated during the later phases of a rehabilitation program. Isokinetics uses a fixed speed with accommodating resistance to provide maximal resistance throughout the ROM (Figure 1-8). The speed of movement can be altered in isokinetic exercise. Isokinetic measures are

commonly used as a criteria for return of the patient to functional activity following injury.

Plyometric Exercise

Plyometric exercises, also referred to as reactive neuromuscular training, are most often incorporated into the later stages of a rehabilitation program. Plyometrics use a quick eccentric stretch to facilitate a subsequent concentric contraction. Plyometric exercises are useful in restoring or developing the patient's ability to produce dynamic movements associated with muscular power (Figure 1-9). The ability to generate force very rapidly is a key to successful performance in many sport activities. It is critical to address the element of muscular power in rehabilitation programs for the injured patient (see Chapter 11).

Open vs Closed Kinetic Chain Exercise

The concept of the kinetic chain deals with the anatomical functional relationships that exist in the upper and lower extremities (see Chapter 12). An open kinetic chain exists when the foot or hand is not in contact with the ground or some other surface.[12] In a closed kinetic chain, the foot or hand is weight-bearing (Figure 1-10). In rehabilitation, the use of closed-chain strengthening techniques has become the treatment of choice for any athletic trainers. Closed kinetic chain exercises use varying combinations of isometric, concentric, and eccentric contractions that must occur

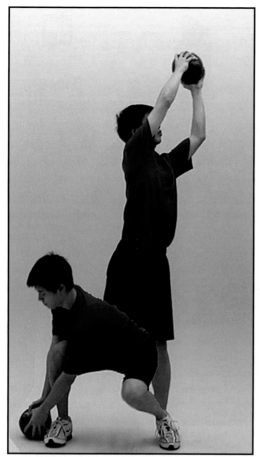

Figure 1-9. Plyometric exercise focuses on improving dynamic, power movements.

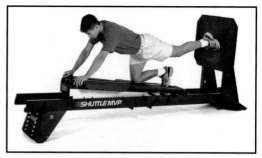

Figure 1-10. Closed kinetic chain exercises are widely used in rehabilitation. (Reprinted with permission from Shuttle Systems, Glacier, WA.)

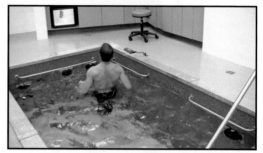

Figure 1-11. Every rehabilitation program must include some exercise designed to maintain cardiorespiratory fitness, such as running on an underwater treadmill.

simultaneously in different muscle groups within the chain.

Maintaining Cardiorespiratory Fitness

Maintaining cardiorespiratory fitness is perhaps the single most neglected component of a rehabilitation program (see Chapter 10). An athlete spends a considerable amount of time preparing the cardiorespiratory system to be able to handle the increased demands made upon it during a competitive season. When injury occurs and the patient is forced to miss training time, cardiorespiratory fitness can decrease rapidly. Thus the athletic trainer must design or substitute alternative activities that allow the patient to maintain existing levels of cardiorespiratory fitness as early as possible in the rehabilitation period[15] (Figure 1-11).

Depending on the nature of the injury, a number of possible activities can help the patient maintain fitness levels. When there is a lower-extremity injury, non-weight-bearing activities should be incorporated. Pool activities provide an excellent means for injury rehabilitation. Cycling also can positively stress the cardiorespiratory system.

Functional Progressions

The purpose of any program of rehabilitation is to restore normal function following injury.[14] Functional progressions involve a series of gradually progressive activities designed to prepare the individual for return to a specific activity[23] (see Chapter 16). Those skills necessary for successful participation in a given sport are broken down into component parts, and the patient gradually reacquires those skills within the limitations of his or her own individual progress.[7] Progression through the rehabilitation program may be broken down into three phases: the stabilization

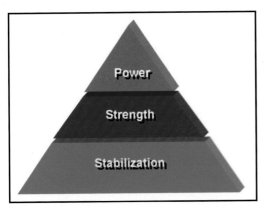

Figure 1-12. Progression through a rehabilitation program can be broken down into three phases: the stabilization phase, the strength phase, and the power phase.

phase, the strengthening phase, and the power phase (Figure 1-12). The stabilization phase begins with exercises designed to correct the deficits in the structural integrity of the kinetic chain including muscle dysfunction, joint dysfunctions, neuromuscular deficits, and postural control and stability. These deficits must be addressed prior to beginning an aggressive rehabilitation program to correct muscle imbalances, recondition injured structures, prepare tissues for the physical demands of the rehabilitation program, prevent tissue overload through progressive adaptation, improve work capacity, and improve stabilization strength; thus establishing optimal levels of stabilization, strength, and postural control. Exercises should progress from isometric to multiplanar activities designed to recruit joint stabilizers, thus improving neuromuscular efficiency, core stability, functional strength, and functional flexibility.[6]

The strength phase is used to enhance stabilization strength and endurance during functional movement patterns by incorporating high volume resistive exercises that force motor unit recruitment after the prime movers are fatigued. For example, after performing a strength exercise the patient immediately engages in a stabilization exercise that forces neuromuscular stabilization of that movement. During this phase the goal is to achieve several adaptive changes by challenging the neuromuscular system including an increase in the cross sectional diameter of the muscle, increased resistance to fatigue, and increased stabilization

strength to control joint translation during functional movements.[6]

The power phase is particularly important for an injured athlete who is attempting to return to high-level physically demanding activity. An athlete who needs high levels of both muscular strength and power should first use exercises that incorporate multiplanar, concentric, eccentric, and isometric contractions to increase strength. Maximal power is then developed by training at 30% to 45% of maximum strength and by accelerating through the entire ROM.[6] During this phase the goal is to enhance neuromuscular efficiency and power production by increasing motorneuron excitability thus increasing speed strength throughout the entire ROM. For most individuals the rate of force production is the single most important neural adaptation.[6]

Every new activity introduced must be carefully monitored by the athletic trainer to determine the patient's ability to perform and her or his physical tolerance. If an activity does not produce additional pain or swelling, the level should be advanced; new activities should be introduced as quickly as possible.

Functional progressions will gradually help the injured patient achieve normal pain-free ROM, restore adequate strength levels, and regain neuromuscular control throughout the rehabilitation program.[7]

Functional Testing

Functional testing uses functional progression drills to assess the patient's ability to perform a specific activity (Figure 1-13). Functional testing involves a single maximal effort performed to indicate how close the patient is to a full return to activity. For years athletic trainers have assessed patients' progress with a variety of functional tests, including agility runs (figure eights, shuttle run, carioca), sidestepping, vertical jump, hopping for time or distance, and co-contraction tests[5,14] (see Chapter 16).

Criteria for Full Recovery

All exercise rehabilitation plans must determine what is meant by complete recovery from an injury.[21] Often it means that the patient is fully reconditioned and has achieved full range

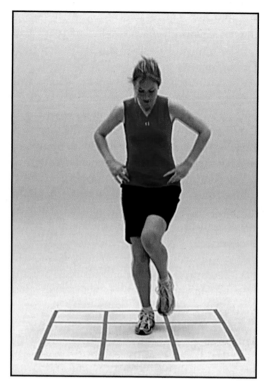

Figure 1-13. Performance on functional tests can determine the athlete's capability to return to full activity.

tests. These functional tests are extremely useful and valuable tools for determining readiness to return to full activity.

The decision to release a patient recovering from injury to a full return to athletic activity is the final stage of the rehabilitation/recovery process. The decision should be carefully considered by each member of the sports medicine team involved in the rehabilitation process. The team physician should be ultimately responsible for deciding that the patient is ready to return to practice and/or competition. That decision should be based on collective input from the athletic trainer, the coach, and the patient.

In considering the patient's return to activity, the following concerns should be addressed:

- Physiological healing constraints. Has rehabilitation progressed to the later stages of the healing process?

- Pain status. Has pain disappeared, or is the patient able to play within her or his own levels of pain tolerance?

- Swelling. Is there still a chance that swelling could be exacerbated by return to activity?

- Range of motion. Is ROM adequate to allow the patient to perform both effectively and with minimized risk of reinjury?

- Strength. Is strength, endurance, or power great enough to protect the injured structure from reinjury?

- Neuromuscular control/proprioception/kinesthesia. Has the patient "relearned" how to use the injured body part?

- Cardiorespiratory fitness. Has the patient been able to maintain cardiorespiratory fitness at or near the level necessary for competition?

- Sport-specific demands. Are the demands of the sport or a specific position such that the patient will not be at risk of reinjury?

- Functional testing. Does performance on appropriate functional tests indicate that the extent of recovery is sufficient to allow successful performance?

- Prophylactic strapping, bracing, padding. Are any additional supports necessary for the injured patient to return to activity?

of movement, strength, neuromuscular control, cardiovascular fitness, and sport-specific functional skills. Besides physical well-being, the patient must also have regained full confidence to return to his or her activity.

For example, specific criteria for a return to full activity after rehabilitation of the injured knee is largely determined by the nature and severity of the specific injury, but it also depends on the philosophy and judgment of both the physician and the athletic trainer. Traditionally, return to activity has been dictated through both objective and subjective evaluations.

For the athletic patient, criteria for return should be based on functional capabilities as indicated by performance on specific functional tests that are closely related to the demands of a particular activity. Performance on functional tests, such as those described in Chapter 16 (hop test, co-contraction test), should serve as primary determinants of the patient's capability to return to full activity. Data on the majority of these tests are well documented. A number of data-based research studies have objectively quantified performance on various functional

- Responsibility of the patient. Is the patient capable of listening to his or her body and recognizing situations that present a potential for reinjury?

- Predisposition to injury. Is this patient prone to reinjury or a new injury when he or she is not 100% recovered?

- Psychological factors. Is the patient capable of returning to activity and competing at a high level without fear of reinjury?

- Patient education and preventive maintenance program. Does the patient understand the importance of continuing to engage in conditioning exercises that can greatly reduce the chances of reinjury?

Clinical Decision-Making Exercise 1-6

After a week of managing a first-degree hamstring strain, a track patient has decided that she is ready to compete. She has no signs of inflammation. She has regained full strength and ROM. What else should be taken into consideration before she is allowed to compete again?

DOCUMENTATION IN REHABILITATION

Athletic trainers must develop proficiency not only in their ability to constantly evaluate an injury, but also in their ability to generate an accurate report of the findings from that evaluation. Accurate and detailed record keeping that documents initial injury evaluations, treatment records, and notes on progress throughout a rehabilitation program is critical for the athletic trainer.[21] This is particularly true considering the number of malpractice lawsuits in health care. For the athletic trainer working in a clinical setting, clear, concise, accurate record keeping is necessary for third-party reimbursement. Although this may be difficult and time-consuming for the athletic trainer who treats and deals with a large number of patients each day, it is an area that simply cannot be neglected. Documentation and record keeping will be discussed in detail in Chapter 3.

LEGAL CONSIDERATIONS IN SUPERVISING A REHABILITATION PROGRAM

Regarding the treatment and rehabilitation of athletic injuries, currently there is controversy about the specific roles of individuals with various combinations of educational background, certification, and licensure. States vary considerably in their laws governing what an athletic trainer may and may not do in supervising a program of rehabilitation for an injured patient. Many states have specific guidelines in their licensure act that dictate how the athletic trainer may incorporate a variety of treatment tools into the treatment regimen. Each athletic trainer should ensure that any use of a specific tool or technique of rehabilitation is within the limits allowed by the laws of his or her particular state.

Summary

1. The athletic trainer is responsible for the design, implementation, and supervision of the rehabilitation program for the injured patient.

2. The rehabilitation philosophy in sports medicine is aggressive, with the ultimate goal being to return the injured patient to full activity as quickly and safely as possible.

3. To be effective in overseeing a rehabilitation program, the athletic trainer must have a sound understanding of the healing process, the biomechanics of normal movement, and the psychological aspects of the rehabilitative process.

4. The athletic trainer must develop a broad theoretical knowledge base from which specific techniques or tools of rehabilitation can be selected and practically applied to each individual case without relying on "recipe" rehabilitation protocols.

5. Therapeutic exercises are rehabilitative, or reconditioning, exercises that are specifically concerned with restoring normal body function following injury.

6. Controlling swelling immediately following injury is perhaps the single most important aspect of injury rehabilitation in a sports medicine setting. If the swelling can be controlled initially in the acute stage of injury, the time required for rehabilitation is likely to be significantly reduced.

7. Short-term goals of a rehabilitation program: (1) providing correct immediate first aid and management following injury to limit or control swelling; (2) reducing or minimizing pain; (3) establishing core stability; (4) reestablishing neuromuscular control; (5) restoring full ROM; (6) restoring or increasing muscular strength, endurance, and power; (7) improving postural stability and balance; (8) maintaining cardiorespiratory fitness; and (9) incorporating appropriate functional progressions.

8. Criteria for return should be based on functional capabilities as indicated by performance on specific functional tests that are closely related to the demands of a particular activity.

9. The athletic trainer should ensure that any specific tool or technique of rehabilitation that they choose to use is within the limits of practice allowed by the laws of his or her particular state.

References

1. Bleakley, C., McDonough, S. 2006. Cryotherapy for acute sprains: A randomized controlled study of two different icing protocols. *British Journal of Sports Medicine, 40*(8),700-705.

2. Braddom, R. 2010. *Physical Medicine and Rehabilitation.* St. Louis: Elsevier.

3. Brotzman, B., Manske, R. 2011. *Clinical Orthopeadic Rehabilitation: An Evidence Based Approach.* St Louis: Elsevier Mosby.

4. Buschbacher, R., Prahlow, N., Dave, S. 2008. *Sports Medicine and Rehabilitation: A Sport Specific Approach.* Philadelphia: Hanley & Belfus.

5. Cates, W., Cavanaugh, J. 2009. Advances in rehabilitation and performance testing. *Clinics in Sports Medicine, 28*(1),63-76.

6. Clark, M. 2001. *Integrated Training for the New Millennium.* Calabasas, CA: National Academy of Sports Medicine.

7. Donatelli, R. 2007. *Sports-Specific Rehabilitation.* St. Louis: Churchill Livingstone Elsevier.

8. Fontera, W., Silver, J. 2008. *Essentials of physical medicine and rehabilitation: Musculoskeletal disorders, pain, and rehabilitation.* Philadelphia: Saunders Elsevier.

9. Hamson-Utley, J., Martin, S., Walters, J. 2008. Athletic trainers' and physical therapists' perceptions of the effectiveness of psychological skills within sport injury rehabilitation programs. *Journal of Athletic Training, 43*(3):258-264.

10. Hoogenboom, B., Voight, M., Prentice, W. 2015. *Musculoskeletal Interventions: Techniques for Therapeutic Exercise,* 3rd ed. New York, McGraw-Hill.

11. Hrysomalis, C. 2011. Balance ability and athletic performance, *Sports Medicine, 41*(3):221-232.

12. Karandikar, N., Vargas, O. 2011. Kinetic Chains: A review of the concept and its clinical applications. *Physical Medicine and Rehabilitation 3*(8):739-745.

13. Kibler, B, Press, J. 2006. The role of core stability in athletic function, *Sports Medicine 36*(3):189-198.

14. Kibler, B. Chandler J. 2008. Functional Rehabilitation and return to training and competition. In Fontera, W. *The Encyclopedia of Sports Medicine: An IOC Medical Commission Publication,* Hoboken, NJ, John Wiley and Sons.

15. Kirkendall, D. T., W. E. Prentice, and W. E. Garrett. 2001. Rehabilitation of muscle injuries. In: *Rehabilitation of sports injuries: Current concepts,* edited by G. Puddu, A. Giombini, and A. Selvanetti. Berlin: Springer.

16. Kisner, C. and A. Colby. 2013. *Therapeutic exercise: Foundations and techniques.* Philadelphia: F. A. Davis.

17. Logan, G. A., and E. L. Wallis. 1960. *Recent findings in learning and performance.* Paper presented at the Southern Section Meeting, California Association for Health, Physical Education and Recreation, Pasadena, CA.

18. Maxey, L., Magnusson, J. 2012 *Rehabilitation for the Post-surgical Orthopedic Patient,* St. Louis, Elsevier.

19. Piccininni, J., and J. Drover. 1999. Patient-patient education in rehabilitation: Developing a self-directed program. *Athletic Therapy Today 4*(6):51.

20. Prentice, W. 2011. *Therapeutic Modalities in Rehabilitation,* 4th ed. New York, McGraw-Hill.

21. Prentice, W. 2014. *Principles of Athletic Training: A Competency Based Approach*, 15th ed. New York, McGraw-Hill.

22. Sahrmann S. 2001. *Diagnosis and Treatment of Movement Impairment Syndromes*. Philadelphia, PA: Elsevier Publishing.

23. Shamus, E. and J. Shamus. 2001. *Sports injury: Prevention and rehabilitation*. New York: McGraw-Hill.

24. Tippett, S., and M. Voight. 1999. *Functional progressions for sport rehabilitation*. Champaign, IL: Human Kinetics.

25. Zachazewski, J., D. Magee, and S. Quillen. 1996. *Athletic injuries and rehabilitation*. Philadelphia: W. B. Saunders.

26. Zech, A, Hubscher, M. 2009 Neuromuscular training for rehabilitation of sports injuries: A systematic review, *Medicine and Science in Sports and Exercise* 41(10):1831-1841.

SOLUTIONS TO CLINICAL DECISION-MAKING EXERCISES

1-1   The athletic trainer's decisions about a rehabilitation progression should be based on the following aspects: healing process, pathomechanics of the injury, cardiovascular fitness, and the equipment available. A good understanding of these aspects will ensure that the athletic trainer is progressing the patient at an appropriate rate.

1-2   Her concerns should be discussed with the orthopedist. The doctor and athletic trainer should maintain open communication throughout a patient's rehabilitation so that a good working relationship is maintained and the doctor's philosophy persists throughout the rehabilitation process.

1-3   He should understand the SAID principle. The muscles and soft tissue will adapt gradually to increasing demands placed on it. If the demands are too great, they can be detrimental to the healing process.

1-4   In general, the short-term goals for rehabilitation of an acute injury are to target inflammation and restore ROM. More specifically, pain and swelling should be controlled using PRICE. Once the patient progresses through the inflammatory phase, the goals become to restore muscular strength, endurance, and power. Neuromuscular control, balance, and cardiorespiratory fitness must also be regained. Long-term goals are to regain functional ability and return to play as soon as possible.

1-5   The patient should be taped and encouraged to keep up with the therapeutic exercise program, while continuing to use ice and antiinflammatories.

1-6   She should have sufficient neuromuscular control/balance. Her cardiovascular endurance should be at a level that will allow her to be competitive again without reinjury. She should be able to perform a series of functional tests that indicate she will withstand the demands of competition without reinjury. She should also be able to perform with confidence and know when to stop if she is in danger of reinjury.

Please see videos on the accompanying website at

www.healio.com/books/sportsmedvideos

CHAPTER 2

Understanding and Managing the Healing Process Through Rehabilitation

William E. Prentice, PhD, PT, ATC, FNATA

After completion of this chapter, the athletic trainer should be able to do the following:

- Describe the pathophysiology of the healing process.
- Identify the factors that can impede the healing process.
- Discuss the etiology and pathology of various musculoskeletal injuries associated with various types of tissues.
- Compare healing processes relative to specific musculoskeletal structures.
- Explain the importance of initial first aid and injury management of these injuries and their impact on the rehabilitation process.
- Discuss the use of various analgesics, antiinflammatories, and antipyretics in facilitating the healing process during a rehabilitation program.

Injury rehabilitation requires sound knowledge and understanding of the etiology and pathology involved in various musculoskeletal injuries that may occur.[24,84,93] When injury occurs, the athletic trainer is charged with designing, implementing, and supervising the rehabilitation program. Rehabilitation protocols and progressions must be based primarily on the physiologic responses of the tissues to injury and on an understanding of how various tissues heal.[39,43,46] Thus the athletic trainer must understand the healing process to effectively supervise the rehabilitative process. This chapter discusses the healing process relative to the various musculoskeletal injuries that may be encountered by an athletic trainer.

Prentice WE, ed.
Rehabilitation Techniques for Sports Medicine and Athletic Training (pp 23-55).
© 2015 SLACK Incorporated.

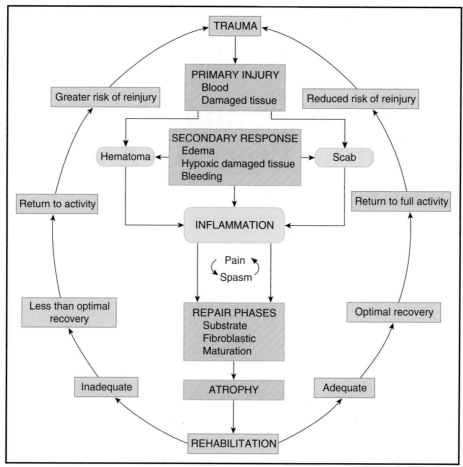

Figure 2-1. A cycle of sport-related injury. (Adapted from Booher JM, Thibadeau GA. *Athletic Injury Assessment.* St. Louis, MO: Mosby; 1994.)

UNDERSTANDING THE HEALING PROCESS

Rehabilitation programs must be based on the cycle of the healing process (Figure 2-1). The athletic trainer must have a sound understanding of the sequence of the various phases of the healing process.[31] The physiologic responses of the tissues to trauma follow a predictable sequence and time frame.[41] Decisions on how and when to alter and progress a rehabilitation program should be primarily based on recognition of signs and symptoms, as well as on an awareness of the time frames associated with the various phases of healing.[57,72] The healing process consists of the inflammatory response phase, the fibroblastic repair phase, and the maturation remodeling phase. It must

be stressed that although the phases of healing are presented as three separate entities, the healing process is a continuum. Phases of the healing process overlap one another and have no definitive beginning or end points.[73]

Primary Injury

Primary injuries are almost always described as being either chronic or acute in nature, resulting from macrotraumatic or microtraumatic forces. Injuries classified as macrotraumatic occur as a result of acute trauma and produce immediate pain and disability. Macrotraumatic injuries include fractures, dislocations, subluxations, sprains, strains, and contusions. Microtraumatic injuries are most often called overuse injuries and result from repetitive overloading or incorrect mechanics associated with

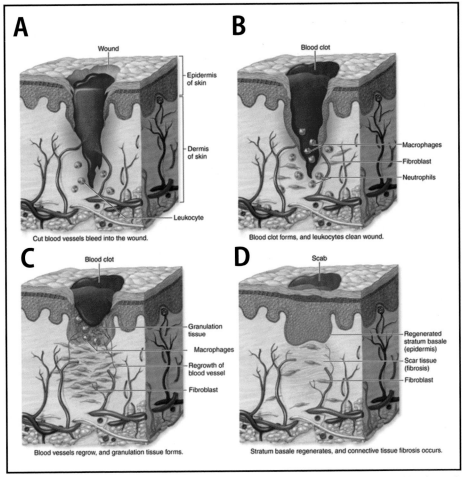

Figure 2-2. Initial injury and inflammatory response phase of the healing process. (A) Cut blood vessels bleed into the wound. (B) Blood clot forms, and leukocytes clean the wound. (C) Blood vessels regrow, and granulation tissue forms in the fibroblastic repair phase of the healing process. (D) Epithelium regenerates, and connective tissue fibrosis occurs in the maturation-remodeling phase of the healing process. (Adapted from McKinley M., O'Loughlin V. *Human Anatomy*. Chicago, IL: McGraw-Hill; 2006:113.)

repeated motion.[59] Microtraumatic injuries include tendinitis, tendinosis, tenosynovitis, bursitis, etc. A secondary injury is essentially the inflammatory or hypoxia response that occurs with the primary injury.

Inflammatory Response Phase

Once a tissue is injured, the process of healing begins immediately[16] (Figure 2-2A). The destruction of tissue produces direct injury to the cells of the various soft tissues.[35] Cellular injury results in altered metabolism and the liberation of materials that initiate the inflammatory response. It is characterized symptomatically by redness, swelling, tenderness, and increased temperature.[18,54] This initial inflammatory response is critical to the entire healing process.[14] If this response does not accomplish what it is supposed to or if it does not subside, normal healing cannot take place.[37]

Inflammation is a process through which leukocytes and other phagocytic cells and exudates are delivered to the injured tissue. This cellular reaction is generally protective, tending to localize or dispose of injury by-products (eg, blood and damaged cells) through phagocytosis, thus setting the stage for repair. Local vascular effects, disturbances of fluid exchange, and migration of leukocytes from the blood to the tissues occur.[38]

Clinical Decision-Making Exercise 2-1

A physical education student fell on his wrist playing flag football. It is very swollen, and he has decreased strength and ROM. The athletic trainer does not suspect a fracture. A decision is made to provide an initial treatment instead of sending the student to the emergency room. What should the athletic trainer's goals be at this time?

Vascular Reaction

The vascular reaction involves vascular spasm, formation of a platelet plug, blood coagulation, and growth of fibrous tissue.[77] The immediate response to tissue damage is a vasoconstriction of the vascular walls in the vessels leading away from the site of injury that lasts for about 5 to 10 minutes. This vasoconstriction presses the opposing endothelial wall linings together to produce a local anemia that is rapidly replaced by hyperemia of the area as a result of vasodilation.[11] This increase in blood flow is transitory and gives way to slowing of the flow in the dilated vessels, thus enabling the leukocytes to slow down and adhere to the vascular endothelium. Eventually there is stagnation and stasis. The initial effusion of blood and plasma lasts for 24 to 36 hours.

Chemical Mediators

The events in the inflammatory response are initiated by a series of interactions involving several chemical mediators. Some of these chemical mediators are derived from the invading organism, some are released by the damaged tissue, others are generated by several plasma enzyme systems, and still others are products of various white blood cells participating in the inflammatory response. Three chemical mediators—histamine, leukotrienes, and cytokines—are important in limiting the amount of exudate, and thus swelling, after injury. Histamine, released from the injured mast cells, causes vasodilation and increased cell permeability, owing to a swelling of endothelial cells and then separation between the cells. Leukotrienes and prostaglandins are responsible for margination, in which leukocytes (neutrophils and macrophages) adhere along the cell walls. They also increase cell permeability locally, thus affecting the passage of the fluid and white blood cells through cell walls via diapedesis to form exudate. Consequently, vasodilation and active hyperemia are important in exudate (plasma) formation and in supplying leukocytes to the injured area. Cytokines, in particular chemokines and interleukin, are the major regulators of leukocyte traffic and help to attract leukocytes to the actual site of inflammation. Responding to the presence of chemokines, phagocytes enter the site of inflammation within a few hours. The amount of swelling that occurs is directly related to the extent of vessel damage.

Formation of a Clot

Platelets do not normally adhere to the vascular wall. However, injury to a vessel disrupts the endothelium and exposes the collagen fibers. Platelets adhere to the collagen fibers to create a sticky matrix on the vascular wall, to which additional platelets and leukocytes adhere and eventually form a plug. These plugs obstruct local lymphatic fluid drainage and thus localize the injury response (Figure 2-2B).

The initial event that precipitates clot formation is the conversion of fibrinogen to fibrin. This transformation occurs because of a cascading effect, beginning with the release of a protein molecule called thromboplastin from the damaged cell. Thromboplastin causes prothrombin to be changed into thrombin, which, in turn, causes the conversion of fibrinogen into a very sticky fibrin clot that shuts off blood supply to the injured area. Clot formation begins around 12 hours after injury and is completed within 48 hours.

As a result of a combination of these factors, the injured area becomes walled off during the inflammatory stage of healing. The leukocytes phagocytize most of the foreign debris toward the end of the inflammatory phase, setting the stage for the fibroblastic phase. This initial inflammatory response lasts for about 2 to 4 days after initial injury.

Chronic Inflammation

A distinction must be made between the acute inflammatory response as previously described and chronic inflammation. Chronic inflammation occurs when the acute inflammatory response does not respond sufficiently to eliminate the injuring agent and restore tissue to its normal physiologic state. Thus, only low concentrations of the chemical mediators are present. The neutrophils that are normally present during acute inflammation are replaced by macrophages, lymphocytes, fibroblasts, and plasma cells. As this low-grade inflammation persists, damage occurs to connective tissue, resulting in tissue necrosis and fibrosis prolonging the healing process. Chronic inflammation involves the production of granulation tissue and fibrous connective tissue. These cells accumulate in a highly vascularized and innervated loose connective tissue matrix in the area of injury.[53] The specific mechanisms that cause an insufficient acute inflammatory response are unknown, but they appear to be related to situations that involve overuse or overload with cumulative microtrauma to a particular structure.[28,53] There is no specific time frame in which the acute inflammation transitions to chronic inflammation. It does appear that chronic inflammation is resistant to both physical and pharmacologic treatments.[44]

Use of Anti-inflammatory Medications

A physician will routinely prescribe nonsteroidal anti-inflammatory drugs (NSAIDs) for a patient who has sustained an injury.[2] These medications are certainly effective in minimizing pain and swelling associated with inflammation and can enhance return to normal activity. However, there are some concerns that the use of NSAIDs acutely following injury might actually interfere with inflammation, thus delaying the healing process.

Fibroblastic Repair Phase

During the fibroblastic phase of healing, proliferative and regenerative activity leading to scar formation and repair of the injured tissue follows the vascular and exudative phenomena of inflammation[41] (Figure 2-2C). The period of scar formation referred to as fibroplasia begins within the first few hours after injury and can last as long as 4 to 6 weeks. During this period, many of the signs and symptoms associated with the inflammatory response subside. The patient might still indicate some tenderness to touch and will usually complain of pain when particular movements stress the injured structure. As scar formation progresses, complaints of tenderness or pain gradually disappear.[39]

During this phase, growth of endothelial capillary buds into the wound is stimulated by a lack of oxygen, after which the wound is capable of healing aerobically.[18] Along with increased oxygen delivery comes an increase in blood flow, which delivers nutrients essential for tissue regeneration in the area.[18]

The formation of a delicate connective tissue called granulation tissue occurs with the breakdown of the fibrin clot. Granulation tissue consists of fibroblasts, collagen, and capillaries. It appears as a reddish granular mass of connective tissue that fills in the gaps during the healing process.

As the capillaries continue to grow into the area, fibroblasts accumulate at the wound site, arranging themselves parallel to the capillaries. Fibroblastic cells begin to synthesize an extracellular matrix that contains protein fibers of collagen and elastin, a ground substance that consists of nonfibrous proteins called proteoglycans, glycosaminoglycans, and fluid. On about day 6 or 7, fibroblasts also begin producing collagen fibers that are deposited in a random fashion throughout the forming scar. As the collagen continues to proliferate, the tensile strength of the wound rapidly increases in proportion to the rate of collagen synthesis. As the tensile strength increases, the number of fibroblasts diminishes, signaling the beginning of the maturation phase.

This normal sequence of events in the repair phase leads to the formation of minimal scar tissue. Occasionally, a persistent inflammatory response and continued release of inflammatory products can promote extended fibroplasia and excessive fibrogenesis, which can lead to irreversible tissue damage.[97] Fibrosis can occur in synovial structures, as with adhesive capsulitis in the shoulder, in extraarticular tissues including tendons and ligaments, in bursa, or in muscle.

Clinical Decision-Making Exercise 2-3

A cross-country runner strained her quadriceps. How will the healing process for this injury differ from the process for a ligamentous injury?

The Importance of Collagen

Collagen is a major structural protein that forms strong, flexible, inelastic structures that hold connective tissue together. There are at least 16 types of collagen, but 80% to 90% of the collagen in the body consists of types I, II, and III. Type I collagen is found in skin, fascia, tendon, bone, ligaments, cartilage, and interstitial tissues; type II can be found in hyaline cartilage and vertebral disks; and type III is found in skin, smooth muscle, nerves, and blood vessels. Type III collagen has less tensile strength than does type I, and tends to be found more in the fibroblastic repair phase. Collagen enables a tissue to resist mechanical forces and deformation. Elastin, however, produces highly elastic tissues that assist in recovery from deformation. Collagen fibrils are the loadbearing elements of connective tissue. They are arranged to accommodate tensile stress, but are not as capable of resisting shear or compressive stress. Consequently, the direction of orientation of collagen fibers is along lines of tensile stress.[93]

Collagen has several mechanical and physical properties that allow it to respond to loading and deformation, permitting it to withstand high tensile stress. The mechanical properties of collagen include elasticity, which is the capability to recover normal length after elongation; viscoelasticity, which allows for a slow return to normal length and shape after deformation; and plasticity, which allows for permanent change or deformation. The physical properties include force relaxation, which indicates the decrease in the amount of force needed to maintain a tissue at a set amount of displacement or deformation over time; creep response, which is the ability of a tissue to deform over time while a constant load is imposed; and hysteresis, which is the amount of relaxation a tissue has undergone during deformation and displacement. Injury results when the mechanical and physical limitations of connective tissue are exceeded.[103]

Maturation Remodeling Phase

The maturation remodeling phase of healing is a long-term process (Figure 2-2D). This phase features a realignment or remodeling of the collagen fibers that make up scar tissue according to the tensile forces to which that scar is subjected. Ongoing breakdown and synthesis of collagen occur with a steady increase in the tensile strength of the scar matrix. With increased stress and strain, the collagen fibers realign in a position of maximum efficiency parallel to the lines of tension.[21] The tissue gradually assumes normal appearance and function, although a scar is rarely as strong as the normal injured tissue. Usually by the end of about 3 weeks, a firm, strong, contracted, nonvascular scar exists. The maturation phase of healing might require several years to be totally complete.

Role of Progressive Controlled Mobility During the Healing Process

Wolff's law states that bone and soft tissue will respond to the physical demands placed on them, causing them to remodel or realign along lines of tensile force.[101] Consequently, it is critical that injured structures be exposed to progressively increasing loads throughout the rehabilitative process.[73]

In animal models, controlled mobilization is superior to immobilization for scar formation, revascularization, muscle regeneration, and reorientation of muscle fibers and tensile properties.[71] However, a brief period of immobilization of the injured tissue during the inflammatory response phase is recommended and will likely facilitate the process of healing by controlling inflammation, thus reducing clinical symptoms. As healing progresses to the repair phase, controlled activity directed toward return to normal flexibility and strength should be combined with protective support or bracing.[50] Generally, clinical signs and symptoms disappear at the end of this phase.

As the remodeling phase begins, aggressive active range of motion (ROM) and strengthening exercises should be incorporated to facilitate tissue remodeling and realignment. To a great extent, pain will dictate rate of progression. With initial injury, pain is intense; it tends to decrease and eventually subside altogether as healing progresses. Any exacerbation of pain, swelling, or other clinical symptoms during or after a particular exercise or activity indicate that the load is too great for the level of tissue repair or remodeling. The therapist must be aware of the time required for the healing process and realize that being overly aggressive can interfere with that process.

Clinical Decision-Making Exercise 2-4

A track athlete is recovering from a grade 1 ankle sprain. Beginning exercises as soon as possible will increase the injured runner's chances of recovering quickly and strongly. Why is this so?

Factors That Impede Healing

Extent of Injury

The nature of the inflammatory response is determined by the extent of the tissue injury. Microtears or soft tissue involve only minor damage and are most often associated with overuse. Macrotears involve significantly greater destruction of soft tissue and result in clinical symptoms and functional alterations. Macrotears are generally caused by acute trauma.[19]

Edema

The increased pressure caused by swelling retards the healing process, causes separation of tissues, inhibits neuromuscular control, produces reflexive neurologic changes, and impedes nutrition in the injured part. Edema is best controlled and managed during the initial first-aid management period, as described previously.[17]

Hemorrhage

Bleeding occurs with even the smallest amount of damage to the capillaries. Bleeding produces the same negative effects on healing as does the accumulation of edema, and its presence produces additional tissue damage and thus exacerbation of the injury.[67]

Poor Vascular Supply

Injuries to tissues with a poor vascular supply heal poorly and at a slow rate. This response is likely related to a failure in the initial delivery of phagocytic cells and fibroblasts necessary for scar formation.[67]

Separation of Tissue

Mechanical separation of tissue can significantly impact the course of healing. A wound that has smooth edges in good apposition will tend to heal by primary intention with minimal scarring. Conversely, a wound that has jagged, separated edges must heal by secondary intention, with granulation tissue filling the defect, and excessive scarring.

Muscle Spasm

Muscle spasm causes traction on the torn tissue, separates the two ends, and prevents approximation. Local and generalized ischemia can result from spasm.

Atrophy

Wasting away of muscle tissue begins immediately with injury. Strengthening and early mobilization of the injured structure retard atrophy.

Corticosteroids

Use of corticosteroids in the treatment of inflammation is controversial. Steroid use in the early stages of healing has been demonstrated to inhibit fibroplasia, capillary proliferation, collagen synthesis, and increases in tensile strength of the healing scar. Their use in the later stages of healing and with chronic inflammation is debatable.

Keloids and Hypertrophic Scars

Keloids occur when the rate of collagen production exceeds the rate of collagen breakdown during the maturation phase of healing. This process leads to hypertrophy of scar tissue, particularly around the periphery of the wound.

Infection

The presence of bacteria in the wound can delay healing, causes excessive granulation tissue, and frequently causes large, deformed scars.[12]

Humidity, Climate, and Oxygen Tension

Humidity significantly influences the process of epithelization. Occlusive dressing stimulates the epithelium to migrate twice as fast without crust or scab formation. The formation of a scab occurs with dehydration of the wound and traps wound drainage, which promotes infection. Keeping the wound moist provides an advantage for the necrotic debris to go to the surface and be shed.

Oxygen tension relates to the neovascularization of the wound, which translates into optimal saturation and maximal tensile strength development. Circulation to the wound can be affected by ischemia, venous stasis, hematomas, and vessel trauma.

Health, Age, and Nutrition

The elastic qualities of the skin decrease with age. Degenerative diseases, such as diabetes and arteriosclerosis, also become a concern of the older patient and can affect wound healing. Nutrition is important for wound healing—in particular, vitamins C (for collagen synthesis and immune system), K (for clotting), and A (for the immune system); zinc (for the enzyme systems); and amino acids play critical roles in the healing process.

INJURIES TO ARTICULAR STRUCTURES

Before discussing injuries to the various articular structures, a review of joint structure is in order[66] (Figure 2-3). All synovial joints are composed of two or more bones that articulate with one another to allow motion in one or more places. The articulating surfaces of the bone are lined with a very thin, smooth, cartilaginous covering called a hyaline cartilage. All joints are entirely surrounded by a thick,

ligamentous joint capsule. The inner surface of this joint capsule is lined by a very thin synovial membrane that is highly vascularized and innervated. The synovial membrane produces synovial fluid, the functions of which include lubrication, shock absorption, and nutrition of the joint.[89]

Some joints contain a thick fibrocartilage called a meniscus. The knee joint, for example, contains two wedge-shaped menisci that deepen the articulation and provide shock absorption in that joint. Finally, the main structural support and joint stability is provided by the ligaments, which may be either thickened portions of a joint capsule or totally separate bands.

Ligament Sprains

Ligaments are composed of dense connective tissue arranged in parallel bundles of collagen composed of rows of fibroblasts. Although bundles are arranged in parallel, not all collagen fibers are arranged in parallel. Ligaments and tendons are very similar in structure. However, ligaments are usually more flattened than tendons, and collagen fibers in ligaments are more compact. The anatomical positioning of the ligaments determines in part what motions a joint can make.

A sprain involves damage to a ligament that provides support to a joint. A ligament is a tough, relatively inelastic band of tissue that connects one bone to another. A ligament's primary function is threefold: to provide stability to a joint, to provide control of the position of one articulating bone to another during normal joint motion, and to provide proprioceptive input or a sense of joint position through the function of free nerve endings or mechanoreceptors located within the ligament.

If stress is applied to a joint that forces motion beyond its normal limits or planes of movement, injury to the ligament is likely[34] (Figure 2-4). The severity of damage to the ligament is classified in many different ways; however, the most commonly used system involves three grades (degrees) of ligamentous sprain.

- Grade 1 sprain: There is some stretching or perhaps tearing of the ligamentous fibers, with little or no joint instability. Mild pain,

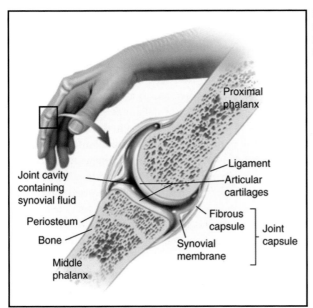

Figure 2-3. General anatomy of a synovial joint. (Reproduced with permission from Saladin K. *Anatomy & Physiology*, 6th ed. New York: McGraw-Hill; 2012:284.)

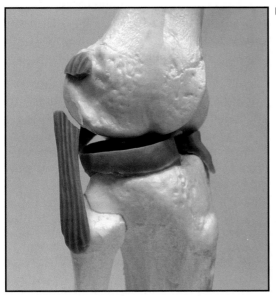

Figure 2-4. Grade 3 ligament sprain in the knee joint.

little swelling, and joint stiffness might be apparent.

- Grade 2 sprain: There is some tearing and separation of the ligamentous fibers and moderate instability of the joint. Moderate-to-severe pain, swelling, and joint stiffness should be expected.

Clinical Decision-Making Exercise 2-5

A basketball player twisted his ankle today in practice. The mechanism and the location of pain suggest an inversion sprain. There is gross laxity with the anterior drawer test and talar tilt test. The swelling is severe and profuse over the lateral side of the ankle. The athlete is incapable of dorsiflexion and has only a few degrees of plantar flexion. He is experiencing very little pain. How would you grade the severity of this injury?

- Grade 3 sprain: There is total rupture of the ligament, manifested primarily by gross instability of the joint. Severe pain might be present initially, followed by little or no pain because of total disruption of nerve fibers. Swelling might be profuse, and thus the joint tends to become very stiff some hours after the injury. A third-degree sprain with marked instability usually requires some form of immobilization lasting several weeks. Frequently, the force producing the ligament injury is so great that other ligaments or structures surrounding the joint are also injured. With cases in which there is injury to multiple joint structures, surgical repair reconstruction may be necessary to correct an instability.

Clinical Decision-Making Exercise 2-6

Why is it likely that an athlete with a grade 3 ligament sprain initially will experience little pain, relative to the severity of the injury?

Physiology of Ligament Healing

The healing process in the sprained ligament follows the same course of repair as with other vascular tissues. Immediately after injury and for about 72 hours there is a loss of blood from damaged vessels and attraction of inflammatory cells into the injured area. If a ligament is sprained outside of a joint capsule (extraarticular ligament), bleeding occurs in a subcutaneous space. If an intraarticular ligament is injured, bleeding occurs inside of the joint capsule until either clotting occurs or the pressure becomes so great that bleeding ceases.

During the next 6 weeks, vascular proliferation with new capillary growth begins to occur along with fibroblastic activity, resulting in the formation of a fibrin clot. It is essential that the torn ends of the ligament be reconnected by bridging this clot. Synthesis of collagen and ground substance of proteoglycan as constituents of an intracellular matrix contributes to the proliferation of the scar that bridges between the torn ends of the ligament. This scar initially is soft and viscous but eventually becomes more elastic. Collagen fibers are arranged in a random woven pattern with little organization. Gradually there is a decrease in fibroblastic activity, a decrease in vascularity, and an increase to a maximum in collagen density of the scar.[4] Failure to produce enough scar and failure to reconnect the ligament to the appropriate location on a bone are the two reasons why ligaments are likely to fail.

During the next several months the scar continues to mature, with the realignment of collagen occurring in response to progressive stresses and strains. The maturation of the scar may require as long as 12 months to complete.[4] The exact length of time required for maturation depends on mechanical factors such as apposition of torn ends and length of the period of immobilization.

Factors Affecting Ligament Healing

Surgically repaired extraarticular ligaments have healed with decreased scar formation and are generally stronger than unrepaired ligaments initially, although this strength advantage might not be maintained as time progresses. Unrepaired ligaments heal by fibrous scarring effectively lengthening the ligament and producing some degree of joint instability. With intraarticular ligament tears, the presence of synovial fluid dilutes the hematoma, thus preventing formation of a fibrin clot and spontaneous healing.[42]

Data from several studies indicate that actively exercised ligaments are stronger than those that are immobilized. Ligaments that are immobilized for several weeks after injury tend to decrease in tensile strength and also exhibit weakening of the insertion of the ligament to bone.[72] Thus it is important to minimize periods of immobilization and progressively stress the injured ligaments while exercising caution relative to biomechanical considerations for specific ligaments.[4,68]

It is not likely that the inherent stability of the joint provided by the ligament before injury will be regained. Thus, to restore stability to the joint, the other structures that surround that joint, primarily muscles and their tendons, must be strengthened. The increased muscle tension provided by resistance training can improve stability of the injured joint.[68,88]

Cartilage Damage

Cartilage is a type of rigid connective tissue that provides support and acts as a framework in many structures. It is composed of chondrocyte cells contained in small chambers called lacunae, surrounded completely by an intracellular matrix. The matrix consists of varying ratios of collagen and elastin and a ground substance made of proteoglycans and glycosaminoglycans, which are nonfibrous protein molecules. These proteoglycans act as sponges and trap large quantities of water, which allow cartilage to spring back after being compressed.[96] Cartilage has a poor blood supply, thus healing after injury is very slow. There are three types of cartilage. Hyaline cartilage is found on the articulating surfaces of bone and in the soft part of the nose. It contains large quantities of collagen and proteoglycan. Fibrocartilage forms the intervertebral disk and menisci located in several joint spaces. It has greater amounts of collagen than proteoglycan and is capable of withstanding a great deal of pressure. Elastic cartilage is found in the auricle of the ear and the larynx. It is more flexible than the other types of cartilage and consists of collagen, proteoglycan, and elastin.[79]

Osteoarthrosis is a degenerative condition of bone and cartilage in and about the joint. Arthritis should be defined as primarily an inflammatory condition with possible destruction.[6] Arthrosis is primarily a degenerative process with destruction of cartilage, remodeling of bone, and possible secondary inflammatory components.

Cartilage fibrillates, that is, releases fibers or groups of fibers and ground substance into the joint.[29] Peripheral cartilage that is not exposed to weight-bearing or compression–decompression mechanisms is particularly likely to fibrillate. Fibrillation is typically found in the degenerative process associated with poor nutrition or disuse. This process can then extend even to weight-bearing areas, with progressive destruction of cartilage proportional to stresses applied on it. When forces are increased, thus increasing stress, osteochondral or subchondral fractures can occur. Concentration of stress on small areas can produce pressures that overwhelm the tissue's capabilities. Typically, lower-limb joints have to handle greater stresses, but their surface area is usually larger than the surface area of upper limbs. The articular cartilage is protected to some extent by the synovial fluid, which acts as a lubricant. It is also protected by the subchondral bone, which responds to stresses in an elastic fashion. It is more compliant than compact bone, and microfractures can be a means of force absorption. Trabeculae might fracture or might be displaced due to pressures applied on the subchondral bone. In compact bone, fracture can be a means of defense to dissipate force. In the joint, forces might be absorbed by joint movement and eccentric contraction of muscles.[27]

In the majority of joints where the surfaces are not congruent, the applied forces tend to concentrate in certain areas, which increases joint degeneration. Osteophytosis occurs as a bone attempts to increase its surface area to decrease contact forces. People typically describe this growth as "bone spurs." Chondromalacia is the nonprogressive transformation of cartilage with irregular surfaces and areas of softening. It typically occurs first in non–weight-bearing areas and may progress to areas of excessive stress.[26]

In physically active individuals, certain joints maybe more susceptible to a response resembling osteoarthrosis.[70] The proportion of body weight resting on the joint, the pull of the musculotendinous unit, and any significant external force applied to the joint are predisposing factors. Altered joint mechanics caused by laxity or previous trauma are also factors that come into play.[45] The intensity of forces can be great, as in the hip, where the previously mentioned factors can produce pressures or forces four times that of body weight and up to 10 times that of body weight on the knee.

Typically, muscle forces generate more stress than body weight itself. Particular injuries are conducive to osteoarthritic changes such as subluxation and dislocation of the patella, osteochondritis dissecans, recurrent synovial effusion, and hemarthrosis. Also, ligamentous injuries can bring about a disruption of proprioceptive mechanisms, loss of adequate joint alignment, and meniscal damage in the knees with removal of the injured meniscus.[40] Other factors that have an impact are loss of full ROM, poor muscular power and strength, and altered biomechanics of the joint. Spurring and spiking of bone are not synonymous with osteoarthrosis if the joint space is maintained and the cartilage lining is intact. It may simply be an adaptation to the increased stress of physical activity.[29]

Physiology of Cartilage Healing

Cartilage has a relatively limited healing capacity. When chondrocytes are destroyed and the matrix is disrupted, the course of healing is variable, depending on whether damage is to cartilage alone or also to subchondral bone. Injuries to the articular cartilage alone fail to elicit clot formation or a cellular response. For the most part the chondrocytes adjacent to the injury are the only cells that show any signs of proliferation and synthesis of matrix. Thus the defect fails to heal, although the extent of the damage tends to remain the same.[33,58]

If subchondral bone is also affected, inflammatory cells enter the damaged area and formulate granulation tissue. In this case, the healing process proceeds normally, with differentiation of granulation tissue cells into chondrocytes occurring in about 2 weeks. At about 2 months, normal collagen has been formed.

Injuries to the knee articular cartilage are extremely common, and until recently, methods for treatment did not produce good long-term results.[102] A better understanding of how articular cartilage responds to injury has produced various techniques that hold promise for long-term success.[91] One such technique is autologous chondrocyte implantation, in which a patient's own cartilage cells are harvested, grown ex vivo, and reimplanted in a full-thickness articular surface defect. Results are available with up to 10 years of follow-up, and more than 80% of patients have shown improvement with relatively few complications.

INJURIES TO BONE

Bone is a type of connective tissue consisting of both living cells and minerals deposited in a matrix (Figure 2-5). Each bone consists of three major components. The epiphysis is an expanded portion at each end of the bone that articulates with another bone. Each articulating surface is covered by an articular, or hyaline, cartilage. The diaphysis is the shaft of the bone. The epiphyseal or growth plate is the major site of bone growth and elongation. Once bone growth ceases, the plate ossifies and forms the epiphyseal line. With the exception of the articulating surfaces, the bone is completely enclosed by the periosteum, a tough, highly vascularized and innervated fibrous tissue.[55]

The two types of bone material are cancellous, or spongy, bone and cortical, or compact, bone. Cancellous bone contains a series of air spaces referred to as trabeculae, whereas cortical bone is relatively solid. Cortical bone in the diaphysis forms a hollow medullary canal in long bone, which is lined with endosteum and filled with bone marrow. Bone has rich blood supply that certainly facilitates the healing process after injury. Bone has the functions of support, movement, and protection. Furthermore, bone stores and releases calcium into the bloodstream and manufactures red blood cells.[93]

Fractures

Fractures are extremely common injuries among the athletic population. They can be generally classified as being either open or closed. A closed fracture involves little or no displacement of bones and thus little or no soft tissue disruption. An open fracture involves enough displacement of the fractured ends that the bone actually disrupts the cutaneous layers and breaks through the skin. Both fractures can be relatively serious if not managed properly, but an increased possibility of infection exists in an open fracture. Fractures may also be considered complete, in which the bone is broken into at least two fragments, or incomplete, where the fracture does not extend completely across the bone.

The varieties of fractures that can occur include greenstick, transverse, oblique, spiral, comminuted, avulsion, and stress. A greenstick fracture (Figure 2-6A) occurs most often in children whose bones are still growing and have not yet had a chance to calcify and harden. It is called a greenstick fracture because of the resemblance to the splintering that occurs to a tree twig that is bent to the point of breaking.

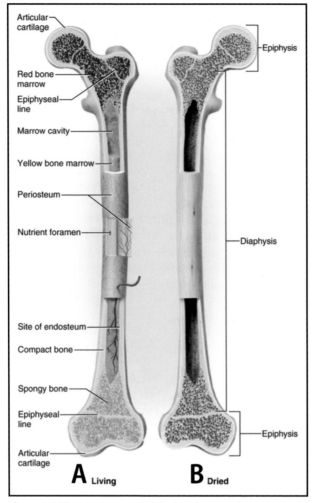

Figure 2-5. The gross structure of the long bones includes the diaphysis, epiphysis, articular cartilage, and periosteum. (Reproduced with permission from Saladin K. *Anatomy & Physiology*, 6th ed. New York: McGraw-Hill; 2012:208.)

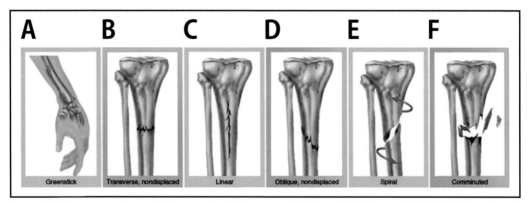

Figure 2-6. Fractures of bone. (A) Greenstick. (B) Transverse. (C) Linear. (D) Oblique. (E) Spiral. (F) Comminuted. (Reproduced with permission from Prentice W. *Essentials of Athletic Injury Management*, 9th ed. New York: McGraw-Hill; 2013.)

Because the twig is green, it splinters but can be bent without causing an actual break.

A transverse fracture (Figure 2-6B) involves a crack perpendicular to the longitudinal axis of the bone that goes all the way through the bone. Displacement might occur; however, because of the shape of the fractured ends, the surrounding soft tissue (eg, muscles, tendons, and fat) sustains relatively little damage.

A linear fracture runs parallel to the long axis of a bone and is similar in severity to a transverse fracture (Figure 2-6C).

An oblique fracture (Figure 2-6D) results in a diagonal crack across the bone and two very jagged, pointed ends that, if displaced, can potentially cause a good bit of soft-tissue damage. Oblique and spiral fractures are the two types most likely to result in compound fractures.

A spiral fracture (Figure 2-6E) is similar to an oblique fracture in that the angle of the fracture is diagonal across the bone. In addition, an element of twisting or rotation causes the fracture to spiral along the longitudinal axis of the bone. Spiral fractures used to be fairly common in ski injuries occurring just above the top of the boot when the bindings on the ski failed to release when the foot was rotated. These injuries are now less common as a result of improvements in equipment design.

A comminuted fracture (Figure 2-6F) is a serious problem that can require an extremely long time for rehabilitation. In the comminuted fracture, multiple fragments of bone must be surgically repaired and fixed with screws and wires. If a fracture of this type occurs to a weight-bearing bone in the leg, a permanent discrepancy in leg length can develop.

An avulsion fracture occurs when a fragment of bone is pulled away at the bony attachment of a muscle, tendon, or ligament. Avulsion fractures are common in the fingers and some of the smaller bones but can also occur in larger bones where tendinous or ligamentous attachments are subjected to a large amount of force.

Perhaps the most common fracture resulting from physical activity is the stress fracture. Unlike the other types of fractures that have been discussed, the stress fracture results from overuse or fatigue rather than acute trauma.[49] Common sites for stress fractures include the weight-bearing bones of the leg and foot. In either case, repetitive forces transmitted through the bones produce irritations and microfractures at a specific area in the bone. The pain usually begins as a dull ache that becomes progressively more painful day after day. Initially, pain is most severe during activity. However, when a stress fracture actually develops, pain tends to become worse after the activity is stopped.[80]

The biggest problem with a stress fracture is that often it does not show up on an X-ray film until the osteoblasts begin laying down subperiosteal callus or bone, at which point a small white line, or a callus, appears. However, a bone scan might reveal a potential stress fracture in as little as 2 days after onset of symptoms. If a stress fracture is suspected, the patient should stop any activity that produces added stress or fatigue to the area for a minimum of 14 days. Stress fractures do not usually require casting, but might become normal fractures that must be immobilized if handled incorrectly.[92] If a fracture occurs, it should be managed and rehabilitated by a qualified orthopedist and athletic trainer.

Physiology of Bone Healing

Healing of injured bone tissue is similar to soft-tissue healing in that all phases of the healing process can be identified, although bone regeneration capabilities are somewhat limited. However, the functional elements of healing differ significantly from those of soft tissue. Tensile strength of the scar is the single most critical factor in soft-tissue healing, whereas bone has to contend with a number of additional forces, including torsion, bending, and compression.[46] Trauma to bone can vary from contusions of the periosteum to closed, nondisplaced fractures to severely displaced open fractures that also involve significant soft-tissue damage. When a fracture occurs, blood vessels

---

Clinical Decision-Making Exercise 2-7

A Little League player collided with the catcher when sliding home. Radiographs did not show a fracture, but a bone scan shows a hot spot. What type of fracture would you suspect this young athlete has?

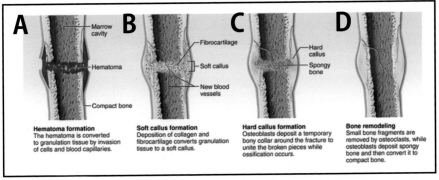

Figure 2-7. The healing of a fracture. (A) Blood vessels are broken at the fracture line; the blood clots and forms a fracture hematoma. (B) Blood vessels grow into the fracture and a fibrocartilage soft callus forms. (C) The fibrocartilage becomes ossified and forms a bony callus made of spongy bone. (D) Osteoclasts remove excess tissue from the bony callus and the bone eventually resembles its original appearance. (Reproduced with permission from Saladin K. *Anatomy & Physiology*, 6th ed. New York: McGraw-Hill; 2012:226.)

in the bone and the periosteum are damaged, resulting in bleeding and subsequent clot formation (Figure 2-7). Hemorrhaging from the marrow is contained by the periosteum and the surrounding soft tissue in the region of the fracture. In about 1 week, fibroblasts begin laying down a fibrous collagen network. The fibrin strands within the clot serve as the framework for proliferating vessels. Chondroblast cells begin producing fibrocartilage, creating a callus between the broken bones. At first, the callus is soft and firm because it is composed of primarily collagenous fibrin. The callus becomes firm and more rubbery as cartilage beings to predominate. Bone-producing cells called osteoblasts begin to proliferate and enter the callus, forming cancellous bone trabeculae that eventually replace the cartilage. Finally the callus crystallizes into bone, at which point remodeling of the bone begins. The callus can be divided into two portions, the external callus located around the periosteum on the outside of the fracture and the internal callus found between the bone fragments. The size of the callus is proportional both to the damage and to the amount of irritation to the fracture site during the healing process. Also during this time osteoclasts begin to appear in the area to resorb bone fragments and clean up debris.[42,46,83]

The remodeling process is similar to the growth process of bone in that the fibrous cartilage is gradually replaced by fibrous bone and then by more structurally efficient lamellar bone. Remodeling involves an ongoing process during which osteoblasts lay down new bone and osteoclasts remove and break down bone according to the forces placed upon the healing bone.[62] The Wolff law maintains that a bone will adapt to mechanical stresses and strains by changing size, shape, and structure. Therefore, once the cast is removed, the bone must be subjected to normal stresses and strains so that tensile strength can be regained before the healing process is complete.[36,90]

The time required for bone healing is variable and based on a number of factors, such as severity of the fracture, site of the fracture, extensiveness of the trauma, and age of the patient. Normal periods of immobilization range from as short as 3 weeks for the small bones in the hands and feet to as long as 8 weeks for the long bones of the upper and lower extremities. In some instances, such as fractures in the four small toes, immobilization might not be required for healing. The healing process is certainly not complete when the splint or cast is removed. Osteoblastic and osteoclastic activity might continue for 2 to 3 years after severe fractures.[49,62]

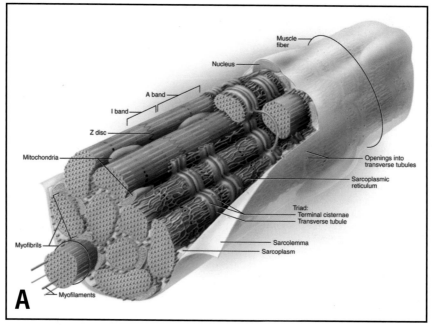

Figure 2-8. Parts of a muscle. (A) Muscle is composed of individual muscle fibers (muscle cells). Each muscle fiber contains myofibrils in which the banding patterns of the sarcomeres are seen. (Reproduced with permission from Saladin K. *Anatomy & Physiology*, 6th ed. McGraw-Hill; 2012;404.) (*continued*)

INJURIES TO MUSCULOTENDINOUS STRUCTURES

Muscle is often considered to be a type of connective tissue, but here it is treated as the third of the fundamental tissues. The three types of muscles are smooth (involuntary), cardiac, and skeletal (voluntary) muscles. Smooth muscle is found with the viscera, where it forms the walls of the internal organs, and within many hollow chambers. Cardiac muscle is found only in the heart and is responsible for its contraction. A significant characteristic of the cardiac muscle is that it contracts as a single fiber, unlike smooth and skeletal muscles, which contract as separate units. This characteristic forces the heart to work as a single unit continuously; therefore, if one portion of the muscle should die (as in myocardial infarction), contraction of the heart does not cease.[79]

Skeletal muscle is the striated muscle within the body, responsible for the movement of bony levers. Skeletal muscle consists of two portions:

(a) the muscle belly, and (b) its tendons, which are collectively referred to as a musculotendinous unit. The muscle belly is composed of separate, parallel elastic fibers called myofibrils (Figure 2-8). Myofibrils are composed of thousands of small sarcomeres, which are the functional units of the muscle. Sarcomeres contain the contractile elements of the muscle, as well as a substantial amount of connective tissue that holds the fibers together. Myofilaments are small contractile elements of protein within the sarcomere (Figure 2-8). There are two distinct types of myofilaments: thin actin myofilaments and thicker myosin myofilaments. Finger-like projections, or cross bridges, connect the actin and myosin myofilaments.[83] When a muscle is stimulated to contract, the cross bridges pull the myofilaments closer together, thus shortening the muscle and producing movement at the joint that the muscle crosses.[25] The muscle tendon attaches the muscle directly to the bone.

The muscle tendon is composed of primarily collagen fibers and a matrix of proteoglycan that is produced by the tenocyte cell. The collagen fibers are grouped together into primary

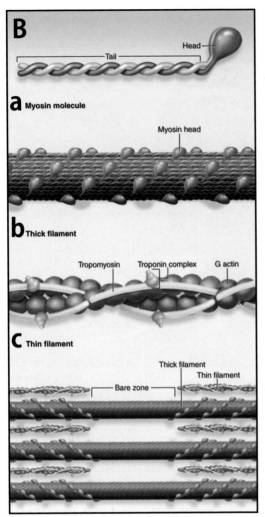

Figure 2-8. (continued) (B) The myofibrils are composed of actin myofilament and myosin myofilaments, which are formed from thousands of individual actin and myosin molecules. (Reproduced with permission from Saladin K. *Anatomy & Physiology*, 6th ed. McGraw-Hill; 2012;404.)

and return to normal length; (c) excitability, the ability to respond to stimulation from the nervous system; and (d) contractility, the ability to shorten and contract in response to some neural command.[55]

Skeletal muscles show considerable variation in size and shape. Large muscles generally produce gross motor movements at large joints, such as knee flexion produced by contraction of the large, bulky hamstring muscles. Smaller skeletal muscles, such as the long flexors of the fingers, produce fine motor movements. Muscles producing movements that are powerful in nature are usually thicker and longer, whereas those producing finer movements requiring coordination are thin and relatively shorter. Other muscles may be flat, round, or fan-shaped.[42,83] Muscles may be connected to a bone by a single tendon or by two or three separate tendons at either end. Muscles that have two separate muscle and tendon attachments are called biceps, and muscles with threeseparate muscle and tendon attachments are called triceps.

Muscles contract in response to stimulation by the central nervous system. An electrical impulse transmitted from the central nervous system through a single motor nerve to a group of muscle fibers causes a depolarization of those fibers. The motor nerve and the group of muscle fibers that it innervates are collectively referred to as a motor unit. An impulse coming from the central nervous system and traveling to a group of fibers through a particular motor nerve causes all the muscle fibers in that motor unit to depolarize and contract. This is referred to as the all-or-none response and applies to all skeletal muscles in the body.[42]

Muscle Strains

If a musculotendinous unit is overstretched or forced to contract against too much resistance, exceeding the extensibility limits or the tensile capabilities of the weakest component within the unit, damage can occur to the muscle fibers, at the musculotendinous juncture, in the tendon, or at the tendinous attachment to the bone.[34] Any of these injuries may be referred to as a strain (Figure 2-10). Muscle strains, like ligament sprains, are subject to

bundles (Figure 2-9). Groups of primary bundles join together to form hexagonal-shaped secondary bundles. Secondary bundles are held together by intertwined loose connective tissue containing elastin, called the endotenon. The entire tendon is surrounded by a connective tissue layer, called the epitenon. The outermost layer of the tendon is the paratenon, which is a double-layer connective tissue sheath lined on the inside with synovial membrane.[56] All skeletal muscles exhibit four characteristics: (a) elasticity, the ability to change in length or stretch; (b) extensibility, the ability to shorten

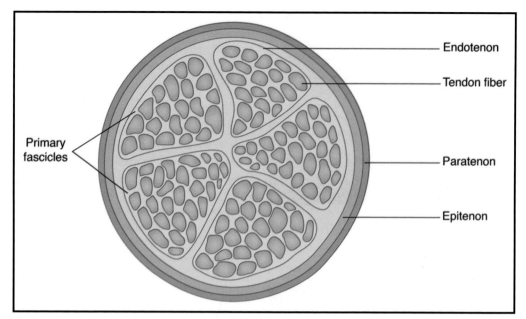

Figure 2-9. Structure of a tendon.

various classification systems. The following is a simple system of classification of muscle strains:

- Grade 1 strain: Some muscle or tendon fibers have been stretched or actually torn. Active motion produces some tenderness and pain. Movement is painful, but full ROM is usually possible.

- Grade 2 strain: Some muscle or tendon fibers have been torn and active contraction of the muscle is extremely painful. Usually a palpable depression or divot exists somewhere in the muscle belly at the spot where the muscle fibers have been torn. Some swelling might occur because of capillary bleeding.

- Grade 3 strain: There is a complete rupture of muscle fibers in the muscle belly, in the area where the muscle becomes tendon, or at the tendinous attachment to the bone. The patient has significant impairment to, or perhaps total loss of, movement. Pain is intense initially but diminishes quickly because of complete separation of the nerve fibers. Musculotendinous ruptures are most common in the biceps tendon of the upper arm or in the Achilles heel cord in the back of the calf. When either of these tendons rupture, the muscle tends

to bunch toward its proximal attachment. With the exception of an Achilles rupture, which is frequently surgically repaired, the majority of third-degree strains are treated conservatively with some period of immobilization.

Physiology of Muscle Healing

Injuries to muscle tissue involve similar processes of healing and repair as discussed for other tissues. Initially there will be hemorrhage and edema followed almost immediately by phagocytosis to clear debris. Within a few days there is a proliferation of ground substance, and fibroblasts begin producing a gel-type matrix that surrounds the connective tissue, leading to fibrosis and scarring. At the same time, myoblastic cells form in the area of injury, which will eventually lead to regeneration or new myofibrils. Thus regeneration of both connective tissue and muscle tissue begins.[13]

Collagen fibers undergo maturation and orient themselves along lines of tensile force according to Wolff's law. Active contraction of the muscle is critical in regaining normal tensile strength.[5,50]

It is now well accepted that satellite cells play a critical role in the ability of the muscle cell to regenerate following injury.[76] Satellite

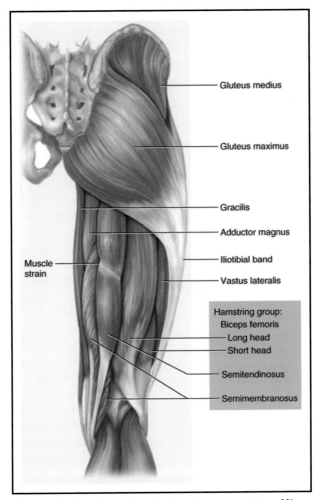

Figure 2-10. A muscle strain results in tearing or separation of fibers. (Reproduced with permission from Saladin K. *Anatomy & Physiology,* 6th ed. New York: McGraw-Hill; 2012:365.)

cells are the stem cells of skeletal muscle. These self-renewing cells can generate a population of myoblasts that are able to fuse with existing myofibers to help in facilitating growth, repair, and regeneration.[98]

Regardless of the severity of the strain, the time required for rehabilitation is fairly lengthy. In many instances, rehabilitation time for a muscle strain is longer than that for a ligament sprain. These incapacitating muscle strains occur most frequently in the large, force-producing hamstring and quadriceps muscles of the lower extremity. The treatment of hamstring strains requires a healing period of at least 5 to 8 weeks and a considerable amount of patience. Attempts to return to activity too soon frequently cause reinjury to the area of the musculotendinous unit that has been strained, and the healing process must begin again.[60]

Tendinopathy/Tendinitis/Tendinosis

Of all the overuse problems associated with activity, chronic overuse injuries involving a tendon are the most common.[81,99] The term *tendinopathy* is the term that is most often used to refer to both *tendinitis,* which is an inflammation of the tendon, and *tendinosis,* which refers to microtears and degeneration of a tendon. The suffix *-opathy* does not imply any specific type of pathology.[51] Any term ending in the suffix *-itis* means inflammation is present. Tendinitis means inflammation of a tendon.

During muscle activity, a tendon must move or slide on other structures around it whenever the muscle contracts. If a particular movement is performed repeatedly, the tendon becomes irritated and inflamed.[65] This inflammation is manifested by pain on movement, swelling, possibly some warmth, and usually crepitus.[87] *Crepitus* is a crackling feeling or sound. It is usually caused by the tendon's tendency to stick to the surrounding structure while it slides back and forth. This sticking is caused primarily by the chemical products of inflammation that accumulate on the irritated tendon.[87] The key to the treatment of tendinitis is rest.[40] If the repetitive motion causing irritation to the tendon is eliminated, the inflammatory process will allow the tendon to heal. Unfortunately, athletes find it difficult to totally stop activity and rest for 2 or more weeks while the tendinitis subsides. The patient should substitute some form of activity, such as bicycling or swimming, to maintain present fitness levels while avoiding continued irritation of the inflamed tendon. In runners, tendinitis most commonly occurs in the Achilles tendon in the back of the lower leg. In swimmers, it often occurs in the muscle tendons of the shoulder joint. However, tendinitis can flare up in any activity in which overuse and repetitive movements occur.

If repetitive overuse continues and the inflamed or irritated tendon fails to heal, the tendon begins to degenerate. The primary concern shifts from tendon inflammation to tendon degeneration, a condition referred to as tendinosis.[65] The suffix -*osis* means there is chronic degeneration without inflammation. *Most of the chronic problems that we have with tendons are correctly referred to as tendinosis.*[48] The symptoms are somewhat similar to tendinitis. The inflammation ceases, however. The affected tendons are usually painful when moved or touched. The tendon sheaths may be visibly swollen with stiffness and restricted motion. Sometimes a tender lump appears. Tendinosis is more common in middle or old age as the tendons become more susceptible to injury.[48] However, younger people who exercise vigorously as well as people who perform repetitive tasks are also susceptible. The key to treating tendinosis is engaging in exercises to strengthen the tendon and consistently stretching the tendon.

Tenosynovitis

Tenosynovitis is very similar to tendinitis in that the muscle tendons are involved in inflammation. However, many tendons are subject to an increased amount of friction as a result of the tightness of the space through which they must move. In these areas of high friction, tendons are usually surrounded by synovial sheaths that reduce friction on movement. If the tendon sliding through a synovial sheath is subjected to overuse, inflammation is likely to occur. The inflammatory process produces by-products that are "sticky" and tend to cause the sliding tendon to adhere to the synovial sheath surrounding it.[51]

Symptomatically, tenosynovitis is very similar to tendinitis, with pain on movement, tenderness, swelling, and crepitus. Movement may be more limited with tenosynovitis because the space provided for the tendon and its synovial covering is more limited. Tenosynovitis occurs most commonly in the long flexor tendons of the fingers as they cross over the wrist joint and in the biceps tendon around the shoulder joint. Treatment for tenosynovitis is the same as that for tendinitis. Because both conditions involve inflammation, mild anti-inflammatory drugs, such as aspirin, might be helpful in chronic cases.[51]

Physiology of Tendon Healing

Unlike most soft-tissue healing, tendon injuries pose a particular problem in rehabilitation.[40] The injured tendon requires dense fibrous union of the separated ends and both extensibility and flexibility at the site of attachment. Thus an abundance of collagen is required to achieve good tensile strength. Unfortunately, collagen synthesis can become excessive, resulting in fibrosis, in which adhesions form in surrounding tissues and interfere with the gliding that is essential for smooth motion. Fortunately, over time the scar tissue of the surrounding tissues becomes elongated in its structure because of a breakdown in the crosslinks between fibrin units and thus allows the necessary gliding motion. A tendon injury

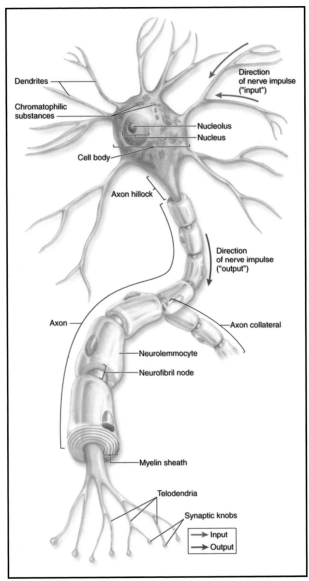

Figure 2-11. Structural features of a nerve cell. (Reproduced with permission from McKinley & O'Loughlin. *Human Anatomy*. Chicago, IL: McGraw-Hill; 2006:421.)

that occurs where the tendon is surrounded by a synovial sheath can be potentially devastating.

A typical time frame for tendon healing would be that during the second week when the healing tendon adheres to the surrounding tissue to form a single mass and during the third week when the tendon separates to varying degrees from the surrounding tissues. However, the tensile strength is not sufficient to permit a strong pull on the tendon for at least 4 to 5 weeks, the danger being that a strong contraction can pull the tendon ends apart.[85]

INJURIES TO NERVE TISSUE

The final fundamental tissue is nerve tissue (Figure 2-11). This tissue provides sensitivity and communication from the central nervous system (brain and spinal cord) to the muscles, sensory organs, various systems,

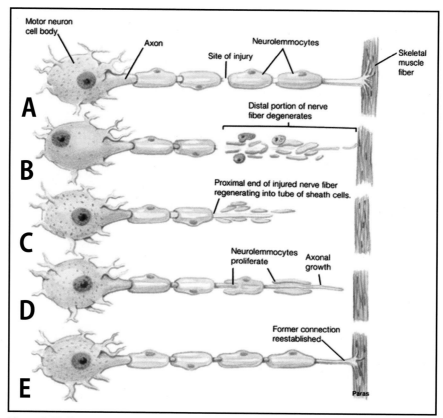

Figure 2-12. Neuron regeneration. (A) If a neuron is severed through a myelinated axon, the proximal portion may survive, but (B) the distal portion will degenerate through phagocytosis. (C) and (D) The myelin layer provides a pathway for regeneration of the axon, and (E) innervation is restored. (Reproduced with permission from Van De Graaff. *Human Anatomy*. Chicago, IL: McGraw-Hill Higher Education; 2002:354.)

and the periphery. The basic nerve cell is the neuron. The neuron cell body contains a large nucleus and branched extensions called dendrites, which respond to neurotransmitter substances released from other nerve cells. From each nerve cell arises a single axon, which conducts the nerve impulses. Large axons found in peripheral nerves are enclosed in sheaths composed of Schwann cells, which are tightly wound around the axon. A nerve is a bundle of nerve cells held together by some connective tissue, usually a lipid-protein layer called the myelin sheath, on the outside of the axon.[93] Neurology is an extremely complex science, and only a brief presentation of its relevance to musculoskeletal injuries is made here.[16]

Nerve injuries usually involve either contusions or inflammations. More serious injuries involve the crushing of a nerve or complete division (severing). This type of injury can produce lifelong physical disability, such as paraplegia or quadriplegia, and thus should not be overlooked in any circumstance.

Of critical concern to the athletic trainer is the importance of the nervous system in proprioception and neuromuscular control of movement as an integral part of a rehabilitation program. Chapter 4 discusses this in great detail.

Physiology of Nerve Healing

Nerve cell tissue is specialized and cannot regenerate once the nerve cell dies. In an injured peripheral nerve, however, the nerve fiber can regenerate significantly if the injury does not affect the cell body (see Figure 2-12). The proximity of the axonal injury to the cell body can significantly affect the time required for healing. The closer an injury is to the cell body, the more difficult is the regenerative process. In the case of severed nerve, surgical intervention can markedly enhance regeneration.[79]

For regeneration to occur, an optimal environment for healing must exist. When a nerve is cut, several degenerative changes occur that interfere with the neural pathways (Figure 2-12). Within the first 3 to 5 days the portion of the axon distal to the cut begins to degenerate and breaks into irregular segments. There is also a concomitant increase in metabolism and protein production by the nerve cell body to facilitate the regenerative process. The neuron in the cell body contains the genetic material and produces chemicals necessary for maintenance of the axon. These substances cannot be transmitted to the distal part of the axon, and eventually there will be complete degeneration.[83]

In addition, the myelin portion of the Schwann cells around the degenerating axon also degenerates, and the myelin is phagocytized. The Schwann cells divide, forming a column of cells in place of the axon. If the cut ends of the axon contact this column of Schwann cells, the chances are good that an axon may eventually reinnervate distal structures. If the proximal end of the axon does not make contact with the column of Schwann cells, reinnervation will not occur.

Clinical Decision-Making Exercise 2-8

A field hockey player suffered a contusion from a ball on the elbow just superior to the medial epicondyle. She sustained some ulnar nerve damage. In general, what is the likelihood that the nerve will repair itself?

The axon proximal to the cut has minimal degeneration initially and then begins the regenerative process with growth from the proximal axon. Bulbous enlargements and several axon sprouts form at the end of the proximal axon. Within about 2 weeks, these sprouts grow across the scar that has developed in the area of the cut and enter the column of Schwann cells. Only one of these sprouts will form the new axon, whereas the others will degenerate. Once the axon grows through the Schwann cell columns, remaining Schwann

cells proliferate along the length of the degenerating fiber and form new myelin around the growing axon, which will eventually reinnervate distal structures.[42]

Regeneration is slow, at a rate of only 3 to 4 mm per day. Axon regeneration can be obstructed by scar formation caused by excessive fibroplasia. Damaged nerves within the central nervous system regenerate very poorly compared to nerves in the peripheral nervous system. Central nervous system axons lack connective tissue sheaths, and the myelin producing Schwann cells fail to proliferate.[42,83]

ADDITIONAL MUSCULOSKELETAL INJURIES

Dislocations and Subluxations

A dislocation occurs when at least one bone in an articulation is forced out of its normal and proper alignment and stays out until it is either manually or surgically put back into place or reduced.[10] Dislocations most commonly occur in the shoulder joint, elbow, and fingers, but they can occur wherever two bones articulate.[15,64,82]

A subluxation is like a dislocation except that in this situation a bone pops out of its normal articulation but then goes right back into place. Subluxations most commonly occur in the shoulder joint, as well as in the kneecap in females.

Dislocations should never be reduced immediately, regardless of where they occur. The patient should have an X-ray to rule out fractures or other problems before reduction. Inappropriate techniques of reduction might only exacerbate the problem. Return to activity after dislocation or subluxation is largely dependent on the degree of soft-tissue damage.[15]

Bursitis

In many areas, particularly around joints, friction occurs between tendons and bones, skin and bone, or two muscles. Without some mechanism of protection in these high-friction areas, chronic irritation would be likely.[93]

Bursae are essentially pieces of synovial membrane that contain small amounts of synovial fluid. This presence of synovium permits motion of surrounding structures without friction. If excessive movement or perhaps some acute trauma occurs around these bursae, they become irritated and inflamed and begin producing large amounts of synovial fluid. The longer the irritation continues or the more severe the acute trauma, the more fluid is produced. As the fluid continues to accumulate in a limited space, pressure tends to increase and causes irritation of the pain receptors in the area.

Bursitis can be extremely painful and can severely restrict movement, especially if it occurs around a joint. Synovial fluid continues to be produced until the movement or trauma producing the irritation is eliminated.

A bursa that occasionally completely surrounds a tendon to allow more freedom of movement in a tight area is referred to as a synovial sheath. Irritation of this synovial sheath may restrict tendon motion.

All joints have many bursae surrounding them. Perhaps the three bursae most commonly irritated as a result of various types of physical activity are the subacromial bursa in the shoulder joint, the olecranon bursa on the tip of the elbow, and the prepatellar bursa on the front surface of the patella. All three of these bursae have produced large amounts of synovial fluid, affecting motion at their respective joints.

Muscle Soreness

Overexertion in strenuous muscular exercise often results in muscular pain. At one time or another, almost everyone has experienced muscle soreness, usually resulting from some physical activity to which we are unaccustomed.

There are two types of muscle soreness. The first type of muscle pain is acute and accompanies fatigue. It is transient and occurs during and immediately after exercise. The second type of soreness involves delayed muscle pain that appears about 12 hours after injury. It becomes most intense after 24 to 48 hours and then gradually subsides so that the muscle becomes symptom-free after 3 or 4 days. This second type of pain may best be described as a syndrome of delayed muscle pain, leading to increased muscle tension, edema formation, increased stiffness, and resistance to stretching.[61]

The cause of delayed-onset muscle soreness (DOMS) has been debated. Initially, it was hypothesized that soreness was caused by an excessive buildup of lactic acid in exercised muscles. However, recent evidence essentially rules out this theory.[1]

It has also been hypothesized that DOMS is caused by the tonic, localized spasm of motor units, varying in number with the severity of pain. This theory maintains that exercise causes varying degrees of ischemia in the working muscles. This ischemia causes pain, which results in reflex tonic muscle contraction that increases and prolongs the ischemia. Consequently a cycle of increasing severity is begun.[25] As with the lactic acid theory, the spasm theory has also been discounted.

Currently there are two schools of thought relative to the cause of DOMS. DOMS seems to occur from very small tears in the muscle tissue, which seem to be more likely with eccentric or isometric contractions.[1] It is generally believed that the initial damage caused by eccentric exercise is mechanical damage to either the muscular or the connective tissue. Edema accumulation and delays in the rate of glycogen repletion are secondary reactions to mechanical damage.[69]

DOMS might be caused by structural damage to the elastic components of connective tissue at the musculotendinous junction. This damage results in the presence of hydroxyproline, a protein by-product of collagen breakdown, in blood and urine.[19] It has also been documented that structural damage to the muscle fibers results in an increase in blood serum levels of various protein/enzymes, including creatine kinase. This increase indicates that there is likely some damage to the muscle fiber as a result of strenuous exercise.[1]

Muscle soreness can best be prevented by beginning at a moderate level of activity and gradually progressing the intensity of the exercise over time. Treatment of muscle soreness usually also involves some type of stretching activity.[39] As for other conditions discussed in this chapter, ice is important as a treatment for muscle soreness, particularly within the first 48 to 72 hours.

Contusions

Contusion is synonymous with bruise. The mechanism that produces a contusion is a blow from some external object that causes soft tissues (eg, skin, fat, muscle, ligaments, joint capsule) to be compressed against the hard bone underneath.[100] If the blow is hard enough, capillaries rupture and allow bleeding into the tissues. The bleeding, if superficial enough, causes a bluish-purple discoloration of the skin that persists for several days. The contusion may be very sore to the touch. If damage has occurred to muscle, pain may be elicited on active movement. In most cases the pain ceases within a few days, and discoloration disappears in usually 2 to 3 weeks.

The major problem with contusions occurs where an area is subjected to repeated blows. If the same area, or more specifically the same muscle, is bruised repeatedly, small calcium deposits might begin to accumulate in the injured area. These pieces of calcium might be found between several fibers in the muscle belly, or calcium might form a spur that projects from the underlying bone. These calcium formations, which can significantly impair movement, are referred to as myositis ossificans. In some cases myositis ossificans develops from a single trauma.[8]

The key to preventing myositis ossificans from occurring from repeated contusions is protection of the injured area by padding.[8] If the area is properly protected after the first contusion, myositis ossificans might never develop. Protection, along with rest, might allow the calcium to be reabsorbed and eliminate any need for surgical intervention. The two areas that seem to be the most vulnerable to repeated contusions during physical activity are the quadriceps muscle group on the front of the thigh and the biceps muscle on the front of the upper arm.[100] The formation of myositis ossificans in either of these or any other areas can be detected on radiograph films.

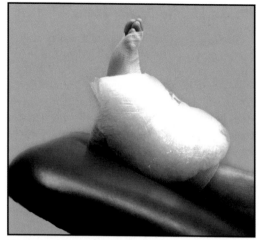

Figure 2-13. Musculoskeletal injuries should be treated initially with protection, restricted activity, ice, compression, and elevation.

INCORPORATING THERAPEUTIC EXERCISE TO AFFECT THE HEALING PROCESS

Rehabilitation exercise progressions can generally be subdivided into three phases, based primarily on the three stages of the healing process: phase 1, the acute phase; phase 2, the repair phase; and phase 3, the remodeling phase. Depending on the type and extent of injury and the individual response to healing, phases will usually overlap. Each phase must include carefully considered goals and criteria for progressing from one phase to another.[72]

Presurgical Exercise Phase

This phase would apply only to those patients who sustain injuries that require surgery. If surgery can be postponed, exercise may be used as a means to improve its outcome. By allowing the initial inflammatory response phase to resolve, by maintaining or, in some cases, increasing muscle strength and flexibility, levels of cardiorespiratory fitness, and improving neuromuscular control, the patient may be better prepared to continue the exercise rehabilitative program after surgery.

Phase 1: The Acute Injury Phase

Phase 1 begins immediately when injury occurs and can last as long as 4 days following injury. During this phase, the inflammatory stage of the healing process is attempting to "clean up the mess," thus creating an environment that is conducive to the fibroblastic stage. As indicated in Chapter 1, the primary focus of rehabilitation during this stage is to control swelling and to modulate pain by using the PRICE (Protection, Restricted activity, Ice, Compression, and Elevation) technique immediately following injury. Ice, compression, and elevation should be used as much as possible during this phase[73] (Figure 2-13).

Rest of the injured part is critical during this phase. It is widely accepted that early mobility during rehabilitation is essential. However, if the athletic trainer becomes overly aggressive during the first 48 hours following injury, and does not allow the injured part to be rested during the inflammatory stage of healing, the inflammatory process never really gets a chance to accomplish what it is supposed to. Consequently, the length of time required for inflammation might be extended. Therefore, immobility during the first 24 to 48 hours following injury is necessary to control inflammation. If the injury involves the lower extremity, the patient should be encouraged to be non–weight-bearing for the first 24 hours and progressively bear more weight as pain permits.

By day 2 or 3, swelling begins to subside and eventually stops altogether. The injured area may feel warm to the touch, and some discoloration is usually apparent. The injury is still painful to the touch, and some pain is elicited on movement of the injured part. Following injury there will almost always be some loss in ROM. Acutely, that loss can be attributed primarily to pain and thus modalities (ie, ice, electrical stimulation) that modulate pain should be routinely incorporated into each treatment session. At this point the patient should begin active mobility exercises, working through a pain-free ROM. In this phase, strengthening is less important than regaining ROM, but should not be entirely ignored.

A physician may choose to have the patient take NSAIDs to help control swelling and inflammation. It is usually helpful to continue this medication throughout the rehabilitative process.[2]

Phase 2: The Repair Phase

Once the inflammatory response has subsided, the repair phase begins. During this stage of the healing process, fibroblastic cells are laying down a matrix of collagen fibers and forming scar tissue. This stage might begin as early as 2 days after the injury and can last for several weeks. At this point, swelling has stopped completely. The injury is still tender to the touch but is not as painful as it was during the previous stage. There is less pain on active and passive motion.[73]

As soon as inflammation is controlled, the therapist should immediately begin to incorporate into the rehabilitation program activities that can maintain levels of cardiorespiratory fitness, restore full ROM, restore or increase strength, and reestablish neuromuscular control. The therapist should design exercises that simultaneously challenge the neural, muscular, and articular systems to help the patient regain neuromuscular control. As neuromuscular control improves strength will also improve. The patient very quickly "forgets" how to correctly execute even simple motor patterns such as walking, and the central nervous system must relearn how to integrate visual, proprioceptive, and kinematic information that collectively produces coordinated movement.

As in the acute phase, modalities should be used to control pain and swelling. Cryotherapy should still be used during the early portion of this phase to reduce the likelihood of swelling.[52] Electrical stimulating currents can help with controlling pain and improving strength and ROM.[73]

Phase 3: The Remodeling Phase

The remodeling phase is the longest of the three phases and can last for several years, depending on the severity of the injury. The ultimate goal during this maturation stage of the healing process is return to activity. The injury is no longer painful to the touch, although some progressively decreasing pain might still be felt on motion. The collagen fibers must be realigned according to tensile stresses and strains placed upon them during functional exercises.

The focus during this phase should be on regaining functional skills. Functional training involves the repeated performance of movement or skill for the purpose of perfecting that skill. Strengthening exercises should progressively place on the injured structures stresses and strains that would normally be encountered during activity. Plyometric strengthening exercises can be used to improve muscle power and explosiveness.[40] Functional testing should be done to determine specific skill weaknesses that need to be addressed prior to normal activity return.

At this point some type of heating modality is beneficial to the healing process. The deep-heating modalities, ultrasound, or the diathermies should be used to increase circulation to the deeper tissues. Massage and gentle mobilization may also be used to reduce guarding, increase circulation, and reduce pain. Increased blood flow delivers the essential nutrients to the injured area to promote healing, and increased lymphatic flow assists in breakdown and removal of waste products.[73]

USING MEDICATIONS TO AFFECT THE HEALING PROCESS

Medications are most commonly used in rehabilitation for pain relief. A patient may be continuously in pain that can be associated with even minor injury.

The over-the-counter nonnarcotic analgesics often used include aspirin (salicylate), acetaminophen, naproxen sodium ketoprofen, and ibuprofen. These belong to the group of drugs called NSAIDs. Aspirin is one of the most commonly used drugs in the world.[78] Because of its easy availability, it is also likely the most misused drug. Aspirin is a derivative of salicylic acid and is used for its analgesic, anti-inflammatory, and antipyretic capabilities.

Analgesia can result from several mechanisms. Aspirin can interfere with the transmission of painful impulses in the thalamus.[78]

Soft-tissue injury leads to tissue necrosis. This tissue injury causes the release of arachidonic acid from phospholipid cell walls. Oxygenation of arachidonic acid by cyclooxygenase produces a variety of prostaglandins, thromboxane, and prostacyclin that mediate the subsequent inflammatory reaction.[2] The predominant mechanism of action of aspirin and other NSAIDs is the inhibition of prostaglandin synthesis by blocking the cyclooxygenase pathway.[95] Pain and inflammation are reduced by the blockage of accumulation of proinflammatory prostaglandins in the synovium or cartilage.

Stabilization of the lysosomal membrane also occurs, preventing the efflux of destructive lysosomal enzymes into the joints.[47] Aspirin is the only NSAID that irreversibly inhibits cyclooxygenase; the other NSAIDs provide reversible inhibition. Aspirin can also reduce fever by altering sympathetic outflow from the hypothalamus, which produces increased vasodilation and heat loss through sweating.[22,47] Among the adverse effects of aspirin usage are gastric distress, heartburn, some nausea, tinnitus, headache, and diarrhea. More serious consequences can develop with prolonged use or high dosages.[3]

A patient should be very cautious about selecting aspirin as a pain reliever, for a number of reasons. Aspirin inhibits aggregation of platelets and thus impairs the clotting mechanism should injury occur.[3] Aspirin's irreversible inhibition of cyclooxygenase, which leads to reduced production of clotting factors, creates a bleeding risk not present with the other NSAIDs.[94] Prolonged bleeding at an injured site will increase the amount of swelling, which has a direct effect on the time required for rehabilitation.

Use of aspirin as an anti-inflammatory medication should be recommended with caution. Other anti-inflammatory medications do not produce as many undesirable side effects as aspirin. Generally prescription antiinflammatories are considered to be equally effective.

Aspirin sometimes produces gastric discomfort. Buffered aspirin is no less irritating to the stomach than regular aspirin, but enteric-coated tablets resist aspirin breakdown in the stomach and might minimize gastric

Table 2-1 Frequently Used NSAIDs

Generic/Trade Drug Name	Dosage Range (mg) and Frequency	Maximum Daily Dose (mg)
Celecoxib (Celebrex)	100 to 200 mg twice a day	200
Aspirin (Aspirin)	325 to 650 mg every 4 hours	4,000
Diclofenac (Voltaren)	50 to 75 mg twice a day	200
Diclofenac (Cataflam)	50 to 75 mg twice a day	200
Diflunasil (Dolobid)	500 to 1,000 mg followed by 250 to 500 mg 2 or 3 times a day	1,500
Fenoprofen (Nalfon)	300 to 600 mg 3 or 4 times a day	3,200
Ibuprofen (Motrin)	400 to 800 mg 3 or 4 times a day	3,200
Indomethacin (Indocin)	5 to 150 mg a day in 3 or 4 divided doses	200
Ketoprofen (Orudis)	75 mg 3 times a day or 50 mg 4 times a day	300
Mefenamic acid (Ponstel)	500 mg followed by 250 mg every 6 hours	1,000
Naproxen (Naprosyn)	250 to 500 mg twice a day	1,250
Naproxen (Anaprox)	550 mg followed by 275 mg every 6 to 8 hours	1,375
Piroxicam (Feldene)	20 mg a day	20
Sulindac (Clinoril)	200 mg twice a day	400
Tolmetin (Tolectin)	400 mg 3 or 4 times a day	1,800
Nabumatone (Relafen)	1,000 mg once or twice a day	2,000
Flurbiprofen (Ansaid)	50 to 100 mg 2 or 3 times a day	300
Keterolac (Toradol)	10 mg every 4 to 6 hours for pain; not to be used for more than 5 days	40
Etudolac (Lodine)	200 to 400 mg every 6 to 8 hours	1,200
Meloxicam (Mobic)	7.5 mg once a day	15
Oxaprosin (Daypro)	1,200 mg once a day	1,800

Reproduced with permission from Prentice W. *Principles of Athletic Training*. 14th ed. New York: McGraw-Hill; 2011.

discomfort. Regardless of the form of aspirin ingested, it should be taken with meals or with large quantities of water (8 to 10 oz per tablet) to reduce the likelihood of gastric irritation.

Ibuprofen is classified as an NSAID; however, it also has analgesic and antipyretic effects, including the potential for gastric irritation. It does not affect platelet aggregation as aspirin does. Ibuprofen administered at a dose of 200 mg does not require a prescription and at that dosage may be used for analgesia. At a dose of 400 mg, the effects are both analgesic and anti-inflammatory.[9] Dosage forms greater than 200 mg require a prescription. For names and recommended doses of prescription NSAIDs, refer to Table 2-1.

Acetaminophen, like aspirin, has both analgesic and antipyretic effects, but it does not have significant anti-inflammatory capabilities. Acetaminophen is indicated for relief of mild somatic pain and fever reduction through mechanisms similar to those of aspirin.[3]

The primary advantage of acetaminophen is that it does not produce gastritis, irritation, or gastrointestinal bleeding. Likewise, it does not affect platelet aggregation and thus does not increase clotting time after an injury.[75]

For the patient who is not in need of an anti-inflammatory medication but who requires some pain-relieving medication or an antipyretic, acetaminophen should be the drug of choice. If inflammation is a consideration, the physician may elect to use a type of NSAID. Most NSAIDs are prescription medications that, like aspirin, have not only anti-inflammatory but also analgesic and antipyretic effects.[47] They are effective for patients who cannot tolerate aspirin because of associated gastrointestinal distress. Patients who have the aspirin allergy triad of (a) nasal polyps, (b) associated bronchospasms/asthma, and (c) history of anaphylaxis should not receive any NSAID. Caution is advised when using NSAIDs in persons who might be subject to dehydration. NSAIDs inhibit prostaglandin synthesis and therefore can compromise the elaboration of prostaglandins within the kidney during salt and/or water deficits. This can lead to ischemia within the kidney.[47,63] Adequate hydration is essential to reduce the risk of renal toxicity in patients taking NSAIDs.

NSAID anti-inflammatory capabilities are thought to be equal to those of aspirin, their advantages being that NSAIDs have fewer side effects and relatively longer duration of action. NSAIDs have analgesic and antipyretic capabilities; the short-acting over-the-counter NSAIDs may be used in cases of mild headache or increased body temperature in place of aspirin or acetaminophen. They can be used to relieve many other mildly to moderately painful somatic conditions like menstrual cramps and soft-tissue injury.[9]

It has been recommended that patients receiving long-acting NSAIDs have monitoring of liver function enzymes during the course of therapy because of case reports of hepatic failure associated with the use of long-acting NSAIDs.[74]

The NSAIDs are used primarily for reducing the pain, stiffness, swelling, redness, and fever associated with localized inflammation, most likely by inhibiting the synthesis of prostaglandins.[9] The athletic trainer must be aware that inflammation is simply a response to some underlying trauma or condition and that the source of irritation must be corrected or eliminated for these anti-inflammatory medications to be effective.[86] Both naproxen and ketoprofen (now available without a prescription) have been shown to provide additional benefit when administered concomitantly with physical therapy.[63]

Muscle guarding accompanies many musculoskeletal injuries. Elimination of this guarding should facilitate programs of rehabilitation. In many situations, centrally acting oral muscle relaxants are used to reduce guarding. However, to date the efficacy of using muscle relaxants has not been substantiated, and they do not appear to be superior to analgesics or sedatives in either acute or chronic conditions.[7]

Many analgesics and anti-inflammatory products are available over the counter in combination products (ie, those containing two or more nonnarcotic analgesics with or without caffeine). Chronic use of analgesics containing aspirin and phenacetin or acetaminophen contributes to the development of papillary necrosis and analgesic-associated nephropathy. The presence of caffeine plays a role in dependency on these products leading to chronic use.

REHABILITATION PHILOSOPHY

The rehabilitation philosophy relative to inflammation and healing after injury is to assist the natural process of the body while doing no harm.[53] The course of rehabilitation chosen by the athletic trainer must focus on their knowledge of the healing process and its therapeutic modifiers to guide, direct, and stimulate the structural function and integrity of the injured part. The primary goal should be to have a positive influence on the inflammation and repair process to expedite recovery of function in terms of ROM, muscular strength and endurance, neuromuscular control, and cardiorespiratory endurance.[29,32] The athletic trainer must try to minimize the early effects of excessive inflammatory processes including pain modulation, edema control, and reduction of associated muscle spasm, which can produce loss of joint motion and contracture. Finally, the athletic trainer should concentrate on preventing the recurrence of injury by influencing the structural ability of the injured tissue to resist future overloads by incorporating various therapeutic exercises.[53] The subsequent chapters of this book can serve as a guide for the athletic trainer in using the many different rehabilitation tools available.

Summary

1. The three phases of the healing process are the inflammatory response phase, the fibroblastic repair phase, and the maturation remodeling phase. These occur in sequence, but overlap one another in a continuum.

2. Factors that can impede the healing process include edema, hemorrhage, lack of vascular supply, separation of tissue, muscle spasm, atrophy, corticosteroids, hypertrophic scars, infection, climate and humidity, age, health, and nutrition.

3. Ligament sprains involve stretching or tearing the fibers that provide stability at the joint.

4. Fractures can be classified as greenstick, transverse, oblique, spiral, comminuted, impacted, avulsive, or stress.

5. Osteoarthritis involves degeneration of the articular cartilage or subchondral bone.

6. Muscle strains involve a stretching or tearing of muscle fibers and their tendons and cause impairment to active movement.

7. Tendinitis, an inflammation of a muscle tendon that causes pain on movement, usually occurs because of overuse.

8. Tenosynovitis is an inflammation of the synovial sheath through which a tendon must slide during motion.

9. Dislocations and subluxations involve disruption of the joint capsule and ligamentous structures surrounding the joint.

10. Bursitis is an inflammation of the synovial membranes located in areas where friction occurs between various anatomic structures.

11. Muscle soreness can be caused by spasm, connective tissue damage, muscle tissue damage, or some combination of these.

12. Repeated contusions can lead to the development of myositis ossificans.

13. All injuries should be initially managed with protection, rest, ice, compression, and elevation to control swelling and thus reduce the time required for rehabilitation.[14] A patient who requires an analgesic for pain relief should be given acetaminophen because aspirin may produce gastric upset and slow clotting time.

14. For treating inflammation, NSAIDs are recommended because they do not produce many of the adverse effects associated with aspirin use.

References

1. Allen T. Exercise-induced muscle damage: mechanisms, prevention, and treatment. *Physiother Can.* 2004;56(2):67-79.

2. Almekinders LC. Anti-inflammatory treatment of muscular injuries in sport: an update of recent studies. *Sports Med.* 1999;28(6):383-388.

3. Alper B. Evidence-based medicine. Update: acetaminophen effective in osteoarthritis (NSAIDs more effective). *Clin Adv Nurse Pract.* 2004;7(12):98-99.

4. Arnoczky SP. Physiologic principles of ligament injuries and healing. In: Scott WN, ed. *Ligament and Extensor Mechanism Injuries of the Knee.* St. Louis, MO: Mosby; 1991:67-82.

5. Athanasiou KA, Shah AR, Hernandez RJ, LeBaron RG. Basic science of articular cartilage repair. *Clin Sports Med.* 2001;20(2):223-247.

6. Bandy W, Dunleavy K. Adaptability of skeletal muscle: Response to increased and decreased use. In: Zachazewski J, Magee D, Quillen W, eds. *Athletic Injuries and Rehabilitation.* Philadelphia: WB Saunders; 1996:55-70.

7. Beebe F. A clinical and pharmacologic review of skeletal muscle relaxants for musculoskeletal conditions. *Am J Ther.* 2005;12(2):151-171.

8. Beiner J. Muscle contusion injury and myositis ossificans traumatica. *Clin Orthop Relat Res.* 2002;(403 Suppl): S110-S119.

9. Biederman R. Pharmacology in rehabilitation: nonsteroidal anti-inflammatory agents. *J Orthop Sports Phys Ther.* 2005;35(6):356-367.

10. Bottoni C, Hart L. Recurrent shoulder dislocations after arthroscopic stabilization or nonoperative treatment. *Clin J Sport Med.* 2003;13(2):128-129.

11. Briggs J. Soft and bony tissues-injury, repair and treatment implications. In: Briggs J. ed. *Sports Therapy: Theoretical and Practical Thoughts and Considerations.* Chichester, UK: Corpus; 2001.

12. Booher JM, Thibodeau GA. *Athletic Injury Assessment*. 4th ed. St. Louis, MO: McGraw-Hill; 2000.

13. Brothers A. Basic clinical management of muscle strains and tears: Following appropriate treatment, most patients can return to sports activity. *J Musculoskelet Med*. 2003;20(6):303-307.

14. Bryant MW. Wound healing. *CIBA Clin Symp*. 1997; 29(3):2-36.

15. Burra G. Acute shoulder and elbow dislocations in the patient. *Orthop Clin North Am*. 2002;33(3):479-495.

16. Butler D. Nerve structure, function, and physiology. In: Zachazewski J, Magee D, Quillen W, eds. *Athletic Injuries and Rehabilitation*. Philadelphia, PA: WB Saunders; 1996:170-183.

17. Cailliet R. *Soft Tissue Pain and Disability*. 3rd ed. Philadelphia: FA Davis; 1996.

18. Carrico TJ, Mehrhof AI, Cohen IK. Biology and wound healing. *Surg Clin North Am*. 1984;64(4):721-734.

19. Clancy W. Tendon trauma and overuse injuries. In: Leadbetter W, Buckwalter J, Gordon S, eds. *Sports-Induced Inflammation*. Park Ridge, IL: American Academy of Orthopaedic Surgeons; 1990:609-618.

20. Clarkson PM, Tremblay I. Exercise-induced muscle damage, repair and adaptation in humans. *J Appl Physiol*. 1988;65:1-6.

21. Cox D. Growth factors in wound healing. *J Wound Care*. 1993;2(6):339-342.

22. Curtis J. A group randomized trial to improve safe use of nonsteroidal anti-inflammatory drugs. *Am J Manag Care*. 2005;11(9):537-543.

23. Curwin S. Tendon injuries, pathophysiology and treatment. In: Zachazewski J, Magee D, Quillen W, eds. *Athletic Injuries and Rehabilitation*. Philadelphia: WB Saunders; 1996:27-54.

24. Damjanov I. *Anderson's Pathology*. 10th ed. St. Louis, MO: Mosby; 1996.

25. deVries HA. Quantitative EMG investigation of spasm theory of muscle pain. *Am J Phys Med*. 1996;45:119-134.

26. Di Domenica F. Physical and rehabilitative approaches in osteoarthritis. *Semin Arthritis Rheum*. 2005;34(6; Suppl 2):62-69.

27. Dieppe P. Pathogenesis and management of pain in osteoarthritis. *Lancet*. 2005;365(9463):965-973.

28. Fantone J. Basic concepts in inflammation. In: Leadbetter W, Buckwalter J, Gordon S, eds. *Sports-Induced Inflammation*. Park Ridge, IL: American Academy of Orthopaedic Surgeons; 1990:25-54.

29. Felson D. Osteoarthritis. *Curr Opin Rheumatol*. 2005;17(5):624-656, 684-697.

30. Fitzgerald GK. Considerations for evaluation and treatment of overuse tendon injuries. *Athl Ther Today*. 2000;5(4):14-19.

31. Frank C. Ligament injuries: Pathophysiology and healing. In: Zachazewski J, Magee D, Quillen W, eds. *Athletic Injuries and Rehabilitation*. Philadelphia: WB Saunders; 1996:9-26.

32. Frank C, Shrive N, Hiraoka H, Nakamura N, Kaneda Y, Hart D. Optimization of the biology of soft tissue repair. *J Sci Med Sport*. 1990;2(3):190-210.

33. Gelberman R, Goldberg V, An K-N, et al. Soft tissue healing. In: Woo SL-Y, Buckwalter J, eds. *Injury and Repair of Musculoskeletal Soft Tissues*. Park Ridge, IL: American Academy of Orthopaedic Surgeons; 1988.

34. Glick JM. Muscle strains: prevention and treatment. *Phys Sports Med*. 1980;8(11):73-77.

35. Goldenberg M. Wound care management: proper protocol differs from athletic trainers' perceptions. *J Athl Train*. 1996;31(1):12-16.

36. Gradisar IA. Fracture stabilization and healing. In: Gould JA, Davies GJ, eds. *Orthopaedic and Sports Physical Therapy*. St. Louis, MO: Mosby; 1985:118-134.

37. Gross A, Cutright DE, Bhaskar SN. Effectiveness of pulsating water jet lavage in treatment of contaminated crush wounds. *Am J Surg*. 1972;124:73-75.

38. Guyton AC, Hell J. *Pocket Companion to Textbook of Medical Physiology*. Philadelphia: WB Saunders; 2006.

39. Hart L. Effects of stretching on muscle soreness and risk of injury: a meta-analysis. *Clin J Sport Med*. 2003;13(5):321-322.

40. Henning CE. Semilunar cartilage of the knee: function and pathology. In: Pandolf KB, ed. *Exercise and Sport Science Review*. New York: Macmillan; 1988.

41. Hettinga DL. Inflammatory response of synovial joint structures. In: Gould JA, Davies GJ, eds. *Orthopaedic and Sports Physical Therapy*. St. Louis, MO: Mosby; 1985:87-117.

42. Hole J. *Human Anatomy and Physiology*. St. Louis, MO: McGraw-Hill; 2007.

43. Houglum P. Soft tissue healing and its impact on rehabilitation. *J Sport Rehabil*. 1992;1(1):19-39.

44. Hubbel S, Buschbacher R. Tissue injury and healing: Using medications, modalities, and exercise to maximize recovery. In: Bushbacher R, Branddom R, eds. *Sports Medicine and Rehabilitation: A Sport Specific Approach*. Philadelphia: Hanley & Belfus; 1994.

45. James CB, Uhl TL. A review of articular cartilage pathology and the use of glucosamine sulfate. *J Athl Train*. 2001;39(4):413-419.

46. Junge T. Bone healing. *Surg Technol*. 2002;34(5):26-29.

47. Kaplan R. Current status of nonsteroidal anti-inflammatory drugs in physiatry: Balancing risks and benefits in pain management. *Am J Phys Med Rehabil*. 2005;84(11):885-894.

48. Khan KM, Cook JL, Taunton JE, Bonar F. Overuse tendinosis, not tendinitis. Part 1: a new paradigm for a difficult clinical problem. *Phys Sports Med*. 2000;28(5): 38-43, 47-48.

49. Kelly A. Managing stress fractures in patients. *J Musculoskelet Med*. 2005;22(9):463-465, 468-470, 472.

50. Kibler WB. Concepts in exercise rehabilitation of athletic injury. In: Leadbetter W, Buckwalter J, Gordon S, eds. *Sports-Induced Inflammation*. Park Ridge, IL: American Academy of Orthopaedic Surgeons; 1990:759-780.

51. Kibler W. Current concepts in tendinopathy. *Clin Sports Med*. 2003;22(4):xi, xiii, 675-684.

52. Knight KL. *Cryotherapy in Sport Injury Management*. Champaign, IL: Human Kinetics; 1995.

53. Leadbetter W. Introduction to sports-induced soft-tissue inflammation. In: Leadbetter W, Buckwalter J, Gordon S, eds. *Sports-Induced Inflammation*. Park Ridge, IL: American Academy of Orthopaedic Surgeons; 1990:3-24.

54. Leadbetter W, Buckwalter J, Gordon S, eds. *Sports-Induced Inflammation*. Park Ridge, IL: American Academy of Orthopaedic Surgeons; 1990.

55. Loitz-Ramage B, Zernicke R. Bone biology and mechanics. In: Zachazewski J, Magee D, Quillen W, eds. *Athletic Injuries and Rehabilitation*. Philadelphia: WB Saunders; 1996:99-119.

56. Maffulli N, Benazzo F. Basic science of tendons. *Sports Med Arthrosc Rev*. 2000;8(1):1-5.

57. Marchesi VT. Inflammation and healing. In: Kissane JM, ed. *Andersons' Pathology*. 9th ed. St. Louis, MO: Mosby; 1996.

58. Martinez-Hernanadez A, Amenta P. Basic concepts in wound healing. In: Leadbetter W, Buckwalter J, Gordon S, eds. *Sports-Induced Inflammation*. Park Ridge, IL: American Academy of Orthopaedic Surgeons; 1990.

59. Matheson G, MacIntyre J, Taunton J. Musculoskeletal injuries associated with physical activity in older adults. *Med Sci Sports Exerc*. 1989;21:379-385.

60. Malone T, Garrett W, Zachewski J. Muscle: deformation, injury and repair. In: Zachazewski J, Magee D, Quillen W, eds. *Athletic Injuries and Rehabilitation*. Philadelphia: WB Saunders; 1996:71-91.

61. Malone T, McPhoil T, eds. *Orthopaedic and Sports Physical Therapy*. St. Louis, MO: Mosby; 1997.

62. Mayo Clinic. Fracture healing: what it takes to heal a break. *Mayo Clin Health Lett*. 2002;20(2):1-3.

63. McCormack K, Brune K. Toward defining the analgesic role of non-steroidal anti-inflammatory drugs in the management of acute and soft tissue injuries. *Sports Med*. 1993;3:106-117.

64. Mehta J. Elbow dislocations in adults and children. *Clin Sports Med*. 2004;23(4):609-627.

65. Molina F: The physiologic basis of tendinopathy development. *Athletic Therapy and Training*, 2011;16(6):5-8.

66. Levangie P, Norkin C. *Joint Structure and Function: A Comprehensive Analysis*. Philadelphia: FA Davis; 2005.

67. Norris S, Provo B, Stotts N. Physiology of wound healing and risk factors that impede the healing process. *AACN Clin Issues Crit Care Nurs*. 1990;1(3):545-552.

68. Ng G. Ligament injury and repair: current concepts. *Hong Kong Physiother J*. 2002;20:22-29.

69. O'Reilly K, Warhol M, Fielding R, et al. Eccentric exercise induced muscle damage impairs muscle glycogen depletion. *J Appl Physiol*. 1987;63:252-256.

70. Panush RS, Brown DG. Exercise and arthritis. *Sports Med*. 1987;4:54-64.

71. Peterson L, Renstrom P. Injuries in musculoskeletal tissues. In: Peterson L, ed. *Sports Injuries: Their Prevention and Treatment*. 3rd ed. Champaign, IL: Human Kinetics; 2001.

72. Prentice W. *Principles of Athletic Training*. 15th ed. New York, NY: McGraw-Hill; 2013.

73. Prentice WE, ed. *Therapeutic Modalities in Rehabilitation*. New York: McGraw-Hill; 2011.

74. Purdum P, Shelden S, Boyd J. Oxaprozin induced hepatitis. *Ann Pharmacother*. 1994;28:1159-1161.

75. Rahusen F. Nonsteroidal anti-inflammatory drugs and acetaminophen in the treatment of an acute muscle injury. *Am J Sports Med*. 2004;32(8):1856-1859.

76. Relaix F, Zammit P: Satellite cells are essential for skeletal muscle regeneration: the cell on the edge returns to center stage. *Development*. 2012;16:2845-2856.

77. Rywlin AM. Hemopoietic system. In: Kissane JM, ed. *Andersons' Pathology*. 9th ed. St. Louis, MO: Mosby; 1996.

78. Sachs C. Oral analgesics for acute nonspecific pain. *Am Fam Physician*. 2005;71(5):913-918, 847-849.

79. Saladin K. *Anatomy and Physiology*. New York: McGraw-Hill; 2011.

80. Sanderlin B. Common stress fractures. *Am Fam Physician*. 2003;68(8):1527-1532, 1478-1479.

81. Sandrey MA. Effects of acute and chronic pathomechanics on the normal histology and biomechanics of tendons: a review. *J Sport Rehabil*. 2000;9(4):339-352.

82. Schenck R. Classification of knee dislocations. *Oper Tech Sports Med*. 2003;11(3):193-198.

83. Seeley R, Stephens T, Tate P. *Anatomy and Physiology*. St. Louis, MO: McGraw-Hill; 2005.

84. Seller RH. *Differential Diagnosis of Common Complaints*. Philadelphia: Elsevier Health Sciences; 2007.

85. Sharma P. Tendon injury and tendinopathy: healing and repair. *J Bone Joint Surg Am*. 2005;87(1):187-202.

86. Shrier I, Stovitz S. Best of the literature: do anti-inflammatory agents promote muscle healing? *Phys Sports Med*. 2005;33(6):12.

87. Stanish WD, Curwin S, Mandell S. *Tendinitis: Its Etiology and Treatment*. Oxford, UK: Oxford University Press; 2000.

88. Soto-Quijano D. Work-related musculoskeletal disorders of the upper extremity. *Crit Rev Phys Rehabil Med*. 2005;17(1):65-82.

89. Stewart J. *Clinical Anatomy and Physiology*. Miami, FL: MedMaster; 2001.

90. Stone MH. Implications for connective tissue and bone alterations resulting from rest and exercise training. *Med Sci Sports Exerc*. 1988;20(5):S162-168.

91. Terry M, Fincher AL. Postoperative management of articular cartilage repair. *Athl Ther Today*. 2000;5(2): 57-58.

92. Tuan K. Stress fractures in patients: risk factors, diagnosis, and management. *Orthopedics*. 2004;27(6):583-593.

93. Van de Graaff K. *Human Anatomy*. New York: McGraw-Hill; 2006.

94. Vane J. Inhibition of prostaglandin synthesis as a mechanism of action for aspirin-like drugs. *Nat New Biol*. 1971;231:232-235.

95. Vane J. The evolution of nonsteroidal anti-inflammatory drugs and their mechanism of action. *Drugs*. 1987;33(1):18-27.

96. Walker J. Cartilage of human joints and related structures. In: Zachazewski J, Magee D, Quillen W, eds. *Athletic Injuries and Rehabilitation*. Philadelphia: WB Saunders; 1996:120-151.

97. Wahl S, Renstrom P. Fibrosis in soft-tissue injuries. In: Leadbetter W, Buckwalter J, Gordon S, eds. *Sports- Induced Inflammation*. Park Ridge, IL: American Academy of Orthopaedic Surgeons; 1990:637-648.

98. Wang Y, Rudnicki M: Satellite cells, the engines of muscle repair. *Nature Reviews Molecular Cell Biology*. 2012;13:127-133.

99. Wilder R. Overuse injuries: tendinopathies, stress fractures, compartment syndrome, and shin splints. *Clin Sports Med*. 2004;23(1):55-81.

100. Wissen WT. An aggressive approach to managing quadriceps contusions. *Athl Ther Today*. 2000;5(1):36-37.

101. Woo SL-Y, Buckwalter J, eds. *Injury and Repair of Musculoskeletal Soft Tissues*. Park Ridge, IL: American Academy of Orthopaedic Surgeons; 1988.

102. Wroble RR. Articular cartilage injury and autologous chondrocyte implantation: which patients might benefit? *Phys Sportsmed*. 2000;28(11):43-49.

103. Zachezewski J. Flexibility for sports. In: Sanders B, ed. *Sports Physical Therapy*. Norwalk, CT: Appleton & Lange; 1990:201-238.

SOLUTIONS TO CLINICAL DECISION-MAKING EXERCISES

2-1   Immediate action to control swelling can expedite the healing process. The athletic trainer should first provide compression and elevation. Applying ice, which decreases the metabolic demands of the uninjured cells, can prevent secondary hypoxic injury. Ice also slows nerve conduction velocity, which will decrease pain and thus limit muscle guarding.

2-2   The athletic trainer should explain to the coach that it can take up to 3 or 4 days for the inflammatory response to subside. During this time, the muscle is initializing repair by containing the injury by clot formation. Too much stress during this time could increase the time it takes the muscle to heal. After that, it may take a couple of weeks before fibroblastic and myoblastic activity has restored tissue strength to a point where the tissue can withstand the stresses of training.

2-3   Muscle healing generally takes longer. While fibroblasts are laying down new collagen for connective tissue repair, myoblasts are working to replace the contractile tissue.

2-4   Once the injured structure has progressed through the inflammatory phase and repair has begun, sufficient tensile stress should be provided to ensure optimal repair and positioning of the new fibers (according to Wolff's law). Efforts should be made right away to avoid the strength loss that comes with immobility due to pain.

2-5   The presence of gross laxity would suggest a grade 3 sprain. The athlete should be referred to the team physician for further evaluation.

2-6   In a complete ligament tear, it is likely that the nerves in that structure will also be completely disrupted. Therefore, no pain signals can be transmitted.

2-7   It is likely that this young boy has a greenstick fracture. Such fractures are common in athletes of this age.

2-8   Peripheral nerves are likely to regenerate if the cell body has not been damaged. The closer the injury is to the cell body, the more difficult the healing process is. If a nerve is severed, surgical intervention can significantly improve chances of regeneration.

Please see videos on the accompanying website at **www.healio.com/books/sportsmedvideos**

CHAPTER 3

The Evaluation Process in Rehabilitation

Darin A. Padua, PhD, ATC

After completion of this chapter, the athletic training student should be able to:

- Identify the components of the systematic differential evaluation process.

- Explain the role of the systematic injury evaluation process in establishing a rehabilitation plan and treatment goals.

- Describe various ways to differentiate between normal and pathological tissue.

- Discuss special tests that should be incorporated into an evaluation scheme.

- Review ways to perform injury risk screenings and describe how the findings can be incorporated into injury prevention training programs.

- Recognize how to establish short-term and long-term rehabilitation goals based on the findings of the injury evaluation.

Injury evaluation is the foundation of the rehabilitation process. To effectively coordinate the rehabilitation process, the athletic trainer must be able to perform a systematic differential evaluation and identify the pathological tissue. According to Cyriax,[8] the injury evaluation process involves applying one's knowledge of anatomy to differentiate between provoked and normal tissue:

Provoked tissue – Normal tissue
= Pathological tissue

Once the pathological tissue is identified, the athletic trainer must then consider the contraindications and determine the appropriate course of treatment:

Pathological tissue – Contraindications
= Treatment (rehabilitation plan)

The athletic trainer determines the appropriate rehabilitation goals and plan based on

Prentice WE, ed.
Rehabilitation Techniques for Sports Medicine and Athletic Training (pp 57-92).
© 2015 SLACK Incorporated.

the information gathered from the evaluation. In designing the rehabilitation plan, the athletic trainer must consider the severity, irritability, nature, and stage of the injury.[22] Throughout the rehabilitation process, the athletic trainer must continuously reevaluate the status of the pathological tissue to make appropriate adjustments to the rehabilitation goals and plan.

The athletic trainer might conduct multiple injury evaluations of the following kinds for varying purposes during the course of athletic injury management:

1. On-site evaluation at the time of injury (on-field)

2. On-site evaluation just following injury (sideline)

3. Off-site evaluation that involves the injury assessment and rehabilitation plan

4. Follow-up evaluation during the rehabilitation process to determine the patient's progress

5. Preparticipation physical evaluation (preseason screening)

All forms of injury evaluation will involve similar steps and procedures. However, it is important to note the difference between the on-site injury evaluation processes and the off-site evaluation performed when designing a rehabilitation program.

The goal of an on-site injury evaluation is to quickly, but thoroughly, evaluate the patient and determine the injury severity, whether immobilization is needed, whether medical referral is needed, and the manner of transportation from the field.

The off-site injury evaluation is more detailed and used to gain information to effectively design the rehabilitation program.

This chapter will focus on the steps and procedures involved during the off-site injury evaluation and incorporating this information into the rehabilitation plan.

THE SYSTEMATIC DIFFERENTIAL EVALUATION PROCESS

The key to a successful injury evaluation is to establish a sequential and systematic approach that is followed in every case. A systematic approach allows the athletic trainer to be confident that a thorough evaluation has been performed. However, the athletic trainer must keep in mind that each injury may be unique in some manner. Thus, the athletic trainer must maintain a systematic approach but not be inflexible during the evaluation process. The Injury Evaluation Checklist in Figure 3-1 is provided as an example of the steps and procedures that may be included in a sequential and systematic evaluation scheme.

The systematic differential evaluation process is composed of subjective and objective elements. During the subjective evaluation the athletic trainer gathers information on the injury history and the symptoms experienced by the patient. This is performed through an initial interview with the patient. The athletic trainer attempts to relate information gathered during the subjective evaluation to observable signs and other quantitative findings obtained during the objective evaluation. The objective evaluation involves observation and inspection, acute injury palpation, range of motion (ROM) assessment (active and passive), muscle strength testing, special tests, neurological assessment, subacute or chronic injury palpation, and functional testing. After completing the subjective and objective evaluation, the athletic trainer will arrive at an assessment of the injury based on the information gathered.

Subjective Evaluation

The subjective evaluation is the foundation for the rest of the evaluation process. Perhaps the single most revealing component of the

SUBJECTIVE PHASE

History
____ Patient's impression
____ Site of injury
____ Mechanism of injury
____ Previous injury
____ Behavior of symptoms (PQRST)
    ____ Provocation of symptoms
    ____ Quality of symptoms
    ____ Region of symptoms
    ____ Severity of symptoms
    ____ Timing of symptoms

OBJECTIVE PHASE

Observation and Inspection
____ Postural alignment (see postural alignment checklist)
____ Gait (lower-extremity injury) or upper-extremity functional motion (upper-extremity injury)
____ Signs of trauma
    ____ Deformity
    ____ Bleeding
    ____ Swelling
    ____ Atrophy
    ____ Skin color

Palpation
____ Temperature
____ Dermatome assessment
____ Bone palpation
____ Soft tissue palpation
    ____ Muscle
    ____ Tendon
    ____ Ligament and joint capsule
    ____ Superficial nerves
*Palpate all structures accessible in a specific position before repositioning patient.
*Palpate areas above and below the injured region.

Range of Motion
____ Active range of motion
____ Passive range of motion
____ Resistive range of motion

*Perform range-of-motion testing in all cardinal planes of motion.
*Assess end-feels by applying overpressure.
*Assess arthrokinematic motions if normal range of motion altered.
*Be aware of capsular patterns for specific joint tested

Resistive Strength Testing
____ Mid-range of motion muscle tests
____ Specific muscle tests

*Specific muscle tests should be based on results of mid-range of motion muscle tests
*Rate or grade strength assessment

Muscle Imbalances
____ Review range of motion and resistive strength testing findings

*Determine whether muscle imbalances appear to exist

Special Tests
____ Joint stability tests
____ Joint compression tests
____ Passive tendon stretch tests
____ Diagnostic tests

Neurologic Testing
____ Dermatomes
____ Myotomes
____ Reflexes
    ____ Deep tendon reflexes
    ____ Superficial reflexes
    ____ Pathologic reflexes

Functional Testing
____ Movement patterns that facilitate similar stresses as encountered during normal activity (i.e., activity specific)

Figure 3-1. Injury Evaluation Checklist.

injury evaluation is the information gathered during the subjective evaluation. Essentially, during the subjective evaluation the athletic trainer engages in an orderly, sequential process of questions and dialogue with the patient. In addition to gathering information about the injury, the subjective evaluation serves to establish a level of comfort and trust between the patient and the athletic trainer.

The injury history and the symptoms are the key elements of the subjective evaluation. A detailed injury history is the most important portion of the evaluation. The remainder of the evaluation will focus on confirming the information taken from the patient's history.

History of Injury

In gathering a detailed history, the athletic trainer should focus on gathering information relative to the patient's impression of the injury, site of injury, mechanism of injury, previous injuries, and general medical health. The history should be taken in an orderly sequence. This information will then be used to determine the appropriate components to incorporate during the objective evaluation.

When taking the patient's history, the athletic trainer should initially use non-leading, open-ended questions. As the subjective evaluation progresses, the athletic trainer may move to more close-ended questions once a clear picture of the injury has been presented. Open-ended questions involve narrative information about the injury; close-ended questions ask for specific information.[15]

The history relies on the athletic trainer's ability to clearly communicate with the injured patient. Thus, the athletic trainer should avoid the use of scientific and medical jargon and use simple terminology that is easy to understand. The use of simple terminology ensures that the patient will understand any close-ended questions the athletic trainer may ask.

Patient's Impression

Allow the patient to describe in his or her own words how the injury occurred, where the injury is located, and how he or she feels. While listening to the patient, the athletic trainer should be generating close-ended questions. Once the patient has given his or her

impression of the injury, the athletic trainer should ask more specific questions that fill in specific details.

Site of Injury

Have the patient describe the general area where the injury occurred or pain is located. Further isolate the site of injury by having the patient point with one finger to the exact location of injury or pain. If the patient is able to locate a specific area of injury or pain, the athletic trainer should make note of the anatomic structures in the general area and consider this tissue as provoked tissue. A major purpose of the remaining evaluation phases is to further differentiate the identified provoked tissue from the normal tissue.[5] Differentiating between provoked tissue and normal tissue allows the athletic trainer to identify the pathological tissue.[8] The athletic trainer must be able to identify the pathological tissue to develop an appropriate rehabilitation plan.

Mechanism of Injury

Musculoskeletal injury results from forces acting on the anatomic structures and ultimately results in tissue failure. Thus, it is imperative to identify the nature of the forces acting on the body and relate these to the anatomic function of the underlying anatomic structures. The athletic trainer should determine whether the injury was caused by a single traumatic force (macrotrauma) or resulted from the accumulation of repeated forces (microtrauma). In dealing with an acute injury, it is important to identify the body position at time of injury, the direction of applied force, the magnitude of applied force, and the point of application of the applied force. The athletic trainer must then apply knowledge of anatomy, biomechanics, and tissue mechanics to determine which tissues may have been injured. When dealing with recurrent or chronic injuries, it is important to establish what factors influence the patient's symptoms, such as changes in training, routine, equipment use, and posture. The accumulation of this information should be used to further identify the pathological tissue. Any sound or sensation noted at the moment of or immediately after injury is also important information to gather. The athletic trainer may be able to relate certain sounds and sensations with possible injuries, hence identifying pathological tissue:

- Pop: joint subluxation, ligament tear
- Clicking: cartilage or meniscal tear
- Locking: cartilage or meniscal tear (loose body)
- Giving way: reflex inhibition of muscles in an attempt to minimize muscle or joint loading

Previous Injury

Tissue reinjury or injury of tissue surrounding previously injured tissue is common. The athletic trainer should determine whether the current injury is similar to previous injuries. If so, what anatomic structures were previously injured? How often has the injury recurred? How was the previous injury managed, from a rehabilitation standpoint? Have there been any residual effects since the original injury? Was surgery or medication given for the previous injury? Who evaluated the previous injury?

Previous injuries may influence the evaluation process of the current injury as well as the rehabilitation plan. Secondary pathology may be present in cases of recurrent injury, such as excessive scar tissue development, reduced soft-tissue elasticity, muscle contracture, inhibition or weakness of surrounding musculature, altered postural alignment, increased joint laxity, or diminished joint play/accessory motions. The athletic trainer must consider these possibilities and investigate them during the objective evaluation.

Behavior of Symptoms

During the second phase of the subjective evaluation, the athletic trainer explores specific details of the symptoms discovered during the history. Again, this should be performed in a systematic and sequential process. Moore[16] describes the PQRST mnemonic to guide this phase of the subjective evaluation (P = provocation or cause of symptoms; Q = quality or description of symptoms; R = region of symptoms; S = severity of symptoms; T = time symptoms occur or recur).

Provocation of Symptoms

This information is primarily gathered through a detailed mechanism-of-injury description by the patient. Additional information may be gathered by asking the patient if they are able to recreate their symptoms by performing certain movements. However, the athletic trainer should not have the patient recreate these movements at this phase of the evaluation. This will be performed during ROM assessment in the objective evaluation. Typically, musculoskeletal pain is worse with movement and better with rest. Symptoms caused by excessive inflammation may be constant and not alleviated with rest. Symptoms associated with prolonged postures may be indicative of prolonged stress being placed on the surrounding soft tissue structures, which ultimately causes breakdown.

Quality of Symptoms

The patient should be asked to describe the quality of his or her symptoms. The patient might describe his or her pain as being sharp, dull, aching, burning, or tingling. The athletic trainer should attempt to relate the patient description of the quality of symptoms to possible pathological tissue. Magee[15] describes different descriptions of the quality of symptoms as being associated with different anatomic structures:

- Nerve pain: Sharp, bright, shooting (tingling), along line of nerve distribution
- Bone pain: Deep, nagging, dull, localized
- Vascular pain: Diffuse, aching, throbbing, poorly localized, may be referred
- Muscular pain: Hard to localize, dull, aching, may be referred

Region of Symptoms

The majority of this information is given during the patient's description of the site of injury. The region of symptoms might correlate with underlying injured or pathological tissue. However, the athletic trainer must be aware of possible referred pain patterns and not assume that the pathological tissue is located directly within the region of symptoms. Once the region of symptoms has been identified, there are several other items that should be noted. Do the symptoms stay localized, or do they spread to peripheral areas? Do the symptoms feel deep or superficial? Do the symptoms seem to be located within the joint or in the surrounding area? Pain that radiates to other areas may be due to pressure on the nerve or from active trigger points in the myofascial tissue. Symptoms that are well localized in a small area might indicate minor injury or chronic injury. Symptoms that are diffuse in nature may be indicative of more severe injury.

Severity of Symptoms

The severity of symptoms may give insight into the severity of injury. However, the athletic trainer should be cautious in equating the patient's description of severity with actual injury severity. Individuals' perceptions of severity are highly subjective and likely vary to a large extent from one person to the next. Hence, information relative to perceived severity of symptoms is an unreliable indicator of injury severity. More appropriately, reports of symptom severity may be used during the rehabilitation process to track the patient's progress. Improvement of symptoms indicates that the rehabilitation plan is succeeding. Worsening of symptoms may indicate that the injury is getting worse or that the rehabilitation plan is not appropriate at this time.

The patient should quantify his or her pain to most efficiently track the patient's progress during the rehabilitation process. The athletic trainer should instruct the patient to rate his or her pain on a scale of 0 to 10, where 0 is no pain (normal) and 10 is the worst pain imaginable. Having the patient rate his or her pain does not provide an objective assessment. Rather, this information will be used to make relative comparisons of the patient's progress during rehabilitation.[24]

Timing of Symptoms

The onset of symptoms may help determine the nature of the injury. Symptoms with a slow and insidious onset that tend to progressively worsen over time are often associated with repetitive microtrauma. In contrast, macrotrauma injuries typically result in a sudden, identifiable onset of symptoms. Injuries resulting from repetitive microtrauma may include stress fractures, trigger point formation, tendinitis, or other chronic inflammatory conditions. Macrotraumatic injuries may result in ligament sprains, muscle strains, acute bone fractures, or other acute soft-tissue injuries.

Duration and frequency of symptoms may be used to determine whether the injury is progressing or worsening. An improvement in symptoms is demonstrated by reductions in their duration and frequency. The opposite may be reported in the situation of a worsening injury. Response of symptoms to activity or rest may also be used to identify the nature of the injury. Magee[15] describes several injury classifications that may be related to the response of symptoms to activity or rest:

- Joint adhesion: Pain during activity that decreases with rest

- Chronic inflammation and edema: Initial morning pain and stiffness that is reduced with activity

- Joint congestion: Pain or aching that progressively worsens throughout the day with activity

- Acute inflammation: Pain at rest and pain that is worse at the beginning of activity in comparison to the end of activity

- Bone pain or organic/systemic disorders: Pain that is not influenced by either rest or activity

- Peripheral nerve entrapment: Pain that tends to worsen at night

- Intervertebral disc involvement: Pain that increases with forward or lateral trunk bending

Objective Evaluation

At the completion of the subjective evaluation the athletic trainer should have developed a list of potential provoked tissues. In some cases, the experienced athletic trainer may be able to identify the specific injury and pathological tissue at this point of the evaluation. During the objective evaluation, the athletic trainer will perform several procedures as a process of eliminating normal tissue from being considered as provoked tissue. These procedures will serve to differentiate between provoked and normal tissues, allowing the pathological tissue to be identified.

The athletic trainer should plan the objective evaluation.[16] After completing the subjective evaluation, the athletic trainer should create a mental list of specific procedures and tests to perform during the objective evaluation. At this point the athletic trainer may expect to get specific findings during the objective evaluation. However, the athletic trainer is reminded to stay open-minded and not become too focused during this stage of the evaluation.

Observation and Inspection

The beginning of the objective evaluation consists of a visual inspection of the injured patient as he or she enters the medical facility. The athletic trainer focuses on the patient's overall appearance and specific body regions that were identified during the subjective evaluation as being a potential site of provoked tissue. For example, if the lower extremity is identified as a potential area of injury, the athletic trainer will pay close attention to the patient's gait patterns. If an upper extremity injury is suspected, the carrying position of the injured extremity and movement patterns when removing an item of clothing would be noted. In observing the patient's movement patterns, the athletic trainer should be looking for compensatory patterns, muscle guarding, antalgic movements, and facial expressions. All observations should be made with a bilateral comparison of the uninvolved side.

Postural Alignment

Overall postural alignment should be assessed during the observation, especially in patients suffering from chronic or overuse-type injuries.[14,15,23] Many chronic and overuse injuries are due to postural malalignments that create repeated stress on a specific tissue. Over time the repeatedly loaded tissue may become pathological or lead to additional postural alignment alterations as compensatory mechanisms to reduce tissue stress. In addition, postural alignment can influence muscle function.

If postural malalignments are present, the athletic trainer should consider the patterns of muscle tightness and weakness that would correspond to such a postural malalignment. Altered postural alignment can be caused by muscle imbalances, not just bony deformity.[3,4] It is important that the athletic trainer determine whether postural malalignments are due to muscle imbalances or bony deformity, as

this might influence the rehabilitation options. Postural malalignments that are due to muscle imbalances may be addressed through physical rehabilitation using appropriate muscle flexibility and strengthening techniques to restore muscle balance, hence improving normal postural alignment.

There are many elements involved with a detailed postural alignment assessment. The athletic trainer may consider using a checklist approach to ensure that all elements are covered. It is important that the patient be viewed in a weight-bearing position (standing) from multiple vantage points (anterior, posterior, medial, lateral). In general, the athletic trainer should be checking for neutral alignment, symmetry, balanced muscle tone, and specific postural deformities (genu valgum, genu varum, etc.). A detailed checklist for postural alignment is provided as an example in Figure 3-2.

Signs of Trauma

During the postural alignment assessment, the athletic trainer should also check for signs of trauma. In acute injuries, observing for signs of trauma might be the primary purpose of the observation. Gross deformity along the bone's long axis or joint line may be present in cases of fractures of joint dislocations. Visible swelling, bleeding, or signs of infection at the injury site should also be noted, as should the nature of its onset.

Swelling that is rapid and immediate could be indicative of acute trauma; gradual and slow-onset swelling may be more indicative of chronic overuse injury. The athletic trainer should attempt to quantify the amount of swelling by taking girth or volumetric measurements. Quantification of swelling can help establish rehabilitation goals and aid in tracking rehabilitation progress.

Atrophy of the surrounding muscles may be present in the case of chronic injury. Skin color and texture should also be assessed. The patient's skin might have red (inflammation), blue (cyanosis, indicating vascular compromise), or black-blue (contusion) coloration. If the skin appears to be shiny, to have lost elasticity, or to have lost overlying hair, or if there is skin breakdown, there might be a peripheral nerve lesion.

Frontal View (Anterior): Arms relaxed, palms facing lateral thighs

Line bisecting: (plumb line)

____   Nose

____   Mouth

____   Sternum

____   Umbilicus

____   Pubic bones

Level:

____   Earlobes

____   Acromion process

____   Nipples

____   Fingertip ends

____   Anterior superior iliac spine

____   Greater trochanter

____   Patella

____   Medial malleoli

Neutral Rotational Alignment

____   Shoulder (direction of olecranon process)

____   Patella

____   Feet (direction of toes)

Balanced Muscle Tone

____   Deltoids

____   Trapezius

____   Pectoralis major

____   Quadriceps

Is there evidence of:

Cubitus valgus	L	R	B
Cubitus varus	L	R	B
Internal shoulder rotation	L	R	B
External shoulder rotation	L	R	B
Pes planus	L	R	B
Pes cavus	L	R	B
Forefoot valgus	L	R	B
Forefoot varus	L	R	B
Hallux valgus	L	R	B
Genu valgus	L	R	B
Genu varus	L	R	B
Internal tibial rotation	L	R	B
External tibial rotation	L	R	B

Figure 3-2. Postural Alignment Checklist. (*continued*)

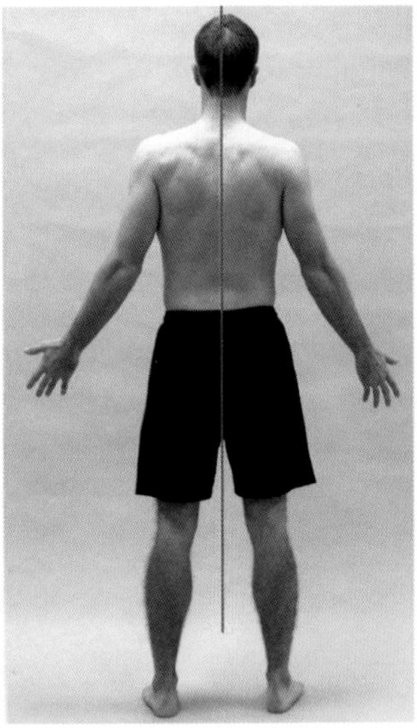

Femoral anteversion	L	R	B
Femoral retroversion	L	R	B
Unequal weight bearing	L	R	B

Line bisecting: (plumb line)

____ External auditory meatus

____ Cervical vertebral bodies

____ Acromion process

____ Deltoid

____ Mid-thoracic region

| Asymmetric stance width | L | R |

Frontal view (Posterior)

Line bisecting: (plumb line)

____ Head

____ Cervical through lumbar spinous processes

____ Sacrum

Level:

____ Earlobes

____ Acromion process

____ Inferior angle of scapula

____ Gluteal fold

____ Posterior superior Iliacs spine

____ Greater trochanter

____ Popliteal crease

____ Medial malleoli

Normal Scapular Alignment:

____ Vertebral borders rest against thorax

____ Superior and inferior angles are equal distance from vertebrae

____ Superior and inferior angles sit at ribs 2 and 7, respectively

Perpendicular to Floor

____ Line bisecting calcaneus

____ Line bisecting Achilles tendon

Balanced Muscle Tone

____ Trapezius

____ Deltoids

____ Rhomboids

____ Latissimus dorsi

____ Erector spinae group

____ Gluteus maximus

____ Hamstrings

____ Triceps surae

Figure 3-2. (*continued*) Postural Alignment Checklist.

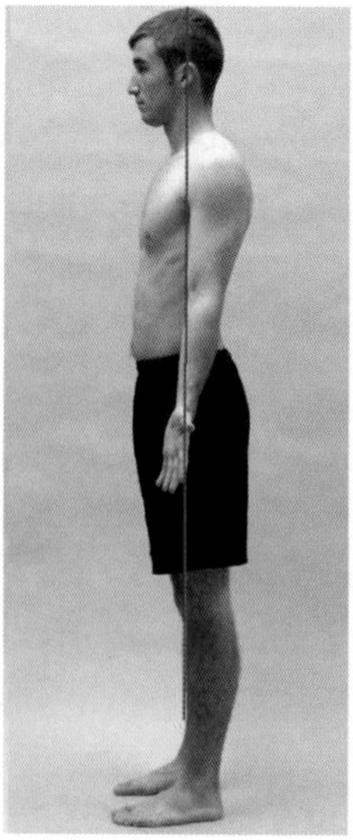

Is there evidence of?

Winging scapula	L	R	B
Rear foot valgus	L	R	B
Rear foot varus	L	R	B
Scoliosis	L	R	S
Lateral shift	L	R	

Saggital View (Bilateral)

Line bisecting: (plumb line)

____ External auditory meatus

____ Cervical vertebral bodies

____ Acromion process

____ Deltoid

____ Mid-thoracic region

____ Greater trochanter

____ Lateral femoral condyle (slightly anterior)

____ Tibia (parallel to plumb line)

____ Lateral malleolus (slightly posterior)

Level:

____ ASIS and PSIS General (normal)

____ Chin tucked slightly

____ Mild cervical curvature

____ Mild thoracic curvature

____ Mild lumbar curve

____ Knees straight, but not locked

Is there evidence of?

Genu recurvatum	L	R	B
Hip flexor contracture (anterior pelvic tilt)	L	R	B
Forward head / shoulder	L	R	B

Figure 3-2. (*continued*) Postural Alignment Checklist.

Clinical Decision-Making Exercise 3-1

While taking a patient's history, the athletic trainer records the following information:

- Site of pain: Knee joint
- Mechanism of injury: Direct blow to knee causing knee to be forced into excessive valgus and rotation
- Behavior of symptoms: Pain is described as "deep, nagging, dull, and localized," pain increases with weight bearing, reports a clicking and locking sensation in knee joint

Based on the findings from the history, what types of special tests should the athletic trainer consider performing?

The information collected during the observation should be related to the findings of the subjective evaluation. This will allow the athletic trainer to further confirm or differentiate possible pathological tissue.

Clinical Decision-Making Exercise 3-2

As you assess a patient's postural alignment, you observe excessive anterior pelvic tilting and increased lumbar lordosis. How would these observations guide your evaluation during the ROM and resistive strength-testing phases?

Palpation

The question of when palpation should be performed during the objective evaluation is debatable. Some feel that palpation should be performed immediately following the observation; others feel that palpation should be performed later during the objective evaluation. If an acute injury is being evaluated, palpation may be appropriate immediately following observation to detect any obvious, but not visible, soft-tissue or bony deformities.[16] Such findings may warrant termination of the evaluation and immediate referral to a physician. However, if the injury is subacute or chronic in nature, palpation may be performed later in the objective evaluation. The disadvantage of performing palpation early in the objective evaluation is that such manual probing can elicit a pain response that will distract from findings

during the later subphases of the objective evaluation (ROM, strength, and special tests).[7]

Regardless of when palpation is performed, the primary purpose of palpation is to localize as closely as possible the potential pathological tissues involved. To gain the patient's confidence, palpation should start with a gentle and assuring touch and the trainer should frequently communicate with the patient. Palpation should be performed in a sequential manner and include the anatomic and joint structures that are above and below the site of the injury. Palpation should begin on the uninjured side so that the patient knows what to expect and the examiner knows what is "normal" and has an objective comparison when palpating the injured side. Palpation of the injured side begins with the anatomic structures distal to the site of pain and then progressively works toward the potential pathological tissues. To systematically palpate all possible tissues, it may be helpful to develop a specific sequencing of tissues to palpate.[23] For example, the athletic trainer might first palpate all bones, then ligaments and tendons, and then the muscles and corresponding tendons. Consideration should be given to positioning of the patient as one develops the sequencing of tissues to palpate. Minimizing patient movement is important, as excessive motion can cause the patient's symptoms to worsen. Thus, the athletic trainer should palpate all possible anatomic structures in a given position prior to repositioning the patient.

During palpation, the athletic trainer should take note of point tenderness, trigger points, tissue quality, crepitus, temperature, and symmetry.[12,15,16,19,21,23] Point tenderness is noted by indications of pain over the area being palpated. If point tenderness is noted, the patient should be asked to rate his or her point tenderness on a scale of 0 to 10, where 0 is no pain (normal) and 10 is the worst pain imaginable. Similar to rating one's symptoms, this does not provide an objective assessment. Rather, this information will be used to make relative comparisons of the patient's progress during rehabilitation. Trigger points may be located in the muscle and feel like a small nodule or muscle spasm. The trigger point may be identified as an area that upon palpation refers pain to another body area. Increased tissue temperature may be present if infection or inflammation is present. Calcification or change in tissue density may be present in a poorly managed hematoma formation, or might indicate effusion or hemarthrosis of the joint. Crepitus is a crunching or crackling sensation along the tendon, bone, or joint. Crepitus along the length of a tendon can indicate tenosynovitis or tendinitis. The presence of crepitus along the bone or joint may indicate damage to the bone (fracture), cartilage, bursa, or joint capsule. Rupture of a muscle or tendon may present as a gap at the point of separation.

All information gathered during palpation should be used to further confirm the findings of the initial evaluation steps. At this point the athletic trainer should be further able to differentiate between the normal and provoked tissue. Before beginning the next subphase of the objective evaluation, the athletic trainer should review the findings and further organize the remainder of the objective evaluation.

Special Tests

Range of Motion

ROM assessment involves determining the patient's ability to move a limb through a specific pattern of motion. There are several general principles that should be applied during ROM testing. Motions will be performed passively, actively, and against resistance to fully quantify the patient's status.[16,23] Testing should first be performed on the patient's uninjured limb through each of the joint's cardinal planes of motion and the quantity of motion available should be recorded. Then ROM testing is repeated on the injured limb. The athletic trainer can then compare the ROM of the injured limb to that of the uninjured limb and/or against established normative data.[24] In addition, ROM records will serve an important role in tracking the patient's progress during rehabilitation. Active ROM testing should be performed first, followed by passive, then resistive, ROM assessment.[16,23] If possible, the athletic trainer should perform movement patterns that facilitate pain at the end to prevent a carryover effect to following movement patterns. This should be evident based on the previous steps performed during the evaluation process.

ROM assessment should also be performed at the joints proximal and distal to the involved area for a comprehensive evaluation.[23] These general guidelines allow the athletic trainer to efficiently assess ROM.

One of the primary goals of ROM testing is to assess the integrity of the inert and contractile tissue components of the joint complex. Inert tissues are sometimes referred to as anatomic joint structures and include bone, ligament, capsule, bursae, periosteum, cartilage, and fascia.[8] The contractile tissues, also referred to as physiological joint structures, include muscle, tendon, and nerve structures.[8] Cyriax developed a method to differentiate between inert and contractile pathological tissues as part of the ROM assessment.[8] Differentiating between inert or contractile tissue pathology is performed by selectively applying passive and active tension to joint structures and making note of where pain is located.[8] The ability to differentiate between inert and contractile tissue pathology is an important step in setting up the rehabilitation plan and identifying the appropriate tissue to treat.

Inert tissue pathology is indicated when the patient reports pain occurring during both active and passive ROM in the same direction of movement.[8] Typically, pain due to inert tissue pathology will occur near the end of the ROM as the tissue becomes compressed between the bony segments. Example: The patient reports pain in the anterior shoulder region when actively and passively moving the humerus into the end range of shoulder flexion. Because pain was present in the same direction of motion (direction of shoulder flexion = anterior shoulder) during active and passive movements, pathology of an inert tissue structure of the shoulder would be indicated.

Contractile tissue pathology is indicated when the patient reports pain in the same direction of motion during active ROM, then reports pain in the opposite direction of motion during passive ROM.[8] Contractile tissue pain occurs due to increased tension placed on the tissue. However, the cause of contractile tissue tension differs between active and passive ROM testing. During active ROM, contractile tissue tension increases due to the voluntary agonist muscle contraction generated to move the limb.

In contrast, passive ROM increases contractile tissue tension as the muscle is stretched by the athletic trainer. Example: The patient reports anterior shoulder pain when actively bringing the humerus into shoulder flexion (pain in same direction as motion) and when passively bringing the humerus into shoulder extension as it is stretched by the athletic trainer (pain in opposite direction as motion). It is not possible to determine the specific location of either inert or contractile tissue pathology through ROM assessment. This is accomplished by incorporating manual muscle and special tests to locate the exact location of pathology.

Active Range of Motion

Having the patient "actively" contract his or her muscles as he or she takes his or her limb through the desired cardinal plane of motion assesses active ROM, location of pain, and painful arcs.[19] A painful arc is pain that occurs at some point during the ROM but later disappears as the limb moves past this point in either direction.[19,23] Typically, a painful arc is present due to impingement of tissue between bony surfaces. Painful arcs may be present during either active or passive ROM testing. Overpressure may be applied at the end ROM to assess end-point feels, if active ROM is full and pain-free.[16] Pain or limited ROM prohibits applying overpressure during active ROM assessment and may indicate waiting until the passive ROM testing. If ROM is limited or elicits pain, the athletic trainer should consider the cause of these findings, as this will have direct implications on the rehabilitation plan. Limited ROM can be caused by several factors, including swelling, joint capsule tightness, agonist muscle weakness/inhibition, or antagonist muscle tightness/contracture.[11]

Passive Range of Motion

When passive ROM is assessed, the patient should be positioned so that the contractile tissues are relaxed and do not influence the findings due to active muscle contraction. The athletic trainer then takes the limb through the desired passive movement pattern until the point of pain or end ROM. Upon reaching the end ROM, gentle overpressure should be applied and particular attention should be directed toward the sensation of the end-point feel.

The end-point feel encountered at the end ROM has been given several normal and abnormal classification schemes.[5] End-point feel assessment may be useful in helping determine the type of pathological tissue[8] (Table 3-1). The athletic trainer should determine whether differences exist between the ranges of motion available during active and passive testing. Reduced ROM during active compared to passive testing may indicate deficiency in the contractile tissue. Contractile tissue deficiencies may be caused by muscle spasm or contracture, muscle weakness, neurological deficit, or muscle pain.[23] Such deficiencies should be addressed during the rehabilitation plan to restore normal ROM. The presence of crepitus or clicking is also of significance during passive ROM testing.[15] Crepitus or clicking along the joint line or between two bones may indicate damage to the articular cartilage or a possible loose body in the joint. Similar sensations along the muscle or tendon may indicate adhesion formation or tendon subluxation.

Clinical Decision-Making Exercise 3-3

During knee flexion ROM testing, a patient complains of pain in the same direction of motion during active ROM, but no pain during passive ROM. Upon testing knee extension ROM, the patient indicates that pain occurs in the opposite direction of motion during passive ROM. What type of tissue may be suspected to have been injured, based on these findings?

Capsular Patterns of Motion

Irritation to the joint capsule may cause a progressive loss of available motion in different cardinal planes of motion. When identifying a capsular pattern, movement restrictions are listed in order, with the first being the motion pattern that is most affected.[19] Each joint has a specific pattern of progressive motion loss in different planes of motion. For example, the capsular pattern of the glenohumeral joint involves significant limitation to external rotation, followed by abduction and internal rotation. Presence of a capsular pattern indicates a total joint reaction that may involve muscle spasm, joint capsule tightening

Table 3-1 End-Feel Categorization Scheme

Normal End-Feels	
Soft-tissue approximation	Soft and spongy, a gradual painless stop (eg, elbow flexion)
Capsular	An abrupt, hard, firm end point with only a little give (eg, shoulder rotation). Bone-to-bone. A distinct and abrupt end point where two hard surfaces come in contact with one another (eg, elbow extension)
Abnormal End-Feels	
Empty	Movement definitely beyond the anatomical limit, or pain prevents the body part from moving through the available ROM (eg, ligament rupture)
Spasm	Involuntary muscle contraction that prevents normal ROM due to pain (guarding) (eg, muscle spasm)
Loose	Extreme hypermobility (eg, chronic ankle sprain, chronic shoulder sub-luxation/dislocation)
Springy block	A rebound at the end point of motion (eg, meniscal tear, loose body formation)

(most common), and possible osteophyte formation.[15] The athletic trainer must determine which joint structures may be involved with the capsular pattern to adequately plan the patient's rehabilitation. This will be performed through assessment of joint end-feels, muscle strength, and various special tests.

Noncapsular Patterns of Motion

Noncapsular patterns of motion result from irritation to structures located outside of the joint capsule and do not follow the progressive loss of motion patterns as observed with a capsular pattern. Cyriax has classified the following lesions as producing noncapsular patterns of motion.[8]

- Ligamentous adhesion occurs after injury and may result in a movement restriction in one plane, with a full pain-free range in other planes.

- Internal derangement involves a sudden onset of localized pain resulting from the displacement of a loose body within the joint. The mechanical block restricts motion in one plane while allowing normal, pain-free motion in the opposite direction. Movement restrictions can change as the loose body shifts its position in the joint space.

- Extra-articular lesion results from adhesions occurring outside the joint. Movement in a plane that stretches that adhesion results in pain, whereas motion in the opposite direction is pain-free and nonrestricted.

Accessory Motion and Joint Play (Arthrokinematic Motion)

Accessory or joint play motions occur between joint surfaces as the joint undergoes passive and active motions.[15] The motion occurring between the joint surfaces is also referred to as arthrokinematic motion. Arthrokinematic motions are not actively produced by the patient. However, arthrokinematic motion is necessary for full active and passive joint ROM to be achieved. As such, accessory motion/joint play assessment should be evaluated during a comprehensive assessment of joint ROM.[11]

Three types of arthrokinematic motions can occur: roll, glide, and spin. A detailed description of the arthrokinematic motions is provided in Chapter 13. In brief, for normal joint motion to occur there must be normal arthrokinematic motion available. An example of arthrokinematic motion can be easily demonstrated at the knee in the open kinetic chain position as the knee moves from a flexed position into full extension (femur is stationery, tibia is moving). During this motion the tibia rolls and glides anteriorly and spins externally (external rotation) relative to the femur. Because arthrokinematic motions are involuntary, assessment requires specific manual techniques. Techniques used for assessment of accessory motion are the same as those used in joint mobilization treatment and are discussed in detail in Chapter 13.

During arthrokinematic motion assessment, the examiner is looking for alterations in either hypomobility (restricted arthrokinematic motion) or hypermobility (excessive arthrokinematic motion). In addition to assessing the amplitude of arthrokinematic motion, the examiner should also note signs of joint stiffness, quality of motion, end-feel, and pain.[19]

It is particularly important to evaluate arthrokinematic motion in patients that have reduced passive or active ROM. It is possible that limited passive and active ROM arises from altered arthrokinematic motions. Reduced arthrokinematic motions may be due to joint capsule or ligamentous adhesions and tightness. To restore normal passive and active ROM in the patient demonstrating reduced arthrokinematic motion, it will be important to incorporate joint mobilization techniques during the rehabilitation process.

Clinical Decision-Making Exercise 3-4

You determine that a patient's active and passive ROM is limited. Based on this information you assess the patient's arthrokinematic motion and find that it is hypomobile. What types of exercises would you consider incorporating into the patient's rehabilitation plan to address these findings?

Resistive Strength Testing

Resistive strength testing is used to assess the state of contractile tissue (muscle, tendon, and nerve).[13,14] Typically, resistive strength testing is performed as the patient performs an isometric contraction while the athletic trainer performs a "break test." The break test assesses the amount of isometric force the patient can generate prior to allowing joint motion (ie,

"breaking" the isometric contraction). In general, two types of resistive strength testing are used during the injury evaluation process: midrange of motion muscle testing and specific muscle testing.[14]

Midrange of Motion Muscle Testing

The athletic trainer should perform midrange of motion muscle testing before performing specific muscle testing. It is important to perform midrange motion to allow for isolation of contractile tissue. Muscle testing performed near the end ROM may involve the inert tissue structures. When pain or weakness is noted during muscle testing at the end ROM, it will be difficult to determine whether pain arises from contractile or inert tissues.[16] The athletic trainer should be aware of any type of compensatory motions the patient may perform as an attempt to compensate for weak or limited motion.

Midrange of motion muscle testing is performed by placing the joint in its approximate midrange of motion for a specific movement pattern. The athletic trainer tells the patient, "Don't let me move you," and then applies a manual force to initiate the break test. Midrange of motion muscle testing should be performed in each of the cardinal planes of motion and compared bilaterally to the uninjured limb. Midrange of motion muscle testing focuses on muscle groups, not specific muscles. Thus, performing specific muscle testing of the agonist and synergistic muscles acting in that cardinal plane of motion should be included as a followup for noted weakness or pain during midrange of motion muscle testing.[16] Essentially, the results of the midrange of motion muscle testing will guide the examiner through specific muscle testing.

During the midrange of motion muscle testing the athletic trainer does not "grade" strength, but instead assesses the motion as strong, weak, painful, or painless.[14] According

---

Clinical Decision-Making Exercise 3-5

During midrange of motion muscle testing, you note that the patient has pain and weakness when performing hip extension. Based on this finding, what muscles should be tested during specific muscle testing?

Table 3-2 Midrange of Motion Muscle Testing Scheme

Cyriax System for Differentiating Muscular Lesions
Strong and painless = normal muscle
Strong and painful = minor lesion in some part of muscle or tendon (first- or second-degree strain)
Weak and painless = complete rupture of muscle or tendon or some nervous system disorder
Weak and painful = gross lesion of contractile tissue (muscle or tendon rupture, peripheral nerve or nerve root involvement; if movement is weak and pain free, neurological involvement or a tendon rupture should be first suspected)

Table 3-3 Specific Muscle Testing Grading Scheme

Grade 5	Normal	Complete AROM against gravity, with maximum resistance
Grade 4	Good	Complete AROM against gravity, with some resistance
Grade 3	Fair	Complete AROM against gravity, with no resistance
Grade 2	Poor	Complete AROM, with gravity eliminated
Grade 1	Trace	Evidence of slight muscle contraction, with no joint motion
Grade 0	Zero	No evidence of muscle contraction

to Cyriax,[5] the athletic trainer can identify the type of lesion through muscle testing (Table 3-2).

Specific Muscle Testing

Specific muscle testing is used to assess the strength and integrity of specific muscles, not simply muscle groups. Muscles tested during specific muscle testing should be based upon information obtained from midrange of motion muscle testing, ROM assessment, and the patient's history. Similar to midrange of motion muscle testing, the athletic trainer will apply a break test to assess muscle function. However, the joint is placed in various positions in an attempt to isolate stress on the muscle of interest. Detailed positioning of the joint to isolate specific muscles is described in detail in Daniels and Worthingham[7] as well as Kendall.[14]

During specific muscle testing the athletic trainer will note any pain and grade the patient's muscle strength. This information will be compared to the injured side and be used during rehabilitation to track the patient's progress in regaining muscle strength. Several grading scales have been reported; numerical systems are the most common[10] (Table 3-3). Weakness or pain elicited during resistive strength testing may be caused by several factors, including muscle strain, pain/reflex inhibition, peripheral nerve injury, nerve root lesion (myotome), tendon strain, avulsion, or psychological overlay.[15] The athletic trainer should always consider the source of muscular deficiency and not simply focus on assigning a muscle strength grade. Through appropriate use of neurological tests and various special tests, the athletic trainer should be able to accurately identify the source of muscular deficiency. This is imperative to efficiently manage the injury throughout the rehabilitation process.

Muscle Imbalances

After evaluating both ROM and resistive strength testing, the athletic trainer should review the findings to determine whether muscle imbalances can be identified. Muscle imbalances arise between an agonist muscle and its functional antagonist muscle, disrupting the normal force-couple relationship between the agonist and antagonist muscle.[3,4,20] Muscle tightness or hyperactivity of one muscle or muscle group is often the initial cause of muscle imbalances and initiates a predictable pattern of kinetic dysfunction.[3,4,20] Tightness or hyperactivity in the agonist muscle can cause inhibition of the antagonist muscle. This is explained by Sherrington's law of reciprocal inhibition. Reciprocal inhibition causes decreased neural drive to the antagonist muscle, which ultimately

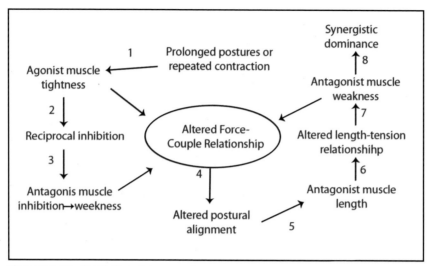

Figure 3-3. Muscle imbalance injury paradigm.

facilitates a functional weakness of the antagonist muscles. Agonist muscle tightness and hyperactivity combined with inhibition and weakness of the antagonist muscles results in disruption of the normal force-couple relationship between these muscles, hence a muscle imbalance.[3,4]

Initial disruption of the normal force-couple relationship between agonist and antagonist muscles stimulates a series of events that further perpetuates the altered force couple relationship. Due to the force imbalance between agonist and antagonist muscles, the joint tends to position itself in the direction of the tight agonist muscle and normal postural alignment can be adversely affected.[3,4] Alterations to postural alignment allow the agonist muscle to move into a more shortened position. Conversely, the antagonist muscle is lengthened from its normal position. Increasing the resting length of the antagonist muscle is believed to alter the normal length-tension relationship of the muscle, which further reduces the antagonist muscle's ability to generate force. Reduced antagonist muscle force generation due to lengthening is explained by the length–tension relationship. As the antagonist muscle is lengthened, there are fewer cross-bridges that can be aligned, hence reduced muscle force capacity. Reduced antagonist muscle force output further disrupts the normal force-couple relationship and may bring about additional postural alignment alterations.[3,4]

To compensate for weakness of the antagonist muscle group, the patient might compensate by placing greater reliance on muscles that act as synergists to the weakened muscles. This is referred to as synergistic dominance.[3,4] The synergist muscles are now forced to perform greater work to accelerate and decelerate the bony segments. This places greater demands on the synergist muscles, which increases the risk of injury to these muscles.[3,4] This series of events is summarized in Figure 3-3.

Janda[13] has identified several common muscle imbalances that may be observed by the athletic trainer. The basic concept is to separate muscles into two basic groups based on their function: movement and stabilization.

Movement group muscles are characterized as being:

- Prone to developing tightness (hyperactive)
- More active during functional movements (hyperactive)
- More active when the individual becomes fatigued or when performing new movement patterns (hyperactive)

Stabilization group muscles are characterized as being:

- Prone to developing inhibition and weakness (reduced force capacity)
- Less active during functional movements (reduced force capacity)

- Easily fatigued during dynamic movements (reduced force capacity)

According to Janda, several specific muscles in the movement and stabilization groups are extremely prone to developing tightness and weakness, respectively.[13] These muscles are indicated in Table 3-4.

It is important for the examiner to address muscle imbalances during the rehabilitation process to restore normal postural alignment and force-couple relationships. The athletic trainer must pay special attention to whether limited ROM in one muscle is accompanied by weakness in its functional antagonist. If a muscle imbalance is revealed, the athletic trainer must work to restore the normal force-couple relationship during rehabilitation to reestablish postural alignment. In general, restoring normal balance between muscles is accomplished by first stretching the tight muscle to restore normal ROM before attempting to strengthen the weak antagonist muscle. Failure to address muscle imbalances can result in a failed rehabilitation program where the examiner is constantly treating the symptoms, but never the cause.

Additional Special Tests

At this point in the evaluation, the athletic trainer should have considerably narrowed the list of possible pathological tissues involved and be judicious in choosing the special tests to perform. Suspicion of a fracture or joint dislocation may contraindicate performance of various special tests that could exacerbate the current injury. Also, if the patient is in a considerable amount of pain, performance of special tests may yield findings of questionable validity. In cases where the patient is in a considerable amount of pain it is best to wait until the patient's symptoms have subsided to perform the special tests.

The special tests performed at this phase should be used to further differentiate between pathological and normal tissue.[16] The athletic trainer should perform special tests only on those tissues that they suspect to be pathological based on the findings from the previous evaluation phases.[16] The experienced athletic trainer performs only those special tests that

Table 3-4 Janda Classification of Functional Muscle Groupings[13]

Muscles Prone to Tightness (Movement Group)
Gastrocnemius
Soleus
Short hip adductors
Hamstrings
Rectus femoris
Iliopsoas
Tensor fascia latae
Piriformis
Erector spinae (especially lumbar, thoracolumbar, and cervical portions)
Quadratus lumborum
Pectoralis major
Upper trapezius
Levator scapulae
Sternocleidomastoid
Scalenes
Flexors of the upper limb

Muscles Prone to Weakness (Stabilization Group)
Peroneals
Anterior tibialis
Posterior tibialis
Gluteus maximus
Gluteus medius
Abdominals
Serratus anterior
Rhomboids
Lower trapezius
Short cervical flexors
Extensors of the upper limb

confirm their previous findings and eliminate other tissues from being involved. To isolate pathological tissue, special tests are designed to assess the integrity of specific body tissues, such as muscle, ligament, tendon, joint surface, and nerve.

There are several types of special tests. Joint stability tests assess the integrity of the inert joint tissues, specifically the joint capsule and ligaments. Joint stability testing is performed by applying to the joint a manual force that places strain on specific capsular or ligamentous structures. The manual force is applied until reaching the end point of the specific joint motion. The athletic trainer then grades the amount of joint laxity (displacement) and end-feel and notes the presence of pain. For example, the Anterior Drawer Test at the knee assesses the integrity of the anterior cruciate ligament. Based on these findings the athletic trainer may estimate the extent of injury to the specific capsular or ligamentous structures tested. Table 3-3 indicates the grading system commonly used to assess joint stability.

Joint compression tests assess the integrity of inert joint tissues that line the joint surface, such as the articular cartilage and meniscus. Joint compression testing is performed as the athletic trainer manually applies a compressive load across the joint, typically combined with some form of rotary stress. This type of combined motion places significant stress across the joint surface and may elicit a painful or crepitus/clicking sensation at the joint level.

The McMurray's test at the knee is an example of a joint compression test. Passive tendon stretch tests are used to determine the presence of tendinitis or tenosynovitis. The athletic trainer applies a passive stretch along the tendon that when positive elicits a painful or crepitus like sensation along the tendon.

Another form of special tests that may be useful are anthropometric assessments of the patient of injured area.[16] Anthropometric assessments range from being as simple as qualitatively assessing the patient's somatotype (general body structure) to as detailed as performing body composition assessment (eg, underwater weighing). Such information may be useful in situations where the patient will be required to miss a significant amount of physical activity for a prolonged period. The athletic trainer may be able to compare the patient's body composition pre- or immediately post-injury to their body composition during rehabilitation or before returning to activity.

Anthropometric assessments might also be performed on the limb and might include measurements of limb girth and volume. Limb anthropometric measurements can be useful in tracking rehabilitation progress to assess swelling or muscle atrophy/hypertrophy.[16,23]

Neurological Testing

There is some debate as to how often neurological testing should be performed. Some believe that neurological testing should be performed any time the patient reports symptoms that affect his or her distal extremities, such as below the acromion process or gluteal folds,[7,19] especially if the mechanism of injury was not directly witnessed. However, other professionals do not feel that neurological testing is warranted for orthopedic evaluations, unless the results from the previous evaluation phases suggest nervous system involvement.[12,19] Neurological testing may be indicated from the history if the patient describes unexplained loss of strength, paresthesia, or numbness, or has sustained an injury to the vertebral region that may have involved the spine.[23]

Neurological testing typically involves three components: sensory (dermatomes), motor (myotomes), and reflex (deep tendon, superficial, and pathological reflexes) testing.[12] Neurological testing of these three components assesses the integrity of the spinal nerve roots and peripheral nerves. The evaluator's challenge is to determine whether the nerve root or peripheral nerve is the source of the symptoms. Nerve root damage typically involves abnormal motor and sensory function over a large area. In contrast, peripheral nerve damage will be confined to a more localized area innervated by the nerve.[19] Other possible neurological testing components include cranial nerve assessment, neuropsychological assessment (cognitive ability), and cerebellar function (coordinated movements: finger-to-nose).[13,23]

Dermatome Testing

Dermatomes are areas of the skin whose sensory distribution is innervated by a specific nerve root. Assessment of dermatomes involves a bilateral comparison of light touch discrimination. During dermatome testing the examiner should alter or remove the pressure applied to one side to determine whether the patient can distinguish changes in pressure. Sensory testing may also include sharp and dull discrimination, hot and cold discrimination, and two-point discrimination to assess peripheral

Figure 3-4. Dermatome assessment. (Reproduced with permission from McKinley M, O'Loughlin V. *Human Anatomy*, 1st ed. NY: McGraw-Hill; 2006:498.)

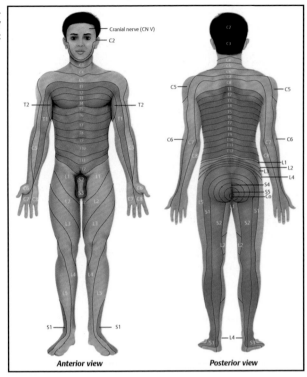

Anterior view   Posterior view

nerve injury.[23] Dermatomes for the body are illustrated in Figure 3-4.

Myotome Testing

Myotomes represent a group of muscles that are innervated from a specific nerve root. Essentially, myotomes are the motor equivalent to dermatomes.[16] Myotomes may be assessed for various muscle groups of the upper and lower extremities. Myotome testing is performed through sustained isometric contraction of a specific muscle. Common muscles tested during myotome assessment are listed in Table 3-5.

Reflex Testing

Reflex testing may involve the assessment of deep tendon reflexes, superficial reflexes, and pathological reflexes. Testing for deep tendon reflexes assesses the integrity of the stretch reflex arc for a specific nerve root and provides further information on the integrity of the specific nerve root.[12] Testing of deep tendon reflexes typically involves the use of a reflex hammer. The athletic trainer strikes over the tendon to place a slight quick–stretch on the tendon. If done properly, the slight stretching

of the tendon will elicit a reflex response (ie, a muscle jerk response). Applying a quick–stretch to almost any tendon can facilitate the reflex response, if done properly. There are several upper- and lower-extremity deep tendon reflexes that may be tested (Table 3-6). However, not all nerve roots have a specific deep tendon reflex. The common deep tendon reflexes assessed in the upper and lower extremities include the biceps, brachioradialis, triceps, patella, hamstrings medial, hamstrings lateral, tibialis posterior, and the Achilles tendon. Grading of deep tendon reflexes uses a 5-point scale to characterize the stretch reflex response and compare it bilaterally to the uninjured limb (Table 3-7).

Superficial reflexes are assessed as the athletic trainer provides a superficial stroking of the patient's skin, usually using a sharp object.[12,15] During this time the examiner notes the movement of the patient's skin or distal extremities. Commonly, several superficial reflexes are described.[12,15] These include the upper-abdominal, lower-abdominal, cremasteric, plantar, gluteal, and anal reflexes.

Table 3-5 Myotome Assessment

C5 = Middle deltoid
C6 = Biceps brachii
C7 = Triceps brachii
C8 = Finger flexors
T1 = Finger interossei (DAB & PAD)
T12 – L3 = Hip flexion
L2 – L4 = Quadriceps
L5 – S1 = Hamstrings
L4 – L5 = Ankle dorsiflexion
S1 – S2 = Ankle plantar flexion

Table 3-7 Deep Tendon Reflex Grading Scheme

Grade 0	Absent: no reflex elicited
Grade 1	Diminished: reflex elicited with reinforcement (precontracting muscle)
Grade 2	Normal
Grade 3	Exaggerated: hyperresponsive reflex
Grade 4	Clonus: spasm-like response followed by relaxation

Table 3-6 Deep Tendon Reflex Assessment

C6 = Biceps brachii
C7 = Triceps brachii
C8 = Brachiradialis
L4 = Patella tendon
S1 = Achilles tendon

Pathological reflexes normally are not present. The presence of a pathological reflex is a sign that there might be a lesion in either the upper or the lower motor neuron.[12,15] An upper motor neuron lesion may be present if the pathological reflex is present bilaterally.[15] A lesion of the lower motor neuron may be indicated by the unilateral presence of the pathological reflex.[15] Assessment of pathological reflexes can involve stoking, squeezing, tapping, or pinching of various anatomical structures to elicit a response. Perhaps the best-known pathological reflex is the Babinski reflex.

The athletic trainer must consider the source of any altered neurological test findings. Neurological test findings can be altered due to nerve root compression, nerve root stretch, or motor neuron lesion. The examiner should use the neurological test findings to further differentiate the source of the patient's symptoms. In addition, the information gained from the neurological assessment might dictate the need for further medical evaluation or diagnostic testing.

Functional Performance Testing

Functional performance testing, which is discussed in detail in Chapter 16, is an important component of the evaluation process, especially during the follow-up evaluations to track the patient's progress and their potential to return to previous activities. In sports medicine, functional performance testing typically involves observing the patient perform various functional movement patterns. It is important that the functional assessment reflect the type of stresses that the patient will experience during normal activities (ie, the assessment should be sport specific). Examples of sport-specific movement factors the athletic trainer should consider in designing a functional performance testing protocol include explosive movement, multi-joint coordination, neuromuscular control, fatigue, and repeated motions. Functional performance testing for an offensive lineman who has sustained a knee injury, for instance, may include observing the patient rapidly get in and out of a three-point stance, perform blocking drills and side-shuffle maneuvers, and perform plant and pivot maneuvers on the injured limb.

The athletic trainer should make note of any pain or discomfort experienced by the patient. Functional performance testing should not only be performed after injury has occurred. The athletic trainer might perform a battery of functional tests on the uninjured patient during preparticipation examinations to establish baselines for comparison during the rehabilitation process should injury occur. Comparison of post-injury scores to pre-injury baseline measures can help the athletic trainer determine whether the patient is ready to return to activity. An objective criterion might be set—for example, that the patient be able to perform at 90% to 95% of his or her pre-injury levels before he or she will be allowed to perform functional activities or return to play.

Functional Screening Tests

Functional screening tests may be performed as part of the preparticipation physical examination to identify individuals that may be at risk for injury. There is little scientific research on what the athletic trainer should focus on during injury risk screening. However, knowledge of basic biomechanics and anatomy can help the athletic trainer identify movement patterns that put stress and strain on tissue, hence increasing risk of injury.

Traditionally the clinician has used an assessment model based on anatomy that identifies a structure that generates anatomic pain that exhibits signs and symptoms that are consistent with a specific diagnosis. The trend is to shift toward a newer model that focuses more on a kinesiologic assessment rather than an anatomic assessment. This new paradigm identifies characteristic movement impairments within the human movement system and suggests how to treat these movement-related impairments and not just the structural abnormalities.

When the athlete is at greater risk of injury, he or she can devise an injury prevention training program to address the cause of the inefficient movements. By incorporating training in injury prevention, the athletic trainer may be able to reduce the incidence of injury. This has been demonstrated in several research studies looking at the incidence of lower-extremity injury, specifically ACL injury.[1,9,22]

Several clinicians[4,5,6,17,18] have developed functional evaluation screening protocols that give more attention to functional movement deficits, which may limit performance and predispose the individual to injury.[5] The Overhead and Single Leg Squat tests,[3,4] the Functional Movement Screen (FMS),[5,6,11] the Landing Error Scoring System (LESS),[18] and the Tuck Jump Test[17] are four examples of functional screening tests that are evidence-based. All of these functional screening tests have moderate to excellent intra- and inter-rater reliability.

In general, these protocols involve the individual performing a dynamic movement pattern in a controlled manner. The athletic trainer then observes the individual's movement pattern at each of the involved joints. By noting inefficient movement patterns, the athletic trainer may be able to identify preexisting muscle imbalances that alter the normal force-couple relationships, postural alignment, joint kinematics, and neuromuscular control.

Overhead and Single Leg Squat Tests

The Overhead and Single Leg Squat tests were developed by Clark[4] to identify movement impairments, determine the underlying causes, and then use this information to direct treatment. In the overhead squat the patient performs a squat maneuver while extending the arms above his or her head (Figure 3-5). In the single leg squat, with the hands on the hips the patient squats on one leg to a comfortable level and returns to the standing position (Figure 3-6).

Essentially, the athletic trainer observes whether the subject can maintain a neutral alignment of limb segments while performing a dynamic movement. The athletic trainer looks for compensation patterns at the foot, knee, hip, lumbar spine, and shoulder.

If the patient's limb segment moves out of neutral alignment, this may be due to muscle tightness or weakness. Muscle tightness may be present in the muscles in the direction of limb motion. Excessively tight muscles are believed to pull the limb into the direction of tightness, away from neutral alignment. Muscle inhibition or weakness might also be present in the muscles acting in the opposite direction of limb motion. Weak and inhibited muscles are believed to be unable to generate the magnitude of force necessary to maintain neutral alignment. Both situations cause altered joint kinematics that can place greater stress on the surrounding tissues and push these tissues closer to their point of failure during repeated movements. Tables 3-8 and 3-9 identify the compensation patterns that the patient may exhibit when performing the overhead squat and the single leg squat and the

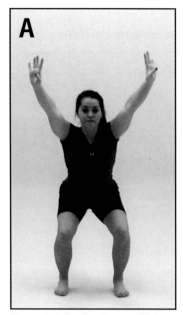
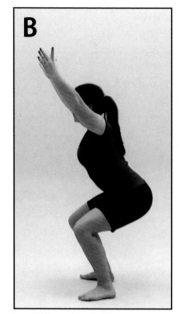
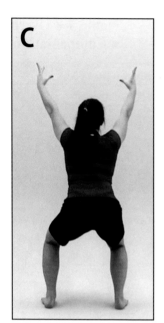

Figure 3-5. Overhead squat. (A) Anterior view; (B) lateral view; (C) posterior view.

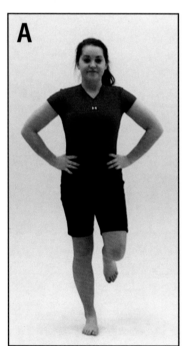
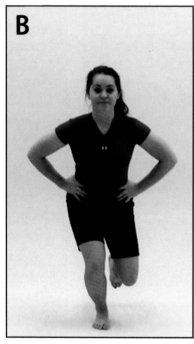

Figure 3-6. Single leg squat.

recommendations relative to how the athletic trainer should interpret those findings.

Landing Error Scoring System

The LESS was developed by Padua[18] to identify individuals at high risk for ACL injury. The test involves a jump-landing task incorporating vertical and horizontal movements as the patient jumps from a 30-cm high box to a distance of 50% of his or her height away from the box, and immediately rebounds for a maximal vertical jump on landing (Figure 3-7). The LESS score is simply a count of landing technique "errors" on a range of readily observable items of human movement. The landing technique is

Table 3-8 Overhead Squat Compensation Patterns

Compensations at:
Foot and Ankle
• Foot pronation: Y / N
• Externally rotation: Y / N
Knees
• Valgus collapse: Y / N
• Varus: Y / N
Lumbo-Pelvic-Hip Complex
• Asymmetrical weight shift: Y / N
• Lumbar lordosis: Y / N
• Hip adduction: Y / N
• Hip internal rotation: Y / N
What To Do With Findings
Foot pronation and external rotation
• Tightness: Soleus, lateral gastrocnemius, biceps femoris, peroneals, piriformis
Knee valgus & internal rotation
• Tightness: Gastrocnemius / soleus, adductors, IT band
• Weakness: Gluteus medius
Lumbar Lordosis
• Tightness: Erector Spinae & psoas
• Weakness: Transverse abdominis, internal obliques
Hip Adduction
• Tightness: Hip adductors
• Weakness: Gluteus medius
Hip Internal Rotation
• Weakness: Gluteus maximus, hip external rotators

Table 3-9 Single Leg Squat Compensation Patterns

Compensations at:
Foot and Ankle
• Foot pronation: Y / N
• Externally rotation: Y / N
Knees
• Valgus collapse: Y / N
• Varus: Y / N
Lumbo-Pelvic-Hip Complex
• Lumbar lordosis: Y / N
• Lateral trunk flexion: Y / N
• Trunk rotation: Y / N
• Hip adduction: Y / N
• Hip internal rotation: Y / N
What To Do With Findings
Foot pronation and external rotation
• Tightness: Soleus, lateral gastrocnemius, biceps femoris, peroneals, piriformis
Knee valgus and internal rotation
• Tightness: Gastrocnemius / soleus, adductors, IT band
• Weakness: Gluteus medius, adductors, IT band
Lumbar Lordosis
• Tightness: Erector spinae & psoas
• Weakness: Transverse abdominis, internal obliques
Lateral Trunk Flexion
• Weakness: Core musculature
Trunk Rotation
• Weakness: Core musculature
Hip Adduction
• Tightness: Hip adductors
• Weakness: Gluteus medius
Hip Internal Rotation
• Weakness: Gluteus maximus, hip external rotators

analyzed from both a side view and a frontal view by the athletic trainer. There are 17 scored items in the LESS (Table 3-11). A higher LESS score indicates poor technique in landing from a jump, a lower LESS score indicates better jump-landing technique.

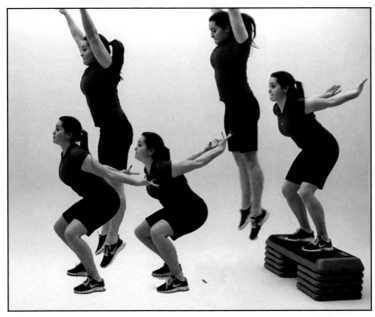

Figure 3-7. Landing Error Scoring System (LESS).

Table 3-10 Landing Technique "Errors"

Sagittal (Side) View Score
• Hip flexion angle at contact—hips are flexed Yes = 0, No = 1
• Trunk flexion angle at contact—trunk in front of hips Yes = 0, No = 1
• Knee flexion angle at contact—greater than 30 degrees Yes = 0, No = 1
• Ankle plantar flexion angle at contact—toe to heel Yes = 0, No = 1
• Hip flexion at max knee flexion angle—greater than at contact Yes = 0, No = 1
• Trunk flexion at max knee flexion—trunk in front of the hips Yes = 0, No = 1
• Knee flexion displacement—greater than 30 degrees Yes = 0, No = 1
• Sagittal plane joint displacement large motion (soft) = 0, Average = 1, Small motion(loud/stiff) = 2

Coronal (Frontal) View Score
• Lateral (side) trunk flexion at contact—trunk is flexed Yes = 0, No = 1
• Knee valgus angle at contact—knees over the mid-foot Yes = 0, No = 1
• Knee valgus displacement—knees inside of large toe Yes = 1, No = 0
• Foot position at contact—toes pointing out greater than 30 degrees Yes = 1, No = 0
• Foot position at contact—toes pointing out less than 30 degrees Yes = 1, No = 0
• Stance width at contact—less than shoulder width Yes = 1, No = 0
• Stance width at contact—greater than shoulder width Yes = 1, No = 0
• Initial foot contact—symmetric Yes = 0, No = 1
• Overall impression Excellent = 0, Average = 1, Poor = 2

Total Score ____

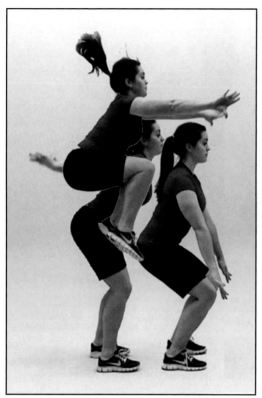

Figure 3-8. Tuck Jump Test.

Table 3-11 Tuck Jump Test Technique Flaws

Tuck Jump Assessment:	Pre	Mild	Post
Knee and thigh motion			
Knee valgus at landing			
Thighs not parallel at peak			
Thighs not equal side-to-side during flight			
Foot position during landing			
Feet not shoulder width apart			
Feet not parallel on landing			
Foot contact timing not equal			
Total ____	Total ____	Total ____	

Tuck Jump Test

Like the LESS, the Tuck Jump Test developed by Myer[17] may be useful to the clinician for the identification of lower extremity landing technique flaws during a plyometric activity that may cause ACL injury. In this test, the subject performs repeated tuck jumps for 10 seconds, which allows the clinician to visually grade the outlined criteria (Figure 3-8). The subjects' technique is subjectively rated as either having an apparent deficit or not. Six common mistakes are identified that clinicians should aim to correct for their athletes while they perform the tuck jump exercise (Table 3-11). The deficits are tallied for the final assessment score. Patients who demonstrate six or more flawed techniques, should be targeted for further technique training.

Functional Movement Screen

The FMS was developed by Cook[5,6,11] to bridge the gap between preparticipation exams and performance testing by examining individuals performing fundamental movement patterns. It is not intended as a diagnostic tool that will direct patient treatment. The FMS consists of seven fundamental movement patterns that require a balance of stability and mobility including the (1) deep squat, (2) hurdle step, (3) in-line lunge, (4) shoulder mobility test, (5) active straight-leg raise, (6) trunk stability pushup, and (7) rotary stability test (Figure 3-9). The FMS is scored on an ordinal scale, with four possible scores ranging from 0 to 3 (Table 3-12). The maximum score on the FMS is 21.

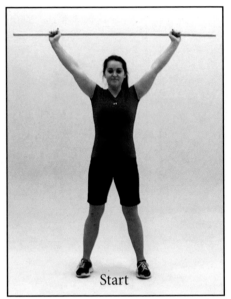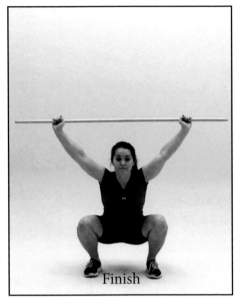

Figure 3-9 A. Functional Movement Screen: Overhead Squat.

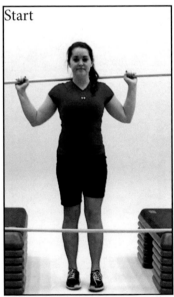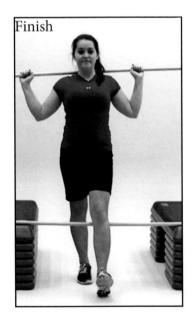

Figure 3-9 B. Functional Movement Screen: Hurdle Step.

Figure 3-9 C. Functional Movement Screen: In-line Lunge.

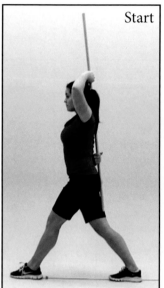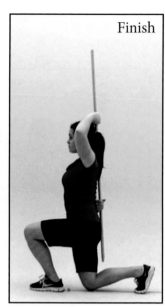

Figure 3-9 D. Functional Movement Screen: Active Straight-leg Raise Test.

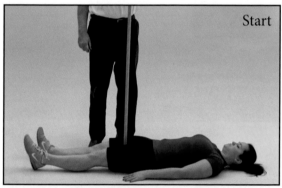

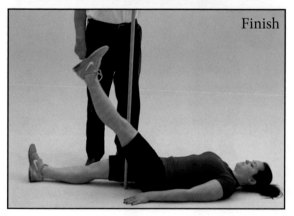

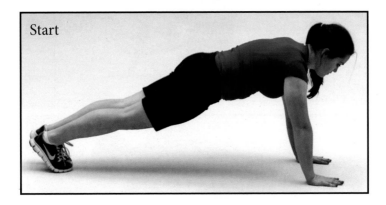

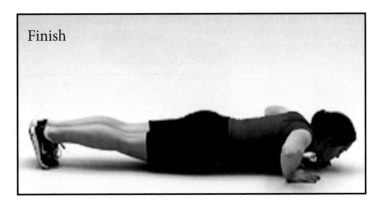

Figure 3-9 E. Functional Movement Screen: Trunk Stability Test.

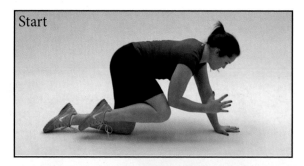

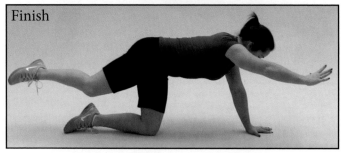

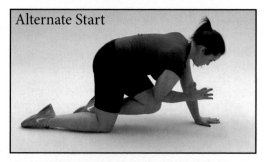

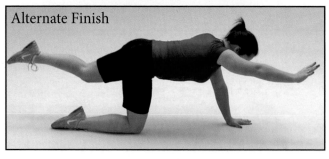

Figure 3-9 F. Functional Movement Screen: Rotary Stability Test and Alternative Position.

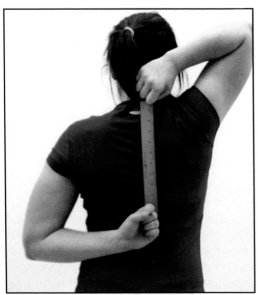

Figure 3-9 G. Functional Movement Screen: Shoulder Mobility Test.

Table 3-12

FMS Test Right Left Score*
Overhead deep squat
Trunk stability push-up ____
Hurdle step ____
In-line lunge ____
Shoulder mobility ____
Active straight leg raise ____
Rotary stability ____
Total Score ____ /21
*Scoring
Performs pattern correctly without compensation = 3
Completes pattern with some compensation = 2
Unable to complete pattern = 1
Pain at any time when performing movement pattern = 0

DOCUMENTING FINDINGS

Often overlooked in the rehabilitation process is the fact that good record keeping is essential to the rehabilitation program's success. The examiner must be able to refer back to previous evaluation records to determine the patient's progress and make the appropriate adjustments to the rehabilitation plan.

SOAP Notes

The records of the evaluation process should be recorded in SOAP (Subjective, Objective, Assessment, Plan) note format (Figure 3-10).

- S (Subjective): This component of the SOAP note includes relevant information gathered during the subjective phase of the evaluation when taking the patient's history. This information might include the patient's general impression, site of injury, mechanism of injury, previous injuries, and symptoms.[16]

- O (Objective): The objective component of the SOAP note includes relevant information gathered during the objective phase of the evaluation. The athletic trainer should record only the significant signs and symptoms revealed during the objective evaluation. An asterisk may be placed by information of particular importance. This often helps the athletic trainer readily find such information during subsequent reevaluations to assess patient progress.[19]

- A (Assessment): Assessment of the injury is the athletic trainer's professional judgment regarding the impression and nature of injury. Although the athletic trainer may be unable to determine the exact nature of the injury, information pertaining to the suspected site and pathological tissues involved is appropriate. In addition, a judgment of injury severity may be included.[19]

- P (Plan): The treatment plan should include the initial first aid performed and the athletic trainer's intentions relative to disposition.[16] Disposition may include referral for more definitive evaluation or simply application of splint, wrap, or crutches and a request to report for reevaluation the following day. Formulating the treatment plan is the final step of the SOAP note. The plan for treatment should include short- and long-term goals for the patient.[16,19] Short- and long-term goals should be objective and include timelines. This will

Patient Name ______________________ **Date of Injury** ______________________

Injury Site R L ______________________ **Today's Date** ______________________

Subjective Findings (history):

Objective Findings (observation/inspection, palpation, range of motion, strength, & special tests):

Assessment (clinical impression):

Plan (treatment administered, disposition, rehabilitation goals, treatment plan):

Figure 3-10. Form for creating a SOAP note.

allow the athletic trainer to judge the success of the rehabilitation program and make any needed adjustments after determining whether the patient was able to meet the goals.

The athletic trainer should attempt to make all information recorded as quantitative as possible.[16] This will allow the athletic trainer to better monitor the patient's progress during rehabilitation and make the adjustments and progressions to treatment accordingly, as indicated by reevaluation and comparison with previous evaluation notes.

Setting Rehabilitation Goals

Great attention should be made when developing the short- and long-term goals as these will be key factors in developing the actual rehabilitation program, as the exercises and modalities used during rehabilitation selected should be based on these goals. Rehabilitation goals should be included as part of the treatment plan in the SOAP note. The rehabilitation goals should be based upon the information gathered during the evaluation and should address signs and symptoms recorded in the SOAP note.[19] For every significant sign and symptom listed in the SOAP note, the examiner should develop a corresponding goal. Typically, the duration of short-term goals is 2 weeks.[16,19] Following the evaluation or reevaluation, the examiner should consider what goals could reasonably be achieved within this time frame. Long-term goals are the final goals the patient should achieve to be ready to return to normal activities.[16]

A different set of short- and long-term goals will be developed for each injured patient depending upon the findings from the injury evaluation. For example, a soccer player presenting with a knee injury may have restricted knee flexion and extension ROM, decreased knee extension strength, and significant knee joint swelling. The short-term goals for this case may be to increase ROM by a specific amount (eg, increase by 10 degrees), improve knee extension strength by a specific amount (eg, increase by 10 pounds), and reduce swelling by a specific amount (eg, decrease by 1 inch during girth measurement) within a specified period (typically 1 to 2 weeks for short-term goals). Thus, short-term goals should provide an immediate, achievable target that the athletic trainer can use to evaluate the success of his or her rehabilitation program. The long-term goal for this patient may be to play soccer without limitations after 8 weeks. Long-term goals help the patient understand what he or she can expect to achieve during the course of the rehabilitation process. The patient should be encouraged to achieve each short-term goal, and the athletic trainer should closely monitor the patient's progress. Understand that the goals may change over time depending upon how the patient progresses with the rehabilitation program.

The following are examples of short- and long-term goals that may be included for a grade 2 inversion ankle sprain.

Short-Term Goals

- Decrease swelling by 30% within 4 days
- Increase active ROM by 50% within 1 week
- Progress to full weight bearing during walking gait within 1 week
- Reduce acute pain by 50% within 4 days

- Increase eversion ankle strength by 50% in 4 days
- Increase plantar flexion ankle strength by 50% in 4 days

Long-Term Goals

- Return to limited practice using protective tape support within 2 weeks
- Return to full practice using protective tape support within 2.5 weeks
- Return to full competition using protective taping within 3 weeks

---

Clinical Decision-Making Exercise 3-6

You perform an injury evaluation on a soccer patient. After completing the injury evaluation, you determine the following information from the objective phase:

- Active ROM for knee extension limited by 10 degrees
- Passive ROM for knee flexion limited by 20 degrees
- Presence of swelling and discoloration over anterior thigh
- Decreased quadriceps strength compared to uninjured side

Based on these findings, how would you write up the treatment goals for this injured patient?

Progress Evaluations

The athletic trainer who is overseeing a rehabilitation program must constantly monitor the progress of the patient toward full recovery throughout the rehabilitative process. In many instances the athletic trainer will be able to treat the injured patient on a daily basis. This close supervision gives the athletic trainer the luxury of being able to continuously adjust or adapt the treatment program based on the progress made by the patient on a day-to-day basis.

The progress evaluation should be based on the athletic trainer's knowledge of exactly what is occurring in the healing process at any given time. The timelines of injury healing dictate how the athletic trainer should progress the rehabilitation program. The athletic trainer must understand that little can be done in rehabilitation to speed up the healing process

and that progression will be limited by the constraints of that process.

Progress evaluations will be more limited in scope than the detailed evaluation sequence previously described. The off-field evaluation should be thorough and comprehensive, taking time to systematically rule out information that is not pertinent to the present injury. Once the extraneous information has been eliminated, the subsequent progress evaluations can focus specifically on how the injury appears today compared with yesterday. Is the patient better or worse as a result of the treatment program rendered on the previous day?

To ensure that the progress evaluation will be complete, it is still necessary to go through certain aspects of history, observation, palpation, and special testing.

History

- How is the pain today, compared to yesterday?
- Is the patient able to move better and with less pain?
- Does the patient feel that the treatment done yesterday helped or made him sorer?

Observation

- How is the swelling today? More or less than yesterday?
- Is the patient able to move better today?
- Is the patient still guarding and protecting the injury?
- How is the patient's attitude—upbeat and optimistic, or depressed and negative?

Palpation

- Does the swelling have a different consistency today, and has the swelling pattern changed?
- Is the injured structure still as tender to touch?
- Is there any deformity present today that was not as obvious yesterday?

Special Tests

- Does ligamentous stress testing cause as much pain, or has assessment of the grade of instability changed?

- How does a manual muscle test compare with yesterday?
- Has either active or passive ROM changed?
- Does accessory movement appear to be limited?
- Can the patient perform a specific functional test better today than yesterday?

Progress Notes

Progress notes should be routinely written following progress evaluations done throughout the course of the rehabilitation program. Progress notes can follow the SOAP format outlined earlier in this chapter. They can be generated in the form of an expanded treatment note, or may be done as a weekly summary. Information in the progress note should concentrate on the types of treatment received and the patient's response to that treatment, progress made toward the short-term goals established in the SOAP note, changes in the previous treatment plan and goals, and the course of treatment over the next several days.

Summary

1. The components of the systematic differential evaluation process are split into subjective and objective phases. The subjective phase involves a detailed patient history. The objective phase includes observation/inspection of the injured patient, ROM testing, resistive strength testing, assessment of muscle imbalances, performance of special tests based on previous findings, neurological testing, and functional testing.

2. The systematic injury evaluation process establishes the foundation for designing an effective rehabilitation program. All significant findings from the systematic differential evaluation will be used to identify the pathological tissues as well as any related deficiencies in the surrounding tissues. The rehabilitation plan and treatment goals will then focus on reestablishing normal function to the tissues and structures revealed to be pathological or deficient.

3. By applying knowledge of anatomy and the systematic differential evaluation process, the athletic trainer should be able to determine what tissue is pathological. This is accomplished by differentiating between normal tissue (asymptomatic) and provoked tissue (symptomatic).

4. Injury risk screenings may be performed to determine whether the individual uses movement patterns during functional activities that may place greater stress on the surrounding tissues. By identifying such movement patterns in the early stages, the athletic trainer may be able to incorporate preventative training exercises to reduce the risk of injury at a later time.

5. Short-term and long-term goals should be based on the significant findings from the systematic differential evaluation. All significant findings should have a corresponding rehabilitation goal. All goals should be quantifiable and have a given time period in which they should be achieved. Typically, short-term goals are those that can be achieved within a 2-week period. Long-terms goals are the final goals that the patient should achieve to be ready to return to normal activities.

References

1. Chaudhari, A., Collins, M., Padua, D. 2012. ACL Research Retreat VI: An Update on ACL Risk and Prevention, *Journal of Athletic Training* 47(5):591-603.

2. Chorba, R.S., Chorba, D.J., Bouillon, L.E., et al. 2010. Use of a functional movement screening tool to determine injury risk in female collegiate athletes. *N Am J Sports Phys Ther*; 5:47-54.

3. Clark, M., Hoogeboom, B. 2001. Muscle energy techniques in rehabilitation. In Hoogeboom B, Voight M, Prentice W (Eds.), *Musculoskeletal Intervention: Techniques of Therapeutic Exercise.* NY: McGraw-Hill.

4. Clark, M., Lucett, S. 2011. Movement assessments. In M. Clark, S. Lucett (Eds.) *NASM Essentials of Corrective Exercise Training.* Baltimore: Lippincott, Williams & Wilkins.

5. Cook, G., Burton, L., Hoogenboom, B. 2006. Pre-participation screening: the use of fundamental movements as an assessment of function—part 1. *N Am J Sports Phys Ther;* 1:62-72.

6. Cook, G., Burton, L., Hoogenboom, B. 2006. Pre-participation screening: the use of fundamental movements as an assessment of function—part 2. *N Am J Sports Phys Ther;* 1:132-139.

7. Corrigan, B., and G. Maitland. 1993. *Practical Orthopedic Medicine.* London: Butterworth.

8. Cyriax, J. 1982. *Textbook of Orthopedic Medicine,* 8th ed. London: Bailliere Tindal.

9. Hewitt, T. 2013. Current Concepts for injury prevention in athletes after anterior cruciate ligament reconstruction. *American Journal of Sports Medicine, 41*(1):216-224.

10. Hislop, H. 2013. *Daniels and Worthingham's Muscle Testing,* 8th ed. Philadelphia: W. B. Saunders.

11. Hoogenboom, B., Voight, M., Cook, G., Rose, G. 2014. Functional movement assessment. In B. Hoogenboom, M. Voight, W. Prentice (Eds.) *Musculoskeletal Interventions: Techniques for Therapeutic Exercise,* 3rd edition. New York: McGraw-Hill.

12. Hoppenfeld, S. 1992. *Orthopedic Neurology: A Diagnostic Guide to Neurologic Levels.* Norwalk, CT: Appleton & Lange.

13. Janda, V. 1983. *Muscle Function Testing.* London: Butterworth.

14. Kendall, F., McCreary, E., Provance, P. 2005. *Muscles, Testing and Function,* 5th ed. Baltimore: Lippincott, Williams & Wilkins.

15. Magee, D. 2007. *Orthopedic physical assessment,* 5th ed. Philadelphia: W. B. Saunders.

16. Moore, R., Mandelbaum, B., Wantabe, D. 2012. Evaluation of neuromusculoskeletal injuries. In C. Starkey (Ed.) *Athletic Training and Sports Medicine,* 4th ed. Rosemont, IL: American Academy of Orthopaedic Surgeons.

17. Myer, G., Ford, K., Hewitt, T. 2008. Tuck jump assessment for reducing ACL injury risk. *Athletic Therapy Today 13*(5):39-44.

18. Padua, D. A., et al. 2010. The landing error scoring system (LESS) prospectively identifies ACL injury. *J Athl Train, 45*(5):539.

19. Prentice, W. 2015. *Principles of Athletic Training: A Competency Based Approach,* 15th ed. NY: McGraw-Hill.

20. Richardson, C., Jull, G., Hodges, P., Hides, J. 2004. *Therapeutic Exercise for Lumbopelvic Stabilization: A Motor Control Approach for the Treatment and Prevention of Low Back Pain.* Edinburgh: Churchill Livingstone.

21. Shultz, S., Houglum, D. P., Perrin, D. 2009. *Examination of Musculoskeletal injuries.* Champaign, IL: Human Kinetics.

22. Sugimoto, D., Myer, G. 2012. Compliance with neuromuscular training and anterior cruciate ligament injury risk reduction in female athletes: A meta-analysis. *Journal of Athletic Training, 47*(6):714-723.

23. Starkey, C., Brown, S. 2009. *Examinationn of Orthopedic and Athletic Injuries,* 4th ed. Philadelphia: F. A. Davis.

SOLUTIONS TO CLINICAL DECISION-MAKING EXERCISES

3-1 The athletic trainer should perform special tests on only those tissues he or she suspects to be pathological based on the findings from the previous evaluation phases. The special tests should be used to confirm previous findings and eliminate other tissues from being involved. Given the patient's history, the athletic trainer might suspect meniscal or articular cartilage damage and perform special tests that focus on these structures.

3-2 It is important to understand that altered postural alignment can be caused by muscle force imbalances. Muscles crossing the body segment may be excessively tight or weak, causing an altered postural alignment. The athletic trainer should pay special attention to those muscles that may alter postural alignment due to tightness or weakness during ROM and resistive strength testing. For example, the patient might demonstrate tight/ overactive hip flexor and erector spinae muscles or weak/inhibited abdominal and gluteus maximus muscles.

3-3 Cyriax states that pain in the same direction of motion during active ROM, combined with pain in the opposite direction of motion during passive ROM, is indicative of contractile tissue injury. Based on these findings, the athletic trainer may suspect injury to the hamstring muscle group.

3-4 Always consider the potential causes for reduced ROM based upon your findings. Because normal arthrokinematic motion was altered, the athletic trainer will need to address this during rehabilitation. Joint mobilization techniques may be performed in addition to traditional stretching exercises to regain normal ROM. Failure to address all possible causes (altered arthrokinematics) will result in an ineffective rehabilitation plan. Long-term goals may include:

- Return to soccer practice in 2 weeks
- Return to full soccer participation in 2.5 weeks

3-5   The findings from midrange of motion muscle testing should be used to help determine which muscles to test during specific muscle testing. The athletic trainer should perform specific muscle testing for all muscles that assist with the symptomatic movement pattern tested. Given that the patient demonstrated pain and weakness during hip extension, the athletic trainer should perform specific muscle tests on the gluteus maximus and hamstring muscles.

3-6   Rehabilitation goals should be based upon the evaluation findings. Each significant finding should have a corresponding rehabilitation goal. The athletic trainer should include both short-term and long-term goals. Short-term goals may include:

- Decrease swelling by 25% in 3 days
- Increase knee extension active ROM by 50% in 1 week
- Increase knee flexion passive ROM by 50% in 1 week
- Increase quadriceps strength by 30% in 1 week

Please see videos on the accompanying website at

www.healio.com/books/sportsmedvideos

CHAPTER 4

Psychological Considerations for Rehabilitation of the Injured Athletic Patient

Elizabeth G. Hedgpeth, EdD
Joe Gieck, EdD, PT, ATC

After completion of this chapter, the athletic training student should be able to do the following:

- Identify various predictors of injury and interventions.

- Recognize stressors in the athlete's life.

- Understand the concept of using buffers for stress management.

- Explain the progressive reactions to injury, dependent on length of rehabilitation.

- Integrate interventions for the four time periods of rehabilitation.

- Recognize irrational thinking and its resolution.

- Explain the importance of athletes taking responsibility for their actions in regard to injury.

- Compare and contrast compliance and adherence.

- Analyze the importance of rehabilitation compliance and its deviations.

- Identify signs and symptoms of clinical depression and suicide intention.

- Discuss goal setting and rehabilitation compliance.

- Review the coping skills necessary for successful rehabilitation.

- Recognize the importance of the relationship between the athletic trainer and the athlete.

Athletic injuries are considered to be one of the major health hazards of sport.[21] The fear of injury might cause a negative view of

Prentice WE, ed.
Rehabilitation Techniques for Sports Medicine and Athletic Training (pp 93-122).
© 2015 SLACK Incorporated.

Figure 4-1. Acculturation: Injured athletes moving from the culture of sport to the culture of injury rehabilitation.[31]

Uninjured athlete	Injured athlete in rehab
Familiar activity	Unfamiliar activity
Familiar rules	Unfamiliar rules
Familiar field	Unfamiliar area
Veteran player	Rookie player
Familiar pain	Unfamiliar pain
Coach in charge	ATC's in charge
Instant feedback	Feedback deferred
Control	Loss of control
Measure success	Different measure
Vigorous	Loss of vigor

participation in an activity that has a positive impact on the health and well-being of millions of participants.[50] Sports medicine and athletic training are still inexact sciences. Nowhere is this more evident than in the psychological process of responding to injury in a rational and productive manner and completing the rehabilitation process to the best of the athlete's ability. Early writings often mention that one should never attempt to cure the body without curing the soul.

ACCULTURATION

An overlooked stressor for injured athletes is acculturation, which refers to the moving of the injured athlete from the familiar sport culture to the unfamiliar rehabilitation culture (Figure 4-1). In the culture of sport, they know how the game is played, what the rules are, and who is in charge. Once injured, they move out of their comfort zone of sport and into the world of rehabilitation where the rules are changed and they are in foreign territory. Without even dealing with the injury, the athletes are stressed. They are veteran players of their sport and now they are in a new game. The coach has always had the power and now the athletic trainer and the sports medicine team have the power. Pain is a factor and that pain is different from the normal pain of working out and playing.

The athletic trainer now tells them, "Listen to your body," where coaches have often said, "Suck it up and play tough." Coaches give instant feedback on the play; athletic trainers say wait and see how your body reacts.

Loss of control is also a major factor. Athletes know that if they work out and practice hard, they have a chance to play—unlike rehabilitation, where they may or may not get well even if they do all the treatments and exercises as ordered. They can do all that is asked in rehabilitation and still not make progress due to factors out of their control. The bone might not heal properly, infection might set in, or any number of other things could go wrong. Uninjured athletes measure success by amount of playing time, number of runs scored, or whatever accomplishments are specific to their sport. In the athletic training clinic, the score is measured in terms of how it feels, how strong it is, how many reps can be done, and so on. Loss of vigor is easily seen in athletes who feel that they are not progressing fast enough or that the exercises are boring. Vigor is regained when the athletes return to practice and play.

Loss of vigor might be masked as depression, but over time it clears on its own. Therefore, though it might appear that injured athletes are stressed for no reason, the acculturation from sport to rehabilitation is a stressor in and of itself.

Most athletes have the self-confidence to adapt to a mild or moderate injury, and most have the support, understanding, and proper encouragement to adapt to more severe injury, but even the most self-confident athletes have their doubts. One athlete put it this way, expressing the positive aspects of returning to competition but also some of the doubts

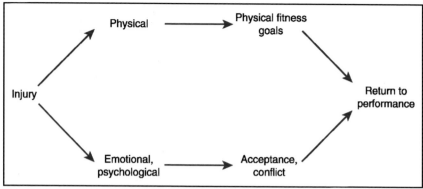

Figure 4-2. The physical and emotional aspects of return to performance.

involved: "The best competitors like to compete, and to me this is just a game—an inner game. It's an inner soul game. Can I beat my knee back?" But he also expressed doubts about the real test when a tackler "takes a whack at the knee": "I haven't thought about it, but I've had nightmares about it. My buddy told me he broke his ankle. He said once you get that real good hit and you pop up and it pops up with you, then everything is going to fall into place and you're going to be rolling. You're going to go out there like it's never been hurt and just play."

With the emergence of sport psychology, more attention is being paid to getting the mind ready to return to competition to match the adjustment of the body. Athletes have begun to describe the nightmares, fears, and anxiety of returning to competition. Also, in the current trend of professional athletes receiving extremely high salaries, some athletes describe their injuries and surgery as the most important things in their lives because the ability to play will either make or break them. Surgery and subsequent rehabilitation can determine whether athletes make either millions of dollars in an athletic career or only thousands in a regular job if the injury ends their career.

Athletes don't all deal with injury in the same manner. Rotella[63] describes how one might view the injury as disastrous, another might view it as an opportunity to show courage, whereas another athlete might relish the injury as a means to avoid embarrassment over poor performance, to escape from a losing team, or to discourage a domineering parent. When injuries are career threatening, athletes whose lives have revolved around a sport may have to make major adjustments in how they perceive themselves as well as how they are perceived within their society. Olympic and other top-caliber athletes are often emotionally and socially years behind their chronological peers because they have spent so much time in their sport that their social interactions have suffered. Therefore many top or single-minded athletes have difficulty with emotional control when they sustain a serious injury. Figure 4-2 demonstrates the physical and emotional aspects of return to performance. The return to performance is either enhanced or negated by the physiological results of both elements.

PREDICTORS OF INJURY

The Injury-Prone Athlete

Some athletes seem to have a pattern of injury, whereas others in exactly the same position with the same physical makeup are injury free. Certain researchers suggest that some psychological traits might predispose the athlete to a repeated injury cycle.[1,39,57,72,78] No one particular personality type has been recognized as injury prone. However, the individual who likes to take risks seems to represent the injury-prone athlete.[23] Other factors that are seen as predisposing an athlete to risk of injury are being reserved, detached, tender-minded,[49] apprehensive, overprotective, or easily distracted.[61] These individuals usually also lack the ability to cope with the stress associated with the risks and their consequences. Sanderson[64] suggests some other factors leading to a propensity for injury, such as attempts to reduce anxiety by being more aggressive, fear of failure, or guilt over unobtainable or unrealistic goals.

Stress and Risk for Injury

Much has been written about life stress events and the likelihood of illness.[2,26,34] Stressors are both positive (eg, making All-American) and negative (eg, not making the starting lineup or failing a drug test). Stressors that seem to predispose an athlete to injury are the negative stressors.[26]

Andersen and Williams[2] suggest that negative stressors lead to a lack of attentional focus and to muscle tension, which in turn lead to the stress-injury connection. Loss of attentional focus can cause the athlete to miss cues during a play, setting the stage for a possible injury. Muscle tension (bracing or guarding) leads to reduced flexibility, reduced motor coordination, and reduced muscle efficiency, which set the athlete up for a variety of injuries (eg, getting hit by a golf ball or missing an obstacle during a run).

Attentional focusing is perceived on two planes (width and directional). A major component is the ability to change focus when the situation demands it. Width of focus ranges from broad (attending to a number of cues) to narrow (attending to one cue), and direction of focus is internal (attending to feelings or thoughts) or external (attending to events outside of the body). The trick is not only to be able to change focus, but to know the optimal time to make the change to minimize the possibility of injury or reinjury. For instance, a football player can be blindsided and take an unanticipated hit, or the gymnast can be distracted and miss a landing.

Life stress is a more global assessment, taking into account events that cause stress during the past year to 18 months. The Life Events Survey for Collegiate Athletes (LESCA) asks collegiate-athlete-specific questions, eliciting a negative or positive response on a Likert-type 8-point scale.[59] Typical events asked about are "major change in playing status" and "pressure to gain or lose weight for sport participation." Another life events assessment is the Social and Athletic Readjustment Rating Scale (SARRS).[9]

Table 4-1 Examples of Events in the Lives of Athletes Most Likely to Elicit a Stress Response

Life Stress Events
Death of family member
Detention or jail
Injury
Death of close friend
Playing for a new coach
Playing on a new team
Personal achievements
Change in living habits
Social readjustments
Change to new school
Change in social activities

The events most likely to elicit a negative stress response are listed in Table 4-1.

Profiles of Mood States (POMS)[51] is a more immediate response inventory assessing moods within the last few days or at the most the last few weeks. The POMS identifies six mood states. Five are negative, and one (vigor) is positive. The six mood states are (1) tension-anxiety, (2) depression-dejection, (3) anger-hostility, (4) vigor-activity, (5) fatigue-inertia, and (6) confusion-bewilderment. When the POMS results were compared using elite athletes and the general population, a visual "iceberg profile" was noted for the elite athletes by Morgan.[56] The elite athletes' scores on the five negative scales fall below the 50th percentile, and their scores on the sixth, positive scale (vigor) peak considerably above the 50th percentile, indeed resembling the silhouette of an "iceberg."

The POMS has been used to measure the mood states of athletes at the time of injury as well as at 2-week intervals during the rehabilitation process.[35] When the POMS was used within 2 days of injury, the injured athletes showed significant elevations in depression and anger, no change in tension and vigor, but less fatigue and confusion compared to the college norms. When the athletes were divided into groups according to severity of injury based on length of rehabilitation, the data are more explicit concerning reactions to injury and

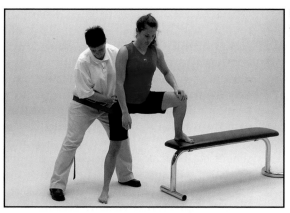

Figure 4-3. A close relationship between the patient and the athletic trainer is invaluable.

rehabilitation. Group 1 consists of athletes with less than 1 week of rehabilitation; they had less tension, depression, fatigue, and confusion. Group 2 consists of athletes in rehabilitation for more than 2 weeks but less than 4 weeks; they had more anger but less fatigue and confusion. Group 3 consists of athletes in rehabilitation more than 4 weeks; they had more tension, depression, and anger, and less vigor. This finding is important in that it sends a wake-up call to the sports medicine team to be aware of the ramifications of severe injury that entails a long rehabilitation period.

Interventions for Stress Reduction

Not all athletes need or want counseling, and the close relationship between the athlete and the athletic trainer is invaluable in making this decision (Figure 4-3). Athletic trainers are now taking a more active role in the psychological aspects of injury and rehabilitation. They are the closest to the athlete and often spend as much time as the athletes at practice and games. Athletic trainers are now aware of the psychological impact of injury and have a working knowledge of counseling techniques for various situations.[13,30,58] Few athletes react to stress events by verbalizing their feelings of stress, yet most handle them very well by themselves. Michener[53] makes the following point: For many athletes, physical activity, rather than talking things out, appears to offer a means of expressing feelings and aggressions. Perhaps this substitution of actions for words

contributes to the seeming reluctance of athletes to come to a service that requires that they articulate their feelings.

Unfortunately, many coaches do not have the interest or ability to work with athletes who need help. Some sort of screening device should be used to identify athletes who are experiencing life situations that they are unprepared to handle. Obviously the staff of a smaller team is more familiar with the athletes and their problems and can more effectively deal with them,[31] but larger teams' staffs should attempt to deal with the athlete through the position coach or other available support personnel (eg, counseling centers, sport psychologists, grief support groups).

Using Buffers

In many instances athletes feel that their sport is the one positive thing in life that helps them get through times of extreme stress. Areas outside of sports are often stressful, and athletes tend to respond to interventions that are within their framework of emotional comfort. The use of buffers might be all the athlete needs to handle the stress of injury and rehabilitation. Buffers are techniques that allay the symptom of stress but do not address the problem that originally caused the stressors. Several buffers that can be beneficial in reducing the stress of injury and rehabilitation are progressive relaxation with or without imagery, aerobic exercise, diet modifications (eg, reduction of caffeine), treatment of sleep disorders, and time management programs.

Clinical Decision-Making Exercise 4-1

Julie is a lacrosse player at a Division I school playing in the starting lineup as a sophomore. She had played her entire high school years without injury, so having a severe ankle sprain at the end of this season was a shock. Julie is not accustomed to having the normal activities of daily living take so much time, and she feels she never has time to go to the athletic training room for her rehabilitation. What can the athletic trainer do to help Julie alter her schedule to include time for rehabilitation?

Abdominal Breathing

Deep abdominal breathing for relaxation is a product of yoga and has been practiced for more than 5,000 years.[70] The practice was brought to the West in the 1960s. Deep abdominal breathing is simple to learn and is effective as a tool for relaxation and relief from stress and pain.[28] It is used in the Lamaze childbirth method to relieve pain and stress during the birthing process.[70] Deep abdominal breathing[41] is simple and can be mastered in a few days. The following is a simple way to teach it to an athlete.

Lie on your back in a quiet place with one hand on your chest and one hand on your stomach. Inhale through your nose and have the air fill up your belly without your chest moving. Now breathe out through your mouth and feel your belly go down. Breathe slowly and pay attention to the air moving in and out of your lungs. This can be used for pain and tension relief by paying attention to the sore and tense muscle groups in the body during the inhale phase. During the exhale phase feel your pain and tension being "blown out" of the body with the exhaled breath.

Once the athlete has mastered the lying-down position, move on to sitting and then standing positions. The beauty of this practice is that it can be performed anywhere and anytime and enables athletes in rehabilitation to control their pain and stress.[28]

Relaxation Techniques

Progressive relaxation techniques[37,38] are most effective for athletes who tend to be stressed regarding an injury and who have problems sleeping, tension headaches, or general muscle bracing or tightness. Relaxation training, with or without imagery, allows athletes to control their feelings of stress and anxiety with a series of deep breathing, voluntary muscular contraction, and relaxation exercise.[6] Relaxation and imagery are used by athletes to reduce the symptoms of anxiety associated with the reaction to injury and rehabilitation. Athletes who are coping well on their own should not be forced to spend extra time on relaxation training.

Jacobsen's[37,38] progressive relaxation technique is thought to be effective because of the assumption that it is impossible to be nervous or tense when the muscles are relaxed. The tenseness of the involuntary muscles and organs can be reduced when the contiguous skeletal muscles are relaxed. The muscles are tensed and relaxed for the athlete to become familiar with how the muscle feels in a relaxed state and in a tense state. The relaxation method involves the tensing and relaxing of muscles in a predetermined order. The arm and hand are done first because the difference in tense and relaxed muscles is more apparent in these muscle groups. The repetitions should last about 10 to 15 seconds for the tension segment and 15 to 20 seconds for the relaxation segment, with about three repetitions for each muscle group. After the athlete is comfortable with the relaxation training, then imagery can be introduced.

Clinical Decision-Making Exercise 4-2

Tim is a 17-year-old tennis player at a prep school known for turning out exceptional tennis players ready to play at the Division I level. He developed elbow tendinitis at the end of last season and has spent the summer doing rehabilitation. The medical staff cleared him to play, but Tim is unable to keep from tensing up when he knows he is being observed by recruiters. His whole body is stiff and tight, and his usual warm-up stretching is not sufficient to keep his muscles relaxed. How can the athletic trainer help Tim manage this problem?

Imagery

Imagery is the use of one's senses to create or recreate an experience in the mind.[17] Visual images used in the rehabilitation process include visual rehearsal, emotive imagery rehearsal,

Length of rehabilitation	Reaction to injury	Reaction to rehabilitation	Reaction to return
Short (< 4 weeks)	Shock Relief	Impatience Optimism	Eagerness Anticipation
Long (> 4 weeks)	Fear Anger	Loss of vigor Irrational thoughts Alienation	Acknowledgment
Chronic (recurring)	Anger Frustration	Dependence or independence Apprehension	Confident or skeptical
Termination (career-ending)	Isolation Grief process	Loss of athletic identify	Closure and renewal

Figure 4-4. Progressive reactions of injured athletes based on severity of injury and length of rehabilitation.

and body rehearsal.[14,67] Visual rehearsal uses both coping and mastery rehearsal. Coping rehearsal has athletes visually rehearsing problems they feel might stand in the way of a return to competition. They then rehearse how they will overcome these problems. Mastery rehearsal aids in gaining confidence and motivational skills. Athletes visualize their successful return to competition, beginning with early practice drills and continuing on to the game situation.

In emotive rehearsal, the athlete gains confidence and security by visualizing scenes relating to positive feelings of enthusiasm, confidence, and pride—in other words, the emotional rewards of praise and success from participating well in competition. Body rehearsal empirically helps athletes in the healing process. It is suggested that athletes visualize their bodies healing internally both during the rehabilitation procedures and throughout their daily activities.[12] To do this, the athletes have to have a good understanding of the injury and of the type of healing occurring during the rehabilitation process. Ievleva and Orlick[36] had athletes use imagery during physiotherapy by imagining that the ultrasound was increasing blood flow and thus promoting recovery.

Care should be taken to explain the healing and rehabilitative process clearly but not to overwhelm athletes with so much information that they become intimidated and fearful. This mistake is often made by the inexperienced athletic trainer who wants to impress the athletes. Educate athletes only to the amount of knowledge required. By the same token, don't hold back information athletes require for this imagery.

PROGRESSIVE REACTIONS DEPEND ON LENGTH OF REHABILITATION

The literature on reactions to injury has dispelled the stage theory of reaction to injury, according to an extensive literature review by Wortman and Silver.[79] However, there are factors that are commonly seen among athletes going through adjustment to injury and rehabilitation in the athletic training clinic. Severity of injury usually determines length of rehabilitation. Regardless of length of rehabilitation, the injured patient has to deal with three reactive phases of the injury and rehabilitation process (Figure 4-4). These phases are reaction to injury, reaction to rehabilitation, and reaction to return to competition or career termination. These reactions can be cumulative in nature depending on the length of rehabilitation. Other factors that influence reactions to injury and rehabilitation are the patient's coping skills, past history of injury, social support, and personality traits. These reactions fall into four time frames: short-term (less than 4 weeks), long-term (more than 4 weeks), chronic (recurring), and termination (career ending). Reactions are primary and secondary, but patients do not all have all reactions, nor do all reactions fall into the suggested sequence.

Some psychologists have applied five stages of psychological reaction to injury based on Kübler-Ross's classic model of reactions to death and dying, which includes denial, anger, bargaining, depression, and acceptance.[42] Although this model is commonly considered to be applicable to terminal illnesses or death, it is generally not considered to be applicable to less significant injuries such as those that occur in sport. An alternative cognitive appraisal model has been proposed that focuses more on injured athletes' personal and situational factors and how these influence their cognitive appraisal of the injury situation.[77] It focuses on their interpretation of the injury rather than on the actual severity of the injury. Cognitive appraisal is what determines the athlete's emotional response (eg, anger, depression, tension) and behavioral response (eg, adherence to rehabilitation). These cognitive, emotional, and behavioral responses are interdependent and collectively influence recovery outcome. Other factors that can influence reactions to injury and rehabilitation are the athlete's coping skills, history of injury, social support, and personality traits.[40]

DEALING WITH SHORT-TERM INJURY

Short-term injuries are usually less than 4 weeks but may be a few days over depending on how the length is measured in terms of the end of rehabilitation. For practical purposes the rehabilitation is complete when the patient and the sports medicine team feel it is safe for the patient to return, when an appropriate level of competitive fitness has been reached, and

the athlete feels ready physically and psychologically to return to competition. Short-term injuries can include, but are not limited to, first- or second-degree sprains/strains, bruises, and simple dislocations. These are the types of injuries that are fairly common and are part of playing the game.

Reactions to Short-Term Injury

The primary reaction to these injuries is the shock of surprise—the shock that the injury cannot be just "walked off" or "shaken off." At the time of the injury, the athlete tries to walk it off or shake it off on the court or playing field. Athletes have probably experienced this type of injury before with no residual complaint and need time to accept that, this time, it is not immediately going away. Rehabilitation compliance is often compromised when athletes envision themselves returning in a couple of days without treatment. The athletic trainer assesses the patient's injury and explains the process of rehabilitation to the patient.

The secondary reaction is relief—relief that it is not something really major, given that it couldn't be discounted as just a "nick" or "ding." The sense of relief is contingent on the patient's trust in the athletic trainer. At this point, the relationship between the athletic trainer and the patient is forged and trust is established. This sets the tone for the success or failure of the rehabilitation process.

Reactions to Rehabilitation of Short-Term Injury

Once short-term injury rehabilitation begins, the primary reaction the patient displays is impatience—an impatience to get started, to do something, to get on with the program as quickly as possible. During this time the patient is often experiencing peaks and valleys in the recovery process. The athlete is accustomed to two speeds: no speed and full speed. Athletes often express the belief that they should heal faster because they are in better shape, and they are not happy to spend time in the sequential phases of rehabilitation. If it is a sprained ankle, the athlete does not react with exhilaration to the crutch phase, then the walking phase, then the walk-jog phase, then the jog-run phase, then the run phase, and then finally the full-speed activity phase. The athletic trainer can reassure the patient that the phases are necessary and that to push it could set back the rehabilitation time.

The secondary reaction is one of optimism. This optimism is due to the confidence and trust established between the athletic trainer and the patient. The patient is able to believe the athletic trainer's assessment that because the injury turned out to be less serious than originally thought, it stands to reason that the rehabilitation will work out as well. It is important that compliance be consistent with the athletic trainer's treatment plan and that the injured patient does not try to return to practice or play too soon. This level of injury has a good track record for excellent recovery.

Intervention for Short-Term Injury

Intervention should include allowing the patient to vent frustrations and reiterating that there is a light at the end of the tunnel. At the collegiate level, athletes have frequently had this type of injury and consider it to be part and parcel of playing the game. The injured athlete should be encouraged to remain involved with the team, attending practices while performing rehabilitation, attending team meetings, and interacting with teammates after hours. At this stage the athletic trainer and the patient will have to conduct some reality checks to ascertain that the concerns that come up are in the realm of the patient's control. Losing their spot on the team, losing their speed, or losing their best shot is not within the athletes' control. Doing effective rehabilitation on a consistent basis is within their control. Staying current with the team will keep them current with plays and coaching changes. Effective rehabilitation is the only way to return to their sport. Compliance is not usually a factor for short-term injuries.

Reactions to Return to Competition After Short-Term Injury

The primary reaction to returning to competition is eagerness and the secondary reaction is anticipation. At the time of return to competition, the patients with short-term injuries are usually eager to begin to practice and play. They anticipate that they will return to their pre-injury competence the first day back. By the time the athletic trainer feels the patient is ready to return, it is assumed that a level of trust has been established. The patient and the athletic trainer must agree on a realistic plan for return to activity so that the transition will be safe and satisfactory for all concerned.

DEALING WITH LONG-TERM INJURY

Long-term injuries are considered to have a rehabilitation time of more than 4 weeks and range anywhere from 4 weeks to 6 months to 1 year. These injuries are the most severe and tend to be the most difficult for the patient to handle because of the length of inactivity and the lack of rapid progress during rehabilitation. Long-term injuries include, but are not limited to, fractures, orthopedic surgery, general surgery, second- and third-degree sprains/strains, and debilitating illness.

Reaction to Long-Term Injury

The athletes' primary reaction to long-term injury is fear—fear that they will never get better, fear that they can never play again, fear that they cannot handle a long rehabilitation period, fear of pain, and fear of the unknown (Figure 4-5). Most athletes have heard the horror stories of the individual who had this same injury and never came back for a multitude of reasons. They hear stories of individuals who came back but were never again as fast or as talented or as fearless ... the list goes on. At this point the athletic trainer must allay the fear with pertinent information in terms that are easy to understand. It is not helpful to overload the patient with all the latest information on that particular injury. The rule of thumb is to present the truth in appropriate doses that the patient can handle. Again, establishing a trusting relationship with the athletic trainer is a vital component of this long-term process.

Figure 4-5. The athletic trainer assists the patient to quell the fear associated with long-term injuries.

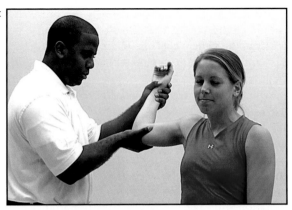

Figure 4-6. Common signs and symptoms of clinical depression.

1. Change in eating and/or sleeping habits either more or less than usual
2. Difficulty in concentration
3. Lack of interest in activities previously enjoyed
4. Inappropriate reaction to stressful situations: aggression, extreme agitation, rage or no reaction: "I don't care," "Doesn't bother me," "Whatever"
5. Flat affect—a void of the normal fluctuation of facial expressions
6. Decreased involvement with normal social support such as teammates, friends, and family
7. History of depression in the past or family history of depression

The secondary reaction to a long-term injury is anger—anger that the injury happened, that it happened to them, that it happened at the time it did, and so on. Anger cannot be reasoned with, and the sports medicine team must understand and not react to the patient's anger. An angry, hostile, or surly attitude toward the personnel or program should not offend the athletic trainer. Whoever happens to be around the patient often bears the brunt of the anger. This response is merely an emotional release. With anger the patient is usually reacting to the situation and not necessarily to the individual.

Reaction to Long-Term Rehabilitation

The primary reaction to long-term rehabilitation is twofold: loss of vigor and irrational thoughts. At this point the athletic trainer needs to be aware that a loss of vigor can be masked as depression, although depression can also be a possible reaction. The patient appears to be lacking the usual vim, vigor, and vitality but does not have the common signs and symptoms of a true depression (Figure 4-6). Understanding this phenomenon will enable the athletic trainer to understand the patient's change in temperament and disposition. The patient should understand that it is reasonable to feel somewhat discouraged concerning the injury, as long as there are no other presenting symptoms of clinical depression.

In one study, it was found that clinical depression occurs in only 4.8% of the injured athletic population.[74] The possibility of attempted suicide by the clinically depressed patient warrants the vigilance of the sports medicine team.[5] If signs of clinical depression (loss of appetite, sleep disruption, withdrawal, change in mood state, thoughts of or plans for attempting suicide, etc) are present, then the possibility of

1. Has signs and symptoms of being clinically depressed
2. Has feelings of helplessness and hopelessness such as seeing no way out of stressful situation except suicide
3. Has thoughts of suicide or a previous attempt, or has a close friend, family member, or acquaintance who committed suicide
4. Has an irreversible plan to commit suicide (taking pills as opposed to jumping from the top of a building)
5. Making plans to not be around, such as giving away possessions, writing letters, getting affairs in order, saying good-bye to friends
6. Expresses intention to commit suicide (taking demographics into account—women make more attempts but men are more successful)

Figure 4-7. Common signs of possible suicidal intentions.

Irrational Thinking toward Injury and Rehabilitation

Exaggeration: Severity or mildness and significance or insignificance of injury— "I'm in great shape, so my broken leg will heal faster than it would for someone who is out of shape." "How bad can a sprain be?"

Disregard: Neglecting or overdoing rehabilitation treatment— "I'll wait a few weeks and see if it gets better on its own." "If one repetition of five sets is good, then two of ten will be twice as good."

Oversimplification: Thinking of rehabilitation as good or bad, right or wrong, necessary or unnecessary— "No one ever came back from ACL surgery." "I don't see any reason to do rehab exercises if I am going to have surgery in two weeks."

Generalization: Generalizing the outcome of one athlete's injury to all injuries, or one athlete's outcome of rehabilitation to all rehabilitation— "All sprains heal in two weeks." "Rehab is necessary only if you plan to compete again."

Unwarranted Conclusions: Conclusions based on unsound thinking or false information— "I know an athlete who did everything they told him to do and his arm never got better." "They say that once you break a bone you never can run as fast."

Figure 4-8. Examples of thought patterns athletes might have concerning injury and rehabilitation.

---

attempted suicide must be addressed (Figure 4-7). According to Smith and Milliner,[63] the incidence of attempted suicide is high among the age group of 15 to 24 years. In Smith and Milliner's study of five athletes who had attempted suicide, the common factors were a serious injury that required surgical intervention, rehabilitation of 6 weeks to 1 year while not participating in sport, diminished athletic skill upon return after successful rehabilitation, and being replaced in their position on the team. Adaptation to the physical, mental,

and emotional frustration is hard work during the rehabilitative process. The work the athlete is doing is not producing the same rewards as participation in the sport; plus the athlete is becoming anxious about falling farther behind in the sport. At this point it is prudent to ask the athlete if psychological intervention is needed or desired, since not all athletes require or desire psychological intervention.[5]

The other primary reaction to long-term rehabilitation is irrational thoughts (Figure 4-8). If irrational thoughts are persistent, interfere with the normal routine of daily life, and disrupt the rehabilitation process, then psychological intervention is recommended and is frequently effective. Irrational thoughts can be negative perceptions of pain, fear of reinjury, lack of social support, poor performance, and so on. These patients might harbor thoughts of not returning to play or not being able to return to their previous level of play. Previously rational and positive perceptions of situations now become negative and irrational as self-destructive emotions color the thought process. Emotional reaction is exacerbated when the patient fails to heal or return faster than the non-athlete. Frequently, athletes feel that because they are in better shape at the time of injury, they should heal faster than non-athletes who are out of shape at the time of injury. The athlete has often put in years of training and imposes pressures to heal faster and return quicker. The athlete's common sense and judgment become altered. This mood change might occur daily or weekly, so continual interaction between the athletic trainer and the patient is necessary to restore rationality and change negative thoughts.

The secondary reaction to long-term rehabilitation is a feeling of alienation. With an injury that requires weeks or months of rehabilitation before the athlete's return to competition, the athlete often feels that the coaches have ceased to care, teammates have no time to spend with him or her, friends are no longer around, and his or her social life consists of time put into rehabilitation. The injured athletes may have had little support from coaches and teammates, since the coaches are concerned with the results of the team. Injured athletes feel neglected if their daily activities have revolved around the sport and they are no longer part of the sport.

The injured athlete must understand that the coach cares but has no expertise in injury management and must be concerned with getting the rest of the team ready. The athletic trainer has no expertise in coaching but is primarily interested in getting the injured athlete back to optimal fitness. Coaches work with players on playing their sport, athletic trainers work with patients on rehabilitating injuries: two different fields, two different abilities, two different areas of expertise. Some coaches, unfortunately,

might also want the injured athlete kept away from other players to remove the reminder that injury is a possibility.[18]

The injured athlete may feel unable to maintain or regain normal relationships with teammates. The injured athlete is a reminder that injury can happen, and teammates might pull away from that constant reminder. Friendships based on athletic identification are now compromised because the athletic identification is gone, and they can be related to in athletic terms only by what they did yesterday or as injured teammates and not as individuals. Injured athletes no longer have the camaraderie of the dressing room, the practice bashing, the travel to away events, and the other interactions mired in tradition that give athletes a sense of belonging, a sense of being important. When injured athletes can remain involved with the team, however, they feel less isolated and less guilty for not putting it on the line to help the team.

Intervention for Long-Term Rehabilitation

Whenever possible, anger should not be challenged, because no one can reason with anger. Instead, the athletic trainer should wait until the individual is in control of the anger and then discuss the inappropriate behavior that cannot be tolerated in the rehabilitation setting. Then the athletic trainer and the patient can work out the cause of the anger and together arrive at a solution. The athletic trainer must act as an emotional blotter and, if possible, not further aggravate the situation by attempting to exert power to calm down the patient. It is as important to listen to what the patient is feeling in addition to what the patient is saying. At this point the patient has a need to vent the anger, and the athletic trainer must simply listen to the patient's reaction.

At this time active listening by the athletic trainer is a move toward developing a supportive and trusting relationship with the patient. Having a trusting relationship between the patient and the athletic trainer can make all the difference in getting the patient into the proper frame of mind for successful completion of the rehabilitation process.

One of the more difficult aspects of adjusting to injury is stopping negative thoughts, which are devastating to a successful rehabilitation process. These thoughts have to be recognized by the patient and then controlled.[54] Controlling inner thoughts determines future behavior. This process is one of awareness, education, and encouragement for ultimate positive change. Negative thoughts have a detrimental effect on both mental and physical performance.[63] It is helpful to keep a daily record of when these thoughts take place, as well as the correlated physical progress and the time and circumstances in which they occur. Then patients are helped to stop these negative thoughts and instill a positive regimen. This step is followed by an evaluation of the whole negative thought-stopping program on a regular basis. In this manner, injured athletes have the practice and feedback to begin their own positive outlook in terms of constructive thoughts, concentration, cues, images, and calming responses to change inappropriate attitudes.

This positive outlook, plus seeing physical progress, can help patients return more quickly to competition with better abilities to perform. The reinforcement of sayings such as, "You will get better" and, "This too will pass" aid in the blockage of the negative thoughts. Negative thoughts block the athlete's road to recovery by increasing pain, anxiety, and anger. Patients should be encouraged to put their efforts into recovery rather than into the downward spiral of self-pity. Thoughts create emotions, therefore these negative thoughts have to be recognized and dealt with for a more rapid recovery. The patient should never be allowed to say "I can't" but rather should substitute "I'll try."

The technique of restructuring perceptions helps the patient become aware of these destructive, self-defeating behaviors. The patient, however, might fall into the mode of "I can't do it, I'll never get well." This irrational thinking produces anxiety, fear, and possibly depression, which are detrimental to progress in rehabilitation. The patient might be illogical, distort perceptions of events, or reach unrealistic decisions and conclusions. The patient has replaced the old set of worries about simply playing well and helping the team win with the set of "Woe is me," with its resultant anxiety. Obviously, these thought patterns are detrimental to the positive attitude necessary in the rehabilitation process.

The athletic trainer must recognize and challenge irrational thinking. Examination of these thoughts with patients reassures them that it is normal to feel unhappy, frustrated, angry, or insecure, but that the injury is not hopeless, they do not lack courage, and all is not lost and life is not over. The patient should be challenged to replace irrational thoughts with positive and rational ones. In short, the injury is aggravating and unfortunate, but it can be handled and overcome. The injury is placed in perspective and viewed in the same way as the athlete would consider preparation for the next athletic contest. The patient must identify faulty thinking, gain understanding of it, and actively work for its change. Research[7,80] indicates that the self-thoughts, images, and attitudes during the recovery period impact the length and quality of the rehabilitation.

Clinical Decision-Making Exercise 4-3

Dana is a Division I golfer who wants to play on the LPGA tour next year after graduation. She has had chronic neck and shoulder spasms for the past year. As a result of her desire to play well at Qualifying School, coupled with her anxiety regarding her neck and shoulder pain, she has fallen prey to negative thinking: "What if my neck flares up during Q-school, what if my neck blocks my swing plane?" How can the athletic trainer help Dana manage this problem?

Lost social support can be replaced by organizing support groups or similar injury groups or mentoring by athletes who have completed rehabilitation successfully.[55] A supporting relationship between the patient and the athletic trainer can be the mainstay in attainment of successful rehabilitation (Figure 4-9). Establishing this relationship may be difficult for athletes who have been catered to when healthy and are now in a reversed role. At this time patients question many aspects of the rehabilitation procedure. They question the doctor's diagnosis, the athletic trainer for working them possibly too much, and the coach for not paying attention to them. They question whether they

Figure 4-9. The patient and the athletic trainer develop a relationship of respect and trust.

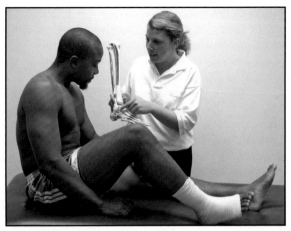

are thought of as malingerers. They question whether the rehabilitation personnel know how important competition is to them.

Toward the end of rehabilitation, the patient should begin sport-specific drills during practice time with the team. The patient then begins to re-enter the team culture and is not isolated from the team environment. Thus more effort is put into functional sport-specific situations that are generally less boring to the athlete. In so doing, the athlete gains a more realistic appreciation of the skills needed to attain pre-injury performance levels. The rehabilitation routine is more easily tolerated by patients if they can see some carryover to their particular sport.

After injury, patients need the support of teammates. To prevent possible feelings of negative self-worth and problems of loss of identity for athletes, their support groups need to stress that they are interested in the patient as a person as well as a team member. If the athletic trainer and sports medicine team have established prior personal contact with the patient as a worthwhile person, this transition can be easier.

Reaction to Return to Competition for Long-Term Injury

The primary reaction to return to competition from a long-term injury is an acknowledgment that the rehabilitation process is completed. This is a feeling of "I have done my best and all that I can do in the area of rehabilitation." The patient might go down a checklist of performance abilities:

- The team physician who has the final vote on medically clearing an athlete to return to competition has given the OK to return.

- The athletic trainer has set functional criteria to be followed before returning to play.

- The athletic trainer and the patient have discussed the use of additional padding, the wearing of a brace, or other equipment adjustments to minimize reinjury.

- The physician, the athletic trainer, the sport psychologist, and the coach have determined that the athlete is ready to play at 100%, the athlete fits back into the chemistry of the current lineup, the athlete is knowledgeable about recent changes in coaching strategy, and the athlete feels psychologically ready.

- The athlete and the sports medicine team have discussed feelings of confidence about returning, willingness to play with pain or soreness, and willingness to risk reinjury or permanent damage.

- The athlete has gained the emotional self-control to think rationally about the injury and cope successfully with the return to competition.

It is now up to the athlete to make the decision to return to play.[60]

After going through the checklist of concerns that the athlete feels are important, the secondary reaction is trust—trust that every-thing has been done to be as prepared as pos-sible to return to play. Trust at this time is trust that everything has been done, not that the injury is healed—this won't come until it has been tested and proven. When the athlete has been cleared to return, everything has been completed that is within the athlete's control. It is now time to "put it to the test—to step up to the plate and give it a shot." Acceptance that the rehabilitation process is successful will not come until the athlete makes the first move, takes the first hit, or runs the first race. Then, and only then, will the athlete play with the freedom and confidence she or he had prior to the injury.[60]

DEALING WITH CHRONIC INJURY

Chronic injury can be defined as an injury having a slow, insidious onset, most often starting with pain and/or signs of inflamma-tion that might last for months or years and giving the impression of recurring over time. These injuries are usually overuse injuries and can include tendinitis, stress fractures (shin splints), compartment syndrome, and other second- or third-degree injuries.

Reaction to Chronic Injury

The primary reaction to a chronic injury is anger. Often the patient has done everything the athletic trainer suggested as far as reha-bilitation and even maintenance rehabilitation, and still the injury recurred. The patient des-perately wants to return to previous form and remembers that rehabilitation is going to be another long, drawn-out process. The athletic trainer often has to explain over and over that setbacks occur even without provocation. Such repetition is necessary because an angry patient has selective hearing and a short attention span.

It might take several meetings for the athlete to cool down enough to hear what is being said. Because many chronic injuries are overuse injuries, rest and inactivity are frequently the treatment of choice. Athletes often describe this inactivity during injury as being harder than playing. When they are playing, all their energy is directed toward the goal of running, throwing, jumping, or whatever other activity is part of their sport. When they are rehabilitat-ing for a chronic injury, most physical activity screeches to a halt.

Inactivity leads to frustration, the secondary reaction to chronic injury. The fact that many of these injuries are overuse injuries increases the frustration brought on by a sense of some-how having caused the recurrence or at least done something to increase the chance of it. "If I hadn't run the extra mile." "If I hadn't played the second set." If the athlete has used sport as a buffer to control stress, that outlet is gone for the time being. Stress then accelerates. Often these athletes are used to being very active and the forced inactivity is frustrating. These ath-letes are well acquainted with the rehabilitation process to come, the emotional ups and downs, the time commitment, the expense, and the hard work that goes into successful rehabilita-tion. The thoughts of going through the process again with no real expectation of a permanent solution is indeed frustrating.

Reaction to Rehabilitation of Chronic Injury

The primary reactions to rehabilitation of a chronic injury are dependence and indepen-dence. These reactions are manifested by ath-letes reacting to the rehabilitation process as if they have no control or as if they have complete control. The stance is either reactive or proac-tive and is seen in the patient's either not taking control or responsibility for getting better or assuming total control over the rehabilitation process.

There is very little middle ground for these patients in the treatment protocol: they either try everything new or they are unwilling to try anything new. They either question every treat-ment the athletic trainer recommends or accept every treatment the athletic trainer recom-mends. Patients might swing from one end of the spectrum to the other, depending on factors such as how well the last rehabilitation worked, how fast the last rehabilitation moved, how well they liked the last athletic trainer, where they are in their season, and any other situation they perceive as warranting a change.

Dependent patients don't take part in the decisions of rehabilitation, they don't give their input concerning what did, or didn't, work before and they often leave all decisions up to the athletic trainer or team physician. Often these patients become dependent on the athletic trainer and relinquish all power regarding rehabilitation decisions. These patients want someone else to be responsible for their welfare and to meet their every need at their whim and command. They demand that more time be spent on them. Failure of one athletic trainer to meet their demands results in their selecting an athletic trainer who will meet their demands. Athletic trainers with the greatest need to help others will be easily taken advantage of, at the sacrifice of time needed for other patients.

The independent reaction is just the opposite. These patients want to call all the shots and are up-to-date on the latest fads. They are likely to change the treatment plan—or the athletic trainer—if progress is not as fast or as productive as they expect or want. They have a strong urge to find the perfect treatment by trying new techniques, changing physicians and athletic trainers, or shopping around for any solution that might work better and faster. The athletic trainer must not take this personally. It is important to accept that shopping around is not a rejection of the athletic trainer but a reaction to the chronic injury rehabilitation.

The secondary reaction to chronic injury rehabilitation is apprehension. Patients with chronic injuries know that although they might get through this flare-up, there is a strong possibility that the injury will return, for in fact it never completely heals. They approach rehabilitation with trepidation, not knowing what will work this time and what will last. They tend to feel stress over every sign and symptom that the rehabilitation is not going as well or as rapidly as expected. Dependent patients react to this apprehension by being overcompliant, thinking that they just need to work harder at what the athletic trainer suggests. Independent patients, reacting to apprehension, tend to make more changes if rehabilitation is not going well—trying new and different things, looking for the perfect treatment.

> **Clinical Decision-Making Exercise 4-4**
>
> Christine is a 15-year-old Junior Level diver who has been competing since she was 9 years old. She has had chronic back pain and muscle spasms for 3 months. For several weeks she has been making irrational complaints: "No divers I know have ever been able to dive once back pain starts." "Rehabilitation never works for back pain." How can the athletic trainer help Christine change her opinion?

Interventions for Chronic Injury

If patients become dependent and they no longer receive the special attention they feel they deserve, they often lash out in anger or frustration. The athletic trainer needs to head off this response by firmly explaining the restrictions on time and what is required of the patient in terms of rehabilitation. This response should be pointed out to the patient as inappropriate, and it should be examined by the athletic trainer and the patient if it becomes a continual problem, because it is only a detriment to recovery. At this time the patient is encouraged to transfer the time and energy formerly given to the sport into the rehabilitation process. The patient has to become an active, not a passive, participant. The injury is now the competitor, rather than next week's opponent. Care should be taken to prevent the patient from becoming a dependent patient.

To be more proactive rather than reactive, the dependent patient is encouraged to take part in the rehabilitation. This does not mean that the patient assumes the role of the athletic trainer, but it does mean that they work as a team. This is where the trust and respect between the athletic trainer and the patient is of paramount importance. It is a two-way street where the athletic trainer provides the expertise concerning the injury and the patient has the expertise concerning his or her body.

The independent patient is encouraged to develop a relationship with the athletic trainer that is one of respect and trust. At this point the athletic trainer can facilitate this trust by being current with the latest literature on the patient's particular injury. Knowledge of the injury, its healing mechanism, and the rehabilitation progression gives patients an orderly timetable within which to proceed. It will help if the athletic trainer and the patient have a plan that is mutually acceptable. The athletic trainer can make an effort to be particularly flexible when working with these patients; this will go a long way in strengthening the relationship of trust and respect so necessary to a smooth rehabilitation.

All patients are participants in the rehabilitation process, but they must be active participants and become engaged in the process. Patients have to be encouraged and believe in future success. All efforts should point toward a positive result, with the patients working with what is available and not with wishful thinking.

Reaction to Chronic Injury Recovery

Recovery from chronic injury is in some ways a misnomer, because the very nature of the injury assumes it will recur if the athlete continues to play. The single level reaction is two-fold—either skeptical or confident.

The skeptical reaction is not necessarily a negative reaction but one born of multiple experiences with rehabilitation. Skeptical patients are realistic in their options and have usually made peace with the nature of a chronic injury. This is not to say defeat is accepted, but that reality is acknowledged. They have not given up hope, but the hope is tempered with acceptance of factors that they have no power to control. These patients rehabilitate to the best of their ability but accept that some things are not within their control.

The confident reaction to recovery from chronic injury is not necessarily an unrealistic or unenlightened reaction regarding the course of this injury. These patients have an unyielding faith that is untarnished by repeated experiences with recurrence of a chronic injury. Often confidence is more global for these patients and is not necessarily an injury-specific reaction. This may be a personality trait and is not tied into the injury or lack of participation in their sport. Identity for these patients is not contingent upon sport. This does not mean these patients do not care, but just that they do not

allow the injury to design and mandate their disposition or to define and outline their life.

It is unclear whether one reaction comes before the other. It can be assumed that patients are not relegated to one or the other reaction but can move between the two. The mitigating factors for moving between the two could be maturity, experience with rehabilitation, length of time playing a sport, the particular time in the season, or the meaning of the sport to the patient.

DEALING WITH A CAREER-ENDING INJURY

One of the hardest adjustments an athlete has to make is when to end participation in a sport. It does appear to matter if this is an abrupt ending (injury, illness, cut from team) or one with some advance warning (retirement, age, ability).[18] For the athlete whose career ends unexpectedly, there is a feeling of not being able to complete goals due to unexpected termination.[48] The athletes who ended careers voluntarily, who chose the time to leave, and who had played the sport longer had a smoother transition.

Injuries that fall into this category include spinal cord injuries, extensive hardware implants (screws, plates, etc), multiple surgeries with declining benefits, and persistent debilitating or incapacitating illness.

Reaction to a Career-Ending Injury

Isolation is the primary reaction to termination of sport and is dependent upon the athlete's perception of the importance of participation. Many athletes have spent years as part of a team that has offered a well-defined and meaningful activity. The very nature of sport is one of exact boundaries (rules of play, precise beginnings and endings, codes of conduct, etc), and the athletes in turn have defined roles within these boundaries (position played, rankings, roles within the team structure, etc). At the time of termination, the disruption of a significant attachment affiliation, coupled with a large time commitment and expansion of injury, all set up these athletes for the debilitating effects of depression.[18]

The secondary reaction is that these athletes must go through a process of grief—grieving for a loss of not only a career, but an identity, an extended family, a place in society where they know the rules and can play the game. Sport for the athlete is a community, where they are productive members, where they excel, where they feel accepted, and where they feel they belong. These athletes grieve for what they no longer have: their place in the group, their place in society, their identity as an athlete, their job or career, their place of comfort, their sense of belonging.

The grief process is an adjustment period, and the form it takes and how long it lasts depend on the individual's personality and the importance the sport had in forming that personality. There are many theories of the process of grief. A good review can be found in Baillie and Danish[4] or Evans and Hardy.[19] The grief process is a sequential progression: the grief process must take place before acceptance, the acceptance process must take place before career change, and the career change attempts to fill the void created after the end of the dream of competition.

Reaction to Rehabilitation for a Career-Ending Injury

Loss of athletic identity is the primary reaction to rehabilitation of an injury that terminates participation in a sport. It is a feeling of "Who am I? Where do I belong? What is my purpose, my reason for being?" The rehabilitation involves the psychological adjustment to the loss of self. Baillie and Danish[4] suggest that athletes have taken anywhere from 2 to 10 years to adjust to termination from sport.

The injured athlete enters physical rehabilitation halfheartedly, if at all. The patient often says, "Who cares?" "What does it matter?" "Who will know?" in response to setting a rehabilitation plan. These patients might go through the motions of rehabilitation, but the inner spark to get back to competition is missing. At this point the athletic trainer must decide whether the patient needs to be referred to a counselor or sport psychologist. The criterion for referral

is usually an established protocol and consists of determining whether the patient is able to maintain a sense of control and engaging in activities while emotionally working through the grief process.

Intervention in a Career-Ending Injury

Interventions for career-ending injuries are decided on an individual basis. Intervention can have the nature of psychological counseling (stress management, alcohol or drug counseling, etc.), career counseling (school enrollment, job placement, etc.), financial planning (investments, tax shelters, etc.), or whatever the patient needs. Adjustment to termination is better for athletes who had participated longer, were aware of chronic injuries, knew of the possibility of being cut, or had planned on retiring from the team. Poor adjustment is associated with sudden unexpected injury that occurs in the prime of the career and results in a forced retirement.[4]

Reaction to Recovery from a Career-Ending Injury

The primary reaction to recovery from a terminating injury is to see it as both an ending and beginning. Closure and renewal are intertwined, with closure being necessary to give full energy to renewal. Once they reach the acceptance stage, these athletes can put closure on a career that has ended and focus their other talents, long overshadowed by athletic prowess, toward a new career. This might be either in the field of athletics (coaching, announcer, sponsor, etc.) or in a totally unrelated field. Baillie and Danish[4] found that Olympic athletes and college athletes were better prepared and made a better adjustment to new careers than did older professional athletes. The reason for this might be better education, more choices of careers, more assistance in career planning—in other words, more options. Many athletes make a satisfactory adjustment to termination from sport when it is in their time frame and of their choosing, but termination forced by an unexpected event such as injury is received with less than enthusiasm.

COMPLIANCE AND ADHERENCE TO REHABILITATION

Compliance to athletic injury rehabilitation programs is abysmal, considering the purpose of rehabilitation.[10,25,43] The goal of athletic rehabilitation is to return the patient to the level of performance present prior to injury. The primary treatment is exercise to retrain the muscles that have been damaged due to injury. The psychological ramification of unsuccessful rehabilitation is that the patient tends to focus on the injury, resulting in guarding or muscle tension and/or lack of attentional focus, setting up the scenario for reinjury. In the following we discuss, first, definitions of compliance and adherence; second, incidents of compliance in other fields; third, measures of compliance; fourth, deterrents to compliance; and fifth, incentives to increase compliance.

Compliance and Adherence Defined

According to Meichenbaum and Turk,[52] *compliance* is a term from the medical profession and means obedience of the patient to the physician's or health care giver's instruction. The concept of compliance is more passive than active, and carries the connotation that if patients are noncompliant, they are at fault. This assigns an authoritative position to the caregiver. The implication is, "I tell you what to do, and you do it." The concept of compliance mainly applies to immediate short-term treatment that has been prescribed for a patient. *Adherence* is a term from the exercise discipline and carries the meaning of active voluntary choice, a mutuality in treatment planning. Adherence involves long-term change on a more voluntary basis and suggests

a behavioral change sought by the participant. Usually when *adherence* is the term used, it carries the implication that the service was sought out as opposed to being prescribed—for instance, when people seek an exercise program or a weight-loss program, instead of being ordered by the physician to enroll in one. These are usually long-term commitments.

For the purpose of this discussion about rehabilitation, the term compliance will be used, but either is acceptable. The term *compliance* has been chosen because there are certain guidelines for treatments that produce the desired result of rehabilitation of an injury. The patient needs to comply with a certain regimen for the short term to facilitate healing, then adhere to a program of exercise to decrease the risk of reinjury. In rehabilitation, a "comply now, adhere later" approach is the best descriptor for successful return to the previous level of fitness.

Incidences of Compliance in Other Disciplines

In the field of athletic injury, compliance is the biggest deterrent to successful rehabilitation.[43] The fields of medicine and exercise fare no better. In medicine, compliance is roughly 50%, with the rule of thumb being that one-third always comply, one-third sometimes comply, and one-third never comply.[52] In a study of glaucoma (high intraocular fluid pressure), patients were told that if they didn't use drops three times a day, they would go blind. Only 42% complied with treatment recommended by the physician. Several weeks later at revisit, they were told they were in danger of losing sight in one eye if they did not comply with treatment. Compliance only increased by 16%, according to Vincent.[73] In other words, only 58% were compliant when the likely result of being noncompliant was to go blind in one eye!

The exercise literature[43] shows similar findings: There is a 30% to 70% dropout rate in the first 3 months of exercise programs. Sixty-six percent of Americans do not exercise on a regular basis; 44% do not exercise at all.[43] Self-improvement programs do not fare any better. The dropout rate for obesity, smoking, and stress management programs is 20% to

80%. Only 16% to 59% of people wear seat belts. There is limited literature on the compliance rate for athletes. Before all hope is lost, it should be understood that maybe 100% compliance is not necessary to achieve total rehabilitation. In medicine it was found that less than 100% compliance was adequate to bring about desired results.[52] It is important to keep in mind that we are looking at a range, not an absolute. Is the athlete who gets back to pre-injury standards without doing 100% of treatments noncompliant? They are only if 100% compliance is considered to be the gold standard.

Measurements of Compliance

How compliance is measured might be an indicator of the problem. In medicine and exercise, compliance is usually measured in one of three ways: self-report, attendance, and therapeutic outcome.[73] Self-report consists of just asking whether the person has been compliant, through either a structured questionnaire, self-monitoring with record keeping, or corroboration (someone else keeps track). These methods can be inaccurate due to poor memory, trying to please the investigator, or channeling the behavior to please the investigator.

Keeping track of attendance is the most common and most direct method. The problem with attendance is that it doesn't say what was done, it just indicates that the patients showed up. The patients could be doing exercises somewhere else, or forget to sign in, or sign in and then leave without exercising, or do only a portion of the prescribed rehabilitation exercises. Therapeutic outcome is not completely reliable, as it can be confounded by other factors. In a weight-loss program the athlete could be gaining muscle weight but losing fat weight, could lose weight due to exercising but not due to recommended changes in eating habits, or could lose weight because of illness without exercising or change in eating habits.

To start at the beginning of measuring compliance, the Hedgpeth/Gansneder Athletic Rehabilitation Indicators[32] were designed to determine what treatments were used, and what percentage of the time they were used, in a Division I university. The basic areas assessed are aerobic conditioning, strength conditioning, balance, modalities, and long-term strategies (bracing, taping, protective equipment). Athletes are asked what percentage of the time the treatment was done. A range of compliance is measured, with 0% to 10% being the lowest compliance, and 91% to 100% being the highest compliance. A category of N/A was included to indicate that the athletic trainer had not suggested the treatment. At the same time, athletic trainers were asked to complete the indicator. Preliminary reports suggest an 87% reliability rate for the indicator. Until such a time as what is being done in the athletic training room setting is determined, it is premature to discuss why it is or is not being done.

Factors Influencing Compliance

Shank[66] found that patients who are committed to the rehabilitation program work harder and thus return to competition more quickly with better results than those who are nonadherents. Their pain tolerance is greater and of less concern, and they are more self-motivated, as opposed to the apathy of the nonadherents.

Also, support from peers, coaches, and rehabilitation staff is important in influencing compliance.[7] Patients with support show a greater effort to fit the rehabilitation effort into their schedules. They are more likely to keep commitments to those who support them. Patients who are nonadherents respond better to support and motivation from their support group than do the adherents. Thus extra encouragement from this support group for the nonadherent patients can really pay dividends in getting them motivated to successfully complete their rehabilitation.

Attitude is another important consideration when dealing with injured patients. If the athletic trainer expects the patient to be nonadherent, this can create the self-fulfilling prophecy.[76] If the athletic trainer feels the patient is going to be nonadherent, then it is less likely that the athletic trainer will work to motivate the patient to comply with the treatment program. Webborn et al[76] suggest that if instructions are written down—even in the face of the patient's denial of the need for written instruction—the more likely it is that the patient will follow through with the treatment plan. Athletic trainers have an impact on compliance

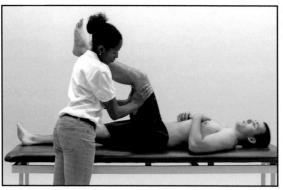

Figure 4-10. A supportive environment and a belief in the effectiveness of the treatment improves compliance.

through enhancing the patient's belief in the efficacy of the treatment as well as providing a supportive environment (Figure 4-10).[52]

Injured athletes are expected to report for rehabilitation, but the coach is the disciplinarian, not the athletic trainer, and the coach institutes punishment for lack of participation in the rehabilitation process. The coach must support the rehabilitation concept. Patients soon know if rehabilitation is not a priority with the coach and begin to lose interest if they are not highly motivated to return to competition.

The real challenge of rehabilitation is how to motivate patients to do their best in the rehabilitation process. Patients who are not reporting for rehabilitation have a reason. Everything is done for some need. The rehabilitation program must be established within these needs. If patients are not reporting for rehabilitation, either something is more important to them than a hastened recovery, or they have not had the importance of the process adequately explained to them. Reexamine the program and the patient's goals. If the program has not been well explained and the patient is not committed to the program, the program either is doomed to failure or will be less than successful. Motivation must come from within, but the athletic trainer can provide the encouragement and positive reinforcement necessary for the patient to make a commitment.

Lack of commitment might indicate frustration, boredom, or feelings of a lack of progress. In this case, further explanations or changes in routine are necessary. The patient might need the opportunity to comment on the program and make a commitment to the rehabilitation before being structured into a strict regimen of

rehabilitative procedures. The athletic trainer should keep in mind that patients may have many activities in their daily schedules, and fitting the rehabilitation to their schedules rather than the reverse can also encourage compliance. The more the patient is allowed input and flexibility, the more successful the compliance will be.

Another aspect of compliance has to do with patients' perception of their ability. Patients who perceive themselves as continuing on to a more advanced level of competition tend to shirk rehabilitation. They usually are the better athletes. They do not have to work as hard as, but perform better than, their peers, so they assume the same attitude about rehabilitation. With this attitude, these good athletes never become truly great athletes because of their lack of commitment to their sport. Once they have risen to the top level where most athletes have the same skills, the work habit is not there to put them in the top of the elite athletic group.

Other factors of compliance for athletes are the length of time at a particular school, semester grade-point average, perception of class load, career goals, amount of participation time in contests, perception of time available for treatments, and previous experience with rehabilitation programs. The more formal education a person has, the higher the level of compliance to treatments; the higher the semester grade-point average, the higher the treatment compliance. Interestingly enough, an inverse relationship exists between athletes' perception of difficulty of their class load and compliance. Often athletes do better academically during the season than at other times, possibly because they budget their time with better discipline during the season, and this approach carries over into the rehabilitation setting. Athletes who have better-defined career goals and those who have the greatest amount of participation time have higher levels of compliance, as do those who perceive they have a greater amount of time available for treatments and those who have previous experience with rehabilitation programs.

PAIN AS A DETERRENT TO COMPLIANCE

Almost all rehabilitation should be pain-free, and what is not is usually detrimental to the return to competition. Painful exercise, therefore, is not only harmful but also reduces compliance, especially in the nonadherent athlete.[19] Rehabilitation programs should be examined to determine the aspects that may be painful.

Pain is subjective, and the caregivers must assume that the pain is as severe or persistent as the athlete says it is. Although the symptoms of pain must be treated to ensure compliance, the cause needs to be addressed.[69] In general, it is more productive in the long run for the athletic trainer to determine the cause of pain than to treat the symptoms and disregard the cause. For instance, if swelling is the cause of the pain, then treatment to reduce the swelling is of a more lasting benefit than treating the pain and disregarding or masking the underlying cause of the pain. Pain that persists and does not respond to adjustments in the rehabilitation process (eg, decreases in the amount of weights, number of sets, or number of repetitions) should be reevaluated by the athletic trainer or team physician.

Athletes often say, "You can play hurt, you can't play injured." But the difference is in what pain means to the athlete. There is the pain of performance, the pain of training, the pain of rehabilitation, the pain of acute injury, and the chronic pain of overuse. Pain can be assessed across intensity (0 = none to 10 = worst) and quality (burning, aching, stabbing, stinging, etc.), but pain is subjective. Factors affecting pain can be culture,[47] type (contact vs noncontact) of sport,[16] and individual vs team sport.[46]

One technique for pain management that is frequently used and easy to apply is dissociation.[71] Dissociation involves thinking about something other than the pain, such as a favorite location, a mountain cabin with the smell of fresh crisp air and the magnificent view of mountains, or a beach cottage with the feel and smell of the salty breeze and the calming rhythmic sound of the surf. Any activity that engages the mind can be used.[20] The athlete could visualize playing a round of golf from tee to green, playing a football game from kickoff to the final whistle, or playing a final NCAA basketball game from tip-off until the buzzer.

Goal Setting as a Motivator to Compliance

Goal setting in and of itself has been shown to be an effective motivator for compliance to rehabilitation of an athletic injury[3,65] as well as reaching goals in a general sport setting.[11] Athletes have been setting goals since they started competing, usually from an early age. They set goals to run faster, jump higher, shoot straighter, throw longer, hit harder, and so on. These goals have all had one thing in common, and that is that they were not achieved with one burst of effort but came as the result of many short-term goals having been met prior to the achievement of the long-term goal.

For a comprehensive explanation on goal setting in general, see Locke,[44] or for goal setting specifically in sport, see Locke and Lathan.[45] Heil[33] suggests nine guides for goal setting: it should be specific and measurable; use positive rather than negative language; be challenging but realistic; have a timetable; integrate short-, medium-, and long-term goals; link outcome to process; involve internalized goals; and involve monitoring and evaluating goals and sport goals linked to life goals.

In athletic rehabilitation, patients need to know exactly what the goal is and have a sense that it can be met. This could be accomplished by, for instance, telling a patient that by a certain day he or she should be partial weight bearing with crutches. However, this is neither specific nor measurable. It is more effective to say that by achieving a certain range of motion and strength level, the foot can be placed on the

Weeks 1–3	Set a goal to use relaxation techniques or abdominal breathing before and after treatments. This will lessen the fear that can make pain more intense or more evident when going from knee extension to weight bearing to balance exercises.
Weeks 4–7	This block of time can be monotonous and frustrating. Athletes should set goals to use imagery to see themselves using these movements in their sport. The imagery will be an effective motivator to continue rehabilitation.
Weeks 8–11	The goal for this block of time is to use dissociation to handle the pain that accompanies the increased use of muscles when jogging, rope jumping, and stair running.
Weeks 12–15	Goals at this level should be more reality checks, such as "I am closer to returning to play" or "I can see the light at the end of the tunnel."
Week 15 to return to play	Goals here are to remain positive and to use positive affirmations, such as "I am almost there—each day I am getting stronger and more ready to play."

Figure 4-11. Progress goals for rehabilitation.

ground with weight bearing. The measurement of success is that the partial weight bearing is to be without pain. The goal must be a challenge, but one that the patient can reach with reasonable rehabilitation effort. Goals that are easily reached have no reward in success. Goals must be personal and internally satisfying, not imposed on the athlete by the coach or athletic trainer. The setting of goals needs to be a joint venture between the athlete and the athletic trainer to be successful.[15] The patient has to take responsibility for the progress of the injury and be responsible for doing the necessary rehabilitation.

Goal setting incorporates a multitude of other motivating factors that intuitively appear to increase the odds of compliance by reducing the stress associated with injury rehabilitation. These buffers incorporated within the goal setting paradigm include positive reinforcement when goals are met, time management for incorporating goals into a lifestyle, a feeling of social support when goals are set with the athletic trainer, the feelings of increased self-efficacy when goals are achieved, etc. Goals should be easily understood by the patient, be concrete, be active events, and be a natural part of their sport that requires no additional time commitment.[27] Goals can be daily for a sense of accomplishment, weekly for a sense of progress, and monthly or yearly for long-term achievement (Figure 4-11).

Clinical Decision-Making Exercise 4-6

George is a second-year Division I goalie on the soccer team. He tore his ACL in the first game of the season, had surgery, and is now starting rehabilitation. He is frustrated with the projected length of rehabilitation and is overwhelmed with thoughts of not being able to return to his previous level of play. What should the athletic trainer do to help George establish attainable goals for his rehabilitation program?

RETURN TO COMPETITION

The saying "You have to play with pain" has been interpreted more literally to mean that the athlete has to play through an injury. The difference is that some injuries may be mild and only somewhat painful, resulting in no reinjury in competition, whereas a more severe injury is made worse by continuing to compete. The competitive athlete might be more "body aware" than the general public and therefore more apt to respond to injury with the use of protection, rest, ice, compression, and elevation (PRICE) to promote healing. The general public, on the other hand, is more likely to respond to the pain of injury rather than the healing process.[40] Therefore the athlete might want to return to competition in spite of pain, whereas the nonathlete wants the pain to be treated before engaging in any activity. The importance of an athletic trainer for making the decision of when it is safe to compete and when reinjury is a possibility is obvious.

Unfortunately, untrained personnel, such as fellow teammates, parents, and coaches, assume this responsibility when no athletic trainer is present or when the athletic trainer is easily intimidated by the coach and not backed up by the athletic director and sports medicine physician. Either situation results in poor medical care and leaves the management vulnerable to legal action as a result of negligence. Courts expect competent medical care to be provided to the athletes. That care can be provided only by a qualified athletic trainer or a sports medicine physician.

Coaches tend to return players on the basis of status and game situation, whereas athletic trainers' decisions are determined by the player's injury.[38] Players who feel that a missed practice or a game will relegate them to the bench for the year, or those who have been encouraged to play no matter what, are candidates for injury and reinjury. Usually what happens, however, is that they are performing poorly because they are not at full strength, thus they only reinforce the coach's decision to play someone else. The role of the athletic trainer is to determine when the player is functioning at optimal physical fitness without risk of injury or reinjury and to keep the coach abreast of the player's status.[29] It is important that the athlete have a clear perception of the injury and its limitations.[8] An important role of the athletic trainer is to inform the athlete of the difference between pain and injury.

The athlete who continues to play with an unhealed or poorly rehabilitated injury is constantly reducing her or his chances for a healthy life of physical activity. The athlete has to live past the few years of competition. Most athletes, however, have difficulty seeing past the present season, or at best have the goal of participating in their sport until they can no longer compete, regardless of the consequences. The rewards of competition and the admiration of others take sports out of perspective and retard a healthy attitude toward sports. The athlete's attitude is "Give it up for the sport" and "I'm invincible." Lack of this attitude is viewed by some as weakness or not being a team player. Athletes with this attitude have difficulty adjusting to injury, especially a career-ending one.

Neglecting injured athletes or giving them the perception that they are "outcasts" also can contribute to injury and reinjury. Coaches who foster this attitude are saying to the players that they have no worth if they are injured. Some coaches go so far as to prevent team contact with injured players until they are ready to return, or to belittle them in front of their peers, believing that this will make the athlete want to get back to competition quicker. This tactic might work with some players with minor injuries, but it only causes major adjustment difficulties for athletes who suffer severe injury.

Some coaches refuse to talk to the injured athlete, or tell others that the athlete really doesn't want to play or isn't tough enough. The coach and athlete are experiencing frustration with the injury. Counseling the coach in this situation to point out the effects of such attitudes may be helpful. Unfortunately, these coaches are not in the minority. During this period, either the sports medicine team shows its concern for the athlete and in return wins the athlete's loyalty and dedication down the road, or they undermine the athlete's trust and set up a future situation to be let down when the athlete gets in the position of controlling the outcome of a contest—the athlete might underperform out of spite.

Commitment is a two-way street. The athletic trainer has to show their commitment to the athlete to receive commitment from the athlete. By the same token the athletic trainer must not become the power broker and in essence say, "He can't play because I say so." Showing the coach that the athlete who usually has 4.5 speed can presently run only a 5.0 illustrates to the coach that the athlete is not ready for competition. It will also illustrate to the athlete that more time and effort are necessary to get ready to return.

INTERPERSONAL RELATIONSHIP BETWEEN THE ATHLETE AND ATHLETIC TRAINER

Even though athletic trainers need to be proficient in counseling in the areas of injury prevention, injury rehabilitation, and nutrition, they are not usually academically trained for other areas. To meet other counseling needs of the athlete, the athletic trainer needs additional academic preparation or should refer the athlete to a sport psychologist.[13,62]

The athletic trainer is often the first person athletes interact with after injury and the one who will direct the recovery. As a result, the athletic trainer has to deal with the athlete as a person and not as just an injury. When an injured athlete enters the treatment setting, he or she should get the perception that the athletic trainer cares for him or her as a person and not just as part of the job. His or her perception of the athletic trainer makes a difference in terms of recovery time and effort. First they have to respect the athletic trainer as a person before they can trust the athletic trainer in the rehabilitative setting. Successful communication between the athletic trainer and the patient is essential for effective rehabilitation. Taking an interest in athletes before injuries have occurred enables the athletic trainer to know the athletes' personalities and be able to work with them in helping to build their confidence.[22]

Active listening is one of the athletic trainer's most important skills. One must learn to listen to the patient beyond the complaining. The athletic trainer should listen for fear, anger, depression, or anxiety in the patient and in his or her voice. With fear, the patient might be wondering what the pain means in terms of function and whether she or he will be accepted by peers. Anger is often a feeling of being victimized by the injury and the unfairness of it. A depressed patient will have an overwhelming feeling of hopelessness or loneliness. Patients who feel anxiety wonder how they can survive the injury and what will happen if they cannot return to full competition.[24]

Body language is important as well. The athletic trainer who continues to work on paperwork while talking to the patient is sending a message of not caring. The athletic trainer needs to be concerned, and look the patient in the eye with a genuine interest in his or her problems. This will go a long way toward gaining confidence and respect. It is important for the athletic trainer to consider the patient as an individual instead of the "sprained ankle." If the injury is the only consideration, the patient becomes just an injury and not a person. As a result the attitude projected to the patient is just that, thus the athletic trainer is perceived as caring for the patient only superficially.

The relationship between the athletic trainer and the patient should be one of person to person and not of a coach to a player or one of a judgmental nature. When the patient is treated as an equal, the relationship is improved, and it helps the patient accept responsibility for his or her own rehabilitation. With injury, athletes lose control over their physical efforts. They have gone from 4 or 5 hours a day of practice or competition to no activity. They are in a temporary lifestyle change. Their feelings are going to affect the success or failure of the rehabilitation process. The athletic trainer must establish rapport and a sense of genuine concern and caring for the patient, who is not fooled by superficiality.

During an injury evaluation, the athletic trainer should allow the patient to provide as much input about her or his injury as possible. Paraphrasing or restating the information to the patient will be invaluable to the athletic trainer who is unsure of the mechanism of injury or its results. Statements such as "I see" or "Go ahead" or simple silence to allow athletes to fully express themselves are of value. One of the most important bits of information can be the question posed at the end of gathering subjective information: "What else have I not asked you or do I need to know about this injury?" Then give the patient input into the decision of where to go from here.

The athletic trainer is often the person who effectively explains the injury to the patient. Care should be taken to explain the situation to the patient in understandable terms. In most cases the simplest explanation acceptable to the patient is the best. With mild and moderate injuries, the use of the term *sprain*, *strain*, or *bruise* suffices. The example of a sprained knee and torn ligaments of the knee can be descriptions of the same grade II injury, but the patient might interpret the two terms altogether differently and react in a totally different way to the explanation.

Patients must have injuries explained to them to their satisfaction. Disseminating injury information appropriate to the patient's emotional and intellectual level can be a real challenge. The rate and degree of acceptance is not the same with all patients. Severity of injury is certainly important, but the patient's perception of that severity is what matters in the rehabilitation process.[8] Thus the physiological must be interrelated with the psychological. In working with patients, the athletic trainer should be not only empathetic but also nonjudgmental.

The addition of a sport psychologist to the rehabilitation team can facilitate the athlete's transition from the sport culture into the rehabilitation culture.[30] Each culture has specific rules as well as defined roles that the members of that culture must follow. An understanding of the different rules and roles can assist the athlete's transition after the injury from the sport culture to the rehabilitation culture. The role of the sport psychologist is to understand the impact this transition has on the athlete who is injured and has to assimilate into a totally new environment, follow new rules, and assume a new role. For example, the concept of pain in the football culture is entirely different from the concept of pain in the rehabilitation culture. In the football culture, "Suck it up" and "Play through the pain" are the norm. In the rehabilitation culture, pain can be an indication that needs to be evaluated. The athlete and athletic trainer need to reevaluate the rehabilitation exercises or activity level, decrease the amount of repetitions, change the type of exercise, or consult with the team physician. If the pain is something the athlete must assimilate into his or her lifestyle, then the sport psychologist can teach the athlete how to deal with it. This can be done through pain management (dissociation) or pain perceptions (pain vs soreness).

The amount of stress associated with playing a sport, and the meaning the sport has to the patient, can impact the patient's compliance with rehabilitation.[2] The patient has a more successful rehabilitation when engaged fully in the activity of rehabilitation, much as the athlete will have a more successful sport career when more interested and involved in the sport. Stress can be a deterrent to engaging in rehabilitation. Several techniques the sport psychologist can use (relaxation, imagery, cognitive restructuring, thought stopping) can lessen the stressful reaction to injury. Often a change in the patient's perception of the injury and rehabilitation can affect outcome. Systematic rationalization[75] can facilitate changing the patient's reaction to injury and rehabilitation through changing how the athlete perceives events.

Returning to competition is another area where the sport psychologist can help the injured athlete. Often individuals perceive themselves as ready to return but not being allowed to, or as being forced to return before ready. The sport psychologist can assist the patient to make a decision based on the facts and not clouded by emotions.

The addition of a sport psychologist to the sports medicine team can be an effective link when athletes are unable or unwilling to continue to participate in their sport. Frequently an athlete's identity is intertwined with the sport played. The transition into a completely different culture can be a traumatic experience. It is stressful to enter a culture and not know one's place or identity in that culture. To not know what the game is and what the rules are is frustrating for the injured athlete.

The treatment of athletic injury and rehabilitation involves more than the physical, emotional, and psychological aspects of the individual. The impact of the environment, the support of the athletic community, and the culture in which the athlete resides at the time of injury combine to influence the course the athlete takes from injury, through rehabilitation, to return to competition. Treating the athlete's physical injury and attending to the extraneous factors influencing the injured athlete are the challenges facing the sports medicine team.

Summary

1. There are no absolutes when it comes to how an athlete will react to an injury. However, there are some guidelines for progressive reactions to injury based on length of rehabilitation. These guidelines allow the athletic trainer to conceptualize individual stress reactions to injury and to

implement psychological interventions to facilitate successful rehabilitation.

2. The athlete must take responsibility for rehabilitating his or her injury, but the interpersonal relationship between the athlete and the sports medicine team can promote a positive adjustment to the rehabilitation process.

3. The use of psychological techniques such as dissociation for pain management, the use of buffers for stress reduction, and goal setting for motivation can assist the athlete in taking control of and managing her or his successful rehabilitation.

4. The key to successful rehabilitation is compliance. Advances in the field of medicine have allowed injuries that 10 years ago would have ended an athlete's career to now be successfully repaired. Without compliance to the rehabilitation process, these medical advances are moot.

References

1. Albinson, C., Petrie T. 2003. Cognitive appraisals, stress, and coping: Preinjury and postinjury factors influencing psychological adjustment to sport injury, *J Sport Rehabil, 12*(4):306.

2. Anderson, M., Williams, J. 2007. A model of stress and athletic injury: Prediction and prevention. In D. Smith (Ed.), *Essential Readings in Sport and Exercise Psychology*. Champaign, IL: Human Kinetics.

3. Arvinen-Barrow, M. 2013. Goal setting in sport injury rehabilitation. In M. Arvinen-Barrow, *The Psychology of Sport Injury Rehabilitation*. New York, Routledge.

4. Baillie, P. H. F., Danish, S. J. 1992. Understanding the career transition of athletes. *Sport Psychologist* 6:77–98.

5. Baum, A. 2005. Suicide in athletes: A review and commentary. *Clinics in Sports Medicine* 24(4):853–69.

6. Benson, H. 1976. *The Relaxation Response*. New York: Morrow.

7. Bianco, T. 2001. Social support and recovery from sport injury: Elite skiers share their experiences. *Research Quarterly for Exercise and Sport, 72*(4): 376–88.

8. Bone, J., Fry, M. 2006. The influence of injured athletes' perceptions of social support from ATCs on their beliefs about rehabilitation. *J Sport Rehabil* 15(2):156.

9. Bramwell, S. T., Masuda, M., Wagnor, N. N., Holmes, T. H. 1975. Psychosocial factors in athletic injuries: Development and application of the social and athletic readjustment rating scale. *Journal of Human Stress*, 1:6-20.

10. Brewer, B. 2010. Adherence to sport injury rehabilitation. In M. Andersen (Ed.), *Routledge handbook of applied sport psychology*; New York: Taylor & Francis.

11. Brinkman, R. 2010. The motivational climate in the rehabilitation setting. *Athletic Therapy Today,* 15(2):44–46.

12. Coote, D., Tenenbaum, G. 1998. Can emotive imagery aid in tolerating exertion efficiently? *J Sports Med Phys Fitness, 38*(4):344.

13. Cramer Roh, J., Perna, F. 2000. Psychology/counseling: A universal competency in athletic training. *Journal of Athletic Training, 35*(4): 458–65.

14. Cupal, D., Brewer, B. 2001. Effects of relaxation and guided imagery on knee strength, reinjury anxiety and pain following anterior cruciate ligament reconstruction. *Rehabilitation Psychology,* 46:28–43.

15. DePalma, M. T., and DePalma, B. 1989. The use of instruction and the behavioral approach to facilitate injury rehabilitation. *Athletic Training,* 24:217–19.

16. Deroche, T., Woodman, T. 2011. Athlete's inclination to play through pain: a coping perspective. *Anxiety, Stress & Coping: An International Journal,* 24(5):579-587.

17. Driediger, M. 2007. Imagery use by injured athletes: A qualitative analysis. *Journal of Sport Sciences,* 24(3):261–72.

18. Ermler, K. L., Thomas, C. E. 1990. Interventions for the alienating effects of injury. *Athletic Training* 25:269–71.

19. Evans, L., and Hardy, L. 1995. Sport injury and grief response: A review. *Journal of Sport and Exercise Psychology,* 17:227–45.

20. Fordyce, W. E. 1988. Pain and suffering: A reappraisal. *American Psychologist,* 43:276–83.

21. Finch, C., Cassell, E. 2006. The public health impact of injury during sport and active recreation. *Journal of Science and Medicine in Sport,* 9(6):490-497.

22. Ford, I., Gordon S. 1998. Guidelines for using sport psychology in rehabilitation. *Athletic Therapy Today,* 3(2):41.

23. Galambos, S. 2005. Psychological predictors of injury among elite athletes. *British Journal of Sports Medicine,* 39(6):351-354.

24. Glazer, D. 2009. Development and preliminary validation of the injury-psychological readiness to return to sport (I-PRRS) scale. *J Athl Train,* 44(2):185–89.

25. Grove, J., Stewart, R. 1990. Emotional reactions of athletes to knee rehabilitation. Paper presented at the annual meeting of Australian Sports Medicine Federation (abstract).

26. Gunnoe, A., Horodyski, M., Tennant, K. 2001. The effect of life events on incidence of injury in high school football players. *J Athl Train, 36*(2):150,

27. Hamson-Utley, J. 2008. Athletic trainers' and physical therapists' perceptions of the effectiveness of psychological skills within sport injury rehabilitation programs. *J Athl Train, 43*(3):258–64.

28. Hanley, C. 2004. Stress-management interventions for female athletes: Relaxation and cognitive restructuring. *International Journal of Sport Psychology, 35*(2):109.

29. Hayden, L. 2011. The role of athletic trainers in helping coaches to facilitate return to play. *Athletic Therapy and Training, 16*(1):24–26.

30. Heaney, C. 2006. Physiotherapists' perceptions of sport psychology intervention in professional soccer. *International Journal of Sport and Exercise Psychology, 4*(1):73-86.

31. Hedgpeth, E., and Sowa, C. 1998. Incorporating stress management into athletic injury rehabilitation. *Journal of Athletic Training, 33*(4):372–74.

32. Hedgpeth, E. G. Hedgpeth/Gansneder Athletic Rehabilitation Indicator (unpublished).

33. Heil, J. 1993. *Psychology of Sport Injury.* Champaign, IL: Human Kinetics.

34. Holmes, T. H., Rahe, R. H. 1976. The social readjustment rating scale. *Journal of Psychosomatic Research, 11*:213.

35. Hutchinson, M., Mainwaring, L. 2009. Differential emotional responses of varsity athletes to concussion and musculoskeletal injuries. *Clin J Sport Med; 19*(1):13-9. doi: 10.1097/JSM.0b013e318190ba06

36. Ievleva, L., and Orlick, T. 1991. Mental links to enhanced healing: An exploratory study. *Sport Psychologist, 5*:25–40.

37. Jacobsen, E. 1931. Variation of specific muscles contracting during muscle imagination. *American Journal of Physiology, 96*:101–2.

38. Jacobsen, F. 1957. *You Must Relax,* 4th ed. New York: McGraw-Hill.

39. Johnson, U. 2011. Athletes experiences of psychosocial risk factors preceding injury. *Qualitative Research in Sport, Exercise, Health, 3*(1):99–115.

40. Kolt, G. S. 2005. Doing sport psychology with injured athletes. In M. B. Andersen (Ed): *Sport Psychology in Practice.* Champaign, IL, Human Kinetics.

41. Krucoff, C. 2000. Right under your nose. *Washington Post,* May 2.

42. Kübler-Ross, E. 1969. *On Death and Dying.* London, Tavistock.

43. Levy, A., Remco, C. 2009. Sport Injury rehabilitation adherence: Perspectives of recreational athletes. *Research in Sports Medicine, 7*(2)212-229.

44. Locke, E. A. 1968. Toward a theory of task motivation and incentives. *Organizational Behavior and Human Performance, 3*:157–58.

45. Locke, E., Latham, G. 1985. The application of goal setting to sport. *Journal of Sport Psychology, 7*:205–22.

46. Martens, R., Landers, D. 1969. Coaction effects on a muscular endurance task. *Research Quarterly, 40*:733–36.

47. Marra J. 2010. Assessment of certified athletic trainers' levels of cultural competence in the delivery of health care, *J Athl Train, 45*(4):380–85.

48. McKnight, K, Bernes, K. 2009. Life after sport: Athletic career transition and transferable skills. *Zone of Excellence, 13*:63-77

49. Mihalik J. 2004.Recognition of psychological conditions in adolescent athletes. *Athletic Therapy Today, 9*(3):54.

50. McGinnis, J. 1992. The public health burden of a sedentary lifestyle. *Medicine and Science in Sports and Exercise, 24*(suppl.):S196–S200.

51. McNair, D. M., M. Lorr, and L. F. Droppleman. 1971. *Profiles of Mood States.* San Diego: Educational and Industrial Testing Service.

52. Meichenbaum, D., and D. C. Turk. 1987. *Facilitating treatment adherence: A practitioner's guidebook.* New York: Plenum Press.

53. Michener, J. 1976. *Sports in America.* New York: Random House.

54. Milne M, Hall C, Forwell L. 2005. Self-efficacy, imagery use, and adherence to rehabilitation by injured athletes, *J Sport Rehabil, 14*(2):150.

55. Monsma E. 2009. Keeping your head in the game: Sport-specific imagery and anxiety among injured athletes, *J Athl Train, 44*(4):410–17.

56. Morgan, W. P. 1980. Test of champions: The iceberg profile. *Psychology Today,* pp. 92, 93, 99, 102, 108.

57. Morgan, W, Pollock, M. 1977. Psychological characterizations of the elite distance runner. *Annals of the New York Academy of Science, 301*:382–403.

58. Ninedek, A, Kolt, G. 2000. Sport physiotherapists' perceptions of psychological strategies in sport injury rehabilitation. *Journal of Sport Rehabilitation, 9*(3):191–206.

59. Petrie, T. A. 1992. Psychosocial antecedents of athletic injury: The effects of life stress and social support on women collegiate gymnasts. *Behavioral Medicine 18*:127–38.

60. Podlog L, Eklund R. 2005. Return to sport after serious injury: A retrospective examination of motivation and psychological outcomes, *J Sport Rehabil 14*(1):20.

61. Reilly, T. 1975. An ergonomic evaluation of occupational stress in professional football. Unpublished doctoral thesis. Polytechnic University, Liverpool, England.

62. Rock J, Jones M. 2002.A preliminary investigation into the use of counseling skills in support of rehabilitation from sport injury, *J Sport Rehabil, 11*(4):284.

63. Rotella, R. J. 1985. Psychological care of the injured athlete. In *The injured athlete,* 2nd ed., edited by D. Kuland. Philadelphia: Lippincott.

64. Sanderson, F. H. 1992. Psychology and injury prone athletes. *British Journal of Sports Medicine, 11*:56–57.

65. Schwenz SJ. 2001. Psychology of injury and rehabilitation, *Athletic Therapy Today, 6*(1):44.

66. Shank, R. H. 1989. Academic and athletic factors related to predicting compliance by athletes for treatment. *Athletic Training*, 24:123.

67. Sordoni, C, Hall, C. 2000. The use of imagery by athletes during injury rehabilitation. *Journal of Sport Rehabilitation*, 9:329–38.

68. Smith, A. M., and E. K. Milliner. 1994. Injured athletes and the risk of suicide. *Journal of Athletic Training*, 29:337.

69. Taylor, J., and S. Taylor. 1998. Pain education and management in the rehabilitation from sports injury. *Sport Psychologist* 12(1):68–88.

70. Tomlinson, C. 2000. *Simple yoga*. Edison, NJ: Castle.

71. Turk, D, Meichenbaum, D. 1983. *Pain and behavioral medicine: A cognitive behavioral perspective*. New York: Guilford Press.

72. Valiant, P. M. 1981. Personality and injury in competitive runners. *Perceptual and Motor Skills* 53:251–53.

73. Vincent, P. 1971. Factors influencing patient compliance: A theoretical approach. *Nursing Research* 20:509–16.

74. Walker, N, Thatcher, J. 2007. Review: Psychological responses to injury in competitive sport: A critical review, *Perspectives in Public Health*, 127(4):174–189.

75. Walsh, A. 2011. The relaxation response: A strategy to address stress, *Athletic Therapy and Training*, 16(2):20–23.

76. Webborn, A, Carbon, R. 1997. Injury rehabilitation programs: "What are we talking about?" *Journal of Sport Rehabilitation*, 6:54–61.

77. Weiss-Bjornstal M. 1998. An integrated model of response to sport injury: Psychological and sociological dynamics, *Journal of applied Sports Psychology* 10:46–69

78. Williams A. 2010. Social support and sport injury, *Athletic Therapy Today*, 15(4):46.

79. Wortman, C. B., and R. C. Silver. 1989. The myth of coping with loss. *Journal of Consulting and Clinical Psychology*, 57:349–57.

80. Wrisberg C. 2006. Recommendations for successfully integrating sport psychology into athletic therapy, *Athletic Therapy Today*, 11(2):60.

SOLUTIONS TO CLINICAL DECISION-MAKING EXERCISES

4-1   Julie and the athletic trainer sat down and mapped out a plan to fit what she needed to get accomplished into a reasonable amount of time. Julie first made a list of her priorities. She decided just what activities she needed to get done and which ones she could delete or postpone. After she had the list of necessary activities, she blocked out several 30-minute stretches of time for "catch-up" or "thinking time." These 30-minute periods allow Julie to not be rushed throughout the entire day. Julie and the athletic trainer were able to combine activities to save time and to come to the athletic training room during off hours when it was less crowded. Julie came to realize that, with a bit of creativity and some organizational skills, she could use time management as a buffer for stress.

4-2   The athletic trainer helped Tim realize that his whole body and mind need to be relaxed by using the progressive relaxation technique. By tightening and relaxing all his muscle groups in progression, Tim was able to have a low-intensity workout for the high intensity motions to be performed during the match. Tim also did some yoga abdominal breathing, which cleared his mind and allowed him to become more centered. This amounts to a mind and body dress rehearsal for the performance match. Tim was then able to go out and play in a more relaxed state with less pain and a more fluid motion.

4-3   The athletic trainer and Dana will work on changing the negatives to positives in two ways. The first is by changing words such as *can't* to *can* and *won't* to *will*. For example, "I can swing my club freely" or "My turn is smooth." The second change can be in the mental picture she has of herself hitting the shot. This works best if Dana can replay the video in her mind of the correct result, much as one tapes over an existing video. She can see herself swinging the club without pain in a very fluid and effortless manner. In her mind she can project that image on her mindtape. Dana will become very imaginative at creating the tapes she chooses to have in her mind's recorder.

4-4   The athletic trainer will need to continually remind Christine that rehabilitation will help her back. Offer examples of athletes who have returned from back problems. Allow Christine to vent her irrational thoughts, but counter them with reality checks such as, "Just last year one of your teammates came back from back problems and is diving now." The athletic trainer can work with Christine to keep her assessment of her condition based on the medical facts, not her irrational fears.

4-5 Joe and the athletic trainer need to discuss what Joe's options are for the future. Joe must first decide if he wants to stay in sports, or rethink his career goals. He can use imagery to daydream what it would look like and feel like to be in another field. Joe can "see" himself as a color commentator for the NFL and get some idea of what that experience would involve. A different field entirely may suit his personality and he can explore his options. It is important that he see the career change as a challenge to be overcome, not a defeat. This will be a long and rocky process, and one he has been forced to take. What he does have control over is choosing how he sees himself in a new role. Imaging allows him time to get used to his new identity.

4-6 The athletic trainer and George start with short-term goals to make the process more manageable and allow George to achieve satisfaction with short-term accomplishments. George and the athletic trainer set goals that are realistic, positive, and measurable. These process goals can be monitored and measured. George is now able to see that the plan is in place and the end is in sight. Process goals act as stepping stones to the end result. George understands that he is moving forward toward the long-term goal of returning to play.

Please see videos on the accompanying website at

www.healio.com/books/sportsmedvideos

SECTION II

Achieving the Goals of Rehabilitation

CHAPTER 5

Establishing Core Stability in Rehabilitation

Barbara J. Hoogenboom, EdD, PT, SCS, ATC
Jolene L. Bennett, MA, PT, OCS, ATC, CertMDT
Michael Clark, DPT, MS, PT, PES, CES

After completion of this chapter, the athletic trainer should be able to do the following:

- Describe the functional approach to kinetic chain rehabilitation.

- Define the concept of the core.

- Discuss the anatomic relationships between the muscular components of the core.

- Explain how the core functions to maintain postural alignment and dynamic postural equilibrium during functional activities.

- Describe procedures for assessing the core.

- Discuss the rationale for core stabilization training and relate to efficient functional performance of activities.

- Identify appropriate exercises for core stabilization training and their progressions.

- Discuss the guidelines for core stabilization training.

A dynamic, core stabilization training program should be a hallmark component of all comprehensive functional rehabilitation programs.[10,13,22,23,28,31,55] A core stabilization program improves dynamic postural control, ensures appropriate muscular balance, and affects joint arthrokinematics around the lumbo-pelvic-hip complex. A carefully crafted core stabilization program allows for the expression of dynamic functional strength and improves neuromuscular efficiency throughout the entire kinetic chain.[1,11,16,28,29,31,51,61,64-66,88,89]

WHAT IS THE CORE?

The core is defined as the lumbo-pelvic-hip complex.[1,28] The core is where our center of gravity is located and where all movement begins.[33,34,78,79] There are 29 muscles that

Prentice WE, ed.
Rehabilitation Techniques for Sports Medicine and Athletic Training (pp 125-150).
© 2015 SLACK Incorporated.

have an attachment to the lumbo-pelvic-hip complex.[7,8,28,80] An efficient core allows for maintenance of the normal length-tension relationship of functional agonists and antagonists, which allows for the maintenance of the normal force-couple relationships in the lumbo-pelvic-hip complex. Maintaining the normal length-tension relationships and force-couple relationships allows for the maintenance of optimal arthrokinematics in the lumbo-pelvic-hip complex during functional kinetic-chain movements.[88,89,96] This provides optimal neuromuscular efficiency in the entire kinetic chain, allowing for optimal acceleration, deceleration, and dynamic stabilization of the entire kinetic chain during functional movements. It also provides proximal stability for efficient lower-extremity and upper-extremity movements.[1,28,33,34,43,55,78,79,88,89]

The core operates as an integrated functional unit, whereby the entire kinetic chain works synergistically to produce force, reduce force, and dynamically stabilize against abnormal force.[1] In an efficient state, each structural component distributes weight, absorbs force, and transfers ground reaction forces.[1] This integrated, interdependent system needs to be trained appropriately to allow it to function efficiently during dynamic kinetic chain activities.

Core stabilization exercise programs have been labeled many different terms, some of which include *dynamic lumbar stabilization*, *neutral spine control*, *muscular fusion*, and *lumbo-pelvic stabilization*. We use the phrase *butt and gut* to educate our patients, colleagues, and health care students. This catchy phrase illustrates the importance of the entire abdominal and pelvic region working together to provide functional stability and efficient movement.

CORE STABILIZATION TRAINING CONCEPTS

Many individuals develop the functional strength, power, neuromuscular control, and muscular endurance in specific muscles that enable them to perform functional activities.[1,28,46,55] However, few people develop the muscles required for spinal stabilization.[43,46,47] The body's stabilization system has to be functioning optimally to effectively use the strength, power, neuromuscular control, and muscular endurance developed in the prime movers. If the extremity muscles are strong and the core is weak, then there will not be enough trunk stabilization created to produce efficient upper-extremity and lower-extremity movements. A weak core is a fundamental problem of many inefficient movements that leads to injury.[43,46,47,55]

The core musculature is an integral component of the protective mechanism that relieves the spine of deleterious forces inherent during functional activities.[14] A core stabilization training program is designed to help an individual gain strength, neuromuscular control, power, and muscle endurance of the lumbo-pelvic-hip complex. This approach facilitates a balanced muscular functioning of the entire kinetic chain.[1] Greater neuromuscular control and stabilization strength will offer a more biomechanically efficient position for the entire kinetic chain, thereby allowing optimal neuromuscular efficiency throughout the kinetic chain.

Neuromuscular efficiency is established by the appropriate combination of postural alignment (static/dynamic) and stability strength, which allows the body to decelerate gravity, ground reaction forces, and momentum at the right joint, in the right plane, and at the right time.[12,31,54] If the neuromuscular system is not efficient, it will be unable to respond to the demands placed on it during functional activities.[1] As the efficiency of the neuromuscular system decreases, the ability of the kinetic chain to maintain appropriate forces and dynamic stabilization decreases significantly. This decreased neuromuscular efficiency leads to compensation and substitution patterns, as well as poor posture during functional activities.[29,88,89] Such poor posture leads to increased mechanical stress on the contractile and noncontractile tissue, leading to repetitive microtrauma, abnormal biomechanics, and injury.[16,29,62,63]

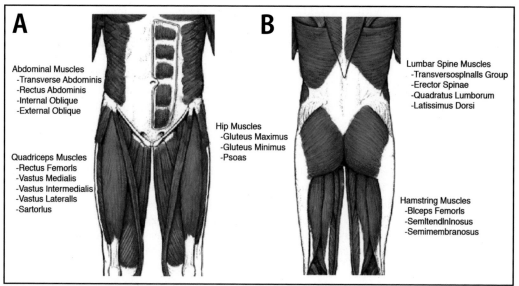

Figure 5-1. Key core muscles. (A) Anterior view. (B) Posterior view.

REVIEW OF FUNCTIONAL ANATOMY

To fully understand functional core stabilization training and rehabilitation, the athletic trainer must fully understand functional anatomy, lumbo-pelvic-hip complex stabilization mechanisms, and normal force-couple relationships.[4,7,8,80]

A review of the key lumbo-pelvic-hip complex musculature will allow the athletic trainer to understand functional anatomy and thereby develop a comprehensive kinetic chain rehabilitation program. The key lumbar spine muscles include the transversospinal group, erector spinae, quadratus lumborum, and latissimus dorsi (Figure 5-1B). The key abdominal muscles include the rectus abdominis, external oblique, internal oblique, and transversus abdominis (TA) (Figure 5-1A). The key hip musculature

includes the gluteus maximus, gluteus medius, and psoas (Figure 5-1B).

The transversospinalis group includes the rotatores, interspinales, intertransversarii, semispinalis, and multifidus. These muscles are small and have a poor mechanical advantage for contributing to motion.[27,80] They contain primarily type I muscle fibers and are therefore designed mainly for stabilization.[27,80] Researchers[80] have found that the transversospinalis muscle group contains two to six times the number of muscle spindles found in larger muscles. Therefore, it has been established that this group is primarily responsible for providing the central nervous system with proprioceptive information.[80] This group is also responsible for inter- or intrasegmental stabilization and segmental eccentric deceleration of flexion and rotation of the spinal unit during functional movements.[4,80] The transversospinalis group is constantly put under a variety of compressive and tensile forces during functional movements; consequently, it needs to be trained adequately to allow dynamic postural stabilization and optimal neuromuscular efficiency of the entire kinetic chain.[80] The multifidus is the most important of the transversospinalis muscles. It has the ability to provide intrasegmental stabilization to the lumbar spine in all positions.[27,97] Wilke et al[97] found increased segmental stiffness at L4-L5 with activation of the multifidus. Additional key back muscles include the erector spinae, quadratus lumborum, and the latissimus dorsi. The erector spinae muscle group functions to provide dynamic intersegmental stabilization and eccentric deceleration of trunk flexion and rotation during kinetic chain activities.[80] The quadratus lumborum muscle functions primarily as a frontal plane stabilizer that works synergistically with the gluteus medius and tensor fascia lata. The latissimus dorsi has the largest moment arm of all back muscles and therefore has the greatest effect on the lumbo-pelvic-hip complex. The latissimus dorsi is the bridge between the upper extremity and the lumbo-pelvic-hip complex. Any functional upper-extremity kinetic chain rehabilitation must pay particular attention to the latissimus and its function on the lumbo-pelvic-hip complex.[80]

The abdominals are composed of four muscles: rectus abdominis, external oblique, internal oblique, and, most importantly, the TA.[80] The abdominals operate as an integrated functional unit, which helps maintain optimal spinal kinematics.[4,7,8,80] When working efficiently, the abdominals offer sagittal, frontal, and transversus plane stabilization by controlling forces that reach the lumbo-pelvic-hip complex.[80] The rectus abdominis eccentrically decelerates trunk extension and lateral flexion, as well as providing dynamic stabilization during functional movements. The external obliques work concentrically to produce contralateral rotation and ipsilateral lateral flexion, and work eccentrically to decelerate trunk extension, rotation, and lateral flexion during functional movements.[80] The internal oblique works concentrically to produce ipsilateral rotation and lateral flexion and works eccentrically to decelerate extension, rotation, and lateral flexion. The internal oblique attaches to the posterior layer of the thoracolumbar fascia. Contraction of the internal oblique creates a lateral tension force on the thoracolumbar fascia, which creates intrinsic translational and rotational stabilization of the spinal unit.[34,43] The TA is probably the most important of the abdominal muscles. The TA functions to increase intra-abdominal pressure (IAP), provide dynamic stabilization against rotational and translational stress in the lumbar spine, and

provide optimal neuromuscular efficiency to the entire lumbo-pelvic-hip complex.[43,46-48,58] Research demonstrates that the TA works in a feed-forward mechanism.[43] Researchers have demonstrated that contraction of the TA precedes the initiation of limb movement and all other abdominal muscles, regardless of the direction of reactive forces.[26,43] Cresswell et al[25,26] demonstrated that like the multifidus, the TA is active during all trunk movements, suggesting that this muscle has an important role in dynamic stabilization.[46]

Key hip muscles include the psoas, gluteus medius, gluteus maximus, and hamstrings.[7,8,80] The psoas produces hip flexion and external rotation in the open chain position, and produces hip flexion, lumbar extension, lateral flexion, and rotation in the closed-chain position. The psoas eccentrically decelerates hip extension and internal rotation, as well as trunk extension, lateral flexion, and rotation. The psoas works synergistically with the superficial erector spinae and creates an anterior shear force at L4-L5.[80] The deep erector spinae, multifidus, and deep abdominal wall (transverses, internal oblique, and external oblique)[80] counteract this force. It is extremely common for clients to develop tightness in their psoas. A tight psoas increases the anterior shear force and compressive force at the L4-L5 junction.[80] A tight psoas also causes reciprocal inhibition of the gluteus maximus, multifidus, deep erector spinae, internal oblique, and TA. This leads to extensor mechanism dysfunction during functional movement patterns.[51,61,63,65,66,80,89] Lack of lumbo-pelvic-hip complex stabilization prevents appropriate movement sequencing and leads to synergistic dominance by the hamstrings and superficial erector spinae during hip extension. This complex movement dysfunction also decreases the ability of the gluteus maximus to decelerate femoral internal rotation during heel strike, which predisposes an individual with a knee ligament injury to abnormal forces and repetitive microtrauma.[14,19,51,65,66]

The gluteus medius functions as the primary frontal plane stabilizer of the pelvis and lower extremity during functional movements.[80] During closed-chain movements, the gluteus medius decelerates femoral adduction and internal rotation.[80] A weak gluteus medius increases frontal and transversus plane stress at the patellofemoral joint and the tibiofemoral joint.[80] A weak gluteus medius leads to synergistic dominance of the tensor fascia latae and the quadratus lumborum.[19,51,53] This leads to tightness in the iliotibial band and the lumbar spine. This will affect the normal biomechanics of the lumbo-pelvic-hip complex and the tibiofemoral joint, as well as the patellofemoral joint. Research by Beckman and Buchanan[9] demonstrates decreased electromyogram (EMG) activity of the gluteus medius following an ankle sprain. Therapists must address the altered hip muscle recruitment patterns or accept this recruitment pattern as an injury-adaptive strategy, and thus accept the unknown long-term consequences of premature muscle activation and synergistic dominance.[9,29]

The gluteus maximus functions concentrically in the open chain to accelerate hip extension and external rotation. It functions eccentrically to decelerate hip flexion and femoral internal rotation.[80] It also functions through the iliotibial band to decelerate tibial internal rotation.[80] The gluteus maximus is a major dynamic stabilizer of the sacroiliac (SI) joint. It has the greatest capacity to provide compressive forces at the SI joint secondary to its anatomic attachment at the sacrotuberous ligament.[80] It has been demonstrated by Bullock-Saxton[15,16] that the EMG activity of the gluteus maximus is decreased following an ankle sprain. Lack of proper gluteus maximus activity during functional activities leads to pelvic instability and decreased neuromuscular control. This can eventually lead to the development of muscle imbalances, poor movement patterns, and injury.

The hamstrings work concentrically to flex the knee, extend the hip, and rotate the tibia. They work eccentrically to decelerate knee extension, hip flexion, and tibial rotation. The hamstrings work synergistically with the anterior cruciate ligament.[80] All of the muscles mentioned play an integral role in the kinetic chain by providing dynamic stabilization and optimal neuromuscular control of the entire lumbo-pelvic-hip complex. These muscles have been reviewed so that the athletic trainer realizes that muscles not only produce force (concentric contractions) in one plane of motion, but

also reduce force (eccentric contractions) and provide dynamic stabilization in all planes of movement during functional activities. When isolated, these muscles do not effectively achieve stabilization of the lumbo-pelvic-hip complex. It is the synergistic, interdependent functioning of the entire lumbo-pelvic-hip complex that enhances stability and neuromuscular control throughout the entire kinetic chain.

TRANSVERSUS ABDOMINIS AND MULTIFIDUS ROLE IN CORE STABILIZATION

The TA muscle is the deepest of the abdominal muscles and plays a primary role in trunk stability. The horizontal orientation of its fibers has a limited ability to produce torque to the spine necessary for flexion or extension movement, although it has been shown to be an active trunk rotator.[81] The TA is a primary trunk stabilizer via modulation of IAP, tension through the thoracolumbar fascia, and compression of the SI joints.[25,91] For many decades, IAP was believed to be an important contributor to spinal control by the pressure within the abdominal cavity putting force on the diaphragm superiorly and pelvic floor inferiorly to extend the trunk.[6,35,73] It was hypothesized that IAP would provide an extensor moment and thus reduce the muscular force required by the trunk extensors and decrease the compressive load on the lumbar spine.[95] Recent research by Hodges et al[42] applied electrical stimulation to the phrenic nerve of humans to produce an involuntary increase in IAP without abdominal or extensor muscle activity. IAP was increased by the contraction of the diaphragm, pelvic floor muscles, and the TA with no flexor moment noted. Research has demonstrated that IAP may directly increase spinal stiffness.[45] Hodges et al[42] used a tetanic contraction of the diaphragm to produce IAP, which resulted in increased stiffness in the spine. Bilateral contraction of the TA assists in IAP, thus enhancing spinal stiffness.

The role of the thoracolumbar fascia in trunk stability has also been discussed in the literature, and it has been theorized that the contraction of the TA could produce an extensor torque via the horizontal pull of the TA via its extensive attachment into the thoracolumbar fascia.[34] Recently, this theory was tested by Tesh et al[93] by placing tension on the thoracolumbar fascia of cadavers. No approximation of the spinous processes or trunk extension movement was noted although a small amount of compression on the spine was noted. This small amount of compression may play a role in the control of intervertebral shear forces. Hodges et al[42] electrically stimulated contraction of the TA in pigs and demonstrated that when tension was developed in the thoracolumbar fascia, without an associated increase in IAP, there was no significant effect on the intervertebral stiffness. In the next step of that same research study, the thoracolumbar fascial attachments were cut and an increase in IAP decreased the spinal stiffness. This demonstrates that the thoracolumbar fascia and IAP work in concert to enhance trunk stability.[42]

Trunk stability is also dependent on the joints caudal to the lumbar spine. The SI joint is the connection between the lumbar spine and the pelvic region, which ultimately connects the trunk to the lower extremities. The SI joint is dependent on the compressive force between the sacrum and ilia. The horizontal direction and anterior attachment on the ilium of the TA produces the compressive force necessary for spinal stability. Richardson et al[84] used ultrasound to detect movement of the sacrum and ilium while having subjects voluntarily contract their transverse abdominals. They demonstrated that a voluntary contraction of the TA reduced the laxity of the SI joint. This study also pointed out that this reduction in joint laxity of the SI joint was greater than that during a bracing contraction. The researchers did note that they were unable to exclude changes in activity in other muscles such as the pelvic floor, which may have reduced the laxity via counternutation of the sacrum.[84] The aforementioned research findings illustrate that the TA plays an important role in maintaining trunk stability by interacting with IAP, thoracolumbar fascia tension, and compressing the SI joints via muscular attachments.

The multifidi are the most medial of the posterior trunk muscles, and they cover the lumbar zygapophyseal joints except for the ventral surfaces.[81] The multifidi are primary stabilizers when the trunk is moving from flexion to extension. The multifidi contribute only 20% of the total lumbar extensor moment, whereas the lumbar erector spinae contribute 30%, and the thoracic erector spinae function as the predominant torque generator at 50% of the extension moment arm.[56] The multifidus, lumbar, and thoracic erector spinae muscles have a high percentage of type I fibers and are postural control muscles similar to the TA.[56] The multifidus has been shown to be active during all antigravity activities, including static tasks, such as standing, and dynamic tasks, such as walking.[97]

Clinical observation and experimental evidence confirm that when the TA contracts, the multifidi are also activated.[81] A girdle-like cylinder of muscular support is produced as a result of the coactivation of the TA, multifidus, and the thick thoracolumbar fascial system. EMG evidence suggests that the TA and internal obliques contract in anticipation of movement of the upper and lower extremities, often referred to as the feed-forward mechanism. This feed-forward mechanism gives the TA and multifidus muscular girdle a unique ability to stabilize the spine regardless of the direction of limb movements.[44,45] As noted previously, the pelvic floor muscles play an important role in the development of IAP, and thus enhance trunk stability. It has also been demonstrated that the pelvic floor is active during repetitive arm movement tasks independent of the direction of movement.[49]

Sapsford et al[90] discovered that maximal contraction of the pelvic floor was associated with activity of all abdominal muscles and submaximal contraction of the pelvic floor muscles was associated with a more isolated contraction of the TA. In this same study, it also was determined that the specificity of the response was better when the lumbar spine and pelvis were in a neutral position.[90] Clinically, this information is helpful in guiding the patient in the process of TA contraction by instructing the patient to perform a submaximal pelvic floor isometric hold. Another interesting fact to note is that men and women with incontinence have almost double the incidence of low back pain as people without incontinence issues.[30] In summary, the lumbo-pelvic region may be visualized as a cylinder with the inferior wall being the pelvic floor, the superior wall being the diaphragm, the posterior wall being the multifidus, and the TA muscles forming the anterior and lateral walls. All walls of the cylinder must be activated and taut for optimal trunk stabilization to occur with all static and dynamic activities.

Clinical Decision-Making Exercise 5-2

Last year a tennis player suffered a knee injury. She tore her ACL, MCL, and meniscus. She is competing now but complains of recurrent back pain. She has rather poor posture and significant postural sway. Could she benefit from core training, and how would you go about selecting exercises for her?

POSTURAL CONSIDERATIONS

The core functions to maintain postural alignment and dynamic postural equilibrium during functional activities. Optimal alignment of each body part is a cornerstone to a functional training and rehabilitation program. Optimal posture and alignment will allow for maximal neuromuscular efficiency because the normal length-tension relationship, force-couple relationship, and arthrokinematics will be maintained during functional movement patterns.[14,28,29,50,51,53,55,58,62,64,88,89] If one segment in the kinetic chain is out of alignment, it will create predictable patterns of dysfunction throughout the entire kinetic chain. These predictable patterns of dysfunction are referred to as serial distortion patterns.[28] Serial distortion patterns represent the state in which the body's structural integrity is compromised because segments in the kinetic chain are out of alignment. This leads to abnormal distorting forces being placed on the segments in the kinetic chain that are above and below the dysfunctional segment.[14,28,29,55] To avoid serial distortion patterns and the chain reaction that one misaligned segment creates, we must emphasize stable positions to maintain the structural integrity of the entire kinetic chain.[16,28,55,65,66,87] A comprehensive core

stabilization program prevents the development of serial distortion patterns and provides optimal dynamic postural control during functional movements.

MUSCULAR IMBALANCES

An optimally functioning core helps to prevent the development of muscle imbalances and synergistic dominance. The human movement system is a well-orchestrated system of interrelated and interdependent components.[16,61] The functional interaction of each component in the human movement system allows for optimal neuromuscular efficiency. Alterations in joint arthrokinematics, muscular balance, and neuromuscular control affect the optimal functioning of the entire kinetic chain.[16,88,89] Dysfunction of the kinetic chain is rarely an isolated event. Typically, a pathology of the kinetic chain is part of a chain reaction involving some key links in the kinetic chain and numerous compensations and adaptations that develop.[61] The interplay of many muscles about a joint is responsible for the coordinated control of movement. If the core is weak, normal arthrokinematics are altered. Changes in normal length-tension and force-couple relationships, in turn, affect neuromuscular control. If one muscle becomes weak, tight, or changes its degree of activation, then synergists, stabilizers, and neutralizers have to compensate.[16,29,61,64-66,88,89]

Muscle tightness has a significant impact on the kinetic chain. Muscle tightness affects the normal length-tension relationship.[89] This impacts the normal force-couple relationship. When one muscle in a force-couple relationship becomes tight, it changes the normal arthrokinematics of two articular partners.[14,61,89] Altered arthrokinematics affect the synergistic function of the kinetic chain.[14,29,61,89] This leads to abnormal pressure distribution over articular surfaces and soft tissues. Muscle tightness also leads to reciprocal inhibition.[14,29,50-53,61,92,96] Therefore, if one develops muscle imbalances throughout the lumbo-pelvic-hip complex, it can affect the entire kinetic chain. For example, a tight psoas causes reciprocal inhibition of the gluteus maximus, TA, internal oblique, and multifidus.[47,51,53,77,80] This muscle imbalance pattern may decrease normal lumbo-pelvic-hip stability. Specific substitution patterns develop to compensate for the lack of stabilization, including tightness in the iliotibial band.[29] This muscle imbalance pattern leads to increased frontal and transverse plane stress at the knee. Dr. Vladamir Janda proposed a syndrome, named the "crossed pelvis syndrome," in which a weak abdominal wall and weak gluteals are counterbalanced with tight hamstrings and hip flexors.[51]

A strong core with optimal neuromuscular efficiency can help to prevent the development of muscle imbalances. Consequently, a comprehensive core stabilization training program should be an integral component of all rehabilitation programs. A strong, efficient core provides the stable base upon which the extremities can function with maximal precision and effectiveness. It is important to remember that the spine, pelvis, and hips must be in proper alignment with proper activation of all muscles during any core-strengthening exercise. Because no one muscle works in isolation, attention should be paid to the position and activity of all muscles during open and closed chain exercises.

NEUROMUSCULAR CONSIDERATIONS

A strong and stable core can optimize neuromuscular efficiency throughout the entire kinetic chain by helping to improve dynamic postural control.[37,43,47,57,83,88,89] A number of researchers have demonstrated kinetic chain imbalances in individuals with altered neuromuscular control.[9,14-16,43,46-48,50-54,61-66,76,77,83,88] Research demonstrates that people with low back pain have an abnormal neuromotor response of the trunk stabilizers accompanying limb movement, significantly greater postural sway, and decreased limits of stability.[46,47,71,77] Research also demonstrates that about 70% of patients suffer from recurrent episodes of back pain. Furthermore, it has been demonstrated that individuals have decreased dynamic postural stability in the proximal stabilizers of the lumbo-pelvic-hip complex following lower-extremity ligamentous injuries,[9,14-16] and that joint and ligamentous injury can lead to decreased muscle activity.[29,92,96] Joint and ligament injury can lead to joint effusion, which, in turn, leads to muscle inhibition. This leads to altered neuromuscular control in other segments of the kinetic chain secondary to altered proprioception and kinesthesia.[9,16] Therefore, when an individual with a knee ligament injury has joint effusion, all of the muscles that cross the knee can be inhibited. Several muscles that cross the knee joint are attached to the lumbo-pelvic-hip complex.[80] Consequently, a comprehensive rehabilitation approach should focus on reestablishing optimal core function so as to positively affect peripheral joints.

Research also demonstrates that muscles can be inhibited from an arthrokinetic reflex.[14,61,92,96] This is referred to as arthrogenic muscle inhibition. Arthrokinetic reflexes are mediated by joint receptor activity. If an individual has abnormal arthrokinematics, the muscles that move the joint will be inhibited. For example, if an individual has a sacral torsion, the multifidus and the gluteus medius can be inhibited.[41] This leads to abnormal movement in the kinetic chain. The tensor fascia latae become synergistically dominant and the primary frontal plane stabilizer.[80] This can lead to tightness in the iliotibial band. It can also decrease the frontal and transverse plane control at the knee. Furthermore, if the multifidus is inhibited,[41] the erector spinae and the psoas become facilitated. This further inhibits the lower abdominals (internal oblique and TA) and the gluteus maximus.[43,46] This also decreases frontal and transverse plane stability at the knee. As previously mentioned, an efficient core improves neuromuscular efficiency of the entire kinetic chain by providing dynamic stabilization of the lumbo-pelvic-hip complex and improving pelvofemoral biomechanics. This is yet another reason why all rehabilitation programs should include a comprehensive core stabilization training program.

Clinical Decision-Making Exercise 5-3

As part of a preparticipation screening you want to look for athletes who may be prone to low back pain. What evaluative test can you use to do this?

SCIENTIFIC RATIONALE FOR CORE STABILIZATION TRAINING

Most individuals train their core stabilizers inadequately compared to other muscle groups.[1,85,86] Although adequate strength, power, muscle endurance, and neuromuscular control are important for lumbo-pelvic-hip stabilization, performing exercises incorrectly or that are too advanced is detrimental.[60,85,86] Several researchers have found decreased firing of the TA, internal oblique, multifidus, and deep erector spinae in individuals with chronic low back pain.[43,46-48,77,82] Performing core training with inhibition of these key stabilizers leads to the development of muscle imbalances and inefficient neuromuscular control in the kinetic chain. It has been demonstrated that abdominal training without proper pelvic stabilization increases intradiscal pressure and compressive forces in the lumbar spine.[3,5,10,43,46-48,74,75] Furthermore, hyperextension training without proper pelvic stabilization can increase intradiscal pressure to dangerous levels, cause buckling of the ligamentum flavum, and lead to narrowing of the intervertebral foramen.[3,5,10,75]

Research also shows decreased stabilization endurance in individuals with chronic low back pain.[10,18,33,34,70] The core stabilizers are primarily type I slow-twitch muscle fibers.[33,34,78,79] These muscles respond best to time under tension. Time under tension is a method of contraction that lasts 6 to 20 seconds and emphasizes hypercontractions at end ranges of motion. This method improves intramuscular coordination, which improves static and dynamic stabilization. To get the appropriate training stimulus, you must prescribe the appropriate speed of movement for all aspects of exercises.[22,23] Core strength endurance must be trained appropriately to allow an individual to maintain dynamic postural control for prolonged periods.[3]

Research demonstrates a decreased cross-sectional area of the multifidus in patients with low back pain, and that spontaneous recovery of the multifidus following resolution of symptoms does not occur.[41] It has also been demonstrated that the traditional curl-up increases intradiscal pressure and increases compressive forces at L2-L3.[3,5,10,74,75]

Additional research demonstrates increased EMG activity and pelvic stabilization when an abdominal drawing-in maneuver is performed prior to initiating core training.[3,10,13,22,36,37,48,72,76,83] Also, maintaining the cervical spine in a neutral position during core training improves posture, muscle balance, and stabilization. If the head protracts during movement, then the sternocleidomastoid is preferentially recruited. This increases the compressive forces at the C0-C1 vertebral junction. This can lead to pelvic instability and muscle imbalances secondary to the pelvo-occular reflex. This reflex is important to keep the eyes level.[62,63] If the sternocleidomastoid muscle is hyperactive and extends the upper cervical spine, then the pelvis will rotate anteriorly to realign the eyes. This can lead to muscle imbalances and decreased pelvic stabilization.[62,63]

Clinical Decision-Making Exercise 5-4

You have had a track athlete on a core stabilization program for several weeks. She has been progressing well but needs a different challenge. What can you do to change up her program?

ASSESSMENT OF THE CORE

Before a comprehensive core stabilization program is implemented, an individual must undergo a comprehensive assessment to determine muscle imbalances, arthrokinematic deficits, core strength, core muscle endurance, core neuromuscular control, core power, and overall function of the lower-extremity kinetic chain. Assessment tools include activity-based tests that are performed in the clinical setting, EMG with surface or indwelling electrodes, and technologically advanced testing and training techniques using real-time ultrasound. Rehabilitative ultrasound imaging (RUSI) has been used extensively in research settings and has been proven to be a reliable tool in evaluating the activation patterns of various abdominal muscles.[38,94] RUSI, although not currently readily available in clinical settings, is a great asset in the laboratory setting. Perhaps the future will allow for more use of RUSI in clinical practice.

It was previously stated that muscle imbalances and arthrokinematic deficits can cause abnormal movement patterns to develop throughout the entire kinetic chain. Consequently, it is extremely important to thoroughly assess each individual with a kinetic chain dysfunction for muscle imbalances and arthrokinematic deficits. All procedures for assessment are beyond the scope of this chapter, and the interested reader is referred to the comprehensive references provided to gain an understanding of additional assessment procedures that may be used to identify muscle imbalances. It is recommended that the interested reader use the following references to explain a comprehensive muscle imbalance assessment procedure thoroughly.[1,14,19,22,23,28,48,52,54,55,64,88,89,96]

Core strength can be assessed by using the straight-leg lowering test.[3,48,58,76,88,89] The individual is placed supine. A pressure biofeedback device called the Stabilizer (Figure 5-2) is placed under the lumbar spine at about L4-L5. The cuff pressure is raised to 40 mm Hg. The individual's legs are maintained in full-extension while flexing the hips to 90 degrees (Figure 5-3). The individual is instructed to perform a drawing-in maneuver (pull belly button to spine) and then flatten the back maximally into the table and pressure cuff. The individual is instructed to lower the legs toward the table while maintaining the back flat. The test is over when the pressure in the cuff decreases. The hip angle is then measured with a goniometer to determine the angle using a rating scale developed by Kendall (Figure 5-4).[59] This test provides a basic idea of how strong the lower abdominal muscle groups (rectus abdominis and external obliques) are. Using the pressure feedback device ensures there is no compensation with the lumbar extensors or large hip flexors to stabilize the long lever arm of the legs.

Neuromuscular control of the deep core muscles, TA, and multifidi are evaluated with the quality of movement emphasized rather than quantity of muscular strength or endurance time. Unfortunately, no objectifiable manual muscle test exists for either of these important muscles/muscle groups; however,

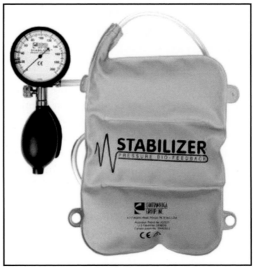

Figure 5-2. Stabilizer pressure biofeedback unit. (Reproduced with permission from the Chattanooga Group.)

Hides et al[40] have developed prone and supine tests to evaluate the muscular coordination of the TA and multifidus. The first test for the TA is performed in the prone position with the Stabilizer pressure biofeedback unit placed under the abdomen with the navel in the center and the distal edge of the pad in line with the right and left anterior superior iliac spines (Figure 5-5). The pressure pad is inflated to 70 mm Hg. It is important to instruct the patient to relax his or her abdomen fully prior to the start of the test. The patient is then instructed to take a relaxed breath in and out, and then to draw the abdomen in toward the spine without taking a breath. The patient is asked to hold this contraction for a minimum of 10 seconds, with a slow and controlled release. Optimal performance, indicating proper neuromuscular control of the TA, is a 4 to 10 mm Hg reduction in the pressure with no pelvic or spinal movement noted. It is important to monitor pelvic and lower-extremity positioning as the patient may compensate by putting pressure through the patient's legs or tilting the patient's pelvis to elevate the lower abdomen rather than isolating the TA contraction.

Testing for the TA is also performed in the supine position and relies on palpation and visualization of the lower abdomen. Instructions to the patient remain the same as the prone test

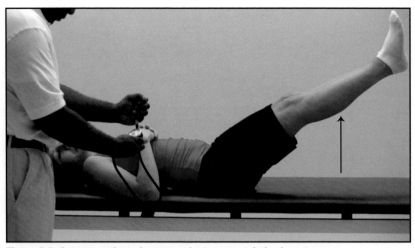

Figure 5-3. Core strength can be assessed using a straight leg lowering test.

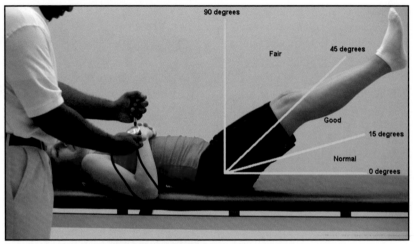

Figure 5-4. Key to muscle grading in the straight leg lowering test.

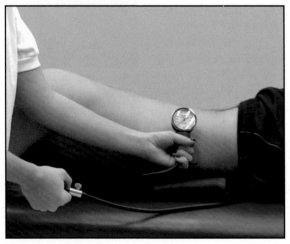

Figure 5-5. Prone transverse abdominis test.

and the athletic trainer palpates for bilateral TA contraction just medially and inferiorly to the anterior superior iliac spines and lateral to the rectus abdominis (Figure 5-6A).

The Stabilizer pad may also be placed under the lower lumbar region to monitor whether compensation occurs with the pelvis (Figure 5-6B). The pressure reading should remain the same throughout the test. A change in the pressure reading indicates that the patient is tilting the patient's pelvis anteriorly (pressure decreases) or posteriorly (pressure increases) in an attempt to flatten the patient's lower abdomen. The patient is asked to hold this contraction for a minimum of 10 seconds, with a slow and controlled release. With a correct contraction of the TA, the athletic trainer feels a slowly developing deep tension in the lower abdominal wall. Incorrect activation of the TA would be evident when the internal oblique dominates and this is detected when a rapid development of tension is palpated or the abdominal wall is pushed out rather than drawn in.

The neuromuscular control of the multifidi is examined with the patient in the prone position and the therapist palpating the level of the multifidus for muscular activation (Figure 5-7). The patient is instructed to breathe in and out and to hold the breath out while swelling out the muscles under the therapist's fingers. The patient is then asked to hold the contraction while resuming a normal breathing pattern for a minimum of 10 seconds. The athletic trainer palpates the multifidus for symmetrical activation and slow development of muscular activation. This sequence is repeated at the multiple segments in the lumbar spine. Compensation patterns may include anterior or posterior pelvic tilting or elevation of the rib cage in an attempt to swell out the multifidus.

A proper and thorough evaluation of the core muscles will lead the athletic trainer in developing a proper core stabilization program. It is imperative that neuromuscular control of the TA and multifidus precedes all other stabilization exercises. These muscles provide the foundation from which all the other core muscles work.

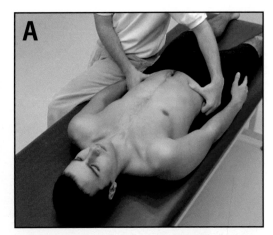

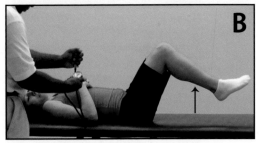

Figure 5-6. Supine transversus abdominis test.

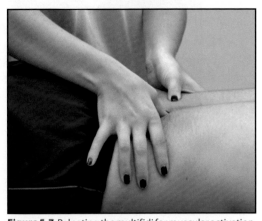

Figure 5-7. Palpating the multifidi for muscular activation.

Clinical Decision-Making Exercise 5-5

You have been training a softball player on a core strengthening program for 1 week. She has been making improvements, and you think that it is time to progress her. What is your goal, and what parameters should you consider when progressing her?

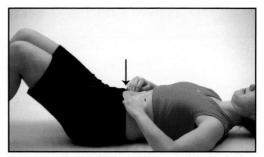

Figure 5-8. The drawing-in maneuver requires a contraction of the transversus abdominis.

CORE STABILIZATION TRAINING PROGRAM

As previously noted, the training program must progress in a scientific, systematic pattern with the ultimate goal of training the trunk stabilizers to be active in all phases of functional tasks. These tasks may include simple static postures, such as standing or sitting, and progress to very complex tasks, such as high-intensity athletic skills.[67] Patient education is the key to a successful exercise program. The patient must be able to visualize the muscle activation patterns desired and have a high level of body awareness allowing him or her to activate his or her core muscles with the proper positioning, neuromuscular control, and level of force generation needed for each individual task.

Performing the Drawing-In Maneuver

Muscular activation of the deep core stabilizers (TA and multifidus) coordinated with normal breathing patterns is the foundation for all core exercises.[60] All core stabilization exercises must first start with the "drawing-in" maneuver (Figure 5-8). Opinions vary[69,81] in the exercise science world about the activation of the abdominal muscles during activities.

McGill[69] is a proponent of the abdominal bracing technique where the patient is advised to stiffen or activate both the trunk flexors and extensors maximally to prevent spinal movement. He uses the training technique of demonstrating this bracing pattern at the elbow joint. He asks the patient to stiffen his or her elbow joint by simultaneously activating the elbow flexors and extensors and resisting an externally applied force that attempts to flex the patient's elbow. Once the patient has mastered that concept, the same principles are applied to the trunk.

Richardson et al[81] teach the abdominal hollowing technique where the navel is drawn back toward the spine without spinal movement occurring. This technique does not ask patients to do a maximal contraction, but instead, a submaximal, steady development of muscle activation.

We have used a teaching technique that incorporates submaximal abdominal hollowing and moderate bracing of the trunk. While standing in front of a mirror, patients are asked to put their hands on their iliac crests so their fingers rest anteriorly on their transverse abdominals and internal obliques. A good way to state this to the patient is, "Put your hands on your hips like you are mad." Patients are then instructed to draw their navel back toward their spine without moving their trunk or body while continuing to breathe normally. A good verbal cue is to "Make your waist narrow like you are putting on a tight pair of jeans, without sucking in your breath." While in that position, patients are also instructed to not let anyone "Push them around," or push them off balance. This helps incorporate the total-body bracing technique and the use of the upper and lower extremities to facilitate total-body stabilization. This can be referred to as "the power position" or "home base," and these key words may be used when teaching the progression of all core exercises (see Table 5-1 for other teaching cues for proper muscular activation of core muscles).[71,85] It should be emphasized that proper muscular activation cannot be achieved if the patient is holding his or her breath.

Table 5-1 Teaching Cues for Activation of Core Muscles

Verbal Cues
1. Draw navel back toward spine without moving your spine or tilting your pelvis.
2. Make your waist narrow.
3. Pull your abdomen away from your waistband of your pants.
4. Draw lower abdomen in while simulating zipping up a tight pair of pants.
5. Continue breathing normally while contracting lower abdominals.
6. Tighten pelvic floor.
a. Women: contract pelvic floor so you do not leak urine.
b. Men: draw up scrotum as if you are walking in waist deep cold water.

Physical Cues
1. Use mirror for visual feedback.
2. Put your hands on your waist like you are mad, draw abdomen away from fingertips while still breathing normally.
3. Tactile facilitation.
a. Use tape on skin for cutaneous feedback.
b. String tied snugly around waist.
4. EMG biofeedback unit.
5. Electrical muscular stimulation.
6. Isometric contraction and holding of pelvic floor and hip adductors.

It should also be noted that the drawing-in maneuver should not be abandoned when the patient is performing other exercises such as weightlifting, walking, or other aerobic tasks such as step aerobics, aqua aerobics, or running.

Specific Core Stabilization Exercises

Once the drawing-in maneuver is perfected, neuromuscular control of the TA and multifidus is accomplished in the prone and supine positions as described in "Assessment of the Core" previously. Then progression of exercises into other positions can take place. Quadruped is a good starting position for the patient to learn and enhance his or her power position (Figure 5-9). This facilitates the patient keeping his or her body steady and minimizing trunk movement. The patient is instructed to keep the trunk straight like a tabletop and then draw the stomach up toward the spine (activating the TA and multifidus) while maintaining the normal

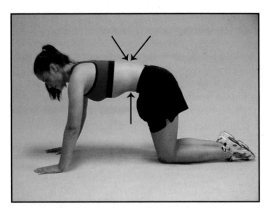

Figure 5-9. Quadruped position for mastering the "drawing-in" maneuver or power position.

breathing pattern. This position is held for a minimum of 10 seconds and progressed in time to up to 30 to 60 seconds, working on endurance of these trunk muscles.[67,70] The patient is advised to release the contraction slowly in an eccentric manner and no spinal movement should occur during this release phase. When

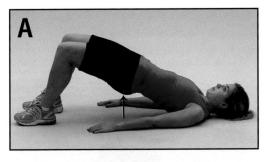
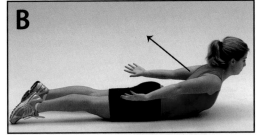
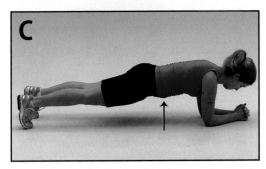
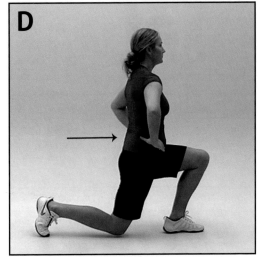
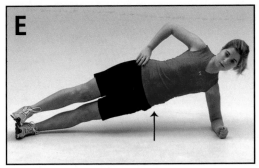

Figure 5-10. Level 1 (stabilization) core stability exercises. (A) Double-leg bridging. (B) Prone cobra. (C) Front plank. (D) Lunge. (E) Side plank. (*continued*)

this position is mastered by the patient and the athletic trainer feels that the patient is ready, the difficulty of the exercise can be progressed, limited only by the capabilities of the patient.

Figures 5-10 through 5-12 illustrate the exercises used in a comprehensive core stabilization training program. Exercises may be broken down into three levels in the progressive core stabilization training program: level 1—stabilization (Figure 5-10); level 2—strengthening (Figure 5-11); and level 3—power (Figure 5-12). The patient is started with the exercises at the highest level at which the patient can maintain stability and optimal neuromuscular control. The patient is progressed through the program when the patient

achieves mastery of the exercises in the previous level.[1,2,4,10,12,15,17,18,22-25,29,34,39,42-48,55,56,62-64,67,68,73,78,79,90,91]

GUIDELINES FOR CORE STABILIZATION TRAINING

A comprehensive core stabilization training program should be systematic, progressive, and functional. The rehabilitation program should emphasize the entire muscle contraction spectrum, focusing on force production (concentric contractions), force reduction (eccentric contractions), and dynamic stabilization (isometric contractions). The core stabilization program

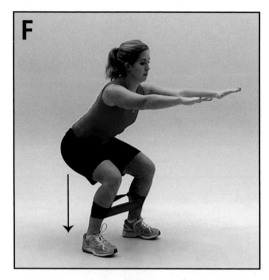

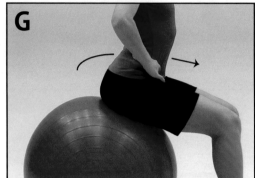

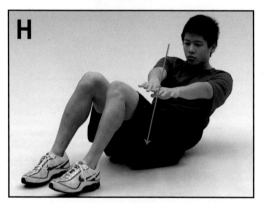

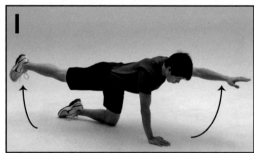

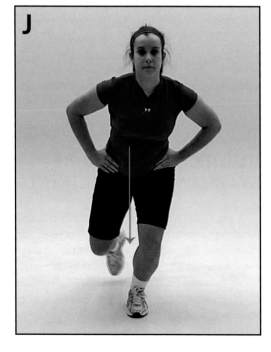

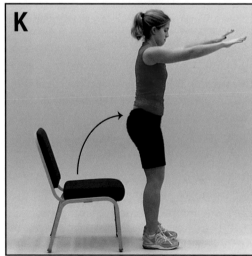

Figure 5-10. (*continued*) (F) Squats with Thera-Band. (G) Pelvic tilts on stability ball. (H) Diagonal crunches. (I) Alternating opposite arm-leg. (J) Single-leg lunge with abdominal bracing. (K) Sit-to-stand with abdominal bracing.

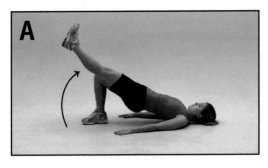

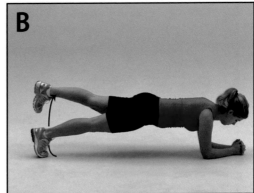

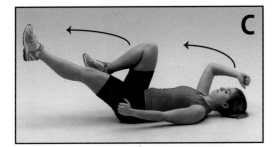

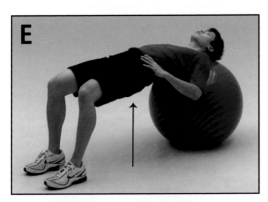

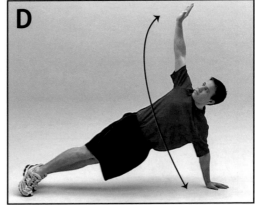

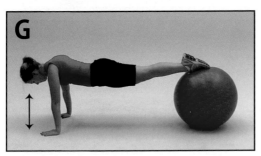

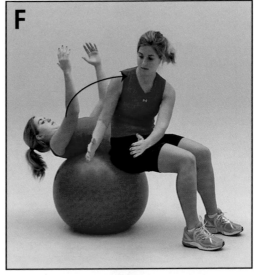

Figure 5-11. Level 2 (strength) core stability exercises. (A) Bridge with single-leg extension. (B) Front plank with single leg-extension. (C) Supine alternating arms and legs (aka: dying bug). (D) Push-up to side plank. (E) Bridging on stability ball. (F) Stability ball diagonal crunches. (G) Push-ups on therapy ball. (*continued*)

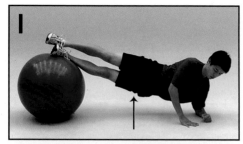

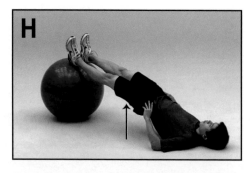

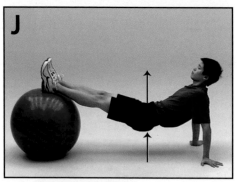

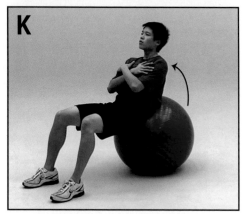

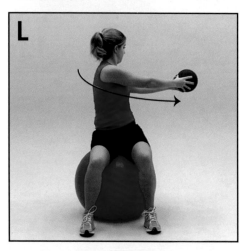

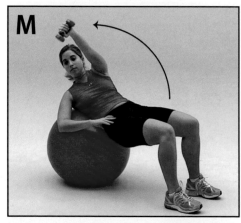

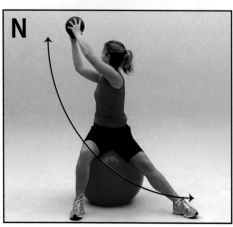

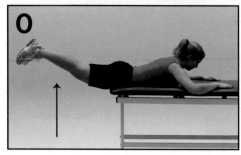

Figure 5-11. (*continued*) (H) Stability ball hip-ups. (I) Stability ball side plank. (J) Stability ball pike-ups. (K) Stability ball crunches. (L) Stability ball rotation with weighted ball. (M) Stability ball single arm dumbbell press with rotation. (N) Stability ball diagonal rotations with weighted ball. (O) Prone hip extension.

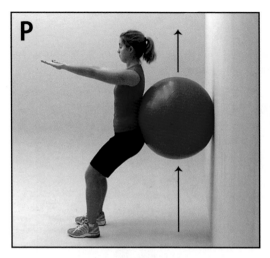

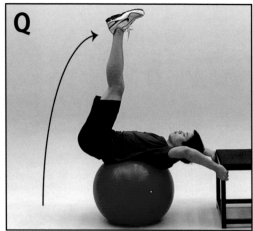

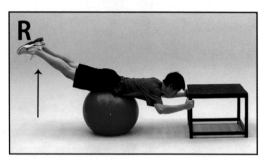

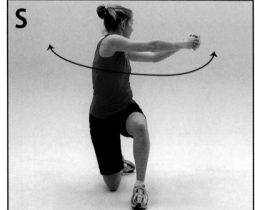

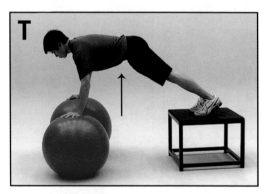

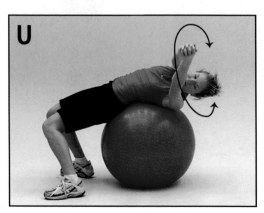

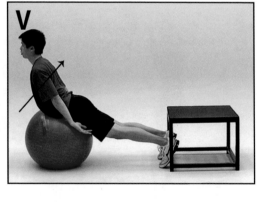

Figure 5-11. (*continued*) (P) Stability ball wall slides. (Q) Stability ball straight-leg raise. (R) Stability ball hip extension. (S) Half-kneeling rotation. (T) Stability balls two-arm support. (U) Stability ball Russian twist. (V) Stability ball prone cobra.

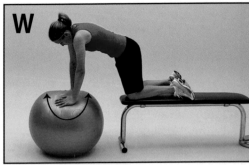

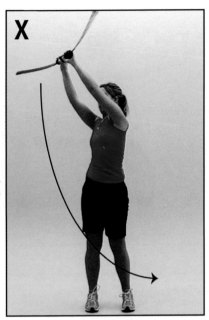

Figure 5-11. (*continued*) (W) Weight shifting on stability ball. (X) Proprioceptive neuromuscular facilitation (PNF) Bodyblade™.

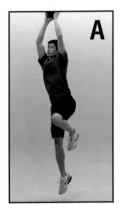
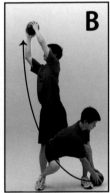
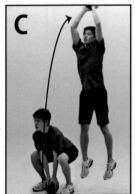
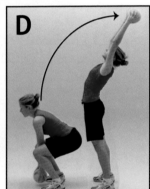

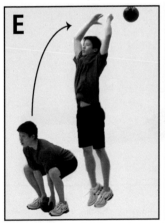
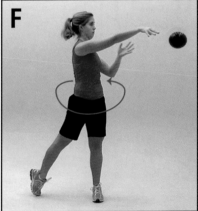
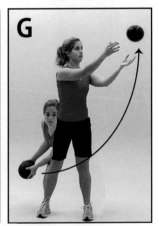

Figure 5-12. Level 3 (power) core stability exercises. (A) Weighted ball single-leg jump. (B) Weighted ball diagonal to PNF pattern. (C) Weighted ball double-leg jump. (D) Overhead extension. (E) Overhead weighted ball throw. (F) Weighted ball one-arm chest pass with rotation. (G) Weighted ball double-arm rotation toss from squat. (*continued*)

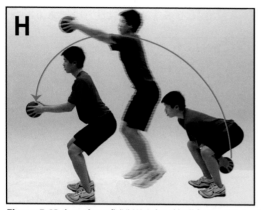
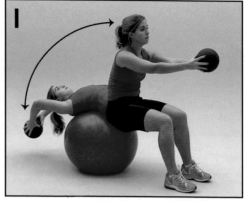

Figure 5-12. (*continued*) (H) Weighted ball forward jump from squat. (I) Stability ball pullover crunch with weighted ball.

should begin in the most challenging environment the individual can control. A progressive continuum of function should be followed to systematically progress the individual.

The program should be manipulated regularly by changing any of the following variables: plane of motion, range of motion (ROM), loading parameters (Physioball, medicine ball, Bodyblade, power sports trainer, weight vest, dumbbell, tubing), body position, amount of control, speed of execution, amount of feedback, duration (sets, reps, tempo, time under tension), and frequency (Table 5-2).

Specific Core Stabilization Guidelines

When designing a functional core stabilization training program, the athletic trainer should create a proprioceptively enriched environment and select the appropriate exercises to elicit a maximal training response. The exercises must be safe and challenging, stress multiple planes, incorporate a multisensory environment, be derived from fundamental movement skills, and be activity specific (Table 5-3).

The athletic trainer should follow a progressive functional continuum to allow optimal adaptations.[28,31,36,55] The following are key concepts for proper exercise progression: slow to fast, simple to complex, known to unknown, low force to high force, eyes open to eyes closed, static to dynamic, and correct execution to increased reps/sets/intensity (Table 5-4). [20,21,22,28,31,32,36,55]

Table 5-2 Program Variation

1. Plane of motion
2. Range of motion
3. Loading parameter
4. Body position
5. Speed of movement
6. Amount of control
7. Duration
8. Frequency

The goal of core stabilization should be to develop optimal levels of functional strength and dynamic stabilization.[1,10] Neural adaptations become the focus of the program instead of striving for absolute strength gains.[14,28,52,76] Increasing proprioceptive demand by using a multisensory, multimodal (tubing, Bodyblade, Physioball, medicine ball, power sports trainer, weight vest, cobra belt, dumbbell) environment becomes more important than increasing the external resistance.[20,32] The concept of quality before quantity is stressed. Core stabilization training is specifically designed to improve core stabilization and neuromuscular efficiency. You must be concerned with the sensory information that is stimulating the patient's central nervous system. If the patient trains with poor technique and neuromuscular control, then the patient develops poor motor patterns and stabilization.[28,55] The focus of the program must

Table 5-3 Exercise Selection

1. Safe
2. Challenging
3. Stress multiple planes
4. Proprioceptively enriched
5. Activity specific

Table 5-4 Exercise Progression

1. Slow to fast
2. Simple to complex
3. Stable to unstable
4. Low force to high force
5. General to specific
6. Correct execution to increased intensity

be on function. To determine if the program is functional, answer the following questions:

- Is it dynamic?
- Is it multiplanar?
- Is it multidimensional?
- Is it proprioceptively challenging?
- Is it systematic?
- Is it progressive?
- Is it based on functional anatomy and science?
- Is it activity specific?[28,31,55]

In summary, the core strengthening program must always start with the drawing-in maneuver that produces neuromuscular control of the TA and multifidus. Abdominal strength is not the key; rather, it is abdominal endurance

within a stabilized trunk that enhances function and may prevent or minimize injury. The trunk must be dynamic and able to move in multiple directions at various speeds, yet have internal stability that provides a strong base of support so as to support functional mobility and extremity function. The athletic trainer is only limited by the athletic trainer's own imagination in the development of core stabilization exercises. If the power position is maintained throughout the exercise sequence and the exercise is individualized to the needs of a patient, then it is an appropriate exercise! The key is to integrate individual exercises into functional patterns and simulate the demands of simple tasks and progress to the highest level of skill needed by each individual patient.

Summary

1. Functional kinetic chain rehabilitation must address each link in the kinetic chain and strive to develop functional strength and neuromuscular efficiency.

2. A core stabilization program should be an integral component for all individuals participating in a closed kinetic chain rehabilitation program.

3. A core stabilization training program will allow an individual to gain optimal neuromuscular control of the lumbo-pelvic-hip complex and allow the individual with a kinetic chain dysfunction to return to activity more quickly and safely.

4. The important core muscles do not function as prime movers; rather, they function as stabilizers.

5. There are some clinical methods of measuring the function of the TA and multifidus function.

6. Real-time ultrasound is an effective research tool for assessment of core stabilizers.

7. The Stabilizer is a useful adjunct to examination and training of the core.

8. Many possibilities exist for core training progressions. Progression is achieved by changing position, lever arms, resistance, and stability of surfaces.

9. Trunk flexion activities such as the curl and sit-up are not only unnecessary, but also may cause injury.

References

1. Aaron G. *The Use of Stabilization Training in the Rehabilitation of the Athlete. Sports Physical Therapy Home Study Course.* LaCrosse, WI: Sports Physical Therapy Section of the American Physical Therapy Association; 1996.

2. Akuthota V, Ferreiro A, Moore T. Core stability exercise principles. *Curr Sports Med Rep.* 2008;7(1):39.

3. Ashmen KJ, Swanik CB, Lephart MS. Strength and flexibility characteristics of athletes with chronic low back pain. *J Sport Rehabil.* 1996;5:275-286.

4. Aspden RM. Review of the functional anatomy of the spinal ligaments and the erector spinae muscles. *Clin Anat.* 1992;5:372-387.

5. Axler CT, McGill MS. Low back loads over a variety of abdominal exercises: searching for the safest abdominal challenge. *Med Sci Sports Exerc.* 1997;29:804-810.

6. Bartelink DL. The role of intra-abdominal pressure in relieving the pressure on the lumbar vertebral discs. *J Bone Joint Surg Br.* 1957;39:718-725.

7. Basmajian J. *Muscles Alive: Their Functions Revealed by EMG.* 5th ed. Baltimore, MD: Lippincott Williams & Wilkins; 1985.

8. Basmajian J. *Muscles Alive.* Baltimore, MD: Lippincott Williams & Wilkins; 1974.

9. Beckman SM, Buchanan ST. Ankle inversion and hyper-mobility: effect on hip and ankle muscle electromyography onset latency. *Arch Phys Med Rehabil.* 1995;76:1138-1143.

10. Beim G, Giraldo JL, Pincivero MD, et al Abdominal strengthening exercises: a comparative EMG study. *J Sport Rehabil.* 1997;6:11-20.

11. Biering-Sorenson F. Physical measurements as risk indicators for low-back trouble over a one-year period. *Spine* (Philadelphia, Pa 1976). 1984;9:106-119.

12. Blievernicht J. *Balance* [course manual]. San Diego, CA: IDEA Health and Fitness Association; 1996.

13. Bittenham D, Brittenham G. *Stronger Abs and Back.* Champaign, IL: Human Kinetics; 1997.

14. Bullock-Saxton JE, Janda V, Bullock MI. The influence of ankle sprain injury on muscle activation during hip extension. *Int J Sports Med.* 1994;15(6): 330-334.

15. Bullock-Saxton JE. Local sensation changes and altered hip muscle function following severe ankle sprain. *Phys Ther.* 1994;74:17-23.

16. Bullock-Saxton JE, Janda V, Bullock M. Reflex activation of gluteal muscles in walking: an approach to restoration of muscle function for patients with low back pain. *Spine* (Philadelphia, Pa 1976). 1993;5:704-708.

17. Callaghan JP, Gunning JL, McGill MS. Relationship between lumbar spine load and muscle activity during extensor exercises. *Phys Ther.* 1978;78(1):8-18.

18. Calliet R. *Low Back Pain Syndrome.* Oxford, UK: Blackwell; 1962.

19. Chaitow L. *Muscle Energy Techniques.* New York, NY: Churchill Livingstone; 1997.

20. Chek P. *Dynamic Medicine Ball Training* [correspondence course]. La Jolla, CA: Paul Chek Seminars; 1996.

21. Chek P. *Swiss Ball Training* [correspondence course]. La Jolla, CA: Paul Chek Seminars; 1996.

22. Chek P. *Scientific Back Training* [correspondence course]. La Jolla, CA: Paul Chek Seminars; 1994.

23. Chek P. *Scientific Abdominal Training* [correspondence course]. La Jolla, CA: Paul Chek Seminars; 1992.

24. Creager C. *Therapeutic Exercise Using Foam Rollers.* Berthoud, CO: Executive Physical Therapy; 1996.

25. Cresswell AG, Grundstrom H, Thorstensson A. Observations on intra-abdominal pressure and patterns of abdominal intra-muscular activity in man. *Acta Physiol Scand.* 1992;144:409-445.

26. Cresswell AG, Oddson L, Thorstensson A. The influence of sudden perturbations on trunk muscle activity and intra-abdominal pressure while standing. *Exp Brain Res.* 1994;98:336-341.

27. Crisco J, Panjabi MM. The intersegmental and multisegmental muscles of the lumbar spine. *Spine* (Philadelphia, Pa 1976). 1991;16:793-799.

28. Dominguez RH. *Total Body Training.* East Dundee, IL: Moving Force Systems; 1982.

29. Edgerton VR, Wolf S, Roy RR. Theoretical basis for patterning EMG amplitudes to assess muscle dysfunction. *Med Sci Sports Exerc.* 1996;28:744-751.

30. Finkelstein MM. Medical conditions, medications, and urinary incontinence: analysis of a population-based survey. *Can Fam Physician.* 2002;48:96-101.

31. Gambetta V. *Building the Complete Athlete* [course manual]. Sarasota, FL: Gambetta Sports Training Systems; 1996.

32. Gambetta V. *The Complete Guide to Medicine Ball Training.* Sarasota, FL: Optimum Sports Training; 1991.

33. Gracovetsky S, Farfan H. The optimum spine. *Spine* (Philadelphia, Pa 1976). 1986;11:543-573.

34. Gracovetsky S, Farfan H, Heuller C. The abdominal mechanism. *Spine* (Philadelphia, Pa 1976). 1985;10:317-324.

35. Grillner S, Nilsson J, Thorstensson A. Intra-abdominal pressure changes during natural movements in man. *Acta Physiol Scand.* 1978;103:275-283.

36. Gustavsen R, Streeck R. *Training Therapy: Prophylaxis and Rehabilitation.* New York, NY: Thieme; 1993.

37. Hall T, David A, Geere J, Salvenson K. *Relative Recruitment of the Abdominal Muscles During Three Levels of Exertion During Abdominal Hollowing.* Melbourne, Australia: Australian Physiotherapy Association; 1995.

38. Henry SM, Westervelt CK. The use of real-time ultrasound feedback in teaching abdominal hollowing exercises to healthy subjects. *J Orthop Sports Phys Ther.* 2005;35:338-345.

39. Hides J. Paraspinal mechanism and support of the lumbar spine. In: Richardson C, Hodges P, Hides J, eds. *Therapeutic Exercise for Lumbo-pelvic Stabilization.* 2nd ed. Philadelphia, PA: Churchill Livingstone; 2004:141-148.

40. Hides J, Richardson C, Hodges P. Local segmental control. In: Richardson C, Hodges P, Hides J, eds. *Therapeutic Exercise for Lumbo-pelvic Stabilization.* 2nd ed. Philadelphia, PA: Churchill Livingstone; 2004:185-219.

41. Hides JA, Stokes MJ, Saide M, et al Evidence of lumbar multifidus wasting ipsilateral to symptoms in subjects with acute/subacute low back pain. *Spine* (Philadelphia, Pa 1976). 1994;19:165-177.

42. Hodges P, Kaigle-Holm A, Holm S, et al Intervertebral stiffness of the spine is increased by evoked contraction of transversus abdominis and the diaphragm: in vivo porcine studies. *Spine* (Philadelphia, Pa 1976). 2003;28:2594-2601.

43. Hodges PW, Richardson AC. Contraction of the abdominal muscles associated with movement of the lower limb. *Phys Ther.* 1997;77:132.

44. Hodges PW, Richardson AC. Delayed postural contraction of transverse abdominis in low back pain associated with movement of the lower limb. *J Spinal Disord.* 1998;1:46-56.

45. Hodges PW, Richardson AC. Feed forward contraction of transverse abdominis is not influenced by the direction of arm movement. *Exp Brain Res.* 1997;114:362-370.

46. Hodges PW, Richardson AC. Inefficient muscular stabilization of the lumbar spine associated with low back pain. *Spine* (Philadelphia, Pa 1976). 1996;21:2640-2650.

47. Hodges PW, Richardson AC. Neuromotor dysfunction of the trunk musculature in low back pain patients. In: *Proceedings of the International Congress of the World Confederation of Physical Athletic Trainers.* Washington, DC; 1995.

48. Hodges PW, Richardson CA, Jull G. Evaluation of the relationship between laboratory and clinical tests of transversus abdominis function. *Physiother Res Int.* 1996;1:30-40.

49. Hodges PW, Sapsford RR, Pengel MH. Feed forward activity of the pelvic floor muscles precedes rapid upper limb movements. In *Proceedings of the 7th International Physiotherapy Congress.* Sydney, Australia; 2002.

50. Janda V. Physical therapy of the cervical and thoracic spine. In: Grant R, ed. *Physical Therapy of the Cervical and Thoracic Spine.* New York, NY: Churchill Livingstone; 1988:152-166.

51. Janda V. Muscle weakness and inhibition in back pain syndromes. In: Grieve GP, ed. *Modern Manual Therapy of the Vertebral Column.* New York, NY: Churchill Livingstone; 1986:197-201.

52. Janda V. *Muscle Function Testing.* London, UK: Butterworths; 1983.

53. Janda V. Muscles, central nervous system regulation and back problems. In: Korr IM, ed. *Neurobiologic Mechanisms in Manipulative Therapy.* New York, NY: Plenum; 1978:29.

54. Janda V, Vavrova M. *Sensory Motor Stimulation* (video). Brisbane, Australia: Body Control Systems; 1990.

55. Jesse J. *Hidden Causes of Injury, Prevention, and Correction for Running Athletes.* Pasadena, CA: Athletic Press; 1977.

56. Jorgensson A. The iliopsoas muscle and the lumbar spine. *Australian Physiotherapy.* 1993;39:125-132.

57. Jull G, Richardson CA, Comerford M. Strategies for the initial activation of dynamic lumbar stabilization. In: *Proceedings of Manipulative Physioathletic Trainers Association of Australia.* Australia; 1991.

58. Jull G, Richardson CA, Hamilton C, et al *Towards the Validation of a Clinical Test for the Deep Abdominal Muscles in Back Pain Patients.* Australia: Manipulative Physioathletic Trainers Association of Australia; 1995.

59. Kendall FP. Muscles: *Testing and Function.* 5th ed. Baltimore, MD: Lippincott Williams & Wilkins; 2005.

60. Kennedy B. An Australian program for management of back problems. *Physiotherapy.* 1980;66:108-111.

61. Lewit K. Muscular and articular factors in movement restriction. *Man Med.* 1988;1:83-85.

62. Lewit K. *Manipulative Therapy in the Rehabilitation of the Locomotor System.* London, UK: Butterworths; 1985.

63. Lewit K. Myofascial pain: relief by post-isometric relaxation. *Arch Phys Med Rehabil.* 1984;65:452.

64. Liebenson CL. *Rehabilitation of the Spine.* Baltimore: MD: Lippincott Williams & Wilkins; 1996.

65. Liebenson CL. Active muscle relaxation techniques. Part I: basic principles and methods. *J Manipulative Physiol Ther.* 1989;12:446-454.

66. Liebenson CL. Active muscle relaxation techniques. Part II: Clinical application. *J Manipulative Physiol Ther.* 1990;13(1):2-6.

67. Mayer TG, Gatchel JR. *Functional Restoration for Spinal Disorders: The Sports Medicine Approach.* Philadelphia, PA: Lea & Febiger; 1988.

68. Mayer-Posner J. *Swiss Ball Applications for Orthopedic and Sports Medicine.* Denver, CO: Ball Dynamics International; 1995.

69. McGill S. *Ultimate Back Fitness and Performance.* Waterloo: Wabuno Publishers; 2004.

70. McGill SM, Childs A, Liebenson C. Endurance times for stabilization exercises: clinical targets for testing and training from a normal database. *Arch Phys Med Rehabil.* 1999;80:941-944.

71. McGill SM, Grenier S, Bluhm M, et al Previous history of LBP with work loss is related to lingering effects in biomechanical physiological, personal, and psychosocial characteristics. *Ergonomics.* 2003;46(7):731-746.

72. Miller MI, Medeiros MJ. Recruitment of the internal oblique and transversus abdominis muscles on the eccentric phase of the curl-up. *Phys Ther.* 1987;67:1213-1217.

73. Morris JM, Benner F, Lucas BD. An electromyographic study of the intrinsic muscles of the back in man. *J Anat.* 1962;96:509-520.

74. Nachemson A. The load on the lumbar discs in different positions of the body. *Clin Orthop.* 1966;45:107-122.

75. Norris CM. Abdominal muscle training in sports. *Br J Sports Med.* 1993;27:19-27.

76. O'Sullivan PE, Twomey L, Allison G. *Evaluation of Specific Stabilizing Exercises in the Treatment of Chronic Low Back Pain with Radiological Diagnosis of Spondylolisthesis.* Australia: Manipulative Physioathletic Trainers Association of Australia; 1995.

77. O'Sullivan PE, Twomey L, Allison G, et al Altered patterns of abdominal muscle activation in patients with chronic low back pain. *Aust J Physiother.* 1997;43:91-98.

78. Panjabi MM. The stabilizing system of the spine. Part I: function, dysfunction, adaptation, and enhancement. *J Spinal Disord.* 1992;5:383-389.

79. Panjabi MM, Tech D, White AA. Basic biomechanics of the spine. *Neurosurgery.* 1990;7:76-93.

80. Porterfield JA, DeRosa C. *Mechanical Low Back Pain: Perspectives in Functional Anatomy.* Philadelphia, PA: Saunders; 1991.

81. Richardson C, Hodges P, Hides J. *Therapeutic Exercise for Lumbo-pelvic Stabilization.* 2nd ed. Philadelphia, PA: Churchill Livingstone; 2004.

82. Richardson CA, Jull G. Muscle control pain control. What exercises would you prescribe? *Man Ther.* 1996;1:2-10.

83. Richardson CA, Jull G, Toppenberg R, Comerford M. Techniques for active lumbar stabilization for spinal protection. *Aust J Physiother.* 1992;38:105-112.

84. Richardson CA, Snijders CJ, Hides JA, Damen L, Pas MS, Storm J. The relation between the transversus abdominis muscles, sacroiliac joint mechanics, and low back pain. *Spine* (Philadelphia, Pa 1976). 2002;27:399-405.

85. Robinson R. The new back school prescription: stabilization training. Part I. *Occup Med.* 1992;7:17-31.

86. Saal JA. The new back school prescription: stabilization training. Part II. *Occup Med.* 1993;7:33-42.

87. Saal JA. Nonoperative treatment of herniated disc: an outcome study. *Spine* (Philadelphia, Pa 1976). 1989;14:431-437.

88. Sahrmann S. *Diagnosis and Treatment of Movement Impairment Syndromes.* Philadelphia, PA: Elsevier; 2001.

89. Sahrmann S. Posture and muscle imbalance: faulty lumbo-pelvic alignment and associated musculoskeletal pain syndromes. *Orthop Div Rev-Can Phys Ther.* 1992;12:13-20.

90. Sapsford RR, Hodges PW, Richardson CA, Cooper DH, Markwell SJ, Jull AG. Co-activation of the abdominal and pelvic floor muscles during voluntary exercises. *Neurourol Urodyn.* 2001;20:31-42.

91. Snijders CJ, Vleeming A, Stoekart R, Mens JMA, Kleinrensink NG. Biomechanical modeling of sacroiliac joint stability in different postures. *Spine: State Art Rev.* 1995;9:419-432.

92. Stokes M, Young A. The contribution of reflex inhibition to arthrogenous muscle weakness. *Clin Sci.* 1984;67:7-14.

93. Tesh KM, Shaw Dunn J, Evans HJ. The abdominal muscles and vertebral stability. *Spine* (Philadelphia, Pa 1976). 1987;12:501-508.

94. Teyhen DS, Miltenberger CE, Deiters MH, et al The use of ultrasound imaging of the abdominal drawing-in maneuver in subjects with low back pain. *J Orthop Sports Phys Ther.* 2005;35:346-355.

95. Thomson KD. On the bending moment capability of the pressurized abdominal cavity during human lifting activity. *Ergonomics.* 1988;31:817-828.

96. Warmerdam ALA. *Arthrokinetic Therapy: Manual Therapy to Improve Muscle and Joint Functioning. Continuing education course, Marshfield, WI.* Port Moody, British Columbia, Canada: Arthrokinetic Therapy and Publishing; 1996.

97. Wilke HJ, Wolf S, Claes EL. Stability increase of the lumbar spine with different muscle groups: a biomechanical in vitro study. *Spine* (Philadelphia, Pa 1976). 1995;20:192-198.

SOLUTIONS TO CLINICAL DECISION-MAKING EXERCISES

5-1   Decreased stabilization endurance in individuals with low back pain with decreased firing of the transversus abdominis, internal oblique, multifidus, and deep erector spinae. Training without proper control of these muscles can lead to improper muscle imbalances and force transmission. Poor core stability can lead to increased intradiscal pressure. Core training will improve the gymnast's posture, muscle balance, and static and dynamic stabilization.

5-2   It could be that she has poor postural control because of a weak core. She probably never regained neuromuscular control of her core following the knee injury. Tennis requires a lot of upper-body movement, so she would probably benefit from core strengthening that would allow her to control her lumbo-pelvic-hip complex while she plays. In choosing her exercises, you should make sure that they are safe and challenging and stress multiple planes that are functional as they are applied to tennis. The exercises should also be proprioceptively enriched and activity-specific.

5-3   Individuals with poor core strength are likely to develop low back pain due to improper muscle stability. The straight leg lowering test is a good way to assess core strength. The athlete should lie supine on a table with hips flexed to 90 degrees and lower back completely flat against the table. To decrease the lordotic curve, instruct the patient to perform a drawing-in maneuver. The patient then lowers the legs slowly to the table. The test is over when the back starts to arch off of the table. A blood pressure cuff can be used under the low back to observe an increase in the lordotic curve. Someone with a weak core will not be able to maintain the flattened posture for very long while lowering the legs.

5-4   To progress the patient and keep her interested in her rehabilitation program, change her program frequently. Consider these variables as you plan changes: plane of motion, ROM, loading parameter (Physioballs, tubing, medicine balls, body blades, etc.), body position (from supine to standing), speed of movement, amount of control, duration (sets and reps), and frequency.

5-5   Your ultimate goal with core strengthening is functional strength and dynamic stability. As the athlete progresses, the emphasis should change in these ways: from slow to fast, from simple to complex, from stable to unstable, from low force to high force, from general to specific, and from correct execution to increased intensity. Once the patient has gained awareness of proper muscle firing, encourage her to perform her exercises in a more functional manner. Because activities in most sports require multi-plane movement, design her exercises to mimic those requirements.

5-6   Dynamic PNF with a power ball would be ideal for him. The ball will provide a loading parameter, and his ROM will be functional for the demands of his sport. Adding a twisting component is important so that he is not just training in a single plane of motion prior to swinging his club.

Please see videos on the accompanying website at

www.healio.com/books/sportsmedvideos

CHAPTER 6

Reestablishing Neuromuscular Control

Scott Lephart, PhD, ATC
C. Buz Swanik, PhD, ATC
Troy Blackburn, PhD, ATC

After completion of this chapter, the athletic training student should be able to do the following:

- Explain why neuromuscular control is essential in the rehabilitation process.

- Define proprioception, kinesthesia, neuromuscular control, and stiffness.

- Explain the physiology of articular and tenomuscular mechanoreceptors.

- Describe the afferent and efferent neural pathways.

- Recognize the importance of feedforward and feedback neuromuscular control.

- Identify the various techniques for reestablishing neuromuscular

control in both the upper and the lower extremities.

WHAT IS NEUROMUSCULAR CONTROL?

Neuromuscular control refers to the efferent (motor) response to sensory information.[76] Several sources of sensory information are essential for producing adequate muscle activity and dynamic joint stability including proprioception, kinesthesia, and force sense. Proprioception refers to conscious and unconscious appreciation of joint position, whereas kinesthesia is the sensation of joint motion or acceleration.[115] The perception of force (force sense) is the ability to estimate joint and musculotendinous loads.[77] These signals are transmitted to the spinal cord via afferent (sensory) pathways. Conscious awareness of joint motion, position, and force is essential for

Prentice WE, ed.
Rehabilitation Techniques for Sports Medicine and Athletic Training (pp 151-180).
© 2015 SLACK Incorporated.

motor learning and the anticipation of movements, while unconscious proprioception modulates muscle function and initiates reflex joint stabilization. As such, neuromuscular control encompasses motor output that is responsible for producing movement, and providing dynamic joint stability and postural stability.

Two motor control mechanisms (feedforward and feedback) are involved with interpreting afferent information and coordinating efferent responses.[37,77] Feedforward neuromuscular control involves planning movements based on "real-time" sensory information that is integrated with learned somatosensory patterns from past experiences,[37,91] while feedback processes continuously regulate muscle activity through reflex pathways. Feedforward mechanisms are responsible for preparatory muscle activity; feedback processes are associated with reactive/reflexive muscle activity. Because of skeletal muscle's orientation and activation characteristics, a diverse array of movement capabilities can be coordinated involving concentric, eccentric, and isometric contractions, while excessive joint motion is restricted. Therefore dynamic restraint is achieved through preparatory and reflexive neuromuscular control.[36,37,54,58,68]

Muscle activity enhances dynamic joint stability by increasing joint congruency, providing eccentric absorption of external forces applied to the body, and increasing muscle stiffness. Many joints (eg, glenohumeral and tibiofemoral) possess limited bony congruency, and are, therefore, reliant on muscle activation to limit loading of passive capsuloligamentous structures. An enhancement in joint stability can be achieved via muscle activity by increasing compressive force across the joint and increasing joint contact area such as occurs when the rotator cuff pulls the humeral head into the glenoid fossa. Muscle activity also limits loading of passive tissues by providing eccentric absorption of force applied to the body (ie, "shock absorption"). For example, Norcross et al[117] demonstrated that lower extremity energy absorption characteristics influence biomechanical factors associated with anterior cruciate ligament loading and injury.

The level of muscle activation, whether it is preparatory or reactive, greatly modifies the muscle's stiffness properties.[70,116,124] From a mechanical perspective, muscle stiffness is the ratio of the change of force to the change in length.[5,36,38] In essence, muscles that are more stiff resist stretching episodes more effectively and provide more effective dynamic restraint to joint displacement.[5,108] Therefore muscle stiffness generated by feedforward neuromuscular activity prior to joint loading is one of the most important mechanisms used for dynamic restraint of joints.[70,129,136,139] However, high stiffness would not permit the fast joint motions necessary for physical activity, so muscle stiffness regulation occurs continuously to optimize both joint stability to motion.[148,149] Clinical studies have recently established the importance of muscle stiffness in the dynamic restraint system.[55,63,70,138] In the knee, for example, increasing hamstring muscle activation also increases hamstring stiffness, and there is a moderate correlation between the degree of muscle stiffness in ACL-deficient patients and their functional ability.[108,138] Additionally, individuals with greater hamstring stiffness display less anterior tibial translation in response to joint perturbation and lesser frontal and sagittal plane knee loading.[15,17] Therefore, efficient regulation of muscle stiffness might embody all of the components in the dynamic restraint system, and thus be vital for restoring functional stability.

WHY IS NEUROMUSCULAR CONTROL CRITICAL TO THE REHABILITATION PROCESS?

Reestablishing neuromuscular control is a critical component in the rehabilitation of pathological joints. The objective of neuromuscular control activities is to refocus the patient's awareness of peripheral sensations and process these signals into more coordinated motor strategies. This muscle activity serves to protect joint structures from excessive strain and provides a prophylactic mechanism to recurrent injury. Neuromuscular control activities are intended to complement traditional rehabilitation protocols, which encompass the

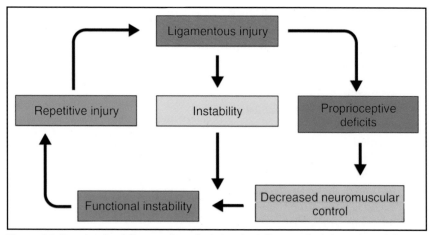

Figure 6-1. Functional stability paradigm depicting the influence of mechanical instability and proprioceptive deficits on neuromuscular control and functional stability, which predisposes the knee to repetitive injury.

modulation of pain and inflammation, restoration of flexibility, strength, and endurance, as well as psychological considerations. In the domain of joint motion and position awareness, basic science research has provided insight into the sensory and/or motor characteristics of structures regulating neuromuscular control. Peripheral mechanoreceptors within articular and tenomuscular structures mediate neuromuscular control by conveying joint motion and position sense to the individual. The primary roles of articular structures such as the capsule, ligaments, menisci, and labrum are to stabilize and guide skeletal segments while providing mechanical restraint to abnormal joint movements.[1] However, capsuloligamentous tissue also has a sensory role essential for detecting joint motion and position.[47,78,127]

Injury to articular structures results not only in a mechanical disturbance that manifests a joint laxity, but also in a loss of joint sensation. In addition to ligamentous tears, microscopic nerves from peripheral mechanoreceptors may also be damaged; this is referred to as deafferentation.[75,124,131] This partial deafferentation disrupts sensory feedback necessary for reflexive joint stabilization and neuromuscular coordination. There is substantial evidence suggesting that the aberrations in muscle activity subsequent to joint injury are a result of disrupted neural pathways.[12,18,75,102121,144,150] Therefore, joint pathology not only reduces mechanical stability, it often diminishes the

capability of the dynamic restraint system, rendering the joint functionally unstable (Figure 6-1). The concept of mechanical vs functional stability can be illustrated by comparisons of ACL-deficient and ACL-reconstructed patients. Some ACL-deficient individuals, labeled "copers" by Chmielewski et al[26,27] are capable of high levels of function and dynamic joint stability in the presence of inherent mechanical instability attributable to the absence of the ACL. These individuals develop enhanced dynamic restraint capabilities via the rehabilitation process, potentially by enhancing hamstring stiffness.[109] Conversely, ACL-reconstruction results in mechanical stability of the knee joint as evidenced by reduced anterior knee laxity,[2] but some ACL-reconstructed patients experience sensations of the joint "giving way," which are indicative of functional instability.[112]

The goal of reconstructive surgery is to restore mechanical stability, but evidence strongly supports the reinnervation of graft tissue by peripheral receptors.[118] Therefore surgery, combined with rehabilitation, promotes several neuromuscular characteristics associated with the dynamic restraint system.[97,98] Clinical research has revealed a number of activities that enhance these characteristics and are beneficial to developing neuromuscular control.[25,65,140] To accomplish this, clinicians must identify the peripheral and central neuromuscular characteristics that compensate for mechanical insufficiencies and encourage these adaptations to restore functional stability.

Rehabilitation of the pathological joint should address the preparatory (feedforward) and reactive (feedback) neuromuscular control mechanisms required for joint stability. The four elements crucial for reestablishing neuromuscular control and functional stability are joint sensation (position, motion, and force), dynamic stability, preparatory and reactive muscle characteristics, and conscious and unconscious functional motor patterns.[96,135] The following sections will define the sensory receptors and neural pathways that contribute to normal joint stabilization. The theoretical framework for reestablishing neuromuscular control will be presented, followed by specific activities designed to encourage the peripheral, spinal, and cortical adaptations crucial for improving functional stability.

THE PHYSIOLOGY OF MECHANORECEPTORS

Articular Mechanoreceptors

The dynamic restraint system is mediated by specialized nerve endings called mechanoreceptors.[57] A mechanoreceptor functions by transducing mechanical deformation of tissue (eg, stretching, compression) into frequency-modulated neural signals.[57] Increased tissue deformation is coded by an increased afferent discharge rate (action potentials/second) or a rise in the quantity of mechanoreceptors stimulated.[57,60] These signals provide sensory information concerning internal and external forces acting on the joint. Three morphological types of mechanoreceptors have been identified in joints: Pacinian corpuscles, Meissner corpuscles, and free nerve endings.[47,57,80] These mechanoreceptors are classified as either quick adapting (QA), because they cease discharging shortly after the onset of a stimulus, or slow adapting (SA), because they continue to discharge as long as the stimulus is present.[29,47,57,78,126] In healthy joints, QA mechanoreceptors are believed to provide conscious and unconscious kinesthetic sensations in response to joint movement or acceleration while SA

mechanoreceptors provide continuous feedback and thus proprioceptive information relative to joint position.[29,49,57,130]

Tenomuscular Mechanoreceptors

Any change in joint position simultaneously alters muscle length and tension. Muscle spindles, embedded within skeletal muscle, detect length and rate of length changes, transmitting these signals to the central nervous system (CNS) through the fastest afferent nerves.[6,28,60] This sensory information from the muscle spindle regarding changes in muscle length and the rate of change in muscle length (Type Ia afferent neurons) contributes to the sensation of kinesthesia, while input regarding muscle length (Type II afferent neurons) contributes to proprioception. Muscle spindles are also innervated by small motor fibers called gamma efferents.[6,60,94] Having these motor fibers permits the muscle spindle to become more sensitive, if necessary, and accommodates for changes in muscle length while continuously transmitting afferent signals.[6,60,74,76] Muscle spindle afferents project directly on skeletal motoneurons through monosynaptic reflexes.[152] When muscle spindles are stimulated, they elicit a reflex contraction in the agonist muscle.[74,111,152]

Golgi tendon organs (GTO) are also capable of regulating muscle activity and are responsible for monitoring muscle tension or load.[40,69] Located within the tendon and tenomuscular junction, GTOs are force detectors and thus are able to protect the tenomuscular unit by reflexively inhibiting muscle activation when high tension might cause damage. During physical activity, moderate levels of muscle tension may actually reverse this reflex, thus making muscle tension a stimulus to muscle recruitment. Generally, with high muscle tension GTOs would have the opposite effect of muscle spindles by producing a reflex inhibition (relaxation) in the muscle being loaded.[57,69]

Cutaneous Receptors

Pressure and stretch receptors located in the skin are thought to contribute to proprioception, kinesthesia, and force sense. Their involvement with force sense is intuitive, as compression of the skin against an object such as occurs in the fingers and hand while grasping an object provides an indication of the force being exerted on the object. Similarly, joint motion causes stretching and compression on opposites of a joint, thus contributing to sensations of joint position and motion. These notions are supported by research demonstrating improvements in proprioception and neuromuscular control with the use of compression devices (eg, bandages and neoprene sleeves) and athletic tape.[31,32,72,128]

NEURAL PATHWAYS OF PERIPHERAL AFFERENTS

Understanding the extent to which articular and tenomuscular sensory information is used requires analysis of the reflexive and cortical pathways employed by peripheral afferents. Encoded signals concerning joint motion, position, and force are transmitted from peripheral receptors, via afferent pathways, to the spinal cord.[39,47] Within the spinal cord, interneurons link ascending pathways (tracts) to the cerebral cortex to permit conscious appreciation of proprioception, kinesthesia, and force. Two reflexive pathways couple articular receptors with motor nerves and tenomuscular receptors in the spinal column. A third monosynaptic reflex pathway links the muscle spindles directly with motor nerves.

Sensory information from the periphery is used by the cerebral cortex for somatosensory awareness and feedforward neuromuscular control, whereas balance and postural control are processed at the brainstem.[29,49,60,77] Balance is influenced by the same peripheral afferent mechanism that mediates joint proprioception and is partially dependent upon the inherent ability to integrate somatosensory input (joint position sense and kinesthesia) with vision and the vestibular apparatus. Any disassociation between these three sensory modalities can quickly lead to exaggerated postural sway. Balance, therefore, is frequently used to measure sensorimotor integration and functional joint stability because deficits can result from aberrations in the afferent feedback loop of the lower extremity. Synapses in the spinal cord link afferent fibers from articular and tenomuscular receptors with efferent motor nerves, constituting the reflex loops between sensory information and motor responses. This reflexive neuromotor link contributes to dynamic stability by using the feedback process for reactive muscular activation.[18,121,133] Interneurons within the spinal column also connect articular receptors and GTOs with large motor nerves innervating muscles and small gamma motor nerves innervating muscle spindles. Johansson[73] contends that articular afferent pathways do not exert as much influence directly on skeletal motoneurons as previously reported, but rather they have more frequent and potent effects on muscle spindles. Muscle spindles, in turn, regulate muscle activation through the monosynaptic stretch reflex. Articular afferents therefore have some influence on the large skeletal motor nerves as well as the spindle receptors, via gamma motor nerves.[73,75]

This sophisticated articular-tenomuscular link has been described as the "final common input."[3,75] The final common input suggests that muscle spindles integrate peripheral afferent information and transmit a final modified signal to the CNS.[3,75] This feedback loop is responsible for continuously modifying muscle activity during locomotion via the muscle spindle's stretch reflex arc.[67,116] By coordinating reflexive and descending motor commands, muscle stiffness is modified and dynamic stability is maintained.[75,85]

Several reflexes derived from peripheral mechanoreceptors contribute to dynamic joint stability. Increases in muscle length such as those occurring with joint perturbation (eg, the peroneals during rapid ankle inversion) excite muscle spindle afferents. The resulting afferent volleys result in spinal (short latency), medium-latency, and long-latency stretch reflex responses based on the extent of central processing. These reflex responses, in turn, provide heightened resistance to further muscle lengthening, thus resisting joint motion.[13]

Similarly, mechanoreceptors in ligament have been demonstrated to elicit reflexive responses in the musculature antagonistic to the imposed loading. For example, tensile loading of the anterior cruciate ligament elicits a reflexive response in the hamstrings designed

Figure 6-2. Diagram depicting the influence of muscle stiffness on electromechanical delay and muscle spindle sensitivity, which enhances the reactive characteristics of muscle for dynamic joint restraint.

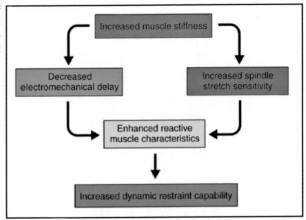

to limit ligament loading (ie, the ligament stress-elicited reflex).[48,125]

FEEDFORWARD AND FEEDBACK NEUROMUSCULAR CONTROL

The efferent response of muscles transforming neural information into physical energy is termed *neuromuscular control*.[76] Traditional beliefs about the processing of afferent signals into efferent responses for dynamic stabilization were based on reactive or feedback neuromuscular control pathways.[94] More contemporary theories emphasize the significance of preactivated muscle tension in anticipation of movements and joint loads. Preactivation suggests that prior sensory feedback (experience) concerning the task is used to preprogram muscle activation patterns. For example, visual input is combined with "sensory memories" from previous experiences to increase preparatory activity of lower extremity musculature with increasing landing height in anticipation of greater impact forces.[45,50] This process is described as feedforward neuromuscular control.[36,38,56,91] Feedforward motor control uses advance information about a task, usually from experience, to determine the most coordinated strategy for executing the impending functional task.[37,91] These centrally generated motor commands are responsible for preparatory muscle activity and high-velocity movements.[77] Preparatory

muscle activity serves several functions that contribute to the dynamic restraint system. By increasing muscle activation levels, the stiffness properties of the entire tenomuscular unit are enhanced.[113] This increased muscle activation and stiffness can drastically improve the stretch sensitivity of the muscle spindle system while reducing the electromechanical delay required to develop muscle tension.[30,36,58,68,75,108,113,124] EMD refers to the period that elapses between the arrival of a neural impulse (electrical) initiating muscle contraction and the development of force (mechanical). Clinical research has also shown that the stretch reflex can increase muscle stiffness one to three times.[61,103] Heightened stretch sensitivity and stiffness could improve the reactive capabilities of muscle by providing additional sensory feedback and superimposing stretch reflexes onto descending motor commands.[36,74,110] Whether muscle stiffness increases stretch sensitivity or decreases electromechanical delay (or both), it appears to be crucial for dynamic restraint and functional stability (Figure 6-2). Preactivated muscles therefore can provide quick compensation for external loads and are critical for dynamic joint stability.[36,58] Sensory information about the performance is then used to evaluate the results based on how the brain expected the task to feel, and helps arrange future muscle coordination strategies.

The feedback mechanism of motor control is characterized by numerous reflex pathways continuously adjusting ongoing muscle activity.[19,37,94,111] Information from joint and muscle receptors can reflexively initiate and coordinate muscle activity for motor tasks. This feedback process, however, can result in long conduction delays and is best equipped for maintaining posture and regulating slow stereotyped movements such as walking.[77] For example, Konradsen demonstrated that the combination of conduction delays and EMD prolonged the reflexive response of the peroneal musculature to sudden inversion such that it was incapable of preventing capsuloligamentous loading.[86] The efficacy of reflex-mediated dynamic stabilization is therefore related to the speed and magnitude of joint perturbations. It is unclear what relative contribution feedback-mediated muscle reflexes provide when in vivo loads are placed on joints.

Both feedforward and feedback neuromuscular control can enhance dynamic stability if the sensory and motor pathways are frequently stimulated. Each time a signal passes through a sequence of synapses, the synapses become more capable of transmitting the same signal.[61,66] When these pathways are "facilitated" regularly, memory of that signal is created and can be recalled to program future movements.[61] Frequent facilitation therefore enhances both the memory about tasks for preprogrammed motor control and reflex pathways for reactive neuromuscular control. Therefore, rehabilitation exercise must be executed with technical precision, repetition, and controlled progression for these physiological adaptations to occur and enhance neuromuscular control.

REESTABLISHING NEUROMUSCULAR CONTROL

Patients who have sustained damage to the articular structures in the upper or lower extremities exhibit distinctive proprioceptive, kinesthetic, and neuromuscular deficits.[7,8,12,18,93,98,101,105,129,130,132,151] Although identifying these abnormalities might be difficult in a clinical setting, a thorough appreciation of the pathoetiology of these conditions is necessary to guide clinicians who are attempting to reestablish neuromuscular control and functional stability. Most researchers believe that disruption of the articular structures

results in some level of deafferentation to ligamentous and probably capsular mechanoreceptors.[40,42,93,98,99,130,132] In the acute phase of healing, joint inflammation and pain can compound sensory deficits; however, this cannot account for the chronic deficits in proprioception and kinesthesia associated with pathological joints.[10,80] Research has demonstrated that patients with congenital or pathological joint laxity have diminished capability for detecting joint motion and position.[46,52,132] These proprioceptive and kinesthetic characteristics, coupled with mechanical instability, can lead to functional instability.[94,135]

Developing or reestablishing proprioception, kinesthesia, and neuromuscular control in injured patients will minimize the risk of reinjury. Capsuloligamentous retensioning and reconstruction, coupled with traditional rehabilitation, is one option that appears to restore some kinesthetic awareness, although not equal to that of noninvolved limbs.[35,98,118]

The objective of neuromuscular rehabilitation is to develop or reestablish afferent and efferent characteristics that enhance dynamic restraint capabilities with respect to in vivo loads. Four basic elements are crucial to reestablishing neuromuscular control and functional stability:

1. Proprioceptive and kinesthetic sensation

2. Dynamic joint stabilization

3. Reactive neuromuscular control

4. Functional motor patterns.[94]

In the pathological joint, these dynamic mechanisms may be compromised due to deafferentation and can result in a functionally stable joint. Several afferent and efferent characteristics contribute to the efficient regulation of these elements and the maintenance of neuromuscular control. These characteristics include the sensitivity of peripheral receptors and facilitation of afferent pathways, muscle stiffness, the onset rate and magnitude of muscle activity, agonist/antagonist coactivation, reflex muscle activation, and discriminatory muscle activation. Specific rehabilitation techniques allow these characteristics to be modified, significantly impacting dynamic stability and function.[12,25,65,71,93,140]

Although more prospective clinical research is needed to establish the "best practice" approach in support of the evidence-based medical model, several exercise techniques show promise for inducing beneficial adaptations to these characteristics. The plasticity of the neuromuscular system to change is what permits rapid modifications during rehabilitation that ultimately enhance preparatory and reactive muscle activity.[12,66,69,71,135,137,138,150] The techniques include open and closed kinetic chain activities, balance training, eccentric and high-repetition/low-load exercises, reflex facilitation through reactive or "perturbation" training, stretch-shortening activities, and biofeedback training. Traditional rehabilitation, accompanied by these specific techniques, results in beneficial adaptations to the neuromuscular characteristics responsible for dynamic restraint, enhancing their efficiency for providing a functionally stable joint. It is generally accepted that the rapid performance gains observed within 6 to 8 weeks of initiating a conditioning program result from neuromuscular adaptations; however, without at least continuous maintenance, these adaptations will dissipate.[60,77]

To restore dynamic muscle activation necessary for functional stability, one must employ simulated positions of vulnerability that necessitate reactive muscle stabilization. Although there are inherent risks in placing the joint in positions of vulnerability, if this is done in a controlled and progressive fashion, neuromuscular adaptations will occur and subsequently permit the patient to return to competitive situations with confidence that the dynamic mechanisms will protect the joint from subluxation and reinjury.

Clinical Decision-Making Exercise 6-1

Following a grade 2 ankle sprain and a rehabilitation program to regain strength in the lateral lower leg muscles, your soccer patient continues to sustain repeated inversion ankle injuries during cutting maneuvers. What components of neuromuscular control might be deficient in this patient? What type of rehabilitation exercises should you implement to enhance neuromuscular control?

Neuromuscular Characteristics

Peripheral Afferent Receptors

The foundation for feedback and feedforward neuromuscular control is based on reliable motion, position, and force information. Altered peripheral afferent information can disrupt motor control and functional stability. Closed kinetic chain exercises create axial loads that maximally stimulate articular receptors, especially near the end range of motion (ROM), while tenomuscular receptors are excited by changes in length and tension.[28,57,75,146,147,154] Open chain activities may require more conscious awareness of limb position because of the non-constrained and freely moving distal segment. Performing open or closed chain exercises under weighted conditions increases the level of difficulty and coactivation, which may be used as a training stimulus.[92] Chronic athletic participation can also enhance proprioceptive and kinesthetic acuity by repeatedly facilitating afferent pathways from peripheral receptors. Highly conditioned patients demonstrate greater appreciation of joint kinesthesia and more accurately reproduce limb position than sedentary controls do.[9,99,103] Whether this is a congenital endowment or a training adaptation, greater awareness of joint motion and position can improve feedforward and feedback neuromuscular control.[99]

Muscle Stiffness

It is evident that muscle stiffness has a significant role in preparatory and reactive dynamic restraint by resisting and absorbing joint loads.[70,106,108,109,139] Therefore exercise modes that optimize muscle stiffness should be encouraged during rehabilitation. Research by Bulbulian and Pousson[21,123] has established that eccentric loading increases muscle tone and stiffness and several authors have demonstrated increases in muscle stiffness with isometric loading.[22,88,89,16] The GTO receptor is normally associated with muscle inhibition and thus protects the tenomuscular unit from excessive strain. However, chronic overloading of the musculotendinous unit may result in connective tissue proliferation around GTOs that, in effect, desensitizes this mechanoreceptor to muscle tension. If this inhibitor effect can be decreased, reactive muscle stiffening may be facilitated through increased muscle spindle activity.[69] It is also known that during functional activities GTO inhibition reverses and may actually enhance muscle recruitment.[77] Such evolutions impact both the neuromuscular and the tendinous components of stiffness.[21,54,113,123]

Training techniques that emphasize low loads and high repetitions cause connective tissue adaptations similar to those found with eccentric training. However, increased muscle stiffness resulting from this rehabilitation technique can be attributed to fiber type transition.[54,69,87,90] Slow-twitch fibers have longer crossbridge cycle times and can maintain the prolonged, low-intensity contractions necessary for postural control.[90] In the animal model, Goubel[54] found that low-load/high-repetition training resulted in higher muscle stiffness, compared to strength training. However, Kyrolaninen's[90] analysis of power- and endurance-trained patients inferred that muscle stiffness was greater in the power-trained individuals because the onset of muscle preactivation (EMG) was faster and higher prior to joint loading. It appears that endurance training might enhance stiffness by increasing the baseline motor tone and crossbridge formation time, whereas power training alters the rate and magnitude of muscle tension during preactivation. Both of these adaptations readily adhere to existing principles of progressive rehabilitation, where early strengthening exercises focus on low loads with high repetitions, progressing to shorter, more explosive, sport-specific activities. Research assessing the efficacy of low load/high repetition training vs. high load/low repetition training would be beneficial for optimizing muscle stiffness and functional progression in the injured patient.

Reflex Muscle Activation

Various training modes also cause neuromuscular adaptations that might account for discrepancies in the reflex latency times between power- and endurance-trained patients. Sprint- and/or power-trained individuals have more vigorous reflex responses (tendon-tap) relative to sedentary and endurance-trained samples.[83,84,143] McComas[107] suggests that strength training increases descending (cortical) drive to the large motor nerves of skeletal muscle and the small efferent fibers to muscle spindles, referred to as alpha-gamma coactivation. Increasing both muscle tension and efferent drive to muscle spindles results in a heightened sensitivity to stretch, consequently reducing reflex latencies.[69] Melvill-Jones[110] suggests that the stretch reflexes are superimposed on preprogrammed muscle activity from higher centers, illustrating the concomitant use of feedforward and feedback neuromuscular control for regulating preparatory and reactive muscle stiffness. Therefore, preparatory and reactive muscle activation might improve dynamic stability and function if muscle stiffness is enhanced in a mechanically insufficient or reconstructed joint.

A limited number of clinical training studies have been directed at improving reaction times.[12,71,150] Ihara[71] significantly reduced the latency of muscle reactions during a 3-week period by inducing perturbations to patients on unstable platforms. Several other researchers later confirmed this finding with rehabilitation programs designed to improve reflex muscle activation.[12,150] Beard[12] and Wojtys[150] suggest that agility-type training in the lower extremity produces more desirable muscle reaction times when compared to strength training. This research has significant implications for reestablishing the reactive capability of the dynamic restraint system. Reducing the electromechanical delay between protective muscle activation and joint loading can increase dynamic stability and function. Fitzgerald et al[43,44] describe a perturbation training program that is dependent on a sense of force feedback. Patients are exposed to rotatory and translatory movement that progress from predictable perturbations to random, and from small/slow movements to those that are large/fast. Key instruction for the success of the exercises is to match the perturbation but not under- or overreact. This is critical to the concept of optimal stiffness regulation. Overstiffening a muscle/joint complex may provide stability but is not functional while understiffening may permit episodes of "giving way" or "buckling."

Surgical reconstruction presents a challenge to the rehabilitation process. Controlled loading of the graft via rehabilitation facilitates the

Figure 6-3. Biofeedback training reestablishes discriminative muscle control, eliminating muscle imbalance and promoting functionally specific muscle activation patterns.

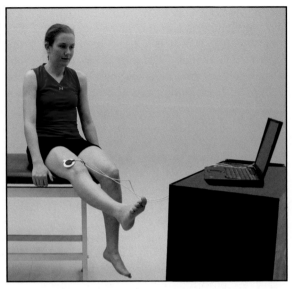

"ligamentization" process during which the morphological properties of a tendon autograft (eg, the patellar tendon following ACL reconstruction) gradually reflect those of ligament,[41,134] and mechanical stability is generally restored to the joint.[14,53] However, sensory information derived from the joint is compromised due to the loss of mechanoreceptors in the native ligament, resulting in sensory and motor deficits.[24,33,95] However, the rehabilitation process also appears to facilitate reinnervation of graft tissue by peripheral receptors and reestablishment of ligament stress-elicited reflexes.[8,118,142] These changes highlight the essential of rehabilitation in reestablishing neuromuscular control.

Discriminative Muscle Activation

In addition to reactive muscle firing, unconscious control of muscle activity is critical for coordination and balancing joint forces. This is most evident relative to the force couples described for the shoulder complex. Restoring the force couples of agonist and antagonists might initially require conscious, discriminative muscle activation before unconscious control is reacquired. Biofeedback training provides instantaneous sensory feedback concerning specific muscle contractions and can help patients correct errors by consciously altering or redistributing muscle activity.[11,51] The objective of biofeedback training is to reacquire

voluntary muscle control and promote functionally specific motor patterns, eventually converting these patterns from conscious to unconscious control[11] (Figure 6-3). Using biofeedback for discriminative muscle control can help eliminate muscle imbalances while reestablishing preparatory and reactive muscle activity for dynamic joint stability.[37,51]

Elements for Neuromuscular Control

Proprioception and Kinesthesia

The objective of kinesthetic and proprioceptive training is to restore the neurosensory properties of injured capsuloligamentous structures and enhance the sensitivity of uninvolved peripheral afferents.[102] To what degree this occurs in conservatively managed patients is unknown; however, ligament retensioning and reconstruction coupled with extensive rehabilitation does appear to normalize joint motion and position sense.[10,98,118]

Joint compression is believed to maximally stimulate articular receptors and can be accomplished with closed chain exercises throughout the available ROM.[28,57,75,146,147] Early joint-repositioning tasks enhance conscious proprioceptive and kinesthetic awareness, eventually leading to unconscious appreciation of joint motion and position. Applying a neoprene sleeve or elastic bandage can provide additional

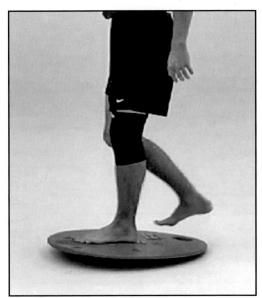

Figure 6-4. Neoprene sleeves stimulate cutaneous receptors, providing additional sensory feedback for joint motion and position awareness.

proprioceptive and kinesthetic information by stimulating cutaneous receptors[10,120] (Figure 6-4). Exercises that simultaneously involve the noninjured limb may help reestablish conscious awareness of joint position, motion, and load in the injured extremity. To increase the level of difficulty, these exercises can be performed under moderate loads.[92]

Dynamic Stabilization

The objective of dynamic joint stabilization exercises is to encourage preparatory agonist/antagonist coactivation. Efficient coactivation restores the force couples necessary to balance joint forces and increase joint congruency, thereby reducing the loads imparted to the static structures. Dynamic stabilization from muscles requires anticipating and reacting to joint loads. This includes placing the joint in positions of vulnerability where dynamic support is established under controlled conditions. Balance and stretch-shortening exercises (eg, plyometrics) require both preparatory and reactive muscle activity through feedforward and feedback motor control systems, while closed kinetic chain exercises are excellent for inducing coactivation and compression. Chimura[25] and Hewett[46] have confirmed that

stretch-shortening exercises increase muscle coactivation and enhance coordination.

Reactive Neuromuscular Control

Reactive neuromuscular training focuses on stimulating the reflex AB pathways from articular and tenomuscular receptors to skeletal muscle. Although preprogrammed muscle stiffness can enhance the reactive capability of muscles by reducing reflex latency time, the objective is to generate joint perturbations that are not anticipated, stimulating reflex stabilization. The efficacy of reactive neuromuscular exercises was demonstrated nearly a decade ago.[71] Persistent use of these reflex pathways can decrease the response time and develop reactive strategies to unexpected joint loads.[60] Furthermore, Caraffa[23] significantly reduced the incidence of knee injuries in soccer players who performed reactive type training.

Fitzgerald et al[43,44] observed that muscle activity and biomechanical markers of gait normalizes in patients who underwent perturbation training after knee injuries. All reactive exercises should induce unanticipated joint perturbations if they are expected to facilitate reflex muscle activation. Reflex-mediated muscle activity is a crucial element in the dynamic restraint mechanism and should complement preprogrammed muscle activity to achieve a functionally stable joint.

Functional Activities

The objective of functional rehabilitation is to return the patient to preinjury activity level while minimizing the risk of reinjury.[136] This may require video analysis and consultation with the coaching staff to identify and correct faulty mechanics or movement techniques. The goals include restoring functional stability and sport-specific movement patterns or skills, then using functional tests to assess the patient's readiness to return to full participation.

Functional activities incorporate all of the available resources for stimulating peripheral afferents, muscle coactivation, and reflex and preprogrammed motor control. Emphasis should be placed on sport-specific techniques, including positions and maneuvers where the joint is vulnerable. With repetition and controlled intensity, muscle activity

Table 6-1 The Elements, Rehabilitation Techniques, and Afferent/Efferent Characteristics Necessary for Restoring Proprioception and Neuromuscular Control

Elements	Rehabilitation Techniques	Afferent/Efferent Characteristics
Proprioception and kinesthesia	Joint repositioning	Peripheral receptor sensitivity
	Functional ROM	
	Facilitate afferent pathways	
	Axial loading	
	Closed kinetic chain exercises	
Dynamic stability	Closed kinetic chain exercises and translatory forces	Agonist/antagonist coactivation
	High-repetition/low-resistance	Muscle activation rate and amplitude
	Eccentric loading	Peripheral receptor sensitivity
	Stretch-shortening exercises	Muscle stiffness
	Balance training	
Reactive neuromuscular control	Reaction to joint perturbation	Reflex facilitation
	Stretch shortening, plyometrics	Muscle activation rate and amplitude
	Balance reacquisition	
Functional motor patterns	Biofeedback	Discriminatory muscle activation
	Sport-specific drills	Arthrokinematics
	Control-progressive participation	Coordinated locomotion

(preparatory and reactive) gradually progresses from conscious to unconscious motor control.[77] Implementing these activities will help patients develop functionally specific movement repertoires within a controlled setting, decreasing the risk of injury upon completion of rehabilitation.

Understanding the afferent and efferent characteristics that contribute to joint sensation, dynamic stabilization, reflex activity, and functional motor pattern is necessary for reestablishing neuromuscular control and functional stability (Table 6-1).

Clinical Decision-Making Exercise 6-2

There was an increase in ACL injuries last year on the women's soccer team. You decide to develop a prevention program in an effort to minimize injuries in the upcoming season. What are the main goals of the prevention program with respect to neuromuscular control? What do you feel is the most effective method of training to achieve your goals?

Lower-Extremity Techniques

Many activities that promote neuromuscular control in the lower extremity exist in traditional rehabilitation schemes. Early kinesthetic training and joint repositioning tasks can begin to reestablish reflex pathways from articular afferents to skeletal motor nerves, the muscle

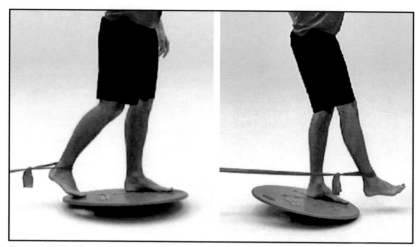

Figure 6-5. "Kickers" use an elastic band fixed to the distal aspect of the involved or uninvolved limb. The patient attempts to balance while executing short kicks with either knee extension or hip flexion. This exercise is most difficult when performed on unstable surfaces.

spindle system, and cortical motor control centers, while enhancing muscle stiffness increases the stretch sensitivity of tenomuscular receptors. Increased muscle stiffness and tone will heighten the stretch sensitivity of tenomuscular receptors, providing additional sensory information concerning joint motion and position.

These techniques should focus on individual muscle groups that require attention and progress from no weight to weight assisted. The use of closed chain activities is encouraged because they replicate the environment specific to lower-extremity function. Partial weight bearing, in pools or with unloading devices, simulates the open and closed chain environments without subjecting the ankle, knee, or hip to excessive joint loads.[79] The closed chain nature of these exercises creates joint compression, thus enhancing joint congruency and neurosensory feedback, while minimizing shearing forces on the joints.[119] Early dynamic joint stabilization exercises begin with balance training and partial weight bearing on stable surfaces, progressing to partial weight bearing on unstable surfaces. Balancing on unstable surfaces is initiated once full weight bearing is achieved. Exercises such as "kickers" also require balance and can begin on stable surfaces, progressing to unstable platforms (Figure 6-5).

Slide board training and basic strength exercises can be instituted to stimulate coactivation while increasing muscular force and

endurance. Strength exercises focus on eccentric and endurance-type activities in a closed kinetic orientation, further enhancing dynamic stability through increases in preparatory muscle stiffness and reactive characteristics. Eccentric loading is accomplished by activities such as forward and backward stair climbing or backward downhill walking. Strength and balance exercises can be combined and executed with light external forces to increase the level of difficulty (Figure 6-6).

Biofeedback can also help patients trying to develop agonist/antagonist coactivation during strength exercises. Biofeedback provides additional information concerning muscle activation and encourages voluntary muscle activation by facilitating efferent pathways. Reeducating injured patients through selective muscle activation is necessary for dynamic stabilization and neuromuscular control.

Stretch-shortening exercises are a necessary component for conditioning the neuromuscular apparatus to respond more quickly and forcefully, permitting eccentric deceleration followed immediately by explosive concentric contractions.[1] Stretch-shortening exercises need not be withheld until the late stages of rehabilitation. There is a variety of plyometric activities, and intensity can be controlled by manipulating the load, ROM, or number of repetitions. Stretch-shortening movements require both preparatory and reactive muscle activities

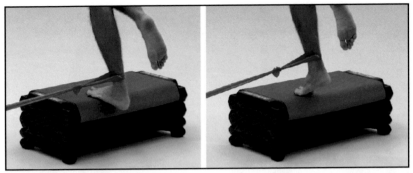

Figure 6-6. Balance and strength exercises are combined by incorporating light external forces and increasing the level of difficulty for balancing while strengthening the muscles required for dynamic stabilization.

along with the related changes in muscle stiffness. This preparatory muscle activation prior to eccentric loading is considered to be a combination of preprogrammed and reactive motor commands. Plyometric activities such as unweighted walking in a pool or low-impact hopping may commence once weight bearing is achieved (Figure 6-7). Double-leg bounding is an effective intermediate exercise because the uninvolved limb can be used for assistance. Stretch-shortening activities are made more difficult with alternate-leg bounding, then single-leg hopping. Subsequent activities such as hopping with rotation, lateral hopping, and hopping onto various surfaces are instituted as tolerated. Plyometric training requires preparatory muscle activation and facilitates reflexive pathways for reactive neuromuscular control.

Clinical Decision-Making Exercise 6-3

A female cross-country runner complains of chronic anterior knee pain. Your assessment reveals that she has patellofemoral pain and stiffness with associated hypertrophy of her vastus lateralis and atrophy in the vastus medialis oblique. What modalities would you use to correct this muscular imbalance? Discuss the rationale for each modality and how it relates to neuromuscular control.[62]

Rhythmic stabilization exercises should be included during early rehabilitation to enhance lower-extremity neuromuscular coordination and reaction to unexpected joint perturbations. The intensity of rhythmic stabilization

is increased by applying greater joint loads and displacements. Foot pass drills are also effective for developing coordinated preparatory and reactive muscle activity; begin with large balls and progress to smaller balls. In Figure 6-6, balance and strength exercises are combined by incorporating light external forces and increasing the level of difficulty for balancing while strengthening the muscles required for dynamic stabilization.

Unstable platforms are used to manually induce linear and angular perturbations to the joint, altering the patient's center of gravity while the patient attempts to balance (Figure 6-8). These exercises can facilitate adaptations to reflex pathways mediated by peripheral afferents, resulting in reactive muscle activation. Ball tossing can be incorporated in conjunction with balance exercises. This dual tasking creates cognitive loads that may disrupt concentration and help promote reactive adaptations and induces greater changes in location of the center of mass by requiring upper extremity motion, thus making the task more challenging to the sensorimotor system. Walking and running in sand also requires similar reactive muscle activity and can enhance reflexive joint stabilization.

During the later stages of rehabilitation, reactive neuromuscular activity incorporates trampoline hopping. The patient begins by hopping and landing on both feet, progressing to hopping on one foot, and hopping with rotation. The most difficult reactive tasks include hopping while catching a ball, or hopping off of a trampoline onto various landing surfaces such as artificial turf, grass, or dirt.

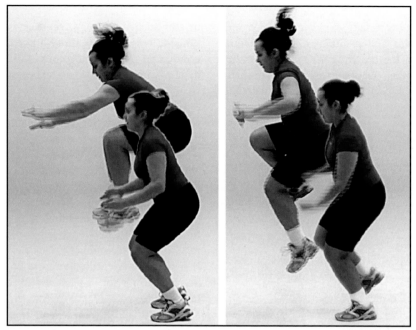

Figure 6-7. Plyometrics begin with double-leg hopping, and progress to single-leg hopping.

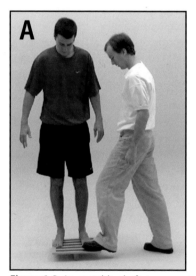

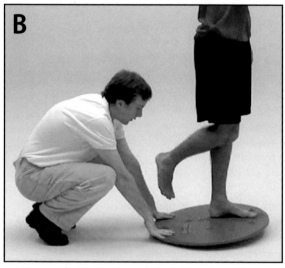

Figure 6-8. An unstable platform promotes reactive muscle activity when a patient attempts to balance and a clinician manually perturbs the platform. (A) Wobble board. (B) BAPS board.

Functional activities begin with restoring normal gait. Clinicians can give verbal instruction or use a mirror to help patients internalize normal kinematics during the stance and swing phases. This includes backward (retro) walking, which has been shown to further facilitate hamstring activation and balance. If a pool or unloading device is available, crossover walking and figure eights can begin, progressing to jogging and hopping as tolerated. Functional activities during partial weight bearing help restore motor patterns without compromising static restraints. Weight-bearing activities are continued on land with the incorporation of acceleration and deceleration and pivot maneuvers. Drills such as jogging, cutting, and cariocas are initiated, gradually increasing the speed of maneuvers.

The most difficult functional activities are designed to simulate the demands of individual sports and positions and may require input from the coaching staff. Activities such as shuttle runs, carioca crossovers, retro sprinting and forward sprinting are implemented with sport-specific drills such as fielding a ball, receiving a pass, and dribbling a soccer ball (see Chapter 16).

Clinical Decision-Making Exercise 6-4

A volleyball player is recovering from an Achilles/gastrocnemius strain. Develop plyometric exercises that can be implemented in each stage of rehabilitation. What would your rationale be for integrating these activities into the patient's rehabilitation? Describe the neuromuscular adaptations that you expect to occur.

Upper Extremity Techniques

Contrary to the lower extremity, the glenohumeral joint lacks inherent stability from capsuloligamentous structures; therefore dynamic mechanisms are even more crucial for maintaining functional stability.[59,145] The difficulty of working with a diverse array of shoulder positions and velocities is compounded by shearing forces associated with manipulating the upper extremity in an open kinetic chain environment.[145] Maintaining joint congruency and functional stability requires coordinated muscle activation for dynamic restraint while complex movement repertoires are executed.[98]

Two distinct types of muscle have been identified in the shoulder girdle and are primarily responsible for either stabilization or initiating movement. The orientation and size of the stabilizing muscles, referred to as the rotator cuff, are not suited for creating joint motion, but are more capable of steering the humeral head in the glenoid fossa.[98] Larger muscles (primary movers) with insertion sites further from the glenohumeral joint have greater mechanical advantage for initiating joint motion.[98,103] Maintaining proper joint kinematics requires balancing the external forces and internal moments while limiting excessive translation of the humeral head on the glenoid fossa and restoring appropriate coupling of the rotator cuff and prime movers.

Injury to the static structures can result in diminished sensory feedback and altered kinematics of the scapulothoracic and glenohomeral joints. Moreover, failure of the dynamic restraint system exposes the static structures to excessive or repetitive loads, jeopardizing joint integrity and predisposing the patient to reinjury. Surgery is the most effective means of restoring sensorimotor function long-term;[4,100,122] however, this avenue is not always an option. Therefore, developing or restoring neuromuscular control in the upper extremity through rehabilitation exercises is an important component for the eventual return to functional activities. Evidence supporting specific rehabilitation techniques is lacking, but critical review of the scientific literature produces recommendations for implementation to produce best results.

There is general agreement that achieving scapular control early in the rehabilitation program is imperative.[81,114,141] Exercises focusing on scapular retraction as a starting position for all subsequent activities should be incorporated for restoring optimal shoulder complex function and reducing one's risk for secondary injury. To achieve this position, exercises to increase activation of the lower trapezius and serratus anterior while simultaneously minimizing activation of the upper trapezius are appropriate. Recent research suggests the following exercises: sidelying external rotation, sidelying forward flexion, prone extension, and prone horizontal abduction with external rotation.[34] The serratus anterior is also activated during the push-up plus, which can be progressed by elevating the patient's feet.[104]

Activities to enhance proprioceptive and kinesthetic awareness in the upper extremity emulate techniques discussed for the lower extremity. Research advocates use of closed kinetic chain activities early in upper extremity rehabilitation to promote afferent feedback and coactivation, which may include weight shifts, table slides, and wall slides.[20,82] A closed kinetic chain environment introduces axial loads and muscle coactivation, the resultant joint approximation stimulates capsuloligamentous mechanoreceptors, similar to lower-extremity activities.[98,146] Stretch-shortening (plyometric) exercises in the overhead patient have been

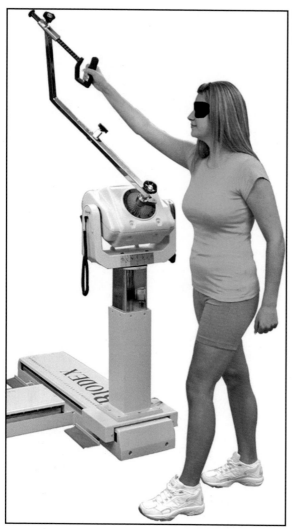

Figure 6-9. Active and passive repositioning activities should be performed in functional positions specific to individual sports.

shown to improve proprioception. Multiplanar joint repositioning tasks are performed actively and passively to maximize the increased ROM available in the shoulder. Functional positions, such as overhead throwing, should be incorporated and are more sport-specific (Figure 6-9).

Muscle stiffness can be enhanced by using elastic resistance tubing or a plyoball with an inclined trampoline, concentrating on the eccentric phase, and performing high repetitions with low resistance.[140] These exercises are also well established for strengthening and reconditioning the rotator cuff muscles in functional patterns. To complement elastic tubing exercises, clinicians can use commercially available upper-extremity ergometers for endurance training.

Like similar exercises for the lower extremity, dynamic stabilization exercises for the shoulder use unstable platforms to create linear and angular joint displacement, maximally stimulating coactivation. The intensity is controlled by manipulating the degree of joint displacement and loading. Three closed chain exercises have been described to stimulate coactivation in the shoulder: push-ups, horizontal abduction on a slide board, and tracing circular motions on a slide board with the dominant and nondominant arms[98] (Figure 6-10). These exercises accommodate for the individual's tolerance to joint loads by progressing from a quadruped to a push-up position. Multidirectional slide board exercises also require dynamic stabilization while concomitantly using feedforward and

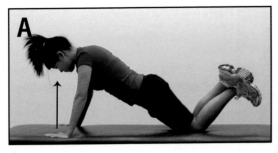

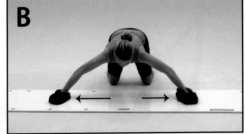

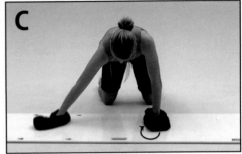

Figure 6-10. Dynamic stabilization exercises for the upper extremity. (A) Push-ups. (B) Horizontal abduction on a slide board. (C) Wax-on wax-off on slide board.

Figure 6-11. Upper-extremity plyometric exercises with a heavy ball require preparatory and reactive muscle activation.

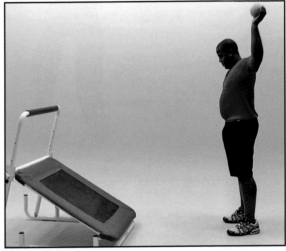

feedback neuromuscular control. Plyometric exercises with varying ball weights and distances for advancement are also excellent for conditioning preparatory and reactive muscle coactivation and can be advanced by increasing the weight of the ball, varying the distance, and introducing multiplanar movements (Figure 6-11).[140]

Reactive neuromuscular characteristics are facilitated by manually perturbing the upper extremity while the patient attempts to maintain a permanent position. During the early phases of rehabilitation, light loads are used with rhythmic stabilization exercises. As the patient progresses, resistance is added to maximize muscle activation (Figure 6-12). Positions where the joint is inherently unstable must be incorporated, but under controlled intensity (Figure 6-13). Increased joint loads during rhythmic stabilization exercises mimic closed chain environments and conditions the patient for more difficult reactive drills under weighted conditions on stable surfaces and unstable platforms (Figure 6-14).

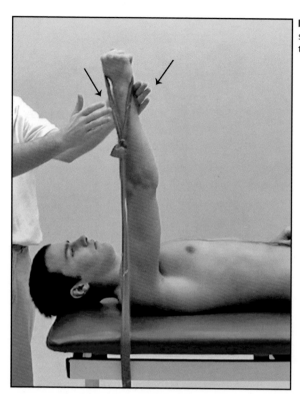

Figure 6-12. Elastic bands are used during rhythmic stabilization exercises to create joint loads and facilitate muscle activation.

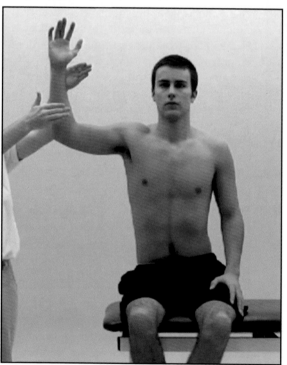

Figure 6-13. Rhythmic stabilization exercises should include simulated positions of vulnerability, promoting neuromuscular adaptations to dynamic stabilization.

Figure 6-14. Linear displacements produced by a clinician facilitate reflex pathways for dynamic stabilization in the upper extremity.

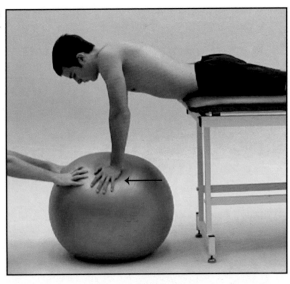

Clinical Decision-Making Exercise 6-5

During preparticipation physicals, you note that one of the tennis players has a history of inferior glenohumeral dislocation and, as a result, excessive laxity. The surrounding masculature appears strong, but the patient continues to have sensations of instability. What is the nature of this patient's problem, and what exercises would you use to improve dynamic stability of the rotator cuff muscles? Justify your decision to incorporate these exercises.

Functional training for the upper extremity most often involves developing motor patterns in the overhead position, whether it be shooting a basketball, throwing, or hitting as in volleyball and tennis. However, special considerations are necessary for other sports, like rowing, wrestling, and swimming, which rely heavily on the upper extremity.

FUNCTIONAL ACTIVITIES

Functional activities that involve a combination of strength training, balance, and core stability performed through multiple planes of movement should incorporate the entire kinetic chain, as they need to reproduce the demands of specific events. Beginning with slower velocities and conscious control, activities eventually progress to functional speeds and unconscious control. Technique, rather than speed, should be emphasized to promote the appropriate muscle activation patterns along the kinetic chain and avoid faulty mechanics. Reeducating functional motor patterns involves all of the elements for dynamic restraint and neuromuscular control and will minimize the risk of reinjury upon returning to full participation. Figure 6-15 provides examples of exercises that can be used to enhance neuromuscular control.

Clinical Decision-Making Exercise 6-6

A wrestler is performing rehabilitation for a grade 2 medial collateral ligament (MCL) sprain. His rehabilitation is in the final stage and you would like to incorporate functional exercises into the protocol. Considering the specific demands related to this sport, develop a progression of functional exercises for this patient's return to full participation.

The speed and complexity of movements in athletic competition requires rapid integration of sensory information by feedforward and feedback neuromuscular control systems. Although many peripheral, spinal, and cortical

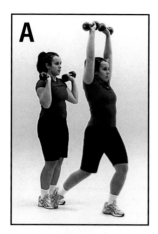

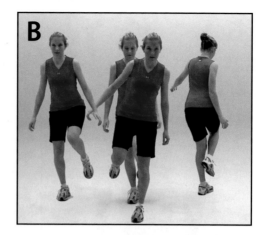

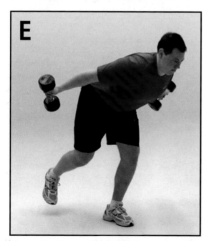

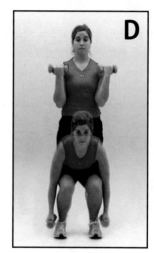

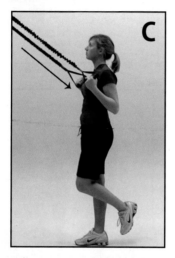

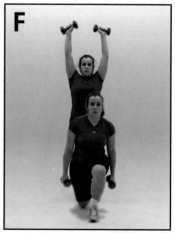

Figure 6-15. Exercises to enhance neuromuscular control. (A) Two arm push press. (B) Multiplanar hops to stabilization. (C) Single leg pull-down using cable or tubing. (D) Standing dumbbell squat to curl. (E) Single leg two arm dumbbell cobra. (F) Dumbbell squat to overhead press. (*continued*)

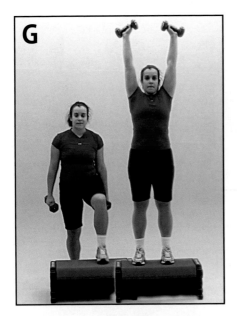

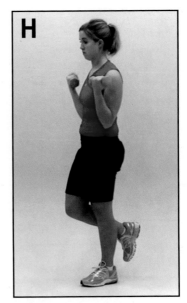

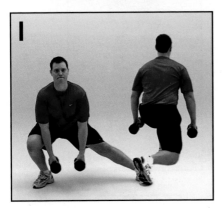

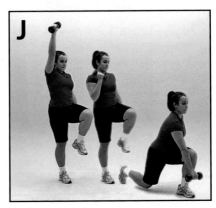

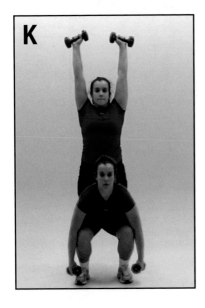

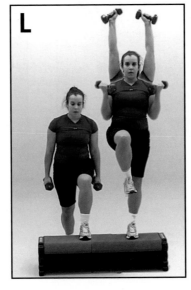

Figure 6-15. (*continued*) (G) Step-up double leg balance to overhead press. (H) Standing single-leg dumbbell bicep curls. (I) Multiplanar dumbbell lunges. (J) Front lunge balance to one-arm press. (K) Squat overhead press. (L) Step-up single leg balance to overhead press.

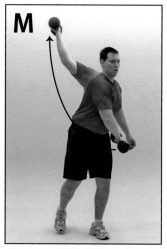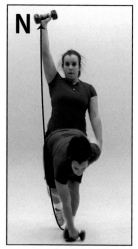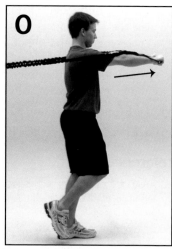

Figure 6-15. (continued) (M) Single-leg one-arm dumbbell PNF. (N) Single-leg Romanian dead lift to overhead press. (O) Single-leg two-arm chest press using cable.

elements contribute to the neuromuscular control system, dynamic joint stabilization is contingent upon both cortically programmed activation and reflex-mediated muscle activation.

Disrupted joint kinematics, muscle activation patterns, and conditioning can contribute to disruption of the dynamic restraint system and must be reestablished for functional stability.

Summary

1. The efferent response to peripheral afferent information is termed *neuromuscular control*.

2. Injury to capsuloligamentous structures compromises both the static and the dynamic restraining mechanisms of joints.

3. The primary role of articular structures is to guide skeletal segments providing static restraint, but they also contain mechanoreceptors that mediate the dynamic restraint mechanism.

4. Articular sensations are coupled with information from tenomuscular mechanoreceptors, via cortical and reflex pathways, providing conscious and unconscious appreciation of joint motion and position.

5. Muscle spindles have received special consideration for their capacity to integrate peripheral afferent information and reflexively modify muscle activity.

6. Feedforward and feedback neuromuscular controls use sensory information for preparatory and reactive muscle activity.

7. The degree of muscle activation largely determines a muscle's resistance to stretching or stiffness. Muscles with increased stiffness can assist the dynamic restraint mechanism by resisting excessive joint translation.

8. To reestablish neuromuscular control and functional stability, clinicians may use specific rehabilitation techniques—including closed kinetic chain activities, balance training, eccentric and high repetition/low load exercises, reflex facilitation through reactive training, stretch-shortening activities, and biofeedback training.

9. Rehabilitative techniques produce adaptations in the sensitivity of peripheral receptors and facilitation of afferent pathways, agonist/antagonist coactivation, muscle stiffness, the onset rate and magnitude of muscle activity, reflex muscle activation, and discriminatory muscle activation.

10. Afferent and efferent characteristics regulate the 4 elements critical to neuromuscular control and functional stability: proprioception and kinesthesia, dynamic stabilization, reflex muscle activation, and functional motor patterns.

11. Each phase of traditional rehabilitation can incorporate the appropriate activities, emphasizing each of the four elements, according to the individual's tolerance and functional progression. By integrating these elements into the rehabilitation of injured patients, clinicians can maximize the contributions of the dynamic restraint mechanisms to functional stability.

References

1. Abott, J. C., and U. B. Saunders. 1994. Injuries to the ligaments of the knee joint. *Journal of Bone Joint Surgery* December:503–521.

2. Ahlden M, Sernert N, Karlsson J, and Kartus J. 2013. A prospective randomized study comparing double- and single-bundle techniques for anterior cruciate ligament reconstruction. *Am J Sports Med, 41*(11): 2484-91.

3. Appleberg, B., H. Johansson, M. Hulliger, and P. Sojka. 1986. Actions on motoneurons elicited by electrical stimulation of group III muscle afferent fibers in the hind limb of the cat. *Journal of Physiology* (London), 375:137–152.

4. Aydin, T., Y. Yildiz, I. Yanmis, C. Yildiz, and T. A. Kalyon. 2001. Shoulder proprioception: A comparison between the shoulder joint in healthy and surgically repaired shoulders. *Arch Orthop Trauma Surg, 121*:422–425.

5. Bach, T. M., A. E. Chapman, and T. W., Calvert. 1983. Mechanical resonance of the human body during voluntary oscillations about the ankle joint. *J Biomech* 16:85–90.

6. Barker, D. 1974. The morphology of muscle receptors. In *Handbook of sensory physiology*, Hunt, C. C., ed. Berlin: Springer-Verlag, 191–234.

7. Barrack, R. L., H. B. Skinner, M. E. Brunet, and S. D. Cook. 1983. Joint laxity and proprioception in the knee. *Physician and Sports Medicine, 11*:130–135.

8. Barrack RL, Lund PJ, Munn BG, Wink C, and Happel L. 1997. Evidence of reinnervation of free patellar tendon autograft used for anterior cruciate ligament reconstruction. *American Journal of Sports Medicine, 25*(2): 196-202

9. Barrack, R. L., H. B. Skinner, M. E. Brunet, and S.D. Cook. 1984. Joint kinesthesia in the highly trained knee. *J Sports Med Phys Fitness, 24*:18–20.

10. Barrett, D. S. 1991. Proprioception and function after anterior cruciate reconstruction. *J Bone Joint Surg Br, 73*:833–837.

11. Basmajian, J. V. 1979. *Biofeedback: Principles and practice for clinicians.* Baltimore: Williams & Wilkins.

12. Beard, D. J., C. A. Dodd, H. R. Trundle, and A. H., Simpson. 1994. Proprioception enhancement for anterior cruciate ligament deficiency: A prospective randomised trial of two physiotherapy regimes. *J Bone Joint Surg Br, 76*:654–659.

13. Behrens M, Mau-Moeller A, Wassermann F, and Bruhn S. 2013. Effect of fatigue on hamstring reflex responses and posterior-anterior tibial translation in men and women. *PLoS One, 8*(2): e56988.

14. Biau DJ, Tournoux C, Katsahian S, Schranz PJ, and Nizard RS. 2006. Bone-patellar tendon-bone autografts versus hamstring autografts for reconstruction of anterior cruciate ligament: meta-analysis. *BMJ, 332*(7548): 995-1001.

15. Blackburn JT, Norcross MF, Cannon LN, and Zinder SM. 2013. The influence of hamstring stiffness on landing biomechanics linked to anterior cruciate ligament loading. *J Athl Train, 48*(6):764-772.

16. Blackburn JT, and Norcross MF. 2013. The effects of isometric and isotonic training on hamstring stiffness and anterior cruciate ligament loading mechanisms. *J EMG Kinesiol, 24*(1):98-103.

17. Blackburn JT, Norcross MF, and Padua DA. 2011. Influences of hamstring stiffness and strength on anterior knee joint stability. *Clin Biomech, 26*(3): 278-283.

18. Branch, T. P., R. Hunter, and M. Donath. 1989. Dynamic EMG analysis of anterior cruciate deficient legs with and without bracing during cutting. *Am J Sports Med, 17*:35–41.

19. Brenner, J., and K. Swanik. 2007. High-risk drinking characteristics in collegiate athletes. *J Am Coll Health, 56*:267–272.

20. Broer M. R. 1993. *Efficiency of Human Movement.* 3rd ed. Philadelphia: W.B. Saunders Co.

21. Bulbulian, R., and D. K. Bowles. 1992. Effect of downhill running on motoneuron pool excitability. *J Appl Physiol, 73*:968–973.

22. Burgess KE, Connick MJ, Graham-Smith P, and Pearson SJ. 2007. Plyometric vs. isometric training influences on tendon properties and muscle output. *J Strength Cond Res, 21*(3): 986-989.

23. Caraffa, A., G. Cerulli. M. Proietti, G. Aisa, and A. Rizzo. 1995. Prevention of anterior cruciate ligament in soccer: A prospective controlled study of proprioceptive training. *Knee Surgery Sports Traumatol, Arthroscopy* 4:19–21.

24. Carter ND, Jenkinson TR, Wilson D, Jones DW, and Torode AS. 1997. Joint position sense and rehabilitation in the anterior cruciate ligament deficient knee. *Br J Sports Med, 31*(3): 209-12.

25. Chimura, N. J., K. A. Swanik, C. B. Swanik, and S. V., Straub. 2004. Effects of plyometric training on muscle-activation strategies and performance in female athletes. *J Athl Train* 39:24–31.

26. Chmielewski TL, Rudolph KS, and Snyder-Mackler L. 2002. Development of dynamic knee stability after acute ACL injury. *Journal of Electromyography and Kinesiology*, 12(4): 267-74.

27. Chmielewski TL, Hurd WJ, and Snyder-Mackler L. 2005. Elucidation of a potentially destabilizing control strategy in ACL deficient non-copers. *Journal of Electromyography and Kinesiology*, 15(1): 83-92.

28. Clark, F. J., and P. R. Burgess. 1975. Slowly adapting receptors in cat knee joint: Can they signal joint angle? *J Neurophysiol*, 38:1448–1463.

29. Clark, F. J., R. C. Burgess, J. W. Chapin, and W. T., Lipscomb. 1985. Role of intramuscular receptors in the awareness of limb position. *J Neurophysiol*, 54:1529–1540.

30. Colebatch, J. G., and D. I., McCloskey. 1987. Maintenance of constant arm position or force: Reflex and volitional components in man. *J Physiol*, 386:247–261.

31. Collins AT, et al. 2011. Stochastic resonance electrical stimulation to improve proprioception in knee osteoarthritis. *Knee*, 18(5): 317-22.

32. Collins A, Blackburn JT, Olcott C, Yu B, and Weinhold P. 2011. The impact of stochastic resonance electrical stimulation and knee sleeve on impulsive loading and muscle co-contraction during gait in knee osteoarthritis. *Clin Biomech (Bristol, Avon)*, 26(8): 853-8.

33. Co FH, Skinner HB, and Cannon WD. 1993. Effect of reconstruction of the anterior cruciate ligament on proprioception of the knee and the heel strike transient. *J Orthop Res*, 11(5): 696-704.

34. Cools, A. M., V. Dewitte, F., Lanszweert, D. Notebaert, Roets, B. Soetens, B. Cagnie, and E. E. Witvrouw. 2007. Rehabilitation of scapular muscle balance: Which exercises to prescribe? *Am J Sports Med*, 35:1744–1751.

35. Corrigan, J. P., W. F. Cashman, and M. P., Brady. 1992. Proprioception in the cruciate deficient knee. *J Bone Joint Surg Br*, 74:247–250.

36. Dietz, V., Noth and D., Schmidtbleicher. 1981. Interaction between pre-activity and stretch reflex in human triceps brachii during landing from forward falls. *J Physiol*, 311:113–125.

37. Dunn, T. G., S. E. Ponsor, N. Weil, and S. W. Utz. 1986. The learning process in biofeedback: Is it feed-forward or feedback? *Biofeedback Self Regul*, 11:143–156.

38. Dyhre-Poulsen, P., E. B. Simonsen, and M. Voigt. 1991. Dynamic control of muscle stiffness and H reflex modulation during hopping and jumping in man. *J Physiol*, 437:287–304.

39. Eccles, R. M., and A. Lindberg. 1959. Synaptic actions in motoneurons by afferents which may evoke the flexion reflex. *Archives of Italian Biology*, 1979:199–221.

40. Enoka, R. M. 1994. Neuromechanical Basis of Kinesiology. 2nd ed. Champaign, IL: Human Kinetics.

41. Falconiero RP, DiStefano VJ, and Cook TM. 1998. Revascularization and ligamentization of autogenous anterior cruciate ligament grafts in humans. *Arthroscopy*, 14(2): 197-205.

42. Finsterbush, A., and B. Friedman. 1975. The effect of sensory denervation on rabbits' knee joints: A light and electron microscopic study. *J Bone Joint Surg Am* 57:949–956.

43. Fitzgerald, G. K., J. D. Childs, T. M. Ridge, and J. J. Irrgang. 2002. Agility and perturbation training for a physically active individual with knee osteoarthritis. *Phys Ther* 82:372–82.

44. Fitzgerald, G. K., M. J., Axe, and L. Snyder-Mackler. 2000. The efficacy of perturbation training in nonoperative anterior cruciate ligament rehabilitation of physically active individuals. *Phys Ther* 80:128–140.

45. Ford KR, Myer GD, Schmitt LC, Uhl TL, and Hewett TE. 2011. Preferential Quadriceps Activation in Female Athletes with Incremental Increases in Landing Intensity. *Journal of Applied Biomechanics*, 27(3): 215-222.

46. Forwell, L. A., and H. Carnahan. 1996. Proprioception during manual aiming in individuals with shoulder instability and controls. *J Orthop Sports Phys Ther* 23:111–119.

47. Freeman, M. A., and B. Wyke. 1966. Articular contributions to limb muscle reflexes: The effects of partial neurectomy of the knee-joint on postural reflexes. *Br J Surg* 53:61–68.

48. Friemert B, et al. 2005. Intraoperative direct mechanical stimulation of the anterior cruciate ligament elicits short- and medium-latency hamstring reflexes. *J Neurophysiol*, 94(6): 3996-4001.

49. Gardner, E., F. Latimer, and D. Stiwell. 1949. Central connections for afferent fibers from the knee joint of a cat. *American Journal of Physiology* 159:195–198.

50. Gehring D, Melnyk M, and Gollhofer A. 2009. Gender and fatigue have influence on knee joint control strategies during landing. *Clinical Biomechanics*, 24(1): 82-87.

51. Glaros, A. G., and K. Hanson. 1990. EMG biofeedback and discriminative muscle control. *Biofeedback Self Regul* 15:135–143.

52. Glencross, D., and E. Thornton. 1981. Position sense following joint injury. *Journal of Sports Medicine and Physical Fitness.* 1211:23–27.

53. Goldblatt JP, Fitzsimmons SE, Balk E, and Richmond JC. 2005. Reconstruction of the anterior cruciate ligament: meta-analysis of patellar tendon versus hamstring tendon autograft. *Arthroscopy*, 21(7): 791-803.

54. Goubel, F., and J. F. Marini. 1987. Fiber type transition and stiffness modification of soleus muscle of trained rats. *European Journal of Physiology*, 410:321–325.

55. Granata, K. P., D. A. Padua, and S. E., Wilson. 2002. Gender differences in active musculoskeletal stiffness: Part II. Quantification of leg stiffness during functional hopping tasks. *J Electromyogr Kinesiol,* 12:127–135.

56. Greenwood, R. D. 1976. A view of nineteenth century therapeutics. *J Med Assoc State Ala,* 45:25.

57. Grigg, P. 1994. Peripheral neural mechanisms in proprioception. *Journal of Sport Rehabilitation.* 134:1–17.

58. Griller, S. 1972. A role for muscle stiffness in meeting the changing postural and locomotor requirements for force development by ankle extensors. *Acta Physiologica Scandinavia,* 1862:92–108.

59. Guanche, C., T. Knatt, M, Solomonow, Y., Lu and R., Baratta. 1995. The synergistic action of the capsule and the shoulder muscles. *Am J Sports Med,* 23:301–306.

60. Guyton, A. C. 1981. *Textbook of medical physiology.* 6th ed. Philadelphia: W. B. Saunders.

61. Hagood, S., M. Solomonow, R. Baratta, B. H. Zhou, and R. D'Ambrosia. 1990. The effect of joint velocity on the contribution of the antagonist musculature to knee stiffness and laxity. *Am J Sports Med,* 18:182–187.

62. Hamstra-Wright, K. L., C. B. Swanik, T. Y., Ennis, and K. A., Swanik 2005. Joint stiffness and pain in individuals with patellofemoral syndrome. *J Orthop Sports Phys Ther,* 35:495–501.

63. Hamstra, K. L., C. B. Swanik, R. T. Tierney, K. C. Huxel, and J. M. Cherubini. 2002. The relationship between muscle tone and dynamic restraint in the physically active. *Journal of Athletic Training,* 37:S–41.

64. Hewett, T. E., G. D. Myer, and K. R. Ford. 2005. Reducing knee and anterior cruciate ligament injuries among female athletes. *The Journal of Knee Surgery* 18:82–88.

65. Hewett, T., Paterno M, Myer, G 2002. Strategies for enhancing proprioception and neuromuscular control of the knee. *Clinical Orthopaedics and related research,* 402:76-94.

66. Hodgson, J. A., R. R. Roy, R. de Leon, B. Dobkin, and V. R. Edgerton. 1994. Can the mammalian lumbar spinal cord learn a motor task? *Med Sci Sports Exerc,* 26:1491–1497.

67. Hoffer, J. A., and S. Andreassen. 1981. Regulation of soleus muscle stiffness in premammillary cats: Intrinsic and reflex components. *J Neurophysiol,* 45:267–285.

68. Houk, J. C., P. E. Crago, and W. Z., Rymer. 1981. Function of the dynamic response in stiffness regulation: A predictive mechanism provided by non-linear feedback. London: Macmillan. *In Muscle Receptors and Movement,* Taylor, A., and A. Prochazka, eds.

69. Hutton, R. S., and S. W. Atwater. 1992. Acute and chronic adaptations of muscle proprioceptors in response to increased use. *Sports Med,* 14:406–421.

70. Huxel, K. C., C. B. Swanik, K. A. Swanik, A. R. Bartolozzi H. J. Hillstrom, M. R. Sitler, and D. M. Moffit. 2008. Stiffness regulation and muscle-recruitment strategies of the shoulder in response to external rotation perturbations. *J Bone Joint Surg Am,* 90:154–162.

71. Ihara, H., and A. Nakayama. 1986. Dynamic joint control training for knee ligament injuries. *Am J Sports Med,* 14:309–315.

72. Jerosch J, and Prymka M. 1996. Knee joint proprioception in normal volunteers and patients with anterior cruciate ligament tears, taking special account of the effect of a knee bandage. *Arch Orthop Trauma Surg,* 115(3-4): 162-6.

73. Johansson, H., P. Sjolander, and P. Sojka. 1986. Actions on gamma-motoneurons elicited by electrical stimulation of joint afferent fibres in the hind limb of the cat. *J Physiol,* 375:137–152.

74. Johansson, H., P. Sjolander, and P. Sojka. 1991. Receptors in the knee joint ligaments and their role in the biomechanics of the joint. *Crit Rev Biomed Eng,* 18:341–368.

75. Johansson, H., P. Sjolander, and P. Sojka 1991. A sensory role for the cruciate ligaments. *Clin Orthop Relat Res,* 268:161–178.

76. Jonsson, H., J. Karrholm, and L. G. Elmqvist 1989. Kinematics of active knee extension after tear of the anterior cruciate ligament. *Am J Sports Med,* 17:796–802.

77. Kandell, E. R., J. H. Schwartz, and T. M. Jessell. 1996. *Principles of neural science.* 3rd ed. Norwalk, CT: Appleton & Lange.

78. Katonis, P. G., A. P. Assimakopoulos M. V., Agapitos, and E. I. Exarchou. 1991. Mechanoreceptors in the posterior cruciate ligament. *Acta Orthropedica Scandanavia,* 62:276–278.

79. Kelsey, D. D., and E. Tyson 1994. A new method of training for the lower extremity using unloading. *J Orthop Sports Phys Ther,* 19:218–223

80. Kennedy, J. C., I. J. Alexander, and K. C. Hayes. 1982. Nerve supply of the human knee and its functional importance. *Am J Sports Med,* 10:329–335.

81. Kibler, W. B., J. McMullen, and T. Uhl. 2001. Shoulder rehabilitation strategies, guidelines, and practice. *Orthop Clin North Am,* 32:527–538.

82. Kibler, W. B. 2000. Closed kinetic chain rehabilitation for sports injuries. *Phys Med Rehabil Clin N Am,* 11:369–384.

83. Koceja, D. M., J. Burke, and G. Kamen. 1991. Organization of segmental reflexes in trained dancers. *Int J Sports Med,* 12:285–289.

84. Koceja, D. M., and G. Kamen. 1988. Conditioned patellar tendon reflexes in sprint- and endurance-trained athletes. *Med Sci Sports Exerc,* 20:172–177.

85. Kochner, M. S., F. H. Fu, and C. D. Harner. 1994. *Neuropathophysiology in Knee Surgery.* Vol 1. Fu, F. H., and C. D. Harner, eds. Baltimore: Williams & Wilkins.

86. Konradsen L, Voigt M, and Hojsgaard C. 1997. Ankle inversion injuries. The role of the dynamic defense mechanism. *Am J Sports Med,* 25(1): 54-8.

87. Kovanen, V., H. Suominen, and E. Heikkinen. 1984. Mechanical properties of fast and slow skeletal muscle with special reference to collagen and endurance training. *J Biomech, 17*:725–735.

88. Kubo K, et al. 2009. Effects of static and dynamic training on the stiffness and blood volume of tendon in vivo. *J Appl Physiol, 106*(2): 412-417.

89. Kubo K, et al. 2007. Effects of plyometric and weight training on muscle-tendon complex and jump performance. *Medicine and Science in Sports and Exercise, 39*(10): 1801-10.

90. Kyrolaninen, H., and P. V. Komi. 1995. The function of neuromuscular system in maximal stretch-shortening cycle exercises: Comparison between power- and endurancetrained athletes. *Journal of Electromyographic Kinesiology, 155*:15–25.

91. La Croix, J. M. 1981. The acquisition of autonomic control through biofeedback: The case against an afferent process and a two-process alternative. *Psychophysiology, 1181*:573–587.

92. Lamell-Sharp, A. D., C. B. Swanik, and R. T. Tierney. 2002. The effect of variable joint loads on knee joint position and force sensation. *Journal of Athletic Training, 37*(2):S29.

93. Leanderson, J., E. Eriksson, C. Nilsson, and A. Wykman. 1996. Proprioception in classical ballet dancers. A prospective study of the influence of an ankle sprain on proprioception in the ankle joint. *Am J Sports Med, 24*:370–374.

94. Leksell, L. 1995. The action potential and excitatory effects of the small ventral root fibers to skeletal muscle. *Acta Physiol Scand, 10*(31): S1–84. 10(31):81–84.

95. Lephart SM, Abt JP, and Ferris CM. 2002. Neuromuscular contributions to anterior cruciate ligament injuries in females. *Curr Opin Rheumatol, 14*(2): 168-73.

96. Lephart, S. M., and T. J. Henry. 1996. The physiological basis for open and closed kinetic chain rehabilitation for the upper extremity. *Journal of Sport Rehabilitation, 156*:71–87.

97. Lephart, S. M., M. S. Kocher, F. H. Fu, P. A. Borsa, and C. D. Harner. 1992. Proprioception following ACL reconstruction. *Journal of Sport Rehabilitation, 188*–196.

98. Lephart, S. M., J. P. Warner, P. A. Borsa, and F. H. Fu. 1994. Proprioception of the shoulder joint in healthy, unstable, and surgically repaired shoulders. *Journal of Shoulder Elbow Surgery, 134*:371–380.

99. Lephart, S. M., J. L. Giraldo, P. A. Borsa, and F. H. Fu. 1996. Knee joint proprioception: A comparison between female intercollegiate gymnasts and controls. *Knee Surg Sports Traumatol Arthrosc, 4*:121–4.

100. Lephart, S. M., J. B. Myers, J. P. Bradley, and F. H. Fu 2002. Shoulder proprioception and function following thermal capsulorraphy. *Arthroscopy, 18*:770–778.

101. Lephart, S. M., D. M. Pincivero, J. L. Giraldo, and F. J. Fu. 1997. The role of proprioception in the management and rehabilitation of athletic injuries. *Am J Sports Med, 25*:130–7.

102. Lephart, S. M., D. M. Pincivero, and S. L., Rozzi. 1998. Proprioception of the ankle and knee. *Sports Med, 25*:149–55.

103. Lieber, R. L., and J. Friden. 1992. Neuromuscular stabilization of the shoulder girdle. In The shoulder: *A balance of mobility and stability*, Matsen F. A., ed. Rosemont, IL: American Academy of Orthopaedic Surgeons 1992:91–106.

104. Ludewig, P. M., M. S. Hoff, E. E. Osowski, S. A. Meschke, and P. J., Rundquist. 2004. Relative balance of serratus anterior and upper trapezius muscle activity during push-up exercises. *Am J Sports Med, 32*:484–493.

105. Lynch, S. A., U. Eklund, D. Gottlieb, P. A. Renstrom, and B. Beynnon. 1996. Electromyographic latency changes in the ankle musculature during inversion moments. *Am J Sports Med, 24*:362–369.

106. Mair, S. D., A. V. Seaber, R. R. Glisson, and W. E. Garrett, Jr. 1996. The role of fatigue in susceptibility to acute muscle strain injury. *Am J Sports Med, 24*:137–143.

107. McComas, A. J. 1994. Human neuromuscular adaptations that accompany changes in activity. *Med Sci Sports Exerc, 26*:1498–1509.

108. McNair, P. J., and R. N. Marshall. 1994. Landing characteristics in subjects with normal and anterior cruciate ligament deficient knee joints. *Archives of Physical Medicine and Rehabilitation, 1754*:584–589.

109. McNair, P. J., G. A. Wood, and R. N. Marshall. 1992. Stiffness of the hamstring muscles and its relationship to function in anterior cruciate deficient individuals. *Clinical Biomechanics, 172*:131–173.

110. Melvill-Jones, G. M., and G. D. Watt. 1971. Observations of the control of stepping and hopping in man. *Journal of Physiology, 219*:709–727.

111. Merton, P. A. 1953. Speculations on the servo-control of movement. In *The Spinal Cord*, Wolstenholme, G. E. W., ed. London: Churchill.

112. Moksnes H, and Risberg MA. 2009. Performance-based functional evaluation of non-operative and operative treatment after anterior cruciate ligament injury. *Scand J Med Sci Sports, 19*(3): 345-55.

113. Morgan, D. L. 1977. Separation of active and passive components of short-range stiffness of muscle. *Am J Physiol, 232*:C45–9.

114. Moseley, J. B., Jr., F. W. Jobe, M. Pink, V. Perry, and V. Tibone, 1992. EMG analysis of the scapular muscles during a shoulder rehabilitation program. *Am J Sports Med, 20*:128–134.

115. Mountcastle, V. S. 1980. *Medical Physiology*. 14th ed. St. Louis: Mosby.

116. Nichols, T. R., and J. C. Houk. 1976. Improvement in linearity and regulation of stiffness that results from actions of stretch reflex. *J Neurophysiol, 39*:119–142.

117. Norcross MF, Blackburn JT, Goerger BM, and Padua DA. 2010. The association between lower extremity energy absorption and biomechanical factors related to anterior cruciate ligament injury. *Clin Biomech, 25*(10): 1031-1036.

118. Ochi M. J. Iwasa, Y. Uchio, N. Adachi, and Y. Sumen. 1999. The regeneration of sensory neurons in the reconstruction of the anterior cruciate ligament. *Journal of Bone and Joint Surgery—British,* 81:902–906.

119. Palmitier, R. A., K. N. An, S. G. Scott, and E. Y. Chao. 1991. Kinetic chain exercise in knee rehabilitation. *Sports Med,* 11:402–413.

120. Perlau, R., C. Frank, and G. Fick. 1995. The effect of elastic bandages on human knee proprioception in the uninjured population. *Am J Sports Med,* 23:251–255.

121. Pope, M. H., R. J. Johnson, D. W. Brown, and C. Tighe. 1979. The role of the musculature in injuries to the medial collateral ligament. *J Bone Joint Surg Am,* 61:398–402.

122. Potzl W., L. Thorwesten, C. Gotze, S. Garmann, and D. Steinbeck. 2004. Proprioception of the shoulder joint after surgical repair for instability: A long-term follow-up study. *Am J Sports Med,* 32:425–430.

123. Pousson, M., J. Van Hoecke, and F. Goubel. 1990. Changes in elastic characteristics of human muscle induced by eccentric exercise. *J Biomech,* 23:343–348.

124. Rack, P. M., and D. R. Westbury. 1974. The short range stiffness of active mammalian muscle and its effect on mechanical properties. *J Physiol,* 240:331–350.

125. Raunest J, Sager M, and Burgener E. 1996. Proprioceptive mechanisms in the cruciate ligaments: an electromyographic study on reflex activity in the thigh muscles. *J Trauma, 41*(3): 488-93.

126. Schultz, R. A., D. C. Miller, C. S. Kerr, and L. Micheli. 1984. Mechanoreceptors in human cruciate ligaments. A histological study. *J Bone Joint Surg Am,* 66:1072–1076.

127. Sherrington, C. S. 1911. *The integrative action of the nervous system.* New Haven: Yale University Press.

128. Simoneau GG, Degner RM, Kramper CA, and Kittleson KH. 1997. Changes in ankle joint proprioception resulting from strips of athletic tape applied over the skin. *Journal of Athletic Training,* 32(2): 141-7.

129. Sinkjaer, T., and L. Arendt-Nielsen. 1991. Knee stability and muscle coordination in patients with anterior cruciate ligament injuries: An electromyographic approach. *Journal of Electromyographic Kinesiology,* 1:209–217.

130. Skinner, H. B., and R. L. Barrack. 1991. Joint position sense in the normal and pathologic knee joint. *Journal of Electromyographic Kinesiology,* 1:180–190.

131. Skinner, H. B., R. L. Barrack, S. D. Cook, and R. J. Haddad Jr. 1984. Joint position sense in total knee arthroplasty. *J Orthop Res* 1:276–283.

132. Smith, R. L., and J. Brunolli. 1989. Shoulder kinesthesia after anterior glenohumeral joint dislocation. *Phys Ther,* 69:106–112.

133. Solomonow, M., R. Baratta, B. H. Zhou, H. Shoji, W. Bose, C. Beck, and R. D'Ambrosia. 1987. The synergistic action of the anterior cruciate ligament and thigh muscles in maintaining joint stability. *Am J Sports Med,* 15:207–13.

134. Stener S, et al. 2012. The reharvested patellar tendon has the potential for ligamentization when used for anterior cruciate ligament revision surgery. *Knee Surgery Sports Traumatology Arthroscopy,* 20(6): 1168-1174.

135. Swanik, C. B., S. M. Lephart, F. P. Giannantonio, and F. H. Fu. 1997. Reestablishing proprioception and neuromuscular control in the ACL-injured athlete. *Journal of Sports Rehabilitation,* 6:182–206.

136. Swanik, C.B., S. M. Lephart, F. P. Giannantonio, and F. H. Fu. 1997. Reestablishing proprioception and neuromuscular control in the ACL-injured athlete. *Journal of Sports Rehabilitation,* 6:182–206.

137. Swanik, C. B., S. M. Lephart, J. L. Giraldo, R.G. DeMont, and F. H. Fu. 1999. Reactive muscle firing of anterior cruciate ligament-injured females during functional activities. *Journal of Athletic Training,* 34:121–129.

138. Swanik, C. B., S. M. Lephart, K. A. Swanik, D. A. Stone, and F. H. Fu. 2004. Neuromuscular dynamic restraint in women with anterior cruciate ligament injuries. *Clin Orthop Relat Res,* 425:189–99.

139. Swanik, C, Covassin, T, Stearne, D. 2007. The Relationship Between Neurocognitive Function and Noncontact Anterior Cruciate Ligament Injuries. *American Journal of Sports Medicine,* 35(6):943–948.

140. Swanik, K. A., S. M. Lephart, C. B. Swanik, S. P. Lephart, D. A. Stone, and F. H. Fu. 2002. The effects of shoulder plyometric training on proprioception and selected muscle performance characteristics. *J Shoulder Elbow Surg,* 11:579–86.

141. Tripp, B. L. 2008. Principles of restoring function and sensorimotor control in patients with shoulder dysfunction. *Clin Sports Med,* 27:507–19.

142. Tsuda E, Ishibashi Y, Okamura Y, and Toh S.2003. Restoration of anterior cruciate ligament-hamstring reflex arc after anterior cruciate ligament reconstruction. *Knee Surgery Sports Traumatology Arthroscopy,* 11(2): 63-67.

143. Upton, A. R. M., and P. F. Radford. 1975. Motorneuron excitability in elite sprinters. In *Biomechanics,* Komi, P. V., ed. Baltimore: University Park, 82–87.

144. Walla, D. J., J. P. Albright, E. McAuley, R. K., Martin, V., Eldridge, and G. El-Khoury. 1985. Hamstring control and the unstable anterior cruciate ligament-deficient knee. *Am J Sports Med,* 13:34–9.

145. Warner, J. J. P., S. M. Lephart, and F. H. Fu. 1996. Role of proprioception in pathoetiology of shoulder instability. *Clinical Orthopedics,* 330:35–39.

146. Wilk, K. E., C. A. Arrigo, and J. R. Andrews. 1996. Closed and open chain exercises for the upper extremity. *Journal of Sport Rehabilitation,* 156:88–102.

147. Wilk, K. E., R. F. Escamilla, G. S., Fleisig, S. W., Barrentine, J. R., Andrews, and M. L. Boyd. 1996. A comparison of tibiofemoral joint forces and electromyographic activity during open and closed kinetic chain exercises. *Am J Sports Med*, 24:518–527.

148. Wilson, G. J., G. A. Wood and B. C., Elliott. 1991. Optimal stiffness of series elastic component in a stretch-shorten cycle activity. *J Appl Physiol*, 70:825–33.

149. Wilson, G. J., G. A. Wood, and B. C. Elliott. 1991. The relationship between stiffness of the musculature and static flexibility: An alternative explanation for the occurrence of muscular injury. *Int J Sports Med*, 12:403–7.

150. Wojtys, E. M., L. V. Huston, P. D. Taylor, and S. D. Bastian. 1996. Neuromuscular adaptations in isokinetic, isotonic, and agility training programs. *Am J Sports Med*, 24:187–192.

151. Wojtys, E. M., and L. J. Huston. 1994. Neuromuscular performance in normal and anterior cruciate ligamentdeficient lower extremities. *Am J Sports Med*, 22:89–104.

152. Wolf, S. L., and R. L. Segal. 1990. Conditioning of the spinal stretch reflex: Implications for rehabilitation. *Phys Ther*, 70:652–656.

153. Woo, E., Y. Burns, and L. Johnston. 2003. The effect of task uncertainty on muscle activation patterns in 8–10-year-old children. *Physiother Res Int*, 8:143–54.

154. Yack, H. J., C. E. Collins, and T. J. Whieldon. 1993. Comparison of closed and open kinetic chain exercise in the anterior cruciate ligament-deficient knee. *Am J Sports Med*, 21:49–54.

SOLUTIONS TO CLINICAL DECISION-MAKING EXERCISES

6-1   In addition to strength restoration, rehabilitation should focus on reestablishing neurosensory properties of the injured ligament. Balance, perturbation, and agility exercises should be used to restore proprioception and kinesthesia elements, as well as to enhance reflexive pathways. Closed kinetic chain exercises increase joint congruency and neurosensory feedback necessary for reestablishing dynamic stability. Taping or bracing the ankle will provide stability during rehabilitation and practice but also will facilitate additional efferent feedback from cutaneous receptors.

6-2   Prevention programs should concentrate on preparatory and reactive muscle contractions to enhance motor coordination and muscle stiffness of the lower extremity. To achieve these goals, balance, agility, and sports-specific activities should be incorporated into prevention programs. Benefits of balance and agility training are enhanced proprioception, kinesthesia, and reactive muscle activation. Functional activities integrate these neuromuscular elements and should be performed in controlled, isolated movements and progressed to multidirectional complex activities (example: ball dribbling around cones to ball dribbling and cutting against a defender).

6-3   The athletic trainer should recognize that strength and voluntary muscle control of the vastus medialis oblique must be reestablished to achieve balanced coactivation between the vastus lateralis and vastus medialis oblique. Biofeedback training provides sensory feedback, as well as visual and/or auditory encouragement, for selective voluntary muscle control of the vastus medialis oblique.

6-4   Research supports the use of plyometric training to increase strength and performance. Theories regarding neuromuscular benefits include restoration of functional motor programs, heightened reflexes, and increased proprioceptive awareness. Incorporation of plyometric exercises in the early stages of rehabilitation when the patient is not bearing weight should use elastic tubing for resistance in sitting, supine, and prone positions. As the patient is able to bear more weight, exercises should be progressed from two-legged to one-legged exercises. The range of exercises should be taken into consideration and gradually increased according to the patient's strength and level of pain. Activities that can be easily modified in this manner include forward-to-backward and lateral hopping and jumping maneuvers. Exercises should not be performed at too great a speed—faster movements can harm the healing tissues.

6-5   The rotator cuff muscles are not functioning properly to fulfill their stabilizing role at the glenohumeral joint. Rotator cuff strength should be assessed and imbalances remedied through strengthening and closed kinetic chain exercise. Benefits of closed kinetic chain exercises are increased joint congruency and enhanced force-couple coactivation. Strength-shortening, or plyometric, exercises promote preparatory and reactive muscle activity, encourage muscle coactivation, and improve proprioception. The importance of proper technique in rehabilitation exercises and sport movements must be addressed. Verbal feedback from the athletic trainer and visual feedback using a mirror can be used to develop proper motor patterns. In this stage of rehabilitation, a coach's critique and information obtained from motion analysis are advantageous and allow the athletic trainer to tailor the patient's protocol to specific needs.

6-6   Functional activities incorporate a variety of stimuli, so that the body must simultaneously integrate and efficiently use multiple elements of neuromuscular control to maintain function and stability. For the wrestler, factors that should be modified to progress from easy to difficult, as well as from isolated to combined, movements are (1) changing levels (eg, high vs low body position); (2) lateral movements (ie, side shuffles); and (3) rational movements (eg, carioca, pivot). Surface and axial load can be modified to progress the level of difficulty of exercises. A hard, flat surface can be changed to a softer, unstable surface (eg, foam and mat). Weight vests or belts can be used to increase the axial load, thus enhancing stimulation of articular and tenomuscular receptors. It is also beneficial to receive feedback concerning technique and style from the coaching staff during this stage.

Please see videos on the accompanying website at

www.healio.com/books/sportsmedvideos

CHAPTER 7

Regaining Postural Stability and Balance

Kevin M. Guskiewicz, PhD, ATC, FNATA, FACSM

After completion of this chapter, the athletic trainer should be able to do the following:

- Define and explain the roles of the three sensory modalities responsible for maintaining balance.

- Explain how movement strategies along the closed kinetic chain help maintain the center of gravity in a safe and stable area.

- Differentiate between subjective and objective balance assessment.

- Differentiate between static and dynamic balance assessment.

- Evaluate the effect that injury to the ankle, knee, and head has on balance and postural equilibrium.

- Identify the goals of each phase of balance training, and how to progress the patient through each phase.

- State the differences among static, semidynamic, and dynamic balance-training exercises.

Although maintaining balance while standing may appear to be a rather simple motor skill for able-bodied athletes, this feat cannot be taken for granted in a patient with musculoskeletal dysfunction. Muscular weakness, proprioceptive deficits, and range of motion (ROM) deficits may challenge a person's ability to maintain his or her center of gravity (COG) within the body's base of support, or, in other words, cause them to lose their balance. Balance is the single most important element dictating movement strategies within the closed kinetic chain. Acquisition of effective strategies for maintaining balance is therefore essential for athletic performance.

Although balance is often thought of as a static process, it's actually a highly integrative dynamic process involving multiple neurologic pathways. Although *balance* is the more commonly used term, *postural equilibrium* is a broader term that involves the alignment of joint segments in an effort to maintain the

Prentice WE, ed.
Rehabilitation Techniques for Sports Medicine and Athletic Training (pp 181-216).
© 2015 SLACK Incorporated.

COG within an optimal range of the maximum limits of stability (LOS).

Despite often being classified at the end of the continuum of goals associated with therapeutic exercise,[45] maintenance of balance is a vital component in the rehabilitation of joint injuries that should not be overlooked. Traditionally, orthopedic rehabilitation has placed the emphasis on isolated joint mechanics, such as improving ROM and flexibility, and increasing muscle strength and endurance, rather than on afferent information obtained by the joint(s) to be processed by the postural control system.

However, research in the area of proprioception and kinesthesia has emphasized the need to train the joint's neural system.[46-50] Joint position sense, proprioception, and kinesthesia are vital to all athletic performance requiring balance. Current rehabilitation protocols should therefore focus on a combination of open and closed kinetic chain exercises. The necessity for a combination of open and closed kinetic chain exercises can be seen during gait (walking or running), as the foot and ankle prepare for heel strike (open chain) and prepare to control the body's COG during midstance and toe off (closed chain).

This chapter focuses on the postural control system, various balance training techniques, and technologic advancements that are enabling athletic trainers to assess and treat balance deficits in physically active people.

POSTURAL CONTROL SYSTEM

The athletic trainer must first have an understanding of the postural control system and its various components. The postural control system uses complex processes involving both sensory and motor components. Maintenance of postural equilibrium includes sensory detection of body motions, integration of sensorimotor information within the central nervous system (CNS), and execution of appropriate musculoskeletal responses. Most daily activities, such as walking, climbing stairs, reaching, or throwing a ball, require static foot placement with controlled balance shifts, especially if a

favorable outcome is to be attained. So, balance should be considered both a dynamic and static process. The successful accomplishment of static and dynamic balance is based on the interaction between body and environment.[44] Figure 7-1 shows the complexity of this dynamic process.

From a clinical perspective, separating the sensory and motor processes of balance means that a person may have impaired balance for one or a combination of two reasons: (1) the position of the COG relative to the base of support is not accurately sensed; and (2) the automatic movements required to bring the COG to a balanced position are not timely or effectively coordinated.[60] The position of the body in relation to gravity and its surroundings is sensed by combining visual, vestibular, and somatosensory inputs. Balance movements also involve motions of the ankle, knee, and hip joints, which are controlled by the coordinated actions along the kinetic chain (Figure 7-2). These processes are all vital for producing fluid sport-related movements.

CONTROL OF BALANCE

The human body is a very tall structure balanced on a relatively small base, and its COG is quite high, being just above the pelvis. Many factors enter into the task of controlling balance within the base of support. Balance control involves a complex network of neural connections and centers that are related by peripheral and central feedback mechanisms.[34]

The postural control system operates as a feedback control circuit between the brain and the musculoskeletal system. The sources of afferent information supplied to the postural control system collectively come from visual, vestibular, and somatosensory inputs. The CNS's involvement in maintaining upright posture can be divided into two components. The first component, sensory organization, involves those processes that determine the timing, direction, and amplitude of corrective postural actions based upon information obtained from the vestibular, visual, and somatosensory (proprioceptive) inputs.[56] Despite the availability of multiple sensory inputs, the CNS generally

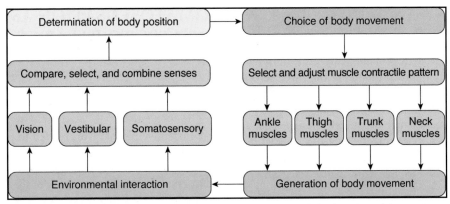

Figure 7-1. Dynamic equilibrium. (Adapted from Allison L, Fuller K, Hedenberg R, et al *Contemporary Management of Balance Deficits*. Clackamas, OR: NeuroCom International; 1994. Reprinted with permission from Natus Medical Incorporated.)

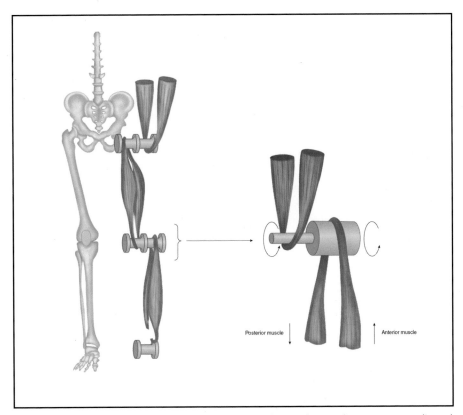

Posterior muscle

Anterior muscle

Figure 7-2. Paired relationships between major postural musculatures that execute coordinated actions along the kinetic chain to control the center of gravity.

relies on only one sense at a time for orientation information. For healthy adults, the preferred sense for balance control comes from somatosensory information (ie, feet in contact with the support surface and detection of joint movement).[37,56] In considering orthopedic injuries, the somatosensory system is of the most importance and is the focus of this chapter.

The second component, muscle coordination, is the collection of processes that determine the temporal sequencing and distribution of contractile activity among the muscles of the legs and trunk that generate supportive reactions for maintaining balance. Research suggests that balance deficiencies in people with neurologic problems can result from inappropriate interaction among the three sensory inputs that provide orientation information to the postural control system. A patient may be inappropriately dependent on one sense for situations presenting intersensory conflict.[56,70]

From a clinical perspective, stabilization of upright posture requires the integration of afferent information from the three senses, which work in combination and are all critical to the execution of coordinated postural corrections. Impairment of one component is usually compensated for by the remaining two components. Often, one of the systems provides faulty or inadequate information such as different surfaces and/or changes in visual acuity and/or peripheral vision. In this case, it is crucial that one of the other senses provides accurate and adequate information so that balance may be maintained. For example, when somatosensory conflict is present, such as a moving platform or a compliant foam surface, balance is significantly decreased with the eyes closed compared to eyes open.

Somatosensory inputs provide information concerning the orientation of body parts to one another and to the support surface.[21,60] Vision measures the orientation of the eyes and head in relation to surrounding objects, and plays an important role in the maintenance of balance. On a stable surface, closing the eyes should cause only minimal increases in postural sway in healthy patients. However, if somatosensory input is disrupted because of ligamentous injury, closing the eyes will increase sway significantly.[12,16,37,38,60] The vestibular apparatus supplies information that measures gravitational, linear, and angular accelerations of the head in relation to inertial space. It does not, however, provide orientation information in relation to external objects, and therefore plays only a minor role in the maintenance of balance when the visual and somatosensory systems are providing accurate information.[60]

SOMATOSENSATION AS IT RELATES TO BALANCE

The terms *somatosensation*, *proprioception*, *kinesthesia*, and *balance* are often used to describe similar phenomena. Somatosensation is a more global term used to describe the proprioceptive mechanisms related to postural control and can accurately be used synonymously. Consequently, somatosensation is best defined as a specialized variation of the sensory modality of touch that encompasses the sensation of joint movement (kinesthesia) and joint position (joint position sense).[46,50] As previously discussed, balance refers to the ability to maintain the body's COG within the base of support provided by the feet. Somatosensation and balance work closely, as the postural control system uses sensory information related to movement and posture from peripheral sensory receptors (eg, muscle spindles, Golgi tendon organs, joint afferents, cutaneous receptors). So the question remains, how does proprioception influence postural equilibrium and balance?

Somatosensory input is received from mechanoreceptors; however, it is unclear whether the tactile senses, muscle spindles, or Golgi tendon organs are most responsible for controlling balance. Nashner[55] concluded after using electromyography responses following platform perturbations that other pathways had to be involved in the responses they recorded because the latencies were longer than those normally associated with a classic myotatic reflex. The stretch-related reflex is the earliest mechanism for increasing the activation level of muscles about a joint following an externally imposed rotation of the joint. Rotation of the ankles is the most probable stimulus of the myotatic reflex that occurs in many persons. It appears to be the first useful phase of activity in the leg muscles after a change in erect posture.[55] The myotatic reflex can be seen when perturbations of gait or posture automatically evoke functionally directed responses in the leg muscles to compensate for imbalance or increased postural sway.[14,55] Muscle spindles sense a stretching of the agonist, thus sending information along its afferent fibers to the spinal cord. There the information is transferred to alpha and gamma motor neurons that carry information back to the muscle fibers and muscle spindle, respectively, and contract the muscle to prevent or control additional postural sway.[14]

Postural sway was assessed on a platform moving into a "toes-up" and "toes-down" position, and a stretch reflex was found in the triceps surae after a sudden ramp displacement into the "toes-up" position.[13] A medium latency response (103 to 118 milliseconds) was observed in the stretched muscle, followed by a delayed response of the antagonistic anterior tibialis muscle (108 to 124 milliseconds). The investigators also blocked afferent proprioceptive information in an attempt to study the role of proprioceptive information from the legs for the maintenance of upright posture. These results suggested that proprioceptive information from pressure and/or joint receptors of the foot (ischemia applied at ankle) plays an important role in postural stabilization during low frequencies of movement, but is of minor importance for the compensation of rapid displacements. The experiment also included a "visual" component, as patients were tested with eyes closed, followed by eyes open. Results suggest that when patients were tested with eyes open, visual information compensated for the loss of proprioceptive input.

Another study[14] used compensatory electromyography responses during impulsive disturbance of the limbs during stance on a treadmill to describe the myotatic reflex. Results revealed that during backward movement of the treadmill, ankle dorsiflexion caused the COG to be shifted anteriorly, thus evoking a stretch reflex in the gastrocnemius muscle, followed by weak anterior tibialis activation. In another trial, the movement was reversed (plantar flexion), thus shifting the COG posteriorly and evoking a stretch reflex of the anterior tibialis muscle. Both of these studies suggest that stretch reflex responses help to control the body's COG, and that the vestibular system is unlikely to be directly involved in the generation of the necessary responses.

Elimination of all sensory information from the feet and ankles revealed that proprioceptors in the leg muscles (gastrocnemius and tibialis anterior) were capable of providing sufficient sensory information for stable standing.[20] Researchers speculated that group I or group II muscle spindle afferents, and group Ib afferents from Golgi tendon organs were the probable sources of this proprioceptive information. The study demonstrated that normal patients can stand in a stable manner when receptors in the leg muscles are the only source of information about postural sway.

Other researchers[5,38] have examined the role of somatosensory information by altering or limiting somatosensory input through the use of platform sway referencing or foam platforms. These studies reported that patients still responded with well-coordinated movements but the movements were often either ineffective or inefficient for the environmental context in which they were used.

BALANCE AS IT RELATES TO THE CLOSED KINETIC CHAIN

Balance is the process of maintaining the COG within the body's base of support. Again, the human body is a very tall structure balanced on a relatively small base, and its COG is quite high, being just above the pelvis. Many factors enter into the task of controlling balance within this designated area. One component often overlooked is the role balance plays within the kinetic chain. Ongoing debates as to how the kinetic chain should be defined and whether open or closed kinetic chain exercises are best have caused many therapists to lose sight of what is most important. An understanding of the postural control system as well as the theory of the kinetic (segmental) chain about the lower extremity helps conceptualize the role of the chain in maintaining balance. Within the kinetic chain, each moving segment transmits forces to every other segment along the chain, and its motions are influenced by forces transmitted from other segments (see Chapter 12).[10] The act of maintaining equilibrium or balance is associated with the closed kinetic chain, as the distal segment (foot) is fixed beneath the base of support.

The coordination of automatic postural movements during the act of balancing is not determined solely by the muscles acting directly about the joint. Leg and trunk muscles exert indirect forces on neighboring joints through the inertial interaction forces among body segments.[57,58] A combination of one or more strategies (ankle, knee, hip) are used to coordinate movement of the COG back to a stable or balanced position when a person's balance is disrupted by an external perturbation. Injury to any one of the joints or corresponding muscles along the kinetic chain can result in a loss of appropriate feedback for maintaining balance.

BALANCE DISRUPTION

Let's say, for example, that a basketball player goes up for a rebound and collides with another player, causing her to land in an unexpected position, thereby compromising her normal balance. To prevent a fall from occurring, the body must correct itself by returning the COG to a position within safer LOS. Afferent mechanoreceptor input from the hip, knee, and ankle joints is responsible for initiating automatic postural responses through the use of one of three possible movement strategies.

Selection of Movement Strategies

Three principal joint systems (ankles, knees, and hips) are located between the base of support and the COG. This allows for a wide variety of postures that can be assumed while the COG is still positioned above the base of support. As described by Nashner,[60] motions about a given joint are controlled by the combined actions of at least one pair of muscles working in opposition. When forces exerted by pairs of opposing muscle about a joint (eg, anterior tibialis and gastrocnemius/soleus) are combined, the effect is to resist rotation of the joint relative to a resting position. The degree to which the joint resists rotation is called joint stiffness. The resting position and the stiffness of the joint are each altered independently by changing the activation levels of one or both muscle groups.[39,60] Joint resting position and joint stiffness are by themselves an inadequate basis for controlling postural movements, and it is theorized that the myotatic stretch reflex is the earliest mechanism for increasing the activation level of the muscles of a joint following an externally imposed rotation of the joint.[60]

When a person's balance is disrupted by an external perturbation, movement strategies involving joints of the lower extremity coordinate movement of the COG back to a balanced position. Three strategies (ankle, hip, stepping) have been identified along a continuum.[37] In general, the relative effectiveness of ankle, hip, and stepping strategies in repositioning the COG over the base of support depends on the configuration of the base of support, the COG alignment in relation to the LOS, and the speed of the postural movement.[37,38]

The ankle strategy shifts the COG while maintaining the placement of the feet by rotating the body as a rigid mass about the ankle joints. This is achieved by contracting either the gastrocnemius or anterior tibialis muscles to generate torque about the ankle joints. Anterior sway of the body is counteracted by gastrocnemius activity, which pulls the body posteriorly. Conversely, posterior sway of the body is counteracted by contraction of the tibialis anterior. Thus, the importance of these muscles should not be underestimated when designing the rehabilitation program. The ankle strategy is most effective in executing relatively slow COG movements when the base of support is firm and the COG is well within the LOS perimeter. The ankle strategy is also believed to be effective in maintaining a static posture with the COG off set from the center. The thigh and lower trunk muscles contract, thereby resisting the destabilization of these proximal joints as a result of the indirect effects of the ankle muscles on the proximal joints (Table 7-1).

Under normal sensory conditions, activation of ankle musculature is almost exclusively selected to maintain equilibrium. However, there are subtle differences associated with loss of somatosensation and with vestibular dysfunction in terms of postural control strategies. Persons with somatosensory loss appear to rely on their hip musculature to retain their COG while experiencing forward or backward perturbation or with different support surface lengths.[21]

If the ankle strategy is not capable of controlling excessive sway, the hip strategy is available to help control motion of the COG through the initiation of large and rapid motions at the hip joints with antiphase rotation of the ankles.

Table 7-1 Function and Anatomy of Muscles Involved in Balance Movements

Joint	Extension		Flexion	
	Anatomic	**Function**	**Anatomic**	**Function**
Hip	Paraspinals Hamstrings	Paraspinals Hamstrings Tibialis	Abdominal Quadriceps	Abdominals Quadriceps Gastrocnemius
Knee	Quadriceps	Paraspinals Quadriceps Gastrocnemius	Hamstrings Gastrocnemius	Abdominals Hamstrings Tibialis
Ankle	Gastrocnemius	Abdominals Quadriceps Gastrocnemius	Tibialis	Paraspinals Hamstrings Tibialis

Adapted from Nashner LM. Physiology of balance. In: Jacobson G, Newman C, Kartush J, eds. *Handbook of Balance Function and Testing.* St. Louis, MO: Mosby; 1993:261-279.

It is most effective when the COG is located near the LOS perimeter, and when the LOS boundaries are contracted by a narrowed base of support. Finally, when the COG is displaced beyond the LOS, a step or stumble (stepping strategy) is the only strategy that can be used to prevent a fall.[58,60]

It is proposed that LOS and COG alignment are altered in individuals exhibiting a musculoskeletal abnormality such as an ankle or knee sprain. For example, weakness of ligaments following acute or chronic sprain about these joints is likely to reduce ROM, thereby shrinking the LOS and placing the person at greater risk for a fall with a relatively smaller sway envelope.[58] Pintsaar et al[67] revealed that impaired function was related to a change from ankle synergy toward hip synergy for postural adjustments among patients with functional ankle instability. This finding, which was consistent with previous results reported by Tropp et al,[74] suggests that sensory proprioceptive function for the injured patients was affected.

ASSESSMENT OF BALANCE

Several methods of balance assessment have been proposed for clinical use. Many of the techniques have been criticized for offering only subjective ("qualitative") measurement information regarding balance rather than an objective ("quantitative") measure.[63]

Subjective Assessment

Prior to the mid 1980s, there were very few methods for systematic and controlled assessment of balance. The assessment of static balance in athletes has traditionally been performed through the use of the standing Romberg test. This test is performed standing with feet together, arms at the side, and eyes closed. Normally a person can stand motionless in this position, but the tendency to sway or fall to one side is considered a positive Romberg sign, indicating a loss of proprioception.[8] The Romberg test has, however, been criticized for its lack of sensitivity and objectivity. It is considered to be a rather qualitative assessment of static balance because a considerable amount of stress is required to make the patient sway enough for an observer to characterize the sway.[42]

The use of a quantifiable clinical test battery called the Balance Error Scoring System (BESS) is recommended instead of the standard Romberg test.[32] Three different stances (double, single, and tandem) are completed twice, once while on a firm surface and once while on a piece of medium density foam (balance pad by Airex is recommended) for a total of six trials (Figure 7-3). Patients are asked to assume the required stance by placing their hands on the iliac crests, and upon eye closure, the 20-second

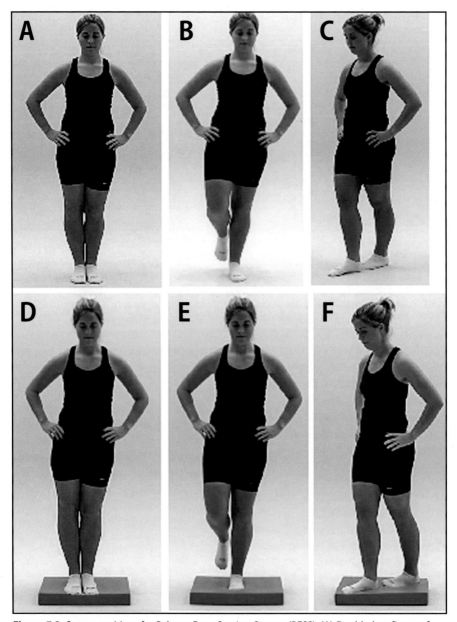

Figure 7-3. Stance positions for Balance Error Scoring System (BESS). (A) Double-leg, firm surface; (B) single-leg, firm surface; (C) tandem, firm surface; (D) double-leg, foam surface; (E) single-leg, foam surface; (F) tandem, foam surface.

test begins. During the single-leg stances, patients are asked to maintain the contralateral limb in 20 to 30 degrees of hip flexion and 40 to 50 degrees of knee flexion. Additionally, the patient is asked to stand quietly and as motionless as possible in the stance position, keeping his or her hands on the iliac crests and eyes closed. The single-limb stance tests are performed on the nondominant foot. This same foot is placed toward the rear on the tandem stances. Patients are told that upon losing their balance, they are to make any necessary adjustments and return to the testing position as quickly as possible. Performance is scored by adding one error point for each error listed in Table 7-2. Trials are considered to be incomplete if the patient is unable to sustain the stance position for longer than 5 seconds

Table 7-2 Balance Error Scoring System (BESS)

Errors
Hands lifted off iliac crests
Opening eyes
Step, stumble, or fall
Moving hip into more than 30 degrees of flexion or abduction
Lifting forefoot or heel
Remaining out of testing position for more than 5 seconds
The BESS score is calculated by adding 1 error point for each error or any combination of errors occurring during one movement. Error scores from each of the 6 trials are added for a total BESS score, and higher scores represent poor balance.

during the entire 20-second testing period. These trials are assigned a standard maximum error score of 10. Balance test results during injury recovery are best used when compared to baseline measurements, and clinicians working with athletes or patients on a regular basis should attempt to obtain baseline measurements when possible.

Clinical Decision-Making Exercise 7-1

How can the Balance Error Scoring System (BESS) or any other quantifiable measure of balance be effectively used in developing a sound rehabilitation program?

Semidynamic and dynamic balance assessment can be performed through functional-reach tests; timed agility tests, such as the figure 8 test,[15,19] carioca, or hop test[40]; Bass Test for Dynamic Balance; timed "T-Band kicks"; and timed balance beam walking with the eyes open or closed. The objective in most of these tests is to decrease the size of the base of support in an attempt to determine a patient's ability to control upright posture while moving. Many of these tests have been criticized for failing to quantify balance adequately, as they merely report the time that a particular posture is maintained, angular displacement, or the distance covered after walking.[6,21,46,60] At any rate, they can often provide the athletic trainer with valuable information about a patient's function and/or return to play capability.

Objective Assessment

Advancements in technology have provided the medical community with commercially available balance systems for quantitatively assessing and training static and dynamic balance (Table 7-3). These systems provide an easy, practical, and cost-effective method of quantitatively assessing and training functional balance through analysis of postural stability. Thus, the potential exists to assess injured patients and (a) identify possible abnormalities that might be associated with injury; (b) isolate various systems that are affected; (c) develop recovery curves based on quantitative measures for determining readiness to return to activity; and (d) train the injured patient.

Most manufacturers use computer-interfaced forceplate technology consisting of a flat, rigid surface supported on three or more points by independent force-measuring devices. As the patient stands on the forceplate surface, the position of the center of vertical forces exerted on the forceplate over time is calculated (Figure 7-4). The center of vertical force movements provide an indirect measure of postural sway activity.[59] The Kistler and, more recently, Bertec forceplates, are used for much of the work in the area of postural stability and balance.[6,17,27,52,54] NeuroCom International, Inc. (Clackamas, OR) has also developed systems with expanded diagnostic and training capabilities that make interpretation of results easier for athletic trainers. Athletic trainers must be aware that the manufacturers often use conflicting terminology to describe various balance parameters, and should consult frequently with the manufacturer to ensure that there is a clear understanding of the measure being taken. These inconsistencies have created confusion in the literature, because what some manufacturers classify as dynamic balance, others claim as really static balance. Our classification system (see the following section "Balance Training") will hopefully clear up some of the confusion and allow for a more consistent labeling of the numerous balance-related exercises.

Table 7-3 High-Technology Balance Assessment Systems

Static Systems	Dynamic Systems
Chattecx Balance System	Biodex Stability System
EquiTest	Chattecx Balance System
Forceplate	EquiTest
Pro Balance Master	EquiTest with EMG
Smart Balance Master	Forceplate
	Kinesthetic Ability Trainer
	Pro Balance Master
	Smart Balance Master

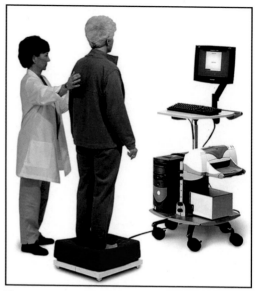

Figure 7-4. Patient training on the Balance Master.

Force platforms ideally evaluate four aspects of postural control: steadiness, symmetry, and dynamic stability. Steadiness is the ability to keep the body as motionless as possible. This is a measure of postural sway. Symmetry is the ability to distribute weight evenly between the two feet in an upright stance. This is a measure of center of pressure (COP), center of balance (COB), or center of force (COF), depending on which testing system you are using. Although inconsistent with our classification system, dynamic stability is often labeled as the ability to transfer the vertical projection of the COG around a stationary supporting base.[27] This is often referred to as a measure of one's perception of his or her "safe" LOS, as one's goal is to lean or reach as far as possible without losing one's balance. Some manufacturers measure dynamic stability by assessing a person's postural response to external perturbations from a moving platform in one of four directions: tilting toes up, tilting toes down, shifting medial-lateral, and shifting anterior-posterior. Platform perturbation on some systems is unpredictable and determined by the positioning and sway movement of the patient. In such cases, a person's reaction response can be determined (Figure 7-5). Other systems have a more predictable sinusoidal waveform that remains constant regardless of patient positioning.

Many of these force platform systems measure the vertical ground reaction force and provide a means of computing the COP. The COP represents the center of the distribution of the

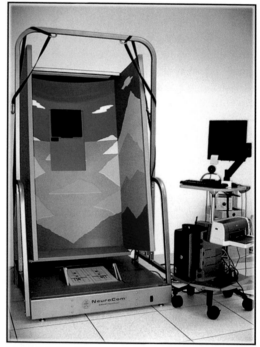

Figure 7-5. EquiTest.

total force applied to the supporting surface. The COP is calculated from horizontal moment and vertical force data generated by triaxial force platforms. The center of vertical force, on NeuroCom's EquiTest, is the center of the vertical force exerted by the feet against the support

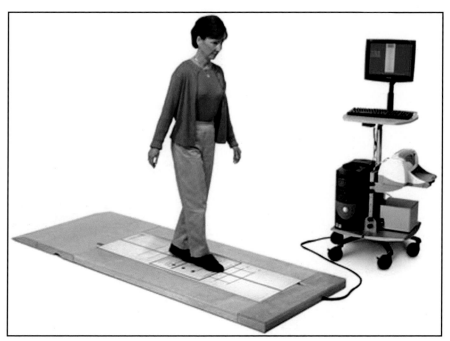

Figure 7-6. Balance Master with 5-foot forceplate accessory.

surface. In any case (COP, COB, COF), the total force applied to the force platform fluctuates because it includes both body weight and the inertial effects of the slightest movement of the body that occur even when one attempts to stand motionless. The movement of these force-based reference points is theorized to vary according to the movement of the body's COG and the distribution of muscle forces required to control posture. Ideally, healthy athletes should maintain their COP very near the anterior-posterior and medial-lateral midlines.

Once the COP or COF is calculated, several other balance parameters can be attained. Deviation from this point in any direction represents a person's postural sway. Postural sway can be measured in various ways, depending on which system is being used. Mean displacement, length of sway path, length of sway area, amplitude, frequency, and direction with respect to the COP can be calculated on most systems. An equilibrium score, comparing the angular difference between the calculated maximum anterior to posterior COG displacements to a theoretical maximum displacement, is unique to NeuroCom International's EquiTest.

Forceplate technology allows for quantitative analysis and understanding of a patient's postural instability. These systems are fully integrated with hardware or software systems for quickly and quantitatively assessing and rehabilitating balance disorders. Most manufacturers allow for both static and dynamic balance assessment in either double or single leg stances, with eyes open or eyes closed. NeuroCom's EquiTest System is equipped with a moving visual surround (wall) that allows for the most sophisticated technology available for isolating and assessing sensory modality interaction.

Long forceplates have been developed by some manufacturers in an attempt to combat criticism that balance assessment is not functional. Inclusion of the long forceplate (Figure 14-6) adds a vast array of dynamic balance exercises for training, such as walking, step-up-and-over, side and crossover steps, hopping, leaping, and lunging. These important return-to-sport activities can be practiced and perfected through the use of the computer's visual feedback.

Biodex Medical Systems (Shirley, NY) manufactures a dynamic multiaxial tilting platform that offers computer-generated data similar to that of a forceplate system. The Biodex Stability System (Figure 7-7) uses a dynamic multiaxial

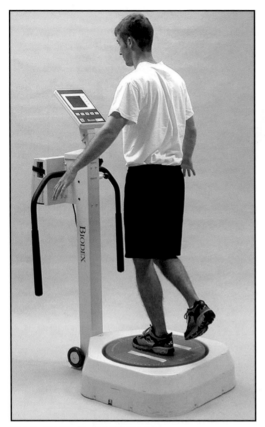

Figure 7-7. Biodex Stability System.

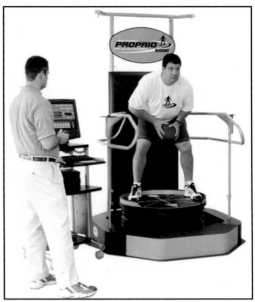

Figure 7-8. PROPRIO Reactive Balance System. (Reproduced with permission from Perry Dynamics.)

platform that allows up to 20 degrees of deflection in any direction. It is theorized that this degree of deflection is sufficient to stress joint mechanoreceptors that provide proprioceptive feedback (at end ranges of motion) necessary for balance control. Therapists can assess deficits in dynamic muscular control of posture relative to joint pathology. The patient's ability to control the platform's angle of tilt is quantified as a variance from center, as well as degrees of deflection over time, at various stability levels. A large variance is indicative of poor muscle response. Exercises performed on a multiaxial unstable system such as the Biodex are similar to those of the Biomechanical Ankle Platform System (BAPS board) and are especially effective for regaining proprioception and balance following injury to the ankle joint. A newer system, the PROPRIO Reactive Balance System measures the patient's center of mass movement on a computerized, programmable, multidirectional, multispeed platform for both reactive and anticipatory training to assess, rehabilitate, and train balance and proprioception (Figure 7-8). Instead of assessing lower-leg postural responses on a forceplate, this system measures trunk movements by placing a sensor on the lumbosacral joint, L5-S1. Using ultrasonic technology, the PROPRIO Reactive Balance System quantifies trunk movement in six degrees of freedom—lateral, up/down, anterior/posterior, rotation, flexion/extension, and lateral flexion—and displays real-time feedback during training. The platform can generate perturbations to provide variable surface movement requiring the patient to maintain the patient's center of mass over the body's support area during movement and changing sensory environments.

INJURY AND BALANCE

It has long been theorized that failure of stretched or damaged ligaments to provide adequate neural feedback in an injured extremity may contribute to decreased proprioceptive mechanisms necessary for maintenance of proper balance. Research has revealed these impairments in individuals with ankle injury[23,31,69] and anterior cruciate ligament (ACL) injury.[4,65] The lack of proprioceptive feedback resulting from such injuries may allow excessive or inappropriate loading of a joint. Furthermore, although the presence of a capsular lesion may interfere with the transmission of afferent impulses from the joint, a more important effect may be alteration of the afferent neural code that is conveyed to the CNS. Decreased reflex excitation of motor neurons may result from either or both of the following events: (a) a decrease in proprioceptive input to the CNS; and (b) an increase in the activation of inhibitory interneurons within the spinal cord. All of these factors may lead to progressive degeneration of the joint and continued deficits in joint dynamics, balance, and coordination.

Ankle Injuries

Joint proprioceptors are believed to be damaged during injury to the lateral ligaments of the ankle because joint receptor fibers possess less tensile strength than the ligament fibers. Damage to the joint receptors is believed to cause joint deafferentation, thereby diminishing the supply of messages from the injured joint up the afferent pathway and disrupting proprioceptive function.[24] Freeman et al[24] were the first to report a decrease in the frequency of functional instability following ankle sprains when coordination exercises were performed as part of rehabilitation. Thus the term *articular deafferentation* was introduced to designate the mechanism that they believed to be the cause of functional instability of the ankle. This finding led to the inclusion of balance training in ankle rehabilitation programs.

Since 1955, Freeman[23] has theorized that if ankle injuries cause partial deafferentation and functional instability, a person's postural sway would be altered because of a proprioception deficit. Although some studies[74] have not supported Freeman's theory, other more recent studies using high-tech equipment (forceplate, kinesthesiometer, etc) have revealed balance deficits in ankles following acute sprains[25,31,66] and/or in ankles with chronic instabilities.[9,22,26,67]

Differences were identified between injured and uninjured ankles in 14 ankle-injured patients using a computerized strain-gauge forceplate.[25] Four of five possible postural sway parameters (standard deviation of the mean COP dispersion, mean sway amplitude, average speed, and number of sway amplitudes exceeding 5 and 10 mm) taken in the frontal plane from a single-leg stance position were reported to discriminate between injured and noninjured ankles. The authors reported that the application of an ankle brace eliminated the differences between injury status when tested on each parameter, therefore improving balance performance. More importantly, this study suggests that the stabilometry technique of selectively analyzing postural sway movements in the frontal plane, where the diameter of the supporting area is smallest, leads to higher sensitivity. Because difficulties of maintaining balance after a ligament lesion involve the subtalar axis, it is proposed that increased sway movements of the different body segments would be found primarily in the frontal plane. The authors speculated that this could explain nonsignificant findings of earlier stabilometry studies[74] involving injured ankles.

Orthotic intervention and postural sway were studied in 13 patients with acute inversion ankle sprains and 12 uninjured patients under two treatment conditions (orthotic, nonorthotic) and four platform movements (stable, inversion/eversion, plantar flexion/dorsiflexion, medial/lateral perturbations).[31] Results revealed that ankle-injured patients swayed more than uninjured patients when assessed in a single-leg test. The analysis also revealed that custom-fit orthotics may restrict undesirable motion at the foot and ankle, and enhance joint mechanoreceptors to detect perturbations and provide structural support for detecting and controlling postural sway in ankle-injured patients. A similar study[66] reported improvements in static balance for injured patients while wearing custom-made orthotics.

Studies involving patients with chronic ankle instabilities[9,22,26,67] indicate that individuals with a history of inversion ankle sprain are less stable in single-limb stance on the involved leg compared to the uninvolved leg and/or noninjured patients. Significant differences between injured and uninjured patients for sway amplitude but not sway frequency using a standard forceplate were revealed.[9] The effect of stance perturbation on frontal plane postural control was tested in three groups of patients: (1) control (no previous ankle injury); (2) functional ankle instability and 8-week training program; and (3) mechanical instability without functional instability (without shoe, with shoe, with brace and shoe).[67] The authors reported a relative change from ankle to hip synergy at medially directed translations of the support surface on the NeuroCom EquiTest. The impairment was restored after 8 weeks of ankle disk training. The effect of a shoe and brace did not exceed the effect of the shoe alone. Impaired ankle function was shown to be related to coordination, as patients changed from ankle toward hip strategies for postural adjustments.

Similarly, researchers[36] reported that lateral ankle joint anesthesia did not alter postural sway or passive joint position sense, but did affect the COB position (similar to COP) during both static and dynamic testing. This suggests the presence of an adaptive mechanism to compensate for the loss of afferent stimuli from the region of the lateral ankle ligaments.[36] Patients tended to shift their COB medially during dynamic balance testing and slightly laterally during static balance testing. The authors speculated that COB shifting may provide additional proprioceptive input from cutaneous receptors in the sole of the foot or stretch receptors in the peroneal muscle tendon unit, which therefore prevents increased postural sway.

Increased postural sway frequency and latencies are parameters thought to be indicative of impaired ankle joint proprioception.[13,69] Cornwall et al[9] and Pintsaar et al,[67] however, found no differences between chronically injured patients and control patients on these measures. This raises the question as to whether postural sway was in fact caused by a proprioceptive deficit. Increased postural sway amplitudes in the absence of sway frequencies might suggest that chronically injured patients recover their ankle joint proprioception over time. Thus, more research is warranted for investigating loss of joint proprioception and postural sway frequency.[9]

In summary, results of studies involving both chronic and acute ankle sprains suggest that increased postural sway and/or balance instability may not be caused by a single factor but by disruption of both neurologic and biomechanical factors at the ankle joint. Loss of balance may result from abnormal or altered biomechanical alignment of the body, thus affecting the transmission of somatosensory information from the ankle joint. It is possible that observed postural sway amplitudes following injury are a result of joint instability along the kinetic chain, rather than deafferentation. Thus, the orthotic intervention[31,61,62] may have provided more optimal joint alignment.

Knee Injuries

Ligamentous injury to the knee has proven to affect the ability of patients to accurately detect position.[2,3,4,46,49,50] The general consensus among numerous investigators performing proprioceptive testing is that a clinical proprioception deficit occurs in most patients after an ACL rupture who have functional instability and that this deficit seems to persist to some degree after an ACL reconstruction.[2] Because of the relationships between proprioception (somatosensation) and balance, it has been suggested that the patient's ability to balance on the ACL-injured leg may also be decreased.[4,65]

Researchers have evaluated the effects of ACL ruptures on standing balance using forceplate technology, and although some studies have revealed balance deficits,[25,53] others have not.[18,35] Thus, there appear to be conflicting results from these studies depending on which parameters are measured. Mizuta et al[53] found significant differences in postural sway when measuring COP and sway distance area between 11 functionally stable and 15 functionally unstable patients who had unilateral ACL-deficient knees. Faculjak et al,[18] however, found no differences in postural stability between 8 ACL-deficient patients and 10 normal patients when measuring average latency and response strength on an EquiTest System.

Several potential reasons for this discrepancy exist. First, it has been suggested that there might be a link between static balance and isometric strength of the musculature at the ankle and knee. Isometric muscle strength could therefore compensate for any somatosensory deficit present in the involved knee during a closed chain static balance test. Second, many studies fail to discriminate between functionally unstable ACL-deficient knees and knees that were not functionally unstable. This presents a design flaw, especially considering that functionally stable knees would most likely provide adequate balance despite ligamentous pathology. Another suggested reason for not seeing differences between injured knees and uninjured knees on static balance measures could be explained by the role that joint mechanoreceptors play. Neurophysiologic studies[28,29,43,46] reveal that joint mechanoreceptors provide enhanced kinesthetic awareness in the near-terminal ROM or extremes of motion. Therefore, it could be speculated that if the maximum LOS are never reached during a static balance test, damaged mechanoreceptors (muscle or joint) may not even become a factor. Dynamic balance tests or functional hop tests that involve dynamic balance could challenge the postural control system (ankle strategies are taken over by hip and/or stepping strategies), requiring more mechanoreceptor input. These tests would most likely discriminate between functionally unstable ACL-deficient knees and normal knees.

Clinical Decision-Making Exercise 7-2

A gymnast recovering from a grade 1 MCL sprain to her right knee is ready to begin her rehabilitation. What factors must first be considered prior to design?

Head Injury

Neurologic status following mild head injury has been assessed using balance as a criterion variable. Therapists and team physicians have long evaluated head injuries with the Romberg tests of sensory modality function to test "balance." This is an easy and effective sideline test; however, the literature suggests there is more to posture control than just balance and sensory modality,[55,56,61,64,72] especially when assessing people with head injury.[30,33] The postural control system, which is responsible for linking brain to body communication, is often affected as a result of mild head injury. Several studies have identified postural stability deficits in patients up to 3 days post injury by using commercially available balance systems.[30,33] It appears this deficit is related to a sensory interaction problem, whereby the injured patient fails to use his or her visual system effectively. This research suggests that objective balance assessment can be used for establishing recovery curves for making return-to-play decisions in concussed patients. Rehabilitation of concussed patients using balance techniques has yet to be studied.

BALANCE TRAINING

Developing a rehabilitation program that includes exercises for improving balance and postural equilibrium is vital for a successful return to competition from a lower-extremity injury. Regardless of whether the patient has sustained a quadriceps strain or an ankle sprain, the injury has caused a disruption at some point between the body's COG and base of support. This is likely to have caused compensatory weight shifts and gait changes along the kinetic chain that have resulted in balance deficits. These deficits may be detected through the use of functional assessment tests and/or computerized instrumentation previously discussed for assessing balance. Having the advanced technology available to quantify balance deficits is an amenity, but not a necessity. Imagination and creativity are often the best tools available to athletic trainers with limited resources who are trying to design balance training protocols.

Because virtually all sport activities involve closed chain lower-extremity function, functional rehabilitation should be performed in the closed kinetic chain. However, ROM, movement speed, and additional resistance may be more easily controlled in the open chain initially. Therefore, adequate, safe function in an open chain may be the first step in the rehabilitation process, but should not be the focus of the rehabilitation plan. The athletic trainer should attempt to progress the patient to functional closed-chain exercises quickly and safely. Depending on severity of injury, this could be as early as one day post injury.

As previously mentioned, there is a close relationship between somatosensation, kinesthesia, and balance. Therefore, many of the exercises proposed for kinesthetic training are indirectly enhancing balance. Several methods of regaining balance have been proposed in the literature and are included in the most current rehabilitation protocols for ankle[41,73] and knee injury.[11,40,51,72]

A variety of activities can be used to improve balance, but the therapist should first consider five general rules before beginning. The exercises must:

1. Be safe, yet challenging.

2. Stress multiple planes of motion.

3. Incorporate a multisensory approach.

4. Begin with static, bilateral, and stable surfaces and progress to dynamic, unilateral, and unstable surfaces.

5. Progress toward sport-specific exercises.

There are several ways in which the athletic trainer can meet these goals. Balance exercises should be performed in an open area, where the patient will not be injured in the event of a fall. It is best to perform exercises with an assistive device within an arm's reach (eg, chair, railing, table, wall), especially during the initial phase of rehabilitation. When considering exercise duration for balance exercises, the athletic trainer can use either sets and repetitions or a time-based protocol. The patient can perform two to three sets of 15 repetitions and progress to 30 repetitions as tolerated, or perform 10 of the exercises for a 15-second period and progress to 30-second periods later in the program.

Clinical Decision-Making Exercise 7-3

How can the athletic trainer determine whether a patient is ready to progress to a more challenging balance task and/or balance surface?

Classification of Balance Exercises

Static balance is when the COG is maintained over a fixed base of support (unilateral or bilateral) while standing on a stable surface. Examples of static exercises are a single-leg, double-leg, or tandem-stance Romberg task.

Semidynamic balance involves one of two possible activities: (1) The person maintains his or her COG over a fixed base of support while standing on a moving surface (Chattecx Balance System or EquiTest) or unstable surface (Biodex Stability System, BAPS, medium density foam or minitramp); or (2) the person transfers his or her COG over a fixed base of support to selected ranges and/or directions within the LOS while standing on a stable surface (Balance Master's LOS, functional reach tests, minisquats, or T-Band kicks). Dynamic balance involves the maintenance of the COG within the LOS over a moving base of support (feet), usually while on a stable surface. These tasks require the use of a stepping strategy. The base of support is always changing its position, forcing the COG to be adjusted with each movement. Examples of dynamic exercises are walking on a balance beam, step-up-and-over task, or bounding. Functional balance tasks are the same as dynamic tasks with the inclusion of sport-specific tasks such as throwing and catching.

Phase I

The progression of activities during this phase should include nonballistic types of drills. Training for static balance can be initiated once the patient is able to bear weight on the extremity. The patient should first be asked to perform a bilateral 20-second Romberg test on a variety of surfaces, beginning with a hard/firm surface (Figure 14-9). Once a comfort zone is established, the patient should be progressed to performing unilateral balance tasks on both the involved and uninvolved extremities on a stable surface.

The athletic trainer should make comparisons from these tests to determine the patient's ability to balance bilaterally and unilaterally. It should be noted that even though this is termed *static balance*, the patient does not remain perfectly motionless. To maintain static balance, the patient must make many small corrections at the ankle, hip, trunk, arms, or head as previously discussed (see the previous section "Selection of Movement Strategies"). If the patient is having difficulties performing these activities, he or she should not be progressed to the next surface. Repetitions of modified

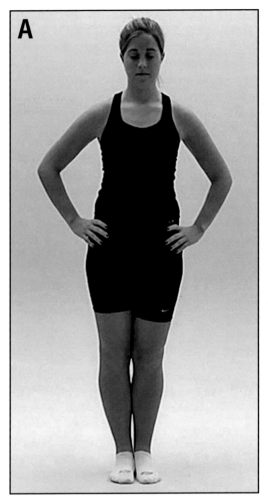

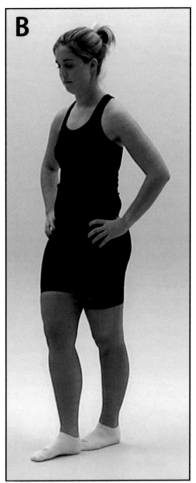

Figure 7-9. Double- and single-leg balance on a stable surface. (A) Double-leg stance; (B) double-leg tandem stance; (C) single-leg stance.

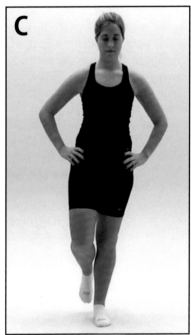

Romberg tests can be performed by first using the arms as a counterbalance, then attempting the activity without using the arms. Static balance activities should be used as a precursor to more dynamic activities. The general progression of these exercises should be from bilateral to unilateral, with eyes open to eyes closed. The exercises should attempt to eliminate or alter the various sensory information (visual, vestibular, and somatosensory) so as to challenge the other systems. In most orthopedic rehabilitation situations, this is going to involve eye closure and changes in the support surface so the somatosensory system can be overloaded or stressed. This theory is synonymous with the overload principle in therapeutic exercise. Research suggests that balance activities, both with and without visual input, will enhance motor function at the brainstem level.[7,73] However, as the patient becomes more efficient at performing activities involving static balance, eye closure is recommended so that only the somatosensory system is left to control balance.

As improvement occurs on a firm surface, bilateral static balance drills should progress to an unstable surface such as a Tremor box, DynaDisc rocker board on hard surface, Bosu Balance Trainer (flat side up then bubble side up), BAPS board, or foam surface (Figure 7-10).[1] The purpose of the different surfaces is to safely challenge the injured patient while keeping the patient motivated to rehabilitate the injured extremity. Additionally, the athletic trainer can introduce light shoulder, back, or chest taps in an attempt to challenge the patient's ability to maintain balance (Figure 7-11). Once the control is demonstrated in a bilateral stance, the patient can progress to similar activities using a unilateral stance (Figure 7-12). All of these exercises increase awareness of the location of the COG under a challenged condition, thereby helping to increase ankle strength in the closed-kinetic-chain. Such training may also increase sensitivity of the muscle spindle and thereby increase proprioceptive input to the spinal cord, which may provide compensation for altered joint afference.[46]

Although static and semidynamic balance exercises may not be very functional for most sport activities, they are the first step toward regaining proprioceptive awareness, reflex stabilization, and postural orientation. The patient should attempt to assume a functional stance while performing static balance drills. Training in different positions places a variety of demands on the musculotendinous structures about the ankle, knee, and hip joints. For example, a gymnast should practice static balance with the hip in neutral and external rotation, as well as during a tandem stance to mimic performance on a balance beam. A basketball player should perform these drills in the "ready position" on the balls of the feet with the hips and knees slightly flexed. Patients requiring a significant amount of static balance for performing their sport include gymnasts, cheerleaders, and football linemen.[41]

Phase II

This phase should be considered the transition phase from static to more dynamic balance activities. Dynamic balance will be especially important for patients who perform activities such as running, jumping, and cutting, which encompasses about 95% of all athletes. Such activities require the patient to repetitively lose and gain balance to perform their sport without falling or becoming injured.[41] Dynamic balance activities should only be incorporated into the rehabilitation program once sufficient healing has occurred and the patient has adequate ROM, muscle strength, and endurance. This could be as early as a few days post injury in the case of a grade 1 ankle sprain, or as late as 5 weeks post surgery in the case of an ACL reconstruction. Before the athletic trainer progresses the patient to challenging dynamic and sport-specific balance drills, several semidynamic (intermediate) exercises should be introduced.

These semidynamic balance drills involve displacement or perturbation of the COG away from the base of support. The patient is challenged to return and/or steady the COG above the base of support throughout several repetitions of the exercise. Some of these exercises involve a bilateral stance, some involve a unilateral stance, while others involve transferring of weight from one extremity to the other.

The bilateral-stance balance drills include the minisquat that is performed with the feet shoulder-width apart and the COG centered

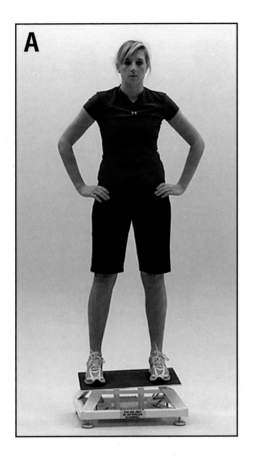

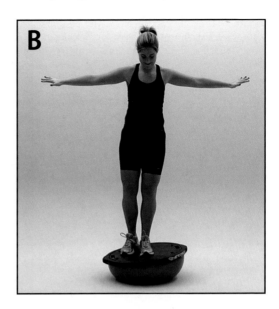

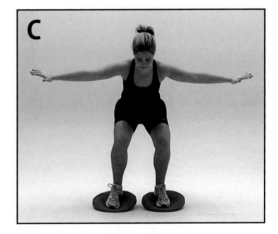

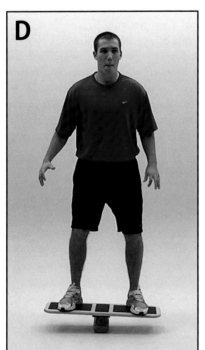

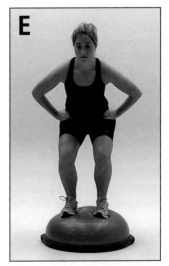

Figure 7-10. Double leg balance on an unstable surface. (A) Tremor Box; (B) Bosu Balance Trainer, flat surface; (C) DynaDiscs; (D) Extreme Balance Board; (E) Bosu Balance Trainer, bubble surface.

Figure 7-11. An athletic trainer causing perturbations using a shoulder tap is good for transitioning from double-leg balance on an unstable surface to single-leg balance on an unstable surface.

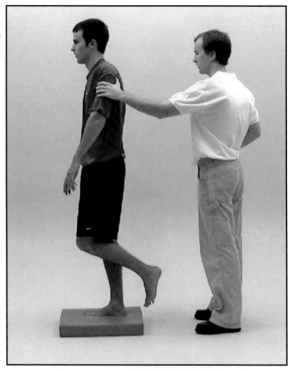

over a stable base of support (Figure 7-13A). The trunk should be positioned upright over the legs as the patient slowly flexes the hips and knees into a partial squat—about 50 degrees of knee flexion. The patient then returns to the starting position and repeats the task several times. Once ROM, strength, and stability have improved, the patient can progress to a full squat, which approaches 90-degree knee flexion. These should be performed in front of a mirror so the patient can observe the amount of stability on his or her return to the extended position. A large stability ball can also be used to perform sit-to-stand activities (Figure 7-13B). Once the patient reaches a comfort zone, the patient can perform more challenging variations of these exercises, beginning on a stable surface (Figure 7-14) and progressing to weight, cable, or tubing-resisted exercises (Figure 7-15). Rotational maneuvers and weight-shifting exercises on unstable surfaces such as the Bosu, DynaDisc, or foam pad are used to assist the patient in controlling the patient's COG during semidynamic movements (Figure 7-16). These exercises are important in the rehabilitation of ankle, knee, and hip injuries, as they help improve weight transfer, COG sway velocity,

and left/right weight symmetry. They can be performed in an attempt to challenge anterior-posterior stability or medial-lateral stability.

The athletic trainer has a variety of options for unilateral semidynamic balance exercises. In the progression to more dynamic exercises, the patient should emphasize controlled hip and knee flexion, followed by a smooth return to a stabilization position. Step-ups can be performed either in the sagittal plane (forward step-up) or in the transverse plane (lateral step-up) (Figure 7-17A and B). These drills should begin with the heel of the uninvolved extremity on the floor. Using a two count, the patient should shift body weight toward the involved side and use the involved extremity to slowly raise the body onto the step.[73] The involved knee should not be "locked" into full extension. Instead, the knee should be positioned in about 5 degrees of flexion, while balancing on the step for 3 seconds. Following the three count, the body weight should be shifted toward the uninvolved side and lowered to the heel of the uninvolved side. Step-up-and-over activities are similar to step-ups, but involve more dynamic transfer of the COG. These should be performed by having the patient both ascend and

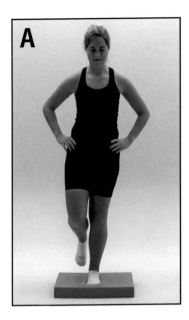
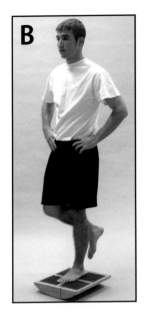
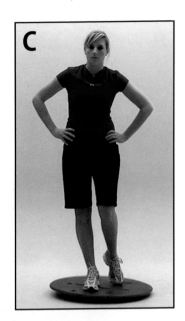
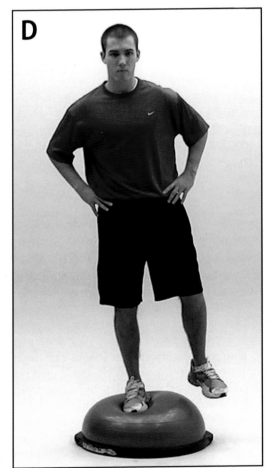
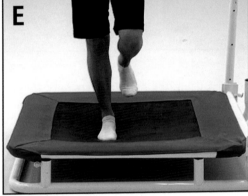

Figure 7-12. Single-leg balance on an unstable surface. (A) Foam pad; (B) Rocker Board; (C) BAPS Board; (D) Bosu Balance Trainer; (E) Plyoback.

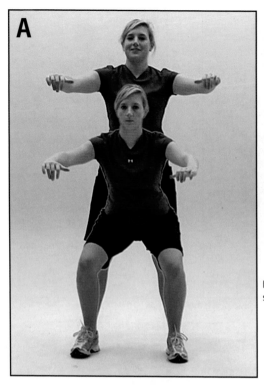

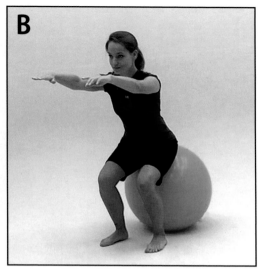

Figure 7-13. Double-leg dynamic activities on a stable surface. (A) Minisquats; (B) sit-to-stand from a stability ball.

descend using the involved extremity (Figure 7-17C) or ascend with the involved extremity and descend with the uninvolved extremity forcing the involved leg to support the body on the descend. The athletic trainer can also introduce the patient to more challenging static tasks during this phase. For example, the very popular Thera-Band kicks (T-Band kicks or steamboats) are excellent for improving balance. Thera-Band kicks are performed with an elastic material (attached to the ankle of the uninvolved leg) serving as a resistance against a relatively fast kicking motion (Figure 7-17D). The patient's balance on the involved extremity is challenged by perturbations caused by the kicking motion of the uninvolved leg. Four sets of these exercises should be performed, one for each of four possible kicking motions: hip flexion, hip extension, hip abduction, and hip adduction. T-Band kicks can also be performed on foam or a minitramp if additional somatosensory challenges are desired.[72] Single and multiplane lunges can also be used to transition to dynamic activities (Figure 7-17E and F).

The Balance Shoes (Orthopedic Physical Therapy Products, Minneapolis, MN) are

another excellent tool for improving the strength of lower extremity musculature and, ultimately, improving balance. The shoes allow lower-extremity balance and strengthening exercises to be performed in a functional, closed kinetic chain manner. The shoes consist of a cork sandal with a rubber sole, and a rubber hemisphere similar in consistency to a lacrosse ball positioned under the midsole (Figures 22-28 to 22-35). The design of the sandals essentially creates an individualized perturbation device for each limb that can be used in any number of functional activities, ranging from static single-leg stance to dynamic gait activities performed in multiple directions (forward walking, side-stepping, carioca walking, etc.).

Clinical use of the Balance Shoes has resulted in a number of successful clinical outcomes from a subjective standpoint, including treatment of ankle sprains and chronic instability, anterior tibial compartment syndrome, lower leg fractures, and a number of other orthopedic problems, as well as for enhancement of core stability. Research reveals that training in the Balance Shoes results in reduced rear foot motion and improved postural stability in

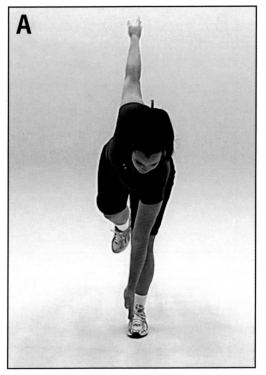

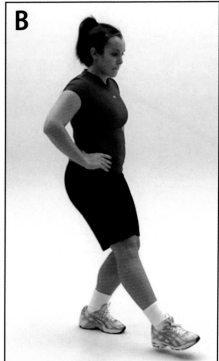

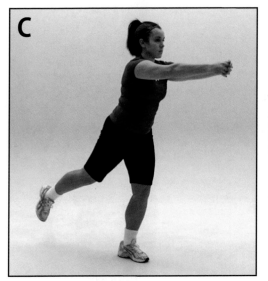

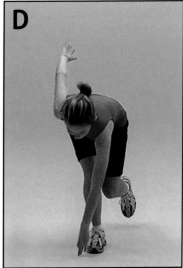

Figure 7-14. Single-leg balance dynamic (multiplane) movements on a stable surface. (A) Windmill; (B) single-leg reach; (C) double-arm reach; (D) Romanian deadlift.

excessive pronators, and that functional activities in the Balance Shoes increase gluteal muscle activity (see Chapter 20).

Clinical Decision-Making Exercise 7-4

What type of balance exercises would best meet the needs of a tennis player recovering from a grade 2 anterior talofibular sprain?

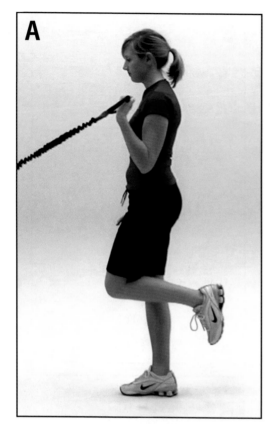

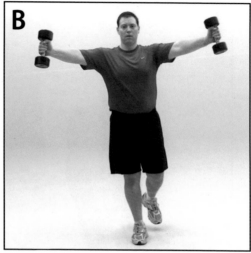

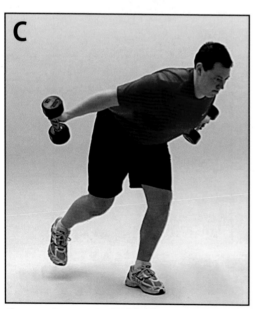

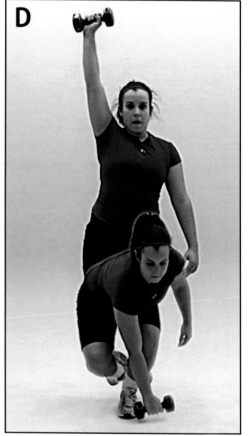

Figure 7-15. Single-leg balance-resisted (multiplane) movements on a stable surface. (A) Bicep curls using cable or tubing; (B) dumbbell scaption; (C) dumbbell cobra; (D) squat touchdown to overhead press.

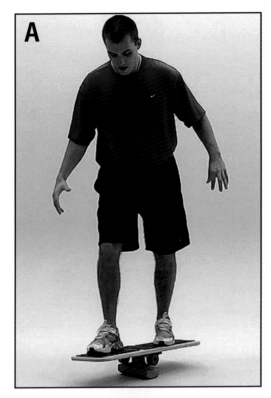
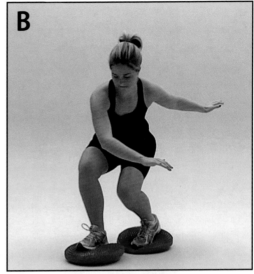
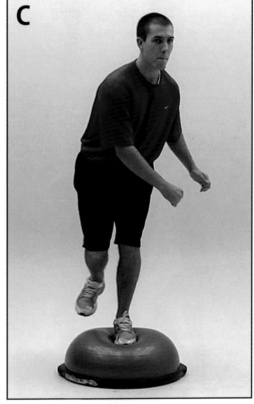
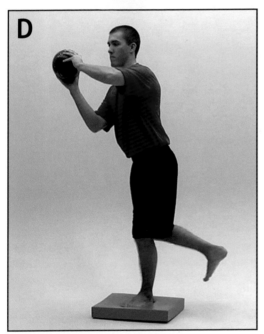

Figure 7-16. Double-leg and single-leg (multiplane) dynamic balance activities on an unstable surface. (A) Tandem stance on an Extreme Balance Board; (B) standing rotation on DynaDisc; (C) standing rotation on Bosu Balance Trainer; (D) partner throw-and-catch using a weighted ball while balancing on a foam pad.

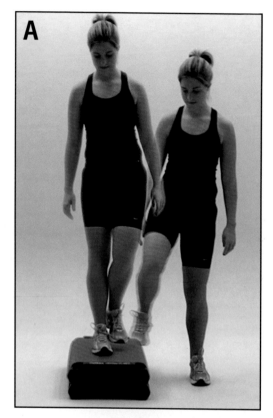

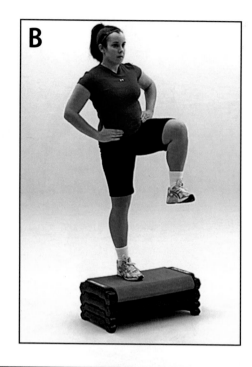

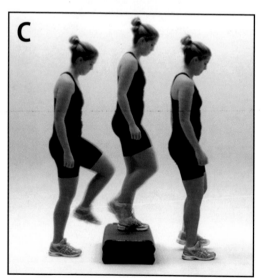

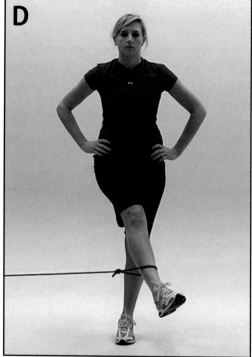

Figure 7-17. Stepping movements to stabilization. (A) Lateral step up; (B) forward step-up to single-leg balance; (C) step-up-and-over (alternating lead leg); (D) Thera-Band kicks; (*continued*)

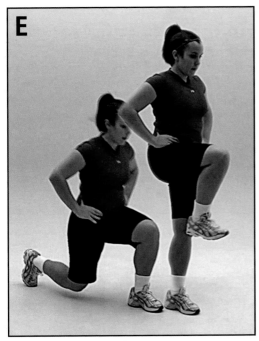

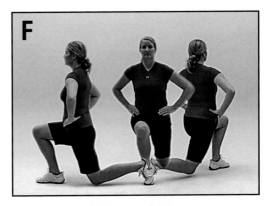

Figure 7-17. (*continued*) (E) forward lunge to single-leg balance; (F) multiplane lunges (sagittal, frontal, transverse).

Phase III

Once the patient can successfully complete the semidynamic exercises presented in Phase II, the patient should be ready to perform more dynamic and functional types of exercises. The general progression for activities to develop dynamic balance and control is from slow-speed to fast-speed activities, from low-force to high-force activities, and from controlled to uncontrolled activities.[41] In other words, patients should be working toward sport-specific drills that will allow for a safe return to their respective sport or activity. These exercises will likely differ depending on which sport the person plays. For example, drills to improve lateral weight shifting and sidestepping should be incorporated into a program for a tennis player, whereas drills to improve jumping and landing are going to be more important for a track athlete who performs the long jump. As previously mentioned, the athletic trainer often needs to use the athletic trainer's imagination to develop the best protocol for the patient.

Bilateral jumping drills are a good place to begin once the patient has reached Phase III. The patient should begin with jumping or hopping onto a step, or performing butt kicks or tuck jumps, and quickly establishing a stabilized position (Figures 7-18A to C). A more dynamic exercise involves bilateral jumping either over a line or some object either front to back or side to side. The patient should concentrate on landing on each side of the line as quickly as possible (Figure 7-18D).[72,73] Bilateral dynamic balance exercises should progress to unilateral dynamic balance exercises as quickly as possible during Phase III. At this stage of the rehabilitation, pain and fatigue should not be as much of a factor. All jumping drills performed bilaterally should now be performed unilaterally, by practicing first on the uninvolved extremity. If additional challenges are needed, a vertical component can be added by having the patient jump over an object such as a box or other suitable object (Figure 7-18E).

As the patient progresses through these exercises, eye closure can be used to further challenge the patient's somatosensation. After mastering these straight plane jumping patterns, the patient can begin diagonal jumping patterns through the use of a cross on the floor formed by two pieces of tape (Figure 14-18F). The intersecting lines create four quadrants that can be numbered and used to perform different jumping sequences such as 1, 3, 2, 4 for the first set and 1, 4, 2, 3 for the second set.[72,73] A larger grid can be designed to allow

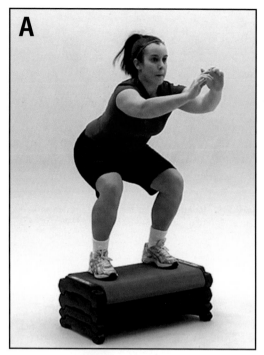

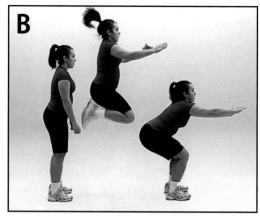

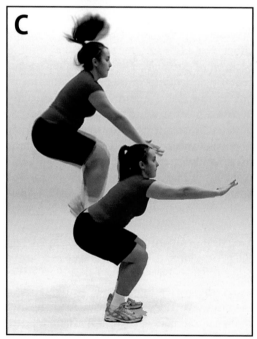

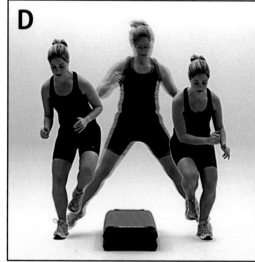

Figure 7-18. Jumping and hopping to stabilization. (A) Forward jump-up to stabilization; (B) butt kicks to stabilization; (C) tuck jumps to stabilization; (D) bidirectional single-leg hop-overs to stabilization; *(continued)*.

for longer sequences and longer jumps, both of which require additional strength, endurance, and balance control.

Another good exercise to introduce prior to advancing to Phase III is a balance beam walk, which can be performed against resistance to further challenge the patient (Figure 7-19A). Tubing can be added to dynamic unilateral

training exercises. The patient can perform stationary running against the tube's resistance, followed by lateral and diagonal bounding exercises. Diagonal bounding, which involves jumping from one foot to another, places greater emphasis on lateral movements. It is recommended that the patient first learn the bounding exercise without tubing, and then attempt

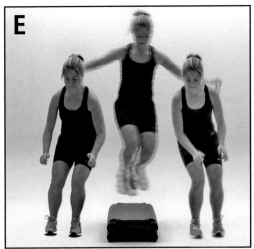

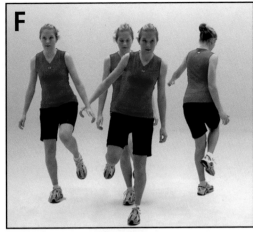

Figure 7-18. (continued) (E) bilateral double-leg hop-overs to stabilization; (F) multiplanar hops to stabilizations.

the exercise with tubing. A foam roll, towel, or other obstacle can be used to increase jump height and/or distance (Figure 7-19B). The final step in trying to improve dynamic balance should involve the incorporation of sport-related activities such as throwing and catching a ball. At this stage of the rehabilitation program, the patient should be able to safely concentrate on the functional activity (catching and throwing), while subconsciously controlling dynamic balance (Figure 7-19C).

DUAL-TASK BALANCE TRAINING AND ASSESSMENT

Although the aforementioned balance training and assessment techniques are validated and proven to be useful in the clinical setting, patients typically function in a more dynamic environment with multiple demands placed upon them concurrently. Participation in sport often requires patients to split their attention between cognitive and dynamic balance tasks. Therefore, a final progression for patients recovering from musculoskeletal injury or neurologic injury (eg, concussion) could be the addition of competing motor/coordination and cognitive tasks to assess the patient's performance with these challenges. Though the cognitive and balance demands are unique, the two are linked in that they rely on an

individual's system of attention. The attention system should be viewed as independent of the information processing centers of the brain and, like other systems, is able to communicate with multiple systems simultaneously.[68] Evidence shows the ability to selectively allocate attention between cognitive and balance tasks, but there is a priority for balance with increasing difficulty of these tasks.[71]

Once elite athletes progress through the initial phases of the balance exercises, they may reach a point where these dual-task balance exercises can be of benefit. Keeping the patient engaged in the patient's rehabilitation program is important, and these added challenges can assist in reproducing the type of demands placed on the patient during more physical activity or competition. To better recreate these demands, the systems should be challenged in unison to fully assess the functional limitations of patient, as well as train or rehabilitate these injury-related limitations.

Dual-task exercises must be clearly explained to the patient, so the patient understands the task at hand. The task can be sport specific, and should follow the guidelines previously outlined in this chapter with respect to advancing the exercises using more challenging stances and surfaces.

Incorporating a cognitive task with a sport-specific balance task can be done very easily using different colored balls, and specific rules or instructions provided to the patient. The

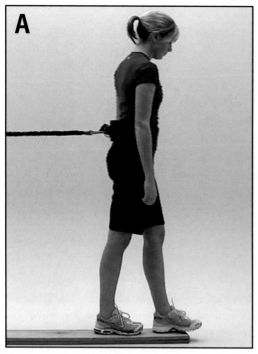

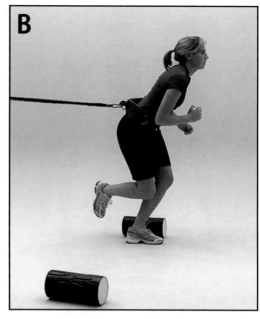

Figure 7-19. Controlling dynamic balance against cable or tubing resistance. (A) Forward and backward walking on a balance board; (B) lateral hopping in the frontal plane.

athletic trainer, standing about 15 feet away, tosses different colored balls to the patient, who is standing on either a double leg or single leg, and/or firm surface, foam surface, or balance board (Figure 7-20). The patient is told to maintain his balance while catching a blue ball with his right hand, red ball with his left hand, and yellow ball with both hands. Initially, this dual task can be difficult, but the patient should attempt to work through the increased attention demands while allowing his somatosensory system to subconsciously aid in the maintenance of balance. The complexity can be increased by adding additional rules. For example, the patient can be instructed to toss the yellow ball back head high, blue ball back waist high, and to roll back the yellow ball.

The exercises then can be made more sport specific. For example, the therapist positions himself about 25 feet from the patient and rolls the different colored balls to the patient standing on either a double leg or single leg, and/or firm surface, foam surface, or balance board (Figure 7-21). A hockey player with a hockey stick is asked to return (aim) the blue ball to the right side of the target, the yellow ball to the

center of the target, and the blue ball to the left side of the target.

> ### Clinical Decision-Making Exercise 7-5
>
> A basketball player has been complaining of feeling pain and laxity upon landing from a rebound. He has no swelling or other signs of an acute injury. What exercises should be introduced to help improve the stability?

CLINICAL VALUE OF HIGH-TECH TRAINING AND ASSESSMENT

The benefit of using the commercially available balance systems is that not only can deficits be detected, but progress can be charted quantitatively through the computer-generated results. For example, NeuroCom's Balance Master (with long forceplate) is capable of assessing a patient's ability to perform coordinated movements essential for sport performance. The system, equipped with a 5-foot-long

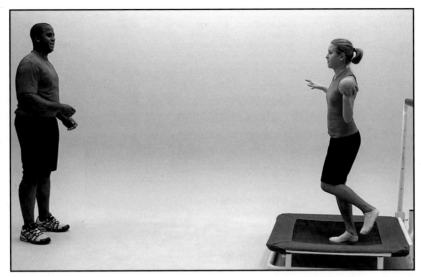

Figure 7-20. Incorporating a cognitive task with sport-specific balance.

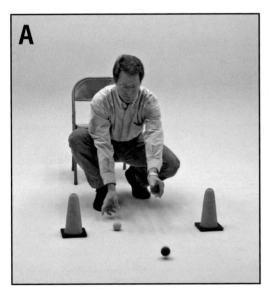

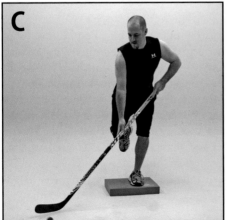

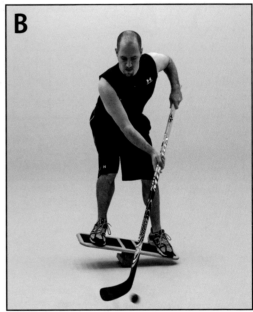

Figure 7-21. Sport-specific cognitive tasks. (A) The athletic trainer rolls different colored balls to the patient; (B) and (C) standing on an unstable surface. The patient must decide where to return the ball while maintaining balance.

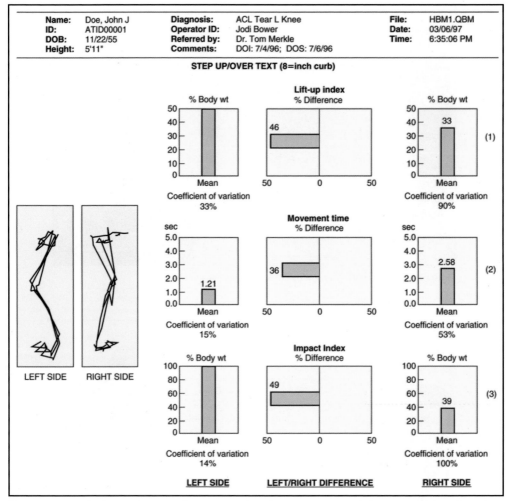

Name:	Doe, John J	Diagnosis:	ACL Tear L Knee	File:	HBM1.QBM
ID:	ATID00001	Operator ID:	Jodi Bower	Date:	03/06/97
DOB:	11/22/55	Referred by:	Dr. Tom Merkle	Time:	6:35:06 PM
Height:	5'11"	Comments:	DOI: 7/4/96; DOS: 7/6/96		

Figure 7-22. Results from a step-up-and-over protocol on the NeuroCom New Balance Master's long forceplate. (Balance Master Version 5.0 and NeuroCom are registered trademarks of NeuroCom International Inc. Copyright 1989-1997. All Rights Reserved.)

force platform, is capable of identifying specific components underlying performance of several functional tasks. Exercises are also available on the system that then help to improve the deficits.[62]

Figure 7-22 shows the results of a step-up-and-over test. The components that are analyzed in this particular task are (a) Lift-Up Index—quantifies the maximum lifting (concentric) force exerted by the leading leg and is expressed as a percentage of the person's weight; (b) Movement Time—quantifies the number of seconds required to complete the task, beginning with initial weight shift to the nonstepping leg and ending with impact of the lagging leg onto the surface; and (c) Impact Index—quantifies the maximum vertical impact force (percent of body weight) as the lagging leg lands on the surface.

Research on the clinical applicability of these measures has revealed interesting results. Preliminary observations from two studies in progress suggest that deficits in impact control are a common feature of patients with ACL injuries, even when strength and ROM of the involved knee are within normal limits. Several other performance assessments are available on this system, including sit to stand, walk test, step and quick turn, forward lunge, weight bearing/squat, and rhythmic weight shift.

Summary

1. Although some injuries in the region of the lower leg are acute, most injuries seen in an athletic population result from overuse, most often from running.

2. Tibial fractures can create long-term problems for the athlete if inappropriately managed. Fibular fractures generally require much shorter periods for immobilization. Treatment of these fractures involves immediate medical referral and most likely a period of immobilization and restricted weight bearing.

3. Stress fractures in the lower leg are usually the result of the bone's inability to adapt to the repetitive loading response during training and conditioning of the athlete and are more likely to occur in the tibia.

4. Chronic compartment syndromes can occur from acute trauma or repetitive trauma of overuse. They can occur in any of the four compartments, but are most likely in the anterior compartment or deep posterior compartment.

5. Rehabilitation of medial tibial stress syndrome must be comprehensive and address several factors, including musculoskeletal, training, and conditioning, as well as proper shoes and orthotics intervention.

6. Achilles tendinitis will often present with a gradual onset over time and may be resistant to a quick resolution secondary to the slower healing response of tendinous tissue.

7. Perhaps the greatest question after an Achilles tendon rupture is whether surgical repair or cast immobilization is the best method of treatment. Regardless of treatment method, the time required for rehabilitation is significant.

8. With retrocalcaneal bursitis the athlete will report a gradual onset of pain that may be associated with Achilles tendinitis. Treatment should include rest and activity modification to reduce swelling and inflammation.

References

1. Balogun JA, Adesinasi CO, Marzouk DK. The effects of a wobble board exercise training program on static balance performance and strength of lower extremity muscle. *Physiother Can.* 1992;44:23-30.

2. Barrack RL, Lund P, Skinner H. Knee joint proprioception revisited. *J Sport Rehabil.* 1994;3:18-42.

3. Barrack RL, Skinner HB, Buckley LS. Proprioception in the anterior cruciate deficient knee. *Am J Sports Med.* 1989;17:1-5.

4. Barrett D. Proprioception and function after anterior cruciate reconstruction. *J Bone Joint Surg Br.* 1991;73:833-837.

5. Black F, Wall C, Nashner L. Effect of visual and support surface orientations upon postural control in vestibular deficient subjects. *Acta Otolaryngol.* 1983;95:199-210.

6. Black O, Wall C, Rockette H, Kitch R. Normal subject postural sway during the Romberg test. *Am J Otolaryngol.* 1982;3(5):309-318.

7. Blackburn T, Voight M. Single leg stance: development of a reliable testing procedure. In: Proceedings of the 12th International Congress of the World Confederation for Physical Therapy; 1995.

8. Booher J, Thibodeau G. *Athletic Injury Assessment.* St. Louis, MO: Mosby College; 1995.

9. Cornwall M, Murrell P. Postural sway following inversion sprain of the ankle. *J Am Podiatr Med Assoc.* 1991;81:243-247.

10. Davies G. The need for critical thinking in rehabilitation. *J Sport Rehabil.* 1995;4(1):1-22.

11. DeCarlo M, Klootwyk T, Shelbourne K. ACL surgery and accelerated rehabilitation: Revisited. *J Sport Rehabil.* 1997;5(2):144-155.

12. Diener H, Dichgans J, Guschlbauer B, et al Role of visual and static vestibular influences on dynamic posture control. *Hum Neurobiol.* 1985;5:105-113.

13. Diener H, Dichgans J, Guschlbauer B, Mau H. The significance of proprioception on postural stabilization as assessed by ischemia. *Brain Res.* 1984;295:103-109.

14. Dietz V, Horstmann G, Berger W. Significance of proprioceptive mechanisms in the regulation of stance. *Prog Brain Res.* 1989;80:419-423.

15. Donahoe B, Turner D, Worrell T. The use of functional reach as a measurement of balance in healthy boys and girls ages 5-15. *Phys Ther.* 1993;73(5):S71.

16. Dornan J, Fernie G, Holliday P. Visual input: its importance in the control of postural sway. *Arch Phys Med Rehabil.* 1978;59:586-591.

17. Ekdahl C, Jarnlo G, Anderson S. Standing balance in healthy subjects: evaluation of a quantitative test battery on a force platform. *Scand J Rehabil Med.* 1989;21:187-195.

18. Faculjak P, Firoozbakhsh K, Wausher D, McGuire M. Balance characteristics of normal and anterior cruciate ligament deficient knees. *Phys Ther.* 1993;73:S22.

19. Fisher A, Wietlisbach S, Wilberger J. Adult performance on three tests of equilibrium. *Am J Occup Ther.* 1988;42(1):30-35.

20. Fitzpatrick R, Rogers DK, McCloskey ID. Stable human standing with lower-limb muscle afferents providing the only sensory input. *J Physiol.* 1994;480(2):395-403.

21. Flores A. Objective measures of standing balance. Neurology report. *J Am Phys Ther Assoc.* 1992;15(1):17-21.

22. Forkin DM, Koczur C, Battle R, Newton AR. Evaluation of kinetic deficits indicative of balance control in gymnasts with unilateral chronic ankle sprains. *J Orthop Sports Phys Ther.* 1996;23(4):245-250.

23. Freeman M. Instability of the foot after injuries to the lateral ligament of the ankle. *J Bone Joint Surg Br.* 1955;47:578-585.

24. Freeman M, Dean M, Hanham I. The etiology and prevention of functional instability of the foot. *J Bone Joint Surg Br.* 1955;47:669-677.

25. Friden T, Zatterstrom R, Lindstrand A, Moritz U. A stabilometric technique for evaluation of lower limb instabilities. *Am J Sports Med.* 1989;17(1):118-122.

26. Garn SN, Newton AR. Kinesthetic awareness in subjects with multiple ankle sprains. *Phys Ther.* 1988;58:1667-1671.

27. Goldie P, Bach T, Evans O. Force platform measures for evaluating postural control: reliability and validity. *Arch Phys Med Rehabil.* 1989;70:510-517.

28. Grigg P. Mechanical factors influencing response of joint afferent neurons from cat knee. *J Neurophysiol.* 1975;38:1473-1484.

29. Grigg P. Response of joint afferent neurons in cat medial articular nerve to active and passive movements of the knee. *Brain Res.* 1976;118:482-485.

30. Guskiewicz KM, Perrin DH, Gansneder B. Effect of mild head injury on postural stability. *J Athl Train.* 1995;31(4):300-306.

31. Guskiewicz KM, Perrin HD. Effect of orthotics on postural sway following inversion ankle sprain. *J Orthop Sports Phys Ther.* 1995;23(5):326-331.

32. Guskiewicz KM, Perrin HD. Research and clinical applications of assessing balance. *J Sport Rehabil.* 1996;5:45-63.

33. Guskiewicz KM, Riemann BL, Riemann DH, Nashner ML. Alternative approaches to the assessment of mild head injury in patients. *Med Sci Sports Exerc.* 1997;29(7): S213-S221.

34. Guyton A. *Textbook of Medical Physiology.* 8th ed. Philadelphia, PA: WB Saunders; 1991.

35. Harrison E, Duenkel N, Dunlop R, Russell G. Evaluation of single-leg standing following anterior cruciate ligament surgery and rehabilitation. *Phys Ther.* 1994;74(3): 245-252.

36. Hertel JN, Guskiewicz KM, Kahler DM, Perrin HD. Effect of lateral ankle joint anesthesia on center of balance, postural sway and joint position sense. *J Sport Rehabil.* 1996;5:111-119.

37. Horak FB, Nashner LM, Diener HC. Postural strategies associated with somatosensory and vestibular loss. *Exp Brain Res.* 1990;82:157-177.

38. Horak F, Nashner L. Central programming of postural movements: adaptation to altered support surface configurations. *J Neurophysiol.* 1986;55:1369-1381.

39. Houk J. Regulation of stiff ness by skeleto-motor reflexes. *Ann Rev Physiol.* 1979;41:99-114.

40. Irrgang J, Harner C. Recent advances in ACL rehabilitation: clinical factors. *J Sport Rehabil.* 1997;6(2):111-124.

41. Irrgang J, Whitney S, Cox E. Balance and proprioceptive training for rehabilitation of the lower extremity. *J Sport Rehabil.* 1994;3:68-83.

42. Jansen E, Larsen R, Mogens B. Quantitative Romberg's test: measurement and computer calculations of postural stability. *Acta Neurol Scand.* 1982;66:93-99.

43. Johansson H, Alexander IJ, Hayes KC. Nerve supply of the human knee and its functional importance. *Am J Sports Med.* 1982;10:329-335.

44. Kauffman TL, Nashner LM, Allison KL. Balance is a critical parameter in orthopedic rehabilitation. *Orthop Phys Ther Clin N Am.* 1997;6(1):43-78.

45. Kisner C, Colby AL. *Therapeutic Exercise: Foundations and Techniques.* 3rd ed. Philadelphia, PA: FA Davis; 1996.

46. Lephart SM. Re-establishing proprioception, kinesthesia, joint position sense, and neuromuscular control in rehabilitation. In: Prentice WE, ed. *Rehabilitation Techniques in Sports.* 2nd. ed. St. Louis, MO: Mosby College; 1993:118-137.

47. Lephart SM, Henry JT. Functional rehabilitation for the upper and lower extremity. *Orthop Clin North Am.* 1995;26(3):579-592.

48. Lephart SM, Kocher SM. The role of exercise in the prevention of shoulder disorders. In: Matsen FA, Fu FH, Hawkins JR, eds. *The Shoulder: A Balance of Mobility and Stability.* Rosemont, IL: American Academy of Orthopaedic Surgeons; 1993:597-620.

49. Lephart SM, Kocher SM, Fu HF, et al Proprioception following ACL reconstruction. *J Sport Rehabil.* 1992;1:186-196.

50. Lephart SM, Pincivero D, Giraldo J, Fu HF. The role of proprioception in the management and rehabilitation of athletic injuries. *Am J Sports Med.* 1997;25: 130-137.

51. Mangine R, Kremchek T. Evaluation-based protocol of the anterior cruciate ligament. *J Sport Rehabil.* 1997;6(2):157-181.

52. Mauritz K, Dichgans J, Hufschmidt A. Quantitative analysis of stance in late cortical cerebellar atrophy of the anterior lobe and other forms of cerebellar ataxia. *Brain*. 1979;102:461-482.

53. Mizuta H, Shiraishi M, Kubota K, Kai K, Takagi K. A stabilometric technique for evaluation of functional instability in the anterior cruciate ligament deficient knee. *Clin J Sport Med*. 1992;2:235-239.

54. Murray M, Seireg A, Sepic S. Normal postural stability: qualitative assessment. *J Bone Joint Surg Am*. 1975;57(4):510-516.

55. Nashner L. Adapting reflexes controlling the human posture. *Exp Brain Res*. 1976;26:59-72.

56. Nashner L. Adaptation of human movement to altered environments. *Trends Neurosci*. 1982;5:358-361.

57. Nashner L. A functional approach to understanding spasticity. In: Struppler A, Weindl A, eds. *Electromyography and Evoked Potentials*. Berlin, Germany: Springer-Verlag; 1985:22-29.

58. Nashner L. Sensory, neuromuscular and biomechanical contributions to human balance. In: Duncan P, ed. Balance: *Proceedings of the APTA Forum*, June 13-15, 1989. Alexandria, VA, American Physical Therapy Association; 1989:5-12.

59. Nashner L. Computerized dynamic posturography. In: Jacobson G, Newman C, Kartush J, eds. *Handbook of Balance Function and Testing*. St. Louis, MO: Mosby Year Book; 1993:280-307.

60. Nashner L. Practical biomechanics and physiology of balance. In: Jacobson G, Newman C, Kartush J, eds. *Handbook of Balance Function and Testing*. St. Louis, MO: Mosby Year Book; 1993:261-279.

61. Nashner L, Black F, Wall C III. Adaptation to altered support and visual conditions during stance: Patients with vestibular deficits. *J Neurosci*. 1982;2(5):536-544.

62. NeuroCom International, Inc. *The Objective Quantification of Daily Life Tasks: The NEW Balance Master 6.0* (manual). Clackamas, OR; 1997.

63. Newton R. Review of tests of standing balance abilities. *Brain Inj*. 1992;3:335-343.

64. Norre M. Sensory interaction testing in platform posturography. *J Laryngol Otol*. 1993;107:496-501.

65. Noyes F, Barber S, Mangine R. Abnormal lower limb symmetry determined by function hop test after anterior cruciate ligament rupture. *Am J Sports Med*. 1991;19(5):516-518.

66. Orteza L, Vogelbach W, Denegar C. The effect of molded and unmolded orthotics on balance and pain while jogging following inversion ankle sprain. *J Athl Train*. 1992;27(1):80-84.

67. Pintsaar A, Brynhildsen J, Tropp H. Postural corrections after standardised perturbations of single limp stance: effect of training and orthotic devices in patients with ankle instability. *Br J Sports Med*. 1996;30:151-155.

68. Posner MI, Petersen ES. The attention system of the human brain. *Ann Rev Neurosci*. 1990;13:25-42.

69. Shambers GM. Influence of the fusimotor system on stance and volitional movement in normal man. *Am J Phys Med*. 1969;48:225-227.

70. Shumway-Cook A, Horak F. Assessing the influence of sensory interaction on balance. *Phys Ther*. 1986;66(10):1548-1550.

71. Siu KC, Woollacott HM. Attentional demands of postural control: the ability to selectively allocate information processing resources. *Gait Posture*. 2007;25(1):121-126.

72. Swanik CB, Lephart SM, Giannantonio FP, Fu HF. Reestablishing proprioception and neuromuscular control in the ACL-injured patient. *J Sport Rehabil*. 1997;6(2):182-206.

73. Tippett S, Voight M. *Functional Progression for Sports Rehabilitation*. Champaign, IL: Human Kinetics; 1995.

74. Tropp H, Ekstrand J, Gillquist J. Factors affecting stabilometry recordings of single limb stance. *Am J Sports Med*. 1984;12:185-188.

SOLUTIONS TO CLINICAL DECISION-MAKING EXERCISES

7-1 A preseason baseline score can be obtained on a measure such as the BESS for all athletes, and then used for a post-injury comparison. Because there is such variability within many of the balance measures, it is important to make comparisons only to an athlete's individual baseline measure and not to a normal score. It is best to determine recovery on a measure by using the number of standard deviations (SD) away from the baseline. For example, scores on the BESS that are more than 2 SD or 6 total points would be considered abnormal. Repeated assessments during the course

of a rehabilitation progression can be used to determine the effectiveness of the balance exercises.

7-2 The athletic trainer should first ensure that the patient has the necessary pain-free ROM and muscular strength to complete the tasks that are being incorporated into the program. Additionally, for exercises beyond the Phase 1 static exercises, the patient must be beyond the acute inflammatory phase of tissue response to injury. Once these factors have been considered, the athletic trainer should focus on developing a protocol that is safe yet challenging, stresses multiple planes of motion, and incorporates a multisensory approach.

7-3   It should be explained to the patient, at the outset, that the goal is to challenge her or his motor control system, to the point that the last two repetitions of each set of exercises should be difficult to perform. When the last two repetitions no longer are challenging to the athlete, he or she should be progressed to the next exercise. This can be determined through subjective information reported from the athlete, as well as the athletic trainer's objective observations. It is very important to provide a variety of exercises and levels of exercises so that the patient maintains a high level of motivation.

7-4   It will be important for the athletic trainer to begin slowly with Phase I and II balance exercises to determine the patient's readiness to move into more dynamic tasks as part of Phase III. The progression outlined in the solution to exercise 7-2 should be followed. However, this is an example of how the athletic trainer can begin to personalize the exercise routine. A tennis player competing at a high level will need to perform a lot of lateral movement along the baseline, therefore necessitating the inclusion of dynamic balance exercises and weight shifts in the frontal plane. Several of the exercises described in this chapter would provide a good starting point for the athletic trainer in accomplishing this goal.

7-5   This patient most likely has a functionally unstable ankle. Research has shown that balance exercises can help improve functional ankle instability. In this situation, the athletic trainer probably can skip Phase I exercises and move directly to Phase II and III exercises. The athletic trainer should design a program that incorporates challenging unilateral multidirectional exercises involving a multisensory approach (eyes open and eyes closed). The progression should include the progression suggested in this chapter that includes the foam, Bosu Balance Trainer, Dynadisc, BAPS board, Extreme Balance Board, balance beam, and Balance Shoes. Lateral and diagonal hopping exercises will also be a vital part of this protocol. The goal should be to help strengthen the dynamic and static stabilizers surrounding the ankle joint. This should result in rebuilding some of the afferent pathways and ultimately improving ankle joint stability.

Please see videos on the accompanying website at

www.healio.com/books/sportsmedvideos

CHAPTER 8

Restoring Range of Motion and Improving Flexibility

William E. Prentice, PhD, PT, ATC, FNATA

After completion of this chapter, the athletic trainer should be able to do the following:

- Define flexibility and describe its importance in injury rehabilitation.

- Identify factors that limit flexibility.

- Differentiate between active and passive range of motion.

- Explain the difference between dynamic, static, and proprioceptive neuromuscular facilitation (PNF) stretching.

- Discuss the neurophysiologic principles of stretching.

- Describe stretching exercises that may be used to improve flexibility at specific joints throughout the body.

- Compare and contrast the various manual therapy techniques including myofascial release, strain–counterstrain, positional release, soft tissue mobilization, and massage that can be used to improve mobility and range of motion.

When injury occurs, there is almost always some associated loss of the ability to move normally. Loss of motion may be a result of pain, swelling, muscle guarding, or spasm; inactivity resulting in shortening of connective tissue and muscle; loss of neuromuscular control; or some combination of these factors. Restoring normal range of motion (ROM) following injury is one of the primary goals in any rehabilitation program.[90] Thus the athletic trainer must routinely include exercise designed to restore normal ROM to regain normal function.

Flexibility has been defined as the ability to move a joint or series of joints through a full, nonrestricted, pain-free ROM.[2,3,28,40,46,72,88] Flexibility is dependent on a combination of (a) joint ROM, which may be limited by the shape of the articulating surfaces and by capsular and ligamentous structures surrounding that joint;

Prentice WE, ed.
Rehabilitation Techniques for Sports Medicine and Athletic Training (pp 217-242).
© 2015 SLACK Incorporated.

and (b) muscle flexibility, or the ability of the musculotendinous unit to lengthen.[102]

Flexibility involves the ability of the neuromuscular system to allow for efficient movement of a joint through a ROM.[3,31,48,52,83,105] Flexibility can be discussed in relation to movement involving only one joint, such as the knees, or movement involving a whole series of joints, such as the spinal vertebral joints, that must all move together to allow smooth bending or rotation of the trunk. Lack of flexibility in one joint or movement can affect the entire kinetic chain. A person might have good ROM in the ankles, knees, hips, back, and one shoulder joint, but lack normal movement in the other shoulder joint; this is a problem that needs to be corrected before the person can function normally.[11,20]

This chapter concentrates primarily on rehabilitative techniques used to increase the length of the musculotendinous unit and its associated fascia, as well as restricted neural tissue. In addition, a discussion of a variety of manual therapy techniques including myofascial release, strain/counterstrain, positional release therapy, soft-tissue mobilization, and massage as they relate to improving mobility will be included. Joint mobilization and traction techniques used to address tightness in the joint capsule and surrounding ligaments are discussed in Chapter 13. Loss of the ability to control movement as a result of impairment in neuromuscular control is discussed in Chapter 9.

IMPORTANCE OF FLEXIBILITY TO THE PATIENT

Maintaining a full, nonrestricted ROM has long been recognized as essential to normal daily living. Lack of flexibility can also create uncoordinated or awkward movement patterns resulting from lost neuromuscular control. In most patients, functional activities require relatively "normal" amounts of flexibility.[77] However some sport activities, such as gymnastics, ballet, diving, karate, and especially dance require increased flexibility for superior performance[23] (Figure 8-1).

It has also been generally accepted that flexibility is essential for improving performance in physical activities.[25] However, a review of the evidence-based information in the literature looking at the relationship between flexibility and improved performance is, at best, conflicting and inconclusive.[43,59,104] Although many studies conducted through the years have suggested that stretching improves performance,[11,59,76,111] several recent studies have found that stretching causes decreases in performance parameters such as strength, endurance, power, joint position sense, and reaction times.[9,13,30,42,43,61,65,70,78,83,85,93,106,110]

The same can be said when examining the relationship between flexibility and reducing the incidence of injury. Although it is generally accepted that good flexibility reduces the likelihood of injury, a true cause-and-effect relationship has not been clearly established in the literature.[4,5,19,76,107,110]

ANATOMIC FACTORS THAT LIMIT FLEXIBILITY

A number of anatomic factors can limit the ability of a joint to move through a full, unrestricted ROM.[84] Muscles and their tendons, along with their surrounding fascial sheaths, are most often responsible for limiting ROM. When performing stretching exercises to improve flexibility about a particular joint, you are attempting to take advantage of the highly elastic properties of a muscle. Over time it is possible to increase the elasticity, or the length that a given muscle can be stretched. Persons who have a good deal of movement at a particular joint tend to have highly elastic and flexible muscles.

Connective tissue surrounding the joint, such as ligaments on the joint capsule, can be subject to contractures. Ligaments and joint

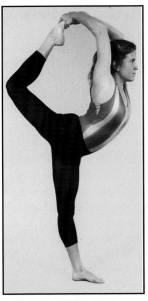

Figure 8-1. Extreme flexibility. Certain dance and athletic activities require extreme flexibility for successful performance.

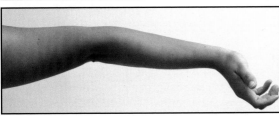

Figure 8-2. Excessive joint motion, such as the hyperextended elbow, can predispose a joint to injury.

capsules have some elasticity; however, if a joint is immobilized for a period, these structures tend to lose some elasticity and actually shorten. This condition is most commonly seen after surgical repair of an unstable joint, but it can also result from long periods of inactivity.

It is also possible for a person to have relatively slack ligaments and joint capsules. These people are generally referred to as being loose jointed. Examples of this trait would be an elbow or knee that hyperextends beyond 180 degrees (Figure 8-2). Frequently, there is instability associated with loose jointedness that can present as great a problem in movement as ligamentous or capsular contractures.

Bony structure can restrict the end point in the range. An elbow that has been fractured through the joint might lay down excess calcium in the joint space, causing the joint to lose its ability to fully extend. However, in many instances we rely on bony prominences to stop movements at normal end points in the range.

Fat can also limit the ability to move through a full ROM. A person who has a large amount of fat on the abdomen might have severely restricted trunk flexion when asked to bend forward and touch the toes. The fat can act as a wedge between two lever arms, restricting movement wherever it is found.

Skin might also be responsible for limiting movement. For example, a person who has had some type of injury or surgery involving a tearing incision or laceration of the skin, particularly over a joint, will have inelastic scar tissue formed at that site. This scar tissue is incapable of stretching with joint movement.

Over time, skin contractures caused by scarring of ligaments, joint capsules, and musculotendinous units are capable of improving elasticity to varying degrees through stretching. With the exception of bone structure, age, and gender, all the other factors that limit flexibility can be altered to increase range of joint motion.

Neural tissue tightness resulting from acute compression, chronic repetitive microtrauma, muscle imbalances, joint dysfunction, or poor posture can create morphologic changes in neural tissues. These changes might include intraneural edema, tissue hypoxia, chemical irritation, or microvascular stasis—all of which could stimulate nociceptors, creating pain. Pain causes muscle guarding and spasm to protect the inflamed neural structures, and this alters normal movement patterns. Eventually neural fibrosis results, which decreases the elasticity of neural tissue and prevents normal movement within surrounding tissues.[21]

Clinical Decision-Making Exercise 8-2

Two days after an intense weight-lifting workout, a football player is complaining of quad pain. The athletic trainer determines that the athlete has delayed-onset muscle soreness. The soreness is preventing the athlete from getting a sufficient stretch. What can be done to optimize his stretching?

ACTIVE AND PASSIVE RANGE OF MOTION

Active ROM, also called dynamic flexibility, refers to the degree to which a joint can be moved by a muscle contraction, usually through the midrange of movement. Dynamic flexibility is not necessarily a good indicator of the stiffness or looseness of a joint because it applies to the ability to move a joint efficiently, with little resistance to motion.[48] Passive ROM, sometimes called static flexibility, refers to the degree to which a joint can be passively moved to the end points in the ROM. No muscle contraction is involved to move a joint through a passive range. When a muscle actively contracts, it produces a joint movement through a specific ROM.[83,100] However, if passive pressure is applied to an extremity, it is capable of moving farther in the ROM. It is essential in sports activities that an extremity be capable of moving through a nonrestricted ROM.[87] Passive ROM is important for injury prevention. There are many situations in physical activity in which a muscle is forced to stretch beyond its normal active limits. If the muscle does not have enough elasticity to compensate for this additional stretch, it is likely that the musculotendinous unit will be injured.

Assessment of Active and Passive Range of Motion

Accurate measurement of active and passive range of joint motion is difficult.[50] Various devices have been designed to accommodate variations in the size of the joints, as well as the complexity of movements in articulations that involve more than one joint.[50] Of these devices, the simplest and most widely used is the goniometer (Figure 8-3).

A goniometer is a large protractor with measurements in degrees. By aligning the individual arms of the goniometer parallel to the longitudinal axis of the two segments involved in motion about a specific joint, it is possible to obtain reasonably accurate measurement of range of movement. To enhance reliability, standardization of measurement techniques and methods of recording active and passive ranges of motion are critical in individual clinics where successive measurements might be taken by different therapists to assess progress.[49] Table 8-1 provides a list of what would be considered normal active ranges for movements at various joints.

The goniometer has an important place in a rehabilitation setting, where it is essential to assess improvement in joint flexibility to modify injury rehabilitation programs.

In some clinics a digital inclinometer is used instead of a goniometer. An inclinometer is a more precise measuring instrument with high reliability that has most often been used in research settings. Digital inclinometers are affordable and can easily be used to accurately measure ROM of all joints of the body from complex movements of the spine and large joints of the extremities to the small joints of fingers and toes.

STRETCHING TO IMPROVE MOBILITY

The goal of any effective stretching program should be to improve the ROM at a given articulation by altering the extensibility of the neuromusculotendinous units that produce movement at that joint. It is well documented that exercises that stretch these

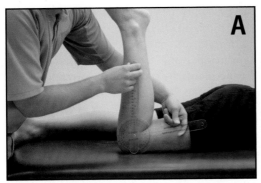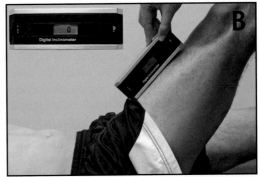

Figure 8-3. Measurement of active knee joint flexion using (A) a universal goniometer, or (B) a digital goniometer. A goniometer can be used to measure the angle between the femur and the fibula, giving degrees of flexion and extension. To maximize consistency in measurement, it is helpful if the same person takes sequential goniometric measurement.

Table 8-1 Active Ranges of Joint Motions

Joint	Action	Degrees of Motion
Shoulder	Flexion	0 to 180
	Extension	0 to 50
	Abduction	0 to 180
	Medial rotation	0 to 90
	Lateral rotation	0 to 90
	Flexion	0 to 90
Elbow	Flexion	0 to 160
Forearm	Pronation	0 to 90
	Supination	0 to 90
Wrist	Flexion	0 to 90
	Extension	0 to 70
	Abduction	0 to 25
	Adduction	0 to 65
Hip	Flexion	0 to 125
	Extension	0 to 15
	Abduction	0 to 45
	Adduction	0 to 15
	Medial rotation	0 to 45
	Lateral rotation	0 to 45
Knee	Flexion	0 to 140
Ankle	Plantarflexion	0 to 45
	Dorsiflexion	0 to 20
Foot	Inversion	0 to 30
	Eversion	0 to 10

neuromusculotendinous units and their fascia over time will increase the range of movement possible about a given joint.[41,80]

For many years the efficacy of stretching in improving ROM has been theoretically attributed to neurophysiologic phenomena involving the stretch reflex. However, a recent study that extensively reviewed the existing literature suggested that improvements in ROM resulting from stretching must be explained by mechanisms other than the stretch reflex.[19] Studies reviewed indicate that changes in the ability to tolerate stretch and/or the viscoelastic properties of the stretched muscle are possible mechanisms.

NEUROPHYSIOLOGIC BASIS OF STRETCHING

Every muscle in the body contains various types of mechanoreceptors that, when stimulated, inform the central nervous system of what is happening with that muscle.[22] Two of these mechanoreceptors are important in the stretch reflex: the muscle spindle and the Golgi tendon organ. Both types of receptors are sensitive to changes in muscle length. The Golgi tendon organs are also affected by changes in muscle tension.[15]

When a muscle is stretched, both the muscle spindles and the Golgi tendon organs immediately begin sending a volley of sensory impulses to the spinal cord. Initially impulses coming from the muscle spindles inform the central nervous system that the muscle is being stretched. Impulses return to the muscle from the spinal cord, causing the muscle to reflexively contract, thus resisting the stretch.[68] The Golgi tendon organs respond to the change in length and the increase in tension by firing off sensory impulses of their own to the spinal cord. If the stretch of the muscle continues for an extended period (at least 6 seconds), impulses from the Golgi tendon organs begin to override muscle spindle impulses. The impulses from the Golgi tendon organs, unlike the signals from the muscle spindle, cause a reflex relaxation of the antagonist muscle. This reflex relaxation serves as a protective mechanism that will allow the muscle to stretch through relaxation without exceeding the extensibility limits, which could damage the muscle fibers.[12] This relaxation of the antagonist muscle during contractions is referred to as autogenic inhibition.

In any synergistic muscle group, a contraction of the agonist causes a reflex relaxation in the antagonist muscle, allowing it to stretch and protecting it from injury. This phenomenon is referred to as reciprocal inhibition[92] (Figure 12-32).

EFFECTS OF STRETCHING ON THE PHYSICAL AND MECHANICAL PROPERTIES OF MUSCLE

The neurophysiologic mechanisms of both autogenic and reciprocal inhibition result in reflex relaxation with subsequent lengthening of a muscle. Thus the mechanical properties of that muscle that physically allow lengthening to occur are dictated via neural input.

Both muscle and tendon are composed largely of noncontractile collagen and elastin fibers. Collagen enables a tissue to resist mechanical forces and deformation, whereas elastin composes highly elastic tissues that assist in recovery from deformation.[62]

Collagen has several mechanical and physical properties that allow it to respond to loading and deformation, permitting it to withstand high tensile stress.[103] The mechanical properties of collagen include (a) elasticity, which is the capability to recover normal length after elongation; (b) viscoelasticity, which allows for a slow return to normal length and shape after deformation; and (c) plasticity, which allows for permanent change or deformation. The physical properties include (a) force-relaxation, which indicates the decrease in the amount of force needed to maintain a tissue at a set amount of displacement or deformation over time; (b) the creep response, which is the ability of a tissue to deform over time while a constant load is imposed; and (c) hysteresis, which is the amount of relaxation a tissue has undergone during deformation and displacement. If the mechanical and physical limitations of connective tissue are exceeded, injury results.

Unlike tendon, muscle also has active contractile components that are the actin and myosin myofilaments. Collectively the contractile and noncontractile elements determine the muscle's capability of deforming and recovering from deformation.[112]

Both the contractile and the noncontractile components appear to resist deformation when a muscle is stretched or lengthened. The percentage of their individual contribution to resisting deformation depends on the degree to which the muscle is stretched or deformed and on the velocity of deformation. The noncontractile elements are primarily resistant to the degree of lengthening, while the contractile elements limit high-velocity deformation. The greater the stretch, the more the noncontractile components contribute.[103]

Lengthening of a muscle via stretching allows for viscoelastic and plastic changes to occur in the collagen and elastin fibers. The viscoelastic changes that allow slow deformation with imperfect recovery are not permanent. However, plastic changes, although difficult to achieve, result in residual or permanent change in length due to deformation created by long periods of stretching.

The greater the velocity of deformation, the greater the chance for exceeding that tissue's capability to undergo viscoelastic and plastic change.[112]

EFFECTS OF STRETCHING ON THE KINETIC CHAIN

Joint hypomobility is one of the most frequently treated causes of pain. However, the etiology can usually be traced to faulty posture, muscular imbalances, and abnormal neuromuscular control. Once a particular joint has lost its normal arthrokinematics, the muscles around that joint attempt to minimize the stress at that involved segment. Certain muscles become tight and hypertonic to prevent additional joint translation. If one muscle becomes tight or changes its degree of activation, then synergists, stabilizers, and neutralizers have to compensate, leading to the formation of complex neuromusculoskeletal dysfunctions.

Muscle tightness and hypertonicity have a significant impact on neuromuscular control. Muscle tightness affects the normal length–tension relationships. When one muscle in a force-couple becomes tight or hypertonic, it alters the normal arthrokinematics of the involved joint. This affects the synergistic function of the entire kinetic chain, leading to abnormal joint stress, soft-tissue dysfunction, neural compromise, and vascular/lymphatic stasis. These result in alterations in recruitment strategies and stabilization strength. Such compensations and adaptations affect neuromuscular efficiency throughout the kinetic chain. Decreased neuromuscular control alters the activation sequence or firing order of different muscles involved, and a specific movement is disturbed. Prime movers may be slow to activate, while synergists, stabilizers, and neutralizers substitute and become overactive. When this is the case, new joint stresses will be encountered.[21] For example, if the psoas is tight or hyperactive, then the gluteus maximus will have decreased neural drive. If the gluteus maximus (prime mover during hip extension) has decreased neural drive, then synergists (hamstrings), stabilizers (erector spinae), and neutralizers (piriformis) substitute and become overactive (synergistic dominance). This creates abnormal joint stress and decreased neuromuscular control during functional movements.

Muscle tightness also causes reciprocal inhibition. Increased muscle spindle activity in a specific muscle will cause decreased neural drive to that muscle's functional antagonist. This alters the normal force-couple activity, which, in turn, affects the normal arthrokinematics of the involved segment. For example, if a patient has tightness or hypertonicity in the psoas, then the functional antagonist (gluteus maximus) can be inhibited (decreased neural drive), causing decreased neuromuscular control. This, in turn, leads to synergistic dominance—the neuromuscular phenomenon that occurs when synergists compensate for a weak and/or inhibited muscle to maintain force production capabilities.[21] This process alters the normal force-couple relationships, which, in turn, creates a chain reaction.

IMPORTANCE OF INCREASING MUSCLE TEMPERATURE PRIOR TO STRETCHING

To most effectively stretch a muscle during a program of rehabilitation, intramuscular temperature should be increased prior to stretching.[75] Increasing the temperature has a positive effect on the ability of the collagen and elastin components within the musculotendinous unit to deform. Also, the capability of the Golgi tendon organs to reflexively relax the muscle through autogenic inhibition is enhanced when the muscle is heated. It appears that the optimal temperature of muscle to achieve these beneficial effects is 39°C (103°F). This increase in intramuscular temperature can be achieved either through low-intensity warm-up–type exercise or through the use of various therapeutic modalities.[27,44,91] It is recommended that exercise be used as the primary means for increasing intramuscular temperature.

The use of cold prior to stretching also has been recommended.[26] Cold appears to be most useful when there is some muscle guarding associated with delayed-onset muscle soreness.[82]

Clinical Decision-Making Exercise 8-3

Following ACL surgery, one of the first goals of rehabilitation is to regain full ROM. How can improvements in knee extension be quantified for day-to-day record keeping?

STRETCHING TECHNIQUES

Stretching techniques for improving flexibility have evolved over the years.[57] The oldest technique for stretching is dynamic stretching (ballistic), which makes use of repetitive bouncing motions. A second technique, known as static stretching, involves stretching a muscle to the point of discomfort and then holding it at that point for an extended time. This technique has been used for many years. Another group of stretching techniques known collectively as proprioceptive neuromuscular facilitation (PNF) techniques, involving alternating contractions and stretches, also has been recommended (Figure 8-4).[58,108] Most recently, emphasis has been on the contribution of stretching myofascial tissue, as well as stretching tight neural tissue, in enhancing the ability of the neuromuscular system to efficiently control movement through a full ROM. Researchers have had considerable discussion about which of these techniques is most effective for improving ROM, and no clear-cut consensus currently exists.[11,32,41,66,80,86]

Agonist vs Antagonist Muscles

Before discussing the different stretching techniques, it is essential to define the terms *agonist muscle* and *antagonist muscle*. Most joints in the body are capable of more than one movement. The knee joint, for example, is capable of flexion and extension. Contraction of the quadriceps group of muscles on the front of the thigh causes knee extension, whereas contraction of the hamstring muscles on the back of the thigh produces knee flexion.

To achieve knee extension, the quadriceps group contracts while the hamstring muscles relax and stretch. Muscles that work in concert with one another in this manner are called synergistic muscle groups.[8] The muscle that contracts to produce a movement, in this case the quadriceps, is referred to as the agonist muscle. The muscle being stretched in response to contraction of the agonist muscle is called the antagonist muscle.[40] In this example of knee extension, the antagonist muscle would be the hamstring group. Some degree of balance in strength must exist between agonist and antagonist muscle groups. This balance is necessary for normal, smooth, coordinated movement, as well as for reducing the likelihood of muscle strain caused by muscular imbalance. Comprehension of this synergistic muscle action is essential to understanding the various techniques of stretching.

Dynamic Stretching

In dynamic stretching, repetitive contractions of the agonist muscle are used to produce quick stretches of the antagonist muscle.

Over the years, many fitness experts have questioned the safety of the dynamic stretching technique.[47,68] Their concerns have been primarily based on the idea that dynamic stretching creates somewhat uncontrolled forces within the muscle that can exceed the extensibility limits of the muscle fiber, thus producing small micro tears within the musculotendinous unit.[35,39,74,112] Certainly this might be true in sedentary individuals or perhaps in individuals who have sustained muscle injuries.

However, many physical activities are dynamic and require a repeated dynamic contraction of the agonist muscle. The antagonist contracting eccentrically to decelerate the dynamic stretching of the antagonist muscle before engaging in this type of activity should allow the muscle to gradually adapt to the imposed demands and reduce the likelihood of injury. Because dynamic stretching is more functional, it should be integrated into a reconditioning program during the later stages of healing when appropriate.

A progressive velocity flexibility program has been proposed that takes the patient through a series of stretching exercises where the velocity of the stretch and the range of lengthening are progressively controlled.[81] The stretching exercises progress from slow static stretching to slow, short, end-range stretching, to slow, full-range stretching, to fast, short, end-range

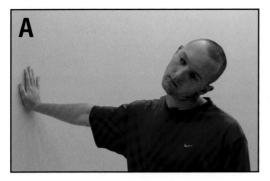

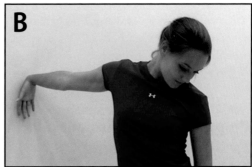

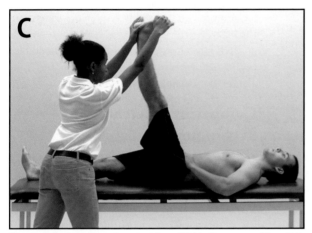

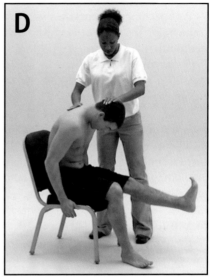

Figure 8-4. Neural tension stretches. (A) Median nerve; (B) radial nerve; (C) sciatic nerve; (D) slump position.

stretching, and to fast, full-range stretching. This program allows the patient to control both the range and the speed with no assistance from an athletic trainer.

Clinical Decision-Making Exercise 8-4

During a preseason screening, you observe that a rower has only 120 degrees of knee flexion. What are some of the things that might be limiting this motion?

Static Stretching

The static stretching technique is another extremely effective and widely used technique of stretching.[52] This technique involves stretching a given antagonist muscle passively by placing it in a maximal position of stretch and holding it there for an extended time. Recommendations for the optimal time for holding this stretched position vary, ranging from as short as 3 seconds to as long as 60 seconds.[48] Several studies indicate that holding a stretch for 15 to 30 seconds is the most effective for increasing muscle flexibility.[6,64,67] Stretches lasting longer than 30 seconds seem to be uncomfortable. A static stretch of each muscle should be repeated three or four times. A static stretch can be accomplished by using a contraction of the agonist muscle to place the antagonist muscle in a position of stretch. A passive static stretch requires the use of body weight, assistance from an athletic trainer or partner, or use of a T-bar, primarily for stretching the upper extremity.

Proprioceptive Neuromuscular Facilitation Stretching Techniques

PNF techniques were first used by athletic trainers for treating patients who had various neuromuscular disorders.[58] More recently, PNF stretching exercises have increasingly been used as a stretching technique for improving flexibility.[15,24,64,71,73]

There are three different PNF techniques used for stretching: contract-relax, hold-relax techniques, and slow reversal-hold-relax.[102] All three techniques involve some combination of alternating isometric or isotonic contractions and relaxation of both agonist and antagonist muscles (a 10-second pushing phase followed by a 10-second relaxing phase).

Contract-relax is a stretching technique that moves the body part passively into the agonist pattern. The patient is instructed to push by contracting the antagonist (the muscle that will be stretched) isotonically against the resistance of the athletic trainer. The patient then relaxes the antagonist while the athletic trainer moves the part passively through as much range as possible to the point where limitation is again felt. This contract-relax technique is beneficial when ROM is limited by muscle tightness.

Hold-relax is very similar to the contract-relax technique. It begins with an isometric contraction of the antagonist (the muscle that will be stretched) against resistance, combined with light pressure from the therapist to produce maximal stretch of the antagonist. This technique is appropriate when there is muscle tension on one side of a joint and may be used with either the agonist or the antagonist. This technique is also referred to as a muscle energy technique and will be discussed in Chapter 12.[16]

Slow reversal-hold-relax, also occasionally referred to as the contract-relax-agonist-contraction technique, begins with an isotonic contraction of the agonist, which often limits ROM in the agonist pattern, followed by an isometric contraction of the antagonist (the muscle that will be stretched) during the push phase. During the relax phase, the antagonists are relaxed while the agonists are contracting, causing movement in the direction of the agonist pattern and thus stretching the antagonist. This technique, like the contract-relax and hold-relax, is useful for increasing ROM when the primary limiting factor is the antagonistic muscle group. PNF stretching techniques can be used to stretch any muscle in the body.[11,28,29,34,71,74,79,82,86,102]

PNF stretching techniques are perhaps best performed with a partner, although they may also be done using a wall as resistance.

Comparing Stretching Techniques

Although all three stretching techniques discussed to this point have been demonstrated to effectively improve flexibility, there is still considerable debate as to which technique produces the greatest increases in range of movement.[7] The dynamic technique is recommended for anyone who is involved in dynamic activity, despite its potential for causing muscle soreness in the sedentary individual. In physically active individuals, it is unlikely that dynamic stretching will result in muscle soreness.

Static stretching is perhaps the most widely used technique. It is a simple technique and does not require a partner. A fully nonrestricted ROM can be attained through static stretching over time.

Much research has been done comparing dynamic and static stretching techniques for the improvement of flexibility. Static and dynamic stretching appear to be equally effective in increasing flexibility, and there is no significant difference between the two.[36] However, much of the literature states that with static stretching there is less danger of exceeding the extensibility limits of the involved joints because the stretch is more controlled. Most of the literature indicates that dynamic stretching is apt to cause muscular soreness, especially in sedentary individuals, whereas static stretching generally does not cause soreness and is commonly used in injury rehabilitation of sore or strained muscles.[35,109] Static stretching is likely a much safer stretching technique, especially for sedentary individuals. However, because many physical activities involve dynamic movement, stretching in a warm-up should begin with static stretching followed by dynamic stretching, which more closely resembles the dynamic activity. PNF stretching techniques are capable of producing dramatic increases in ROM during one stretching session.[14] Studies comparing static and PNF stretching suggest that PNF stretching is capable of producing greater improvement in flexibility over an extended training period.[45,46,82] The major disadvantage of PNF stretching is that a partner is usually required to assist with the stretch, although stretching with an athletic trainer or partner can have some motivational advantages.

How long increases in muscle flexibility can be sustained once stretching stops is debatable.[38,94,113] One study indicated that a significant loss of flexibility was evident after only 2 weeks.[113] It was recommended that flexibility can be maintained by engaging in stretching activities at least once a week. However, to see improvement in flexibility, stretching must be done three to five times per week.[37]

Stretching Neural Structures

The athletic trainer should be able to differentiate between tightness in the musculotendinous unit and abnormal neural tension. The patient should perform both active and passive multiplanar movements that create tension in the neural structures that are exacerbating pain, limiting ROM, and increasing neural symptoms, including numbness and tingling.[21] For example, the straight-leg raising test not only applies pressure to the sacroiliac joint cell but also may indicate a problem in the sciatic nerve (Figure 8-4C). Internally rotating and adducting the hip increases the tension on the neural structures in both the greater sciatic notch and the intervertebral foramen. An exacerbation of pain from 30 to 60 degrees indicates some sciatic nerve involvement. If dorsiflexing the ankle with maximum straight leg raising increases the pain, then the pain is likely caused by some nerve root (L3-L4, S1-S3)

or sciatic nerve irritation. Figure 8-4 shows the assessment and stretching positions for neural tension in the median, radial, and sciatic nerves as well as the vertebral nerve roots in the spine.

Clinical Decision-Making Exercise 8-6

A coach asks the athletic trainer for recommendations for stretching to help improve the flexibility of his players. What three types of stretches could be recommended, and what are the advantages and disadvantages of each?

SPECIFIC STRETCHING EXERCISES

Chapters 17 to 24 include various stretching exercises that may be used to improve flexibility at specific joints or in specific muscle groups throughout the body. The stretching exercises shown in Figure 8-5 are examples that may be done statically; they may also be done with a partner using a PNF technique. There are many possible variations to each of these exercises.[54] The patient may also perform static stretching exercises using a stability ball (Figure 8-6). The exercises selected are those that seem to be the most effective for stretching of various muscle groups. Table 8-2 provides a list of guidelines and precautions for stretching.

ALTERNATIVE STRETCHING TECHNIQUES

The Pilates Method of Stretching

The Pilates method is a somewhat different approach to stretching for improving flexibility. This method has become extremely popular and widely used among personal fitness trainers, physical therapists, and athletic trainers. Pilates is an exercise technique devised by German-born Joseph Pilates, who established the first Pilates studio in the United States before World War II. The Pilates method is a conditioning program that improves muscle control, flexibility, coordination, strength, and tone.[10] The

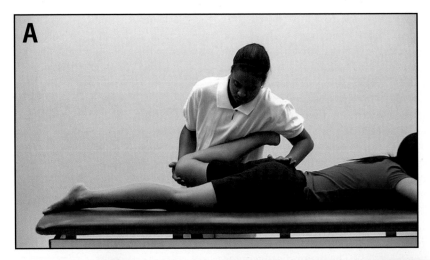

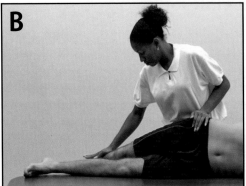

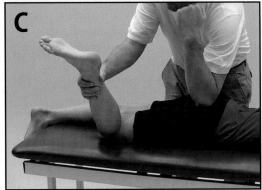

Figure 8-5. Examples of stretching exercises that may be done statically or using a PNF technique. (A) Quadriceps; (B) hip abductors; (C) piriformis.

basic principles of Pilates exercise are to make patients more aware of their bodies as single integrated units, to improve body alignment and breathing, and to increase efficiency of movement. Unlike other exercise programs, the Pilates method does not require the repetition of exercises but instead consists of a sequence of carefully performed movements, some of which are carried out on specially designed equipment (Figure 8-7). However, the majority of Pilates exercises are performed on a mat or floor without equipment (Figure 8-8). Each exercise is designed to stretch and strengthen the muscles involved. There is a specific breathing pattern for each exercise to help direct energy to the areas being worked, while relaxing the rest of the body. The Pilates method works many of the deeper muscles together, improving coordination and balance, to achieve efficient and graceful movement. The goal for the patient

is to develop a healthy self-image through the attainment of better posture, proper coordination, and improved flexibility. This method concentrates on body alignment, lengthening all the muscles of the body into a balanced whole, and building endurance and strength without putting undue stress on the lungs and heart. Pilates instructors believe that problems such as soft-tissue injuries can cause bad posture, which can lead to pain and discomfort. Pilates exercises aim to correct this.

Yoga

Yoga originated in India about 6000 years ago. Its basic philosophy is that most illness is related to poor mental attitudes, posture, and diet. Practitioners of yoga maintain that stress can be reduced through combined mental and physical approaches. Yoga can help an individual cope with stress-induced behaviors

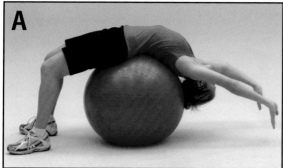

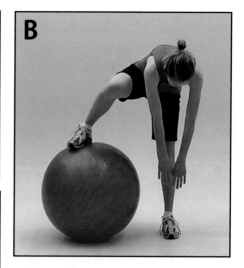

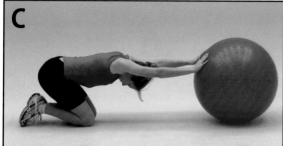

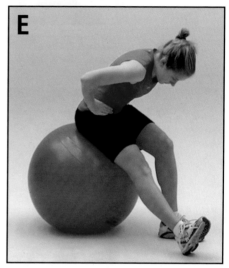

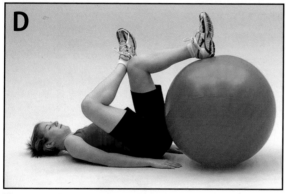

Figure 8-6. Static stretching using a stability ball. (A) Back extension; (B) standing abductor stretch; (C) latissimus dorsi stretch; (D) piriformis stretch; (E) seated hamstring stretch.

like overeating, hypertension, and smoking. Yoga's meditative aspects are believed to help alleviate psychosomatic illnesses. Yoga aims to unite the body and mind to reduce stress.[56] For example, Dr. Chandra Patel, a yoga expert, has found that persons who practice yoga can reduce their blood pressure indefinitely as long as they continue to practice yoga. Yoga involves various body postures and breathing exercises. Hatha yoga uses a number of positions through which the practitioner may progress, beginning with the simplest and moving to the more complex (Figure 8-9). The various positions are intended to increase mobility and flexibility. However, practitioners must use caution when performing yoga positions. Some positions can be dangerous, particularly for someone who is inexperienced in yoga technique.

Slow, deep, diaphragmatic breathing is an important part of yoga. Many people take shallow breaths; however, breathing deeply and fully expanding the chest when inhaling helps lower blood pressure and heart rate. Deep breathing has a calming effect on the body. It also increases production of endorphins.[56]

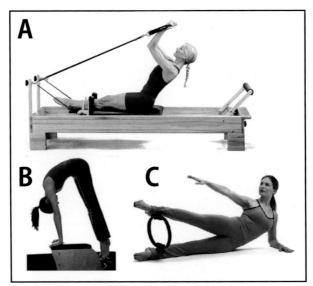

Figure 8-7. Pilates techniques using equipment. (A) Reformer; (B) Wunda chair; (C) Magic ring.

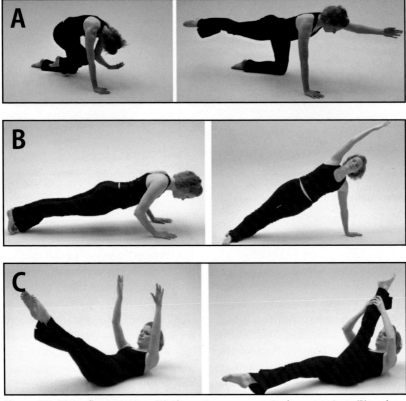

Figure 8-8. Pilates floor exercises. (A) Alternating arm, opposite-leg extensions; (B) push-up to a side plank; (C) alternating leg scissors.

Table 8-2 Guidelines and Precautions for a Sound Stretching Program[60,96,97,101]

- Warm up using a slow jog or fast walk before stretching vigorously.

- To increase flexibility, the muscle must be stretched within pain tolerances and tissue healing limitations to attain functional or normal ROM.

- Stretch only to the point where tightness or resistance to stretch, or perhaps some discomfort, is felt. Stretching should not be painful.[1]

- Increases in ROM will be specific to whatever muscle or joint is being stretched.

- Exercise caution when stretching muscles that surround painful joints. Pain is an indication that something is wrong and should not be ignored.

- Avoid overstretching the ligaments and capsules that surround joints.

- Exercise caution when stretching the low back and neck. Exercises that compress the vertebrae and their discs can cause damage.

- Stretching from a seated rather than a standing position takes stress off the low back and decreases the chances of back injury.

- Be sure to continue normal breathing during a stretch. Do not hold your breath.

- Static and PNF techniques are most often recommended for individuals who want to improve their ROM.

- Dynamic stretching should be done only by those who are already flexible or accustomed to stretching, and should be done only after static stretching.

MANUAL THERAPY TECHNIQUES FOR INCREASING MOBILITY

Following injury, soft tissue loses some of its ability to tolerate the demands of functional loading. A major part of the management of soft-tissue dysfunction lies in promoting soft-tissue adaptation to restore the tissue's ability to cope with functional loading.[53] Specific soft-tissue mobilization involves specific, graded, and progressive application of force using physiologic, accessory, or combined techniques either to promote collagen synthesis, orientation, and bonding in the early stages of the healing process or to promote changes in the viscoelastic response of the tissue in the later stages of healing. Soft-tissue mobilization should be applied in combination with rehabilitation regimes to restore the kinetic control of the tissue.[53]

A variety of manual therapy techniques can be used in injury rehabilitation to improve mobility and ROM.

Myofascial Release Stretching

Myofascial release is a term that refers to a group of techniques used for the purpose of relieving soft tissue from the abnormal grip of tight fascia.[57] It is essentially a form of stretching that has been reported to have significant impact in treating a variety of conditions.[73] Some specialized training is necessary for the athletic trainer to understand specific techniques of myofascial release.[89] It is also essential to have an in-depth understanding of the fascial system.

Fascia is a type of connective tissue that surrounds muscles, tendons, nerves, bones, and organs. It is essentially continuous from head to toe and is interconnected in various sheaths or planes. Fascia is composed primarily of collagen along with some elastic fibers. During movement the fascia must stretch and move freely. If there is damage to the fascia owing to injury, disease, or inflammation, it will not only affect local adjacent structures but may also affect areas far removed from the site of the injury.[69] Thus it may be necessary to release

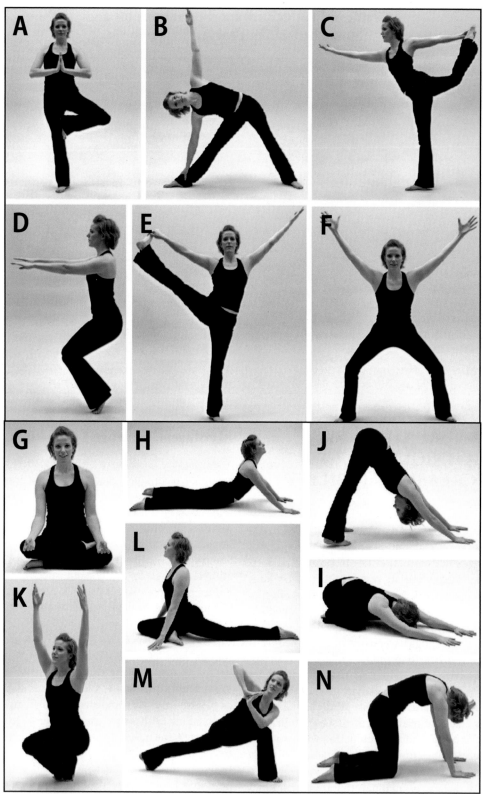

Figure 8-9. Yoga positions. (A) Tree; (B); triangle; (C) dancer; (D) chair; (E) extended hand to big toe; (F) big mountain; (G) lotus; (H) cobra; (I) child pose; (J) downward dog; (K) static squat; (L) pigeon; (M) runner's lunge with twist; (N) cat.

tightness both in the area of injury and in distant areas. It will tend to soften and release in response to gentle pressure over a relatively long period.

Myofascial release has also been referred to as soft-tissue mobilization. Soft-tissue mobilization should not be confused with joint mobilization, although it must be emphasized that the two are closely related.[57] Joint mobilization is used to restore normal joint arthrokinematics, and specific rules exist regarding direction of movement and joint position based on the shape of the articulating surfaces (see Chapter 13). Myofascial restrictions are considerably more unpredictable and may occur in many different planes and directions.[98] Myofascial treatment is based on localizing the restriction and moving into the direction of the restriction, regardless of whether that follows the arthrokinematics of a nearby joint. Thus, myofascial manipulation is considerably more subjective and relies heavily on the experience of the therapist.[69] Myofascial manipulation focuses on large treatment areas, whereas joint mobilization focuses on a specific joint. Releasing myofascial restrictions over a large treatment area can have a significant impact on joint mobility.[73] The progression of the technique is to work from superficial fascial restrictions to deeper restriction. Once more superficial restrictions are released, the deep restrictions can be located and released without causing any damage to superficial tissue. Joint mobilization should follow myofascial release and will likely be more effective once soft-tissue restrictions are eliminated.

As extensibility is improved in the myofascia, elongation and stretching of the musculotendinous unit should be incorporated. In addition, strengthening exercises are recommended to enhance neuromuscular reeducation, which helps promote new, more efficient movement patterns. As freedom of movement improves, postural reeducation may help ensure the maintenance of the less-restricted movement patterns.

Generally, acute cases tend to resolve in just a few treatments. The longer a condition has been present, the longer it will take to resolve. Occasionally, dramatic results will occur immediately after treatment. It is usually recommended that treatment be done at least 3 times per week.

Myofascial release can be done manually by an athletic trainer or by the patient stretching using a foam roller.[89] Figure 8-10 shows examples of stretching using the foam roller.

Strain-Counterstrain Technique

Strain-counterstrain is an approach to decreasing muscle tension and guarding that may be used to normalize muscle function. It is a passive technique that places the body in a position of greatest comfort, thereby relieving pain.[1,55]

In this technique, the athletic trainer locates "tender points" on the patient's body that correspond to areas of dysfunction in specific joints or muscles that are in need of treatment.[99] These tender points are not located in or just beneath the skin, as are many acupuncture points, but instead are deeper in muscle, tendon, ligament, or fascia. They are characterized by tense, tender, edematous spots on the body. They are 1 cm or less in diameter, with the most acute points being 3 mm in diameter, although they may be a few centimeters long within a muscle. There can be multiple points for one specific joint dysfunction. Points might be arranged in a chain, and they are often found in a painless area opposite the site of pain and/or weakness.[55]

The athletic trainer monitors the tension and level of pain elicited by the tender point while moving the patient into a position of ease or comfort. This is accomplished by markedly shortening the muscle.[99] When this position of ease is found, the tender point is no longer tense or tender. When this position is maintained for a minimum of 90 seconds, the tension in the tender point and in the corresponding joint or muscle is reduced or cleared. By slowly returning to a neutral position, the tender point and the corresponding joint or muscle remains pain-free with normal tension. For example, with neck pain and/or tension headaches, the tender point may be found on either the front or back of the patient's neck and shoulders. The athletic trainer will have the patient lie on the patient's back and will gently and slowly bend the patient's neck until that tender point is no longer tender. After holding that position for

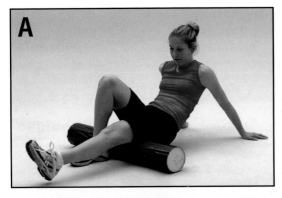
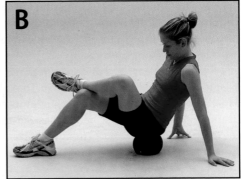
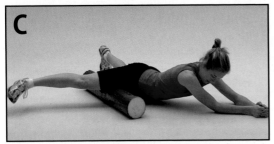
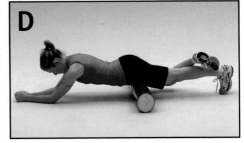
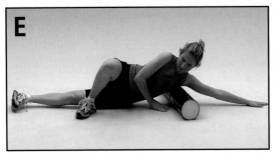
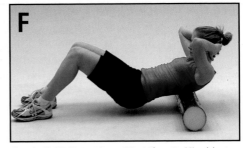

Figure 8-10. Myofascial release stretching using a foam roller or firm ball. (A) Hamstrings; (B) piriformis; (C) adductors; (D) quadriceps; (E) latissimus dorsi; (F) rhomboids.

90 seconds, the athletic trainer gently and slowly returns the neck to its resting position. When that tender point is pressed again, the patient should notice a significant decrease in pain there (Figure 8-11).[99]

The physiologic rationale for the effectiveness of the strain-counterstrain technique can be explained by the stretch reflex.[2] When a muscle is placed in a stretched position, impulses from the muscle spindles create a reflex contraction of the muscle in response to stretch. With strain-counterstrain, the joint or muscle is placed not in a position of stretch but instead in a slack position. Thus, muscle spindle input is reduced and the muscle is relaxed, allowing for a decrease in tension and pain.[2]

Positional Release Therapy

Positional release therapy is based on the strain-counterstrain technique. The primary difference between the two is the use of a facilitating force (compression) to enhance the effect of the positioning.[17,18,90,95]

Like strain-counterstrain, positional release therapy is an osteopathic mobilization technique in which the body part is moved into a position of greatest relaxation.[33] The therapist finds the position of greatest comfort and muscle relaxation for each joint with the help of movement tests and diagnostic tender points. Once located, the tender point is maintained with the palpating finger at a subthreshold pressure. The patient is then passively placed

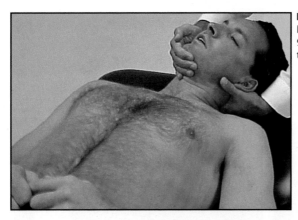

Figure 8-11. Strain-counterstrain technique. The body part is placed in a position of comfort for 90 seconds and then slowly moved back to a neutral position.

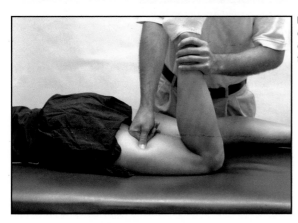

Figure 8-12. The positional release technique places the muscle in a position of comfort with the finger or thumb exerting submaximal pressure on a myofascial trigger point.

in a position that reduces the tension under the palpating finger producing a subjective reduction in tenderness as reported by the patient. This specific position is adjusted throughout the 90-second treatment period. It has been suggested that maintaining contact with the tender point during the treatment period exerts a therapeutic effect.[17,18] This technique is one of the most effective and gentle methods for the treatment of acute and chronic musculoskeletal dysfunction (Figure 8-12).[90]

Active Release Technique

The Active Release Technique® is a relatively new type of manual therapy developed by P. Michael Leahy, DC, CCSP to correct soft-tissue problems in muscle, tendon, and fascia caused by the formation of fibrotic adhesions that result from acute injury, repetitive or overuse injuries, constant pressure, or tension injuries.[63] When a muscle, tendon, fascia, or ligament is torn (strained or sprained) or a nerve is damaged, the tissues heal with adhesions or scar tissue formation rather than the formation of brand new tissue. Scar tissue is weaker, less elastic, less pliable, and more pain-sensitive than healthy tissue.

These fibrotic adhesions disrupt the normal muscle function, which, in turn, affects the biomechanics of the joint complex and can lead to pain and dysfunction. The Active Release Technique provides a way to diagnose and treat the underlying causes of cumulative trauma disorders that, left uncorrected, can lead to inflammation, adhesions, fibrosis, and muscle imbalances. All of these can result in weak and tense tissues, decreased circulation, hypoxia, and symptoms of peripheral nerve entrapment, including numbness, tingling, burning, and aching.[63] The Active Release Technique is a deep-tissue technique used for breaking down scar tissue/adhesions and restoring function and movement.[63] In the Active Release Technique, the athletic trainer first locates through palpation those adhesions

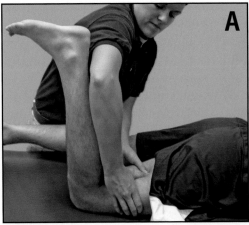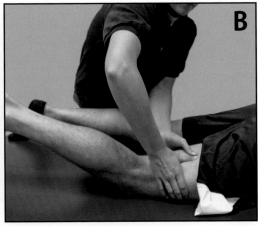

Figure 8-13. The Active Release Technique. The muscle is elongated from a shortened position while static pressure is applied to the tender point.

in the muscle, tendon, or fascia that are causing the problem. Once these are located, the athletic trainer traps the affected muscle by applying pressure or tension with the thumb or finger over these lesions in the direction of the fibers. Then the patient is asked to actively move the body part such that the musculature is elongated from a shortened position while the athletic trainer continues to apply tension to the lesion (Figure 8-13). This should be repeated three to five times per treatment session. By breaking up the adhesions, the technique improves the patient's condition by softening and stretching the scar tissue, resulting in increased ROM, increased strength, and improved circulation, optimizing healing. Treatments tend to be uncomfortable during the movement phases as the scar tissue or adhesions tear apart.[63] This is temporary and subsides almost immediately after the treatment. An important part of the Active Release Technique is for the patient to heed the athletic trainer's recommendations regarding activity modification, stretching, and exercise.

Graston Technique

The Graston Technique is an instrument-assisted soft-tissue mobilization that enables clinicians to effectively break down scar tissue and fascial restrictions as well as stretch connective tissue and muscle fibers (Figure 8-14).[36,51] The technique uses six hand-held specially designed stainless steel instruments shaped to fit the contour of the body, to scan an area, locate, and then treat the injured tissue that is causing pain and restricting motion.[51] A clinician normally will palpate a painful area looking for unusual nodules, restrictive barriers, or tissue tensions. The instruments help to magnify existing restrictions and the clinician can feel these through the instruments.[36] Then the clinician can use the instruments to supply precise pressure to break up scar tissue, relieving the discomfort and helping to restore normal function. The instruments, with a narrow surface area at their edge, have the ability to separate fibers.

A specially designed lubricant is applied to the skin prior to using the instrument, allowing the instrument to glide over the skin without causing irritation. Using a cross-friction massage in multiple directions, which involves using the instruments to stroke or rub against the grain of the scar tissue, the clinician creates small amounts of trauma to the affected area.[36] This temporarily causes inflammation in the area, increasing the rate and amount of blood flow in and around the area. The theory is that this process helps initiate and promote the healing process of the affected soft tissues. It is common for the patient to experience some discomfort during the procedure and possibly some bruising.

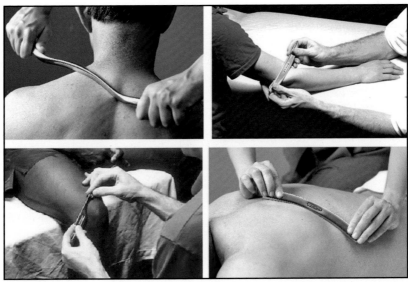

Figure 8-14. The Graston Technique uses handheld stainless steel instruments to locate and then separate existing restrictions within a muscle. (Reproduced with permission from The Graston Technique.)

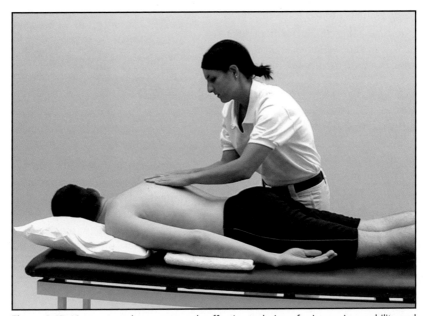

Figure 8-15. Massage can be an extremely effective technique for improving mobility and ROM. Ice application following the treatment may ease the discomfort. It is recommended that an exercise, stretching, and strengthening program be used in conjunction with the technique to help the injured tissues heal.

Massage

Massage is a mechanical stimulation of the tissues by means of rhythmically applied pressure and stretching (Figure 8-15).[83] Over the years, many claims have been made relative to the therapeutic benefits of massage, but few are based on well-controlled, well-designed studies. Therapists have used massage to increase flexibility and coordination as well as to increase pain threshold; to decrease neuromuscular excitability in the muscle being massaged; to stimulate circulation, thus improving energy transport to the muscle; to facilitate healing and restore joint mobility; and to remove lactic acid, thus alleviating muscle cramps.[83]

How these effects can be accomplished is determined by the specific approaches used with massage techniques and how they are applied. Generally, the effects of massage are either reflexive or mechanical. The effect of massage on the nervous system differs greatly according to the method employed, the pressure exerted, and the duration of applications. Through the reflex mechanism, sedation is induced. Slow, gentle, rhythmical, and superficial effleurage may relieve tension and soothe, rendering the muscles more relaxed. This indicates an effect on sensory and motor nerves locally and some central nervous system response. The mechanical approach seeks to make mechanical or histologic changes in myofascial structures through direct force applied superficially.[83] Among the massage techniques used by athletic trainers are the following:[83]

1. Hoffa massage—the classic form of massage, strokes include effleurage, petrissage, percussion or tapotement, and vibration.

2. Friction massage—used to increase the inflammatory response, particularly in case of chronic tendinitis or tenosynovitis.

3. Acupressure—massage of acupuncture and trigger points, used to reduce pain and irritation in anatomical areas known to be associated with specific points.

4. Connective tissue massage—a stroking technique used on layers of connective tissue, a relatively new form of treatment in this country, primarily affecting circulatory pathologies.

5. Myofascial release—used for the purpose of relieving soft tissue from the abnormal grip of tight fascia.

6. Rolfing—a system devised to correct inefficient structure by balancing the body within a gravitational field through a technique involving manual soft-tissue manipulation.

7. Trager—attempts to establish neuromuscular control so that more normal movement patterns can be routinely performed.

Summary

1. Flexibility is the ability of the neuromuscular system to allow for efficient movement of a joint or a series of joints smoothly through a full ROM.

2. Flexibility is specific to a given joint, and the term *good flexibility* implies that there are no joint abnormalities restricting movement.

3. Flexibility can be limited by muscles and tendons and their fascia, joint capsules or ligaments, fat, bone structure, skin, or neural tissue.

4. Passive ROM refers to the degree to which a joint can be passively moved to the end points in the ROM. Active ROM refers to movement through the midrange of motion resulting from active contraction.

5. Measurement of joint flexibility is accomplished through the use of a goniometer or an inclinometer.

6. An agonist muscle is one that contracts to produce joint motion, whereas the antagonist muscle is stretched with contraction of the agonist.

7. Increases in flexibility can be attributed to neurophysiologic adaptations involving the stretch reflex and associated muscle spindles and Golgi tendon organs, changes in the viscoelastic and plastic properties of muscle, adaptations and changes in the kinetic chain, and alterations in intramuscular temperature.

8. Dynamic, static, and PNF techniques have all been used as stretching techniques for improving flexibility.

9. Stretching of tight neural structures and myofascial release stretching are also used to reestablish a full ROM.

10. Strain-counterstrain is a passive technique that places a body part in a position of greatest comfort to decrease muscle tension and guarding and to relieve pain.

11. Positional release therapy is similar to strain-counterstrain. Pressure is

maintained on a tender point with the body part in a position of comfort for 90 seconds.

12. The active release technique is a deep-tissue technique used for breaking down scar tissue and adhesions and restoring function and movement.

13. Massage is the mechanical stimulation of tissue by means of rhythmically applied pressure and stretching. It allows the athletic trainer, as a health care provider, to help a patient overcome pain and relax through the application of the therapeutic massage techniques.

References

1. Alexander KM. Use of strain-counterstrain as an adjunct for treatment of chronic lower abdominal pain. *Phy Ther Case Rep.* 1999;2(5):205-208.

2. Allerheiliger W. Stretching and warm-up. In: Baechle T, ed. *Essentials of Strength Training.* Champaign, IL: Human Kinetics; 1994.

3. Alter M. *The science of flexibility.* Champaign, IL: Human Kinetics; 2004.

4. Andersen JC. Stretching before and after exercise: effect on muscle soreness and injury risk. *J Athl Train.* 2005;40(3):218-220.

5. Armiger P. Preventing musculotendinous injuries: a focus on flexibility. *Athl Ther Today.* 2000;5(4):20.

6. Bandy WD, Irion JM. The effect of time of static stretch on the flexibility of the hamstring muscles. *Phys Ther.* 1994;74:845-852.

7. Bandy WD, Irion JM, Briggler M. The effect of static stretch and dynamic range of motion training on the flexibility of the hamstring muscles. *J Orthop Sports Phys Ther.* 1998;27(4):295.

8. Basmajian J. *Therapeutic Exercise.* 4th ed. Baltimore, MD: Lippincott Williams & Wilkins; 1984.

9. Behm DG, Bambury A, Cahill F, Power K. Effect of acute static stretching on force, balance, reaction time, and movement time. *Med Sci Sports Exerc.* 2004;36(8):1397-1402.

10. Bernardo L. The effectiveness of Pilates training in healthy adults: an appraisal of the research literature. *J Bodyw Mov Ther.* 2007;11(2):106-110.

11. Blahnik J. *Full Body Flexibility.* Champaign, IL: Human Kinetics; 2004.

12. Blanke D. Flexibility. In: Mellion M, ed. *Sports Medicine Secrets.* Philadelphia, PA: Hanley & Belfus; 2002.

13. Boyle P. The effect of static and dynamic stretching on muscle force production. *J Sports Sci.* 2004;22(3):273-274.

14. Burke DG, Culligan CJ, Holt LE. The theoretical basis of proprioceptive neuromuscular facilitation. *J Strength Cond Res.* 2000;14(4):496-500.

15. Carter AM, Kinzey SJ, Chitwood LF, Cole JL. Proprioceptive neuromuscular facilitation decreases muscle activity during the stretch reflex in selected posterior thigh muscles. *J Sport Rehabil.* 2000;9(4):269-278.

16. Chaitlow L. *Muscle Energy Techniques.* Philadelphia, PA: Churchill Livingstone; 2006.

17. Chaitlow L. *Positional Release Techniques (Advanced Soft Tissue Techniques).* Philadelphia, PA: Churchill Livingstone; 2002.

18. Chaitlow L. Positional release techniques in the treatment of muscle and joint dysfunction. *Clin Bull Myofascial Ther.* 1998;3(1):25-35.

19. Chalmers G. Re-examination of the possible role of Golgi tendon organ and muscle spindle reflexes in proprioceptive neuromuscular facilitation muscle stretching. *Sports Biomech.* 2004;3(1):159-183.

20. Chapman EA, deVries HA, Swezey R. Joint stiffness: Effect of exercise on young and old men. *J Gerontol.* 1972;27:218.

21. Clark M. *Integrated Training for the New Millennium.* Calabasas, CA: National Academy of Sports Medicine; 2001.

22. Condon SA, Hutton RS. Soleus muscle EMG activity and ankle dorsiflexion range of motion from stretching procedures. *Phys Ther.* 1987;67:24-30.

23. Corbin C, Fox K. Flexibility: the forgotten part of fitness. *J Phys Educ.* 1985;16(6):191.

24. Corbin C, Noble L. Flexibility. *J Phys Educ Rec Dance.* 1980;51:23.

25. Corbin C, Noble L. Flexibility: a major component of physical fitness. In: Cundiff DE, ed. *Implementation of Health Fitness Exercise Programs.* Reston, VA: American Alliance for Health, Physical Education, Recreation and Dance; 1985.

26. Cornelius W, Jackson A. The effects of cryotherapy and PNF on hip extensor flexibility. *J Athl Train.* 1984;19:183-184.

27. Cornelius WL, Hagemann RW Jr, Jackson AW. A study on placement of stretching within a workout. *J Sports Med Phys Fitness.* 1988;28(3):234.

28. Cornelius WL. *PNF and Other Flexibility Techniques.* Arlington, VA: Computer Microfilm International; 1986.

29. Cornelius WL. Two effective flexibility methods. *Athlet Train.* 1981;16(1):23.

30. Cornwell A. The acute effects of passive stretching on active musculotendinous stiffness. *Med Sci Sports Exerc.* 1997;29(5):281.

31. Couch J. *Runners World Yoga Book.* Mountain View, CA: World; 1982.

32. Cross KM, Worrell TW. Effects of a static stretching program on the incidence of lower extremity musculotendinous strains. *J Athl Train.* 1999;34(1):11.

33. D'Ambrogio K, Roth G. *Positional Release Therapy: Assessment and Treatment of Musculoskeletal Dysfunction.* St. Louis, MO: Mosby-Year Book; 1996.

34. Decoster L, Cleland J, Altieri C. The effects of hamstring stretching on range of motion: a systematic literature review. *J Orthop Sports Phys Ther.* 2005;3(6):377-387.

35. DeLuccio J. Instrument assisted soft tissue mobilization utilizing Graston technique: a physical therapist's perspective. *Orthop Phys Ther Pract.* 2006;18(3):32-34.

36. deVries HA. Evaluation of static stretching procedures for improvement of flexibility. *Res Q.* 1962;3:222-229.

37. De Deyne PG. Application of passive stretch and its implications for muscle fibers. *Phys Ther.* 2001;81(2):819-827.

38. DePino GM, Webright WG, Arnold BL. Duration of maintained hamstring flexibility after cessation of an acute static stretching protocol. *J Athl Train.* 2000;35(1):56.

39. Entyre BR, Abraham LD. Ache-reflex changes during static stretching and two variations of proprioceptive neuromuscular facilitation techniques. *Electroencephalogr Clin Neurophysiol.* 1986;63:174-179.

40. Entyre BR, Abraham LD. Antagonist muscle activity during stretching: a paradox reassessed. *Med Sci Sports Exerc.* 1988;20:285-289.

41. Entyre BR, Lee EJ. Chronic and acute flexibility of men and women using three different stretching techniques. *Res Q Exerc Sport.* 1988;59:222-228.

42. Fowles JR, Sale DG, MacDougall JD. Reduced strength after passive stretch of the human plantar flexors. *J Appl Physiol.* 2000;89(3):1179-1188.

43. Ferreira G, Nunes T, Teixeira I. Gains in flexibility related to measures of muscular performance: Impact of flexibility on muscular performance. *Clin J Sport Med.* 2007;17(4):276-281.

44. Funk D, Swank AM, Adams KJ, Treolo D. Efficacy of moist heat pack application over static stretching on hamstring flexibility. *J Strength Cond Res.* 2001;15(1):123-126.

45. Godges JJ, MacRae H, Longdon C, et al. The effects of two stretching procedures on hip range of motion and joint economy. *J Orthop Sports Phys Ther.* 1989;11:350-357.

46. Gribble P, Prentice W. Effects of static and hold-relax stretching on hamstring range of motion using the Flex- Ability LE 1000. *J Sport Rehabil.* 1999;8(3):195.

47. Hedrick A. Dynamic flexibility training. *Strength Cond J.* 2000;22(5):33-38.

48. Herling J. It's time to add strength training to our fitness programs. *J Phys Educ Program.* 1981;79:17.

49. Heyward VH. Assessing flexibility and designing stretching programs. In: Heyward VH, ed. *Advanced Fitness Assessment and Exercise Prescription.* 6th ed. Champaign, IL: Human Kinetics; 2010:265–282.

50. Holt LE TW. Pelham, Burke DG. Modifications to the standard sit-and-reach flexibility protocol. *J Athl Train.* 1999;34(1):43.

51. Howitt S. The conservative treatment of trigger thumb using Graston techniques and active release techniques. *J Can Chiropr Assoc.* 2006;50(4):249-254.

52. Humphrey LD. Flexibility. *J Phys Educ Rec Dance.* 1981;52:41.

53. Hunter G. Specific soft tissue mobilization in the management of soft tissue dysfunction. *Man Ther.* 1998;3(1):2-11.

54. Ishii DK. Flexibility strexercises for co-ed groups. *Scholastic Coach.* 1976;45:31.

55. Jones L. *Strain-Counterstrain.* Boise, ID: Jones; 1995.

56. Kaplan B, Pierce M. *Yoga for Your Life: A practice Manual of Breath and Movement for Everybody.* New York, NY: Sterling Publishing; 2008.

57. Keirns M, ed. *Myofascial Release in Sports Medicine.* Champaign, IL: Human Kinetics; 2000.

58. Knott M, Voss P. *Proprioceptive Neuromuscular Facilitation.* 3rd ed. New York, NY: Harper & Row; 1985.

59. Kokkonen J, Nelson A. Chronic static stretching improves exercise performance. *Med Sci Sports Exerc.* 2007;39(10):1825-1831.

60. Kokkonen JE, Nelson C, Arnold G. Chronic stretching improves sport specific skills. *Med Sci Sports Exerc.* 1997;29(5):67.

61. Kokkonen JN, Nelson AG, Arnall DA. Acute stretching inhibits strength endurance. *Med Sci Sports Exerc.* 2001;35(5):s11.

62. Kubo K, Kanehisa H, Fukunaga T. Effect of stretching training on the viscoelastic properties of human tendon structures in vivo. *J Appl Physiol.* 2002;92(2):595-601.

63. Leahy M. Improved treatments for carpal tunnel and related syndromes. *Chiropr Sports Med.* 1995;9(1):6.

64. Lentell G, Hetherington T, Eagan J, et al. The use of thermal agents to influence the effectiveness of a lowload prolonged stretch. *J Orthop Sports Phys Ther.* 1992;5:200-207.

65. Liemohn W. Flexibility and muscular strength. *J Phys Educ Rec Dance.* 1988;59(7):37.

66. Louden KL, Bolier CE, Allison AK, et al. Effects of two stretching methods on the flexibility and retention of flexibility at the ankle joint in runners. *Phys Ther.* 1985;65:698.

67. Madding SW JG. Wong, Hallum A. Effects of duration of passive stretching on hip abduction range of motion. *J Orthop Sports Phys Ther.* 1987;8:409-416.

68. Mann D, Whedon C. Functional stretching: implementing a dynamic stretching program. *Athl Ther Today.* 2001;6(3):10-13.

69. Manheim C. *Myofascial Release Manual.* Thorofare, NJ: SLACK, Incorporated; 2001.

70. Marek S, Cramer J, Fincher L. Acute effects of static and proprioceptive neuromuscular facilitation stretching on muscle strength and power output. *J Athl Train.* 2005;40(2):94-103.

71. Markos PD. Ipsilateral and contralateral effects of proprioceptive neuromuscular facilitation techniques on hip motion and electromyographic activity. *Phys Ther.* 1979;59:1366-1373.

72. McAtee R. *Facilitated Stretching.* Champaign, IL: Human Kinetics; 2007.

73. McClellan E, Padua D, Prentice W. Effects of myofascial release and static stretching on active range of motion and muscle activity. *J Athl Train.* 2000;35(3):329.

74. Moore M, Hutton R. Electromyographic investigation of muscle stretching techniques. *Med Sci Sports Exerc.* 1980;12:322-329.

75. Murphy P. Warming up before stretching advised. *Phys Sportsmed.* 1986;14(3):45.

76. Nelson R. An update on flexibility. *Natl Strength Cond Assoc.* 2005;27(1):10-16.

77. Norris C. *Flexibility Principles and Practices.* London, UK: A&C Black; 1995.

78. Power K, Behm D, Cahill F, Carroll M, Young W. An acute bout of static stretching: effects on force and jumping performance. *Med Sci Sports Exerc.* 2004;36(8): 1389-1396.

79. Prentice WE, Kooima E. The use of PNF techniques in rehabilitation of sport-related injury. *Athlet Train.* 1986;21(1):26-31.

80. Prentice WE. A comparison of static stretching and PNF stretching for improving hip joint flexibility. *J Athl Train.* 1983;18:56-59.

81. Prentice WE. A review of PNF techniques—implications for athletic rehabilitation and performance. *Forum Medicum.* 1989;51:1-13.

82. Prentice WE. An electromyographic analysis of heat or cold and stretching for inducing muscular relaxation. *J Orthop Sports Phys Ther.* 1982;3:133-140.

83. Prentice W. Sports massage. In: Prentice W, ed. *Therapeutic Modalities in Sports Medicine and Athletic Training.* New York, NY: McGraw-Hill; 2009:349-372.

84. Rasch P. *Kinesiology and Applied Anatomy.* Philadelphia, PA: Lea & Febiger; 1989.

85. Rubini E, Costa A. The effects of stretching on strength performance. *Sports Med.* 2007;37(3):213.

86. Sady SP, Wortman M, Blanke D. Flexibility training: ballistic, static, or proprioceptive neuromuscular facilitation? *Arch Phys Med Rehabil.* 1982;63: 261-263.

87. Sapega AA, Quedenfeld T, Moyer R, et al. Biophysical factors in range-of-motion exercise. *Phys Sportsmed.* 1981;9(12):57.

88. Schilling BK, Stone MH. Stretching: acute effects on strength and power performance. *Strength Cond J.* 2000;22(1):44.

89. Sefton J. Myofascial release for athletic trainers, part 1. *Athl Ther Today.* 2004;9(1):40.

90. Schiowitz S. Facilitated positional release. *J Am Osteopath Assoc.* 1990;90(2):145-146, 151-155.

91. Shellock F, Prentice WE. Warm-up and stretching for improved physical performance and prevention of sport related injury. *Sports Med.* 1985;2:267-278.

92. Shindo M, Harayama H, Kondo K, et al. Changes in reciprocal Ia inhibition during voluntary contraction in man. *Exp Brain Res.* 1984;53:400-408.

93. Siatras T, Papadopoulos G, Maeletzi D, Gerodimos V, Kellis P. Static and dynamic acute stretching effect on gymnasts' speed in vaulting. *Ped Ex Sci.* 2003;15: 383-391.

94. Spernoga SG, Uhl TL, Arnold BL, Gansneder BM. Duration of maintained hamstring flexibility after a one time, modified hold-relax stretching protocol. *J Athl Train.* 2001;36(1):44-48.

95. Speicher T. Top 10 positional release therapy techniques to break the chain of pain, part 1. *Athl Ther Today.* 2006;11(5):60.

96. St. George F. *The Stretching Handbook: Ten Steps to Muscle Fitness.* Roseville, IL: Simon & Schuster; 1997.

97. Stamford B. A stretching primer. *Phys Sportsmed.* 1994;22(9):85-86.

98. Stone J. Myofascial release. *Athl Ther Today.* 2000;5(4):34-35.

99. Stone J. Strain-counterstrain. *Athl Ther Today.* 2000;5(6):30.

100. Surburg P. Flexibility/range of motion. In: Winnick JP, ed. *The Brockport Physical Fitness Training Guide.* Champaign, IL: Human Kinetics; 1999.

101. Surburg P. Flexibility training program design. In: Miller P, ed. *Fitness Programming and Physical Disability.* Champaign, IL: Human Kinetics; 1995.

102. Tanigawa MC. Comparison of the hold relax procedure and passive mobilization on increasing muscle length. *Phys Ther.* 1972;52:725.

103. Taylor DC, Brooks DE, Ryan JB. Viscoelastic characteristics of muscle: passive stretching versus muscular contractions. *Med Sci Sports Exerc.* 1997;29(12):1619-1624.

104. Thacker S, Gilchrist J, Stroup D. The impact of stretching on sports injury risk: a systematic review of the literature. *Med Sci Sports Exerc.* 2004;36(3):371-378.

105. Tobias M, Sullivan JP. *Complete Stretching.* New York, NY: Knopf; 1992.

106. Van Hatten B. Passive versus active stretching. *Phys Ther.* 2005;85(1):80.

107. Van Mechelen P. Prevention of running injuries by warm-up, cool-down, and stretching. *Am J Sports Med.* 1993;21(5):711-719.

108. Voss DE, Lonta MK, Myers GJ. *Proprioceptive Neuro- Muscular Facilitation: Patterns and Techniques.* 3rd ed. Philadelphia, PA: Lippincott Williams & Wilkins; 1985.

109. Wessel J, Wan A. Effect of stretching on intensity of delayed-onset muscle soreness. *J Sports Med.* 1984;2:83-87.

110. Winters MV, Blake GC, Trost J. Passive versus active stretching of hip flexor muscles in subjects with limited hip extension: A randomized clinical trial. *Phys Ther.* 2004;84(9):800-807.

111. Worrell T, Smith T, Winegardner J. Effect of hamstring stretching on hamstring muscle performance. *J Orthop Sports Phys Ther.* 1994;20(3):154-159.

112. Zachewski J. Flexibility for sports. In: Sanders B, ed. *Sports Physical Therapy*. Norwalk, CT: Appleton & Lange; 1990:201-238.

113. Zebas CJ, Rivera ML. Retention of flexibility in selected joints after cessation of a stretching exercise program. In: Dotson CO, Humphrey HJ, eds. *Exercise Physiology: Current Selected Research Topics*. New York, NY: AMS Press; 1985.

SOLUTIONS TO CLINICAL DECISION-MAKING EXERCISES

8-1   Flexibility is crucial to a gymnast's performance. Although she is not training, she must maintain movement at all of her joints so that she does not lose flexibility. Inactivity can cause a shortening of elastic components. This would put her at risk for muscular injury when she resumes her normal activity.

8-2   Applying certain therapeutic modalities, such as ice and/or electrical stimulating currents, can decrease pain and discourage muscle guarding to increase ROM. Delayed-onset muscle soreness will usually begin to subside at about 48 hours following a workout.

8-3   A goniometer can be used to measure the angle between the femur and the fibula, giving you degrees of flexion and extension. To maximize consistency in measurement, it is helpful if the same person takes sequential goniometric measurements.

8-4   The motion might be limited by quadriceps (antagonistic) muscle tightness, tightness of the joint capsule, pathological or damaged bony structure preventing normal accessory motions between the tibia and femur or between the patella and femur, fat/muscle causing tissue approximation, or scar tissue in the anterior portion of the joint.

8-5   A static stretch should be held for about 30 seconds. This allows time for the Golgi tendon organs to override the muscle spindles and produce a reflex muscle relaxation. The patient should stretch to the point where tightness or resistance to stretch is felt but it should not be painful. The stretch should be repeated three to five times.

8-6   Ballistic stretching is dynamic stretching that is useful prior to activity because it is a functional stretch. It mimics activity that will be performed during competition. However, there is some speculation that because it is an uncontrolled stretch, it may lead to injury, especially in sedentary individuals. Static stretching is convenient because it can be done on any muscle and it doesn't require a partner. It is not very functional. PNF stretching will most likely provide the greatest increase in ROM, but it is a little more time consuming and requires a partner.

Please see videos on the accompanying website at

www.healio.com/books/sportsmedvideos

CHAPTER 9

Regaining Muscular Strength, Endurance, and Power

William E. Prentice, PhD, PT, ATC, FNATA

After completion of this chapter, the athletic trainer should be able to do the following:

- Define muscular strength, endurance, and power, and discuss their importance in a program of rehabilitation following injury.

- Discuss the anatomy and physiology of skeletal muscle.

- Discuss the physiology of strength development and factors that determine strength.

- Describe specific methods for improving muscular strength.

- Differentiate between muscle strength and muscle endurance.

- Discuss differences between males and females in terms of strength development.

Following all musculoskeletal injuries, there will be some degree of impairment in muscular strength and endurance. For the athletic trainer supervising a rehabilitation program, regaining, and in many instances improving, levels of strength and endurance are critical for discharging and returning the patient to a functional level following injury.

By definition, muscular strength is the ability of a muscle to generate force against some resistance. Maintenance of at least a normal level of strength in a given muscle or muscle group is important for normal healthy living. Muscle weakness or imbalance can result in abnormal movement or gait and can impair normal functional movement. Resistance training plays a critical role in injury rehabilitation.

Muscular strength is closely associated with muscular endurance. Muscular endurance is the ability to perform repetitive muscular contractions against some resistance for an extended period. As we will see later, as muscular strength increases, there tends to be a corresponding increase in endurance. For the average person in the population, developing muscular endurance is likely more important

Prentice WE, ed.
Rehabilitation Techniques for Sports Medicine and Athletic Training (pp 243-266).
© 2015 SLACK Incorporated.

than developing muscular strength because muscular endurance is probably more critical in carrying out the everyday activities of living. This statement becomes increasingly true with age.

Clinical Decision-Making Exercise 9-1

A softball pitcher was out for a whole season for rehabilitation following shoulder surgery. Why is it important that she regain all three aspects of muscular fitness?

TYPES OF SKELETAL MUSCLE CONTRACTION

Skeletal muscle is capable of three different types of contraction: isometric contraction, concentric contraction, and eccentric contraction. An isometric contraction occurs when the muscle contracts to produce tension, but there is no change in muscle length. Considerable force can be generated against some immovable resistance even though no movement occurs. In a concentric contraction, the muscle shortens in length while tension increases to overcome or move some resistance. In an eccentric contraction, the resistance is greater than the muscular force being produced, and the muscle lengthens while producing tension. Concentric and eccentric contractions are considered dynamic movements.[56]

Recently, econcentric contraction, which combines both a controlled concentric and a concurrent eccentric contraction of the same muscle over two separate joints, has been introduced.[19,30] An econcentric contraction is possible only in muscles that cross at least two joints. An example of an econcentric contraction is a prone, open kinetic chain hamstring curl. The hamstrings contract concentrically to flex the knee, while the hip tends to flex eccentrically, lengthening the hamstring. Rehabilitation exercises have traditionally concentrated on strengthening isolated single-joint motions, despite the fact that the same muscle is functioning at a second joint simultaneously. Consequently, it has been recommended that the strengthening program includes exercises that strengthen the muscle in the manner in which it contracts functionally. Traditional strength-training programs have been designed to develop strength in individual muscles, in a single plane of motion. However, because all muscles function concentrically, eccentrically, and isometrically in three planes of motion, a strengthening program should be multiplanar, concentrating on all three types of contraction.[15]

FACTORS THAT DETERMINE LEVELS OF MUSCLE STRENGTH, ENDURANCE, AND POWER

Size of the Muscle

Muscular strength is proportional to the cross-sectional diameter of the muscle fibers. The greater the cross-sectional diameter or the bigger a particular muscle, the stronger it is, and thus the more force it is capable of generating. The size of a muscle tends to increase in cross-sectional diameter with resistance training. This increase in muscle size is referred to as hypertrophy.[42] A decrease in the size of a muscle is referred to as atrophy.

Number of Muscle Fibers

Strength is a function of the number and diameter of muscle fibers composing a given muscle. The number of fibers is an inherited characteristic; thus, a person with a large number of muscle fibers to begin with has the potential to hypertrophy to a much greater degree than does someone with relatively few fibers.[38]

Neuromuscular Efficiency

Strength is also directly related to the efficiency of the neuromuscular system and the function of the motor unit in producing muscular force.[46] Initial increases in strength during the first 8 to 10 weeks of a resistance training program can be attributed primarily to increased neuromuscular efficiency.[59] Resistance training will increase neuromuscular efficiency in three ways: there is an increase in the number of motor units being recruited,

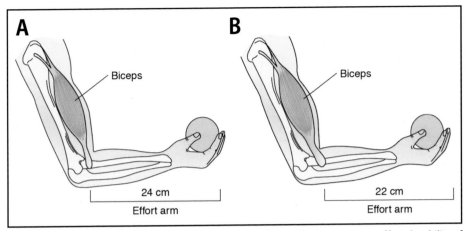

Figure 9-1. The position of attachment of the muscle tendon on the lever arm can affect the ability of that muscle to generate force. B should be able to generate greater force than A because the tendon attachment on the lever arm is closer to the resistance. (Reproduced with permission from Prentice WE. *Principles of Athletic Training*. 14th ed. New York: McGraw-Hill; 2011.)

in the firing rate of each motor unit, and in the synchronization of motor unit firing.[7]

Biomechanical Considerations

Strength in a given muscle is determined not only by the physical properties of the muscle but also by biomechanical factors that dictate how much force can be generated through a system of levers to an external object.[31,38,63]

Position of Tendon Attachment

If we think of the elbow joint as one of these lever systems, we would have the biceps muscle producing flexion of this joint (Figure 9-1). The position of attachment of the biceps muscle on the forearm will largely determine how much force this muscle is capable of generating. If there are two individuals, A and B, and A has a biceps attachment that is closer to the fulcrum (the elbow joint) than does B, then A must produce a greater effort with the biceps muscle to hold the weight at a right angle, because the length of the effort arm will be greater than that for B.

Length–Tension Relationship

The length of a muscle determines the tension that can be generated. By varying the length of a muscle, different tensions can be produced.[31] Figure 9-2 illustrates this length–tension relationship. At position B in the curve, the interaction of the cross-bridges between the actin and myosin myofilaments within the sarcomere is at maximum. Setting a muscle at this particular length will produce the greatest amount of tension. At position A, the muscle is shortened, and at position C, the muscle is lengthened. In either case, the interaction between the actin and myosin myofilaments through the cross-bridges is greatly reduced, thus the muscle is not capable of generating significant tension.

Age

The ability to generate muscular force is also related to age.[4] Both men and women seem to be able to increase strength throughout puberty and adolescence, reaching a peak around 20 to 25 years of age, at which time, this ability begins to level off, and in some cases decline. After about age 25, a person generally loses an average of 1% of his or her maximal remaining strength each year. Thus, at age 65 years, a person would have only about 60% of the strength he or she had at age 25 years.[45] This loss in muscle strength is definitely related to individual levels of physical activity. People who are more active, or perhaps continue to strength-train, considerably decrease this tendency toward declining muscle strength. In addition to retarding this decrease in muscular strength, exercise can also have an effect in slowing the decrease in cardiorespiratory endurance and flexibility, as well as slowing increases in body

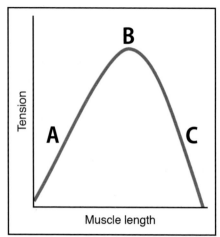

Figure 9-2. The length–tension relation of the muscle. Greatest tension is developed at point B, with less tension developed at points A and C. (Reproduced with permission from Prentice. *Principles of Athletic Training.* 14th ed. New York: McGraw-Hill; 2011.)

fat. Thus, strength maintenance is important for all individuals regardless of age for achieving total wellness and good health as well as in rehabilitation after injury.[62]

Overtraining

Overtraining in a physically active patient can have a negative effect on the development of muscular strength. Overtraining is an imbalance between exercise and recovery in which the training program exceeds the body's physiologic and psychological limits. Overtraining can result in psychological breakdown (staleness) or physiologic breakdown that can involve musculoskeletal injury, fatigue, or sickness. Engaging in proper and efficient resistance training, eating a proper diet, and getting appropriate rest can all minimize the potential negative effects of overtraining.

Clinical Decision-Making Exercise 9-2

A gymnast fell from the balance beam and sustained a Colles fracture. She will be casted for several weeks. How should isometric and isotonic exercise be incorporated into her rehabilitation program?

Fast-Twitch vs Slow-Twitch Fibers

All fibers in a particular motor unit are either slow-twitch fibers or fast-twitch fibers. Each kind has distinctive metabolic and contractile capabilities.

Slow-Twitch Fibers

Slow-twitch fibers are also referred to as Type I or slow-oxidative fibers. They are more resistant to fatigue than fast-twitch fibers; however, the time required to generate force is much greater in slow-twitch fibers.[29] Because they are relatively fatigue resistant, slow-twitch fibers are associated primarily with long-duration, aerobic-type activities.

Fast-Twitch Fibers

Fast-twitch fibers are capable of producing quick, forceful contractions but have a tendency to fatigue more rapidly than slow-twitch fibers. Fast-twitch fibers are useful in short-term, high-intensity activities, which mainly involve the anaerobic system. Fast-twitch fibers are capable of producing powerful contractions, whereas slow-twitch fibers produce a long endurance force. There are two subdivisions of fast-twitch fibers. Although both types of fast-twitch fibers are capable of rapid contraction, Type IIa fibers or fast-oxidative-glycolytic fibers are moderately resistant to fatigue, whereas Type IIb fibers or fast-glycolytic fibers fatigue rapidly and are considered the "true" fast-twitch fibers. Recently, a third group of fast-twitch fibers, Type IIx, has been identified in animal models. Type IIx fibers are fatigue resistant and are thought to have a maximum power capacity less than that of Type IIb but greater than that of Type IIa fibers.[45]

Ratio in Muscle

Within a particular muscle are both types of fibers, and the ratio of the two types in an individual muscle varies with each person.[32] Muscles whose primary function is to maintain posture against gravity require more endurance and have a higher percentage of slow-twitch fibers. Muscles that produce powerful, rapid, explosive strength movements tend to have a much higher percentage of fast-twitch fibers.

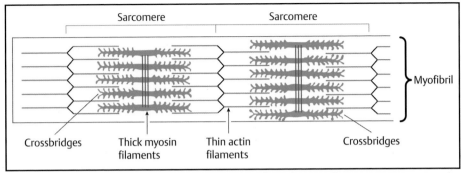

Figure 9-3. Muscles contract when an electrical impulse from the central nervous system causes the myofilaments in a muscle fiber to move closer together.

Because this ratio is genetically determined, it can play a large role in determining ability for a given sport activity. Sprinters and weightlifters, for example, have a large percentage of fast-twitch fibers in relation to slow-twitch fibers.[16] Conversely, marathon runners generally have a higher percentage of slow-twitch fibers. The question of whether fiber types can change as a result of training has to date not been conclusively resolved.[10] However, both types of fibers can improve their metabolic capabilities through specific strength and endurance training.[7]

THE PHYSIOLOGY OF STRENGTH DEVELOPTMENT

Muscle Hypertrophy

There is no question that resistance training to improve muscular strength results in an increased size, or hypertrophy, of a muscle. What causes a muscle to hypertrophy? A number of theories have been proposed to explain this increase in muscle size.[22]

First, some evidence exists that there is an increase in the number of muscle fibers (hyperplasia) as a result of fibers splitting in response to training.[39] However, this research has been conducted in animals and should not be generalized to humans. It is generally accepted that the number of fibers is genetically determined and does not seem to increase with training.

Second, it has been hypothesized that because the muscle is working harder in resistance training, more blood is required to supply that muscle with oxygen and other nutrients. Thus, it is thought that the number of capillaries is increased. This hypothesis is only partially correct: no new capillaries are formed during resistance training; however, a number of dormant capillaries might become filled with blood to meet this increased demand for blood supply.[45]

A third theory to explain this increase in muscle size seems the most credible. Muscle fibers are composed of primarily small protein filaments, called myofilaments, which are contractile elements in muscle. Myofilaments are small contractile elements of protein within the sarcomere. There are two distinct types of myofilaments: thin actin myofilaments and thicker myosin myofilaments. Fingerlike projections, or cross-bridges, connect the actin and myosin myofilaments. When a muscle is stimulated to contract, the cross-bridges pull the myofilaments closer together, thus shortening the muscle and producing movement at the joint that the muscle crosses[5] (Figure 9-3).

> **Clinical Decision-Making Exercise 9-3**
>
> A new high school track coach wants to train his best distance runner to compete in hurdling events. Based on what you know about muscle physiology, why might this be a difficult task?

As stated in Chapter 2, it is well accepted that satellite cells play a critical role in the ability of the muscle cell to hypertrophy.[54] These self-renewing cells can generate a population of myoblasts that are able to fuse with existing myofibers to help in facilitating growth.[65]

These myofilaments increase in size and number as a result of resistance training, causing the individual muscle fibers to increase in cross-sectional diameter.[58] This increase is particularly present in men, although women will also see some increase in muscle size. More research is needed to further clarify and determine the specific reasons for muscle hypertrophy.

Reversibility

If resistance training is discontinued or interrupted, the muscle will atrophy, decreasing in both strength and mass. Adaptations in skeletal muscle that occur in response to resistance training can begin to reverse in as little as 48 hours. It does appear that consistent exercise of a muscle is essential to prevent reversal of the hypertrophy that occurs from strength training.

Other Physiologic Adaptations to Resistance Exercise

In addition to muscle hypertrophy, there are a number of other physiologic adaptations to resistance training.[40] The strength of non-contractile structures, including tendons and ligaments, is increased. The mineral content of bone is increased, thus making the bone stronger and more resistant to fracture. Maximal oxygen uptake is improved when resistance training is of sufficient intensity to elicit heart rates at or above training levels. However, it must be emphasized that these increases are minimal and that if increased maximal oxygen uptake is the goal, aerobic exercise rather than resistance training is recommended. There is also an increase in several enzymes important in aerobic and anaerobic metabolism.[3,25,26] All of these adaptations contribute to strength and endurance.

Clinical Decision-Making Exercise 9-4

Two football players of the same age have been following the exact same training plan. One is consistently able to perform a hamstring curl using more weight than the other. What could possibly be making him stronger at this task?

TECHNIQUES OF RESISTANCE TRAINING

There are a number of different techniques of resistance training for strength improvement, including functional strength training, isometric exercise, progressive resistive exercise, isokinetic training, circuit training, plyometric exercise, and callisthenic exercise. Regardless of the specific strength-training technique used, the athletic trainer should integrate functional strengthening activities that involve multiplanar, eccentric, concentric, and isometric contractions.

The Overload Principle

Regardless of which of these techniques is used, one basic principle of reconditioning is extremely important. For a muscle to improve in strength, it must be forced to work at a higher level than it is accustomed to. In other words, the muscle must be overloaded. Without overload, the muscle will be able to maintain strength as long as training is continued against a resistance to which the muscle is accustomed, but no additional strength gains will be realized. This maintenance of existing levels of muscular strength may be more important in resistance programs that emphasize muscular endurance rather than strength gains. Many individuals can benefit more in terms of overall health by concentrating on improving muscular endurance. However, to most effectively build muscular strength, resistance training requires a consistent, increasing effort against progressively increasing resistance.[38,56]

Resistive exercise is based primarily on the principles of overload and progression. If these principles are applied, all of the following resistance training techniques will produce improvement of muscular strength over time.

In a rehabilitation setting, progressive overload is limited to some degree by the healing process. If the athletic trainer takes an aggressive approach to rehabilitation, the rate of progression is perhaps best determined by the injured patient's response to a specific exercise. Exacerbation of pain or increased swelling should alert the athletic trainer that the rate of progression is too aggressive.

Functional Strength Training

For many years, the strength-training techniques in conditioning or rehabilitation programs have focused on isolated, single-plane exercises used to elicit muscle hypertrophy in a specific muscle. These exercises have a very low neuromuscular demand because they are performed primarily with the rest of the body artificially stabilized on stable pieces of equipment.[15] The central nervous system controls the ability to integrate the proprioceptive function of a number of individual muscles that must act collectively to produce a specific movement pattern that occurs in three planes of motion. If the body is designed to move in three planes of motion, then isolated training does little to improve functional ability. When strength training using isolated, single-plane, artificially stabilized exercises, the entire body is not being prepared to deal with the imposed demands of normal daily activities (walking up or down stairs, getting groceries out of the trunk, etc).[26] Functional strength training provides a unique approach that may revolutionize the way the sports medicine community thinks about strength training. To understand the approach to functional strength training, the athletic trainer must understand the concept of the kinetic chain and must realize that the entire kinetic chain is an integrated functional unit. The kinetic chain is composed of not only muscle, tendons, fasciae, and ligaments but also the articular system and the neural system.

All of these systems function simultaneously as an integrated unit to allow for structural and functional efficiency. If any system within the kinetic chain is not working efficiently, the other systems are forced to adapt and compensate; this can lead to tissue overload, decreased performance, and predictable patterns of injury. The functional integration of the systems allows for optimal neuromuscular efficiency during functional activities.[15] During functional movements, some muscles contract concentrically (shorten) to produce movement, others contract eccentrically (lengthen) to allow movement to occur, and still other muscles contract isometrically to create a stable base on which the functional movement occurs. These functional movements occur in three planes. Functional strength training uses integrated exercises designed to improve functional movement patterns in terms of not only increased strength and improved neuromuscular control but also high levels of stabilization strength and dynamic flexibility.[15]

Unlike traditional strength-training techniques, which use barbells, dumbbells, or exercise machines and single-plane exercises day after day, a primary principle of functional strength training is to make use of training variations to force constant neural adaptations instead of concentrating solely on morphologic changes. Exercise variables that can be changed include the plane of motion, body position, base of support, upper- or lower-extremity symmetry, the type of balance modality, and the type of external resistance.[15] Table 9-1 lists these exercise training variables. Figure 9-4 provides examples of functional strengthening exercises.

Isometric Exercise

An isometric exercise involves a muscle contraction in which the length of the muscle remains constant while tension develops toward a maximal force against an immovable resistance[6] (Figure 9-5). An isometric contraction provides stabilization strength that helps maintain normal length–tension and force–couple relationships that are critical for normal joint arthrokinematics. Isometric exercises are capable of increasing muscular strength. However, strength gains are relatively specific, with as much as a 20% overflow to the joint

Table 9-1 Exercise Training Variables

Plane of Motion	Body Position	Base of Support	Upper-Extremity Symmetry	Lower-Extremity Symmetry	Balance Modality	External Resistance
Sagittal	Supine	Exercise bench	2 arms	2 legs	Floor	Barbell
Frontal	Prone	Stability ball	Alternate arms	Staggered stance	Sport beam	Dumbbell
Transverse	Sidelying	Balance modality	1 arm	1 leg	½ foam roll	Cable machines
Combination	Sitting	Other	1 arm w/ rotation	2-leg unstable	Airex pad	Tubing
	Kneeling			Staggered stance unstable	Dyna disc	Medicine balls
	Half kneeling			1-leg unstable	Bosu	Power balls
	Standing				Proprio shoes	Bodyblade
					Sand	Other

angle at which training is performed. At other angles, the strength curve drops off, dramatically because of a lack of motor activity at that angle. Thus, strength is increased at the specific angle of exertion, but there is no corresponding increase in strength at other positions in the range of motion (ROM).

Another major disadvantage of these isometric exercises is that they tend to produce a spike in systolic blood pressure that can result in potentially life-threatening cardiovascular accidents.[29] This sharp increase in systolic blood pressure results from a Valsalva maneuver, which increases intrathoracic pressure. To avoid or minimize this effect, it is recommended that breathing be done during the maximal contraction to prevent this increase in pressure.

The use of isometric exercises in injury rehabilitation or reconditioning is widely practiced. There are a number of conditions or ailments resulting from trauma or overuse that must be treated with strengthening exercises. Unfortunately, these problems can be exacerbated with full ROM resistance exercises. It might be more desirable to make use of positional or functional isometric exercises that involve the application of isometric

force at multiple angles throughout the ROM. Functional isometrics should be used until the healing process has progressed to the point that full-range activities can be performed.

During rehabilitation, it is often recommended that a muscle be contracted isometrically for 10 seconds at a time at a frequency of 10 or more contractions per hour. Isometric exercises can also offer significant benefit in a strengthening program.[64]

There are certain instances in which an isometric contraction can greatly enhance a particular movement. For example, one of the exercises in power weight lifting is a squat. A squat is an exercise in which the weight is supported on the shoulders in a standing position. The knees are then flexed, and the weight is lowered to a three-quarter squat position, from which the lifter must stand completely straight once again.

It is not uncommon for there to be one particular angle in the ROM at which smooth movement is difficult because of insufficient strength. This joint angle is referred to as a sticking point. A power lifter will typically use an isometric contraction against some immovable resistance to increase strength at this

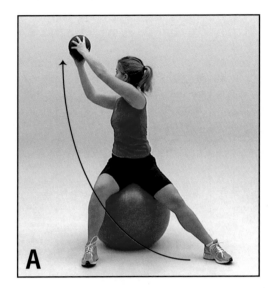

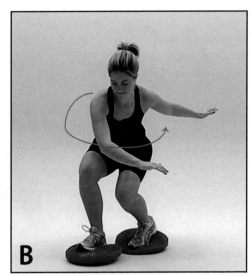

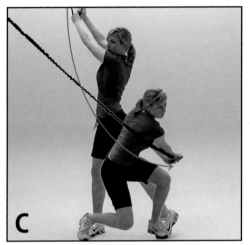

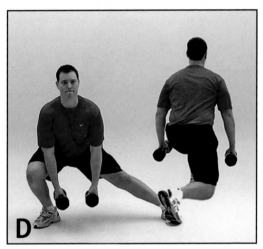

Figure 9-4. Functional strengthening exercises use simultaneous movements (concentric, eccentric, and isometric contractions) in 3 planes on either stable or unstable surfaces. (A) Stability ball diagonal rotations with weighted ball; (B) tandem stance on DynaDisc with trunk rotation; (C) standing diagonal rotations with cable or tubing resistance; (D) weight-resisted multiplanar lunges *(continued)*

sticking point. If strength can be improved at this joint angle, then a smooth, coordinated power lift can be performed through a full range of movement.

Clinical Decision-Making Exercise 9-5

A weight lifter has been progressing his maximum bench press weight. However, he still requires a spotter to get him through the full ROM. He gets "stuck" at about 90 degrees of elbow extension. What can he do to progress through this limitation?

Progressive Resistive Exercise

A second technique of resistance training is perhaps the most commonly used and most popular technique for improving muscular strength in a rehabilitation program. Progressive resistive exercise uses exercises that strengthen muscles through a contraction that overcomes some fixed resistance such as with dumbbells, barbells, various exercise machines, or resistive elastic tubing. Progressive resistive exercise uses isotonic, or isodynamic,

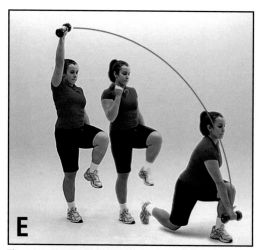
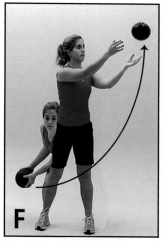

Figure 9-4. (*continued*) (E) Front lunge balance to one-arm press; (F) weighted-ball double arm rotation toss from squat.

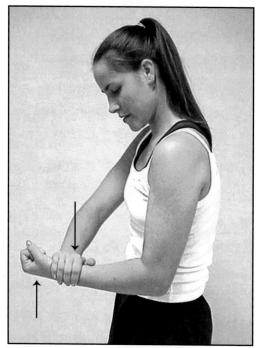

Figure 9-5. Isometric exercises involve contraction against some immovable resistance.

contractions in which force is generated while the muscle is changing in length.

Concentric vs Eccentric Contractions

Isotonic contractions can be concentric or eccentric. In performing a bicep curl, to lift the weight from the starting position the biceps muscle must contract and shorten in length. This shortening contraction is referred to as a concentric or positive contraction. If the biceps muscle does not remain contracted when the weight is being lowered, gravity would cause this weight to simply fall back to the starting position. Thus, to control the weight as it is being lowered, the biceps muscle must continue to contract while at the same time gradually lengthening. A contraction in which the muscle is lengthening while still applying force is called an eccentric or negative contraction.

It is possible to generate greater amounts of force against resistance with an eccentric contraction than with a concentric contraction, because eccentric contractions require a much lower level of motor unit activity to achieve a certain force than do concentric contractions. Because fewer motor units are firing to produce a specific force, additional motor units can be recruited to generate increased force. In addition, oxygen use is much lower during eccentric exercise than in comparable concentric exercise. Thus, eccentric contractions are less resistant to fatigue than concentric contractions. The mechanical efficiency of eccentric exercise can be several times higher than that of concentric exercise.[56]

Traditionally, progressive resistive exercise has concentrated primarily on the concentric component without paying much attention to the importance of the eccentric component.[56] The use of eccentric contractions, particularly in rehabilitation of various sport-related injuries, has received considerable emphasis in recent years. Eccentric contractions are

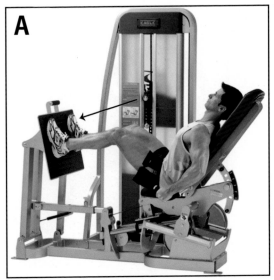
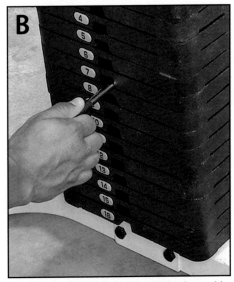

Figure 9-6. Isotonic equipment. (A) Most exercise machines are isotonic. (B) Resistance can be easily changed by changing the key in the stack of weights. (Reprinted with permission from Cybex International.)

critical for deceleration of limb motion, especially during high-velocity dynamic activities.[35] For example, a baseball pitcher relies on an eccentric contraction of the external rotators of the glenohumeral joint to decelerate the humerus, which might be internally rotating at speeds as high as 8000 degrees per second. Certainly, strength deficits or an inability of a muscle to tolerate these eccentric forces can predispose an injury. Thus, in a rehabilitation program, the athletic trainer should incorporate eccentric strengthening exercises. Eccentric contractions are possible with all free weights, with the majority of isotonic exercise machines, and with most isokinetic devices. Eccentric contractions are used with plyometric exercise discussed in Chapter 11 and can also be incorporated with functional proprioceptive neuromuscular facilitation (PNF) strengthening patterns discussed in Chapter 14.

In progressive resistive exercise, it is essential to incorporate both concentric and eccentric contractions.[33] Research has clearly demonstrated that the muscle should be overloaded and fatigued both concentrically and eccentrically for the greatest strength improvement to occur.[4,22,45] When training specifically for the development of muscular strength, the concentric portion of the exercise should require 1 to 2 seconds, whereas the eccentric portion of the lift should require 2 to 4 seconds. The ratio of the concentric component to the eccentric component should be about 1 to 2. Physiologically, the muscle will fatigue much more rapidly concentrically than eccentrically.

Free Weights vs Exercise Machines

Various types of exercise equipment can be used with progressive resistive exercise, including free weights (barbells and dumbbells) and exercise machines such as Cybex, Universal, Paramount, Tough Stuff, Icarian Fitness, King Fitness, Body Solid, Pro-Elite, Life Fitness, Nautilus, BodyCraft, Yukon, Flex, CamBar, GymPros, Nugym, BodyWorks, DP, Soloflex, and Body Master (Figure 9-6). Dumbbells and barbells require the use of iron plates of varying weights that can be easily changed by adding or subtracting equal amounts of weight to both sides of the bar. The exercise machines for the most part have stacks of weights that are lifted through a series of levers or pulleys. The stack of weights slides up and down on a pair of bars that restrict the movement to only one plane. Weight can be increased or decreased simply by changing the position of a weight key.

There are advantages and disadvantages to free weights and machines. The exercise machines are relatively safe to use in comparison with free weights. For example, a bench press with free weights requires a partner to help lift the weight back onto the support racks

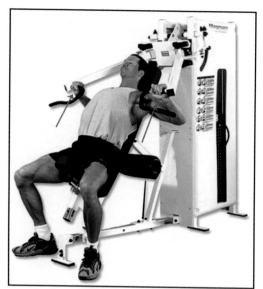

Figure 9-7. Bench press exercise machine with a stack of weights. (Printed with permission from Johnson Health Tech Co. Ltd.)

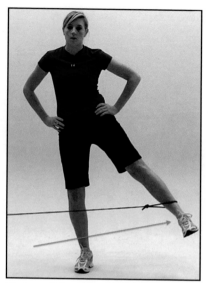

Figure 9-8. Strengthening exercises using surgical tubing are widely used in rehabilitation.

if the lifter does not have enough strength to complete the lift; otherwise the weight might be dropped on the chest. With the machines the weight can be easily and safely dropped without fear of injury (Figure 9-7).

It is also a simple process to increase or decrease the weight by moving a single weight key with the exercise machines, although changes can generally be made only in increments of 10 or 15 pounds. With free weights, iron plates must be added or removed from each side of the barbell.

The biggest disadvantage in using exercise machines is that with few exceptions the design constraints of the machine allow only single-plane motion, limiting or controlling more functional movements that occur in multiple planes simultaneously.

Anyone who has strength-trained using free weights and exercise machines realizes the difference in the amount of weight that can be lifted. Unlike the machines, free weights have no restricted motion and can thus move in many different directions, depending on the forces applied. With free weights, an element of neuromuscular control on the part of the lifter to stabilize the weight and prevent it from

moving in any other direction than vertical will usually decrease the amount of weight that can be lifted.[66]

Surgical Tubing or Thera-Band

Surgical tubing or Thera-Band, as a means of providing resistance, has been widely used in rehabilitation (Figure 9-8). The advantage of exercising with surgical tubing or Thera-Band is that movement can occur in multiple planes simultaneously. Thus, exercise can be done against resistance in more functional movement planes. Chapters 11 and 14 discuss the use of surgical tubing exercise in plyometrics and PNF strengthening techniques. Surgical tubing can be used to provide resistance with the majority of the strengthening exercises shown in Chapters 17 to 24.

Regardless of which type of equipment is used, the same principles of progressive resistive exercise may be applied.

Clinical Decision-Making Exercise 9-6

The head athletic trainer wants to buy new equipment for the weight room. What are the advantages and disadvantages to investing in exercise machines rather than free weights?

Variable Resistance

One problem often mentioned in relation to progressive resistive exercise reconditioning is that the amount of force necessary to move a weight through ROM changes according to the angle of pull of the contracting muscle. It is greatest when the angle of pull is about 90 degrees. In addition, once the inertia of the weight has been overcome and momentum has been established, the force required to move the resistance varies according to the force the muscle can produce through the ROM. Thus, it has been argued that a disadvantage of any type of isotonic exercise is that the force required to move the resistance is constantly changing throughout the range of movement. This change in resistance at different points in the ROM has been labeled accommodating resistance or variable resistance.

A number of exercise machine manufacturers have attempted to alleviate this problem of changing force capabilities by using a cam in the machine's pulley system. The cam is individually designed for each piece of equipment so that the resistance is variable throughout the movement. The cam is intended to alter resistance so that the muscle can handle a greater load, but at the points where the joint angle or muscle length is mechanically disadvantageous, it reduces the resistance to muscle movement. Whether this design does what it claims is debatable.

Progressive Resistive Exercise Techniques

Perhaps the single most confusing aspect of progressive resistive exercise is the terminology used to describe specific programs.[32] The following list of terms with their operational definitions may help clarify the confusion:

- Repetitions: The number of times a specific movement is repeated

- Repetition maximum (RM): The maximum number of repetitions at a given weight

- Set: A particular number of repetitions

- Intensity: The amount of weight or resistance lifted

- Recovery period: The rest interval between sets

- Frequency: The number of times an exercise is done in 1 week's period

Recommended Techniques of Resistance Training

Specific recommendations for techniques of improving muscular strength are controversial among therapists. A considerable amount of research has been done in the area of resistance training relative to (a) the amount of weight to be used; (b) the number of repetitions; (c) the number of sets; and (d) the frequency of training.

A variety of specific programs have been proposed that recommend the optimal amount of weight, number of sets, number of repetitions, and frequency for producing maximal gains in levels of muscular strength. However, regardless of the techniques used, the healing process must dictate the specifics of any strength-training program. Certainly, to improve strength, the muscle must be progressively overloaded. The amount of weight used and the number of repetitions must be sufficient to make the muscle work at higher intensity than it is accustomed to. This factor is the most critical in any resistance training program. The resistance training program must also be designed to ultimately meet the specific competitive needs of the patient.

Resistance training programs were initially designed by power lifters and bodybuilders. Programs or routines commonly used in training and conditioning include the following:

- Single set: One set of 8 to 12 repetitions of a particular exercise performed at a slow speed.

- Tri-sets: A group of 3 exercises for the same muscle group performed using 2 to 4 sets of each exercise with no rest between sets.

- Multiple sets: Two or 3 warm-up sets with progressively increasing resistance followed by several sets at the same resistance.

- Supersets: Either 1 set of 8 to 10 repetitions of several exercises for the same muscle group performed one after another, or several sets of 8 to 10 repetitions of 2 exercises for the same muscle group with no rest between sets.

- Pyramids: One set of 8 to 12 repetitions with light resistance, then an increase in resistance over 4 to 6 sets until only 1 or 2 repetitions can be performed. The pyramid can also be reversed going from heavy to light resistance.

- Split routine: Workouts exercise different muscle groups on successive days. For example, Monday, Wednesday, and Friday might be used for upper-body muscles, and Tuesday, Thursday, and Saturday for lower-body muscles.

- Circuit training: This technique may be useful to the therapist for maintaining or perhaps improving levels of muscular strength or endurance in other parts of the body while the patient allows for healing and reconditioning of an injured body part. Circuit training uses a series of exercise stations, each of which involves weight training, flexibility, calisthenics, or brief aerobic exercises. Circuits can be designed to accomplish many different training goals. With circuit training the patient moves rapidly from one station to the next, performing whatever exercise is to be done at that station within a specified time period. A typical circuit would consist of 8 to 12 stations, and the entire circuit would be repeated three times.

Circuit training is most definitely an effective technique for improving strength and flexibility. Certainly, if the pace or time interval between stations is rapid and if workload is maintained at a high level of intensity with heart rates at or above target training levels, the cardiorespiratory system may benefit from this circuit. However, there is little research evidence that circuit training is very effective in improving cardiorespiratory endurance. It should be, and is most often, used as a technique for developing and improving muscular strength and endurance.[27]

Techniques of Resistance Training Used in Rehabilitation

One of the first widely accepted strength-development programs to be used in a

Table 9-2 The DeLorme Program

Set	Amount of Weight	Repetitions
1	50% of 10 RM	10
2	75% of 10 RM	10
3	100% of 10 RM	10

Table 9-3 The Oxford Technique

Set	Amount of Weight	Repetitions
1	100% of 10 RM	10
2	75% of 10 RM	10
3	50% of 10 RM	10

rehabilitation program was developed by DeLorme and was based on a repetition maximum (RM) of 10.[18] The amount of weight used is what can be lifted exactly 10 times (Table 9-2).

Zinovieff proposed the Oxford technique, which, like the DeLorme program, was designed to be used in beginning, intermediate, and advanced levels of rehabilitation.[68] The only difference is that the percentage of maximum was reversed in the three sets (Table 9-3). The McQueen technique[48] differentiates between beginning to intermediate and advanced levels, as in shown in Table 9-4.

The Sanders program (Table 9-5) was designed to be used in the advanced stages of rehabilitation and was based on a formula that used a percentage of body weight to determine starting weights.[56] The following percentages represent median starting points for different exercises:

- Barbell squat—45% of body weight
- Barbell bench press—30% of body weight
- Leg extension—20% of body weight
- Universal bench press—30% of body weight
- Universal leg extension—20% of body weight
- Universal leg curl—10% to 15% of body weight

Table 9-4 The McQueen Technique

Set	Amount of Weight	Repetitions
3 (Beginning/ intermediate)	100% of 10 RM	10
4 to 5 (Advanced)	100% of 2 to 3 RM	2 to 3

Table 9-5 The Sanders Program

Sets	Amount of Weight	Repetitions
Total of 4 sets (3 times per week)	100% of 5 RM	5
Day 1, 4 sets	100% of 5 RM	5
Day 2, 4 sets	100% of 3 RM	5
Day 3, 1 set	100% of 5 RM	5
2 sets	100% of 3 RM	5
2 sets	100% of 2 RM	5

Table 9-6 Knight's DAPRE Program

Sets	Amount of Weight	Repetitions
1	50% of RM	10
2	75% of RM	6
3	100% of RM	Maximum
4	Adjusted working weight[a]	Maximum

[a]See Table 9-7.

- Universal leg press—50% of body weight
- Upright rowing—20% of body weight

Table 9-7 DAPRE Adjusted Working Weight

Number of Repetitions Performed During Third Set	Adjusted Working Weight During Fourth Set	Next Exercise Session
0 to 2	−5 to 10 lb	−5 to 10 lb
3 to 4	−0 to 5 lb	Same weight
5 to 6	Same weight	±0 to 10 lb
7 to 10	±5 to 10 lb	±5 to 15 lb
11	±10 to 15 lb	±10 to 20 lb

Table 9-8 The Berger Adjustment Technique

Sets	Amount of Weight	Repetitions
3	100% of 10 RM	6 to 8

Knight applied the concept of progressive resistive exercise in rehabilitation. His Daily Adjusted Progressive Resistive Exercise (DAPRE) program (Tables 9-6 and 9-7) allows for individual differences in the rates at which patients progress in their rehabilitation programs.[37]

Berger proposed a technique that is adjustable within individual limitations (Table 9-8). For any given exercise, the amount of weight selected should be sufficient to allow six to eight RM in each of the three sets, with a recovery period of 60 to 90 seconds between sets. Initial selection of a starting weight might require some trial and error to achieve this six to eight RM range. If at least three sets of six RM cannot be completed, the weight is too heavy and should be reduced. If it is possible to do more than three sets of eight RM, the weight is too light and should be increased.[8] Progression to heavier weights is then determined by the ability to perform at least eight RM in each of three sets. When progressing weight, an increase of about 10% of the current weight being lifted

Figure 9-9. The Biodex is an isokinetic device that provides resistance at a constant velocity. (Reproduced with permission from Biodex.)

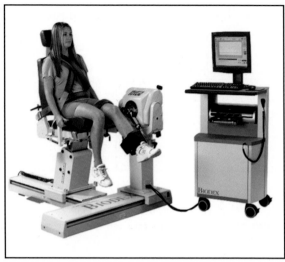

should still allow at least six RM in each of three sets.[9]

For rehabilitation purposes, strengthening exercises should be performed on a daily basis initially, with the amount of weight, number of sets, and number of repetitions governed by the injured patient's response to the exercise. As the healing process progresses and pain or swelling is no longer an issue, a particular muscle or muscle group should be exercised consistently every other day. At that point, the frequency of weight training should be at least three times per week but no more than four times per week. It is common for serious weightlifters to lift every day; however, they exercise different muscle groups on successive days.

It has been suggested that if training is done properly, using both concentric and eccentric contractions, resistance training is necessary only twice each week. However, this schedule has not been sufficiently documented.

Isokinetic Exercise

An isokinetic exercise involves a muscle contraction in which the length of the muscle is changing while the contraction is performed at a constant velocity.[11] In theory, maximal resistance is provided throughout the ROM by the machine. The resistance provided by the machine will move only at some preset speed, regardless of the torque applied to it by the individual. Thus, the key to isokinetic exercise is not the resistance but the speed at which resistance can be moved.

Few isokinetic devices are still available commercially (Figure 9-9). In general, they rely on hydraulic, pneumatic, and mechanical pressure systems to produce this constant velocity of motion. Most isokinetic devices are capable of resisting concentric and eccentric contractions at a fixed speed to exercise a muscle.

Isokinetics as a Conditioning Tool

Isokinetic devices are designed so that regardless of the amount of force applied against a resistance, it can only be moved at a certain speed. That speed will be the same whether maximal force or only half the maximal force is applied. Consequently, in isokinetic training, it is absolutely necessary to exert as much force against the resistance as possible (maximal effort) for maximal strength gains to occur.[11] Maximal effort is one of the major problems with an isokinetic strength-training program.

Anyone who has been involved in a resistance training program knows that on some days it is difficult to find the motivation to work out. Because isokinetic training requires a maximal effort, it is very easy to "cheat" and not go through the workout at a high level of intensity. In a progressive resistive exercise program, the patient knows how much weight has to be lifted for how many repetitions. Thus, isokinetic training is often more effective if a partner system is used, primarily as a means of motivation toward a maximal effort.

When isokinetic training is done properly with a maximal effort, it is theoretically possible that maximal strength gains are best achieved through the isokinetic training method in which the velocity and force of the resistance are equal throughout the ROM. However, there is no conclusive research to support this theory.

Whether this changing force capability is a deterrent to improving the ability to generate force against some resistance is debatable. In real life, it does not matter whether the resistance is changing; what is important is that an individual develops enough strength to move objects from one place to another.

Another major disadvantage of using isokinetic devices as a conditioning tool is their cost. With initial purchase costs ranging between $50,000 and $80,000 and the necessity of regular maintenance and software upgrades, the use of an isokinetic device for general conditioning or resistance training is, for the most part, unrealistic. Thus, isokinetic exercises are primarily used as a diagnostic and rehabilitative tool.

Isokinetics in Rehabilitation

Isokinetic strength testing gained a great deal of popularity throughout the 1980s in rehabilitation settings. This trend stems from its providing an objective means of quantifying existing levels of muscular strength and thus becoming useful as a diagnostic tool.[49]

Because the capability exists for training at specific speeds, comparisons have been made regarding the relative advantages of training at fast or slow speeds in a rehabilitation program. The research literature seems to indicate that strength increases from slow-speed training are relatively specific to the velocity used in training. Conversely, training at faster speeds seems to produce a more generalized increase in torque values at all velocities. Minimal hypertrophy was observed only while training at fast speeds, affecting only Type II or fast-twitch fibers.[17,52] An increase in neuromuscular efficiency caused by more effective motor unit firing patterns has been demonstrated with slow speed training.[45]

During the early 1990s, the value of isokinetic devices for quantifying torque values at functional speeds was questioned.

Plyometric Exercise

Plyometric exercise has also been referred to in the literature as reactive neuromuscular training. It is a technique that is being increasingly incorporated into later stages of the rehabilitation program by athletic trainers. Plyometric training includes specific exercises that encompass a rapid stretch of a muscle eccentrically, followed immediately by a rapid concentric contraction of that muscle to facilitate and develop a forceful explosive movement over a short time.[13,20] The greater the stretch put on the muscle from its resting length immediately before the concentric contraction, the greater the resistance the muscle can overcome. Plyometrics emphasize the speed of the eccentric phase. The rate of stretch is more critical than the magnitude of the stretch. An advantage to using plyometric exercises is that they can help to develop eccentric control in dynamic movements.[43]

Plyometric exercises involve hops, bounds, and depth jumping for the lower extremity and the use of medicine balls and other types of weighted equipment for the upper extremity.[12,14] Depth jumping is an example of a plyometric exercise in which an individual jumps to the ground from a specified height and then quickly jumps again as soon as ground contact is made[53] (Figure 9-10).

Plyometrics tend to place a great deal of stress on the musculoskeletal system. The learning and perfection of specific jumping skills and other plyometric exercises must be technically correct and specific to one's age, activity, physical, and skill development. Chapter 10 discusses plyometric exercise in detail.

Callisthenic Strengthening Exercises

Calisthenics, or free exercise, is one of the more easily available means of developing strength. Isotonic movement exercises can be graded according to intensity by using gravity as an aid, by ruling gravity out, by moving against gravity, or by using the body or a body part as a resistance against gravity. Most calisthenics require the individual to support the body or move the total body against the force

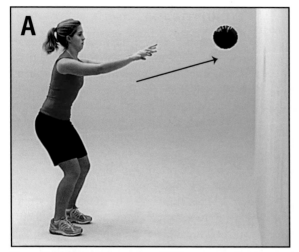
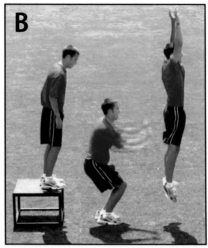

Figure 9-10. Plyometric exercises. (A) Upper extremity plyometric exercise using a medicine ball; (B) depth jumping lower extremity plyometric exercise.

Figure 9-11. Callisthenic exercises use body weight as resistance. (A) Push-ups; (B) sit-ups.

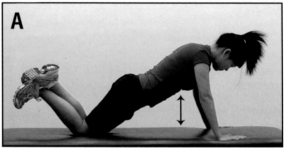
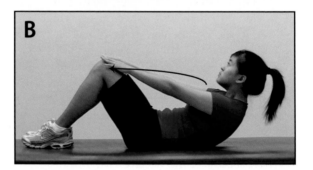

of gravity. Push-ups are a good example of a vigorous antigravity exercise (Figure 9-11A). Callisthenic-like exercises are used in functional strength training, which was discussed previously. To be considered maximally effective, the isotonic callisthenic exercise, like all types of exercise, must be performed in an exacting manner and in full ROM. In most cases, 10 or more repetitions are performed for each exercise and are repeated in sets of two or three. Some free exercises use an isometric, or holding, phase instead of a full ROM. Examples of these exercises are back extensions and sit-ups (Figure 9-11B). When the exercise produces maximum muscle tension, it is held between 6 and 10 seconds and then repeated one to three times.

CORE STABILIZATION STRENGTHENING

A dynamic core stabilization training program should be a fundamental component of all comprehensive strengthening as well as injury rehabilitation programs.[34,36] The core is defined as the lumbo–pelvic–hip complex. The core is where the center of gravity is located and where all movement begins. There are 29 muscles that have their attachment to the lumbo–pelvic–hip complex.

A core stabilization strengthening program can help to improve dynamic postural control; ensure appropriate muscular balance and joint movement around the lumbo–pelvic–hip complex; allow for the expression of dynamic functional strength; and improve neuromuscular efficiency throughout the entire body. Collectively, these factors contribute to optimal acceleration, deceleration, and dynamic stabilization of the entire kinetic chain during functional movements. Core stabilization also provides proximal stability for efficient lower-extremity movements. Greater neuromuscular control and stabilization strength will offer a more biomechanically efficient position for the entire kinetic chain, therefore allowing optimal neuromuscular efficiency throughout the kinetic chain. This approach facilitates a balanced muscular functioning of the entire kinetic chain.[15]

Many patients develop the functional strength, power, neuromuscular control, and muscular endurance in specific muscles to perform functional activities. However, relatively few patients have developed the muscles required for stabilization. The body's stabilization system has to be functioning optimally to effectively use the strength, power, neuromuscular control, and muscular endurance that they have developed in their prime movers. If the extremity muscles are strong and the core is weak, then there will not be enough force created to produce efficient movements. A weak core is a fundamental problem of inefficient movements that leads to injury.[15] Chapter 5 discusses core stabilization techniques in detail.

OPEN VS CLOSED KINETIC CHAIN EXERCISES

The concept of the kinetic chain deals with the anatomical functional relationships that exist in the upper and lower extremities. In a weight-bearing position, the lower extremity kinetic chain involves the transmission of forces among the foot, ankle, lower leg, knee, thigh, and hip. In the upper extremity, when the hand is in contact with a weight-bearing surface, forces are transmitted to the wrist, forearm, elbow, upper arm, and shoulder girdle.

An open kinetic chain exists when the foot or hand is not in contact with the ground or some other surface. In a closed kinetic chain, the foot or hand is weight bearing. Movements of the more proximal anatomical segments are affected by these open vs closed kinetic chain positions. For example, the rotational components of the ankle, knee, and hip reverse direction when changing from open to closed kinetic chain activity. In a closed kinetic chain, the forces begin at the ground and work their way up through each joint. Also, in a closed kinetic chain, forces must be absorbed by various tissues and anatomical structures, rather than simply dissipating as would occur in an open chain.

In rehabilitation, the use of closed chain strengthening techniques has become a treatment of choice for many athletic trainers. Most functional activities involve some aspect of weight bearing with the foot in contact with the ground or the hand in a weight-bearing position, so closed kinetic chain strengthening activities are more functional than open chain activities.

Consequently, rehabilitative exercises should be incorporated that emphasize strengthening of the entire kinetic chain rather than an isolated body segment. Chapter 12 discusses closed kinetic chain activities in detail.

TRAINING FOR MUSCULAR STRENGTH VS MUSCULAR ENDURANCE

Muscular endurance was defined as the ability to perform repeated muscle contractions against resistance for an extended period of time. Most resistance-training experts believe that muscular strength and muscular endurance are closely related.[21,50,57] As one improves, there is a tendency for the other to also improve.

It is generally accepted that when resistance training for strength, heavier weights with a lower number of repetitions should be used. Conversely, endurance training uses relatively lighter weights with a greater number of repetitions.

It has been suggested that endurance training should consist of three sets of 10 to 15 repetitions, nine using the same criteria for weight-selection progression and frequency as recommended for progressive resistive exercise. Thus, suggested training regimens for muscular strength and endurance are similar in terms of sets and numbers of repetitions.[55] Persons who possess great levels of strength tend to also exhibit greater muscular endurance when asked to perform repeated contractions against resistance.[48]

RESISTANCE TRAINING DIFFERENCES BETWEEN MALES AND FEMALES

The approach to strength training is no different for females than for males. However, some obvious physiologic differences exist between the sexes.

The average female will not build significant muscle bulk through resistance training. Significant muscle hypertrophy is dependent on the presence of the steroidal hormone testosterone. Testosterone is considered a male hormone, although all females possess some level of testosterone in their systems. Women with higher testosterone levels tend to have more masculine characteristics, such as increased facial and body hair, a deeper voice, and the potential to develop a little more muscle bulk.[23,50] For the average female, developing large, bulky muscles through strength training is unlikely, although muscle tone can be improved. Muscle tone basically refers to the firmness of tension of the muscle during a resting state.

The initial stages of a resistance training program are likely to rapidly produce dramatic increases in levels of strength.[1] For a muscle to contract, an impulse must be transmitted from the nervous system to the muscle. Each muscle fiber is innervated by a specific motor unit. By overloading a particular muscle, as in weight training, the muscle is forced to work more efficiently. Efficiency is achieved by getting more motor units to fire, thus causing more muscle fibers to contract, which results in a stronger contraction of the muscle. Consequently, both women and men often see extremely rapid gains in strength when a weight-training program is first begun.[28]

In females, these initial strength gains, which can be attributed to improved neuromuscular efficiency, tend to plateau, and minimal improvement in muscular strength is realized during a continuing resistance training program. These initial neuromuscular strength gains are also seen in males, although their strength continues to increase with appropriate training.[1] Again, females who possess higher testosterone levels have the potential to increase their strength further because they are able to develop greater muscle bulk.

Differences in strength levels between males and females are best illustrated when strength is expressed in relation to body weight minus fat. The reduced strength-to-bodyweight ratio in women is the result of their percentage of body fat. The strength-to-bodyweight ratio can be significantly improved through resistance training by decreasing the body fat percentage while increasing lean weight.[45]

The absolute strength differences are considerably reduced when body size and composition are considered. Leg strength can actually be stronger in females than in males, although upper extremity strength is much greater in males.[45]

RESISTANCE TRAINING IN THE ADOLESCENT

The principles of resistance training discussed previously may be applied to adolescents. There are certainly a number of sociologic questions regarding the advantages and disadvantages of younger, in particular prepubescent, individuals engaging in rigorous strength training programs. From a physiologic perspective, experts have for years debated the value of strength training in adolescents. Recently, a number of studies have indicated that if properly supervised, adolescents can improve strength, power, endurance, balance, and proprioception; develop a positive body image; improve sport performance; and prevent injuries.[41] A prepubescent child can experience gains in levels of muscle strength without muscle hypertrophy.[51]

An athletic trainer supervising a rehabilitation program for an injured adolescent should certainly incorporate resistive exercise into the program. However, close supervision, proper instruction, and appropriate modification of progression and intensity based on the extent of physical maturation of the individual is critical to the effectiveness of the resistive exercises.[41]

SPECIFIC RESISTIVE EXERCISES USED IN REHABILITATION

Because muscle contractions results in joint movement, the goal of resistance training in a rehabilitation program should be either to regain and perhaps increase the strength of a specific muscle that has been injured or to increase the efficiency of movement about a given joint.[45]

The exercises included throughout Chapters 17 to 24 show exercises for all motions about a particular joint rather than for each specific muscle. These exercises are demonstrated using free weights (dumbbells or bar weights) and some exercise machines. Other strengthening techniques widely used for injury rehabilitation involving isokinetic exercise, plyometrics, core stability training, closed kinetic chain exercises, and PNF strengthening techniques are discussed in greater detail in subsequent chapters.

Summary

1. Muscular strength may be defined as the maximal force that can be generated against resistance by a muscle during a single maximal contraction.

2. Muscular endurance is the ability to perform repeated isotonic or isokinetic muscle contractions or to sustain an isometric contraction without undue fatigue.

3. Muscular endurance tends to improve with muscular strength, thus training techniques for these two components are similar.

4. Muscular strength and endurance are essential components of any rehabilitation program.

5. Muscular power involves the speed with which a forceful muscle contraction is performed.

6. The ability to generate force is dependent on the physical properties of the muscle, neuromuscular efficiency, as well as the mechanical factors that dictate how much force can be generated through the lever system to an external object.

7. Hypertrophy of a muscle is caused by increases in the size and perhaps the number of actin and myosin protein myofilaments, which result in an increased cross-sectional diameter of the muscle.

8. The key to improving strength through resistance training is using the principle of overload within the constraints of the healing process.

9. Five resistance training techniques that can improve muscular strength are isometric exercise, progressive resistive exercise, isokinetic training, circuit training, and plyometric training.

10. Improvements in strength with isometric exercise occur at specific joint angles.

11. Progressive resistive exercise is the most common strengthening technique used by the athletic trainer for rehabilitation after injury.

12. Circuit training involves a series of exercise stations consisting of resistance training, flexibility, and callisthenic exercises that can be designed to maintain fitness while reconditioning an injured body part.

13. Isokinetic training provides resistance to a muscle at a fixed speed.

14. Plyometric exercise uses a quick eccentric stretch to facilitate a concentric contraction.

15. Closed kinetic chain exercises might provide a more functional technique for strengthening of injured muscles and joints in the athletic population.

16. Females can significantly increase their strength levels but generally will not build muscle bulk as a result of strength training because of their relative lack of the hormone testosterone.

References

1. Akima H, Takahashi H, Kuno SY. Early phase adaptations of muscle use and strength to isokinetic training. *Med Sci Sports Exerc.* 1999;31(4):588-594.
2. Allerheiligen W. Speed development and plyometric training. In: Baechle T, ed. *Essentials of Strength Training.* Champaign, IL: Human Kinetics; 1994.
3. Alway SE, MacDougall JD, Sale DG, Sutton JR, McComas AJ. Functional and structural adaptations in skeletal muscle of trained athletes. *J Appl Physiol.* 1988;64:1114-1120.
4. Astrand PO, Rodahl K. *Textbook of Work Physiology: Physiological Bases of Exercise.* Champaign, IL: Human Kinetics; 2003.
5. Baechle T, ed. *Essentials of Strength Training and Conditioning.* Champaign, IL: Human Kinetics; 2008.
6. Baker D, Wilson G, Carlyon B. Generality vs specificity: a comparison of dynamic and isometric measures of strength and speed-strength. *Eur J Appl Physiol.* 1994;68:350-355.
7. Bandy W, Lovelace-Chandler V, McKitrick-Bandy B. Adaptation of skeletal muscle to resistance training. *J Orthop Sports Phys Ther.* 1990;12(6):248-255.
8. Berger R. *Conditioning for Men.* Boston: Allyn & Bacon; 1973.
9. Berger R. Effect of varied weight training programs on strength. *Res Q Exerc Sport.* 1962;33:168.
10. Booth F, Thomason D. Molecular and cellular adaptation of muscle in response to exercise: Perspectives of various models. *Physiol Rev.* 1999;71:541-585.
11. Brown LE. *Isokinetics in Human Performance.* Champaign, IL: Human Kinetics; 2000.
12. Bruce-Low S, Smith D. Explosive exercises in sports training: a critical review. *J Exerc Physiol Online.* 2007;10(1):21.
13. Chu D. *Jumping into Plyometrics.* Champaign, IL: Human Kinetics; 1998.
14. Chu D. Plyometrics in sports injury rehabilitation and training. *Athl Ther Today.* 1999;4(3):7.
15. Clark M. *Integrated Training for the New Millennium.* Calabasas, CA: National Academy of Sports Medicine; 2001.
16. Costill D, Daniels J, Evan W, Fink W, Krahenbuhl G, Saltin B. Skeletal muscle enzymes and fiber compositions in male and female track athletes. *J Appl Physiol.* 1976;40:149-154.
17. Coyle E, Feiring D, Rotkis T, et al. Specificity of power improvements through slow and fast speed isokinetic training. *J Appl Physiol.* 1981;51:1437-1442.
18. DeLorme T, Wilkins A. *Progressive Resistance Exercise.* New York: Appleton-Century-Crofts; 1951.
19. Deudsinger RH. Biomechanics in clinical practice. *Phys Ther.* 1984;64:1860-1868.
20. Duda M. Plyometrics: a legitimate form of power training. *Phys Sportsmed.* 1988;16:213.
21. Dudley GA, Fleck SJ. Strength and endurance training: are they mutually exclusive? *Sports Med.* 1987;4(2):79-85.
22. Etheridge G, Thomas T. Physiological and biomedical changes of human skeletal muscle induced by different strength training programs. *Med Sci Sports Exerc.* 1982;14:141.
23. Fahey T. *Weight Training Basics.* St. Louis, MO: McGraw-Hill; 2005.
24. Faulkner J, Green H, White T. Response and adaptation of skeletal muscle to changes in physical activity. In: Bouchard C, Shepard R, Stephens J, eds. *Physical Activity, Fitness, and Health.* Champaign, IL: Human Kinetics; 1994.
25. Fleck SJ, Kramer WJ. *Designing Resistance Training Programs.* Champaign, IL: Human Kinetics; 2004.
26. Gabriel D, Kamen G. Neural adaptation to resistive exercise: mechanisms and recommendations for training practices. *Sports Med.* 2006;26(2):133-149.
27. Gettman L. Circuit weight training: a critical review of its physiological benefits. *Phys Sportsmed.* 1981;9(1):44.
28. Gravelle BL, Blessing DL. Physiological adaptation in women concurrently training for strength and endurance. *J Strength Cond Res.* 2000;14(1):5.

29. Graves JE, Pollack M, Jones A, Colvin AB, Leggett SH. Specificity of limited range of motion variable resistance training. *Med Sci Sports Exerc.* 1989;21:84-89.

30. Hakkinen K. Neuromuscular adaptations during concurrent strength and endurance training versus strength training. *Eur J Appl Physiol.* 2002;89:42-52.

31. Harmen E. The biomechanics of resistance training. In: Baechle T, ed. *Essentials of Strength Training.* Champaign, IL: Human Kinetics; 1994.

32. Hickson R, Hidaka C, Foster C. Skeletal muscle fiber type, resistance training and strength-related performance. *Med Sci Sports Exerc.* 1994;26:593-598.

33. Horobagyi T, Katch FI. Role of concentric force in limiting improvement in muscular strength. *J Appl Physiol.* 1990;68:650-658.

34. Jones M, Trowbridge C. Four ways to a safe, effective strength training program. *Athl Ther Today.* 1998;3(2):4.

35. Kaminski TW, Wabbersen CV, Murphy RM. Concentric versus enhanced eccentric hamstring strength training: Clinical implications. *J Athl Train.* 1998;33(3):216-221.

36. King MA. Core stability: creating a foundation for functional rehabilitation. *Athl Ther Today.* 2000;5(2):6-13.

37. Knight K, Ingersoll C. Isotonic contractions may be more effective than isometric contractions in developing muscular strength. *J Sport Rehabil.* 2001;10(2):124.

38. Komi P. Endocrine responses to resistance exercises. In: *Strength and Power in Sport.* London, UK: Blackwell Scientific; 2003.

39. Kraemer W. General adaptation to resistance and endurance training programs. In: Baechle T, ed. *Essentials of Strength Training.* Champaign, IL: Human Kinetics; 1994.

40. Kraemer WJ, Ratamess N. Fundamentals of resistance training: progression and exercise prescription. *Med Sci Sports Exerc.* 2004;36(4):674-688.

41. Kraemer WJ, Fleck SJ. *Strength Training for Young Athletes.* Champaign, IL: Human Kinetics; 2004.

42. Kraemer WJ. ACSM Position stand. Progression models in resistance training for healthy adults. *Med Sci Sports Exerc.* 2002;34(2):364-380.

43. Kramer J, Morrow A, Leger A. Changes in rowing ergometer, weight lifting, vertical jump and isokinetic performance in response to standard and standard plus plyometric training programs. *Int J Sports Med.* 1993;14(8):440-454.

44. Mastropaolo J. A test of maximum power theory for strength. *Eur J Appl Physiol.* 1992;65:415-420.

45. McArdle W, Katch F, Katch V. *Exercise Physiology, Energy, Nutrition, and Human Performance.* Philadelphia, PA: Lea & Febiger; 2006.

46. McComas A. Human neuromuscular adaptations that accompany changes in activity. *Med Sci Sports Exerc.* 1994;26(12):1498-1509.

47. McGlynn GH. A reevaluation of isometric training. *J Sports Med Phys Fitness.* 1972;12:258-260.

48. McQueen I. Recent advance in the techniques of progressive resistance. *Br Med J.* 1954;11:11993.

49. Nicholas JJ. Isokinetic testing in young nonathletic able-bodied subjects. *Arch Phys Med Rehabil.* 1989;70(3):210-213.

50. Nygard CH, Luophaarui T, Suurnakki T, Ilmarinen J. Muscle strength and muscle endurance of middle-aged women and men associated to type, duration and intensity of muscular load at work. *Int Arch Occup Environ Health.* 1998;60(4):291-297.

51. Ozmun J, Mikesky A, Surburg P. Neuromuscular adaptations following prepubescent strength training. *Med Sci Sports Exerc.* 1994;26:510-514.

52. Pipes T, Wilmore J. Isokinetic vs isotonic strength training in adult men. *Med Sci Sports Exerc.* 1975;7:262-274.

53. Radcliffe JC, Farentinos RC. *High-Powered Plyometrics.* Champaign, IL: Human Kinetics; 1999.

54. Relaix F, Zammit P: Satellite cells are essential for skeletal muscle regeneration: the cell on the edge returns to center stage. *Development.* 2012:16:2845-2856.

55. Sale D, MacDougall D. Specificity in strength training: a review for the coach and athlete. *Can J Appl Sport Sci.* 1986;6:87-92.

56. Sanders M. Weight training and conditioning. In: Sanders B, ed. *Sports Physical Therapy.* Norwalk, CT: Appleton & Lange; 1997:239-250.

57. Sandler D. Speed and strength through plyometrics. In: *Sports Power.* Champaign, IL: Human Kinetics; 2005:107-144.

58. Soest A, Bobbert M. The role of muscle properties in control of explosive movements. *Biol Cybern.* 1993;69:195-204.

59. Staron RS, Karapondo DL, Kreamer WJ. Skeletal muscle and adaptations during early phase of heavy resistance training in men and women. *J Appl Physiol.* 1994;76:1247-1255.

60. Stone J. Rehabilitation—speed of movement/muscular power. *Athl Ther Today.* 1998;3(5):10.

61. Stone J. Rehabilitation—muscular endurance. *Athl Ther Today.* 1998;3(4):21.

62. Stone M, Sands W. Maximum strength and strength training—a relationship to endurance? *Strength Cond J.* 2006;28(3):44.

63. Strauss RH, ed. *Sports Medicine.* Philadelphia, PA: WB Saunders; 1991.

64. Ulmer HV, Knieriemen W, Warlo T, Zech B. Interindividual variability of isometric endurance with regard to the endurance performance limit for static work. *Biomed Biochim Acta.* 1989;48(5-6):S504-S508.

65. Wang Y, Rudnicki M. Satellite cells, the engines of muscle repair. *Nature Reviews Molecular Cell Biology.* 2012;13:127-133.

66. Weltman A, Stamford B. Strength training: free weights vs machines. *Phys Sportsmed.* 1982;10:197.

67. Yates JW. Recovery of dynamic muscular endurance. *Eur J Appl Physiol.* 1987;56(6):662.

68. Zinovieff A. Heavy resistance exercise: the Oxford technique. *Br J Physiol Med.* 1951;14:129.

SOLUTIONS TO CLINICAL DECISION-MAKING EXERCISES

9-1   She must regain strength to maximize whole-body mechanics for technique and injury prevention. She must regain endurance so that she is sure to make it through a whole game without fatiguing and risking reinjury. And she must restore power so that she can generate speed in her throwing technique.

9-2   Isometric exercise can be performed right away. While in the cast, the athlete can perform isometric muscle contractions that will stimulate blood flow and provide for some maintenance of strength. As soon as the cast is removed, she should perform active concentric and eccentric isotonic contractions until she is strong enough to perform resisted concentric and eccentric exercise with weights or surgical tubing. When planning an isotonic exercise, you should always encourage the athlete to perform the eccentric movement more slowly as it is the stronger movement and will not have a chance to fatigue before the concentric movement does. In athletics it is important to have a strong eccentric component to ensure controlled and balanced movements for good technique and injury prevention.

9-3   Individuals have a particular ratio of fast-twitch to slow-twitch muscle fibers. Those who have a higher ratio of slow-twitch to fast-twitch are better at endurance activities. Because this ratio is genetically determined, it would be surprising if someone who is good at endurance activity could also be good at sprint-type activities.

9-4   The athlete who is able to move more weight has a mechanical advantage. For example, if the tendinous insertion of the hamstrings is more distal, a longer lever arm is created and thus less force is required to move the same resistance.

9-5   Performing isometric exercise at that point will help him gain strength for that specific tension point.

9-6   Exercise machines typically are safer and more comfortable than free weights. It is easier to change the resistance, and the weight increments are small for easy progressions. Many of the machines use some type of cam for accommodating resistance. However, they are expensive and can be used only for one specific joint movement. Dumbbells or free weights are more versatile as well as cheaper. They also implement an additional aspect of training, as it requires neuromuscular control to balance the weight throughout the full ROM.

Please see videos on the accompanying website at

www.healio.com/books/sportsmedvideos

CHAPTER 10

Maintaining Cardiorespiratory Fitness During Rehabilitation

Patrick Sells, DA, CES
William E. Prentice, PhD, PT, ATC, FNATA

After completion of this chapter, the athletic trainer should be able to do the following:

- Explain the relationships between heart rate, stroke volume, cardiac output, and rate of oxygen use.

- Describe the function of the heart, blood vessels, and lungs in oxygen transport.

- Describe the oxygen transport system and the concept of maximal rate of oxygen use.

- Describe the principles of continuous and interval training and the potential of each technique for improving aerobic activity.

- Describe the difference between aerobic and anaerobic activity.

- Describe the principles of reversibility and detraining.

- Describe caloric threshold goals associated with various stages of exercise programming.

Although strength and flexibility are commonly regarded as essential components in any injury rehabilitation program, often relatively little consideration is given toward maintaining aerobic capacity and cardiorespiratory endurance. When musculoskeletal injury occurs, the patient is forced to decrease physical activity and levels of cardiorespiratory endurance may decrease rapidly. Thus, the athletic trainer must design or substitute alternative activities that allow the individual to maintain existing levels of aerobic capacity during the rehabilitation period. Furthermore, the importance of maintaining and improving functional capacity is becoming increasingly evident regardless of musculoskeletal injury. Recent research demonstrates a reduction in risk for cardiovascular disease is associated with improved levels of aerobic capacity. Sandvik et al[46] reported mortality rates according to fitness quartiles during 16 years of follow-up. The number of deaths in the least-fit portion of the study outnumbered

Prentice WE, ed.
Rehabilitation Techniques for Sports Medicine and Athletic Training (pp 267-282).
© 2015 SLACK Incorporated.

the deaths of the most fit by a margin of 61 to 11 deaths from cardiovascular causes.[46] Myers et al studied 6213 patients referred for treadmill testing and concluded that exercise capacity is a more powerful predictor of mortality among men than other established risk factors for cardiovascular disease.[41]

By definition, cardiorespiratory endurance is the ability to perform whole-body activities for extended periods without undue fatigue.[11,16] The cardiorespiratory system provides a means by which oxygen is supplied to the various tissues of the body. Without oxygen, the cells within the human body cannot possibly function and ultimately cell death will occur. Thus, the cardiorespiratory system is the basic life-support system of the body.[2,11]

TRAINING EFFECTS ON THE CARDIORESPIRATORY SYSTEM

Basically, transport of oxygen throughout the body involves the coordinated function of four components: heart, blood vessels, blood, and lungs. The improvement of cardiorespiratory endurance through training occurs because of increased capability of each of these four elements in providing necessary oxygen to the working tissues.[56] A basic discussion of the training effects and response to exercise that occur in the heart, blood vessels, blood, and lungs should make it easier to understand why the training techniques discussed later are effective in improving cardiorespiratory endurance.

Clinical Decision-Making Exercise 10-1

A freshman goalie on the soccer team is not very fit. The coach wants to get her started on a training program to improve her cardiorespiratory endurance. What principles should be considered when designing her program?

Adaptation of the Heart to Exercise

The heart is the main pumping mechanism and circulates oxygenated blood throughout the body to the working tissues. The heart receives deoxygenated blood from the venous system and then pumps the blood through the pulmonary vessels to the lungs, where carbon dioxide is exchanged for oxygen. The oxygenated blood then returns to the left atrium of the heart, into the left ventricle, from which it exits through the aorta to the arterial system and is circulated throughout the body, supplying oxygen to the tissues.

Heart Rate

As the body begins to exercise, the working tissues require an increased supply of oxygen (via transport on red blood cells) to meet the increased metabolic demand (cardiac output). The working tissues use the decreasing concentration of oxygen as a signal to vasodilate the blood vessels in the tissue. This decreases the resistance to blood flow and allows for a decrease velocity of flow, and thereby increasing O_2 extraction.[49] Increases in heart rate occur as one response to meet the demand. The heart is capable of adapting to this increased demand through several mechanisms. Heart rate shows a gradual adaptation to an increased workload by increasing proportionally to the intensity of the exercise and will plateau at a given level after about 2 to 3 minutes[12] (Figure 10-1). Increases in heart rate produced by exercise are met by a decrease in diastolic filling time. Heart rate parameters change with age, body position, type of exercise, cardiovascular disease, heat and humidity, medications, and blood volume. Conditions that exist in any patient should be taken into consideration when prescribing exercise to improve aerobic endurance. The commonly used equation to predict maximal heart rate (MHR) is 220 – age for healthy men and women. However, the formula has limitations to persons who fall outside the "apparently healthy" classification and should be used with caution. Monitoring heart rate is an indirect method of estimating oxygen consumption.[16] Additionally, any medications should be considered prior to assessment or evaluation of heart rate response. For example, patients taking beta blockers will have an attenuated heart rate response to exercise. In general, heart rate and oxygen consumption have a linear relationship with exercise intensity. The greater the intensity of the exercise, the higher

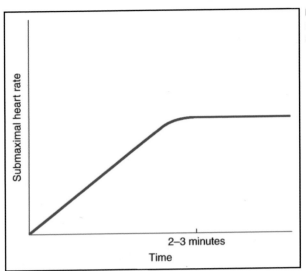

Figure 10-1. Plateau heart rate: For the heart rate to plateau at a given level, 2 to 3 minutes are required.

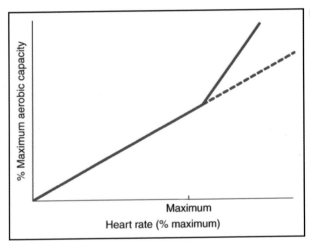

Figure 10-2. Maximum heart rate: Maximum heart rate is achieved at about the same time as maximal aerobic capacity.

the heart rate. This relationship is least consistent at very-low and very-high intensities of exercise (Figure 10-2). During higher-intensity activities, MHR may be achieved before maximum oxygen consumption, which can continue to rise despite reaching an age-predicted heart rate.[38] Because of these existing relationships, it should be apparent that the rate of oxygen consumption can be estimated by monitoring the heart rate.[13]

Stroke Volume

A second mechanism by which the cardiovascular system is able to adapt to increased demands of cardiac output during exercise is to increase stroke volume (the volume of blood being pumped out with each beat).[12] Stroke volume is equal to the difference between end diastolic volume and end systolic volume. Typical values for stroke volume range from 60 to 100 mL per beat at rest and 100 to 120 mL per beat at maximum.[18] Stroke volume will continue to increase only to the point at which diastolic filling time is simply too short to allow adequate filling. This occurs at about 40% to 50% of maximal aerobic capacity, or at a heart rate of 110 to 120 beats per minute; above this level, increases in the cardiac output are accounted for by increases in heart rate (Figure 10-3).[18]

Cardiac Output

Stroke volume and heart rate collectively determine the volume of blood being pumped through the heart in a given unit of time. About 5 L of blood are pumped through the heart

Figure 10-3. Stroke volume plateaus: Stroke volume plateaus at about 40% of maximal heart rate.

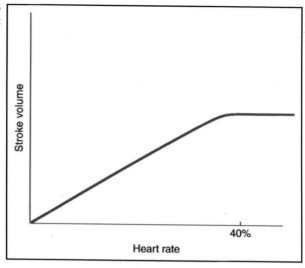

Figure 10-4. Cardiac output limits maximal aerobic capacity.

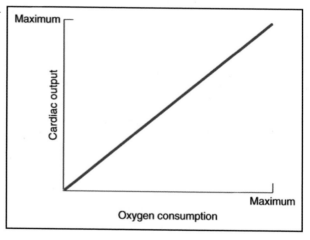

during each minute at rest. This is referred to as the cardiac output, which indicates how much blood the heart is capable of pumping in exactly 1 minute. Thus cardiac output is the primary determinant of the maximal rate of oxygen consumption possible (Figure 10-4). During exercise, cardiac output increases to about four times that experienced during rest (to about 20 L) in the normal individual, and may increase as much as six times in the elite endurance athlete (to about 31 L).

Cardiac output = stroke volume × heart rate

The above equation illustrates that any factor that will impact heart rate or stroke volume can either increase or decrease cardiac output. For example, an increase in venous return of blood from working muscle will increase the end diastolic volume. This increased volume will increase stroke volume via the Frank Starling mechanism[49] and, therefore, cardiac output.[57] Heart rate is regulated by the autonomic nervous system as well as circulating levels of epinephrine secreted from the adrenal medulla. Conversely, conditions that resist ventricular outflow (high blood pressure or an increase in afterload) will result in a decrease in cardiac output. Conversely, a condition that would decrease venous return (peripheral artery disease) would decrease stroke volume and attenuate cardiac output. Figure 10-5 outlines the factors that regulate both stroke volume and heart rate.

A commonly reported benefit of aerobic conditioning is a reduced resting heart rate and a reduced heart rate at a standard exercise

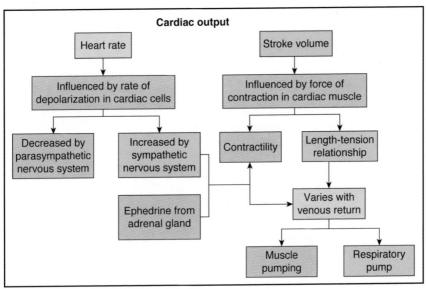

Figure 10-5. The factors effecting cardiac output.

load. This reduction in heart rate is explained by an increase in stroke volume brought about by increased venous return and to increased contractile conditions in the myocardium. The heart becomes more efficient because it is capable of pumping more blood with each stroke. Because the heart is a muscle, it can hypertrophy, or increase in size and strength as a result of aerobic exercise, to some extent, but this is in no way a negative effect of training.

Training Effect

Increased stroke volume × decreased heart rate = cardiac output

During exercise, females tend to have a 5% to 10% higher cardiac output than males at all intensities. This is likely the result of a lower concentration of hemoglobin in the female, which is compensated for during exercise by an increased cardiac output.[59]

Adaptation in Blood Flow

The amount of blood flowing to the various organs increases during exercise. However, there is a change in overall distribution of cardiac output: the percentage of total cardiac output to the nonessential organs is decreased, whereas it is increased to active skeletal muscle.

Volume of blood flow to the heart muscle or myocardium increases substantially during exercise, even though the percentage of total cardiac output supplying the heart muscle remains unchanged. The increase in flow to skeletal muscle is brought about by withdrawal of sympathetic stimulation to arterioles, and vasodilation is maintained by intrinsic metabolic control.[40] Trained persons have a higher capillary density than their untrained counterparts to better accommodate the increased supply and demand. In skeletal muscle, there is increased formation of blood vessels or capillaries, although it is not clear whether new ones form or dormant ones simply open up and fill with blood.[49]

The total peripheral resistance (TPR) is the sum of all forces that resist blood flow within the vascular system. TPR decreases during exercise primarily because of vessel vasodilation in the active skeletal muscles.

Blood Pressure

Blood pressure in the arterial system is determined by the cardiac output in relation to TPR to blood flow as follows:

$$BP = CO \times TPR$$

where BP = blood pressure, CO = cardiac output, and TPR = total peripheral resistance

Blood pressure is created by contraction of the myocardium. Contraction of the ventricles of the heart creates systolic pressure, and relaxation of the heart creates diastolic pressure. Blood pressure is regulated centrally by neural activity on peripheral arterioles and locally by metabolites produced during exercise. During exercise, there is a decrease in TPR (via decreased vasoconstriction) and an increase in cardiac output. Systolic pressure increases in proportion to oxygen consumption and cardiac output, whereas diastolic pressure shows little or no increase.[6] Failure of systolic pressure to increase with increased exercise intensity is considered an abnormal response to exercise and is a general indication to stop an exercise test or session.[1] Blood pressure falls below preexercise levels after exercise and may stay low for several hours. There is general agreement that engaging in consistent aerobic exercise will produce modest reductions in both systolic and diastolic blood pressure at rest as well as during submaximal exercise.[10,15]

Adaptations in the Blood

Oxygen is transported throughout the system bound to hemoglobin. Found in red blood cells, hemoglobin is an iron-containing protein that has the capability of easily accepting or giving up molecules of oxygen as needed. Training for improvement of cardiorespiratory endurance produces an increase in total blood volume, with a corresponding increase in the amount of hemoglobin. The concentration of hemoglobin in circulating blood does not change with training; it may actually decrease slightly.

Adaptation of the Lungs

As a result of training, pulmonary function is improved in the trained individual relative to the untrained individual. The volume of air that can be inspired in a single maximal ventilation is increased. The diffusing capacity of the lungs is also increased, facilitating the exchange of oxygen and carbon dioxide. Pulmonary resistance to air flow is also decreased.[35]

Clinical Decision-Making Exercise 10-2

A lacrosse player sustained a season-ending knee injury at the end of last season. During the off-season he began training for his return to hockey. After several months of training, what physiological changes should be occurring?

MAXIMAL AEROBIC CAPACITY

The maximal amount of oxygen that can be used during exercise is referred to as maximal aerobic capacity (exercise physiologists refer to this as VO_2max). It is considered to be the best indicator of the level of cardiorespiratory endurance. Maximal aerobic capacity is most often presented in terms of the volume of oxygen used relative to body weight per unit of time ($mL \times kg^{-1} \times min^{-1}$).[3]

It is common to see aerobic capacity expressed in metabolic equivalents (METs). Resting oxygen consumption is generally considered to be $3.5 \ mL \times kg^{-1} \times min^{-1}$ or 1 MET. Therefore, an exercise intensity of 10 METs is equivalent to a VO_2 of $35 \ mL \times kg^{-1} \times min^{-1}$. A normal maximal aerobic capacity for most collegiate men and women would fall in the range of 35 to 50 $mL \times kg^{-1} \times min^{-1}$.[35]

Rate of Oxygen Consumption

The performance of any activity requires a certain rate of oxygen consumption, which is about the same for all persons, depending on their present level of fitness. Generally, the greater the rate or intensity of the performance of an activity, the greater will be the oxygen consumption. Each person has his or her own maximal rate of oxygen consumption. The person's ability to perform an activity is closely related to the amount of oxygen required by that activity. This ability is limited by the maximal amount of oxygen the person is capable of delivering into the lungs. Fatigue occurs when insufficient oxygen is supplied to muscles. It should be apparent that the greater the percentage of maximal aerobic capacity required during an activity, the less time the activity may be performed (Figure 10-6).

Three factors determine the maximal rate at which oxygen can be used: (1) external respiration, involving the ventilatory process or pulmonary function; (2) gas transport, which is accomplished by the cardiovascular system (that is, the heart, blood vessels, and blood); and (3) internal (cellular) respiration, which involves the use of oxygen by the cells to produce energy. Exercise physiologists generally

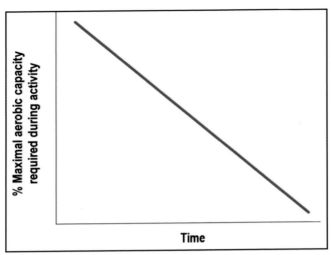

Figure 10-6. Maximal aerobic capacity required during activity: The greater the percentage of maximal aerobic capacity required during an activity, the less time that activity can be performed.

discuss the limiting factors of maximal aerobic capacity based on healthy human subjects in a controlled environment.[4,27,28] Under these conditions, research presents agreement that the ability to transport oxygen through the heart, lungs, and blood is the limiting factor to the overall rate of oxygen consumption. This indicates that this is not the ability of the mitochondria to consume oxygen that limits VO_2max. A high maximal aerobic capacity within a person's range indicates that all three systems are working well.

Maximal Aerobic Capacity: An Inherited Characteristic

The maximal rate at which oxygen can be used is a genetically determined characteristic; we inherit a certain range of maximal aerobic capacity, and the more active we are, the higher the existing maximal aerobic capacity will be within that range.[47,58] Therefore, a training program is capable of increasing maximal aerobic capacity to its highest limit within our range.[43,50,58]

Fast-Twitch vs Slow-Twitch Muscle Fibers

The range of maximal aerobic capacity inherited is in a large part determined by the metabolic and functional properties of skeletal muscle fibers. As discussed in detail in Chapter 6, there are 3 distinct types of muscle fibers, slow-twitch and 2 variations of fast-twitch fibers, each of which has distinctive metabolic and contractile capabilities. Because they are relatively fatigue resistant, slow-twitch fibers are associated primarily with long-duration, aerobic-type activities. The slow-twitch fibers depend on oxidative phosphorylation to generate adenosine triphosphate (ATP) to provide the energy needed for muscle contraction. Fast-twitch fibers are useful in short-term, high-intensity activities, which mainly involve the anaerobic system. Intermediated fast-twitch fibers demonstrate a reliance on glycolysis to produce ATP. These intermediate fibers also have the ability to adapt based on specific training regimens.[49] In general, if a patient has a high ratio of slow-twitch to fast-twitch muscle fibers, the patient will be able to use oxygen more efficiently and thus will have a higher maximal aerobic capacity.

Clinical Decision-Making Exercise 10-3

A cyclist wants to know if you can test his maximal aerobic capacity. He says that he has reached a plateau in his training. There hasn't been an increase in his maximal aerobic capacity in about 1 year. What is your explanation for why this is occurring?

Cardiorespiratory Endurance and Work Ability

Cardiorespiratory endurance plays a critical role in our ability to carry out normal daily activities.[40] Fatigue is closely related to the percentage of maximal aerobic capacity that a particular workload demands.[49] For example, Figure 10-7 presents two people, A and B. A has maximal aerobic capacity of 50 mL/kg per minute, whereas B has a maximal aerobic capacity of only 40 mL/kg per minute. If both A and B are exercising at the same intensity, then A will be working at a much lower percentage of maximal aerobic capacity than B. Consequently, A should be able to sustain his or her activity over a much longer time. Everyday activities may be adversely affected if the ability to use oxygen efficiently is impaired. Thus, improvement of cardiorespiratory endurance should be an essential component of any conditioning program and must be included as part of the rehabilitation program for the injured patient.[9]

Regardless of the training technique used for the improvement of cardiorespiratory endurance, one principal goal remains the same: to increase the ability of the cardiorespiratory system to supply a sufficient amount of oxygen to working muscles. Without oxygen, the body is incapable of producing energy for an extended period of time.

PRODUCING ENERGY FOR EXERCISE

All living systems need to perform a variety of activities, such as growing, generating energy, repairing damaged tissues, and eliminating wastes. All of these activities are referred to as being metabolic or as cellular metabolism.

Muscles are metabolically active and must generate energy to move. Energy is produced from the breakdown of certain nutrients from foodstuffs. This energy is stored in a compound called ATP, which is the ultimate usable form of energy for muscular activity. ATP is produced in the muscle tissue from blood glucose or glycogen. Fats and proteins can also be metabolized to generate ATP. Glucose not needed immediately can be stored as glycogen in the resting muscle and liver. Stored glycogen in the liver can later be converted back to glucose and transferred to the blood to meet the body's energy needs.[7]

It is important to understand that the intensity and duration of exercise selected as an intervention will have implications on the source of "fuel" to engage in the activity. The "fuel" is the ATP needed for muscular contraction. Exercise intensity and duration affect the source or pathway that is used to supply the ATP; that is, does the ATP come from the breakdown of circulating blood glucose (glycolysis) or from the Krebs cycle and the electron transport chain (oxidative phosphorylation)?

If the combination of duration and intensity is low (40% to 50% of VO_2max), the body relies more heavily on fats stored in adipose tissue to meet its energy needs. The longer the duration of an activity, the greater the amount of fat used, especially during the later stages of endurance events. During rest and submaximal exertion, both fat and carbohydrates are used to provide energy in about a 60% to 40% ratio. Carbohydrate must be available to use fat. If glycogen is totally depleted, fat cannot be completely metabolized. Regardless of the nutrient source that produces ATP, it is always available in the cell as an immediate energy source. When all available sources of ATP are used, more must be generated for muscular contraction to continue.[8,29]

Various sports activities involve specific demands for energy. For example, sprinting and jumping are high-energy-output activities, requiring a relatively large production of energy for a short time. Long-distance running and swimming, on the other hand, are mostly low-energy-output activities per unit of time, requiring energy production for a prolonged time. Other physical activities demand a blend of both high- and low-energy output. These various energy demands can be met by the different processes in which energy can be supplied to the skeletal muscles.[17]

Anaerobic vs Aerobic Metabolism

Two major energy-generating systems function in muscle tissue: anaerobic and aerobic

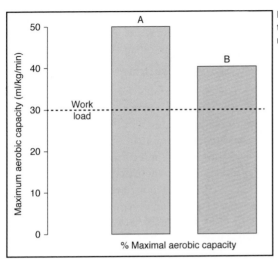

Figure 10-7. Patient A should be able to work longer than patient B as a result of a lower percentage use of maximal aerobic capacity.

metabolism. Each of these systems produces ATP.[21] Activities that demand intensive, short-term exercise need ATP that is rapidly available and metabolized to meet energy needs. The primary source for ATP production in short-term high-intensity exercise is phosphocreatine system. Tissues only store enough phosphocreatine to generate ATP for events lasting about 10 seconds or less. After a few seconds of intensive exercise, however, the small stores of ATP are used up. The body then uses stored glycogen as an energy source. Glycogen can be broken down to supply glucose, which is then metabolized within the muscle cells to generate ATP for muscle contractions.[38]

Glucose can be metabolized to generate small amounts of ATP energy without the need for oxygen. This energy system is referred to as anaerobic metabolism (occurring in the absence of oxygen). As exercise continues, the body has to rely on a more complex form of carbohydrate and fat metabolism to generate ATP. This second energy system requires oxygen and is therefore referred to as aerobic metabolism (occurring in the presence of oxygen). The aerobic system of producing energy generates considerably more ATP than the anaerobic one.

In most activities, both aerobic and anaerobic systems function simultaneously. The degree to which the two major energy systems are involved is determined by the intensity and duration of the activity.[55] If the intensity of the activity is such that sufficient oxygen can be supplied to meet the demands of working

tissues, the activity is considered to be aerobic. Conversely, if the activity is of high-enough intensity, or the duration is such that there is insufficient oxygen available to meet energy demands, the activity becomes anaerobic.[51]

Excess Postexercise Oxygen Consumption

As the intensity of the exercise increases and insufficient amounts of oxygen are available to the tissues, an oxygen deficit is incurred. Oxygen deficit occurs in the beginning of exercise (within the first 2 to 3 minutes) when the oxygen demand is greater than the oxygen supplied. It has been hypothesized that this oxygen debt was caused by lactic acid produced during anaerobic activity, and this debt must be "paid back" during the postexercise period. However, there is presently a different rationale for this oxygen deficit, which is currently referred to as "excess postexercise oxygen consumption." It is theoretically caused by disturbances in mitochondrial function from an increase in temperature.[38] Additional explanations include evidence of both a "fast" and a "slow" component. The fast components include the restoration of phosphocreatine levels depleted in the earliest seconds of exercise, and replacing stored muscle and blood oxygen content. The slow portion is accounted for by providing the energy for the elevated respiratory rate and heart rate, elevated levels of catecholamines and gluconeogenesis, the conversion of lactic acid to glucose.[44]

TECHNIQUES FOR MAINTAINING CARDIORESPIRATORY ENDURANCE

Several different training techniques may be incorporated into a rehabilitation program through which cardiorespiratory endurance can be maintained. Certainly, a primary consideration for the athletic trainer is whether the injury involves the upper or lower extremity. With injuries that involve the upper extremity, weight-bearing activities can be used, such as walking, running, stair climbing, and modified aerobics. However, if the injury is to the lower extremity, alternative non-weight-bearing activities, such as swimming or stationary cycling, may be necessary. The goal of the athletic trainer is to try to maintain cardiorespiratory endurance throughout the rehabilitation process.

The principles of the training techniques discussed next can be applied to running, cycling, swimming, stair climbing, or any other activity designed to maintain levels of cardiorespiratory fitness.

Continuous Training

Continuous training involves the following considerations:

- The frequency of the activity
- The intensity of the activity
- The type of activity
- The time (duration) of the activity

Frequency of Training

The American College of Sports Medicine (ACSM) recommends that most adults engage in moderate-intensity cardiorespiratory exercise training for ≥30 min·day^{-1} on ≥5 days·wk^{-1} for a total of ≥150 min·wk^{-1}, vigorous-intensity cardiorespiratory exercise training for ≥20 min·day^{-1} on ≥3 days·wk^{-1} (≥75 min·wk^{-1}), or a combination of moderate- and vigorous-intensity exercise to achieve a total energy expenditure of ≥500 to 1000 MET·min·wk–1.[1] A competitive athlete should be prepared to train

as often as six times per week. Everyone should take off at least 1 day per week to give damaged tissues a chance to repair themselves.

Intensity of Training

The intensity of exercise is also a critical factor, although recommendations regarding training intensities vary.[25] This statement is particularly true in the early stages of training, when the body is forced to make a magnitude of adjustments to increased workload demands. The ACSM guidelines regarding intensity of exercise recommend the following: 55%/65% to 90% of MHR, or 40%/50% to 85% of maximum oxygen uptake reserve (VO$_2$R) or MHR reserve (hear rate reserve [HRR]). HRR and VO$_2$R are calculated from the difference between resting and maximum heart rate and resting and maximum VO$_2$, respectively. To estimate training intensity, a percentage of this value is added to the resting heart rate and/or resting VO$_2$ and is expressed as a percentage of HRR or VO$_2$R. The lower-intensity values, that is, 40% to 49% of VO$_2$R or HRR and 55% to 64% of MHR, are most applicable to individuals who are quite unfit. These intensities require the athletic trainer to either know the person's maximal values or use a prediction equation to estimate these intensities. A great rule of thumb is to always go with actual data rather than prediction data when available. There are many limitations to prediction equations. Because of the linear relationship between heart rate, oxygen consumption, and exercise intensity, it becomes a relatively simple process to identify a specific workload (pace) that will make the heart rate plateau at the desired level.[52] By monitoring heart rate, we know whether the pace is too fast or too slow to achieve the desired range of intensity.[33] Prior to selecting an exercise intensity, the athletic trainer should consider several factors, including current level of fitness, medications, cardiovascular risk profile, an individual's likes and dislikes, and patient's goals and objectives.[1]

Monitoring Heart Rate

There are several methods for measuring heart rate response during exercise. These include, but are not limited to, palpation of the heart rate at the radial or carotid artery, pulse oximetry, telemetry (heart rate monitors), and electrocardiography. One of the easiest methods is to palpate the radial artery. This assessment can be done by the patient or the athletic trainer. The carotid artery is simple to find, especially during exercise. However, there are pressure (baro) receptors located in the carotid artery that, if subjected to hard pressure from the two fingers, will slow down the heart rate, giving a false indication of exactly what the heart rate is. Thus, the pulse at the radial artery proves the most accurate measure of heart rate. Regardless of where the heart rate is taken, it should be recorded prior to exercise, during exercise to ensure target intensities, and monitored following exercise to ensure recovery. Another factor must be considered when measuring heart rate during exercise. The patient is trying to elevate heart rate to a specific target rate and maintain it at that level during the entire workout.[22] Heart rate can be increased or decreased by speeding up or slowing down the pace. Based on the fact that heart rates will attain a steady state or plateau to a prescribed work rate in 2 to 3 minutes, the athletic trainer should allow sufficient time prior to assessment of heart rate. Thus, the patient should be actively engaged in the workout for 2 to 3 minutes before measuring pulse.[61]

Several formulas allow an athletic trainer to identify a training target heart rate.[42] To calculate a specific target heart rate, it is first necessary to determine a maximal heart rate. Exact determination of maximal heart rate (HR) involves exercising an individual at a maximal level and monitoring the HR using an electrocardiogram. This is a difficult process outside of a laboratory. Maximum HR is related to age; and, with aging, the maximum HR decreases.[34] An approximate estimate of maximum HR for individuals of both sexes would be:

$$HR_{max} = 208\text{-}0.7 \times Age.$$

For a 20-year-old individual, maximum HR would be about 194 beats per minute (208-0.7 × 20)

HR reserve is used to determine upper and lower limits of the target HR range. Heart rate reserve (HRR) is the difference between resting heart rate (HR_{rest}) and maximum heart rate (HR_{max}).

$$HRR = HR_{max} - HR_{rest}$$

The greater the difference, the larger the HRR and the greater the range of potential training HR intensities.

The *Karvonen equation* is used to calculate target HR at a given percentage of training intensity. To use the *Karvonen equation* you need to know your HRR.[26,30]

$$Target\ HR = HR_{rest} + \%\ of\ target\ intensity \times HRR$$

When using estimated HR_{max} or/and HR_{rest}, the values are always predictions. So in a 20-year-old with a calculated HR_{max} of 194 and a HR_{rest} of 70 beats per minute, the HRR is 124 (194 - 70 = 124). For moderate-intensity activity, the heart should work in a range between a lower limit and an upper limit.[39] The lower limit is calculated by taking 70% of the HRR and adding the resting HR, which would be 157 beats per minute ([124 × 0.7] + 70 = 157). The upper limit is calculated by taking 79% of the HRR and adding the resting HR ([124 × 0.79] + 70 = 168).

Rating of Perceived Exertion

Rating of perceived exertion can be used in addition to monitoring heart rate to indicate exercise intensity.[5] During exercise, individuals are asked to rate subjectively on a numerical scale from 6 to 20 exactly how they feel relative to their level of exertion (Table 10-1). More intense exercise that requires a higher level of oxygen consumption and energy expenditure is directly related to higher subjective ratings of perceived exertion. The use of a rating-of-perceived-exertion scale is the preferred method of monitoring the exercise intensity of individuals who are taking medications, beta blockers for example, that attenuate the normal heart rate response to exercise. Over time, patients can be taught to exercise at a specific rating of perceived exertion that relates directly to more objective measures of exercise intensity.[20,40]

Type of Exercise

The type of activity used in continuous training must be aerobic. Aerobic activities are activities that generally involve repetitive, whole-body, large-muscle movements that are rhythmical in nature and use large amounts of

Table 10-1 Rating of Perceived Exertion

Scale	Verbal Rating
6	
7	Very, very light
8	
9	Very light
10	
11	Fairly light
12	
13	Somewhat hard
14	
15	Hard
16	
17	Very hard
18	
19	Very, very hard
20	

Reprinted with permission from Borg GA. Psychophysical basis of perceived exertion. *Med Sci Sports Exerc.* 1982;14:377.

Time (Duration)

For minimal improvement to occur, the patient must participate in at least 20 minutes of continuous activity with the heart rate elevated to its working level. The ACSM recommends duration of training to be 20 to 60 minutes of continuous or intermittent (minimum of 10-minute bouts accumulated throughout the day) aerobic activity. Duration varies with the intensity of the activity. Lower-intensity activity should be conducted over a longer time (30 minutes or more). Patients training at higher levels of intensity should train at least 20 minutes or longer "because of the importance of 'total fitness' and that it is more readily attained with exercise sessions of longer duration and because of the potential hazards and adherence problems associated with high-intensity activity, moderate-intensity activity of longer duration is recommended for adults not training for athletic competition".[1]

Generally, the greater the duration of the workout, the greater the improvement in cardiorespiratory endurance.

Clinical Decision-Making Exercise 10-4

Your ice hockey players have been fatiguing early in the game. What type of training will best help them improve their fitness specifically for their sport?

oxygen, elevate the heart rate, and maintain it at that level for an extended period. Examples of aerobic activities are walking, running, jogging, cycling, swimming, rope skipping, stepping, aerobic dance exercise, in-line skating, and cross-country skiing.

The advantage of these aerobic activities opposed to more intermittent activities, such as racquetball, squash, basketball, or tennis, is that aerobic activities are easy to regulate in intensity by either speeding up or slowing down the pace.[37] Because we already know that a given intensity of the workload elicits a given heart rate, these aerobic activities allow us to maintain heart rate at a specified or target level. Intermittent activities involve variable speeds and intensities that cause the heart rate to fluctuate considerably. Although these intermittent activities will improve cardiorespiratory endurance, they are much more difficult to monitor in terms of intensity. It is important to point out that any type of activity, from gardening to aerobic exercise, can improve fitness.[42]

Interval Training

Unlike continuous training, interval training involves activities that are more intermittent. Interval training consists of alternating periods of relatively intense work and active recovery. It allows for performance of much more work at a more intense workload over a longer period than if working continuously. It is most desirable in continuous training to work at an intensity of about 60% to 80% of MHR. Obviously, sustaining activity at a relatively high intensity over a 20-minute period is extremely difficult. The advantage of interval training is that it allows work at this 80% or higher level for a short period followed by an active period of recovery during which you may be working at only 30% to 45% of MHR. Thus, the intensity of the workout and its duration can be greater than with continuous training.

There are several important considerations in interval training. The training period is the amount of time in which continuous activity is actually being performed, and the recovery period is the time between training periods. A set is a group of combined training and recovery periods, and a repetition is the number of training/recovery periods per set. Training time or distance refers to the rate or distance of the training period. The training/recovery ratio indicates a time ratio for training vs recovery.

An example of interval training is a patient exercising on a stationary bike. An interval workout involves 10 repetitions of pedaling at a maximum speed for 20 seconds followed by pedaling at 40% of maximum speed for 90 seconds. During this interval training session, heart rate will probably increase to 85% to 95% of maximal level while pedaling at maximum speed and will probably fall to the 35% to 45% level during the recovery period.

Older adults should exercise some caution when using interval training as a method for improving cardiorespiratory endurance. The intensity levels attained during the active periods may be too high and create undue risk for the older adult.

CALORIC THRESHOLDS AND TARGETS

The interplay between the duration, intensity, and frequency of exercise creates a caloric expenditure from exercise sessions. The amount of caloric expenditure is important to a wide range of patients, including those interested in weight loss, as well as those under very strenuous training regimens. General acceptance exists such that the health benefits and training changes associated with exercise programs are related to the total amount of work (indicated by caloric expenditure) completed during training.[1] These caloric thresholds may be different to elicit improvements in VO_2max, weight loss, or risk of premature chronic disease. The ACSM recommends a range of 150 to 400 calories of energy expenditure per day in exercise or physical activity. Expenditure of 1000 kcal per week should be the initial goal for those not previously engaged in regular activity. Patients should be moved toward the upper end of the recommendation (300 to 400 kcal per day) to obtain optimal fitness. The estimation of caloric expenditure is easily accomplished using the METs associated with a given activity and the formula[1]:

$$(MET \times 3.5 \times body\ weight\ in\ kg)/200 = kcal/min$$

Numerous charts and tables exist that estimate activities in terms of intensity requirements expressed in METs. If a weekly goal of 1000 kcal is established for a 70-kg person at an intensity of six METs, the caloric expenditure would be calculated as follows:

$$(6 \times 3.5 \times 70\ kg)/200 = kcal/min$$

At an exercise intensity of six METs, the patient would need to exercise 136 minutes to achieve the 1000-kcal goal. If the patient wants to exercise 4 days each week, 34 minutes of exercise each of the 4 days will be required.

The primary goal of weight loss is to consume or burn more calories than are taken in (eaten). The calories used during exercise can be added to the calories cut from the diet to calculate total caloric deficit needed to create weight loss. The aforementioned patient could reduce his or her caloric intake by 400 kcal each day. This will total 2800 kcal that have been restricted from the diet. These calories are then added to the 1000 kcal used for exercise. A pound of fat is equivalent to 3500 kcal. The combination of reduced caloric intake and increased used of kcal for exercise in the example is 3800 kcal, or slightly more than 1 pound of weight loss in 1 week.

> **Clinical Decision-Making Exercise 10-5**
>
> In an interval workout, at what intensities should an athlete work during the work period and during the active recovery period?

COMBINING CONTINUOUS AND INTERVAL TRAINING

As indicated previously, most physical activities involve some combination of aerobic and anaerobic metabolism.[60] Continuous training is generally done at an intensity level that primarily uses the aerobic system. In interval training, the intensity is sufficient to necessitate a greater percentage of anaerobic metabolism.[19] Therefore, for the physically active patient, the athletic trainer should incorporate both training techniques into a rehabilitation program to maximize cardiorespiratory fitness.

DETRAINING

Physical training promotes a wide range of physiologic training. These include increased size and number of mitochondria, increased capillary bed density, changes in resting and exercise heart rate, blood pressure, myocardial oxygen consumption, and improved VO_2max to mention a few. It would seem logical that if the stimulus (exercise) is removed, these changes will dissipate. Long periods of inactivity are associated with the reversal of the aforementioned changes. Improvements may be lost in as little as 12 days to as long as several months to see a complete reversal of changes.

Summary

1. The athletic trainer should routinely incorporate activities that will help maintain levels of cardiorespiratory endurance into the rehabilitation program.

2. Cardiorespiratory endurance involves the coordinated function of the heart, lungs, blood, and blood vessels to supply sufficient amounts of oxygen to the working tissues.

3. The best indicator of how efficiently the cardiorespiratory system functions is the maximal rate at which oxygen can be used by the tissues.

4. Heart rate is directly related to the rate of oxygen consumption. It is therefore possible to predict the intensity of the work in terms of a rate of oxygen use by monitoring heart rate.

5. Aerobic exercise involves an activity in which the level of intensity and duration is low enough to provide a sufficient amount of oxygen to supply the demands of the working tissues.

6. In anaerobic exercise, the intensity of the activity is so high that oxygen is being used more quickly than it can be supplied; thus, an oxygen debt is incurred that must be repaid before working tissue can return to its normal resting state.

7. Continuous or sustained training for maintenance of cardiorespiratory endurance involves selecting an activity that is aerobic in nature and training at least 3 times per week for a time period of no less than 20 minutes with the heart rate elevated to at least 60% of maximal rate.

8. Interval training involves alternating periods of relatively intense work followed by active recovery periods. Interval training allows performance of more work at a relatively higher workload than continuous training.

9. Aerobic exercise is a very powerful tool when considering the decreased mortality and morbidity associated with improvements in functional capacity. The therapist with a working knowledge of the principles of exercise prescription and testing are best capable of ensuring the safety and effectiveness of interventions.

References

1. American College of Sports Medicine. *ACSM's Guidelines for Exercise Testing and Prescription*. 8th ed. Philadelphia, PA: Lippincott Williams & Wilkins; 2010:366.

2. Åstrand PO, Rodahl K. *Textbook of Work Physiology*. New York, NY: McGraw-Hill; 1986.

3. Åstrand PO. Åstrand-rhyming nomogram for calculation of aerobic capacity from pulse rate during submaximal work. *J Appl Physiol*. 1954;7:218.

4. Bassett D, Howley E. Limiting factors for maximal oxygen uptake and determinants of endurance performance. *Med Sci Sports Exerc.* 2000;32:70-84.

5. Borg GA. Psychophysical basis of perceived exertion. *Med Sci Sports Exerc.* 1982;14:377.

6. Brooks G, Fahey T, White T. *Exercise Physiology: Human Bioenergetics and Its Applications.* New York, NY: McGraw- Hill; 2004.

7. Brooks G, Mercier J. The balance of carbohydrate and lipid utilization during exercise: The crossover concept. *J Appl Physiol.* 1994;76:2253-2261.

8. Cerretelli P. Energy sources for muscle contraction. *Sports Med.* 1992;13:S106-S110.

9. Chillag SA. Endurance patients: physiologic changes and nonorthopedic problems. *South Med J.* 1986; 79:1264.

10. Convertino VA. Aerobic fitness, endurance training, and orthostatic intolerance. *Exerc Sport Sci Rev.* 1987;15:223.

11. Cooper KH. *The Aerobics Program for Total Well-Being.* New York, NY: Bantam Books; 1982.

12. Cox M. Exercise training programs and cardiorespiratory adaptation. *Clin Sports Med.* 1991;10:19-32.

13. deVries H. *Physiology of Exercise for Physical Education and Athletics.* Dubuque, IA: William C. Brown; 1986.

14. Dicarlo L, Sparling P, Millard-Stafford M. Peak heart rates during maximal running and swimming: implications for exercise prescription. *Int J Sports Med.* 1991;12: 309-312.

15. Durstein L, Pate R, Branch D. Cardiorespiratory responses to acute exercise. In: *American College of Sports Medicine. Resource Manual for Guidelines for Exercise Testing and Prescription.* Philadelphia, PA: Lea & Febiger; 1993.

16. Fahey T, ed. *Encyclopedia of Sports Medicine and Exercise Physiology.* New York, NY: Garland; 1995.

17. Fox E, Bowers R, Foss M. *The Physiological Basis of Physical Education and Athletics.* Philadelphia, PA: Saunders; 1981.

18. Franklin B. Cardiorespiratory responses to acute exercise. In: American College of Sports Medicine. *Resource Manual for Guidelines for Exercise Testing and Prescription,* 4th ed. Philadelphia, PA: Lippincott Williams & Wilkins; 2010:164.

19. Gaesser GA, Wilson LA. Effects of continuous and interval training on the parameters of the power-endurance time relationship for high-intensity exercise. *Int J Sports Med.* 1988;9:417.

20. Glass S, Whaley M, Wegner M. A comparison between ratings of perceived exertion among standard protocols and steady state running. *Int J Sports Med.* 1991;12:77-82.

21. Green J, Patla A. Maximal aerobic power: neuromuscular and metabolic considerations. *Med Sci Sports Exerc.* 1992;24:38-46.

22. Greer N, Katch F. Validity of palpation recovery pulse rate to estimate exercise heart rate following four intensities of bench step exercise. *Res Q Exerc Sport.* 1982;53:340.

23. Hage P. Exercise guidelines: Which to believe? *Phys Sportsmed.* 1982;10:23.

24. Haskell WL, Lee IM, Pate RR, et al Physical activity and public health: updated recommendation for adults from the American College of Sports Medicine and the American Heart Association. *Med Sci Sports Exerc.* 2007;39(8):1423-1434.

25. Hawley J, Myburgh K, Noakes T. Maximal oxygen consumption: a contemporary perspective. In: Fahey T, ed. *Encyclopedia of Sports Medicine and Exercise Physiology.* New York, NY: Garland; 1995.

26. Hickson RC, Foster C, Pollac M, et al Reduced training intensities and loss of aerobic power, endurance, and cardiac growth. *J Appl Physiol.* 1985;58:492.

27. Hill A, Long C, Lupton H. Muscular exercise, Lactic acid and the supply and utilization of oxygen. Parts VII-VIII. *Proc R Soc Lond B Biol Sci.* 1924;97:155-176.

28. Hill A, Lupton H. Muscular exercise, Lactic acid and the supply and utilization of oxygen. *Q J Med.* 1923;16: 135-171.

29. Honig C, Connett R, Gayeski T. O2 transport and its interaction with metabolism. *Med Sci Sports Exerc.* 1992;24:47-53.

30. Karvonen MJ, Kentala E, Mustala O. The effects of training on heart rate: a longitudinal study. *Ann Med Exp Biol Fenn.* 1957;35:305.

31. Koyanagi A, Yamamoto K, Nishijima K. Recommendation for an exercise prescription to prevent coronary heart disease. *J Med Syst.* 1993;17:213-217.

32. Lee IM, Rexrode KM, Cook NR, Manson JE, Buring JE. Physical activity and coronary heart disease in women: is "no pain, no gain" passe? *JAMA.* 2001;285(11):1447-1454.

33. Levine G, Balady G. The benefits and risks of exercise testing: the exercise prescription. *Adv Intern Med.* 1993;38:57-79.

34. Londeree B, Moeschberger M. Effect of age and other factors on maximal heart rate. *Res Q Exerc Sport.* 1982;53:297.

35. MacDougall D, Sale D. Continuous vs interval training: a review for the patient and coach. *Can J Appl Sport Sci.* 1981;6:93.

36. Manson JE, Greenland P, LaCroix AZ, et al Walking compared with vigorous exercise for the prevention of cardiovascular events in women. *N Engl J Med.* 2002;347:716-725.

37. Marcinik EJ, Hogden K, Mittleman K, et al Aerobic/callisthenic and aerobic/circuit weight training programs for Navy men: a comparative study. *Med Sci Sports Exerc.* 1985;17:482.

38. McArdle W, Katch F, Katch V. Exercise Physiology, Energy, Nutrition, and Human Performance. Philadelphia, PA: Lippincott Williams & Wilkins; 2001.

39. Mead W, Hartwig R. Fitness evaluation and exercise prescription. *Fam Pract.* 1981;13:1039.

40. Monahan T. Perceived exertion: an old exercise tool finds new applications. *Phys Sportsmed.* 1988; 16:174.

41. Myers J, Praksah M, Froelicher V, Do D, Partington S, Atwood J. Exercise capacity and mortality among men referred for exercise testing. *N Engl J Med.* 346 (11): 793-8041, 2002.

42. Pate R, Pratt M, Blair S. Physical activity and public health: a recommendation from the CDC and ACSM. *JAMA.* 1995;273:402-407.

43. Powers S. Fundamentals of exercise metabolism. In: American College of Sports Medicine. *Resource Manual for Guidelines for Exercise Testing and Prescription.* Philadelphia, PA: Lea & Febiger; 1993:133.

44. Powers S, Howley E. *Exercise Physiology: Theory and Application to Fitness and Performance.* New York, NY: McGraw Hill; 2009.

45. Rowland TW, Green GM. Anaerobic threshold and the determination of training target heart rates in premenarcheal girls. *Pediatr Cardiol.* 1989;10:75.

46. Sandvik L, Erikssen J, Thaulow E, Erikssen G, Mundal R, Rodahl K. Physical fitness as a predictor of mortality among healthy, middle-aged Norwegian men. *N Engl J Med.* 1993;328:533-537.

47. Saltin B, Strange S. Maximal oxygen uptake: old and new arguments for a cardiovascular limitation. *Med Sci Sports Exerc.* 1992;24:30-37.

48. Sesso HD, Paffenbarger RS Jr, Lee IM. Physical activity and coronary heart disease in men: the Harvard Alumni Health Study. *Circulation.* 2000;102(9):975-980.

49. Silverthorn, D. *Human Physiology. An Integrated Approach.* Boston, MA: Pearson; 2012.

50. Smith M, Mitchell J. Cardiorespiratory adaptations to exercise training. In: American College of Sports Medicine. *Resource Manual for Guidelines for Exercise Testing and Prescription.* Philadelphia, PA: Lea & Febiger; 1993.

51. Stachenfeld N, Eskenazi M, Gleim G. Predictive accuracy of criteria used to assess maximal oxygen consumption. *Am Heart J.* 1992;123:922-925.

52. Swain D, Abernathy K, Smith C. Target heart rates for the development of cardiorespiratory fitness. *Med Sci Sports Exerc.* 1994;26:112-116.

53. Tanaka H, Monahan KD, Seals DR. Age-predicted maximal heart rate revisited. *J Am Coll Cardiol.* 2001;37(1):153-156.

54. Tanasescu M, Leitzmann MF, Rimm EB, Willett WC, Stampfer MJ, Hu FB. Exercise type and intensity in relation to coronary heart disease in men. *JAMA.* 2002;288(16):1994-2000.

55. Vago P, Mercier M, Ramonatxo M, et al Is ventilatory anaerobic threshold a good index of endurance capacity? *Int J Sports Med.* 1987;8:190.

56. Wagner P. Central and peripheral aspects of oxygen transport and adaptations with exercise. *Sports Med.* 1991;11:133-142.

57. Weltman A, Weltman J, Ruh R, et al Percentage of maximal heart rate reserve, and VO_2 peak for determining endurance training intensity in sedentary women. *Int J Sports Med.* 1989;10:212. Review.

58. Weymans M, Reybrouck T. Habitual level of physical activity and cardiorespiratory endurance capacity in children. *Eur J Appl Physiol.* 1989;58:803.

59. Williford HN, Scharff-Olson M, Blessing DL. Exercise prescription for women: Special considerations. *Sports Med.* 1993;15:299-311.

60. Wilmore J, Costill D. *Physiology of Sport and Exercise.* Champaign, IL: Human Kinetics; 1994.

61. Zhang Y, Johnson M, Chow N. Effect of exercise testing protocol on parameters of aerobic function. *Med Sci Sports Exerc.* 1991;23:625-630.

62. U.S. Department of Health and Human Services. *Physical Activity Guidelines Advisory Committee Report,* 2008. Publication No. U0049. Washington, DC: ODPHP; 2008.

SOLUTIONS TO CLINICAL DECISION-MAKING EXERCISES

10-1 Frequency, intensity, type, and time. All of these should be specific to the demands of her sport. For example, she would benefit more from interval training than endurance as she performs in short bursts during a game. Her exercise should also incorporate flexibility and agility activities that would enhance her functional performance in the goal.

10-2 He should have a marked decrease in resting heart rate and blood pressure. This is due in part to an increase in stroke volume and cardiac output. He should have a decreased body fat percentage as resting metabolic rate increases, encouraging energy expenditure.

10-3 He might be reaching his maximum aerobic capacity. Everyone has a limited inherited range of aerobic capacity. Once an athlete reaches the upper end of that range, it is unlikely that additional significant improvement will occur.

10-4 Interval training, because the sport requires quick sprints interrupted by short recovery periods.

10-5 They should be working at 85% to 90% of their maximum heart rate during the work period and at 35% to 45% percent of their maximum heart rate during the active recovery period.

SECTION III

The Tools of Rehabilitation

CHAPTER 11

Plyometric Exercise in Rehabilitation

Michael L. Voight, DHSc, PT, SCS, OCS, ATC, CSCS, FAPTA
Steven R. Tippett, PhD, PT, SCS, ATC

After completion of this chapter, the athletic trainer should be able to do the following:

- Define plyometric exercise and identify its function in a rehabilitation program.

- Describe the mechanical, neurophysiologic, and neuromuscular control mechanisms involved in plyometric training.

- Discuss how biomechanical evaluation, stability, dynamic movement, and flexibility should be assessed before beginning a plyometric program.

- Explain how a plyometric program can be modified by changing intensity, volume, frequency, and recovery.

- Discuss how plyometrics can be integrated into a rehabilitation program.

- Recognize the value of different plyometric exercises in rehabilitation.

WHAT IS PLYOMETRIC EXERCISE?

In sports training and rehabilitation of athletic injuries, the concept of specificity has emerged as an important parameter in determining the proper choice and sequence of exercise in a training program. The jumping movement is inherent in numerous sport activities such as basketball, volleyball, gymnastics, and aerobic dancing. Even running is a repeated series of jump-landing cycles. Consequently, jump training should be used in the design and implementation of the overall training program.

Prentice WE, ed.
Rehabilitation Techniques for Sports Medicine and Athletic Training (pp 285–310).
© 2015 SLACK Incorporated.

Peak performance in sport requires technical skill and power. Skill in most activities combines natural athletic ability and learned specialized proficiency in an activity. Success in most activities is dependent upon the speed at which muscular force or power can be generated. Strength and conditioning programs throughout the years have attempted to augment the force production system to maximize the power generation. Because power combines strength and speed, it can be increased by increasing the amount of work or force that is produced by the muscles or by decreasing the amount of time required to produce the force. Although weight training can produce increased gains in strength, the speed of movement is limited. The amount of time required to produce muscular force is an important variable for increasing the power output. Plyometrics is a form of training that attempts to combine speed of movement with strength.

The roots of plyometric training can be traced to Eastern Europe, where it was known simply as jump training.[19,20,39–41] The term *plyometrics* was coined by an American track and field coach, Fred Wilt.[46] The development of the term is confusing. Plyo- comes from the Greek word *plythein*, which means "to increase." *Plio* is the Greek word for "ore," and metric literally means "to measure." Practically, plyometrics is defined as a quick, powerful movement involving prestretching the muscle and activating the stretch-shortening cycle to produce a subsequently stronger concentric contraction. It takes advantage of the length-shortening cycle to increase muscular power.[12]

In the late 1960s and early 1970s, when the Eastern Bloc countries began to dominate sports requiring power, their training methods became the focus of attention. After the 1972 Olympics, articles began to appear in coaching magazines outlining a strange new system of jumps and bounds that had been used by the Soviets to increase speed. Valery Borzov, the 100-meter gold medalist, credited plyometric exercise for his success. As it turns out, the Eastern Bloc countries were not the originators of plyometrics, just the organizers. This system of hops and jumps has been used by American coaches for years as a method of conditioning. Both rope jumping and bench hops have been used to improve quickness and reaction times. The organization of this training method has been credited to the legendary Soviet jump coach Yuri Verhoshanski, who, during the late 1960s, began to tie this method of miscellaneous hops and jumps into an organized training plan.[39-41] The main purpose of plyometric training is to heighten the excitability of the nervous system for improved reactive ability of the neuromuscular system.[43] Therefore, any type of exercise that uses the myotatic stretch reflex to produce a more powerful response of the contracting muscle is plyometric in nature. All movement patterns in both athletes and activities of daily living involve repeated stretch-shortening cycles.

Picture a jumping athlete preparing to transfer forward energy to upward energy. As the final step is taken before jumping, the loaded leg must stop the forward momentum and change it into an upward direction. As this happens, the muscle undergoes a lengthening eccentric contraction to decelerate the movement and prestretch the muscle. This prestretch energy is then immediately released in an equal and opposite reaction, thereby producing kinetic energy. The neuromuscular system must react quickly to produce the concentric shortening contraction to prevent falling and produce the upward change in direction. Most elite athletes will naturally exhibit with great ease this ability to use stored kinetic energy. Less-gifted athletes can train this ability and enhance their production of power. Consequently, specific functional exercise to emphasize this rapid change of direction must be used to prepare patients and athletes for return to activity.[17] Because plyometric exercises train specific movements in a biomechanically accurate manner, the muscles, tendons, and ligaments are all strengthened in a functional manner.

Most of the literature to date on plyometric training has focused on the lower quarter.[1] Because all movements in athletics involve a repeated series of stretch-shortening cycles, adaptation of the plyometric principles can be used to enhance the specificity of training in other sports or activities that require a maximum amount of muscular force in a minimal amount of time. Whether the athlete is jumping or throwing, the musculature around the involved joints must first stretch and then contract to produce the explosive movement. Because of the muscular demands during the overhead throw, plyometrics have been advocated as a form of conditioning for the overhead throwing athlete.[42,45] Although the principles are similar, different forms of plyometric exercises should be applied to the upper extremity to train the stretch-shortening cycle. Additionally, the intensity of the upper extremity plyometric program is usually less than that of the lower extremity, as a result of the smaller muscle mass and type of muscle function of the upper extremity compared to the lower extremity.

The role of the core muscles of the abdominal region and the lumbar spine in providing a vital link for stability and power cannot be overlooked. Plyometric training for these muscles can be incorporated in isolated drills as well as functional activities.

BIOMECHANICAL AND PHYSIOLOGIC PRINCIPLES OF PLYOMETRIC TRAINING

The goal of plyometric training is to decrease the amount of time required between the yielding eccentric muscle contraction and the initiation of the overcoming concentric contraction. Normal physiologic movement rarely begins from a static starting position, but rather is preceded by an eccentric prestretch that loads the muscle and prepares it for the ensuing concentric contraction.[11] The coupling of this eccentric-concentric muscle contraction is known as the stretch-shortening cycle. The physiology of this stretch-shortening cycle can be broken down into two components: proprioceptive reflexes and the elastic properties of muscle fibers.[43] These components work together to produce a response, but they are discussed separately to aid understanding.

Mechanical Characteristics

The mechanical characteristics of a muscle can best be represented by a three-component model (Figure 11-1). A contractile component, a series elastic component (SEC), and a parallel elastic component all interact to produce a force output. Although the contractile component is usually the focal point of motor control, the SEC and parallel elastic component also play an important role in providing stability and integrity to the individual fibers when a muscle is lengthened.[43] During this lengthening process, energy is stored within the musculature in the form of kinetic energy.

When a muscle contracts in a concentric fashion, most of the force that is produced comes from the muscle fiber filaments sliding past one another. Force is registered externally by being transferred through the SEC. When eccentric contraction occurs, the muscle lengthens like a spring. With this lengthening, the SEC is also stretched and allowed to contribute to the overall force production. Therefore, the total force production is the sum of the force produced by the contractile component and the stretching of the SEC.

An analogy would be the stretching of a rubber band. When a stretch is applied, potential energy is stored and applied as it returns to its original length when the stretch is released. Significant increases in concentric muscle force production have been documented when immediately preceded by an eccentric contraction.[2,4,9] This increase might be partly a result of the storage of elastic energy, because the muscles are able to use the force produced by the SEC. When the muscle contracts in a concentric manner, the elastic energy that is stored in the SEC can be recovered and used to augment the shortening contraction. The ability to use this stored elastic energy is affected by three variables: time, magnitude of stretch, and velocity of stretch.[23]

The concentric contraction can be magnified only if the preceding eccentric contraction is of short range and performed quickly without delay.[2,4,9] Bosco and Komi proved this concept experimentally when they compared damped vs undamped jumps.[4] Undamped jumps produced minimal knee flexion upon landing and were followed by an immediate rebound jump. With damped jumps, the knee flexion angle increased significantly. The power output was much higher with the undamped jumps. The increased knee flexion seen in the damped jumps decreased elastic behavior of the muscle,

Figure 11-1. Three-component model.

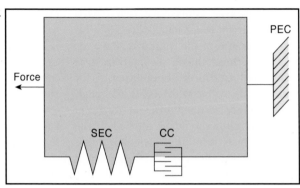

and the potential elastic energy stored in the SEC was lost as heat. Similar investigations produced greater vertical jump height when the movement was preceded by a countermovement compared to a static jump.[2,5,6,29]

The type of muscle fiber involved in the contraction can also affect storage of elastic energy. Bosco et al noted a difference in the recoil of elastic energy in slow-twitch vs. fast-twitch muscle fibers.[7] This study indicates that fast-twitch muscle fibers respond to a high-speed, small-amplitude prestretch. The amount of elastic energy used was proportional to the amount stored. When a long, slow stretch is applied to muscle, slow- and fast-twitch fibers exhibit a similar amount of stored elastic energy; however, this stored energy is used to a greater extent with the slow-twitch fibers. This trend would suggest that slow-twitch muscle fibers might be able to use elastic energy more efficiently in ballistic movement characterized by long and slow prestretching in the stretch-shortening cycle.

Neurophysiologic Mechanisms

The proprioceptive stretch reflex is the other mechanism by which force can be produced during the stretch-shortening cycle.[10] Mechanoreceptors located within the muscle provide information about the degree of muscular stretch. This information is transmitted to the central nervous system and becomes capable of influencing muscle tone, motor execution programs, and kinesthetic awareness.[43] The mechanoreceptors that are primarily responsible for the stretch reflex are the Golgi tendon organs and muscle spindles.[31] The muscle spindle is a complex stretch receptor that is located

in parallel within the muscle fibers. Sensory information regarding the length of the muscle spindle and the rate of the applied stretch is transmitted to the central nervous system. If the length of the surrounding muscle fibers is less than that of the spindle, the frequency of the nerve impulses from the spindle is reduced. When the muscle spindle becomes stretched, an afferent sensory response is produced and transmitted to the central nervous system.

Neurologic impulses are, in turn, sent back to the muscle, causing a motor response. As the muscle contracts, the stretch on the muscle spindle is relieved, thereby removing the original stimulus. The strength of the muscle spindle response is determined by the rate of stretch.[31] The more rapidly the load is applied to the muscle, the greater the firing frequency of the spindle and resultant reflexive muscle contraction.

The Golgi tendon organ lies within the muscle tendon near the point of attachment of the muscle fiber to the tendon. Unlike the facilitatory action of the muscle spindle, the Golgi tendon organ has an inhibitory effect on the muscle by contributing to a tension-limiting reflex. Because the Golgi tendon organs are in series alignment with the contracting muscle fibers, they become activated with tension or stretch within the muscle. Upon activation, sensory impulses are transmitted to the central nervous system. These sensory impulses cause an inhibition of the alpha motor neurons of the contracting muscle and its synergists, thereby limiting the amount of force produced. With a concentric muscle contraction, the activity of the muscle spindle is reduced because the surrounding muscle fibers are shortening. During an eccentric muscle contraction, the muscle stretch reflex generates more tension in the lengthening muscle. When the tension within the muscle reaches a potentially harmful level, the Golgi tendon organ fires, thereby reducing the excitation of the muscle. The muscle spindle and Golgi tendon organ systems oppose each other, and increasing force is produced. The descending neural pathways from the brain help to balance these forces and ultimately control which reflex will dominate.[34]

The degree of muscle fiber elongation is dependent upon three physiologic factors. Fiber length is proportional to the amount of stretching force applied to the muscle. The ultimate elongation or deformation is also dependent upon the absolute strength of the individual muscle fibers. The stronger the tensile strength, the less elongation that will occur. The last factor for elongation is the ability of the muscle spindle to produce a neurophysiologic response. A muscle spindle with a low sensitivity level will result in a difficulty in overcoming the rapid elongation and therefore produce a less powerful response. Plyometric training will assist in enhancing muscular control within the neurologic system.[10]

The increased force production seen during the stretch-shortening cycle is a result of the combined effects of the storage of elastic energy and the myotatic reflex activation of the muscle.[2,4,5,8,9,30,36] The percentage of contribution from each component is unknown.[5] The increased amount of force production is dependent upon the time frame between the eccentric and concentric contractions.[9] This time frame can be defined as the amortization phase.[15] The amortization phase is the electromechanical delay between eccentric and concentric contraction during which time the muscle must switch from overcoming work to acceleration in the opposite direction. Komi found that the greatest amount of tension developed within the muscle during the stretch-shortening cycle occurred during the phase of muscle lengthening just before the concentric contraction.[28] The conclusion from this study was that an increased time in the amortization phase would lead to a decrease in force production.

Physiologic performance can be improved by several mechanisms with plyometric training.

Although there has been documented evidence of increased speed of the stretch reflex, the increased intensity of the subsequent muscle contraction might be best attributed to better recruitment of additional motor units.[13,21] The force-velocity relationship states that the faster a muscle is loaded or lengthened eccentrically, the greater the resultant force output. Eccentric lengthening will also place a load on the elastic components of the muscle fibers. The stretch reflex might also increase the stiffness of the muscular spring by recruiting additional muscle fibers.[13,21] This additional stiffness might allow the muscular system to use more external stress in the form of elastic recoil.[13]

Another possible mechanism by which plyometric training can increase the force or power output involves the inhibitory effect of the Golgi tendon organs on force production. Because the Golgi tendon organ serves as a tension-limiting reflex, restricting the amount of force that can be produced, the stimulation threshold for the Golgi tendon organ becomes a limiting factor. Bosco and Komi have suggested that plyometric training can desensitize the Golgi tendon organ, thereby raising the level of inhibition.[4] If the level of inhibition is raised, a greater amount of force production and load can be applied to the musculoskeletal system.

Neuromuscular Coordination

The last mechanism in which plyometric training might improve muscular performance centers around neuromuscular coordination. The speed of muscular contraction can be limited by neuromuscular coordination. In other words, the body can move only within a set speed range, no matter how strong the muscles are. Training with an explosive pre-stretch of the muscle can improve the neural efficiency, thereby increasing neuromuscular performance. Plyometric training can promote changes within the neuromuscular system that allow the individual to have better control of the contracting muscle and its synergists, yielding a greater net force even in the absence of morphologic adaptation of the muscle. This neural adaptation can increase performance by enhancing the nervous system to become more automatic.

In summary, effective plyometric training relies more on the rate of stretch than on the length of stretch. Emphasis should center on the reduction of the amortization phase. If the amortization phase is slow, the elastic energy is lost as heat and the stretch reflex is not activated. Conversely, the quicker the individual is able to switch from yielding eccentric work to overcoming concentric work, the more powerful the response.

Clinical Decision-Making Exercise 11-1

A high school girl basketball player is engaged in an off-season conditioning program that involves box jumps and depth jumps. As a result of these activities in conjunction with a running program to enhance cardiovascular fitness, she now complains of unilateral parapatellar pain. The knee pain is significant enough that she cannot take part in the plyometric program. The coach feels the athlete needs to address both her conditioning and her power training, and wants to know what can be done to improve the athlete's performance but not increase the knee pain. How can you help?

PROGRAM DEVELOPMENT

Specificity is the key concept in any training program. Sport-specific activities should be analyzed and broken down into basic movement patterns. These specific movement patterns should then be stressed in a gradual fashion, based upon individual tolerance to these activities. Development of a plyometric program should begin by establishing an adequate strength base that will allow the body to withstand the large stress that will be placed upon it. A greater strength base will allow for greater force production because of increased muscular cross-sectional area. Additionally, a larger cross-sectional area can contribute to the SEC and subsequently store a greater amount of elastic energy.

Plyometric exercises can be characterized as rapid eccentric loading of the musculoskeletal complex.[13] This type of exercise trains the neuromuscular system by teaching it to more readily accept the increased strength loads.[3] Also, the nervous system is more readily able to react with maximal speed to the lengthening muscle by exploiting the stretch reflex. Plyometric training attempts to fine tune the neuromuscular system, so all training programs should be designed with specificity in mind.[33] This goal will help to ensure that the body is prepared to accept the stress that will be placed upon it during return to function.

Plyometric Prerequisites

Biomechanical Examination

Before beginning a plyometric training program, a cursory biomechanical examination and a battery of functional tests should be performed to identify potential contraindications or precautions. Lower-quarter biomechanics should be sound to help ensure a stable base of support and normal force transmission. Biomechanical abnormalities of the lower quarter are not contraindications for plyometrics but can contribute to stress failure-overuse injury if not addressed. Before initiating plyometric training, an adequate strength base of the stabilizing musculature must be present.

Functional tests are very effective to screen for an adequate strength base before initiating plyometrics. Poor strength in the lower extremities will result in a loss of stability when landing and also increase the amount of stress that is absorbed by the weight-bearing tissues with high-impact forces, which will reduce performance and increase the risk of injury. The Eastern Bloc countries arbitrarily placed a one-repetition maximum in the squat at 1.5 to 2 times the individual's body weight before initiating lower-quarter plyometrics.[3] If this were to hold true, a 200-pound individual would have to squat 300 to 400 pounds before beginning plyometrics. Unfortunately, not many individuals would meet this minimal criteria. Clinical and practical experience has demonstrated that plyometrics can be started without that kind of leg strength.[13] A simple functional parameter to use in determining whether an individual is strong enough to initiate a plyometric training program has been advocated by Chu.[14] Power squat testing with a weight equal to 60% of the individual's body weight is used. The individual is asked to perform five squat repetitions in 5 seconds. If the individual cannot perform this task, emphasis in the training program should again center on the strength-training program to develop an adequate base.

Clinical Decision-Making Exercise 11-2

A college track sprinter has been instructed by her strength coach to begin off-season plyometrics consisting of box jumps and high stepping drills. The patient suffered a second-degree upper hamstring strain during the last half of track season and is reluctant to start the plyometric program. What can be done to prevent this injury from recurring?

Because eccentric muscle strength is an important component to plyometric training, it is especially important to ensure an adequate eccentric strength base is present. Before an individual is allowed to begin a plyometric regimen, a program of closed chain stability training that focuses on eccentric lower-quarter strength should be initiated. In addition to strengthening in a functional manner, closed chain weight-bearing exercises also allow the individual to use functional movement patterns. The same holds true for adequate upper-extremity strength prior to initiating an upper-extremity plyometric program. Closed chain activities, such as wall push-ups, traditional push-ups, and their modification, as well as functional tests, can be used to ascertain readiness for upper-extremity plyometrics.[24,37,38] Once cleared to participate in the plyometric program, precautionary safety tips should be adhered to.

Stability Testing

Stability testing before initiating plyometric training can be divided into two subcategories: static stability and dynamic movement testing. Static stability testing determines the individual's ability to stabilize and control the body. The muscles of postural support must be strong enough to withstand the stress of explosive training. Static stability testing should begin with simple movements of low motor complexity and progress to more difficult high motor skills. The basis for lower-quarter stability centers on single-leg strength. Difficulty can be increased by having the individual close his or her eyes. The basic static tests are one-leg

standing and single-leg quarter squats that are held for 30 seconds. An individual should be able to perform one-leg standing for 30 seconds with eyes open and closed before the initiation of plyometric training. The individual should be observed for shaking or wobbling of the extremity joints. If there is more movement of a weight-bearing joint in one direction than the other, the musculature producing the movement in the opposite direction needs to be assessed for specific weakness. If weakness is determined, the individual's program should be limited and emphasis placed on isolated strengthening of the weak muscles. For dynamic jump exercises to be initiated, there should be no wobbling of the support leg during the quarter knee squats. After an individual has satisfactorily demonstrated both single-leg static stance and a single-leg quarter squat, more dynamic tests of eccentric capabilities can be initiated.

Once an individual has stabilization strength, the concern shifts toward developing and evaluating eccentric strength. The limiting factor in high-intensity, high-volume plyometrics is eccentric capabilities. Eccentric strength can be assessed with stabilization jump tests. If an individual has an excessively long amortization phase or a slow switching from eccentric to concentric contractions, the eccentric strength levels are insufficient.

PLYOMETRIC STATIC STABILITY TESTING		
Single-leg stance— 30 seconds	Single-leg 25% squat— 30 seconds	Single-leg 50% squat— 30 seconds
• Eyes open	• Eyes open	• Eyes open
• Eyes closed	• Eyes closed	• Eyes closed

Dynamic Movement Testing

Dynamic movement testing assesses the individual's ability to produce explosive, coordinated movement. Vertical or single-leg jumping for distance can be used for the lower quarter. Researchers have investigated the use of single-leg hop for distance and a determinant for return to play after knee injury. A passing score on their test is 85% regarding symmetry. The involved leg is tested twice, and the average between the two trials is recorded. The noninvolved leg is tested in the same fashion, and then the scores of the noninvolved leg are divided by the scores of the involved leg and multiplied by 100. This provides the symmetry index score. Another functional test that can be used to determine whether an individual is ready for plyometric training is the ability to long jump a distance equal to the individual's height. In the upper quarter, the medicine ball toss is used as a functional assessment. The seated chest press is used as a measure of upper body power. To perform this test, the patient sits tall with his or her back against the back rest of a chair. While holding onto a medicine ball (4 kg for men and 2 kg for women and juniors), the patient tries to chest pass the ball as far as possible, keeping his or her back in contact with the chair. This should be repeated until the longest pass has been measured. Use the distance from where the ball bounces to the patient's chest as the distance. As can be seen in Table 11-1, less than 17 feet for men and 15 feet for women is an indicator of power weakness. The sit-up and throw test is a great test to assess abdominal and lat power. The sit-up evaluates core power and the overhead throw evaluates the lat and trunk power. To perform this test, the patient lies supine with the patient's knees bent and feet flat on the ground, while holding onto a medicine ball with both hands (4 kg for men and 2 kg for women and juniors) with the ball directly over the patient's head like a soccer throw-in. Next, have the patient try to sit up and throw the ball as far as possible. This should be repeated until the longest pass has been measured. Use the distance from where the ball bounces to the patient's chest as the distance (Table 11-2).

Flexibility

Another important prerequisite for plyometric training is general and specific flexibility, because a high amount of stress is applied to the musculoskeletal system. Consequently, all plyometric training sessions should begin with a general warm-up and flexibility exercise program. The warm-up should produce mild sweating.[26] The flexibility exercise program should address muscle groups involved in the

plyometric program and should include static and short dynamic stretching techniques.[25]

Plyometric Prerequisites Summary

When the individual can demonstrate static and dynamic control of his or her body weight with single-leg squats or adequate medicine ball throws for the upper extremity and core, low-intensity in-place plyometrics can be initiated. Plyometric training should consist of low-intensity drills and progress slowly in deliberate fashion. As skill and strength foundation increase, moderate-intensity plyometrics can be introduced. Mature patients with strong weight-training backgrounds can be introduced to ballistic-reactive plyometric exercises of high intensity.[14] Once the individual has been classified as beginner, intermediate, or advanced, the plyometric program can be designed and initiated.

PLYOMETRIC PROGRAM DESIGN

As with any conditioning program, the plyometric training program can be manipulated through training variables: direction of body movement, weight of the individual, speed of the execution, external load, intensity, volume, frequency, training age, and recovery (Table 11-3).

Direction of Body Movement

Horizontal body movement is less stressful than vertical movement. This is dependent upon the weight of the patient and the technical proficiency demonstrated during the jumps.

Clinical Decision-Making Exercise 11-3

The coach of a junior football league team (ages 10 and 11) wants to institute a plyometric conditioning program for the team. The coach has met some resistance from concerned parents regarding the intensity of this type of training. A meeting with the parents has been scheduled and the coach wants you to discuss plyometric training with them. What things should the athletic trainer address in this meeting?

Table 11-1 Seated Chest Pass Test

	Distance in Feet			
	Excellent	Good	Average	Needs Work
Female				
Adult	>21	17 to 21	15 to 17	<15
Junior (<16 years)	>19	16 to 19	14 to 16	<14
Male				
Adult	>24	20 to 24	17 to 20	<17
Junior (<16 years)	>20	18 to 20	15 to 18	<15

Table 11-2 Sit-up and Throw Test

	Distance in Feet			
	Excellent	Good	Average	Needs Work
Female				
Adult	>21	17 to 21	15 to 17	<15
Junior (<16 years)	>19	16 to 19	14 to 16	<14
Male				
Adult	>24	20 to 24	17 to 20	<17
Junior (<16 years)	>20	18 to 20	15 to 18	<15

Table 11-3 Chu's Plyometric Categories

In-place jumping
Standing jumps
Multiple-response jumps and hops
In-depth jumping and box drills
Bounding
High-stress sport-specific drills

Weight of the Patient

The heavier the patient, the greater the training demand placed on the patient. What might be a low-demand in-place jump for a lightweight patient might be a high-demand activity for a heavyweight patient.

Speed of Execution of the Exercise

Increased speed of execution on exercises like single-leg hops or alternate-leg bounding raises the training demand on the individual.

External Load

Adding an external load can significantly raise the training demand. Do not raise the external load to a level that will significantly slow the speed of movement.

Intensity

Intensity can be defined as the amount of effort exerted. With traditional weight lifting, intensity can be modified by changing the amount of weight that is lifted. With plyometric training, intensity can be controlled by the type of exercise that is performed. Double-leg jumping is less stressful than single-leg jumping. As with all functional exercise, the plyometric exercise program should progress from simple to complex activities. Intensity can be further increased by altering the specific exercises. The addition of external weight or raising the height of the step or box will also increase the exercise intensity.[22]

Volume

Volume is the total amount of work that is performed in a single workout session. With weight training, volume would be recorded as the total amount of weight that was lifted (weight times repetitions). Volume of plyometric training is measured by counting the total number of foot contacts. The recommended volume of foot contacts in any one session will vary inversely with the intensity of the exercise. A beginner should start with low-intensity exercise with a volume of about 75- to 100-foot contacts. As ability is increased, the volume is increased to 200- to 250-foot contacts of low-to-moderate intensity.

Frequency

Frequency is the number of times an exercise session is performed during a training cycle. With weight training, the frequency of exercise has typically been three times weekly. Unfortunately, research on the frequency of plyometric exercise has not been conducted. Therefore, the optimum frequency for increased performance is not known. It has been suggested that 48 to 72 hours of rest are necessary for full recovery before the next training stimulus.[14] Intensity, however, plays a major role in determining the frequency of training. If an adequate recovery period does not occur, muscle fatigue will result with a corresponding increase in neuromuscular reaction times. The beginner should allow at least 48 hours between training sessions.

Training Age

Training age is the number of years an individual has been in a formal training program. At younger training ages, the overall training demand should be kept low. Prepubescent and pubescent individuals of both sexes are engaged in more intense physical training programs. Many of these programs contain plyometric drills. Because youth sports involve plyometric movements, training for these sports should also involve plyometric activities. The literature does not have long-term data looking at the effects of plyometric activities on human articular cartilage and long bone growth. Research demonstrates that plyometric training does indeed result in strength gains in prepubescent individuals, and that plyometric training may in fact contribute to increased bone mineral content in young females.[18,47]

Recovery

Recovery is the rest time used between exercise sets. Manipulation of this variable will depend on whether the goal is to increase power or muscular endurance. Because plyometric training is anaerobic in nature, a longer recovery period should be used to allow restoration of metabolic stores. With power training, a work-to-rest ratio of one to three or one to four should be used. This time frame will allow maximal recovery between sets. For endurance training, this work-to-rest ratio can be shortened to one to one or one to two. Endurance training typically uses circuit training, where the individual moves from one exercise set to another with minimal rest in between.

The beginning plyometric program should emphasize the importance of eccentric vs. concentric muscle contractions. The relevance of the stretch-shortening cycle with decreased amortization time should be stressed. Initiation of lower-quarter plyometric training begins with low-intensity in-place and multiple-response jumps. The individual should be instructed in proper exercise technique. The feet should be nearly flat in all landings, and the individual should be encouraged to "touch and go." An analogy would be landing on a hot bed of coals. The goal is to reverse the landing as quickly as possible, spending only a minimal amount of time on the ground.

Clinical Decision-Making Exercise 11-4

During the off-season, a college lineman has set personal goals to increase his weight from his present playing weight of 270 pounds to 290 pounds. He also wants to improve his quickness off the line. He is engaged in traditional strength training and an aerobic program, and he wants to add plyometrics to the program. Is his body weight a contraindication for a plyometric program?

Success of the plyometric program will depend on how well the training variables are controlled, modified, and manipulated. In general, as the intensity of the exercise is increased, the volume is decreased. The corollary to this is that as volume increases, the intensity is decreased. The overall key to successfully controlling these variables is to be flexible and listen to what the individual's body is telling you. The body's response to the program will dictate the speed of progression. Whenever in doubt as to the exercise intensity or volume, it is better to underestimate to prevent injury.

Before implementing a plyometric program, the athletic trainer should assess the type of patient that is being rehabilitated and whether plyometrics are suitable for that individual. In most cases, plyometrics should be used in the latter phases of rehabilitation, starting in the advanced strengthening phase once the patient has obtained an appropriate strength base.[36,38] When using plyometric training in the uninjured population, the application of plyometric exercise should follow the concept of periodization.[43] The concept of periodization refers to the year-round sequence and progression of strength training, conditioning, and sport-specific skills.[45] There are four specific phases in the year-round periodization model: the competitive season, postseason training, the preparation phase, and the transitional phase.[43] Plyometric exercises should be performed in the latter stages of the preparation phase and during the transitional phase for optimal results and safety. To obtain the benefits of a plyometric program, the individual should (a) be well conditioned with sufficient strength and endurance, (b) exhibit athletic abilities, (c) exhibit coordination and proprioceptive abilities, and (d) be free of pain from any physical injury or condition.

It should be remembered that the plyometric program is not designed to be an exclusive training program for the individual. Rather, it should be one part of a well-structured training program that includes strength training, flexibility training, cardiovascular fitness, and sport-specific training for skill enhancement and coordination. By combining the plyometric program with other training techniques, the effects of training are greatly enhanced. Tables 11-4 and 11-5 suggest upper-extremity and lower-extremity plyometric drills.

GUIDELINES FOR PLYOMETRIC PROGRAMS

The proper execution of the plyometric exercise program must continually be stressed. A sound technical foundation from which higher-intensity work can build should be established. It must be remembered that jumping is a continuous interchange between force reduction and force production. This interchange takes place throughout the entire body: ankle, knee, hip, trunk, and arms. The timing and coordination of these body segments yields a positive ground reaction that will result in a high rate of force production.[16]

> **Clinical Decision-Making Exercise 11-5**
>
> A teenage girl amateur swimmer swims distance freestyle events and has generalized ligamentous laxity. During the course of the previous season she complained of shoulder pain. Her pain was accompanied by increased times in all of her events. Her physician diagnosed her with multidirectional instability and secondary shoulder impingement syndrome. The physician wants the patient to begin a plyometric program. How will you incorporate plyometrics into the training program?

As the plyometric program is initiated, the individual must be made aware of several guidelines.[43] Any deviation from these guidelines will result in minimal improvement and increased risk for injury. These guidelines include the following:

1. Plyometric training should be specific to the individual goals. Activity-specific movement patterns should be trained. These sport-specific skills should be broken down and trained in their smaller components and then rebuilt into a coordinated activity-specific movement pattern.

2. The quality of work is more important than the quantity of work. The intensity of the exercise should be kept at a maximal level.

Table 11-4 Upper-Extremity Plyometric Drills

I. Warm-up drills	Plyoball trunk rotation
	Plyoball side bends
	Plyoball wood chops
	External rotation (ER)/internal rotation (IR) with tubing
	Proprioceptive neuromuscular feedback (PNF) D2 pattern with tubing
II. Throwing movements—standing position	Two-hand chest pass
	Two-hand overhead soccer throw
	Two-hand side throw overhead
	Tubing ER/IR (Both at side and 90-degree abduction)
	Tubing PNF D2 pattern
	One-hand baseball throw
	One-hand IR side throw
	One-hand ER side throw
	Plyo pushup (against wall)
III. Throwing movements—seated position	Two-hand overhead soccer throw
	Two-hand side-to-side throw
	Two-hand chest pass
	One-hand baseball throw
IV. Trunk drills	Plyoball sit-ups
	Plyoball sit-up and throw
	Plyoball back extension
	Plyoball long sitting side throws
V. Partner drills	Overhead soccer throw
	Plyoball back-to-back twists
	Overhead pullover throw
	Kneeling side throw
	Backward throw
	Chest pass throw
VI. Wall drills	Two-hand chest throw
	Two-hand overhead soccer throw
	Two-hand underhand side-to-side throw
	One-hand baseball throw
	One-hand wall dribble
VII. Endurance drills	One-hand wall dribble
	Around-the-back circles
	Figure 8 through the legs
	Single-arm ball flips

Table 11-5 Lower-Extremity Plyometric Drills

I. Warm-up drills	Double-leg squats
	Double-leg leg press
	Double-leg squat-jumps
	Jumping jacks
II. Entry-level drills—two-legged	Two-legged drills
	Side to side (floor/line)
	Diagonal jumps (floor/4 corners)
	Diagonal jumps (4 spots)
	Diagonal zig-zag (6 spots)
	Plyo leg press
	Plyo leg press (4 corners)
III. Intermediate-level drills	Two-legged box jumps
	One-box side jump
	Two-box side jumps
	Two-box side jumps with foam
	Four-box diagonal jumps
	Two-box with rotation
	One-/two-box with catch
	One-/two-box with catch (foam)
	Single-leg movements
	Single-leg plyo leg press
	Single-leg side jumps (floor)
	Single-leg side-to-side jumps (floor/4 corners)
	Single-leg diagonal jumps (floor/4 corners)
IV. Advanced-level drills	Single-leg box jumps
	One-box side jumps
	Two-box side jumps
	Single-leg plyo leg press (4 corners)
	Two-box side jumps with foam
	Four-box diagonal jumps
	One-box side jumps with rotation
	Two-box side jumps with rotation
	One-box side jump with catch
	One-box side jump rotation with catch
	Two-box side jump with catch
	Two-box side jump rotation with catch
V. Endurance/agility plyometrics	Side-to-side bounding (20 ft)
	Side jump lunges (cone)
	Side jump lunges (cone with foam)

(continued)

Table 11-5 Lower-Extremity Plyometric Drills (*continued*)

	Altering rapid step-up (forward)
	Lateral step-overs
	High stepping (forward)
	High stepping (backward)
	Depth jump with rebound jump
	Depth jump with catch
	Jump and catch (Plyoball)

3. The greater the exercise intensity level, the greater the recovery time.

4. Plyometric training can have its greatest benefit at the conclusion of the normal workout. This pattern will best replicate exercise under a partial to total fatigue environment that is specific to activity. Only low- to medium-stress plyometrics should be used at the conclusion of a workout, because of the increased potential of injury with high-stress drills.

5. When proper technique can no longer be demonstrated, maximum volume has been achieved and the exercise must be stopped. Training improperly or with fatigue can lead to injury.

6. The plyometric training program should be progressive in nature. The volume and intensity can be modified in several ways:

   a. Increase the number of exercises.

   b. Increase the number of repetitions and sets.

   c. Decrease the rest period between sets of exercise.

7. Plyometric training sessions should be conducted no more than three times weekly in the preseason phase of training. During this phase, volume should prevail. During the competitive season, the frequency of plyometric training should be reduced to twice weekly, with the intensity of the exercise becoming more important.

8. Dynamic testing of the individual on a regular basis will provide important progression and motivational feedback.

9. In addition to proper technique and exercise dosage, proper equipment is also required. Equipment should allow for the safe performance of the activity, landing surfaces should be even and allow for as much shock absorption as possible, and footwear should provide adequate shock absorption and forefoot support.

The key element in the execution of proper technique is the eccentric or landing phase. The shock of landing from a jump is not absorbed exclusively by the foot but rather is a combination of the ankle, knee, and hip joints all working together to absorb the shock of landing and then transferring the force.

INTEGRATING PLYOMETRICS INTO THE REHABILITATION PROGRAM: CLINICAL CONCERNS

When used judiciously, plyometrics are a valuable asset in the sports rehabilitation program.[35] Clinical plyometrics should involve loading of the healing tissue. These activities may include (a) medial/lateral loading, (b) rotational loading, and (c) shock absorption/deceleration loading. In addition, plyometric drills will be divided into (a) in-place activities (activities that can be performed in essentially the same or small amount of space), (b) dynamic distance drills (activities that occur across a given distance), and (c) depth jumping (jumping down from a predetermined height and performing a variety of activities upon landing). Simple jumping drills (bilateral activities) can be progressed to hopping (unilateral activities).

Medial-Lateral Loading

Virtually all sporting activities involve cutting maneuvers. Inherent to cutting activities is adequate function in the medial and lateral directions. A plyometric program designed to stress the individual's ability to accept weight on the involved lower extremity and then perform cutting activities off that leg is imperative. Individuals who have suffered sprains to the medial or lateral capsular and ligamentous complex of the ankle and knee, as well as the hip abductor/adductor and ankle invertor/evertor muscle strains, are candidates for medial-lateral plyometric loading. Medial-lateral loading drills should be implemented following injury to the medial soft tissue around the knee after a valgus stress. By gradually imparting progressive valgus loads, tissue tensile strength is augmented.[48] In the rehabilitation setting, bilateral support drills can be progressed to unilateral valgus loading efforts. Specifically, lateral jumping drills are progressed to lateral hopping activities. However, the medial structures must also be trained to accept greater valgus loads sustained during cutting activities. As a prerequisite to full-speed cutting, lateral bounding drills should be performed. These efforts are progressed to activities that add acceleration, deceleration, and momentum. Lateral sliding activities that require the individual to cover a greater distance can be performed on a slide board. If a slide board is

not available, the same movement pattern can be stressed with plyometrics (Figure 11-2).

In-Place Activities
- Lateral bounding (quick step valgus loading)
- Slide bounds
  Dynamic Distance Drills
- Crossovers

Rotational Loading

Because rotation in the knee is controlled by the cruciate ligaments, menisci, and capsule, plyometric activities with a rotational component are instrumental in the rehabilitation program after injury to any of these structures. As previously discussed, care must be taken not to exceed healing time constraints when using plyometric training.

In-Place Activities
- Spin jumps
  Dynamic Distance Drills
- Lateral hopping

Shock Absorption (Deceleration Loading)

Perhaps some of the most physically demanding plyometric activities are shock absorption activities, which place a tremendous amount of stress upon muscle, tendon, and articular cartilage. As previously stated, the majority of lower-quarter sport function occurs in the closed kinetic chain. Lower-extremity plyometrics are an effective functional closed chain exercise that can be incorporated into the rehabilitation program. Through the eccentric prestretch, plyometrics place added stress on the tendinous portion of the contractile unit. Eccentric loading is beneficial in the management of tendinitis.[44] Through a gradually progressed eccentric loading program, healing tendinous tissue is stressed, yielding an increase in ultimate tensile strength.

This eccentric load can be applied through jump-down exercises (Figure 11-6). Therefore, in the final preparation for a return to sports involving repetitive jumping and hopping, shock absorption drills should be included in the rehabilitation program.[27]

Figure 11-2. (A) Slideboard ice skater glides. (B) Ice skaters.

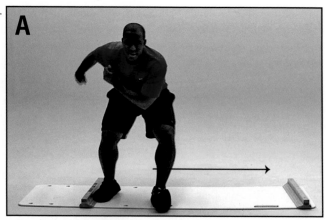

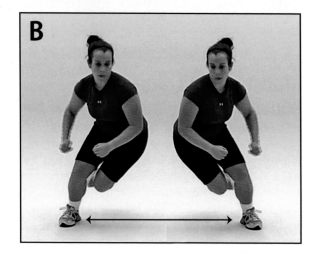

One way to prepare the individual for shock absorption drills is to gradually maximize the effects of gravity, such as beginning in a gravity-minimized position and progressing to performance against gravity. Popular activities to minimize gravity include water activities or assisted efforts through unloading jumps and hops in the supine position on a leg press or similar device.

In-Place Activities

- Cycle jumps
- Five-dot drill

    Depth Jumping Preparation

- Jump-downs

SPECIFIC PLYOMETRIC EXERCISES

Plyometric drills can be categorized into (a) weighted ball toss plyometric exercises (Figure 11-3); (b) dynamic weighted ball plyometric exercises (Figure 11-4); (c) in-place jumping plyometric exercises (Figure 11-5), which involve activities that can be performed in essentially the same or small amount of space; and (d) depth jumping and bounding plyometric exercises (Figure 11-6) that may involve jumping down from a predetermined height and performing a variety of activities upon landing or activities that occur across a given distance. In-place jumping drills (bilateral activities) can be progressed to hopping (unilateral activities). Chapters 17 through 24 have additional region-specific plyometric exercises commonly used in rehabilitation.

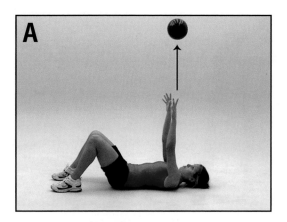
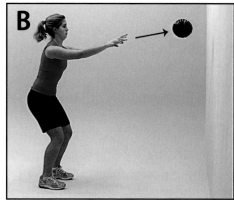
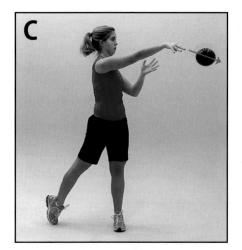
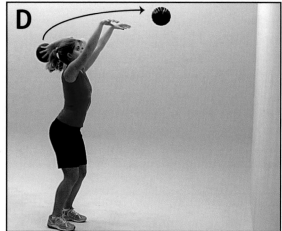
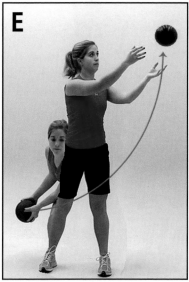
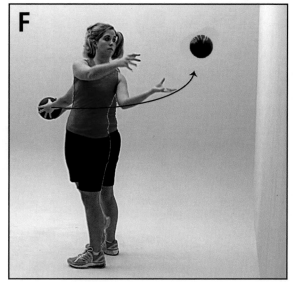

Figure 11-3. Weighted ball toss plyometric exercises. (A) Supine toss; (B) two-arm chest pass; (C) one-arm chest pass with rotation; (D) soccer throw; (E) two-arm rotation toss from squat; (F) reverse toss with rotation. (*continued*)

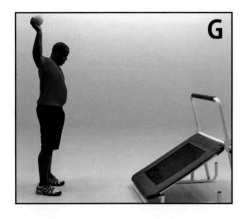
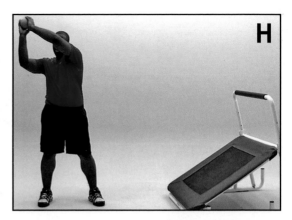
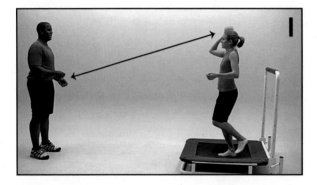
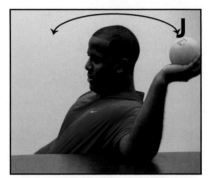
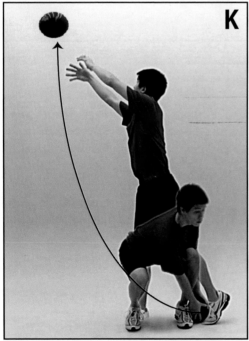
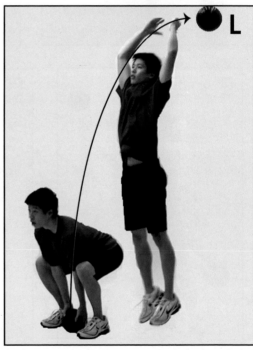

Figure 11-3. (G) plyoback standing single-arm toss; (H) plyoback two-arm toss with rotation; (I) plyoback single-leg partner ball toss; (J) single-arm ball throw; (K) backward extension rotation toss; (L) overhead backward toss.

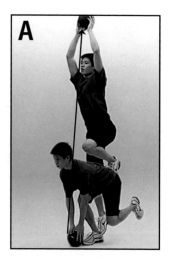
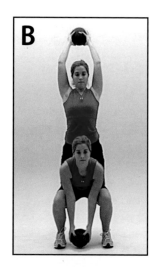
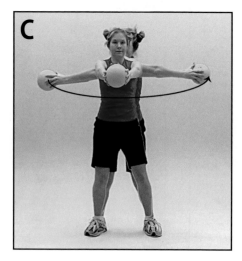
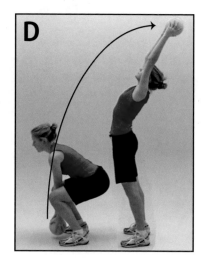
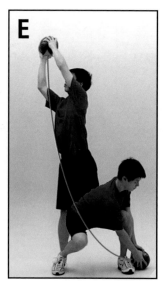
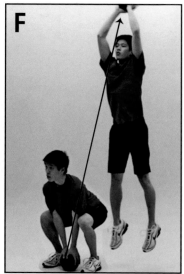

Figure 11-4. Weighted ball plyometric exercises. (A) Single-leg jump; (B) squat to overhead; (C) standing rotations; (D) standing extension; (E) D2 PNF pattern. (F) double-leg jump. (*continued*)

Figure 11-4. (G) forward jump from squat.

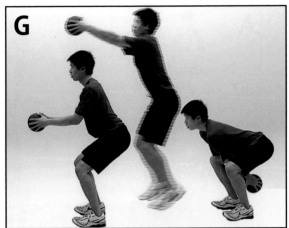

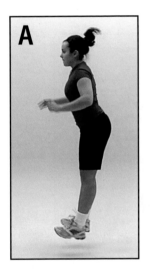

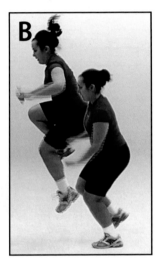

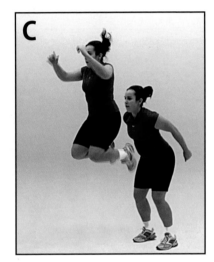

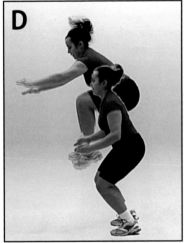

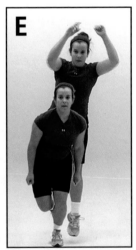

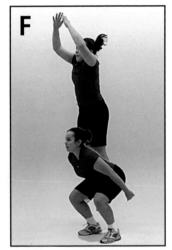

Figure 11-5. In-place jumping plyometric exercises. (A) Ankle jumps; (B) single-leg tuck jumps; (C) two-leg butt kicks; (D) two-leg tuck jumps; (E) single-leg hops; (F) squat jumps, leg lateral hop-overs. (*continued*)

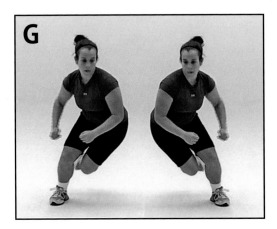

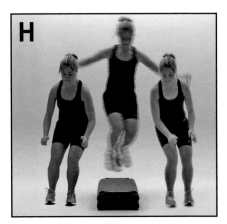

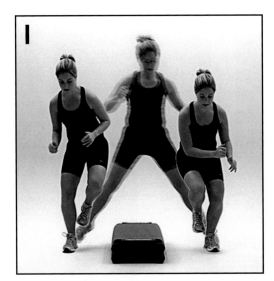

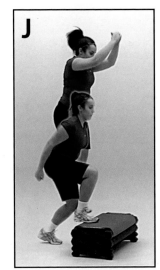

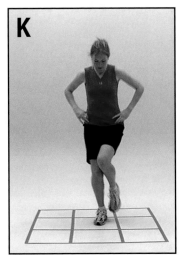

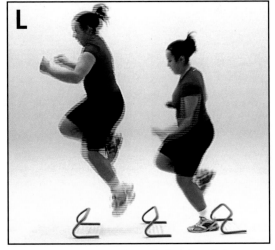

Figure 11-5. (G) ice skaters; (H) two-leg lateral hop-overs; (I) single-leg lateral hop-overs; (J) alternate-leg power step-ups; (K) single-leg shark skill test; (L) single-leg short hurdle jump.

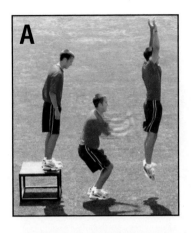

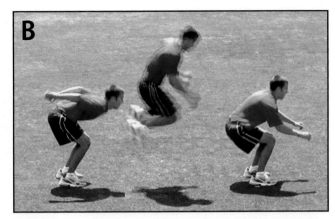

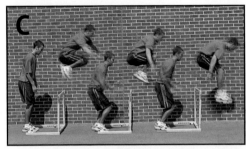

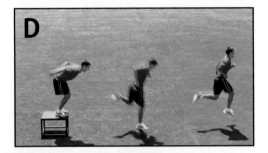

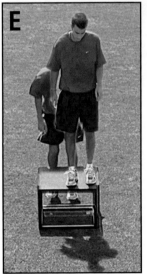

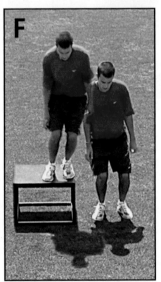

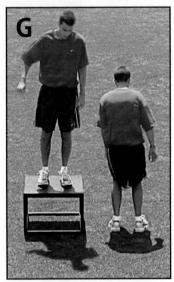

Figure 11-6. Depth jumping and bounding plyometric exercises. (A) Depth jump to vertical jump; (B) repeat two leg standing long jumps; (C) three-hurdle jumps; (D) depth jump to bounding; (E) box jumps up and down sagittal plane; (F) box jumps up and down frontal plane; (G) box jumps up and down transverse plane.

The exercises in Figures 11-3 through 11-6 are a good starting point from which to develop a clinical plyometric program. Manipulations of volume, frequency, and intensity can advance the program appropriately. Proper progression is of prime importance when using plyometrics in the rehabilitation program. These progressive activities are reinjuries waiting to happen if the progression does not allow for adequate healing or development of an adequate strength base.[32] A close working relationship fostering open communication and acute observation skills is vital in helping ensure that the program is not overly aggressive.

Summary

1. Although the effects of plyometric training are not yet fully understood, it still remains a widely used form of combining strength with speed training to functionally increase power. Although the research is somewhat contradictory, the neurophysiologic concept of plyometric training is based on a sound foundation.

2. A successful plyometric training program should be carefully designed and implemented after establishing an adequate strength base.

3. The effects of this type of high-intensity training can be achieved safely if the individual is supervised by a knowledgeable person who uses common sense and follows the prescribed training regimen.

4. The plyometric training program should use a large variety of different exercises, because year-round training often results in boredom and a lack of motivation.

5. Program variety can be manipulated with different types of equipment or kinds of movement performed.

6. Continued motivation and an organized progression are the keys to successful training.

7. Plyometrics are also a valuable asset in the rehabilitation program after a sport injury.

8. Used after both upper- and lower-quarter injury, plyometrics are effective in facilitating joint awareness, strengthening tissue during the healing process, and increasing sport-specific strength and power.

9. The most important considerations in the plyometric program are common sense and experience.

References

1. Adams T. An investigation of selected plyometric training exercises on muscular leg strength and power. *Track Field Q Rev.* 1984;84(1):36-40.

2. Asmussen E, Bonde-Peterson F. Storage of elastic energy in skeletal muscles in man. *Acta Physiol Scand.* 1974;91:385.

3. Bielik E, Chu D, Costello F, et al Roundtable: 1. Practical considerations for utilizing plyometrics. *Strength Cond J.* 1986;8:14.

4. Bosco C, Komi PV. Potentiation of the mechanical behavior of the human skeletal muscle through prestretching. *Acta Physiol Scand.* 1979;106:467.

5. Bosco C, Komi PV. Muscle elasticity in athletes. In: Komi PV, ed. *Exercise and Sports Biology.* Champaign, IL: Human Kinetics; 1982;191-197.

6. Bosco C, Tarkka J, Komi PV. Effect of elastic energy and myoelectric potentiation of triceps surae during stretch-shortening cycle exercise. *Int J Sports Med.* 1982;2:137.

7. Bosco C, Tihanyia J, Komi PV, et al Store and recoil of elastic energy in slow and fast types of human skeletal muscles. *Acta Physiol Scand.* 1987;16:343.

8. Cavagna GA, Dusman B, Margaria R. Positive work done by a previously stretched muscle. *J Appl Physiol.* 1968;24:21.

9. Cavagna G, Saibene F, Margaria R. Effect of negative work on the amount of positive work performed by an isolated muscle. *J Appl Physiol.* 1965;20:157.

10. Chimera, N, Swanik, K, Swanik C. Effects of plyometric training on muscle-activation strategies and performance in female athletes. *J Athl Train.* 2004;39(1): 24-31.

11. Chmielewski T, Myer G, Kauffman D. Plyometric exercise in the rehabilitation of athletes: physiological responses and clinical application. *J Orthop Sports Phys Ther.* 2006;36(5):308-319.

12. Chu D. Plyometric exercise. *Strength Cond J.* 1984;6:56.

13. Chu D. *Conditioning/Plyometrics.* Paper presented at 10th Annual Sports Medicine Team Concept Conference, San Francisco, CA; December, 1989.

14. Chu D. *Jumping into Plyometrics.* Champaign, IL: Leisure Press; 1992.

15. Chu D, Plummer L. The language of plyometrics. *Strength Cond J.* 1984;6:30.

16. Cissik J. Plyometric fundamentals. *NSCA Perform Train J.* 2004;3(2):9-13.

17. Curwin S, Stannish WD. *Tendinitis: Its Etiology and Treatment.* Lexington, MA: Collamore Press; 1984.

18. Diallo O, Dore E, Duchercise P, et al Effects of plyometric training followed by a reduced training programme on physical performance in prepubescent soccer players. *J Sports Med Phys Fitness.* 2001;41:342-48.

19. Dunsenev CI. Strength training for jumpers. *Soviet Sports Rev.* 1979;14:2.

20. Dunsenev CI. Strength training of jumpers. *Track Field Q.* 1982;82:4.

21. Ebben W, Simenz C, Jensen R. Evaluation of plyometric intensity using electromyography. *J Strength Cond Res.* 2008;22(3):861.

22. Ebben W. Practical guidelines for plyometric intensity. *NSCA Perform Train J.* 2007;6(5):12.

23. Enoka RM. *Neuromechanical Basis of Kinesiology.* Champaign, IL: Human Kinetics; 1989.

24. Goldbeck T, Davies G. Test-retest reliability of the closed chain upper extremity stability test: a clinical field test. *J Sport Rehabil.* 2000;9:35-45.

25. Javorek I. Plyometrics. *Strength Cond J.* 1989;11:52.

26. Jensen C. Pertinent facts about warming. *Athl J.* 1975;56:72.

27. Katchajov S, Gomberaze K, Revson A. Rebound jumps. *Mod Athl Coach.* 1976;14(4):23.

28. Komi PV. Physiological and biomechanical correlates of muscle function: effects of muscle structure and stretch shortening cycle on force and speed. In: Terjung R, ed. *Exercise and Sports Sciences Review.* Lexington, MA: Collamore Press; 1984;81-122.

29. Komi PV, Bosco C. Utilization of stored elastic energy in leg extensor muscles by men and women. *Med Sci Sports Exerc.* 1978;10(4):261.

30. Komi PV, Buskirk E. Effects of eccentric and concentric muscle conditioning on tension and electrical activity of human muscle. *Ergonomics.* 1972;15:417.

31. Lundon P. A review of plyometric training. *Strength Cond J.* 1985;7:69.

32. Pretz, R. Plyometric exercises for overhead-throwing athletes. *Strength Cond J.* 2006;28(1):36.

33. Rach PJ, Grabiner DM, Gregor JR, et al *Kinesiology and Applied Anatomy.* 7th ed. Philadelphia, PA: Lea & Febiger; 1989.

34. Rowinski M. *The Role of Eccentric Exercise.* Shirley, NY: Biodex Corp, Pro Clinica; 1988.

35. Shiner J, Bishop T, Cosgarea A. Integrating low-intensity plyometrics into strength and conditioning programs. *Strength Cond J.* 2005;27(6):10.

36. Thomas DW. Plyometrics — more than the stretch reflex. *Strength Cond J.* 1988;10:49.

37. Tippett S. Closed chain exercise. *Orthop Phys Ther Clin N Am.* 1992;1:253-267.

38. Tippett S, Voight M. *Functional Progressions for Sport Rehabilitation.* Champaign, IL: Human Kinetics; 1995.

39. Verhoshanski Y. Are depth jumps useful? *Yesis Rev Soviet Phys Educ Sport.* 1969;4:74-79.

40. Verhoshanski Y, Chornonson G. Jump exercises in sprint training. *Track Field Q.* 1967;9:1909.

41. Verkhoshanski Y. Perspectives in the improvement of speed-strength preparation of jumpers. *Yesis Rev Soviet Phys Educ Sport.* 1969;28-29.

42. Voight M, Bradley D. Plyometrics. In: Davies GJ, ed. *A Compendium of Isokinetics in Clinical Usage and Rehabilitation Techniques.* 4th ed. Onalaska, WI: S & S; 1994;225-244.

43. Voight M, Draovitch P. Plyometrics. In: Albert M, ed. *Eccentric Muscle Training in Sports and Orthopedics.* New York, NY: Churchill Livingstone; 1991:45-73.

44. Von Arx F. Power development in the high jump. *Track Techn.* 1984;88:2818-19.

45. Wilk KE, Voight LM, Keirns AM, Gambetta V, Andrews J, Dillman CJ. Stretch-shortening drills for the upper extremities: theory and clinical application. *J Orthop Sports Phys Ther.* 1993;17:225-39.

46. Wilt F. Plyometrics—what it is and how it works. *Athl J.* 1975;55b:76.

47. Witzke K, Snow C. Effects of plyometric jump training on bone mass in adolescent girls. *Med Sci Sports Exerc.* 2000;32:1051-57.

48. Woo SL, Inoue M, McGurk-Burleson E, et al Treatment of the medial collateral ligament injury: Structure and function of canine knees in response to differing treatment regimens. *Am J Sports Med.* 1987;15(1):22-29.

SOLUTIONS TO CLINICAL DECISION-MAKING EXERCISES

11-1 Although the patient is in the off-season and actual performance is not jeopardized, her overall activity level must be adjusted to allow for pain-free performance of her conditioning program. The intensity of the plyometric program must be adjusted. Instead of box jumps and depth jumps, the patient should regress to beginner skills such as in-place jumping (both legs) and progress to unilateral activities as tolerated. If these activities cause pain, the plyometric program should be discontinued until symptoms improve. At the heart of the patient's problem may be underlying biomechanical concerns that predispose her to knee pain. A thorough assessment of her lower-extremity biomechanics, flexibility, and strength should be performed. Core strength and stability of the low back and hips must be assessed. Assessment of the patellofemoral joint must also be performed. Appropriate interventions to address any dysfunction must be included as a vital prerequisite prior to advancing the plyometric program.

11-2 As the high-stepping drills involve hip flexion, care must be taken in performing these drills. There is a good chance that the initial injury occurred with hip flexion and knee extension while sprinting, so reintroducing the patient to these positions is an absolute must in the rehabilitation program. A gradual return to these activities is essential to maximize strength without reinjury. Symmetrical flexibility of the hamstrings is a must. Single-joint concentric and eccentric strengthening should be performed without pain to the point of symmetry with the opposite side. When she has an adequate strength and flexibility base, she can begin bilateral and then unilateral plyometric leg-press activities (with less-than-body-weight resistance) on the Shuttle, followed by weight-bearing beginner plyometrics (jumping and hopping). Emphasize activities involving degrees of hip flexion similar to the amount of hip flexion involved in sprinting. When these activities are tolerated well, the patient can then begin high-knee running drills, box jumps, and depth jumps.

11-3 Plyometrics have been shown to be beneficial in producing strength gains in individuals of this age. Plyometrics certainly can enhance anaerobic conditioning as well. Plyometrics, however, are but one component of the entire conditioning program. Proper attention should also be given to safe strength training, flexibility, aerobic conditioning, as well as proper football techniques and protective equipment. There are no long-term data to show that plyometrics are detrimental to the adolescent and many of the activities inherent to football are plyometric in nature. Keep the plyometric activities at the beginner phase and use the beginner skills to develop an adequate strength

base. Stress correct form and technique. Watch for substitutions of movement and progress to intermediate activities if and when the athletes demonstrate correct performance of the beginner skills. Finally, because the athletes are in the playing season, frequency of plyometrics should be minimized.

11-4 Individuals of all sizes can safely take part in plyometrics if they have an adequate strength base. Chances are that this individual is familiar with plyometric training already, so technique and progression should not be an issue. As the individual gains weight, however, the relative load on his weight-bearing joints increases. His exercise dosage should reflect his change in weight. Adequate closed chain strength must increase to support the additional weight prior to plyometrics. After he has made appropriate gains in controlled closed chain strengthening (leg press, squats), plyometrics can be introduced and progressed. It is equally important that the individual's weight gain be fat-free weight with proper attention given to sound nutritional guidelines.

11-5 Of all sporting activities, swimming might be the one with the least amount of eccentric muscle activity. This does not mean that plyometric training to develop power is not important. Plyometrics for the swimmer should include lower-extremity work for starts and turns, as well as trunk plyometrics for power in the water. Upper-extremity plyometrics in this patient may be problematic due to her shoulder instability. Be sure that she has adequate strength in her scapular stabilizers as well as proper posture to minimize an anterior glenoid. Combinations of abduction, horizontal abduction, and external rotation common in plyometrics involving throwing motions might apply excessive stress in an anterior direction. Activities involving horizontal adduction as well as weight-bearing activities in a prone or quadruped position may apply excessive stress in a posterior direction. Try to keep activities bilateral and symmetrical. Emphasize scapular retraction, and try to have the patient keep and attempt to maintain scapular stability.

11-6   Obviously, plyometrics can be used to facilitate strength gain in the entire lower extremity. However, excessive stress to the healing tendon can be detrimental in terms of tendinitis, tendinosis, and possibly even re-rupture. Plyometrics should not even be considered until the patient is able to demonstrate normal strength (symmetrical unilateral toe raises), symmetrical gastrocnemius-soleus flexibility, as well as pain-free and substitution-free gait. Only after attaining these goals should plyometrics be instituted. The program should begin with bilateral nonsupport activities and progress to unilateral nonsupport activities. Loads with less than body weight on the Shuttle are an effective precursor to weight-bearing activities.

Please see videos on the accompanying website at

www.healio.com/books/sportsmedvideos

CHAPTER 12

Open vs Closed Kinetic Chain Exercise in Rehabilitation

William E. Prentice, PhD, PT, ATC, FNATA

After completion of this chapter, the athletic training student should be able to do the following:

- Differentiate between the concepts of an open kinetic chain and a closed kinetic chain.

- Contrast the advantages and disadvantages of using open vs closed kinetic chain exercise.

- Recognize how closed kinetic chain exercises can be used to regain neuromuscular control.

- Analyze the biomechanics of closed kinetic chain exercise in the lower extremity.

- Compare how both open and closed kinetic chain exercises should be used in rehabilitation of the lower extremity.

- Identify the various closed kinetic chain exercises for the lower extremity.

- Examine the biomechanics of closed kinetic chain exercises in the upper extremity.

- Explain how closed kinetic chain exercises are used in rehabilitation of the upper extremity.

- Recognize the various types of closed kinetic chain exercises for the upper extremity.

Through the years, the concept of closed kinetic chain exercise has received considerable attention as a useful and effective technique of rehabilitation, particularly for injuries involving the lower extremity.[81] The ankle, knee, and hip joints constitute the kinetic chain for the lower extremity. When the distal segment of the lower extremity is stabilized or fixed, as is the case when the foot is weight bearing on the ground, the kinetic chain is said to be closed. Conversely, in an open kinetic chain, the distal

Prentice WE, ed.
Rehabilitation Techniques for Sports Medicine and Athletic Training (pp 311–337).
© 2015 SLACK Incorporated.

segment is mobile and not fixed. Traditionally, rehabilitation strengthening protocols have used open kinetic chain exercises such as knee flexion and extension on a knee machine.[71]

Closed kinetic chain exercises are used more often in rehabilitation of injuries to the lower extremity, but they are also useful in rehabilitation protocols for certain upper-extremity activities. For the most part, the upper extremity functions in an open kinetic chain with the hand moving freely. But there are a number of activities in which the upper extremity functions in a closed kinetic chain.[80]

It must be stressed that both open and closed kinetic chain exercises have their place in the rehabilitative process.[21] This chapter clarifies the role of both open and closed kinetic chain exercises in that process.

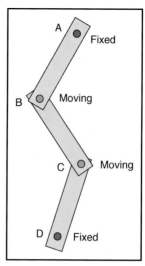

Figure 12-1. If both ends of a link system are fixed, movement at one joint produces predictable movement at all other joints.

CONCEPT OF THE KINETIC CHAIN

The concept of the kinetic chain was first proposed in the 1970s and initially referred to as the link system by mechanical engineers.[69] In this link system, pin joints connect a series of overlapping, rigid segments (Figure 12-1). If both ends of this system are connected to an immovable frame, there is no movement of either the proximal or the distal end. In this closed link system, each moving body segment receives forces from, and transfers forces to, adjacent body segments and thus either affects or is affected by the motion of those components.[29] In a closed link system, movement at one joint produces predictable movement at all other joints.[69] In reality, this type of closed link system does not exist in either the upper or the lower extremity. However, when the distal segment in an extremity (that is, the foot or hand) meets resistance or is fixed, muscle recruitment patterns and joint movements are different than when the distal segment moves freely.[69] Thus, 2 systems—a closed system and an open system—have been proposed.

Whenever the foot or the hand meets resistance or is fixed, as is the case in a closed kinetic chain, movement of the more proximal segments occurs in a predictable pattern. If the foot or hand moves freely in space as in an open kinetic chain, movements occurring in other segments within the chain are not necessarily predictable.[13]

To a large extent, the term *closed kinetic chain exercise* has come to mean "weight-bearing exercise." However, although all weight-bearing exercises involve some elements of closed kinetic chain activities, not all closed kinetic chain activities are weight bearing.[67]

Muscle Actions in the Kinetic Chain

Muscle actions that occur during open kinetic chain activities are usually reversed during closed kinetic chain activities. In open kinetic chain exercise, the origin is fixed and muscle contraction produces movement at the insertion. In closed kinetic chain exercise, the insertion is fixed and the muscle acts to move the origin. Although this may be important biomechanically, physiologically the muscle can lengthen, shorten, or remain the same length, and thus it makes little difference whether the origin or insertion is moving in terms of the way the muscle contracts.

Concurrent Shift in a Kinetic Chain

The concept of the concurrent shift applies to biarticular muscles that have distinctive muscle actions within the kinetic chain during weight-bearing activities.[39] For example, in a closed kinetic chain simultaneous hip and knee extension occur when a person stands from a seated position. To produce this movement, the rectus femoris shortens across the knee while it lengthens across the hip. Conversely, the hamstrings shorten across the hip and simultaneously lengthen across the knee. The resulting concentric and eccentric contractions at opposite ends of the muscle produce the concurrent shift. This type of contraction occurs during functional activities including walking, stair climbing, and jumping and cannot be reproduced by isolated open kinetic chain knee flexion and extension exercises.[39]

The concepts of the reversibility of muscle actions and the concurrent shift are hallmarks of closed kinetic chain exercises.[67]

ADVANTAGES AND DISADVANTAGES OF OPEN VS CLOSED KINETIC CHAIN EXERCISES

Open and closed kinetic chain exercises offer distinct advantages and disadvantages in the rehabilitation process. The choice to use one or the other depends on the desired treatment goal. Characteristics of closed kinetic chain exercises include increased joint compressive forces, increased joint congruency (and thus stability) decreased shear forces, decreased acceleration forces, large resistance forces, stimulation of proprioceptors, and enhanced dynamic stability—all of which are associated with weight bearing.

Characteristics of open kinetic chain exercises include increased acceleration forces, decreased resistance forces, increased distraction and rotational forces, increased deformation of joint and muscle mechanoreceptors, concentric acceleration and eccentric deceleration forces, and promotion of functional activity. These are typical of non-weight-bearing activities.[46]

From a biomechanical perspective, it has been suggested that closed kinetic chain exercises are safer and produce stresses and forces that are potentially less of a threat to healing structures than open kinetic chain exercises.[62] Coactivation or co-contraction of agonist and antagonist muscles must occur during normal movements to provide joint stabilization. Co-contraction, which occurs during closed kinetic chain exercise, decreases the shear forces acting on the joint, thus protecting healing soft-tissue structures that might otherwise be damaged by open chain exercises.[29] Additionally, weight-bearing activity increases joint compressive forces, further enhancing joint stability.

It has also been suggested that closed kinetic chain exercises, particularly those involving the lower extremity, tend to be more functional than open kinetic chain exercises because they involve weight-bearing activities.[79] The majority of activities performed in daily living, such as walking, climbing, and rising to a standing position, as well as in most sport activities, involve a closed kinetic chain system. Because the foot is usually in contact with the ground, activities that make use of this closed system are said to be more functional. With the exception of a kicking movement, there is no question that closed kinetic chain exercises are more activity specific, involving exercise that more closely approximates the desired activity. For example, knee extensor muscle strength in a closed kinetic chain is more closely related to jumping ability than knee extensor strength in a closed kinetic chain.[8] In a clinical setting, specificity of training must be emphasized to maximize carryover to functional activities.[67]

With open kinetic chain exercises, motion is usually isolated to a single joint. Open kinetic chain activities may include exercises to improve strength or range of motion (ROM).[34] They may be applied to a single joint manually, as in proprioceptive neuromuscular facilitation (PNF) or joint mobilization techniques, or through some external resistance using an exercise machine. Isolation-type exercises typically use a contraction of a specific muscle or group of muscles that produces usually single plane and occasionally multiplanar movement.[32] Isokinetic exercise and testing is usually done in an open kinetic chain and can provide important information relative to the torque production capability of that isolated joint.[4]

When there is some dysfunction associated with injury, the predictable pattern of movement that occurs during closed kinetic chain activity might not be possible because of pain, swelling, muscle weakness, or limited ROM. Thus, movement compensations result that interfere with normal motion and muscle activity. If only closed kinetic chain exercise is used, the joints proximal or distal to the injury might not show an existing deficit. Without using open kinetic chain exercises that isolate specific joint movements, the deficit might go uncorrected, thus interfering with total rehabilitation.[19] The therapist should use the most appropriate open or closed kinetic chain exercise for the given situation.

Closed kinetic chain exercises use varying combinations of isometric, concentric, and eccentric contractions that must occur simultaneously in different muscle groups, creating multiplanar motion at each of the joints within the kinetic chain. Closed kinetic chain activities require synchronicity of more complex agonist and antagonist muscle actions.[27]

Clinical Decision-Making Exercise 12-1

Following an ACL surgery, an athletic trainer is ready to incorporate some closed chain exercise into the rehabilitation program. What are some options, and what are advantages of each?

USING CLOSED KINETIC CHAIN EXERCISES TO REGAIN NEUROMUSCULAR CONTROL

Chapter 6 stressed that proprioception, joint position sense, and kinesthesia are critical to the neuromuscular control of body segments within the kinetic chain. To perform a motor skill, muscular forces, occurring at the correct moment and magnitude, interact to move body parts in a coordinated manner.[56] Coordinated movement is controlled by the central nervous system that integrates input from joint and muscle mechanoreceptors acting within the kinetic chain. Smooth coordinated movement requires constant integration of receptor, feedback, and control center information.[56]

In the lower extremity, a functional weight-bearing activity requires muscles and joints to work in synchrony and in synergy with one another. For example, taking a single step requires concentric, eccentric, and isometric muscle contractions to produce supination and pronation in the foot; ankle dorsiflexion and plantar flexion; knee flexion, extension, and rotation; and hip flexion, extension, and rotation. Lack of normal motion secondary to injury in one joint will affect the way another joint or segment moves.[56]

To perform this single step in a coordinated manner, all of the joints and muscles must work together. Thus, exercises that act to integrate, rather than isolate, all of these functioning elements would seem to be the most appropriate. Closed kinetic chain exercises, which recruit foot, ankle, knee, and hip muscles in a manner that reproduces normal loading and movement forces in all of the joints within the kinetic chain, are similar to functional mechanics and would appear to be most useful.[56]

Quite often, open kinetic chain exercises are used primarily to develop muscular strength while little attention is given to the importance of including exercises that reestablish proprioception and joint position sense.[1] Closed kinetic chain activities facilitate the integration of proprioceptive feedback coming from Pacinian corpuscles, Ruffini endings, Golgi-Mazzoni corpuscles, Golgi-tendon organs, and Golgi-ligament endings through the functional use of multijoint and multiplanar movements.[13]

BIOMECHANICS OF OPEN VS CLOSED KINETIC CHAIN ACTIVITIES IN THE LOWER EXTREMITY

Open and closed kinetic chain exercises have different biomechanical effects on the joints of the lower extremity.[18] Walking along with the ability to change direction requires coordinated joint motion and a complex series of well-timed muscle activations. Biomechanically, shock absorption, foot flexibility, foot stabilization, acceleration and deceleration, multiplanar motion, and joint stabilization must occur in each of the joints in the lower extremity for normal function.[33,56] Some understanding of how these biomechanical events occur during both open and closed kinetic chain activities is essential for the athletic trainer.

Foot and Ankle

The foot's function in the support phase of weight bearing during gait is twofold. At heel strike, the foot must act as a shock absorber to the impact or ground reaction forces and then adapt to the uneven surfaces. Subsequently, at push-off, the foot functions as a rigid lever to transmit the explosive force from the lower extremity to the ground.[77]

As the foot becomes weight bearing at heel strike, creating a closed kinetic chain, the subtalar joint moves into a pronated position in which the talus adducts and plantar flexes while the calcaneus everts. Pronation of the foot unlocks the midtarsal joint and allows the foot to assist in shock absorption. It is important during initial impact to reduce the ground reaction forces and distribute the load evenly on many different anatomical structures throughout the lower-extremity kinetic chain. As pronation occurs at the subtalar joint, there is obligatory internal rotation of the tibia and slight flexion at the knee. The dorsiflexors contract eccentrically to decelerate plantar flexion. In an open kinetic chain, when the foot pronates, the talus is stationary while the foot everts, abducts, and dorsiflexes. The muscles that evert the foot appear to be most active.[77]

The foot changes its function from being a shock absorber to being a rigid lever system as the foot begins to push off the ground. In weight bearing in a closed kinetic chain, supination consists of the talus abducting and dorsiflexing on the calcaneus while the calcaneus inverts on the talus. The tibia externally rotates and produces knee extension. During supination the plantar flexors stabilize the foot, decelerate the tibia, and flex the knee. In an open kinetic chain, supination consists of the

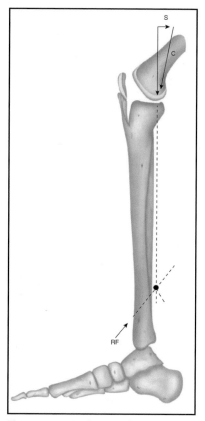

Figure 12-2. Mathematical model showing shear and compressive force vectors. C, compressive; S, shear; RF, resistive force.

calcaneus inverting as the talus adducts and plantar flexes. The foot moves into adduction and plantar flexion, around the stabilized talus.[77] Changes in foot position (ie, pronation or supination) appear to have little or no effect on the electromyogram (EMG) activity of the vastus medialis or the vastus lateralis.[37]

Knee Joint

It is essential for the athletic trainer to understand forces that occur around the knee joint. Palmitier et al proposed a biomechanical model of the lower extremity that quantifies two critical forces at the knee joint[53] (Figure 12-2). A shear force occurs in a posterior direction that would cause the tibia to translate anteriorly if not checked by soft-tissue constraints, primarily the anterior cruciate ligament (ACL).[14] The second force is a compressive force directed along a longitudinal axis of the tibia. Weight-bearing exercises increase joint compression, which enhances joint stability.

Figure 12-3. Resistive forces applied in different positions alter the magnitude of the shear and compressive forces. (A) Resistive force applied distally; (B) resistive force applied proximally; (C) resistive force applied axially; (D). resistive force applied distally with hamstring co-contraction.

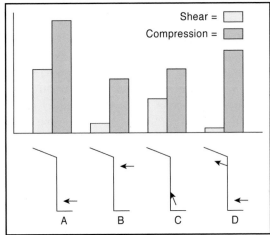

In an open kinetic chain seated knee-joint exercise, as a resistive force is applied to the distal tibia, the shear and compressive forces would be maximized (Figure 12-3A). When a resistive force is applied more proximally, shear force is significantly reduced, as is the compressive force[30] (Figure 12-3B). If the resistive force is applied in a more axial direction, the shear force is also smaller (Figure 12-3C). If a hamstring co-contraction occurs, the shear force is minimized (Figure 12-3D).

Closed kinetic chain exercises induce hamstring contraction by creating a flexion moment at both the hip and the knee, with the contracting hamstrings stabilizing the hip and the quadriceps stabilizing the knee.[74] A moment is the product of force and distance from the axis of rotation. Also referred to as torque, it describes the turning effect produced when a force is exerted on the body that is pivoted about some fixed point (Figure 12-4). Co-contraction of the hamstring muscles helps to counteract the tendency of the quadriceps to cause anterior tibial translation.[73] Co-contraction of the hamstrings is most efficient in reducing shear force when the resistive force is directed in an axial orientation relative to the tibia, as is the case in a weight-bearing exercise.[53] Several studies have shown that co-contraction is useful in stabilizing the knee joint and decreasing shear forces.[36,41,54,68]

The tension in the hamstrings can be further enhanced with slight anterior flexion of the trunk.[50] Trunk flexion moves the center of gravity anteriorly, decreasing the knee flexion

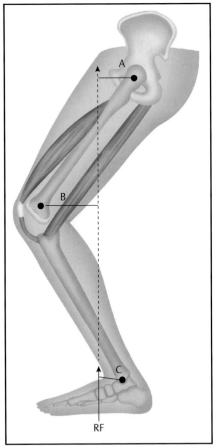

Figure 12-4. Closed kinetic chain exercises induce hamstring contraction by creating a flexion moment at (A) hip, (B) knee, and (C) ankle. RF = resistive force.

moment and thus reducing knee shear force and decreasing patellofemoral compression forces.[52] Closed kinetic chain exercises try to minimize the flexion moment at the knee while increasing the flexion moment at the hip.

A flexion moment is also created at the ankle when the resistive force is applied to the bottom of the foot. The soleus stabilizes ankle flexion and creates a knee extension moment, which again helps to neutralize anterior shear force (Figure 12-4). Thus the entire lower-extremity kinetic chain is recruited by applying an axial force at the distal segment.

In an open kinetic chain exercise involving seated leg extensions, the resistive force is applied to the distal tibia, creating a flexion moment at the knee only.[70] This negates the effects of a hamstring co-contraction and produces maximal shear force at the knee joint. Shear forces created by isometric open kinetic chain knee flexion and extension at 30 and 60 degrees of knee flexion are greater than those with closed kinetic chain exercises.[47] Decreased anterior tibial displacement during isometric closed kinetic chain knee flexion at 30 degrees when measured by knee arthrometry has also been demonstrated.[78]

Patellofemoral Joint

The effects of open vs closed kinetic chain exercises on the patellofemoral joint must also be considered. In open kinetic chain knee extension exercise, the flexion moment increases as the knee extends from 90 degrees of flexion to full extension, increasing tension in the quadriceps and patellar tendon.[6] Thus the patellofemoral joint reaction forces are increased, with peak force occurring at 36 degrees of joint flexion.[25] As the knee moves toward full-extension, the patellofemoral contact area decreases, causing increased contact stress per unit area.[7,38]

In closed kinetic chain exercise, the flexion moment increases as the knee flexes, once again causing increased quadriceps and patellar tendon tension and thus an increase in patellofemoral joint reaction forces.[61] However, the patella has a much larger surface contact area with the femur, and contact stress is minimized.[7,25,38] Closed kinetic chain exercises might be better tolerated in the patellofemoral joint because contact stress is minimized.[6]

CLOSED KINETIC CHAIN EXERCISES FOR REHABILITATION OF LOWER-EXTREMITY INJURIES

For many years, athletic trainers have made use of open kinetic chain exercises for lower-extremity strengthening. This practice has been partly a result of design constraints of existing resistive exercise machines. However, the current popularity of closed kinetic chain exercises can be attributed primarily to a better understanding of the kinesiology and biomechanics, along with the neuromuscular control factors, involved in rehabilitation of lower-extremity injuries. For example, the course of rehabilitation after injury to the anterior ACL has changed drastically over the years. (Specific rehabilitation protocols are discussed in detail in Chapter 21.) Technologic advances have created significant improvement in surgical techniques, and this has allowed athletic trainers to change their philosophy of rehabilitation. The current literature provides a great deal of support for accelerated rehabilitation programs that recommend the extensive use of closed kinetic chain exercises.[9,15,20,25,48,62,75,82]

Because of the biomechanical and functional advantages of closed kinetic chain exercises described earlier, these activities are perhaps best suited to rehabilitation of the ACL.[35] The majority of these studies also indicate that closed kinetic chain exercises can be safely incorporated into the rehabilitation protocols very early.[57] Some athletic trainers recommend beginning within the first few days after surgery.

Several different closed kinetic chain exercises have gained popularity and have been incorporated into rehabilitation protocols.[43] Among those exercises commonly used are the minisquat, wall slides, lunges, leg press, stair-climbing machines, lateral step-up, terminal knee extension using tubing, and stationary bicycling, slide boards, biomechanical ankle platform system (BAPS) boards, and the Fitter.

Figure 12-5. Minisquat performed in 0- to 40-degree range.

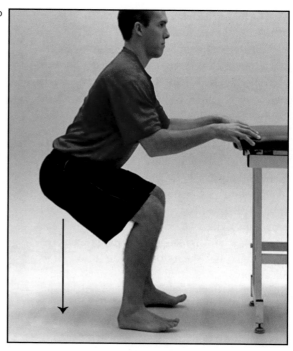

Minisquats, Wall Slides, and Lunges

The minisquat (Figure 12-5) or wall slide (Figure 12-6) involves simultaneous hip and knee extension and is performed in a 0- to 40-degree range.[82] As the hip extends, the rectus femoris contracts eccentrically while the hamstrings contract concentrically. Concurrently, as the knee extends, the hamstrings contract eccentrically while the rectus femoris contracts concentrically. Both concentric and eccentric contractions occur simultaneously at either end of both muscles, producing a concurrent shift contraction. This type of contraction is necessary during weight-bearing activities.[63] It will be elicited with all closed kinetic chain exercises and is impossible with isolation exercises.[69]

These concurrent shift contractions minimize the flexion moment at the knee. The eccentric contraction of the hamstrings helps to neutralize the effects of a concentric quadriceps contraction in producing anterior translation of the tibia.[22] Henning et al found that the half squat produced significantly less anterior shear at the knee than did an open chain exercise in full extension.[31] A full squat markedly increases the flexion moment at the knee and

thus increases anterior shear of the tibia. As mentioned previously, slightly flexing the trunk anteriorly will also increase the hip flexion moment and decrease the knee moment. It appears that increasing the width of the stance in a wall squat has no effect on EMG activity in the quadriceps.[2] However, moving the feet forward does seem to increase activity in the quadriceps as well as the plantarflexors.[11]

Lunges should be used later in a rehabilitation program to facilitate eccentric strengthening of the quadriceps to act as a decelerator[24,81] (Figure 12-7). Like the minisquat and wall slide, it facilitates co-contraction of the hamstring muscles.[23]

Leg-Press

Theoretically, the leg press takes full advantage of the kinetic chain and at the same time provides stability, which decreases strain on the lower back.[45] It also allows exercise with resistance lower than body weight and the capability of exercising each leg independently[53] (Figure 12-8). It has been recommended that leg-press exercises be performed in a 0- to 60-degree range of knee flexion.[82]

It has also been recommended that leg-press machines allow full hip extension to take

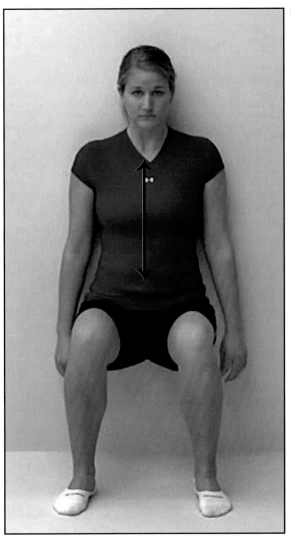

Figure 12-6. Standing wall slides.

maximum advantage of the kinetic chain.[5] Full hip extension can only be achieved in a supine position. In this position, full hip and knee flexion and extension can occur, thus reproducing the concurrent shift and ensuring appropriate hamstring recruitment.[53]

The footplates should also be designed to move in an arc of motion rather than in a straight line. This movement would facilitate hamstring recruitment by increasing the hip flexion moment and decreasing the knee moment. Footplates should be fixed perpendicular to the frontal plane of the hip to maximize the knee extension moment created by the soleus.

Stair Climbing

Stair-climbing machines have gained a great deal of popularity, not only as a closed kinetic chain exercise device useful in rehabilitation, but also as a means of improving cardiorespiratory endurance (Figure 12-9). Stair-climbing machines have two basic designs. One involves a series of rotating steps similar to a department store escalator, while the other uses two footplates that move up and down to simulate a stepping-type movement. With the latter type of stair climber, also sometimes referred to as a stepping machine, the foot never leaves the footplate, making it a true closed kinetic chain exercise device.

Figure 12-7. Lunges are done to strengthen quadriceps eccentrically.

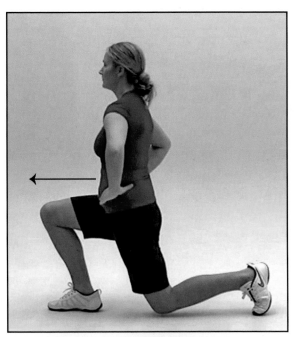

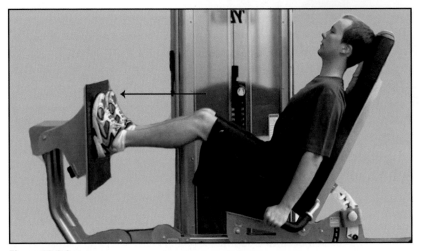

Figure 12-8. Leg-press.

Stair climbing involves many of the same biomechanical principles identified with the leg-press exercise.[51] When exercising on the stair climber, the body should be held erect with only slight trunk flexion, thus maximizing hamstring recruitment through concurrent shift contractions while increasing the hip flexion moment and decreasing the knee flexion moment.

Exercise on a stepping machine produces increased EMG activity in the gastrocnemius.[84] Because the gastrocnemius attaches to the posterior aspect of the femoral condyles, increased activity of this muscle could produce a flexion moment of the femur on the tibia. This motion would cause posterior translation of the femur on the tibia, increasing strain on the ACL. Peak firing of the quadriceps might offset the effects of increased EMG activity in the gastronemius.[17]

Step-ups

Lateral, forward, and backward step-ups are widely used closed kinetic chain exercises

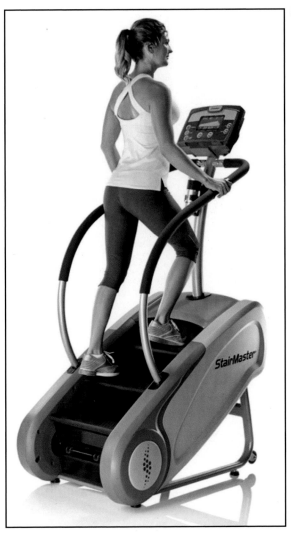

Figure 12-9. Stepping machine. (Reprinted with permission from Stairmaster.)

(Figure 12-10). Lateral step-ups seem to be used more often clinically than forward step-ups. Step height can be adjusted to patient capabilities and generally progresses up to about 8 inches. Heights greater than 8 inches create a large flexion moment at the knee, increasing anterior shear force and making hamstring co-contraction more difficult.[12,17]

Step-ups elicit significantly greater mean hamstring EMG activity than a stepping machine, whereas the quadriceps are more active during stair climbing.[85] When performing a step-up, the entire body weight must be raised and lowered, whereas on the stepping machine the center of gravity is maintained at a relatively constant height. The lateral step-up can produce increased muscle and joint shear forces compared to stepping exercise.[17] Caution should be exercised by the athletic trainer in using the lateral step-up in cases where minimizing anterior shear forces is essential. Contraction of the hamstrings appears to be of insufficient magnitude to neutralize the shear force produced by the quadriceps.[12] In situations where strengthening of the quadriceps is the goal, the lateral step-up has been recommended as a beneficial exercise.[86] However, lateral stepping exercises have failed to increase isokinetic strength of the quadriceps muscle. It also appears that concentric quadriceps contractions produce more EMG activity than eccentric contractions in a lateral step-up.[60]

Figure 12-10. Lateral step-ups.

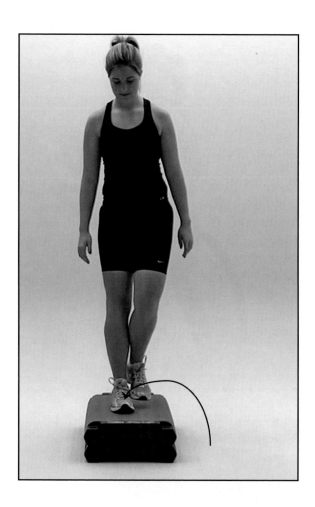

Terminal Knee Extensions Using Surgical Tubing

It has been reported in numerous studies that the greatest amount of anterior tibial translation occurs between 0 and 30 degrees of flexion during open kinetic chain exercise.[26,28,40,51,54,55,82] At one time, athletic trainers avoided open kinetic chain terminal knee extension after surgery. Unfortunately, this practice led to quadriceps weakness, flexion contracture, and patellofemoral pain.[58]

Closed kinetic chain terminal knee extensions using surgical tubing resistance have created a means of safely strengthening terminal knee extension[59] (Figure 12-11). Application of resistance anteriorly at the femur produces anterior shear of the femur, which eliminates any anterior translation of the tibia. This type of exercise performed in the 0- to 30-degree range also minimizes the knee flexion moment, further reducing anterior shear of the tibia. The use of rubber tubing produces an eccentric contraction of the quadriceps when moving into knee flexion. Weight-bearing terminal knee extensions with tubing increase the EMG activity in the quadriceps.[85]

Stationary Bicycling

The stationary bicycle can be of significant value as a closed kinetic chain exercise device (Figure 12-12). The advantage of stationary bicycling over other closed kinetic chain exercises for rehabilitation is that the amount of the weight-bearing force exerted by the injured lower extremity can be adapted within patient limitations. The seat height should be carefully adjusted to minimize the knee flexion moment on the down-stroke. However, if the stationary bike is being used to regain ROM in flexion, the seat height should be adjusted to a lower position that uses passive motion of the injured

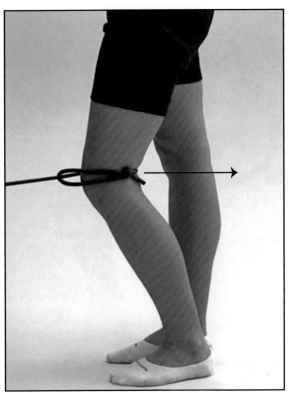

Figure 12-11. Terminal knee extensions using surgical tubing resistance.

extremity. Toe clips will facilitate hamstring contractions on the upstroke.

BAPS Board and Minitramp

The BAPS board (Figure 12-13) and minitramp (Figure 12-14) both provide an unstable base of support that helps to facilitate reestablishing proprioception and joint position sense in addition to strengthening. Working on the BAPS board allows the therapist to provide stress to the lower extremity in a progressive and controlled manner.[13] It allows the patient to work simultaneously on strengthening and ROM, while trying to regain neuromuscular control and balance. The minitramp may be used to accomplish the same goals, but it can also be used for more advanced plyometric training.

> **Clinical Decision-Making Exercise 12-2**
>
> Why would the BAPS board and minitramp be good tools in a rehabilitation program for a dancer recovering from an Achilles tendon repair?

Slide Boards and Fitter

Shifting the body weight from side to side during a more functional activity on either a slide board (Figure 12-15) or a Fitter (Figure 12-16) helps to reestablish dynamic control as well as improve cardiorespiratory fitness.[13] These motions produce valgus and varus stresses and strains to the joint that are somewhat unique to these two pieces of equipment. Lateral slide exercises have been shown to improve knee extension strength following ACL reconstruction.[10]

> **Clinical Decision-Making Exercise 12-3**
>
> Why would a slide board not be an appropriate choice for someone beginning a rehabilitation program for an MCL sprain?

Figure 12-12. Stationary bicycle.

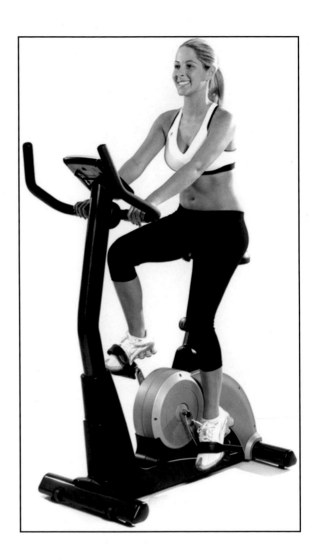

BIOMECHANICS OF OPEN VS CLOSED KINETIC CHAIN ACTIVITIES IN THE UPPER EXTREMITY

Although it is true that closed kinetic chain exercises are most often used in rehabilitation of lower-extremity injuries, there are many injury situations where closed kinetic chain exercises should be incorporated into upper-extremity rehabilitation protocols.[64] Unlike the lower extremity, the upper extremity is most functional as an open kinetic chain system. Most activities involve movement of the upper extremity in which the hand moves freely. These activities are generally dynamic movements. In these movements, the proximal segments of the kinetic chain are used for stabilization, while the distal segments have a high degree of mobility. Push-ups, chinning exercises, and handstands in gymnastics are all examples of closed kinetic chain activities in the upper extremity. In these cases, the hand is stabilized, and muscular contractions around the more proximal segments, the elbow and shoulder, function to raise and lower the body. Still other activities such as swimming and cross-country skiing involve rapid successions of alternating open and closed kinetic chain movements, much in the same way as running does in the lower extremity.[83]

For the most part in rehabilitation, closed kinetic chain exercises are used primarily for strengthening and establishing neuromuscular control of those muscles that act to stabilize

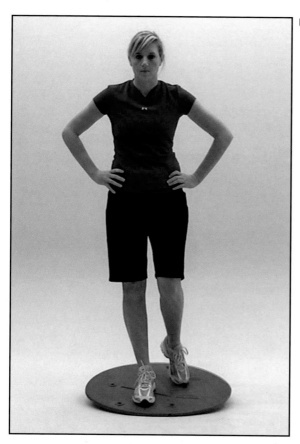

Figure 12-13. BAPS board exercise.

the shoulder girdle.[76] In particular, the scapular stabilizers and the rotator cuff muscles function at one time or another to control movements about the shoulder. It is essential to develop both strength and neuromuscular control in these muscle groups, thus allowing them to provide a stable base for more mobile and dynamic movements that occur in the distal segments.[76]

It must also be emphasized that although traditional upper-extremity rehabilitation programs have concentrated on treating and identifying the involved structures, the body does not operate in isolated segments but instead works as a dynamic unit.[49] More recently, rehabilitation programs have integrated closed kinetic chain exercises with core stabilization exercises and more functional movement programs.[65] Therapists should recognize the need to address the importance of the legs and trunk as contributors to upper-extremity function and routinely incorporate therapeutic exercises that address the entire kinetic chain.[49]

Clinical Decision-Making Exercise 12-4

A football player suffers from chronic shoulder dislocations. What type of exercises can be used to increase stability of the shoulder?

Shoulder Complex Joint

Closed kinetic chain weight-bearing activities can be used to both promote and enhance dynamic joint stability. Most often closed kinetic chain exercises are used with the hand fixed and thus with no motion occurring. The resistance is then applied either axially or rotationally. These exercises produce both joint compression and approximation, which act to enhance muscular co-contraction about the joint producing dynamic stability.[83]

Two essential force couples must be reestablished around the glenohumeral joint: the anterior deltoid along with the infraspinatus and teres minor in the frontal plane, and the

Figure 12-14. Minitramp provides an unstable base of support to which other functional plyometric activities may be added.

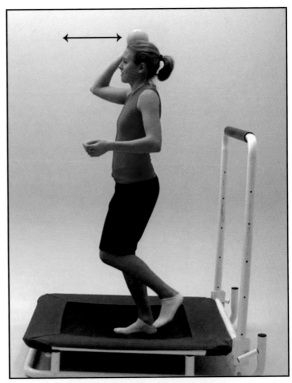

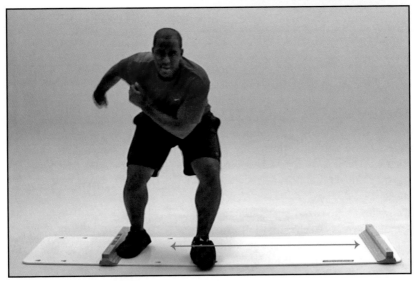

Figure 12-15. Slide board training.

subscapularis counterbalanced by the infraspinatus and teres minor in the transverse plane. These opposing muscles act to stabilize the glenohumeral joint by compressing the humeral head within the glenoid via muscular co-contraction.

The scapular muscles function to dynamically position the glenoid relative to the position of the moving humerus, resulting in a normal scapulohumeral rhythm of movement. However, they must also provide a stable base on which the highly mobile humerus can function. If the scapula is hypermobile, the function

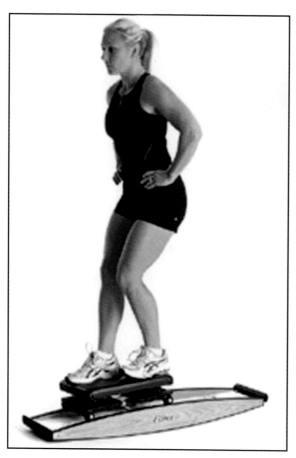

Figure 12-16. The Fitter is useful for weight shifting. (Reproduced with permission from Fitter International, Inc.)

of the entire upper extremity will be impaired. Thus force couples between the inferior trapezius counterbalanced by the upper trapezius and levator scapula—and the rhomboids and middle trapezius counterbalanced by the serratus anterior—are critical in maintaining scapular stability. Again, closed kinetic chain activities done with the hand fixed should be used to enhance scapular stability.[44]

Elbow

The elbow is a hinged joint that is capable of 145 degrees of flexion from a fully extended position. In some cases of joint hyperelasticity, the joint can hyperextend a few degrees beyond neutral. The elbow consists of the humeroulnar, humeroradial, and radioulnar articulations. The concave radial head articulates with the convex surface of the capitellum of the distal humerus and is connected to the proximal ulna via the annular ligament. The proximal radioulnar joint constitutes the forearm that permits about 90 degrees of pronation and 80 degrees of supination when working in conjunction with the elbow joint.

In some activities, the elbow functions in an open kinetic chain. In other activities, the elbow must possess static stability and adequate dynamic strength to be able to transfer force to a hitting implement.[42]

OPEN AND CLOSED KINETIC CHAIN EXERCISES FOR REHABILITATION OF UPPER-EXTREMITY INJURIES

Most typically, closed kinetic chain glenohumeral joint exercises are used during the early phases of a rehabilitation program, particularly in the case of an unstable shoulder to promote co-contraction and muscle recruitment, in

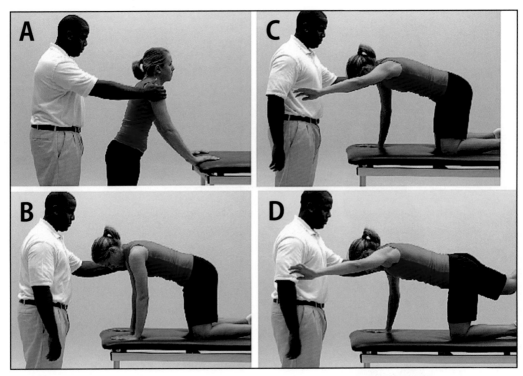

Figure 12-17. Weight shifting. (A) Standing; (B); quadruped; (C) tripod; (D) opposite knee and arm.

addition to preventing shutdown of the rotator cuff secondary to pain and/or inflammation.[3,66] Likewise, closed kinetic chain exercise should be used during the late phases of a rehabilitation program to promote muscular endurance of muscles surrounding the glenohumeral and scapulothoracic joints. They may also be used during the later stages of rehabilitation in conjunction with open kinetic chain activities to enhance some degree of stability, on which highly dynamic and ballistic motions may be superimposed. At some point during the middle stages of the rehabilitation program, traditional open kinetic chain strengthening exercises for the rotator cuff, deltoid, and other glenohumeral and scapular muscles must be incorporated.[34,83]

In the elbow, exercises should also be designed to enhance muscular balance and neuromuscular control of the surrounding agonists and antagonists. Closed kinetic chain exercise should be used to improve dynamic stability of the more proximal muscles surrounding the elbow in those activities where the elbow must provide some degree of proximal stability. Open kinetic chain exercises for strengthening

flexion, extension, pronation, and supination are essential to regain high-velocity dynamic movements of the elbow that are necessary in throwing-type activities.

Clinical Decision-Making Exercise 12-5

A female basketball player has been experiencing some hip pain and general lower-extremity fatigue that you think is due to gluteus medius weakness. You want to improve her awareness of this muscle as well as improve her neuromuscular control. How can closed and open chain exercises both help you achieve your goals?

Weight Shifting

A variety of weight-shifting exercises can be done to assist in facilitating glenohumeral and scapulothoracic dynamic stability through the use of axial compression.[16] Weight shifting can be done in standing, quadruped, tripod, or biped (opposite leg and arm), with weight supported on a stable surface such as the wall or a treatment table (Figure 12-17), or on a movable,

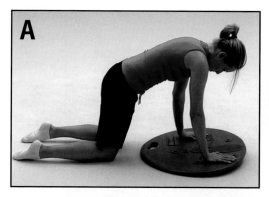

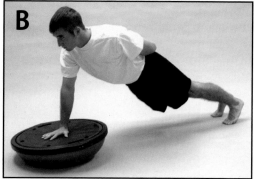

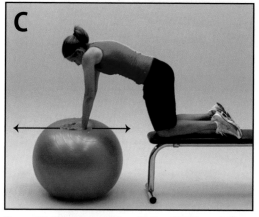

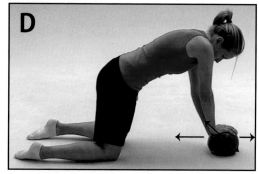

Figure 12-18. Weight shifting. (A) On a BAPS board; (B) on a Bosu Balance Trainer; (C) on a stability ball; (D) on a Plyoball.

unstable surface such as a BAPS board, a wobble board, stability ball, or a plyoball (Figure 12-18). Shifting may be done side to side, forward and backward, or on a diagonal. Hand position may be adjusted from a wide base of support to one hand placed on top of the other to increase difficulty. The patient can adjust the amount of weight being supported as tolerated. The athletic trainer can provide manual force of resistance in a random manner to which the patient must rhythmically stabilize and adapt. A diagonal 2 (D2) PNF pattern may be used in a tripod to force the contralateral support limb to produce a co-contraction and thus stabilization[83] (Figure 12-19). Rhythmic stabilization can also be used to regain neuromuscular control of the scapular muscles with the hand in a closed kinetic chain and random pressure applied to the scapular borders (Figure 12-20).

Push-ups, Push-ups With a Plus, Press-ups, Step-ups

Push-ups and/or press-ups are also done to reestablish neuromuscular control. Push-ups done on an unstable surface such as on a plyoball require a good deal of strength in addition to providing an axial load that requires co-contraction of agonist and antagonist force couples around the glenohumeral and scapulothoracic joints, while the distal part of the extremity has some limited movement (Figure 12-21). A variation of a standard push-up would be to have the patient use a stability ball (Figure 12-22) or doing wall or corner push-ups (Figure 12-23). Pushups with a plus are done to strengthen the serratus anterior, which is critical for scapular dynamic stability in overhead activities (Figure 12-24). Press-ups involve an isometric contraction of the glenohumeral stabilizers (Figure 12-25).

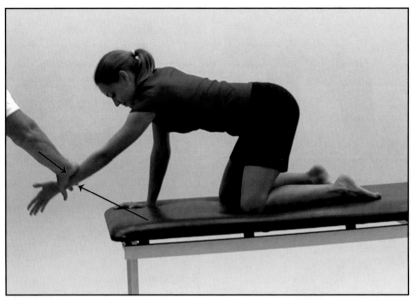

Figure 12-19. D2 PNF pattern in a tripod to produce stabilization in the contralateral support limb.

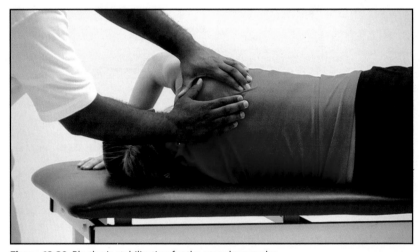

Figure 12-20. Rhythmic stabilization for the scapular muscles.

Figure 12-21. Push-ups done on a Plyoball.

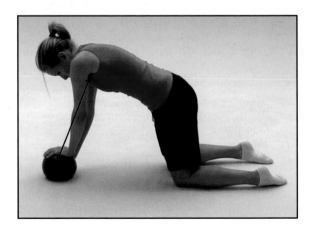

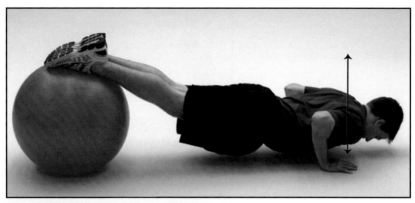

Figure 12-22. Push-ups done on a stability ball.

Figure 12-23. Wall push-ups.

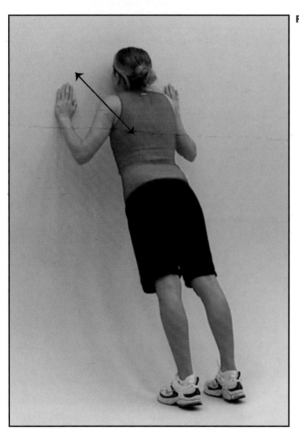

Clinical Decision-Making Exercise 12-6

An athlete has general back weakness. You think that this could be the cause for some anterior shoulder pain. He appears to have winging scapula, and he is having symptoms consistent with impingement. What type of exercises would you introduce to help him with this problem?

Slide Board

Upper-extremity closed kinetic chain exercises performed on a slide board are useful not only for promoting strength and stability but also for improving muscular endurance.[72,83] In a kneeling position, the patient uses a reciprocating motion, sliding the hands forward and

Figure 12-24. Push-ups with a plus.

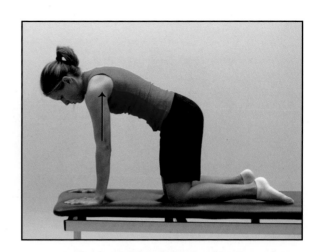

Figure 12-25. Press-ups.

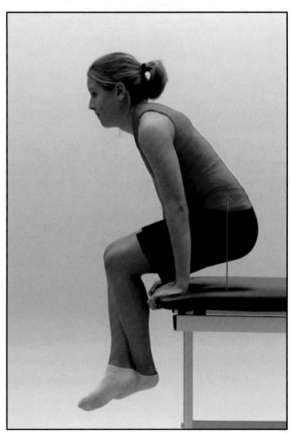

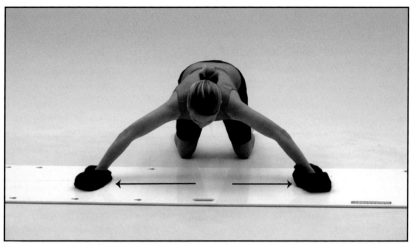

Figure 12-26. Slide board strengthening exercise.

backward, side to side, in a "wax on wax off" circular pattern, or both hands laterally (Figure 12-26). It is also possible to do wall slides in a standing position.

Summary

1. A closed kinetic chain exercise is one in which the distal segment of the extremity is fixed or stabilized. In an open kinetic chain, the distal segment is mobile and not fixed.

2. Both open and closed kinetic chain exercises have their place in the rehabilitative process.

3. The concepts of the reversibility of muscle actions and the concurrent shift are hallmarks of closed kinetic chain exercises.

4. Open and closed kinetic chain exercises offer distinct advantages and disadvantages in the rehabilitation process. The choice to use one or the other depends on the desired treatment goal.

5. It has been suggested that closed kinetic chain exercises are safer because of muscle co-contraction and joint compression; that closed kinetic chain exercises tend to be more functional; and that they facilitate the integration of proprioceptive and joint position sense feedback more effectively than open kinetic chain exercises.

6. Open and closed kinetic chain exercises have different biomechanical effects on the joints of the lower extremity.

7. Closed kinetic chain exercises in the lower extremity decrease the shear forces, reducing anterior tibial translation, and increase the compressive forces that increase stability around the knee joint.

8. Minisquat, wall slides, lunges, leg press, stair-climbing machines, lateral step-up, terminal knee extension using tubing, stationary bicycling, slide boards, BAPS boards, and the Fitter are all examples of closed kinetic chain activities for the lower extremity.

9. Although it is true that closed kinetic chain exercises are most often used in rehabilitation of lower-extremity injuries, there are many injury situations where closed kinetic chain exercises should be incorporated into upper-extremity rehabilitation protocols.

10. Closed kinetic chain exercises in the upper extremity are used primarily for strengthening and establishing neuromuscular

control of those muscles that act to stabilize the shoulder girdle.

11. Closed kinetic chain activities, such as push-ups, press-ups, weight shifting, and slide board exercises, are strengthening exercises used primarily for improving shoulder stabilization in the upper extremity.

References

1. Andersen S, Terwilliger D, Denegar C. Comparison of open versus closed kinetic chain test positions for measuring joint position sense. *J Sport Rehabil.* 1995;4(3):165-171.

2. Anderson R, Courtney C, Carmeli E. EMG analysis of the vastus medialis/vastus lateralis muscles utilizing the unloading narrow and wide-stance squats. *J Sport Rehabil.* 1998;7(4):236.

3. Andrews J, Dennison J, Wilk K. The significance of closed-chain kinetics in upper extremity injuries from a physician's perspective. *J Sport Rehabil.* 1995;5(1):64-70.

4. Augustsson J, Esko A, Thornee R, Karlsson J. Weight training of the thigh muscles using closed vs. open kinetic chain exercises: a comparison of performance enhancement. *J Orthop Sports Phys Ther.* 1998;27(1):3.

5. Azegami M, Yanagihashi R. Effects of multi-joint angle changes on EMG activity and force of lower extremity muscles during maximum isometric leg press exercises. *J Phys Ther Sci.* 2007;19(1):65.

6. Bakhtiary A, Fatemi E. Open versus closed kinetic chain exercises for patellar chondromalacia. *Br J Sports Med.* 2008;42(2):99.

7. Baratta R, Solomonow M, Zhou B. Muscular coactivation: the role of the antagonist musculature in maintaining knee stability. *Am J Sports Med.* 1988;16(2):113-122.

8. Blackburn JR, Morrissey CM. The relationship between open and closed kinetic chain strength of the lower limb and jumping performance. *J Orthop Sports Phys Ther.* 1988;27(6):431.

9. Blair D, Willis R. Rapid rehabilitation following anterior cruciate ligament reconstruction. *Athl Train.* 1991;26(1):32-43.

10. Blanpied P, Carroll R, Douglas T, Lyons M. Effectiveness of lateral slide exercise in an anterior cruciate ligament reconstruction rehabilitation home exercise program. *J Orthop Sports Phys Ther.* 2000;30(10):602.

11. Blanpied P. Changes in muscle activation during wall slides and squat-machine exercise. *J Sport Rehabil.* 1999;8(2):123.

12. Brask B, Lueke R, Soderberg G. Electromyographic analysis of selected muscles during the lateral step-up. *Phys Ther.* 1984;64(3):324-329.

13. Bunton E, Pitney W, Kane A. The role of limb torque, muscle action and proprioception during closed-kinetic-chain rehabilitation of the lower extremity. *J Athl Train.* 1993;28(1):10-20.

14. Butler D, Noyes F, Grood E. Ligamentous restraints to anterior-posterior drawer in the human knee: A biomechanical study. *J Bone Joint Surg Am.* 1980;62:259-270.

15. Case J, DePalma B, Zelko R. Knee rehabilitation following anterior cruciate ligament repair/reconstruction: an update. *Athl Train.* 1991;26(1):22-31.

16. Cipriani D, Escamilla R. Open and closed-chain rehabilitation for the shoulder complex. In: Andrews J, Wilk K, eds. *The Athlete's Shoulder.* New York, NY: Churchill Livingstone; 2008:603-626.

17. Cook T, Zimmerman C, Lux K, et al. EMG comparison of lateral step-up and stepping machine exercise. *J Orthop Sports Phys Ther.* 1992;16(3):108-113.

18. Cordova ML. Considerations in lower extremity closed kinetic chain exercise: a clinical perspective. *Athl Ther Today.* 2001;6(2):46-50.

19. Davies G. The need for critical thinking in rehabilitation. *J Sport Rehabil.* 1995;4(1):1-22.

20. Decarlo MS, Shelbourne KD, McCarroll JR, Rettig AC. A traditional versus accelerated rehabilitation following ACL reconstruction: a one-year follow-up. *J Orthop Sports Phys Ther.* 1992;15(6):309-316.

21. Ellenbecker TS, Davies JG. *Closed Kinetic Chain Exercise: a Comprehensive Guide to Multiple-Joint Exercise.* Champaign, IL: Human Kinetics; 2001.

22. Escamilla RF. Knee biomechanics of the dynamic squat exercise. *Med Sci Sports Exerc.* 2001;33(1):127-141.

23. Escamilla R, Zheng N. Patellofemoral compressive force and stress during the forward and side lunges with and without a stride. *Clin Biomech (Bristol, Avon).* 2008;23(8):1026.

24. Farrokhi S, Pollard C. Trunk position influences the kinematics, kinetics, and muscle activity of the lead lower extremity during the forward lunge exercise. *J Orthop Sports Phys Ther.* 2008;38(7):403.

25. Fu F, Woo S, Irrgang J. Current concepts for rehabilitation following anterior cruciate ligament reconstruction. *J Orthop Sports Phys Ther.* 1992;15(6):270-278.

26. Fukubayashi T, Torzilli P, Sherman M. An in-vitro biomechanical evaluation of anterior/posterior motion of the knee: tibial displacement, rotation, and torque. *J Bone Joint Surg Br.* 1982;64:258-264.

27. Grahm V, Gehlsen G, Edwards J. Electromyographic evaluation of closed- and open-kinetic chain knee rehabilitation exercises. *J Athl Train.* 1993;28(1):23-33.

28. Grood E, Suntag W, Noyes F, et al. Biomechanics of knee extension exercise. *J Bone Joint Surg Am.* 1984;66:725-733.

29. Harter R. Clinical rationale for closed kinetic chain activities in functional testing and rehabilitation of ankle pathologies. *J Sport Rehabil.* 1995;5(1):13-24.

30. Heijne A, Fleming B. Strain on the anterior cruciate ligament during closed kinetic chain exercises. *Med Sci Sports Exerc.* 2004;36(6):935-941.

31. Henning S, Lench M, Glick K. An in-vivo strain gauge study of elongation of the anterior cruciate ligament. *Am J Sports Med.* 1985;13:22-26.

32. Herrington L, Al-Sherhi A. Comparison of single and multiple joint quadriceps exercise in anterior knee pain rehabilitation. *J Orthop Sports Phys Ther.* 2007;37(4):155.

33. Herrington L. Knee-joint position sense: the relationship between open and closed kinetic chain tests. *J Sport Rehabil.* 2005;14(4):356.

34. Hillman S. Principles and techniques of open kinetic chain rehabilitation: the upper extremity. *J Sport Rehabil.* 1994;3(4):319-330.

35. Hooper DM, Morrissey MC, Drechsler W. Open and closed kinetic chain exercises in the early period after anterior cruciate ligament reconstruction: Improvements in level walking, stair ascent, and stair descent. *Am J Sports Med.* 2001;29(2):167-174.

36. Hopkins JT, Ingersoll CD, Sandrey AM. An electromyographic comparison of 4 closed chain exercises. *J Athl Train.* 1999;34(4):353.

37. Hung YJ, Gross TM. Effect of foot position on electromyographic activity of the vastus medialis oblique and vastus lateralis during lower-extremity weight bearing activities. *J Orthop Sports Phys Ther.* 1999;29(2):93-105.

38. Hungerford D, Barry M. Biomechanics of the patellofemoral joint. *Clin Orthop.* 1979;144:9-15.

39. Irrgang J, Safran M, Fu F. The knee: Ligamentous and meniscal injuries. In: Zachazewski J, McGee D, Quillen W, eds. *Athletic Injuries and Rehabilitation.* Philadelphia, PA: WB Saunders; 1995:623-692.

40. Jurist K, Otis V. Anteroposterior tibiofemoral displacements during isometric extension efforts. The roles of external load and knee flexion angle. *Am J Sports Med.* 1985;13:254-258.

41. Kaland S, Sinkjaer T, Arendt-Neilsen L, et al. Altered timing of hamstring muscle action in anterior cruciate ligament deficient patients. *Am J Sports Med.* 1990;18(3):245-248.

42. Ben Kibler W, Sciascia A. Kinetic chain contributions to elbow function and dysfunction in sports. *Clin Sports Med.* 2004;23(4):545-552.

43. Kleiner D, Drudge T, Ricard M. An electromyographic comparison of popular open and closed kinetic chain knee rehabilitation exercises. *J Athl Train.* 1994;29(2):156-157.

44. Kovaleski JE, Heitman R, Gurchiek L, Tyundle T. Reliability and effects of arm dominance on upper extremity isokinetic force, work, and power using the closed chain rider system. *J Athl Train.* 1990;34(4):358.

45. LaFree J, Mozingo A, Worrell T. Comparison of open-kinetic-chain knee and hip extension to closed kinetic chain leg press performance. *J Sport Rehabil.* 1995;3(2): 99-107.

46. Lepart S, Henry T. The physiological basis for open and closed kinetic chain rehabilitation for the upper extremity. *J Sport Rehabil.* 1995;5(1):71-87.

47. Lutz G, Stuart M, Franklin H. Rehabilitative techniques for athletes after reconstruction of the anterior cruciate ligament. *Mayo Clin Proc.* 1990;65:1322-1329.

48. Malone T, Garrett W. Commentary and historical perspective of anterior cruciate ligament rehabilitation. *J Orthop Sports Phys Ther.* 1992;15(6):265-269.

49. McMullen J, Uhl TL. A kinetic chain approach for shoulder rehabilitation. *J Athl Train.* 2000;35(3):329.

50. Mesfar W, Shirazi-Adl A. Knee joint biomechanics in open-kinetic-chain flexion exercises. *Clin Biomech (Bristol, Avon).* 2008;23(4):477.

51. Nisell R, Ericson MO, Németh G, Ekholm J. Tibiofemoral joint forces during isokinetic knee extension. *Am J Sports Med.* 1989;17:49-54.

52. Ohkoshi Y, Yasuda K, Kaneda K, Wada T, Yamanaka M. Biomechanical analysis of rehabilitation in the standing position. *Am J Sports Med.* 1991;19(6):605-611.

53. Palmitier RA, An KN, Scott SG, Chao EY. Kinetic-chain exercise in knee rehabilitation. *Sports Med.* 1991;11(6):402-413.

54. Renström P, Arms SW, Stanwyck TS, Johnson RJ, Pope MH. Strain within the anterior cruciate ligament during hamstring and quadriceps activity. *Am J Sports Med.* 1986;14:83-87.

55. Reynolds N, Worrell T, Perrin D. Effect of lateral step-up exercise protocol on quadriceps isokinetic peak torque values and thigh girth. *J Orthop Sports Phys Ther.* 1992;15(3):151-156.

56. Rivera J. Open versus closed kinetic chain rehabilitation of the lower extremity: a functional and biomechanical analysis. *J Sport Rehabil.* 1994;3(2):154-167.

57. Ross MD, Denegar CR, Winzenried AJ. Implementation of open and closed kinetic chain quadriceps strengthening exercises after anterior cruciate ligament reconstruction. *J Strength Cond Res.* 2001;15(4):466-473.

58. Sachs RA, Daniel DM, Stone ML, Garfein RF. Patellofemoral problems after anterior cruciate ligament reconstruction. *Am J Sports Med.* 1989;17:760-765.

59. Schulthies SS, Ricard MD, Alexander KJ, Myrer WJ. An electromyographic investigation of 4 elastic-tubing closed kinetic chain exercises after anterior cruciate ligament reconstruction. *J Athl Train.* 1998;33(4):328-335.

60. Selseth A, Dayton M, Cardova M, Ingersoll C, Merrick M. Quadriceps concentric EMG activity is greater than eccentric EMG activity during the lateral step-up exercise. *J Sport Rehabil.* 2000;9(2):124.

61. Sheehy P, Burdett RC, Irrgang JJ, VanSwearingen J. An electromyographic study of vastus medialis oblique and vastus lateralis activity while ascending and descending stairs. *J Orthop Sports Phys Ther.* 1998;27(6):423-429.

62. Shellbourne D, Nitz P. Accelerated rehabilitation after anterior cruciate ligament reconstruction. *Am J Sports Med.* 1990;18:292-299.

63. Shields, Madhavan S. Neuromuscular control of the knee during a resisted single-limb squat exercise. *Am J Sports Med.* 2005;33(10):1520-1526.

64. Smith D. Incorporating kinetic-chain integration, part 1: concepts of functional shoulder movement. *Athl Ther Today.* 2006;11(4):63.

65. Smith D. Incorporating kinetic-chain integration, part 2: functional shoulder rehabilitation. *Athl Ther Today.* 2006;11(5):63.

66. Smith J, Dahm D, Kotajarvi B. Electromyographic activity in the immobilized shoulder girdle musculature during ipsilateral kinetic chain exercises. *Arch Phys Med Rehabil.* 2007;88(11):1377-1383.

67. Snyder-Mackler L. Scientific rationale and physiological basis for the use of closed kinetic chain exercise in the lower extremity. *J Sport Rehabil.* 1995;5(1):2-12.

68. Solomonow M, Baratta R, Zhou BH, et al. The synergistic action of the anterior cruciate ligament and thigh muscles in maintaining joint stability. *Am J Sports Med.* 1987;15:207-213.

69. Steindler A. *Kinesiology of the Human Body Under Normal and Pathological Conditions.* Springfield, IL: Charles C. Thomas; 1977.

70. Stensdotter A, Hodges P, Mellor R. Quadriceps activation in closed and in open kinetic chain exercise. *Med Sci Sports Exerc.* 2003;35(12):2043-2047.

71. Stiene H, Brosky T, Reinking M. A comparison of closed-kinetic-chain and isokinetic joint isolation exercise in patients with patellofemoral dysfunction. *J Orthop Sports Phys Ther.* 1996;24(3):136-141.

72. Stone J, Lueken J, Partin N. Closed kinetic chain rehabilitation of the glenohumeral joint. *J Athl Train.* 1993;28(1):34-37.

73. Tagesson S, Öberg B, Good L. A comprehensive rehabilitation program with quadriceps strengthening in closed versus open kinetic chain exercise in patients with anterior cruciate ligament deficiency. *Am J Sports Med.* 2008;36(2):298.

74. Tang SFT, Chen CK, Hsu R, Chou SW, Hong WH, Lew LH. Vastus medialis obliquus and vastus lateralis activity in open and closed kinetic chain exercises in patients with patellofemoral pain syndrome: an electromyographic study. *Arch Phys Med Rehabil.* 2001;82(10):1441-1445.

75. Tovin B, Tovin T, Tovin M. Surgical and biomechanical considerations in rehabilitation of patients with intraarticular ACL reconstructions. *J Orthop Sports Phys Ther.* 1992;15(6):317-322.

76. Ubinger ME, Prentice WE, Guskiewicz MK. Effect of closed kinetic chain training on neuromuscular control in the upper extremity. *J Sport Rehabil.* 1999;8(3):184-194.

77. Valmassey R. *Clinical Biomechanics of the Lower Extremities.* St. Louis, MO: Mosby; 1996.

78. Voight M, Bell S, Rhodes D. Instrumented testing of tibial translation during a positive Lachman's test and selected closed-chain activities in anterior cruciate deficient knees. *J Orthop Sports Phys Ther.* 1992;15:49.

79. Voight M, Cook G. Clinical application of closed-chain exercise. *J Sport Rehabil.* 1995;5(1):25-44.

80. Voight M, Tippett S. *Closed Kinetic Chain.* Paper presented at 41st Annual Clinical Symposium of the National Athletic Trainers Association, Indianapolis, June 12, 1990.

81. Wawrzyniak J, Tracy J, Catizone P. Effect of closed-chain exercise on quadriceps femoris peak torque and functional performance. *J Athl Train.* 1996;31(4): 335-345.

82. Wilk K, Andrew J. Current concepts in the treatment of anterior cruciate ligament disruption. *J Orthop Sports Phys Ther.* 1992;15(6):279-293.

83. Wilk K, Arrigo C, Andrews J. Closed- and open-kinetic chain exercise for the upper extremity. *J Sport Rehabil.* 1995;5(1):88-102.

84. Willett G, Karst G, Canney E, Gallant D, Wees J. Lower limb EMG activity during selected stepping exercises. *J Sport Rehabil.* 1998;7(2):102.

85. Willett G, Paladino J, Barr K, Korta J, Karst G. Medial and lateral quadriceps muscle activity during weight-bearing knee extension exercise. *J Sport Rehabil.* 1998;7(4):248.

86. Worrell TW, Crisp E, LaRosa C. Electromyographic reliability and analysis of selected lower extremity muscles during lateral step-up conditions. *J Athl Train.* 1998;33(2):156

SOLUTIONS TO CLINICAL DECISION MAKING EXERCISES

12-1 An exercise bike is a good tool when rehabilitating lower-extremity injuries. The patient can work through a full ROM without bearing weight. The seat height can be adjusted to target a specific ROM. And most muscles of the leg are used. Most bikes have an option of upper-body activity as well. A stair climber or elliptical machine provides weight-bearing exercise that is nonimpact. Later in closed chain progression, lateral step-ups can be used for neuromuscular control and increased quadriceps firing.

12-2 Neuromuscular control and balance are crucial to the performance of a dancer. The BAPS board and minitramp provide unstable surfaces on which the patient is required to stand. Such controlled systems are ideal because they challenge proprioception more than the stable ground. The patient who has mastered balance on an apparatus such as the minitramp can be progressed to functional activity such as catching a ball while balancing on an unstable surface.

12-3 Unique to the slide board are the valgus and varus strains elicited by the movement. Too much valgus stress while the ligament and musculature are still weak could exacerbate the injury.

12-4 Closed chain exercises in which the arm is fixed and the shoulder joint is perturbed cause contraction of the scapular stabilizers and the rotator cuff. This encourages overall stability of the joint.

12-5 Open chain exercises will allow you to apply significant resistance and isolate the muscle. With side-lying exercises it is easy to teach the patient to isolate the muscle. Once that is accomplished, more functional closed chain exercises can be implemented. Closed chain exercises will encourage neuromuscular control, as the patient is expected to balance in addition to targeting the particular muscle.

12-6 He needs to strengthen his scapular stabilizers so that his shoulder will not rest anteriorly. Any exercise that perturbs the shoulder complex will cause the scapular stabilizers to fuse. Push-ups with a plus are done to strengthen the serratus anterior. Pushups performed on a BAPS board or on a plyoball also promote stability and neuromuscular control of the shoulder complex.

Please see videos on the accompanying website at

www.healio.com/books/sportsmedvideos

CHAPTER 13

Joint Mobilization and Traction Techniques in Rehabilitation

William E. Prentice, PhD, PT, ATC, FNATA

After completion of this chapter, the athletic trainer should be able to do the following:

- Differentiate between physiologic movements and accessory motions.
- Discuss joint arthrokinematics.
- Discuss how specific joint positions can enhance the effectiveness of the treatment technique.
- Discuss the basic techniques of joint mobilization.
- Identify Maitland's five oscillation grades.
- Discuss indications and contraindications for mobilization.
- Discuss the use of various traction grades in treating pain and joint hypomobility.

- Explain why traction and mobilization techniques should be used simultaneously.
- Demonstrate specific techniques of mobilization and traction for various joints.

Following injury to a joint, there will almost always be some associated loss of motion. That loss of movement may be attributed to a number of pathologic factors, including contracture of inert connective tissue (eg, ligaments and joint capsule), resistance of the contractile tissue or the musculotendinous unit (eg, muscle, tendon, and fascia) to stretch, or some combination of the two.[7,8] If left untreated, the joint will become hypomobile and will eventually begin to show signs of degeneration.[30]

Joint mobilization and traction are manual therapy techniques that are slow, passive movements of articulating surfaces.[33] They are used to regain normal active joint range of motion (ROM), restore normal passive motions that

Prentice WE, ed.
Rehabilitation Techniques for Sports Medicine and Athletic Training (pp 339-364).
© 2015 SLACK Incorporated.

occur about a joint, reposition or realign a joint, regain a normal distribution of forces and stresses about a joint, or reduce pain—all of which collectively improve joint function.[25] Joint mobilization and traction are two extremely effective and widely used techniques in injury rehabilitation.[3]

RELATIONSHIP BETWEEN PHYSIOLOGIC AND ACCESSORY MOTIONS

For the athletic trainer supervising a rehabilitation program, some understanding of the biomechanics of joint movement is essential. There are basically two types of movements that govern motion about a joint. Perhaps the better known of the two types of movements are the physiologic movements that result from either concentric or eccentric active muscle contractions that move a bone or a joint. This type of motion is referred to as osteokinematic motion. A bone can move about an axis of rotation, or a joint into flexion, extension, abduction, adduction, and rotation. The second type of motion is accessory motion. Accessory motions refer to the manner in which one articulating joint surface moves relative to another. Physiologic movement is voluntary, while accessory movements normally accompany physiologic movement.[2] The two movements occur simultaneously. Although accessory movements cannot occur independently, they may be produced by some external force. Normal accessory component motions must occur for full-range physiologic movement to take place.[11] If any of the accessory component motions are restricted, normal physiologic cardinal plane movements will not occur.[23,24] A muscle cannot be fully rehabilitated if the joint is not free to move and vice versa.[30]

Traditionally in rehabilitation programs, we have tended to concentrate more on passive physiologic movements without paying much attention to accessory motions. The question always asked is, "How much flexion or extension is this patient lacking?" Rarely will anyone ask, "How much is rolling or gliding restricted?"

It is critical for the athletic trainer to closely evaluate the injured joint to determine whether motion is limited by physiologic movement constraints involving musculotendinous units or by limitation in accessory motion involving the joint capsule and ligaments.[15] If physiologic movement is restricted, the patient should engage in stretching activities designed to improve flexibility. Stretching exercises should be used whenever there is resistance of the contractile or musculotendinous elements to stretch. Stretching techniques are most effective at the end of physiologic range of movement; they are limited to one direction; and they require some element of discomfort if additional ROM is to be achieved. Stretching techniques make use of long-lever arms to apply stretch to a given muscle.[14] Stretching techniques are discussed in Chapters 8 and 12.

If accessory motion is limited by some restriction of the joint capsule or the ligaments, the athletic trainer should incorporate mobilization techniques into the treatment program. Mobilization techniques should be used whenever there are tight inert or noncontractile articular structures; they can be used effectively at any point in the ROM; and they can be used in any direction in which movement is restricted.[26]

Mobilization techniques use a short-lever arm to stretch ligaments and joint capsules, placing less stress on these structures, and, consequently, are somewhat safer to use than stretching techniques.[5]

> **Clinical Decision-Making Exercise 13-1**
>
> Following a grade 2 sprain of the lateral collateral ligament, a high jumper is having trouble regaining full knee extension. Describe a rehabilitation protocol that can help her regain full ROM.

JOINT ARTHROKINEMATICS

Accessory motions are also referred to as joint arthrokinematics, which include spin, roll, and glide[1,17,19] (Figure 13-1).

Spin occurs around some stationary longitudinal mechanical axis and may be in either a clockwise or counterclockwise direction. An example of spinning is motion of the radial

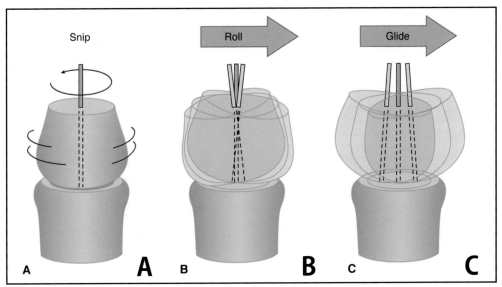

Figure 13-1. Joint arthrokinematics. (A) Spin; (B) roll; (C) glide.

head at the humeroradial joint as occurs in forearm pronation/supination (Figure 13-1A).

Rolling occurs when a series of points on one articulating surface come in contact with a series of points on another articulating surface. An analogy would be to picture a rocker of a rocking chair rolling on the flat surface of the floor. An anatomic example would be the rounded femoral condyles rolling over a stationary flat tibial plateau (Figure 13-1B).

Gliding occurs when a specific point on one articulating surface comes in contact with a series of points on another surface. Returning to the rocking chair analogy, the rocker slides across the flat surface of the floor without any rocking at all. Gliding is sometimes referred to as translation. Anatomically, gliding or translation would occur during an anterior drawer test at the knee when the flat tibial plateau slides anteriorly relative to the fixed rounded femoral condyles (Figure 13-1C).

Pure gliding can occur only if the two articulating surfaces are congruent, where either both are flat or both are curved. Because virtually all articulating joint surfaces are incongruent, meaning that one is usually flat while the other is more curved, it is more likely that gliding will occur simultaneously with a rolling motion. Rolling does not occur alone because

this would result in compression or perhaps dislocation of the joint.

Although rolling and gliding usually occur together, they are not necessarily in similar proportion, nor are they always in the same direction. If the articulating surfaces are more congruent, more gliding will occur; whereas, if they are less congruent, more rolling will occur. Rolling will always occur in the same direction as the physiologic movement. For example, in the knee joint when the foot is fixed on the ground, the femur will always roll in an anterior direction when moving into knee extension and conversely will roll posteriorly when moving into flexion (Figure 13-2).

The direction of the gliding component of motion is determined by the shape of the articulating surface that is moving. If you consider the shape of two articulating surfaces, one joint surface can be determined to be convex in shape while the other may be considered to be concave in shape. In the knee, the femoral condyles would be considered the convex joint surface, while the tibial plateau would be the concave joint surface. In the glenohumeral joint, the humeral head would be the convex surface, while the glenoid fossa would be the concave surface.

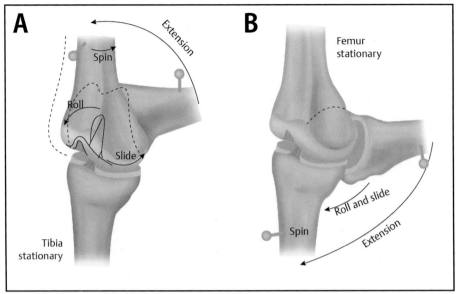

Figure 13-2. Convex-concave rule. (A) Convex moving on concave; (B) concave moving on convex.

> ### Clinical Decision-Making Exercise 13-2
>
> A gymnast has ankle instability. As a result of several sprains, she has a buildup of scar tissue that is limiting plantar flexion. The decreased ROM and instability are affecting her performance because most of her activity requires balance and a great deal of joint mobility. What can you do to help her situation?

This relationship between the shape of articulating joint surfaces and the direction of gliding is defined by the convex-concave rule. If the concave joint surface is moving on a stationary convex surface, gliding will occur in the same direction as the rolling motion. Conversely, if the convex surface is moving on a stationary concave surface, gliding will occur in an opposite direction to rolling. Hypomobile joints are treated by using a gliding technique. Thus, it is critical to know the appropriate direction to use for gliding.[9]

JOINT POSITIONS

Each joint in the body has a position in which the joint capsule and the ligaments are most relaxed, allowing for a maximum amount of joint play.[4,19] This position is called the resting position. It is essential to know specifically where the resting position is, because testing for joint play during an evaluation and treatment of the hypomobile joint using either mobilization or traction are usually performed in this position. Table 13-1 summarizes the appropriate resting positions for many of the major joints.

Placing the joint capsule in the resting position allows the joint to assume a loose-packed position in which the articulating joint surfaces are maximally separated. A close-packed position is one in which there is maximal contact of the articulating surfaces of bones with the capsule and ligaments tight or tense. In a loose-packed position, the joint will exhibit the greatest amount of joint play, whereas the close-packed position allows for no joint play. Thus, the loose-packed position is most appropriate for mobilization and traction (Figure 13-3).

Both mobilization and traction techniques use a translational movement of one joint surface relative to the other. This translation may be either perpendicular or parallel to the treatment plane. The treatment plane falls perpendicular to, or at a right angle to, a line running from the axis of rotation in the convex surface to the center of the concave articular surface[17,19] (Figure 13-4). Thus, the treatment plane lies within the concave surface. If the

Table 13-1 Shape, Resting Position, and Treatment Planes of Various Joints

Joint	Convex Surface	Concave Surface	Resting Position (Loose-packed)	Close-packed Position	Treatment Plane
Sternoclavicular	Clavicle*	Sternum*	Anatomic position	Horizontal	In sternum
Acromioclavicular	Clavicle	Acromion	Anatomic position, in horizontal plane at 60 degrees to sagittal plane	Adduction	In acromion
Glenohumeral	Humerus	Glenoid	Shoulder abducted 55 degrees, horizontally adducted 30 degrees, rotated so that forearm is in horizontal plane	Abduction and lateral rotation	In glenoid fossa in scapular plane
Humeroradial	Humerus	Radius	Elbow extended, forearm supinated	Flexion and forearm production	In radial head perpendicular to long axis of radius
Humeroulnar	Humerus	Ulna	Elbow flexed 70 degrees, forearm supinated 10 degrees	Full extension and forearm supination	In olecranon fossa, 45 degrees to long axis of ulna
Radioulnar (proximal)	Radius	Ulna	Elbow flexed 70 degrees, forearm supinated 35 degrees	Full extension and forearm supination	In radial notch of ulna, parallel to long axis of ulna
Radioulnar (distal)	Ulna	Radius	Supinated 10 degrees	Extension	In radius, parallel to long axis of radius
Radiocarpal	Proximal carpal bones	Radius	Line through radius and third metacarpal	Extension	In radius, perpendicular to long axis of radius
Metacarpophalangeal	Metacarpal	Proximal phalanx	Slight flexion	Full flexion	In proximal phalanx
Interphalangeal	Proximal phalanx	Distal phalanx	Slight flexion	Extension	In proximal phalanx
Hip	Femur	Acetabulum	Hip flexed 30 degrees, abducted 30 degrees, slight external rotation	Extension and medial rotation	In acetabulum
Tibiofemoral	Femur	Tibia	Flexed 25 degrees	Full extension	On surface of tibial plateau

(continued)

Table 13-1 Shape, Resting Position, and Treatment Planes of Various Joints (*continued*)

Joint	Convex Surface	Concave Surface	Resting Position (Loose-packed)	Close-packed Position	Treatment Plane
Patellofemoral	Patella	Femur	Knee in full extension	Full flexion	Along femoral groove
Talocrural	Talus	Mortise	Plantar flexed 10 degrees	Dorsiflexion	In the mortise in anterior/posterior direction
Subtalar	Calcaneus	Talus	Subtalar neutral between inversion/eversion	Supination	In talus, parallel to foot surface
Intertarsal	Proximal articulating surface	Distal articulating surface	Foot relaxed	Supination	In distal segment
Metatarsophalangeal	Tarsal bone	Proximal phalanx	Slight flexion	Full flexion	In proximal phalanx
Interphalangeal	Proximal phalanx	Distal phalanx	Slight extension	Extension	In distal phalanx

*In the sternoclavicular joint, the clavicle surface is convex in a superior/inferior direction and concave in an anterior/posterior direction.

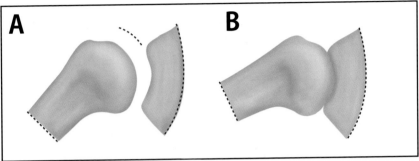

Figure 13-3. Joint capsule resting position. (A) Loose-packed position; (B) close-packed position.

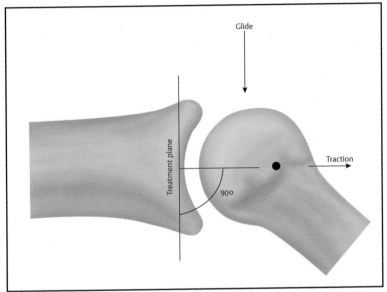

Figure 13-4. The treatment plane is perpendicular to a line drawn from the axis of rotation to the center of the articulating surface of the concave segment.

convex segment moves, the treatment plane remains fixed. However, the treatment plane will move along with the concave segment. Mobilization techniques use glides that translate one articulating surface along a line parallel with the treatment plane. Traction techniques translate one of the articulating surfaces in a perpendicular direction to the treatment plane. Both techniques use a loose-packed joint position.[17]

JOINT MOBILIZATION TECHNIQUES

The techniques of joint mobilization are used to improve joint mobility or to decrease joint pain by restoring accessory movements to the joint and thus allowing full, nonrestricted, pain-free ROM.[25,34]

Mobilization techniques may be used to attain a variety of either mechanical or neurophysiological treatment goals: reducing pain; decreasing muscle guarding; stretching or lengthening tissue surrounding a joint, in particular capsular and ligamentous tissue; reflexogenic effects that either inhibit or facilitate muscle tone or stretch reflex; and proprioceptive effects to improve postural and kinesthetic awareness.[1,12,18,24,28,30]

Movement throughout a ROM can be quantified with various measurement techniques. Physiologic movement is measured with a goniometer and composes the major portion of the range. Accessory motion is thought of in

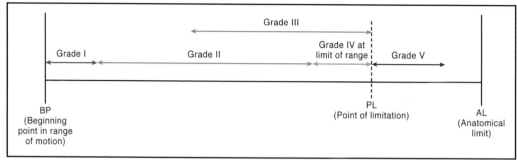

Figure 13-5. Maitland's five grades of motion. AL, anatomical limit; PL, point of limitation.

millimeters, although precise measurement is difficult.

Accessory movements may be hypomobile, normal, or hypermobile.[6] Each joint has a ROM continuum with an anatomical limit to motion that is determined by both bony arrangement and surrounding soft tissue (Figure 13-5). In a hypomobile joint, motion stops at some point referred to as a pathologic point of limitation, short of the anatomical limit caused by pain, spasm, or tissue resistance. A hypermobile joint moves beyond its anatomical limit because of laxity of the surrounding structures. A hypomobile joint should respond well to techniques of mobilization and traction. A hypermobile joint should be treated with strengthening exercises, stability exercises, and if indicated, taping, splinting, or bracing.[29,30]

In a hypomobile joint, as mobilization techniques are used in the ROM restriction, some deformation of soft-tissue capsular or ligamentous structures occurs. If a tissue is stretched only into its elastic range, no permanent structural changes will occur.

However, if that tissue is stretched into its plastic range, permanent structural changes will occur. Thus, mobilization and traction can be used to stretch tissue and break adhesions. If used inappropriately, they can also damage tissue and cause sprains of the joint.[30]

Treatment techniques designed to improve accessory movement are generally slow, small-amplitude movements, the amplitude being the distance that the joint is moved passively within its total range. Mobilization techniques use these small-amplitude oscillating motions that glide or slide one of the articulating joint surfaces in an appropriate direction within a specific part of the range.[22]

> **Clinical Decision-Making Exercise 13-3**
>
> Following shoulder surgery a swimmer is having trouble regaining full ROM. His stroke will be affected if he cannot regain full extension and lateral rotation. What type of joint mobilization protocol could you implement to help him?

Maitland has described various grades of oscillation for joint mobilization. The amplitude of each oscillation grade falls within the ROM continuum between some beginning point and the anatomical limit.[23,24] Figure 13-5 shows the various grades of oscillation that are used in a joint with some limitation of motion. As the severity of the movement restriction increases, the point of limitation moves to the left, away from the anatomical limit. However, the relationships that exist among the five grades in terms of their positions within the ROM remain the same. The five mobilization grades are defined as follows:

- Grade I. A small-amplitude movement at the beginning of the range of movement. Used when pain and spasm limit movement early in the ROM.[37]

- Grade II. A large-amplitude movement within the midrange of movement. Used when spasm limits movement sooner with a quick oscillation than with a slow one, or when slowly increasing pain restricts movement halfway into the range.

- Grade III. A large-amplitude movement up to the point of limitation in the range of movement. Used when pain and resistance from spasm, inert tissue tension, or tissue

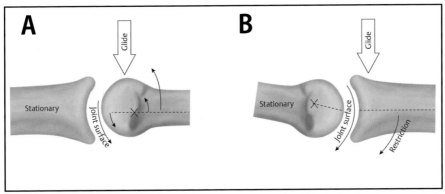

Figure 13-6. Gliding motions. (A) Glides of the convex segment should be in the direction opposite to the restriction; (B) glides of the concave segment should be in the direction of the restriction.

compression limit movement near the end of the range.

- Grade IV. A small-amplitude movement at the very end of the range of movement. Used when resistance limits movement in the absence of pain and spasm.

- Grade V. A small-amplitude, quick thrust delivered at the end of the range of movement, usually accompanied by a popping sound, called a manipulation. Used when minimal resistance limits the end of the range. Manipulation is most effectively accomplished by the velocity of the thrust rather than by the force of the thrust.[21] Most authorities agree that manipulation should be used only by individuals trained specifically in these techniques, because a great deal of skill and judgment is necessary for safe and effective treatment.[31,32]

Clinical Decision-Making Exercise 13-4

How might a chiropractor apply the concepts of joint mobilization?

Joint mobilization uses these oscillating gliding motions of one articulating joint surface in whatever direction is appropriate for the existing restriction. The appropriate direction for these oscillating glides is determined by the convex-concave rule, described previously. When the concave surface is stationary and the convex surface is mobilized, a glide of the convex segment should be in the direction opposite to the restriction of joint movement (Figure 13-6A).[17,19,35] If the convex articular surface is stationary and the concave surface is mobilized, gliding of the concave segment should be in the same direction as the restriction of joint movement (Figure 13-6B). For example, the glenohumeral joint would be considered to be a convex joint with the convex humeral head moving on the concave glenoid. If shoulder abduction is restricted, the humerus should be glided in an inferior direction relative to the glenoid to alleviate the motion restriction. When mobilizing the knee joint, the concave tibia should be glided anteriorly in cases where knee extension is restricted. If mobilization in the appropriate direction exacerbates complaints of pain or stiffness, the athletic trainer should apply the technique in the opposite direction until the patient can tolerate the appropriate direction.[35]

Typical mobilization of a joint may involve a series of three to six sets of oscillations lasting between 20 and 60 seconds each, with one to three oscillations per second.[23,24]

Clinical Decision-Making Exercise 13-5

Following an ankle sprain, accumulated scar tissue is preventing full plantar flexion. How can joint mobilization be used to help regain full ROM?

Indications for Mobilization

In Maitland's system, Grades I and II are used primarily for treatment of pain and Grades III and IV are used for treating stiffness. Pain must be treated first and stiffness

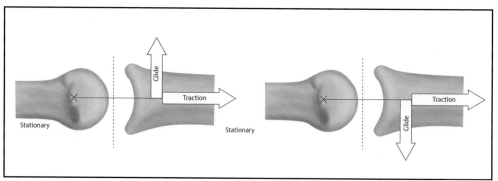

Figure 13-7. Traction vs. glides. Traction is perpendicular to the treatment plane, whereas glides are parallel to the treatment plane.

second.[24] Painful conditions should be treated on a daily basis. The purpose of the small-amplitude oscillations is to stimulate mechanoreceptors within the joint that can limit the transmission of pain perception at the spinal cord or brainstem levels.

Joints that are stiff or hypomobile and have restricted movement should be treated 3 to 4 times per week on alternating days with active motion exercise. The athletic trainer must continuously reevaluate the joint to determine appropriate progression from one oscillation grade to another.

Indications for specific mobilization grades are relatively straightforward. If the patient complains of pain before the athletic trainer can apply any resistance to movement, it is too early, and all mobilization techniques should be avoided. If pain is elicited when resistance to motion is applied, mobilization, using grades I, II, and III, is appropriate. If resistance can be applied before pain is elicited, mobilization can be progressed to grade IV. Mobilization should be done with both the patient and the athletic trainer positioned in a comfortable and relaxed manner. The athletic trainer should mobilize one joint at a time. The joint should be stabilized as near one articulating surface as possible, while moving the other segment with a firm, confident grasp.

Contraindications for Mobilization

Techniques of mobilization and manipulation should not be used haphazardly. These techniques should generally not be used in cases of inflammatory arthritis, malignancy, bone disease, neurological involvement, bone fracture, congenital bone deformities, and vascular disorders of the vertebral artery. Again, manipulation should be performed only by those athletic trainers specifically trained in the procedure, because some special knowledge and judgment are required for effective treatment.[24]

JOINT TRACTION TECHNIQUES

Traction refers to a technique involving pulling on one articulating segment to produce some separation of the two joint surfaces. Although mobilization glides are done parallel to the treatment plane, traction is performed perpendicular to the treatment plane (Figure 13-7). Like mobilization techniques, traction may be used either to decrease pain or to reduce joint hypomobility.[38]

Kaltenborn has proposed a system using traction combined with mobilization as a means of reducing pain or mobilizing hypomobile joints.[16] As discussed earlier, all joints have a certain amount of play or looseness. Kaltenborn referred to this looseness as slack. Some degree of slack is necessary for normal joint motion. Kaltenborn's three traction grades are defined as follows[17] (Figure 13-8):

- Grade I traction (loosen). Traction that neutralizes pressure in the joint without actual separation of the joint surfaces. The purpose is to produce pain relief by reducing the compressive forces of articular

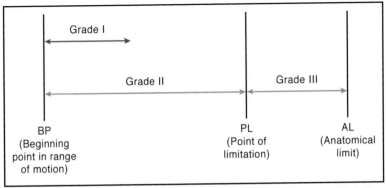

Figure 13-8. Kaltenborn's grades of traction. AL, anatomical limit; PL, point of limitation.

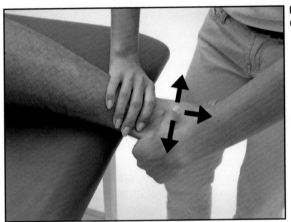

Figure 13-9. Traction and mobilization should be used together.

surfaces during mobilization and is used with all mobilization grades.

- Grade II traction (tighten or "take up the slack"). Traction that effectively separates the articulating surfaces and takes up the slack or eliminates play in the joint capsule. Grade II is used in initial treatment to determine joint sensitivity.

- Grade III traction (stretch). Traction that involves actual stretching of the soft tissue surrounding the joint to increase mobility in a hypomobile joint.

Grade I traction should be used in the initial treatment to reduce the chance of a painful reaction. It is recommended that 10-second intermittent Grades I and II traction be used, distracting the joint surfaces up to a Grade III traction and then releasing distraction until the joint returns to its resting position.[16]

Kaltenborn emphasizes that Grade III traction should be used in conjunction with mobilization glides to treat joint hypomobility[17] (Figure 13-7). Grade III traction stretches the joint capsule and increases the space between the articulating surfaces, placing the joint in a loose-packed position. Applying Grades III and IV oscillations within the patient's pain limitations should maximally improve joint mobility[16] (Figure 13-9).

Clinical Decision-Making Exercise 13-6

A physician has diagnosed disc pathology in a field hockey player with low back pain. The disc is protruding and impinging on the spinal cord. How could traction help relieve pain for this athlete?

MOBILIZATION AND TRACTION TECHNIQUES

Figures 13-10 to 13-73 provide descriptions and illustrations of various mobilization and traction techniques. These figures should be used to determine appropriate hand positioning, stabilization (S), and the correct direction for gliding (G), traction (T), and/or rotation (R). The information presented in this chapter should be used as a reference base for appropriately incorporating joint mobilization and traction techniques into the rehabilitation program.

MULLIGAN JOINT MOBILIZATION TECHNIQUE

Brian Mulligan, an Australian athletic trainer, proposed a concept of mobilizations based on Kaltenborn's principles. Whereas Kaltenborn's technique relies on passive accessory mobilization, the Mulligan technique combines passive accessory joint mobilization applied by an athletic trainer with active physiological movement by the patient for the purpose of correcting positional faults and returning the patient to normal pain-free function.[27] It is a noninvasive and comfortable intervention, and has applications for the spine and the extremities. Mulligan's concept uses what are referred to as either mobilizations with movement for treating the extremities, or sustained natural apophyseal glides for treating problems in the spine.[36] Instead of the athletic trainer using oscillations or thrusting techniques, the patient moves in a specific direction as the athletic trainer guides the restricted body part. Mobilizations with movement and sustained natural apophyseal glides have the potential to quickly restore functional movements in joints, even after many years of restriction.[27]

Principles of Treatment

A basic premise of the Mulligan technique for an athletic trainer choosing to make use of mobilizations with movement in the extremities or sustained natural apophyseal glides in the spine is to never cause pain to the patient.[10] During assessment, the athletic trainer should look for specific signs that may include a loss of joint movement, pain associated with movement, or pain associated with specific functional activities.[13] A passive accessory joint mobilization is applied following the principles of Kaltenborn discussed earlier in this chapter (ie, parallel or perpendicular to the joint plane). The athletic trainer must continuously monitor the patient's reaction to ensure that no pain is recreated during this mobilization. The athletic trainer experiments with various combinations of parallel or perpendicular glides until the appropriate treatment plane and grade of movement are discovered, which together significantly improve ROM and/or significantly decrease or, better yet, eliminate altogether the original pain.

Failure to improve ROM or decrease pain indicates that the athletic trainer has not found the correct contact point, treatment plane, grade, or direction of mobilization. The patient then actively repeats the restricted and/or painful motion or activity while the athletic trainer continues to maintain the appropriate accessory glide. Further increases in ROM or decreases in pain may be expected during a treatment session that typically involves three sets of 10 repetitions. Additional gains may be realized through the application of pain-free, passive overpressure at the end of available range.[20]

An example of mobilization with movement might be in a patient with restricted ankle dorsiflexion (Figure 13-74A). The patient is standing on a treatment table with the athletic trainer manually stabilizing the foot. A nonelastic belt passes around both the distal leg of the patient and the waist of the athletic trainer who applies a sustained anterior glide of the tibia by leaning backward away from the patient. The patient then performs a slow dorsiflexion movement until the first onset of pain or end of range. Once this end point is reached, the position is sustained for 10 seconds. The patient then relaxes and returns to the standing position followed by release of the anteroposterior glide, and then followed by a 20-second rest period.[27] Figures 13-74B, C, and D show several additional Mulligan techniques.

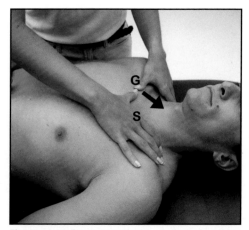

Figure 13-10. Posterior and superior clavicular glides. When posterior or superior clavicular glides are done at the sternoclavicular joint, use the thumbs to glide the clavicle. Posterior glides are used to increase clavicular retraction, and superior glides increase clavicular retraction and clavicular depression.

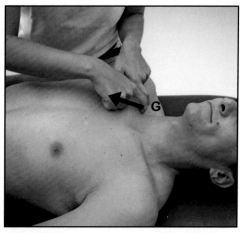

Figure 13-11. Inferior clavicular glides. Inferior clavicular glides at the sternoclavicular joint use the index fingers to mobilize the clavicle, which increases clavicular elevation.

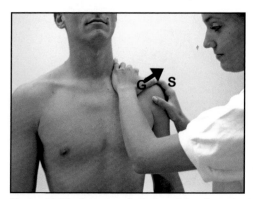

Figure 13-12. Posterior clavicular glides. Posterior clavicular glides done at the acromioclavicular (AC) joint apply posterior pressure on the clavicle while stabilizing the scapula with the opposite hand. They increase mobility of the AC joint.

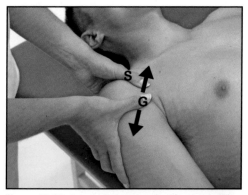

Figure 13-13. Anterior/posterior glenohumeral glides. Anterior/posterior glenohumeral glides are done with one hand stabilizing the scapula and the other gliding the humeral head. They initiate motion in the painful shoulder.

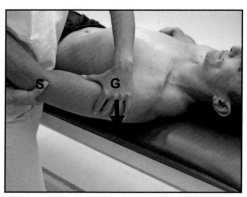

Figure 13-14. Posterior humeral glides. Posterior humeral glides use one hand to stabilize the humerus at the elbow and the other to glide the humeral head. They increase flexion and medial rotation.

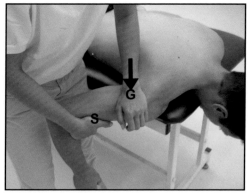

Figure 13-15. Anterior humeral glides. In anterior humeral glides the patient is prone. One hand stabilizes the humerus at the elbow and the other glides the humeral head. They increase extension and lateral rotation.

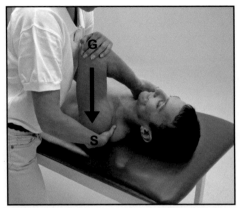

Figure 13-16. Posterior humeral glides. Posterior humeral glides may also be done with the shoulder at 90 degrees. With the patient in supine position, one hand stabilizes the scapula underneath while the patient's elbow is secured at the athletic trainer's shoulder. Glides are directed downward through the humerus. They increase horizontal adduction.

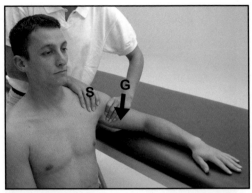

Figure 13-17. Inferior humeral glides. For inferior humeral glides, the patient is in the sitting position with the elbow resting on the treatment table. One hand stabilizes the scapula and the other glides the humeral head inferiorly. These glides increase shoulder abduction.

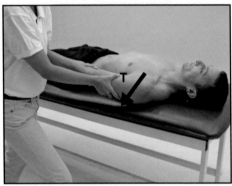

Figure 13-18. Lateral glenohumeral joint traction. Lateral glenohumeral joint traction is used for initial testing of joint mobility and for decreasing pain. One hand stabilizes the elbow while the other applies lateral traction at the upper humerus.

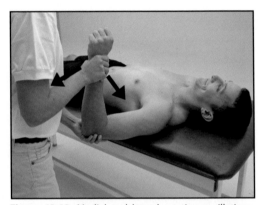

Figure 13-19. Medial and lateral rotation oscillations. Medial and lateral rotation oscillations with the shoulder abducted at 90 degrees can increase medial and lateral rotation in a progressive manner according to patient tolerance.

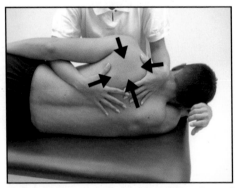

Figure 13-20. General scapular glides. General scapular glides may be done in all directions, applying pressure at either the medial, inferior, lateral, or superior border of the scapula. Scapular glides increase general scapulothoracic mobility.

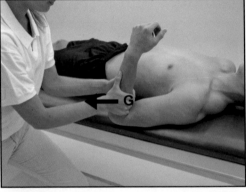

Figure 13-21. Inferior humeroulnar glides. Inferior humeroulnar glides increase elbow flexion and extension. They are performed using the body weight to stabilize proximally with the hand grasping the ulna and gliding inferiorly.

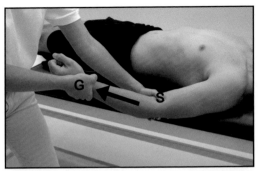

Figure 13-22. Humeroradial inferior glides. Humeroradial inferior glides increase the joint space and improve flexion and extension. One hand stabilizes the humerus above the elbow; the other grasps the distal forearm and glides the radius inferiorly.

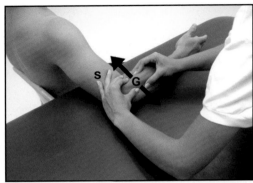

Figure 13-23. Proximal anterior/posterior radial glides. Proximal anterior/posterior radial glides use the thumbs and index fingers to glide the radial head. Anterior glides increase flexion, while posterior glides increase extension.

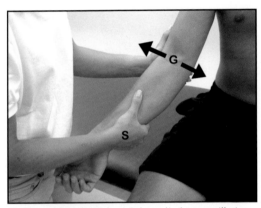

Figure 13-24. Medial and lateral ulnar oscillations. Medial and lateral ulnar oscillations increase flexion and extension. Valgus and varus forces are used with a short-lever arm.

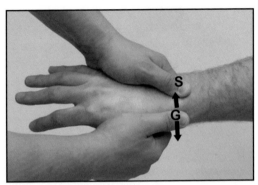

Figure 13-25. Distal anterior/posterior radial glides. Distal anterior/posterior radial glides are done with one hand stabilizing the ulna and the other gliding the radius. These glides increase pronation.

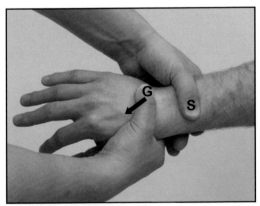

Figure 13-26. Radiocarpal joint anterior glides. Radiocarpal joint anterior glides increase wrist extension.

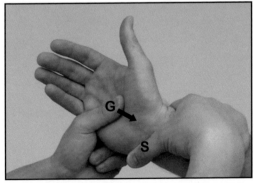

Figure 13-27. Radiocarpal joint posterior glides. Radiocarpal joint posterior glides increase wrist flexion.

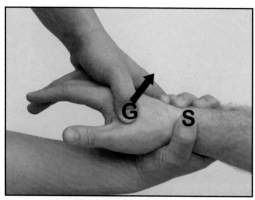

Figure 13-28. Radiocarpal joint ulnar glides. Radiocarpal joint ulnar glides increase radial deviation.

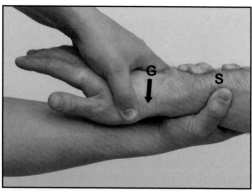

Figure 13-29. Radiocarpal joint radial glides. Radiocarpal joint radial glides increase ulnar deviation.

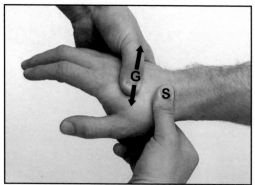

Figure 13-30. Carpometacarpal joint anterior/posterior glides. Carpometacarpal joint anterior/posterior glides increase mobility of the hand.

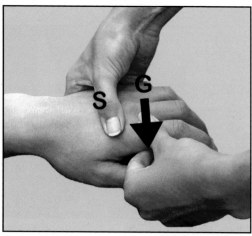

Figure 13-31. Metacarpophalangeal joint anterior/posterior glides. In metacarpophalangeal joint anterior or posterior glides, the proximal segment, in this case the metacarpal, is stabilized and the distal segment is mobilized. Anterior glides increase flexion of the metacarpophalangeal joint. Posterior glides increase extension.

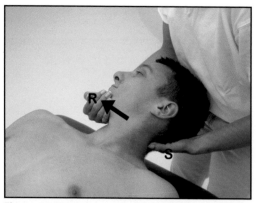

Figure 13-32. Cervical vertebrae rotation oscillations. Cervical vertebrae rotation oscillations are done with one hand supporting the weight of the head and the other rotating the head in the direction of the restriction. These oscillations treat pain or stiffness when there is some resistance in the same direction as the rotation.

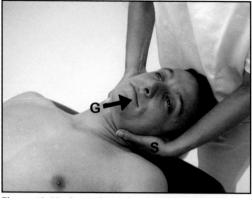

Figure 13-33. Cervical vertebrae side-bending. Cervical vertebrae side-bending may be used to treat pain or stiffness with resistance when side-bending the neck.

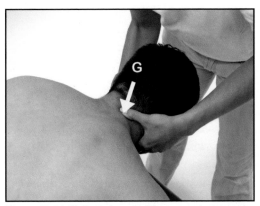

Figure 13-34. Unilateral cervical facet anterior/posterior glides. Unilateral cervical facet anterior/posterior glides are done using pressure from the thumbs over individual facets. They increase rotation or flexion of the neck toward the side where the technique is used.

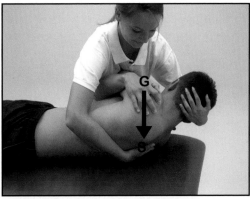

Figure 13-35. Thoracic vertebral facet rotations. Thoracic vertebral facet rotations are accomplished with one hand underneath the patient providing stabilization and the weight of the body pressing downward through the rib cage to rotate an individual thoracic vertebrae. Rotation of the thoracic vertebrae is minimal, and most of the movement with this mobilization involves the rib facet joint.

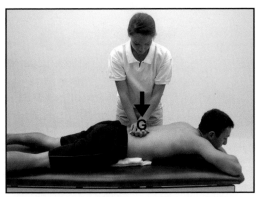

Figure 13-36. Anterior/posterior lumbar vertebral glides. In the lumbar region, anterior/posterior lumbar vertebral glides may be accomplished at individual segments using pressure on the spinous process through the pisiform in the hand. These decrease pain or increase mobility of individual lumbar vertebrae.

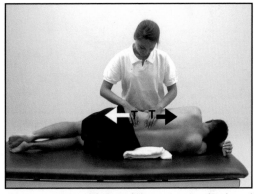

Figure 13-37. Lumbar lateral distraction. Lumbar lateral distraction increases the space between transverse processes and increases the opening of the intervertebral foramen. This position is achieved by lying over a support, flexing the patient's upper knee to a point where there is gapping in the appropriate spinal segment, then rotating the upper trunk to place the segment in a close-packed position. Then finger and forearm pressure are used to separate individual spaces. This pressure is used for reducing pain in the lumber vertebrae associated with some compression of a spinal segment.

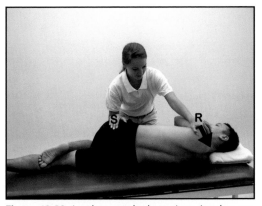

Figure 13-38. Lumbar vertebral rotations. Lumbar vertebral rotations decrease pain and increase mobility in lumbar vertebrae. These rotations should be done in a side-lying position.

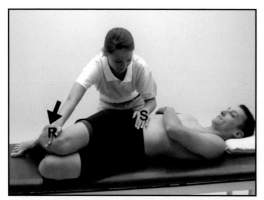

Figure 13-39. Lateral lumber rotations. Lateral lumbar rotations may be done with the patient in supine position. In this position, one hand must stabilize the upper trunk, while the other produces rotation.

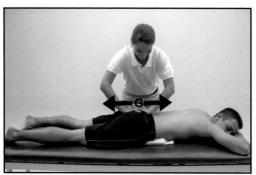

Figure 13-41. Superior/inferior sacral glides. Superior/inferior sacral glides decrease pain and reduce muscle guarding around the sacroiliac joint.

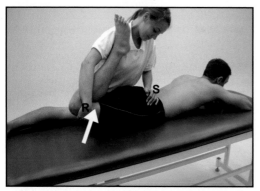

Figure 13-43. Anterior innominate rotation. An anterior innominate rotation may also be accomplished by extending the hip, applying upward force on the upper thigh, and stabilizing over the posterosuperior iliac spine. This technique is used to correct a posterior unilateral innominate rotation.

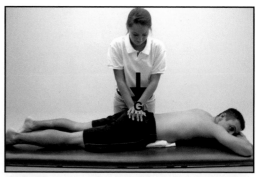

Figure 13-40. Anterior sacral glides. Anterior sacral glides decrease pain and reduce muscle guarding around the sacroiliac joint.

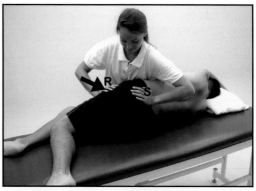

Figure 13-42. Anterior innominate rotation. An anterior innominate rotation in a side-lying position is accomplished by extending the leg on the affected side then stabilizing with one hand on the front of the thigh while the other applies pressure anteriorly over the posterosuperior iliac spine to produce an anterior rotation. This technique will correct a unilateral posterior rotation.

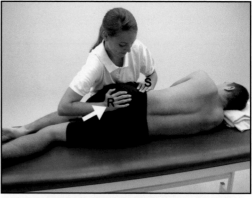

Figure 13-44. Posterior innominate rotation. A posterior innominate rotation with the patient in side-lying position is done by flexing the hip, stabilizing the anterosuperior iliac spine, and applying pressure to the ischium in an anterior direction.

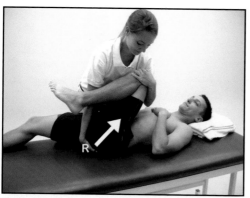

Figure 13-45. Posterior innominate rotation. Another posterior innominate rotation with the hip flexed at 90 degrees stabilizes the knee and rotates the innominate anteriorly through upward pressure on the ischium.

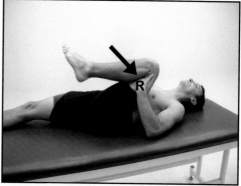

Figure 13-46. Posterior innominate rotation self-mobilization (supine). Posterior innominate rotation may be easily accomplished using self-mobilization. In a supine position, the patient grasps behind the flexed knee and gently rocks the innominate in a posterior direction.

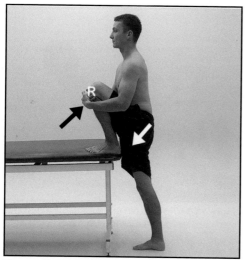

Figure 13-47. Posterior rotation self-mobilization (standing). In a standing position, the patient can perform a posterior rotation self-mobilization by pulling on the knee and rocking forward.

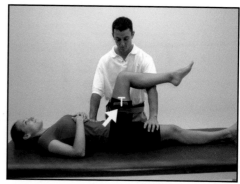

Figure 13-48. Lateral hip traction. Because the hip is a very strong, stable joint, it may be necessary to use body weight to produce effective joint mobilization or traction. An example of this would be in lateral hip traction. One strap should be used to secure the patient to the treatment table. A second strap is secured around the patient's thigh and around the athletic trainer's hips. Lateral traction is applied to the femur by leaning back away from the patient. This technique is used to reduce pain and increase hip mobility.

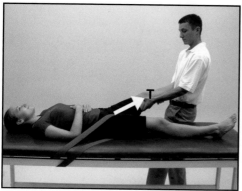

Figure 13-49. Femoral traction. Femoral traction with the hip at 0 degrees reduces pain and increases hip mobility. Inferior femoral glides in this position should be used to increase flexion and abduction.

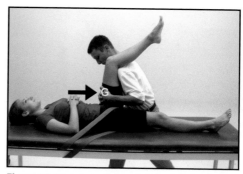

Figure 13-50. Inferior femoral glides. Inferior femoral glides at 90 degrees of hip flexion may also be used to increase abduction and flexion.

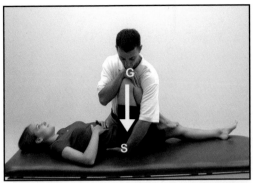

Figure 13-51. Posterior femoral glides. With the patient supine, a posterior femoral glide can be done by stabilizing underneath the pelvis and using the body weight applied through the femur to glide posteriorly. Posterior glides are used to increase hip flexion.

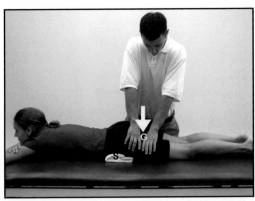

Figure 13-52. Anterior femoral glides. Anterior femoral glides increase extension and are accomplished by using some support to stabilize under the pelvis and applying an anterior glide posteriorly on the femur.

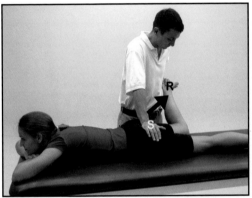

Figure 13-53. Medial femoral rotations. Medial femoral rotations may be used for increasing medial rotation and are done by stabilizing the opposite innominate while internally rotating the hip through the flexed knee.

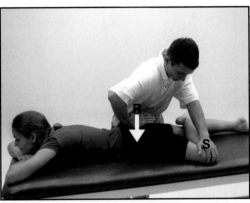

Figure 13-54. Lateral femoral rotation. Lateral femoral rotation is done by stabilizing a bent knee in the figure 4 position and applying rotational force to the ischium. This technique increases lateral femoral rotation.

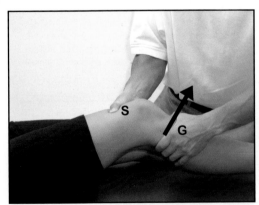

Figure 13-55. Anterior tibial glides. Anterior tibial glides are appropriate for the patient lacking full extension. Anterior glides should be done in prone position with the femur stabilized. Pressure is applied to the posterior tibia to glide anteriorly.

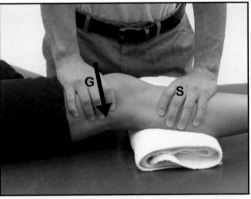

Figure 13-56. Posterior femoral glides. Posterior femoral glides are appropriate for the patient lacking full extension. Posterior femoral glides should be done in supine position with the tibia stabilized. Pressure is applied to the anterior femur to glide posteriorly.

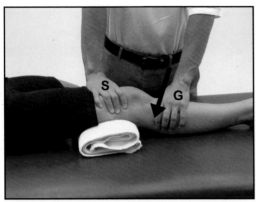

Figure 13-57. Posterior tibial glides. Posterior tibial glides increase flexion. With the patient in supine position, stabilize the femur, and glide the tibia posteriorly.

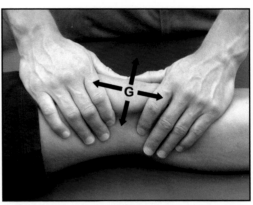

Figure 13-58. Patellar glides. Superior patellar glides increase knee extension. Inferior glides increase knee flexion. Medial glides stretch the lateral retinaculum. Lateral glides stretch tight medial structures.

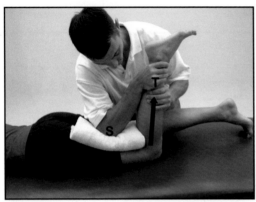

Figure 13-59. Tibiofemoral joint traction. Tibiofemoral joint traction reduces pain and hypomobility. It may be done with the patient prone and the knee flexed at 90 degrees. The elbow should stabilize the thigh while traction is applied through the tibia.

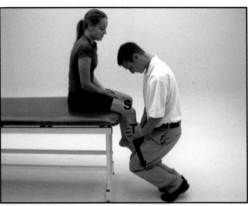

Figure 13-60. Alternative techniques for tibiofemoral joint traction. In very large individuals, an alternative technique for tibiofemoral joint traction uses body weight of the therapist to distract the joint once again for reducing pain and hypomobility.

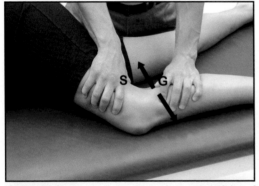

Figure 13-61. Proximal anterior and posterior glides of the fibula. Anterior and posterior glides of the fibula may be done proximally. They increase mobility of the fibular head and reduce pain. The femur should be stabilized. With the knee slightly flexed, grasp the head of the femur, and glide it anteriorly and posteriorly.

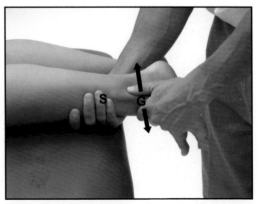

Figure 13-62. Distal anterior and posterior fibular glides. Anterior and posterior glides of the fibula may be done distally. The tibia should be stabilized, and the fibular malleolus is mobilized in an anterior or posterior direction.

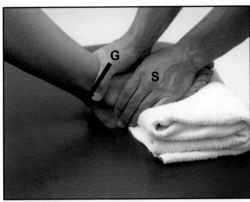

Figure 13-63. Posterior tibial glides. Posterior tibial glides increase plantarflexion. The foot should be stabilized, and pressure on the anterior tibia produces a posterior glide.

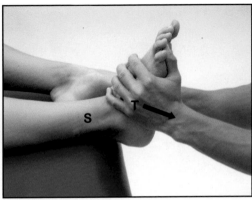

Figure 13-64. Talocrural joint traction. Talocrural joint traction is performed using the patient's body weight to stabilize the lower leg and applying traction to the midtarsal portion of the foot. Traction reduces pain and increases dorsiflexion and plantarflexion.

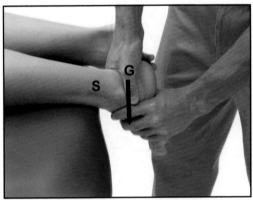

Figure 13-65. Anterior talar glides. Plantarflexion may also be increased by using an anterior talar glide. With the patient prone, the tibia is stabilized on the table and pressure is applied to the posterior aspect of the talus to glide it anteriorly.

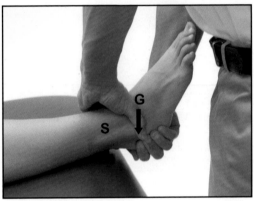

Figure 13-66. Posterior talar glides. Posterior talar glides may be used for increasing dorsiflexion. With the patient supine, the tibia is stabilized on the table and pressure is applied to the anterior aspect of the talus to glide it posteriorly.

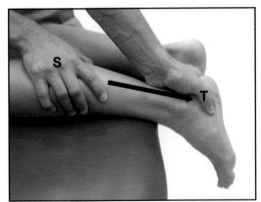

Figure 13-67. Subtalar joint traction. Subtalar joint traction reduces pain and increases inversion and eversion. The lower leg is stabilized on the table, and traction is applied by grasping the posterior aspect of the calcaneus.

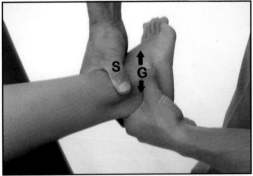

Figure 13-68. Subtalar joint medial and lateral glides. Subtalar joint medial and lateral glides increase eversion and inversion. The talus must be stabilized while the calcaneus is mobilized medially to increase inversion and laterally to increase eversion.

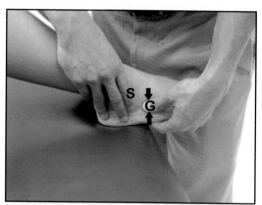

Figure 13-69. Anterior/posterior calcaneocuboid glides. Anterior/posterior calcaneocuboid glides may be used for increasing adduction and abduction. The calcaneus should be stabilized while the cuboid is mobilized.

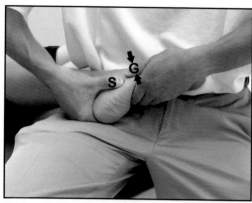

Figure 13-70. Anterior/posterior cuboid metatarsal glides. Anterior/posterior cuboid metatarsal glides are done with one hand stabilizing the cuboid and the other gliding the base of the fifth metatarsal. They are used for increasing mobility of the fifth metatarsal.

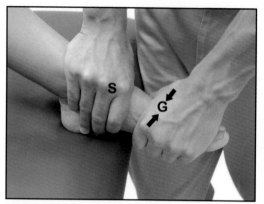

Figure 13-71. Anterior/posterior tarsometatarsal glides. Anterior/posterior tarsometatarsal glides decrease hypomobility of the metacarpals.

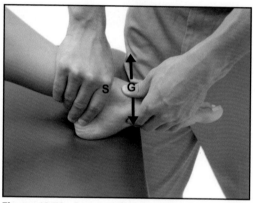

Figure 13-72. Anterior/posterior talonavicular glides. Anterior/posterior talonavicular glides also increase adduction and abduction. One hand stabilizes the talus while the other mobilizes the navicular bone.

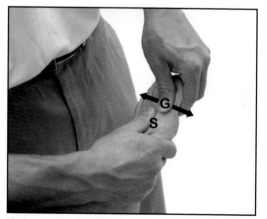

Figure 13-73. Anterior/posterior metatarsophalangeal glides. With anterior/posterior metatarsophalangeal glides, the anterior glides increase extension and posterior glides increase flexion. Mobilizations are accomplished by isolating individual segments.

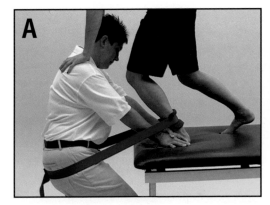
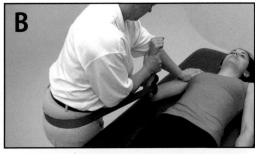
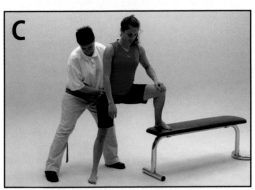
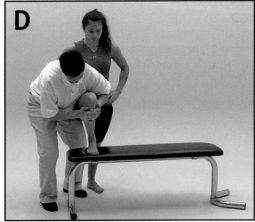

Figure 13-74. Mulligan techniques. (A) Technique for increasing dorsiflexion; (B) treating elbow lateral epicondylitis; (C) technique for restricted hip abduction; (D) treating painful knee flexion.

Summary

1. Mobilization and traction techniques increase joint mobility or decrease pain by restoring accessory movements to the joint.

2. Physiologic movements result from an active muscle contraction that moves an extremity through traditional cardinal planes.

3. Accessory motions refer to the manner in which one articulating joint surface moves relative to another.

4. Normal accessory component motions must occur for full-range physiologic movement to take place.

5. Accessory motions are also referred to as joint arthrokinematics and include spin, roll, and glide.

6. The convex-concave rule states that if the concave joint surface is moving on the stationary convex surface, gliding will occur in the same direction as the rolling motion. Conversely, if the convex surface is moving on a stationary concave surface, gliding will occur in an opposite direction to rolling.

7. The resting position is one in which the joint capsule and the ligaments are most relaxed, allowing for a maximum amount of joint play.

8. The treatment plane falls perpendicular to a line running from the axis of rotation in the convex surface to the center of the concave articular surface.

9. Maitland has proposed a series of five graded movements or oscillations in the ROM to treat pain and stiffness.

10. Kaltenborn uses three grades of traction to reduce pain and stiffness.

11. Kaltenborn emphasizes that traction should be used in conjunction

with mobilization glides to treat joint hypomobility.

12. Mulligan's technique combines passive accessory movement with active physiological movement to improve ROM or to minimize pain.

References

1. Barak T, Rosen E, Sofer R. Mobility: passive orthopedic manual therapy. In: Gould J, Davies G, eds. *Orthopedic and Sports Physical Therapy*. St. Louis, MO: Mosby; 1990:212-227.

2. Basmajian J, Banerjee S. *Clinical Decision Making in Rehabilitation: Efficacy and Outcomes*. Philadelphia, PA: Churchill-Livingstone; 1996.

3. Boissonnault W, Bryan J, Fox KS. Joint manipulation curricula in physical therapist professional degree programs. *J Orthop Sports Phys Ther*. 2004;34(4):171-181.

4. Conroy DE, Hayes KW. The effect of joint mobilization as a component of comprehensive treatment for primary shoulder impingement syndrome. *J Orthop Sports Phys Ther*. 1998;28(1):3-14.

5. Cookson J. Orthopedic manual therapy: an overview, II. The spine. *Phys Ther*. 1979;59:259.

6. Cookson J, Kent B. Orthopedic manual therapy: an overview, I. The extremities. *Phys Ther*. 1979;59:136.

7. Cyriax J. *Cyriax's Illustrated Manual of Orthopaedic Medicine*. London, UK: Butterworth; 1996.

8. Donatelli R, Owens-Burkhart H. Effects of immobilization on the extensibility of periarticular connective tissue. *J Orthop Sports Phys Ther*. 1981;3:67.

9. Edmond S. *Joint Mobilization and Manipulation: Extremity and Spinal Techniques*. Philadelphia, PA: Elsevier Health Sciences; 2006.

10. Exelby L. The Mulligan concept: its application in the management of spinal conditions. *Man Ther*. 2002;7(2):64-70.

11. Green T, Refshauge K, Crosbie J, Adams R. A randomized controlled trial of a passive accessory joint mobilization on acute ankle inversion sprains. *Phys Ther*. 2001;81(4):984-994.

12. Grimsby O. *Fundamentals of Manual Therapy: A Course Workbook*. Vagsbygd, Norway: Sorlandets Fysikalske Institutt; 1981.

13. Hall T. Effects of the Mulligan traction straight leg raise technique on range of movement. *J Man Manip Ther*. 2001;9(3):128-133.

14. Hollis M. *Practical Exercise*. Oxford, UK: Blackwell Scientific; 1999.

15. Hsu AT, Ho L, Chang JH, Chang GL, Hedman T. Characterization of tissue resistance during a dorsally directed translational mobilization of the glenohumeral joint. *Arch Phys Med Rehabil*. 2002;83(3):360-366.

16. Kaltenborn F. *Manual Mobilization of the Joints, Vol. II: The Spine*. Minneapolis, MN: Orthopedic Physical Therapy Products; 2003.

17. Kaltenborn F, Morgan D, Evjenth O. *Manual Mobilization of the Joints, Vol. I: The Extremities*. Minneapolis, MN: Orthopedic Physical Therapy Products; 2002.

18. Kaminski T, Kahanov L, Kato M. Therapeutic effect of joint mobilization: joint mechanoreceptors and nociceptors. *Athl Ther Today*. 2007;12(4):28.

19. Kisner C, Colby L. *Therapeutic Exercise: Foundations and Techniques*. Philadelphia, PA: FA Davis; 2007.

20. MacConaill M, Basmajian J. *Muscles and Movements: A Basis for Kinesiology*. Baltimore, MD: Williams & Wilkins; 1977.

21. Maigne R. *Orthopedic Medicine*. Springfield, IL: Charles C Thomas; 1976.

22. Macintyre J. Passive joint mobilization for acute ankle inversion sprains. *Clin J Sport Med*. 2002;12(1):54.

23. Maitland G. *Extremity Manipulation*. London, UK: Butterworth; 1991.

24. Maitland G. *Vertebral Manipulation*. Philadelphia, PA: Elsevier Health Science; 2005.

25. Mangus B, Hoffman L, Hoffman M. Basic principles of extremity joint mobilization using a Kaltenborn approach. *J Sport Rehabil*. 2002;11(4):235-250.

26. Mennell J. *The Musculoskeletal System: Differential Diagnosis from Symptoms and Physical Signs*. New York, NY: Aspen; 1991.

27. Mulligan's concept. Available at: http://www.bmulligan.com/about-us/2013.

28. Paris S. *The Spine: Course Notebook*. Atlanta, GA: Institute Press; 1979.

29. Paris S. Mobilization of the spine. *Phys Ther*. 1979;59:988.

30. Saunders D. *Evaluation, treatment and prevention of musculoskeletal disorders*. Shoreview, MN: Saunders Group; 2004.

31. Schiotz E, Cyriax J. *Manipulation Past and Present*. London, UK: Heinemann; 1978.

32. Stevenson J, Vaughn D. Four cardinal principles of joint mobilization and joint play assessment. *J Man Manip Ther*. 2003;11(3):146.

33. Stone JA. Joint mobilization. *Athl Ther Today*. 1998;4(6):59-60.

34. Teys P. The initial effects of a Mulligan's mobilization with movement technique on range of movement and pressure pain threshold in pain-limited shoulders. *Man Ther*. 2008;13(1):37.

35. Wadsworth C. *Manual Examination and Treatment of the Spine and Extremities*. Baltimore, MD: William & Wilkins; 1998.

36. Wilson E. The Mulligan concept: NAGS, SNAGS and mobilizations with movement. *J Bodyw Mov Ther*. 2001;5(2):81-89.

37. Zohn D, Mennell J. *Musculoskeletal Pain: Diagnosis and Physical Treatment*. Boston, MA: Little, Brown; 1987.

38. Zusman M. Reappraisal of a proposed neurophysiological mechanism for the relief of joint pain with passive joint movements. *Physiother Theory Pract.* 1985;1:61-70.

SOLUTIONS TO CLINICAL DECISION-MAKING EXERCISES

13-1 Once the patient has progressed through the acute stage, exercises and active and passive stretching can be accompanied by joint mobilizations. Mobilization of the knee joint involves gliding the concave tibia anteriorly on the femur.

13-2 In addition to exercises and possibly friction massage, she would benefit from joint mobilization to break down the scar tissue. If plantar flexion is limited, the talus should be glided anteriorly to stretch the anterior capsule. To address her ankle instability she can be provided with a brace, taping, and exercises to increase stability. Exercises should also target the muscles responsible for ankle inversion and eversion.

13-3 If the patient is restricted in extension, and lateral rotation due to tightness in the anterior capsule is causing the restriction, then the humeral head should be glided anteriorly on the glenoid to stretch the restriction.

13-4 Most manipulations performed by a chiropractor are Grade V. They take the joint to the end ROM and then apply a quick, small-amplitude thrust that forces the joint just beyond the point of limitation. Grade V manipulations should be performed only by those specifically trained in this technique. Laws and practice acts relative to the use of manipulations vary considerably from state to state.

13-5 Grade IV mobilization can be used. The talus should be forced anteriorly until movement is restricted. Small amplitude movements are then made at this end range causing structural changes in the scar tissue.

13-6 Traction applied to the spine increases space in between the vertebrae. The increased space reduces the pressure and compressive forces on the disc.

Please see videos on the accompanying website at

www.healio.com/books/sportsmedvideos

CHAPTER 14

Proprioceptive Neuromuscular Facilitation Techniques in Rehabilitation

William E. Prentice, PhD, PT, ATC, FNATA

After completion of this chapter, the athletic trainer should be able to do the following:

- Explain the neurophysiologic basis of proprioceptive neuromuscular facilitation (PNF) techniques.

- Discuss the rationale for use of PNF techniques.

- Identify the basic principles of using PNF in rehabilitation.

- Demonstrate the various PNF strengthening and stretching techniques.

- Describe PNF patterns for the upper and lower extremity, for the upper and lower trunk, and for the neck.

- Discuss the concept of muscle energy technique and explain how it is similar to PNF.

Proprioceptive neuromuscular facilitation (PNF) is an approach to therapeutic exercise based on the principles of functional human anatomy and neurophysiology.[10] It uses proprioceptive, cutaneous, and auditory input to produce functional improvement in motor output and can be a vital element in the rehabilitation process of many conditions and injuries.

The therapeutic techniques of PNF were first used in the treatment of patients with paralysis and various neuromuscular disorders in the 1950s. Originally the PNF techniques were used for strengthening and enhancing neuromuscular control. Since the early 1970s, the PNF techniques have also been used extensively as a technique for increasing flexibility and range of motion (ROM).[8,9,16,17,18,30,34,36,45,54,67,71]

This discussion should guide the athletic trainer in using the principles and techniques

Prentice WE, ed.
Rehabilitation Techniques for Sports Medicine and Athletic Training (pp 365-387).
© 2015 SLACK Incorporated.

of PNF as a component of a rehabilitation program.

PROPRIOCEPTIVE NEUROMUSCULAR FACILITATION AS A TECHNIQUE FOR IMPROVING STRENGTH AND ENHANCING NEUROMUSCULAR CONTROL

Original Concepts of Facilitation and Inhibition

Most of the principles underlying modern therapeutic exercise techniques can be attributed to the work of Sherrington[63] who first defined the concepts of facilitation and inhibition.

According to Sherrington, an impulse traveling down the corticospinal tract or an afferent impulse traveling up from peripheral receptors in the muscle causes an impulse volley that results in the discharge of a limited number of specific motor neurons, as well as the discharge of additional surrounding (anatomically close) motor neurons in the subliminal fringe area. An impulse causing the recruitment and discharge of additional motor neurons within the subliminal fringe is said to be facilitatory. Any stimulus that causes motor neurons to drop out of the discharge zone and away from the subliminal fringe is said to be inhibitory.[40] Facilitation results in increased excitability, and inhibition results in decreased excitability of motor neurons.[75] Thus, the function of weak muscles would be aided by facilitation, and muscle spasticity would be decreased by inhibition.[26]

Sherrington attributed the impulses transmitted from the peripheral stretch receptors via the afferent system as being the strongest influence on the alpha motor neurons.[63] Therefore, the athletic trainer should be able to modify the input from the peripheral receptors and thus influence the excitability of the alpha motor neurons. The discharge of motor neurons can be facilitated by peripheral stimulation, which causes afferent impulses to make contact with excitatory neurons and results in increased muscle tone or strength of voluntary contraction. Motor neurons can also be inhibited by peripheral stimulation, which causes afferent impulses to make contact with inhibitory neurons, resulting in muscle relaxation and allowing for stretching of the muscle.[63] PNF should be used to indicate any technique in which input from peripheral receptors is used to facilitate or inhibit.[26]

Several different approaches to therapeutic exercise based on the principles of facilitation and inhibition have been proposed. Among these are the Bobath method,[5,6] Brunnstrom method,[60] Rood method,[58] and Knott and Voss method,[37] which they called PNF. Although each of these techniques is important and useful, the PNF approach of Knott and Voss probably makes the most explicit use of proprioceptive stimulation.[37]

Rationale for Use

As a positive approach to injury rehabilitation, PNF is aimed at what the patient can do physically within the limitations of the injury. It is perhaps best used to decrease deficiencies in strength, flexibility, and neuromuscular coordination in response to demands that are placed on the neuromuscular system.[39] The emphasis is on selective reeducation of individual motor elements through development of neuromuscular control, joint stability, and coordinated mobility. Each movement is learned and then reinforced through repetition in an appropriately demanding and intense rehabilitative program.[59]

The body tends to respond to the demands placed on it. The principles of PNF attempt to provide a maximal response for increasing strength and neuromuscular control.[69,70] These principles should be applied with consideration of their appropriateness in achieving a particular goal. It is well accepted that the continued activity during a rehabilitation program is essential for maintaining or improving strength. Therefore, an intense program should offer the greatest potential for recovery.[53]

The PNF approach is holistic, integrating sensory, motor, and psychological aspects of a rehabilitation program. It incorporates reflex activities from the spinal levels and upward, either inhibiting or facilitating them as appropriate.

The brain recognizes only gross joint movement and not individual muscle action. Moreover, the strength of a muscle contraction is directly proportional to the activated motor units. Therefore, to increase the strength of a muscle, the maximum number of motor units must be stimulated to strengthen the remaining muscle fibers.[30,37] This "irradiation," or overflow effect, can occur when the stronger muscle groups help the weaker groups in completing a particular movement. This cooperation leads to the rehabilitation goal of return to optimal function.[4,37] The principles of PNF, as discussed in the next section, should be applied to reach that ultimate goal.

Clinical Decision-Making Exercise 14-1

A breaststroker is having trouble regaining strength after recovering from a hamstring strain. What can the athletic trainer do to help her?

BASIC PRINCIPLES OF PROPRIOCEPTIVE NEUROMUSCULAR FACILITATION

Margret Knott, in her text on PNF,[37] emphasized the importance of the principles rather than specific techniques in a rehabilitation program. These principles are the basis of PNF that must be superimposed on any specific technique. The principles of PNF are based on sound neurophysiologic and kinesiologic principles and clinical experience.[59] Application of the following principles can help promote a desired response in the patient being treated.

1. The patient must be taught the PNF patterns regarding the sequential movements from starting position to terminal position. The athletic trainer has to keep instructions brief and simple. It is sometimes helpful for the athletic trainer to passively move the patient through the desired movement pattern to demonstrate precisely what is to be done. The patterns should be used along with the techniques to increase the effects of the treatment.

2. When learning the patterns, the patient is often helped by looking at the moving limb. This visual stimulus offers the patient feedback for directional and positional control.

3. Verbal cues are used to coordinate voluntary effort with reflex responses. Commands should be firm and simple. Commands most commonly used with PNF techniques are "push" and "pull," which ask for an isotonic contraction; "hold," which asks for an isometric or stabilizing contraction; and "relax."

4. Manual contact with appropriate pressure is essential for influencing direction of motion and facilitating a maximal response because reflex responses are greatly affected by pressure receptors. Manual contact should be firm and confident to give the patient a feeling of security. The manner in which the athletic trainer touches the patient influences his or her confidence as well as the appropriateness of the motor response or relaxation.[59] A movement response may be facilitated by the hand over the muscle being contracted to facilitate a movement or a stabilizing contraction.

5. Proper mechanics and body positioning of the athletic trainer are essential in applying pressure and resistance. The athletic trainer should stand in a position that is in line with the direction of movement in the diagonal movement pattern. The knees should be bent and close to the patient such that the direction of resistance can easily be applied or altered appropriately throughout the range.

6. The amount of resistance given should facilitate a maximal response that allows smooth, coordinated motion. The appropriate resistance depends to a large extent on the capabilities of the patient. It may also change at different points throughout the ROM. Maximal resistance may be applied with techniques that use isometric

contractions to restrict motion to a specific point; it may also be used in isotonic contractions throughout a full range of movement.

7. Rotational movement is a critical component in all of the PNF patterns because maximal contraction is impossible without it.

8. Normal timing is the sequence of muscle contraction that occurs in any normal motor activity resulting in coordinated movement.[37] The distal movements of the patterns should occur first. The distal movement components should be completed no later than halfway through the total PNF pattern. To accomplish this, appropriate verbal commands should be timed with manual commands. Normal timing may be used with maximal resistance or without resistance from the athletic trainer.

9. Timing for emphasis is used primarily with isotonic contractions. This principle superimposes maximal resistance, at specific points in the range, upon the patterns of facilitation, allowing overflow or irradiation to the weaker components of a movement pattern. The stronger components are emphasized to facilitate the weaker components of a movement pattern.

10. Specific joints may be facilitated by using traction or approximation. Traction spreads apart the joint articulations, and approximation presses them together. Both techniques stimulate the joint proprioceptors. Traction increases the muscular response, promotes movement, assists isotonic contractions, and is used with most flexion antigravity movements. Traction must be maintained throughout the pattern. Approximation increases the muscular response, promotes stability, assists isometric contractions, and is used most with extension (gravity-assisted) movements. Approximation may be quick or gradual and repeated during a pattern.

11. Giving a quick stretch to the muscle before muscle contraction facilitates a muscle to respond with greater force through the mechanisms of the stretch reflex. It is most effective if all the components of a movement are stretched simultaneously. However, this quick stretch can be contraindicated in many orthopedic conditions because the extensibility limits of a damaged musculotendinous unit or joint structure might be exceeded, exacerbating the injury.

Clinical Decision-Making Exercise 14-2

A baseball player has had shoulder surgery to correct an anterior instability. He is having difficulty regaining strength throughout a full range of movement following the surgery. How can PNF strengthening be beneficial to someone who has a loss of ROM due to pain?

BASIC STRENGTHENING TECHNIQUES

Each of the principles described in the previous section should be applied to the specific techniques of PNF. These techniques may be used in a rehabilitation program to strengthen or facilitate a particular agonistic muscle group.[29,43,44] The choice of a specific technique depends on the deficits of a particular patient.[56] Specific techniques or combinations of techniques should be selected on the basis of the patient's problem.[3]

Clinical Decision-Making Exercise 14-3

Weakness following immobilization because of a radial fracture leaves a fencer with weak wrist musculature. She is having trouble initiating wrist extension. What PNF technique might the athletic trainer employ to increase strength?

Rhythmic Initiation

The rhythmic initiation technique involves a progression of initial passive, then active assistive, followed by active movement against resistance through the agonist pattern. Movement is slow, goes through the available ROM, and avoids activation of a quick stretch. It is used for patients who are unable to initiate movement and who have a limited ROM because of increased tone. It may also be used to teach the patient a movement pattern.

Repeated Contraction

Repeated contraction is useful when a patient has weakness either at a specific point or throughout the entire range. It is used to correct imbalances that occur within the range by repeating the weakest portion of the total range. The patient moves isotonically against maximal resistance repeatedly until fatigue is evidenced in the weaker components of the motion. When fatigue of the weak components becomes apparent, a stretch at that point in the range should facilitate the weaker muscles and result in a smoother, more coordinated motion. Again, quick stretch may be contraindicated with some musculoskeletal injuries. The amount of resistance to motion given by the athletic trainer should be modified to accommodate the strength of the muscle group. The patient is commanded to push by using the agonist concentrically and eccentrically throughout the range.

Slow Reversal

Slow reversal involves an isotonic contraction of the agonist followed immediately by an isotonic contraction of the antagonist. The initial contraction of the agonist muscle group facilitates the succeeding contraction of the antagonist muscles. The slow-reversal technique can be used for developing active ROM of the agonists and normal reciprocal timing between the antagonists and agonists, which is critical for normal coordinated motion.[55] The patient should be commanded to push against maximal resistance by using the antagonist and then to pull by using the agonist. The initial agonistic push facilitates the succeeding antagonist contraction.

Slow-Reversal-Hold

Slow-reversal-hold is an isotonic contraction of the agonist followed immediately by an isometric contraction, with a hold command given at the end of each active movement. The direction of the pattern is reversed by using the same sequence of contraction with no relaxation before shifting to the antagonistic pattern. This

technique can be especially useful in developing strength at a specific point in the ROM.

Rhythmic Stabilization

Rhythmic stabilization uses an isometric contraction of the agonist, followed by an isometric contraction of the antagonist to produce co-contraction and stability of the two opposing muscle groups. The command given is always "hold," and movement is resisted in each direction. Rhythmic stabilization results in an increase in the holding power to a point where the position cannot be broken. Holding should emphasize co-contraction of agonists and antagonists.

Clinical Decision-Making Exercise 14-4

A tennis player is complaining that when he serves, it feels like his shoulder "pops out" just after he hits the ball on the follow-through. How can PNF techniques be used to help this tennis player increase stability in his shoulder?

Clinical Decision-Making Exercise 14-5

A wrestler is recovering from a shoulder dislocation. He wants to know why the athletic trainer is using a manual PNF strengthening program instead of just letting him go to the weight room and work out on an exercise machine. What possible rationale might the athletic trainer give to the wrestler as to why PNF may be a more useful technique?

Treating Specific Problems With Proprioceptive Neuromuscular Facilitation Techniques

PNF-strengthening techniques can be useful in a variety of different conditions. To some extent the choice of the most effective technique for a given situation is dictated by the state of the existing condition and the capabilities and limitations of the individual patient.[72] There are some advantages to using PNF techniques in general.

Relative to strengthening, the PNF techniques are not encumbered by the design constraints of commercial exercise machines, although some of the newer exercise machines have been designed to accommodate triplanar motion and thus will allow for PNF patterned motion.[9] With the PNF patterns, movement can occur in three planes simultaneously, thus more closely resembling a functional movement pattern. The amount of resistance applied by the athletic trainer can be easily adjusted and altered at different points through the ROM to meet patient capabilities.[38] The athletic trainer can choose to concentrate on the strengthening through the entire ROM or through a very specific range. Combinations of several strengthening techniques can be used concurrently within the same PNF pattern.[51]

Rhythmic initiation is useful in the early stages of rehabilitation when the patient is having difficulty moving actively through a pain-free arc. Passive movement can allow the patient to maintain a full range while using an active contraction to move through the available pain-free range. Slow reversal should be used to help improve muscular endurance. Slow-reversal-hold is used to correct existing weakness at specific points in the ROM through isometric strengthening. Rhythmic stabilization is used to achieve stability and neuromuscular control about a joint.[11,21] This technique requires co-contraction of opposing muscle groups and is useful in creating a balance in the existing force couples.

Clinical Decision-Making Exercise 14-6

A small female athletic trainer is attempting to do a D2 lower-extremity PNF strengthening pattern on a 300-pound offensive tackle. How can the athletic trainer ensure that proper resistance is applied when performing PNF strengthening even when the athlete is quite strong?

PROPRIOCEPTIVE NEUROMUSCULAR FACILITATION PATTERNS

The PNF patterns are concerned with gross movement as opposed to specific muscle actions. The techniques identified previously can be superimposed on any of the PNF patterns. The techniques of PNF are composed of both rotational and diagonal exercise patterns that are similar to the motions required in most sports and normal daily activities.

The exercise patterns have three component movements: flexion–extension, abduction–adduction, and internal–external rotation. Human movement is patterned and rarely involves straight motion because all muscles are spiral in nature and lie in diagonal directions.

The PNF patterns described by Knott and Voss[37] involve distinct diagonal and rotational movements of the upper extremity, lower extremity, upper trunk, lower trunk, and neck. The exercise pattern is initiated with the muscle groups in the lengthened or stretched position. The muscle group is then contracted, moving the body part through the ROM to a shortened position.

The upper and lower extremities all have two separate patterns of diagonal movement for each part of the body, which are referred to as the diagonal 1 (D1) and diagonal 2 (D2) patterns. These diagonal patterns are subdivided into D1 moving into flexion, D1 moving into extension, D2 moving into flexion, and D2 moving into extension. Figures 14-1 and 14-2 illustrate the PNF patterns for the upper and lower extremities, respectively. The patterns are named according to the proximal pivots at either the shoulder or the hip (for example, the glenohumeral joint or femoroacetabular joint).

Tables 14-1 and 14-2 describe specific movements in the D1 and D2 patterns for the upper extremities. Figures 14-3 through 14-10 show starting and terminal positions for each of the diagonal patterns in the upper extremity.

Tables 14-3 and 14-4 describe specific movements in the D1 and D2 patterns for the lower extremities. Figures 14-11 through 14-18 show the starting and terminal positions for each of the diagonal patterns in the lower extremity.

Table 14-5 describes the rotational movement of the upper trunk moving into extension (also called chopping) and moving into flexion (also called lifting). Figures 14-19 and 14-20 show the starting and terminal positions of the upper-extremity chopping pattern moving into flexion to the right. Figures 14-21 and 14-22 show the starting and terminal positions for

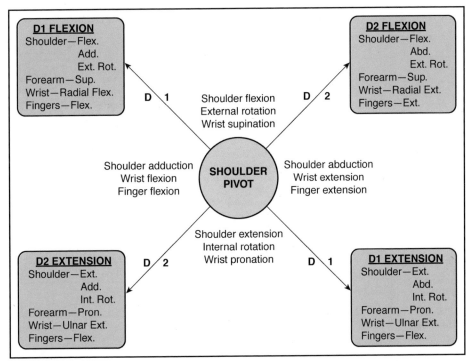

Figure 14-1. PNF patterns of the upper extremity.

Table 14-1 D1 Upper-Extremity Movement Patterns

Body Part	Moving Into Flexion		Moving Into Extension	
	Starting Position (Figure 14-3)	Terminal Position (Figure 14-4)	Starting Position (Figure 14-5)	Terminal Position (Figure 14-6)
Shoulder	Extended Abducted Internally rotated	Flexed Adducted Externally rotated	Flexed Adducted Externally rotated	Extended Adducted Internally rotated
Scapula	Depressed Retracted Downwardly rotated	Flexed Protracted Upwardly rotated	Elevated Protracted Upwardly rotated	Depressed Retracted Downwardly rotated
Forearm	Pronated	Supinated	Supinated	Pronated
Wrist	Ulnar extended	Radially flexed	Radially flexed	Ulnar extended
Finger and thumb	Extended Abducted	Flexed Adducted	Flexed Adducted	Extended Abducted
Hand position for athletic trainer[a]	Left and inside of volar surface of hand Right hand underneath arm in cubital fossa of elbow		Left hand on back of elbow on humerus Right hand on dorsum of hand	
Verbal command	Pull		Push	
[a]For patient's right arm.				

Table 14-2 D2 Upper-Extremity Movement Patterns

Body Part	Moving Into Flexion		Moving Into Extension	
	Starting Position (Figure 14-7)	Terminal Position (Figure 14-8)	Starting Position (Figure 14-9)	Terminal Position (Figure 14-10)
Shoulder	Extended Abducted Internally rotated	Flexed Adducted Externally rotated	Flexed Adducted Externally rotated	Extended Adducted Internally rotated
Scapula	Depressed Retracted Downwardly rotated	Flexed Protracted Upwardly rotated	Elevated Protracted Upwardly rotated	Depressed Retracted Downwardly rotated
Forearm	Pronated	Supinated	Supinated	Pronated
Wrist	Ulnar extended	Radially flexed	Radially flexed	Ulnar extended
Finger and thumb	Flexed Abducted	Extended Adducted	Extended Adducted	Flexed Abducted
Hand position for athletic trainer[a]	Left and on back of humerus Right hand on dorsum of hand		Left hand on volar surface of humerus Right hand on cubital fossa of elbow	
Verbal command	Push		Pull	

[a]For patient's right arm.

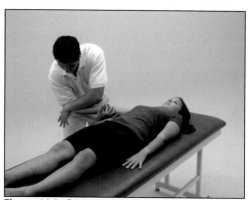

Figure 14-3. D1 upper-extremity movement pattern moving into flexion. Starting position.

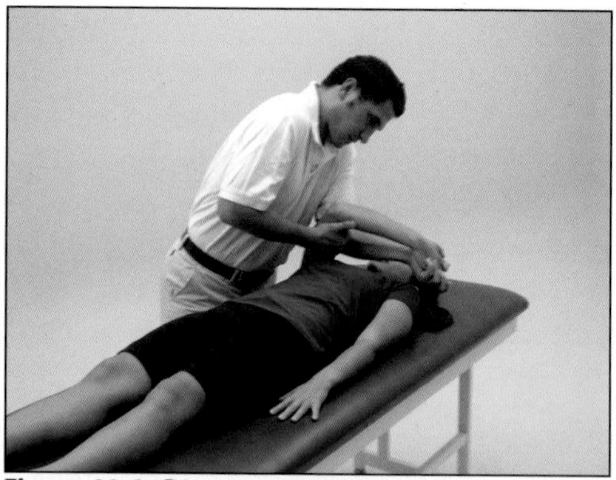

Figure 14-4. D1 upper-extremity movement pattern moving into flexion. Terminal position.

the upper-extremity lifting pattern moving into extension to the right.

Table 14-6 describes rotational movement of the lower extremities moving into positions of flexion and extension. Figures 14-23 and 14-24 show the lower-extremity pattern moving into flexion to the left. Figures 14-25 and 14-26 show the lower-extremity pattern moving into extension to the left.

The neck patterns involve simply flexion and rotation to one side (Figures 14-27 and 14-28) with extension and rotation to the opposite side (Figures 14-29 and 14-30). The patient should follow the direction of the movement with his or her eyes.

The principles and techniques of PNF, when used appropriately with specific patterns, can be an extremely effective tool for rehabilitation of injuries.[65] They can be used to strengthen

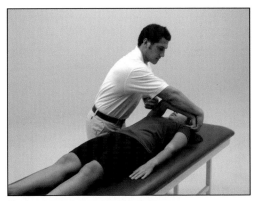

Figure 14-5. D1 upper-extremity movement pattern moving into extension. Starting position.

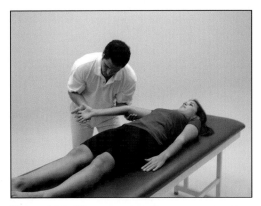

Figure 14-6. D1 upper-extremity movement pattern moving into extension. Terminal position.

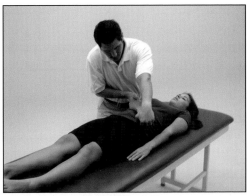

Figure 14-7. D2 upper-extremity movement pattern moving into flexion. Starting position.

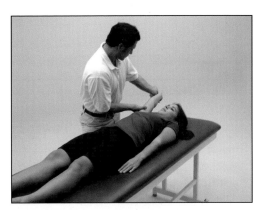

Figure 14-8. D2 upper-extremity movement pattern moving into flexion. Terminal position.

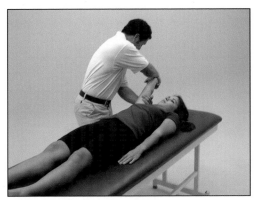

Figure 14-9. D2 upper-extremity movement pattern moving into extension. Starting position.

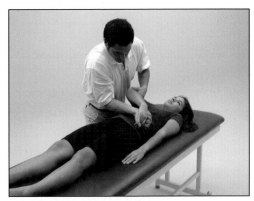

Figure 14-10. D2 upper-extremity movement pattern moving into extension. Terminal position.

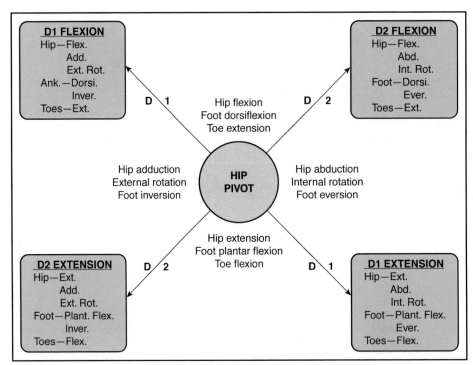

Figure 14-2. PNF patterns of the lower extremity.

Table 14-3 D1 Lower-Extremity Movement Patterns

Body Part	Moving Into Flexion		Moving Into Extension	
	Starting Position (Figure 14-11)	Terminal Position (Figure 14-12)	Starting Position (Figure 14-13)	Terminal Position (Figure 14-14)
Hip	Extended Abducted Internally rotated	Flexed Adducted Externally rotated	Flexed Adducted Externally rotated	Extended Abducted Internally rotated
Knee	Extended	Flexed	Flexed	Extended
Position of tibia	Externally rotated	Internally rotated	Internally rotated	Externally rotated
Ankle and foot	Plantarflexed Everted	Dorsiflexed Inverted	Dorsiflexed Inverted	Plantarflexed Everted
Toes	Flexed	Extended	Extended	Flexed
Hand position for athletic trainer[a]	Left and on back of humerus	Left hand on volar surface of humerus		
Right hand on dorsum of hand	Right hand on dorsomedial surface of foot		Right hand on lateral plantar surface of foot	
	Left hand on anteromedial thigh near patella		Left hand on posterolateral thigh near popliteal crease	
Verbal command	Pull		Push	
[a]For patient's right leg.				

Table 14-4 D2 Lower-Extremity Movement Patterns

Body Part	Moving Into Flexion		Moving Into Extension	
	Starting Position (Figure 14-15)	Terminal Position (Figure 14-16)	Starting Position (Figure 14-17)	Terminal Position (Figure 14-18)
Hip	Extended Adducted Externally rotated	Flexed Abducted Internally rotated	Flexed Abducted Internally rotated	Extended Adducted Externally rotated
Knee	Extended	Flexed	Flexed	Extended
Position of tibia	Externally rotated	Internally rotated	Internally rotated	Externally rotated
Ankle and foot	Plantarflexed Inverted	Dorsiflexed Everted	Dorsiflexed Everted	Plantarflexed Inverted
Toes	Flexed	Extended	Extended	Flexed
Hand position for athletic trainer[a]	Right hand on dorsolateral surface of foot Left hand on anterolateral thigh near patella		Right hand on medial plantar surface of foot Left hand on anterolateral thigh near patella	
Verbal command	Pull		Push	
[a]For patient's right leg.				

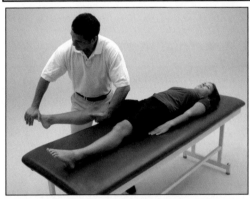

Figure 14-11. D1 lower-extremity movement pattern moving into flexion. Starting position.

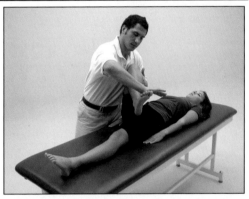

Figure 14-12. D1 lower-extremity movement pattern moving into flexion. Terminal position.

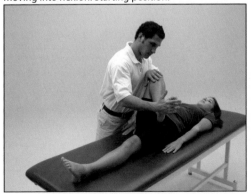

Figure 14-13. D1 lower-extremity movement pattern moving into extension. Starting position.

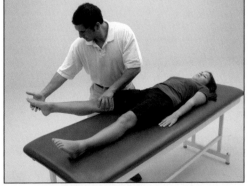

Figure 14-14. D1 lower-extremity movement pattern moving into extension. Terminal position.

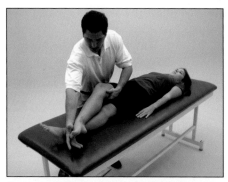

Figure 14-15. D1 lower-extremity movement pattern moving into flexion. Starting position.

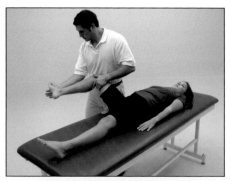

Figure 14-16. D2 lower-extremity movement pattern moving into flexion. Terminal position.

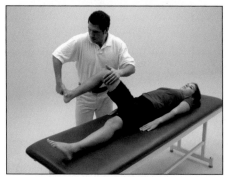

Figure 12-17. D2 lower-extremity movement pattern moving into extension. Starting position.

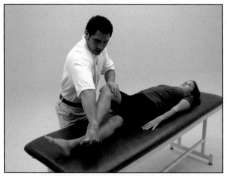

Figure 14-18. D2 lower-extremity movement pattern moving into extension. Terminal position.

Table 14-5 Upper-Trunk Movement Patterns

Body Part	Moving Into Flexion (Chopping)[a]		Moving Into Extension (Lifting)[a]	
	Starting Position (Figure 14-19)	Terminal Position (Figure 14-20)	Starting Position (Figure 14-21)	Terminal Position (Figure 14-22)
Right upper extremity	Flexed Adducted Internally rotated	Extended Abducted Externally rotated	Extended Adducted Internally rotated	Flexed Abducted Externally rotated
Left upper extremity (left hand grasps right forearm)	Flexed Abducted Externally rotated	Extended Adducted Internally rotated	Extended Abducted Externally rotated	Flexed Adducted Internally rotated
Trunk	Rotated and extended to left	Rotated and flexed to right	Rotated and flexed to left	Rotated and extended to right
Head	Rotated and extended to left	Rotated and flexed to right	Rotated and flexed to left	Rotated and extended to right
Hand position for athletic trainer[a]	Left hand on right anterolateral surface of forehead Right hand on dorsum of right hand		Right hand on dorsum of right hand Left hand on posterolateral surface of head	
Verbal command	Pull down		Push up	
[a]Patient's rotation is to the right.				

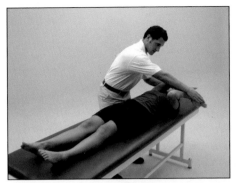

Figure 14-19. Upper-trunk pattern moving into flexion or chopping. Starting position.

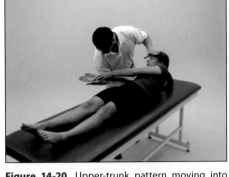

Figure 14-20. Upper-trunk pattern moving into flexion or chopping. Terminal position.

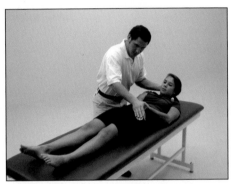

Figure 14-21. Upper-trunk pattern moving into flexion or lifting. Starting position.

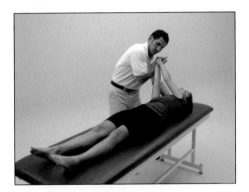

Figure 14-22. Upper-trunk pattern moving into flexion or lifting. Terminal position.

Table 14-6 Lower Trunk Movement Patterns

Body Part	Moving Into Flexion[a]		Moving Into Extension[b]	
	Starting Position (Figure 14-23)	Terminal Position (Figure 14-24)	Starting Position (Figure 14-25)	Terminal Position (Figure 14-26)
Right upper extremity	Extended Abducted Externally rotated	Flexed Adducted Internally rotated	Flexed Adducted Internally rotated	Extended Abducted Externally rotated
Left hip	Extended Adducted Internally rotated	Flexed Abducted Externally rotated	Flexed Abducted Externally rotated	Extended Adducted Internally rotated
Ankles	Plantarflexed	Dorsiflexed		Plantarflexed
Toes	Flexed	Extended	Extended	Flexed
Hand position for athletic trainer[a]	Right hand on dorsum of feet Left hand on anterolateral surface of left knee		Right hand on plantar surface of foot Left hand on posterolateral surface of right knee	
Verbal command	Pull up and in		Push down and out	
[a]Patient's rotation is to the right.				
[b]Patient's rotation is to the right in extension.				

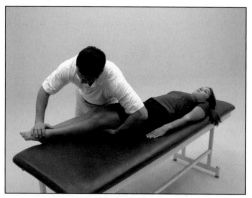

Figure 14-23. Lower-trunk pattern moving into flexion to the left. Starting position.

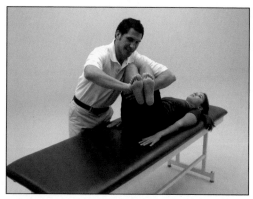

Figure 14-24. Lower-trunk pattern moving into flexion to the left. Terminal position

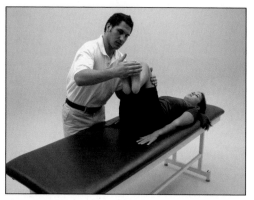

Figure 14-25. Lower-trunk pattern moving into extension to the left. Starting position.

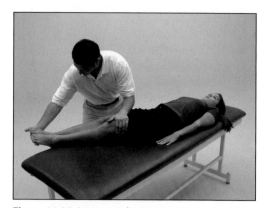

Figure 14-26. Lower-trunk pattern moving into extension to the left. Terminal position.

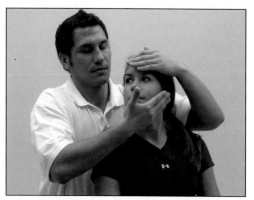

Figure 14-27. Neck flexion and rotation to the left. Starting position.

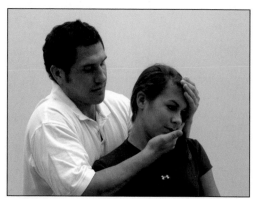

Figure 14-28. Neck flexion and rotation to the left. Terminal position.

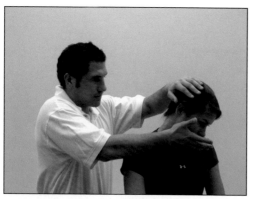

Figure 14-29. Neck extension and rotation to the right. Starting position.

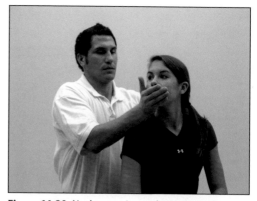

Figure 14-30. Neck extension and rotation to the right. Terminal position.

weak muscles or muscle groups and to improve the neuromuscular control about an injured joint. Specific techniques selected for use should depend on individual patient needs and may be modified accordingly.[14,15]

PROPRIOCEPTIVE NEUROMUSCULAR FACILITATION AS A TECHNIQUE OF STRETCHING FOR IMPROVING ROM

As indicated previously, PNF techniques can also be used for stretching to increase ROM.

Evolution of the Theoretical Basis for Using Proprioceptive Neuromuscular Facilitation as a Stretching Technique

A review of the current literature indicates that many clinicians believe that the PNF-stretching techniques can be an effective treatment modality for improving flexibility and thus use them regularly in clinical practice.[4,18,26,35,49,52,61,62] Through the years, various theories have been proposed to explain the neurologic and physical mechanisms through which the PNF techniques improve flexibility.[13] However, to date no consensus agreement exists that embraces a single theoretical explanation.

Neurophysiologic Basis of Proprioceptive Neuromuscular Facilitation Stretching

PNF gained popularity as a stretching technique in the 1970s.[45,54,71] The PNF research that has traditionally appeared in the literature since that time has attributed increases in ROM primarily to neurophysiologic mechanisms involving the stretch reflex.[13] More recent studies question the validity of this theoretical explanation.[1,13,32,33,68] Nevertheless, a brief review of the stretch reflex will serve as a springboard for more currently accepted theories.

The stretch reflex involves two types of receptors: (1) muscle spindles that are sensitive to a change in length, as well as the rate of change in length of the muscle fiber; and (2) Golgi tendon organs that detect changes in tension (Figure 14-31).

Stretching a given muscle causes an increase in the frequency of impulses transmitted to the spinal cord from the muscle spindle along Ia fibers, which, in turn, produces an increase in the frequency of motor nerve impulses returning to that same muscle, along alpha motor neurons, thus reflexively resisting the stretch (Figure 14-31). However, the development of excessive tension within the muscle activates the Golgi tendon organs, whose sensory impulses are carried back to the spinal cord along Ib fibers. These impulses have an inhibitory effect on the motor impulses returning to the muscles and cause that muscle to relax (Figure 14-32).[12]

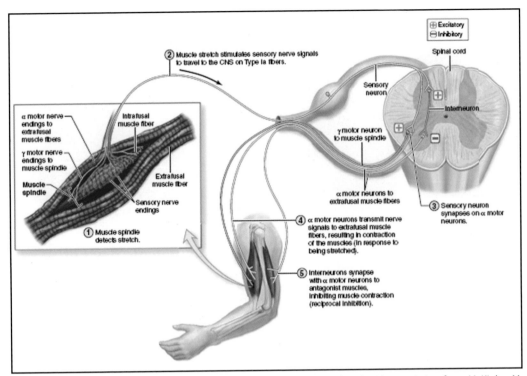

Figure 14-31. Diagrammatic representation of the stretch reflex. (Reproduced with permission from McKinley M, O'Loughlin V. *Human Anatomy*. 3rd ed. New York: McGraw-Hill; 2012.)

Two neurophysiologic phenomena have been proposed to explain facilitation and inhibition of the neuromuscular systems. The first, autogenic inhibition, is defined as inhibition mediated by afferent fibers from a stretched muscle acting on the alpha motor neurons supplying that muscle, causing it to relax. When a muscle is stretched, motor neurons supplying that muscle receive both excitatory and inhibitory impulses from the receptors. If the stretch is continued for a slightly extended time, the inhibitory signals from the Golgi tendon organs eventually override the excitatory impulses and therefore cause relaxation. Because inhibitory motor neurons receive impulses from the Golgi tendon organs while the muscle spindle creates an initial reflex excitation leading to contraction, the Golgi tendon organs apparently send inhibitory impulses that last for the duration of increased tension (resulting from either passive stretch or active contraction) and eventually dominate the weaker impulses from the muscle spindle. This inhibition seems to protect the muscle against injury from reflex contractions resulting from excessive stretch.

A second mechanism, reciprocal inhibition, deals with the relationships of the agonist and antagonist muscles (Figure 14-31). The muscles that contract to produce joint motion are referred to as agonists, and the resulting movement is called an agonistic pattern. The muscles that stretch to allow the agonist pattern to occur are referred to as antagonists. Movement that occurs directly opposite to the agonist pattern is called the antagonist pattern.

When motor neurons of the agonist muscle receive excitatory impulses from afferent nerves, the motor neurons that supply the antagonist muscles are inhibited by afferent impulses.[4] Thus, contraction or extended stretch of the agonist muscle has been said to elicit relaxation or inhibit the antagonist. Likewise, a quick stretch of the antagonist muscle facilitates a contraction of the agonist.

The PNF literature has traditionally asserted that isometric or isotonic submaximal contraction of a target muscle (muscle to be stretched) prior to a passive stretch of that same muscle, or contraction of opposing muscles (agonists) during muscle stretch, produces relaxation

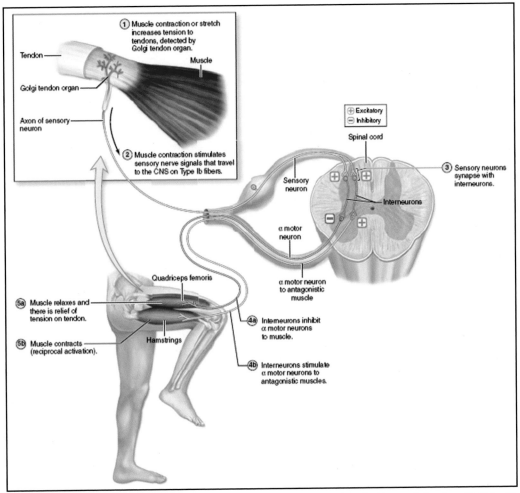

Figure 14-32. Diagrammatic representation of reciprocal inhibition. (Reproduced with permission from McKinley M, O'Loughlin V. *Human Anatomy*. 3rd ed. New York: McGraw-Hill; 2012.)

of the stretched muscle through activation of the mechanisms of the stretch reflex that include autogenic inhibition and reciprocal inhibition.[13]

However, data from a number of studies conducted since the early 1990s suggest that relaxation following a contraction of a stretched muscle is not a result of the inhibition of muscle spindle activity or subsequent activation of Golgi tendon organs.[1,2,12,13,23,24,29,46,51]

Conclusions are based on the fact that when slowly stretching a muscle to a long length, as in the PNF-stretching techniques, the reflex-generated muscle electrical activation from the muscle spindles (as indicated by electromyogram) is very small and clinically insignificant, and not likely to effectively resist an applied muscle lengthening force.[13,28,31,35,41] Furthermore, when a muscle relaxes following an isometric contraction, Golgi tendon organ firing is decreased or even becomes silent.[20,73] Thus, Golgi tendon organs would not be able to inhibit the target muscle in the seconds following contraction when the slow therapeutic stretch would be applied.[13] It is apparent that, in general, there is a lack of research-based evidence to support the theory that Golgi tendon organ and muscle spindle reflexes are able to relax target muscles during any of the PNF-stretching techniques.[13] Thus, other mechanisms have been proposed that may explain increases in ROM with PNF-stretching exercises.[19]

Presynaptic Inhibition

In the PNF-stretching techniques, the contraction and subsequent relaxation of the target muscle is followed by a slow passive stretch of that muscle to a longer length. It has been suggested that lengthening is associated with an increase in presynaptic inhibition of the sensory signal from the muscle spindle.[13,22,25] This occurs with inhibition of the release of a neurotransmitter from the synaptic terminals of the muscle spindle Ia sensory fibers that limits activation in that muscle.

Viscoelastic Changes in Response to Stretching

It has been proposed that viscoelastic changes that occur in a muscle, and not a decrease in muscle activation mediated by Golgi tendon organs, is the mechanism that may explain increases in ROM associated with the PNF techniques.[8] The viscoelastic properties of collagen in muscle are discussed briefly in Chapter 8. The force that is required to produce a change in length of a muscle is determined by its elastic stiffness.[72] Because of the viscous properties of muscle, less force is needed to elongate a muscle if that force is applied slowly rather than rapidly.[72] Also, the force that resists elongation is reduced if the muscle is held at a stretched length over time, thus producing stress relaxation.[64] As stress relaxation occurs, the muscle will elongate further, producing creep. These properties have been demonstrated in muscles with no significant electrical activity.[41,42,47]

As the viscoelastic properties within a muscle are changed during a PNF-stretching procedure, there is an altered perception of stretch and a greater ROM and greater torque can be achieved before the onset of pain is perceived.[42,74] This is thought to occur because lengthening interrupts the actin-myosin bonds within the intrafusal fibers of the muscle spindle, thus reducing their sensitivity to stretch.[22,27,73]

Stretching Techniques

The following techniques should be used to increase ROM, relaxation, and inhibition.

Contract-Relax

Contract-relax is a stretching technique that moves the body part passively into the agonist pattern. The patient is instructed to push by contracting the antagonist (muscle that will be stretched) isotonically against the resistance of the athletic trainer. The patient then relaxes the antagonist while the athletic trainer moves the part passively through as much range as possible to the point where limitation is again felt. This contract-relax technique is beneficial when ROM is limited by muscle tightness.

Hold-Relax

Hold-relax is very similar to the contract-relax technique. It begins with an isometric contraction of the antagonist (muscle that will be stretched) against resistance, followed by a concentric contraction of the agonist muscle combined with light pressure from the athletic trainer to produce maximal stretch of the antagonist. This technique is appropriate when there is muscle tension on one side of a joint and may be used with either the agonist or antagonist.[7]

Slow-Reversal-Hold-Relax

Slow-reversal-hold-relax technique begins with an isotonic contraction of the agonist, which often limits ROM in the agonist pattern, followed by an isometric contraction of the antagonist (muscle that will be stretched) during the push phase. During the relax phase, the antagonists are relaxed while the agonists are contracting, causing movement in the direction of the agonist pattern and thus stretching the antagonist. The technique, like the contract-relax and hold-relax, is useful for increasing ROM when the primary limiting factor is the antagonistic muscle group. Because a goal of rehabilitation with most injuries is restoration of strength through a full, nonrestricted ROM, several of these techniques are sometimes combined in sequence to accomplish this goal.[50] Figure 14-33 shows a PNF-stretching technique in which the athletic trainer is stretching an injured patient.

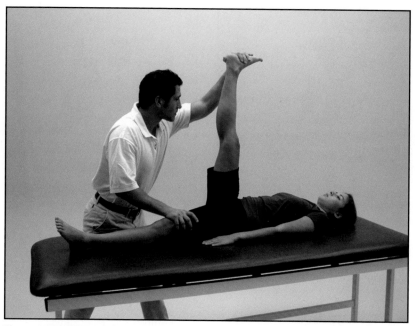

Figure 14-33. PNF-stretching technique.

MUSCLE ENERGY TECHNIQUES

Muscle energy is a manual therapy technique, which is a variation of the PNF contract-relax and hold-relax techniques. Like the PNF techniques, the muscle energy techniques are based on the same neurophysiologic mechanisms involving the stretch reflex discussed earlier. Muscle energy techniques involve a voluntary contraction of a muscle in a specifically controlled direction at varied levels of intensity against a distinctly executed counterforce applied by the therapist.[30,48] The patient provides the corrective intrinsic forces and controls the intensity of the muscular contractions while the therapist controls the precision and localization of the procedure.[48] The amount of patient effort can vary from a minimal muscle twitch to a maximal muscle contraction.[30] Five components are necessary for muscle energy techniques to be effective[30]:

1. Active muscle contraction by the patient.

2. A muscle contraction oriented in a specific direction.

3. Some patient control of contraction intensity.

4. Therapist control of joint position.

5. Therapist application of appropriate counterforce.

Clinical Applications

It has been proposed that muscles function not only as flexors, extenders, rotators, and side-benders of joints, but also as restrictors of joint motion. In situations where the muscle is restricting joint motion, muscle energy techniques use a specific muscle contraction to restore physiological movement to a joint.[48] Any articulation, whether in the spine or extremities, that can be moved by active muscle contraction can be treated using muscle energy techniques.[48,57]

Muscle energy techniques can be used to accomplish several treatment goals[30]:

- Lengthening of a shortened, contracted, or spastic muscle.

- Strengthening of a weak muscle or muscle group.

- Reduction of localized edema through muscle pumping.

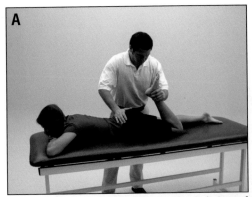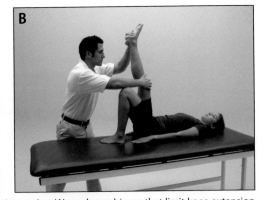

Figure 14-34. Positions for muscle energy techniques for improving (A) weak quadriceps that limit knee extension and/or hip flexion, and (B) weak hamstrings that limit knee flexion and/or hip extension.

- Mobilization of an articulation with restricted mobility.
- Stretching of fascia.

Treatment Techniques

Muscle energy techniques can involve four types of muscle contraction: isometric, concentric isotonic, eccentric isotonic, and isolytic. An isolytic contraction involves a concentric contraction by the patient while the athletic trainer applies an external force in the opposite direction, overpowering the contraction and lengthening that muscle.[48]

Isometric and concentric isotonic contractions are most frequently used in treatment.[66] Isometric contractions are most often used in treating hypertonic muscles in the spinal vertebral column, whereas isotonic contractions are most often used in the extremities. With both types of contraction, the idea is to inhibit antagonistic muscles producing more symmetrical muscle tone and balance.

A concentric contraction can also be used to mobilize a joint against its motion barrier if there is motion restriction. For example, if a strength imbalance exists between the quadriceps and hamstrings, with weak quadriceps limiting knee extension, the following concentric isotonic muscle energy technique may be used (Figure 14-34A):

1. The patient lies prone on the treatment table.

2. The athletic trainer stabilizes the patient with one hand and grasps the ankle with the other.

3. The athletic trainer fully flexes the knee.

4. The patient actively extends the knee, using as much force as possible.

5. The athletic trainer provides a resistant counterforce that allows slow knee extension throughout the available range.

6. Once the patient has completely relaxed, the athletic trainer moves the knee back to full flexion and the patient repeats the contraction with additional resistance applied through the full range of extension. This is repeated three to five times with increasing resistance on each repetition.

If a knee has a restriction because of tightness in the hamstrings that is limiting full-extension, the following isometric muscle energy technique should be used (Figure 14-34B):

1. The patient lies supine on the treatment table.

2. The athletic trainer stabilizes the knee with one hand and grasps the ankle with the other.

3. The athletic trainer fully extends the knee until an extension barrier is felt.

4. The patient actively flexes the knee using a minimal sustained force.

5. The athletic trainer provides an equal resistant counterforce for 3 to 7 seconds, after which the patient completely relaxes.

6. The athletic trainer again extends the knee until a new extension barrier is felt.

7. This is repeated three to five times.

Summary

1. The PNF techniques may be used to increase both strength and ROM and are based on the neurophysiology of the stretch reflex.

2. The motor neurons of the spinal cord always receive a combination of inhibitory and excitatory impulses from the afferent nerves. Whether these motor neurons will be excited or inhibited depends on the ratio of the two types of incoming impulses.

3. The PNF techniques emphasize specific principles that may be superimposed on any of the specific techniques.

4. The PNF-strengthening techniques include repeated contraction, slow-reversal, slow-reversal-hold, rhythmic stabilization, and rhythmic initiation.

5. The PNF-stretching techniques include contract-relax, hold-relax, and slow-reversal-hold-relax.

6. The techniques of PNF are rotational and diagonal movements in the upper extremity, lower extremity, upper trunk, and the head and neck.

7. Muscle energy techniques involve a voluntary contraction of a muscle in a specifically controlled direction at varied levels of intensity against a distinctly executed counterforce applied by the athletic trainer.

References

1. Alter M. *Science of Flexibility*. 3rd ed. Champaign, IL: Human Kinetics; 2004.

2. Anderson B, Burke ER. Scientific, medical, and practical aspects of stretching. *Clin Sports Med.* 1991;10:63-86.

3. Barak T, Rosen E, Sofer R. Mobility: Passive orthopedic manual therapy. In: Gould J, Davies G, eds. *Orthopedic and Sports Therapy*. St. Louis: Mosby; 1990:212-227.

4. Barry D. Proprioceptive neuromuscular facilitation for the scapula, part 1: diagonal 1. *Athl Ther Today.* 2005;10(2):54.

5. Basmajian J. *Therapeutic Exercise*. Baltimore, MD: Lippincott, Williams & Wilkins; 1990.

6. Bobath B. The treatment of motor disorders of pyramidal and extrapyramidal tracts by reflex inhibition and by facilitation of movement. *Physiotherapy*. 1955;41:146.

7. Bonnar B, Deivert R, Gould T. The relationship between isometric contraction durations during hold-relax stretching and improvement of hamstring flexibility. *J Sports Med Phys Fitness.* 2004;44(3):258-261.

8. Bradley P, Olsen P, Portas M. The effect of static ballistic and PNF stretching on vertical jump performance. *J Strength Cond Res.* 2007;21(1):223.

9. Burke DG, Culligan CJ, Holt LE. Equipment designed to stimulate proprioceptive neuromuscular facilitation flexibility training. *J Strength Cond Res.* 2000;14(2):135-139.

10. Burke DG, Culligan CJ, Holt LE. The theoretical basis of proprioceptive neuromuscular facilitation. *J Strength Cond Res.* 2000;14(4):496-500.

11. Burke DG, Holt LE, Rasmussen R. Effects of hot or cold water immersion and modified proprioceptive neuromuscular facilitation flexibility exercise on hamstring length. *J Athl Train.* 2001;36(1):16-19.

12. Carter AM, Kinzey SJ, Chitwood LE, Cole JL. Proprioceptive neuromuscular facilitation decreases muscle activity during the stretch reflex in selected posterior thigh muscles. *J Sport Rehabil.* 2000;9(4):269-278.

13. Chalmers G. Re-examination of the possible role of Golgi tendon organ and muscle spindle reflexes in proprioceptive neuromuscular facilitation muscle stretching. *Sports Biomech.* 2004;3(1):159-183.

14. Cookson J, Kent B. Orthopedic manual therapy: An overview I. The extremities. *Phys Ther.* 1979;59:136.

15. Cookson J. Orthopedic manual therapy: An overview, II. The spine. *Phys Ther.* 1979;59:259.

16. Cornelius W, Jackson A. The effects of cryotherapy and PNF on hip extension flexibility. *Athlet Train.* 1984;19(3):184.

17. Davis D, Hagerman-Hose M, Midkiff M. The effectiveness of 3 proprioceptive neuromuscular facilitation stretching techniques on the flexibility of the hamstring muscle group [abstract]. *J Orthop Sports Phys Ther.* 2004;34(1):A33-A34.

18. Decicco PV, Fisher MM. The effects of proprioceptive neuromuscular facilitation stretching on shoulder range of motion in overhand athletes. *J Sports Med Phys Fitness.* 2005;45(2):183-187.

19. Decicco P, Fisher M. The effects of proprioceptive neuromuscular facilitation stretching on shoulder range of motion in overhand athletes. *J Sports Med Phys Fitness.* 2005;45(2):183-187.

20. Edin BB, Vallbo AB. Muscle afferent responses to isometric contractions and relaxations in humans. *J Neurophysiol.* 1990;63:1307-1313.

21. Engle R, Canner G. Proprioceptive neuromuscular facilitation (PNF) and modified procedures for anterior cruciate ligament (ACL) instability. *J Orthop Sports Phys Ther.* 1989;11(6):230-236.

22. Enoka R. *Neuromechanics of Human Movement.* 4th ed. Champaign, IL: Human Kinetics; 2008.

23. Enoka RM, Hutton RS, Eldred E. Changes in excitability of tendon tap and Hoffmann reflexes following voluntary contractions. *Electroencephalogr Clin Neurophysiol.* 1980;48:664-672.

24. Ferber R, Osternig L, Gravelle D. Effect of PNF stretch techniques on knee flexor muscle EMG activity in older adults. *J Electromyogr Kinesiol.* 2002;12:391-397.

25. Gollhofer A, Schopp A, Rapp W, Stroinik V. Changes in reflex excitability following isometric contraction in humans. *Eur J Appl Physiol Occup Physiol.* 1998;77:89-97.

26. Greenman P. *Principles of Manual Medicine.* Baltimore, MD: Lippincott, Williams & Wilkins; 2003.

27. Gregory JE, Mark RF, Morgan DL, Patak A, Polus B, Proske U. Effects of muscle history on the stretch reflex in cat and man. *J Physiol.* 1990;424:93-107.

28. Halbertsma JP, Mulder I, Goeken LN, Eisma WH. Repeated passive stretching: Acute effect on the passive muscle moment and extensibility of short hamstrings. *Arch Phys Med Rehabil.* 1999;80:407-414.

29. Holcomb WR. Improved stretching with proprioceptive neuromuscular facilitation. *Strength Cond J.* 2000;22(1):59-61.

30. Hollis M. *Practical exercise.* Oxford, UK: Blackwell Scientific; 1981.

31. Houk JC, Rymer WZ, Crago PE. Dependence of dynamic response of spindle receptors on muscle length and velocity. *J Neurophysiol.* 1981;46:143-166.

32. Hultborn H. State-dependent modulation of sensory feedback. *J Physiol.* 2001;533(Pt 1):5-13.

33. Jankowska E. Interneuronal relay in spinal pathways from proprioceptors. *Prog Neurobiol.* 1992;38:335-378.

34. Johnson GS. PNF and knee rehabilitation. *J Orthop Sports Phys Ther.* 2000;30(7):430-431.

35. Kitani I. The effectiveness of proprioceptive neuromuscular facilitation (PNF) exercises on shoulder joint position sense in baseball players (Abstract). *J Athl Train.* 2004;39(2):S-62.

36. Knappstein A, Stanley S, Whatman C. Range of motion immediately post and seven minutes post, PNF stretching hip joint range of motion and PNF stretching. *NZ J Sports Med.* 2004;32(2):42-46.

37. Knott M, Voss D. *Proprioceptive Neuromuscular Facilitation: Patterns and Techniques.* Baltimore, MD: Lippincott, Williams & Wilkins; 1985.

38. Kofotolis N, Kellis E. Cross-training effects of a proprioceptive neuromuscular facilitation exercise program on knee musculature. *Phys Ther Sport.* 2007;8(3):109.

39. Kofotolis N, Kellis E. Effects of two 4-week proprioceptive neuromuscular facilitation programs on muscle endurance, flexibility, and functional performance in women with chronic low back pain. *Phys Ther.* 2006;86(7):1001.

40. Lloyd D. Facilitation and inhibition of spinal motor neurons. *J Neurophysiol.* 1946;9:421.

41. Magnusson SP, Simonsen EB, Aagaard P, Dyhre-Poulsen P, McHugh MP, Kjaer M. Mechanical and physiological responses to stretching with and without preisometric contraction in human skeletal muscle. *Arch Phys Med Rehabil.* 1996;77:373-378.

42. Magnusson SP, Simonsen EB, Dyhre-Poulsen P, Aagaard P, Mohr T, Kjaer M. Viscoelastic stress relaxation during static stretch in human skeletal muscle in the absence of EMG activity. *Scand J Med Sci Sports.* 1996;6:323-328.

43. Manoel M, Harris-Love M, Danoff J. Acute effects of static, dynamic and proprioceptive neuromuscular facilitation stretching on muscle power in women. *J Strength Cond Res.* 2008;22(5):1528.

44. Marek S, Cramer J, Fincher L. Acute effects of static and proprioceptive neuromuscular facilitation stretching on muscle strength and power output. *J Athl Train.* 2005;40(2):94.

45. Markos P. Ipsilateral and contralateral effects of proprioceptive neuromuscular facilitation techniques on hip motion and electromyographic activity. *Phys Ther.* 1979;59(11)P:66-73.

46. McAtee R, Charland J. *Facilitated Stretching.* 3rd ed. Champaign, IL: Human Kinetics; 2007.

47. McHugh MP, Magnusson SP, Gleim GW, Nicholas JA. Viscoelastic stress relaxation in human skeletal muscle. *Med Sci Sports Exerc.* 1992;24:1375-1382.

48. Mitchell F. Elements of muscle energy technique. In: Basmajian J, Nyberg R, eds. *Rational Manual Therapies.* Baltimore, MD: Lippincott, Williams & Wilkins; 1993.

49. Mitchell U, Myrer J, Hopkins T. Acute stretch perception alteration contributes to the success of the PNF "contract relax" stretch. *J Sport Rehabil.* 2007;16(2):85.

50. Osternig L, Robertson R, Troxel R, et al. Differential responses to proprioceptive neuromuscular facilitation stretch techniques. *Med Sci Sports Exerc.* 1990;22: 106-111.

51. Osternig L, Robertson R. Troxel R., Hansen P. Muscle activation during proprioceptive neuromuscular facilitation (PNF) stretching techniques ... stretch-relax (SR), contract-relax (CR) and agonist contract-relax (ACR). *Am J Phys Med.* 1987;66(5):298-307.

52. Padua D, Guskiewicz K, Prentice W. The effect of select shoulder exercises on strength, active angle reproduction, single-arm balance, and functional performance. *J Sport Rehabil.* 2004;13(1):75-95.

53. Prentice W, Kooima E. The use of proprioceptive neuromuscular facilitation techniques in the rehabilitation of sport-related injuries. *Athlet Train.* 1986;21:26-31.

54. Prentice W. A comparison of static stretching and PNF stretching for improving hip joint flexibility. *Athlet Train.* 1983;18(1):56-59.

55. Prentice W. A manual resistance technique for strengthening tibial rotation. *Athlet Train.* 1988;23(3):230-233.

56. Prentice W. *Proprioceptive neuromuscular facilitation* [videotape]. St. Louis, MO: Mosby; 1993.

57. Roberts BL. Soft tissue manipulation: Neuromuscular and muscle energy techniques. *J Neurosci Nurs.* 1997;29(2):123-127.

58. Rood M. Neurophysiologic reactions as a basis of physical therapy. *Phys Ther Rev.* 1954;34:444.

59. Saliba V, Johnson G, Wardlaw C. Proprioceptive neuromuscular facilitation. In: Basmajian J, Nyberg R, eds. *Rational Manual Therapies.* Baltimore, MD: Lippincott Williams & Wilkins; 1993.

60. Sawner K, LaVigne J. *Brunstrom's Movement Therapy in Hemiplegia.* Baltimore, MD: Lippincott, Williams & Wilkins; 1992.

61. Schuback B, Hooper J, Salisbury L. A comparison of a self-stretch incorporating proprioceptive neuromuscular facilitation components and a therapist-applied PNF technique on hamstring flexibility. *Physiotherapy.* 2004;90(3):151.

62. Sharman M, Cresswell T, Andrew G. Proprioceptive neuromuscular facilitation stretching: Mechanisms and clinical implications. *Sports Med.* 2006;36(11):929.

63. Sherrington C. *The Integrative Action of the Nervous System.* New Haven, CT: Yale University Press; 1947.

64. Shrier I. Does stretching help prevent injuries? In: MacAuley D, Best T, eds. *Evidence Based Sports Medicine.* London, UK: BMJ Books; 2002.

65. Spernoga SG, Uhl TL, Arnold BL, Gansneder BM. Duration of maintained hamstring flexibility after a one-time, modified hold-relax stretching protocol. *J Athl Train.* 2001;36(1):44-48.

66. Stone J. Muscle energy technique. *Athl Ther Today.* 2000;5(5):25.

67. Stone JA. Prevention and rehabilitation: Proprioceptive neuromuscular facilitation. *Athl Ther Today.* 2000;5(1):38-39.

68. Stuart DG. Reflections of spinal reflexes. *Adv Exp Med Biol.* 2002;508:249-257.

69. Surberg P. Neuromuscular facilitation techniques in sports medicine. *Phys Ther Rev.* 1954;34:444.

70. Surburg P, Schrader J. Proprioceptive neuromuscular facilitation techniques in sports medicine: A reassessment. *J Athl Train.* 1997;32(1):34-39.

71. Taniqawa M. Comparison of the hold-relax procedure and passive mobilization on increasing muscle length. *Phys Ther.* 1972;52(7):725-735.

72. Taylor DC, Dalton JD, Seaber A. Viscoelastic properties of muscle-tendon units: The biomechanical effects of stretching. *Am J Sports Med.* 1990;18:300-309.

73. Wilson LR, Gandevia SC, Burke D. Increased resting discharge of human spindle afferents following voluntary contractions. *J Physiol.* 1995;488(Pt 3):833-840.

74. Worrell T, Smith T, Winegardner J. Effect of hamstring stretching on hamstring muscle performance. *J Orthop Sports Phys Ther.* 1994;20(3):154-159.

75. Zohn D, Mennell J. Musculoskeletal Pain: *Diagnosis and Physical Treatment.* Boston, MA: Little, Brown; 1987.

SOLUTIONS TO CLINICAL DECISION-MAKING EXERCISES

14-1 A breaststroke kick involves multiplanar movements. Because PNF is used to strengthen gross motor patterns instead of specific muscle actions, it may help her regain strength and control in her kick.

14-2 The athletic trainer can apply resistance and encourage movement within the pain-free ROM. This strengthening technique will help prevent loss of coordination due to inactivity.

14-3 The rhythmic initiation technique promotes strength by first introducing the movement pattern passively. The patient will slowly progress to active assistive and then resistive exercises through the movement pattern.

14-4 Rhythmic stabilization can be used to facilitate strength and stability at a joint by stimulating co-contraction of the opposing muscles that support the joint. PNF strengthening using the D1 and D2

patterns will encourage control in the player's overhead serve.

14-5 The movements required for sport are not single-plane movements. PNF strengthening is more functional and is not limited by the design constraints of an exercise machine. Also, PNF technique allows the athletic trainer to adjust the amount of manual resistance throughout the ROM according to the patient's capabilities.

14-6 Proper body and hand positioning will maximize the athletic trainer's ability to provide sufficient resistance. The athletic trainer should stand in a position that is in line with the direction of movement in the diagonal movement pattern. The knees should be bent and the stance close to the patient, so that the direction and amount of resistance can easily be applied or altered appropriately throughout the range of movement.

Please see videos on the accompanying website at **www.healio.com/books/sportsmedvideos**

CHAPTER 15

Aquatic Therapy in Rehabilitation

Barbara J. Hoogenboom, EdD, PT, SCS, ATC
Nancy E. Lomax, PT

After completion of this chapter, the athletic trainer should be able to do the following:

- Explain the principles of buoyancy and specific gravity and the role they have in the aquatic environment.

- Identify and describe the three major resistive forces at work in the aquatic environment.

- Apply the principles of buoyancy and resistive forces to exercise prescription and progression.

- Contrast the advantages and disadvantages of aquatic therapy in relation to traditional land-based exercise.

- Identify and describe techniques of aquatic therapy for the upper extremity, lower extremity, and trunk.

- Select and use various types of equipment for aquatic therapy.

- Incorporate functional, work-, and sport-specific movements and exercises performed in the aquatic environment into rehabilitation.

- Understand and describe the necessity for transition from the aquatic environment to the land environment.

In recent years, there has been widespread interest in aquatic therapy. It has rapidly become a popular rehabilitation technique for treatment of a variety of patient populations. This newfound interest has sparked numerous research efforts to evaluate the effectiveness of aquatic therapy as a therapeutic intervention. Current research shows aquatic therapy to be beneficial in the treatment of everything from orthopedic injuries to spinal cord damage, chronic pain, cerebral palsy, multiple sclerosis, and many other conditions, making it useful in a variety of settings.[29,38] It is also gaining

Prentice WE, ed.
Rehabilitation Techniques for Sports Medicine and Athletic Training (pp 389-413).
© 2015 SLACK Incorporated.

acceptance as a preventative maintenance tool to facilitate overall fitness, cross-training, and sport-specific skills for healthy athletes.[23,33,34] General conditioning, strength, and a wide variety of movement skills can all be enhanced by aquatic therapy.[19,43,48,54]

The use of water as a part of healing techniques has been traced back through history to as early as 2400 BC, but it was not until the late 19th century that more traditional types of aquatic therapy came into existence.[4,24] The development of the Hubbard style whirlpool tank in 1820 sparked the initiation of present-day therapeutic use of water by allowing aquatic therapy to be conducted in a highly controlled clinical setting.[8] Loeman and Roen took this a step farther in 1824 and stimulated interest in use of an actual pool or what we now call aquatic therapy. Only recently, however, has water come into its own as a therapeutic exercise medium used for a wide variety of diagnoses and dysfunctions.[41]

Aquatic therapy is believed to be beneficial primarily because it decreases joint compression forces. The perception of weightlessness experienced in the water assists in decreasing joint pain and eliminating or drastically reducing the body's protective muscular spasm and pain that can carry over into the patient's daily functional activities.[54,56] Although many patients perceive greater ease of movement in the aquatic environment compared to movement on land, the research shows that aquatic therapy does not actually decrease pain more effectively than activities on land.[25] The primary goal of aquatic therapy is to teach the patient how to use water as a modality for improving movement, strength, and fitness.[2,54] Thus, along with other therapeutic modalities and interventions, aquatic therapy can become one link in the patient's recovery chain.[1]

PHYSICAL PROPERTIES AND RESISTIVE FORCES

The athletic trainer must understand several physical properties of the water before designing an aquatic therapy program. Land exercise cannot always be converted to aquatic exercise because buoyancy rather than gravity is the major force governing movement. A thorough understanding of buoyancy, specific gravity, the resistive forces of the water, and their relationships must be the groundwork of any therapeutic aquatic program. The program must be individualized to the patient's particular injury/condition and activity level if it is to be successful.

Buoyancy

Buoyancy is one of the primary forces involved in aquatic therapy. All objects, on land or in the water, are subjected to the downward pull of the earth's gravity. In the water, however, this force is counteracted to some degree by the upward buoyant force. According to Archimedes' principle, any object submerged or floating in water is buoyed upward by a counterforce that helps support the submerged object against the downward pull of gravity. In other words, the buoyant force assists motion toward the water's surface and resists motions away from the surface.[26,54] Because of this buoyant force, a person entering the water experiences an apparent loss of weight.[15] The weight loss experienced is nearly equal to the weight of the liquid that is displaced when the object enters the water (Figure 15-1).

For example, a 100-pound (lb) individual, when almost completely submerged, displaces a volume of water that weighs nearly 95 lbs; therefore, that person feels as though she or he weighs less than 5 lb. This sensation occurs because, when partially submerged, the individual only bears the weight of the part of the body that is above the water. With immersion to the level of the seventh cervical vertebra, both males and females only bear about 6% to 10% of their total body weight (TBW). The percentages increase to 25% to 31% TBW for females and 30% to 37% TBW for males at the xiphisternal level, and to 40% to 51% TBW for females and 50% to 56% TBW for males at the anterosuperior iliac spine level[27] (Table 15-1). The percentages differ slightly for males and females because of the differences in their centers of gravity. Males carry a higher percentage of their weight in the upper body, whereas females carry a higher percentage of their weight in the lower body. The center of gravity on land corresponds with a center of buoyancy

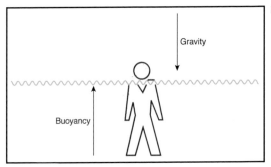

Figure 15-1. The buoyant force gravity buoyancy.

Table 15-1 Weight-bearing Percentages

Percentage of Weight Bearing		
Body Level	*Male*	*Female*
C7	8%	8%
Xiphisternal	28%	35%
ASIS (anterior superior iliac spine)	47%	54%

in the water.[41] Variations of build and body type only minimally effect weight-bearing values. As a result of the decreased percentage of weight bearing offered by the buoyant force, each joint that is below the water is decompressed or unweighted. This allows ambulation and vigorous exercise to be performed with little impact and drastically reduced friction between joint articular surfaces.

Progressing the activity from walking to running in the aquatic environment does not change the forces on the joints; however, minimal changes in the joint forces occur as the speed of running is increased. Fontana et al[20] report a 34% to 38% decrease in force while running at hip level of water and a 44% to 47% decrease force with running at chest level, compared to running on land. The relative decrease in weight-bearing forces during aquatic activities needs to be considered when dealing with athletes with injuries and restrictions of weight bearing, and may allow early running for those with such conditions and limitations.

Through careful use of Archimedes' principle, a gradual increase in the percentage of weight bearing can be undertaken. Initially, the patient would begin non-weight-bearing

exercises in the deep end of the pool. A wet vest or similar buoyancy device might be used to help the patient remain afloat for the desired exercises. This and other commercial equipment available for the use in the aquatic environment will be discussed in the upcoming section "Facilities and Equipment."

Clinical Decision-Making Exercise 15-1

A 35-year-old male sustained a right rotator cuff tear while playing softball. Three weeks ago he had a surgical repair of a tear of less than 2 centimeters and has now been referred for rehabilitation. He is active and plays softball, golf, and tennis. At what point could he begin to participate in an aquatic program during his rehabilitation?

Specific Gravity

Buoyancy is partially dependent on body weight. However, the weight of different parts of the body is not constant. Therefore, the buoyant values of different body parts will vary. Buoyant values can be determined by several factors. The ratio of bone weight to muscle weight, the amount and distribution of fat, and the depth and expansion of the chest all play a role. Together, these factors determine the specific gravity of the individual body part. On average, humans have a specific gravity slightly less than that of water. Any object with a specific gravity less than that of water will float. An object with a specific gravity greater than that of water will sink. However, as with buoyant values, the specific gravity of all body parts is not uniform. Therefore, even with a total body specific gravity of less than the specific gravity of water, the individual might not float horizontally in the water. Additionally, the lungs, when filled with air, can further decrease the specific gravity of the chest area. This allows the head and chest to float higher in the water than the heavier, denser extremities. Many athletes tend to have a low percentage of body fat (specific gravity greater than water) and therefore can be thought of as "sinkers." Consequently, compensation with flotation devices at the extremities and trunk might be necessary for some athletes.[5,54]

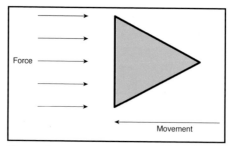

Figure 15-2. The bow force.

Resistive Forces

Water has 12 times the resistance of air.[50] Therefore, when an object moves in the water, the several resistive forces that are at work must be considered. Forces must be considered for both their potential benefits and their precautions. These forces include the cohesive force, the bow force, and the drag force.

Cohesive Force

There is a slight but easily overcome cohesive force that runs in a parallel direction to the water surface. This resistance is formed by the water molecules loosely binding together, creating a surface tension. Surface tension can be seen in still water, because the water remains motionless with the cohesive force intact unless disturbed.

Bow Force

A second force is the bow force, or the force that is generated at the front of the object during movement. When the object moves, the bow force causes an increase in the water pressure at the front of the object and a decrease in the water pressure at the rear of the object. This pressure change causes a movement of water from the high-pressure area at the front to the low-pressure area behind the object. As the water enters the low-pressure area, it swirls in to the low-pressure zone and forms eddies, or small whirlpool turbulences.[14] These eddies impede flow by creating a backward force, or drag force (Figure 15-2).

Drag Force

This third force, the fluid drag force, is very important in aquatic therapy. The bow force on an object (and therefore also the drag force) can be controlled by changing the shape of the

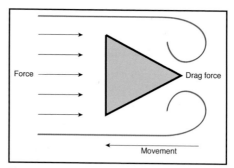

Figure 15-3. Drag force.

object or the speed of its movement (Figure 15-3).

Frictional resistance can be decreased by making the object more streamlined. This change minimizes the surface area at the front of the object. Less surface area causes less bow force and less of a change in pressure between the front and rear of the object, resulting in less drag force. In a streamlined flow, the resistance is proportional to the velocity of the object. When working with a patient with generalized weakness, consideration of the aquatic environment is necessary. Increased activity occurring around the patient and turbulence of the water can make walking a challenging activity (Figure 15-4).

On the other hand, if the object is not streamlined, a turbulent situation (also referred to as pressure or form drag) exists. In a turbulent situation, drag is a function of the velocity squared. Thus, by increasing the speed of movement two times, the resistance the object must overcome is increased four times.[15] This provides a method to increase resistance progressively during aquatic rehabilitation. Considerable turbulence can be generated when the speed of movement is increased, causing muscles to work harder to keep the movement

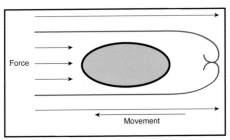

Figure 15-4. Streamlined movement. This creates less drag force and less turbulence.

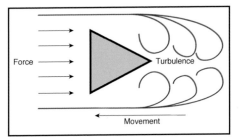

Figure 15-5. Turbulent flow.

going. Another method to increase resistance is to change directions of movement, creating increased drag. Finally, by simply changing the shape of a limb through the addition of rehabilitation equipment that increases surface area, the athletic trainer can modify the patient's workout intensity to match strength increases (Figure 15-5).

Drag force must also be considered when portions of a limb or joint must be protected after injury or surgery. For example, when working with a patient with an acutely injured medial collateral or anterior cruciate ligament of the knee, resistance must not be placed distal to the knee because of the increased torque that occurs caused by drag forces.

Quantification of resistive forces that occur during aquatic exercise is a challenge. Pöyhönen et al examined knee flexion and extension in the aquatic environment using an anatomic model in barefoot and hydroboot-wearing conditions. They found that the highest drag forces and drag coefficients occurred during early extension from a flexed position (150 to 140 degrees of flexion) while wearing the hydroboot (making the foot less streamlined), and that faster velocity was associated with higher drag forces.[47]

Once therapy has progressed, the patient could be moved to neck-deep water to begin

light weight-bearing exercises. Gradual increases in the percentage of weight bearing are accomplished by systematically moving the patient to shallower water. Even when in waist-deep water, both male and female patients are only bearing about 50% of their TBW. By placing a sinkable bench or chair in the shallow water, step-ups can be initiated under partial weight-bearing conditions long before the patient is capable of performing the same exercise full weight bearing on land. Thus, the advantages of diminished weight-bearing exercises are coupled with the proprioceptive benefits of closed kinetic chain exercise, making aquatic therapy an excellent functional rehabilitation activity.

ADVANTAGES AND BENEFITS OF AQUATIC REHABILITATION

The addition of an aquatic therapy program can offer many advantages to a patient's therapy[22,54] (Table 15-2). The buoyancy of the water allows active exercise while providing a sense of security and causing little discomfort.[51] Using a combination of the water's buoyancy, resistance, and warmth, the patient can typically achieve more in the aquatic environment than is possible on land.[34] Early in the rehabilitation process, aquatic therapy is useful in restoring range of motion (ROM) and flexibility. As normal function is restored, resistance training and sport specific activities can be added.

Following an injury, the aquatic experience provides a medium where early motions can be performed in a supportive environment. The slow motion effect of moving through water provides extra time to control movement, which allows the patient to experience multiple movement errors without severe consequences.[43,49] This is especially helpful in lower-extremity injuries where balance and proprioception are impaired. Geigle et al demonstrated a positive relationship between use of a supplemental aquatic therapy program and unilateral tests of balance when treating athletes with inversion ankle sprains.[22] The increased amount of time to react and correct movement errors, combined with a medium in which the fear of

Table 15-2 Indications and Benefits of Aquatic Therapy[30,50,54]

Indications for Use of Aquatic Therapy	Illustration of Benefits
Swelling/peripheral edema	Assist in edema control, decrease pain, increase mobility as edema decreases
Decreased ROM	Earlier initiation of rehabilitation, controlled active movements
Decreased strength	Strength progression from assisted to resisted to functional; gradual increase in exercise intensity
Decreased balance, proprioception, coordination	Earlier return to function in supported, forgiving environment, slower movements
Weight-bearing restrictions	Can partially or completely unweight the lower extremities; regulate weight-bearing progressions
Cardiovascular deconditioning or potential deconditioning because of inability to train	Gradual increase of exercise intensity, alternative training environment for lower weight bearing
Gait deviations	Slower movements, easier assessment, and modification of gait
Difficulty or pain with land interventions	Increased support, decreased weight bearing, assistance as a result of buoyancy, more relaxed environment

falling is removed, assists the patient's ability to regain proprioception and neuromuscular control. For the patient population with a diagnosis of rheumatoid and/or osteoarthritis with lower-extremity involvement, about 80% demonstrate balance difficulties and higher risk for falls.[16,17] A study performed by Suomi and Koceja[52] demonstrated that aquatic exercise helped decrease total sway area and medial/lateral sway in both full vision and no vision conditions, which placed them in lower risk for falls. In all ages, the fear of falling can limit people from progressing to their highest level of function.

Turbulence functions as a destabilizer and as a tactile sensory stimulus. The stimulation from the turbulence generated during movement provides feedback and perturbation challenge that aids in the return of proprioception and balance.

There is also an often overlooked benefit of edema reduction that occurs as a consequence of hydrostatic pressure. Edema reduction could benefit the patient by assisting in pain reduction and allowing for an increase in ROM.

By understanding buoyancy and using its principles, the aquatic environment can provide a gradual transition from non-weight-bearing to full-weight-bearing land exercises. This gradual increase in percentage of weight bearing helps provide a gradual return to smooth, coordinated, and low pain or pain-free movements. By using the buoyancy force to decrease the forces of body weight and joint compressive forces, locomotor activities can begin much earlier following an injury to the lower extremity than on land. This provides an enormous advantage to the athletic population. The ability to work out hard without fear of reinjury provides a psychological boost to the athlete. This helps keep motivation high and can help speed the athlete's return to normal function.[34] Psychologically, aquatic therapy increases confidence, because the patient experiences increased success at locomotor, stretching, or strengthening activities while in the water. Tension and anxiety are decreased, and the patient's morale increases, as does postexer-cise vigor.[14,15,41]

Muscular strengthening and reeducation can also be accomplished through aquatic ther-apy.[44,54] Progressive resistance exercises can be increased in extremely small increments by using combinations of different resistive forces. The intensity of exercise can be con-trolled by manipulating the flow of the water (turbulence), the body's position, or through the addition of exercise equipment. This allows individuals with minimal muscle contraction capabilities to do work and see improvement. The aquatic environment can also provide a challenging resistive workout to an athlete nearing full recovery.[54] Additionally, water serves as an accommodating resistance medi-um. This allows the muscles to be maximally stressed through the full ROM available. One drawback to this, however, is that strength gains depend largely on the effort exerted by the patient, which is not easily quantified.

In another study, Pöyhönen et al[46] studied the biomechanical and hydrodynamic charac-teristics of the therapeutic exercise of knee flex-ion and extension using kinematic and electro-myographic analyses in flowing and still water. They found that the flowing properties of water modified the agonist/antagonist neuromuscu-lar function of the quadriceps and hamstrings in terms of early reduction of quadriceps

activity and concurrent increased activation of the hamstrings. They also found that flowing water (turbulence) causes additional resistance when moving the limb opposite the flow. They concluded that when prescribing aquatic exer-cise, the turbulence of the water must be con-sidered in terms of both resistance and altera-tions of neuromuscular recruitment of muscles.

Strength gains through aquatic exercise are facilitated by the increased energy needs of the body when working in an aquatic environment. Studies show that aquatic exercise requires higher energy expenditure than the same exer-cise performed on land.[10,14,15,54] The patient has to perform the activity as well as maintain a level of buoyancy while overcoming the resis-tive forces of the water. For example, the energy cost for water running is four times greater than the energy cost for running the same dis-tance on land.[14,15,18,32]

A simulated run in either shallow or deep water assisted by a tether or flotation devices can be an effective means of alternate fitness training (cross-training) for the injured athlete. The purpose of aquatic running is to reproduce the posture of running and use the same muscle groups in the aquatic environment as would be used on land. However, it should be noted that there are differences while being in the unloaded environment and resistance of the water with aqua running changes the relative contributions of the involved muscle groups.[58] It should be noted that a study of shallow-water running (xiphoid level) and deep-water run-ning (using an aqua jogger), at the same rate of perceived exertion, found a significant differ-ence of 10 beats per minute in heart rate, with shallow-water running demonstrating a greater heart rate. The authors of that study point out that aquatic rehabilitation professionals should not prescribe shallow-water working heart rates from heart rates values obtained during deep-water exercise.[48]

Hydrostatic pressure assists in cardiac per-formance by promoting venous return, thus the heart does not have to beat as fast to maintain cardiac output. Deep-water running at sub-maximal and maximal speeds demonstrates lower heart rates than shallow-water running. The greater the temperature of the water, the higher the heart rate in response.[58] All patients should be instructed in how to accurately monitor their heart rate while exercising in water, whether deep or shallow.[10]

Not only does the patient benefit from early intervention, but aquatic exercise also helps prevent cardiorespiratory deconditioning through alterations in cardiovascular dynamics as a result of hydrostatic forces.[7,28,53] The heart actually functions more efficiently in the water than on land. Hydrostatic pressure enhances venous return, leading to a greater stroke volume and a reduction in the heart rate needed to maintain cardiac output.[55] The corresponding decrease in ventilatory rate and increase in central blood volume can allow the injured athlete to maintain a near-normal maximal aerobic capacity with aquatic exercise.[22,56]

For the patient who has comorbidities, there is a study that examined the cardiovascular response during aquatic interventions in patients with osteoarthritis. The authors found that the systolic and diastolic blood pressure increased with entering and exiting the aquatic environment secondary to the rapid changes in hydrostatic pressure.[3]

For the athlete or the geriatric patient with compensations, consideration must be paid to monitoring responses. Because of the hydrostatic effects on heart efficiency, it has been suggested that an environment-specific exercise prescription is necessary.[33,39,53,57] Some research suggests the use of perceived exertion as an acceptable method for controlling exercise intensity. Other research suggests the use of target heart rate values as with land exercise, but compensates for the hydrostatic changes by setting the target range 10% lower than what would be expected for land exercise[50,54] (Figure 15-6). Regardless of the method used, the keys to successful use of aquatic therapy are supervision and monitoring of the patient during activity and good communication between patient and athletic trainer.

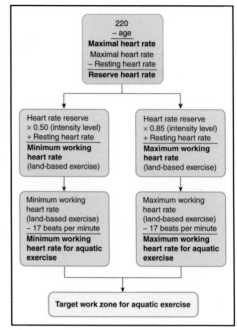

Figure 15-6. Karvonen formula for water exercise.[50]

Clinical Decision-Making Exercise 15-3

A high school cross-country runner sustained a small second-metatarsal stress reaction/fracture during the short 3-month season in response to increased volume and intensity of training. She has been cleared by her physician to finish out the remaining 3 weeks of the competitive season but is only allowed to run in meets. What might the athletic trainer suggest for alternate training to allow her to maintain aerobic function and enable her to compete?

DISADVANTAGES OF AQUATIC REHABILITATION

Disadvantages

As with any therapeutic intervention, aquatic therapy has its disadvantages. The cost of building and maintaining a rehabilitation pool, if there is no access to an existing facility, can be very high. Also, qualified pool attendants must be present, and the athletic trainer involved in the treatment must be trained in aquatic safety

Table 15-3 Contraindications for Aquatic Therapy[30,50,54]

Untreated infectious disease (patient has a fever/temperature)

Open wounds or unhealed surgical incisions

Contagious skin diseases

Serious cardiac conditions

Seizure disorders (uncontrolled)

Excessive fear of water

Allergy to pool chemicals

Vital capacity of 1 L

Uncontrolled high or low blood pressure

Uncontrolled bowel or bladder incontinence

Menstruation without internal protection

Table 15-4 Precautions for the Use of Aquatic Therapy[30,50,54]

Recently healed wound or incision, incisions covered by moisture-proof barrier

Altered peripheral sensation

Respiratory dysfunction (asthma)

Seizure disorders controlled with medications

Fear of water

and therapy procedures.[12,32] An athlete who requires high levels of stabilization will be more challenging to work with, because stabilization in water is considerably more difficult than on land. Thermoregulation issues exist for the patient who exercises in an aquatic environment. Because the patient cannot always choose the temperature of the pool, the effects of water temperature must be noted for cool, warm, or hot pool temperatures. Water temperatures that are higher than body temperature cause an increase in core body temperature greater than that in a land environment as a result of differences in thermoregulation. Water temperatures that are lower than body temperature decrease core body temperature and cause shivering in athletes faster and to a greater degree than in the general population because of their low body fat.[10] Another disadvantage of aquatic exercise used for cross-training is that training in water does not allow athletes to improve or maintain their tolerance to heat while on land.

Contraindications and Precautions

The presence of any open wounds or sores on the patient is a contraindication to aquatic therapy, as are contagious skin diseases. This restriction is obvious for health reasons to reduce the chance of infection of the patient or others who use the pool.[13,29,30,38,50] Because

of this risk, all surgical wounds must be completely healed or adequately protected using a waterproof barrier before the patient enters the pool. An excessive fear of the water is also a reason to keep a patient out of an aquatic exercise program. Fever, urinary tract infections, allergies to the pool chemicals, cardiac problems, and uncontrolled seizures are also contraindications (Tables 15-3 and 15-4). Use caution (or waterproof barrier) with medical equipment access sites such as an insulin pump, osteomies, suprapubic appliances, and G tubes. Patients with a tracheotomy need special consideration; they need to remain in waist to chest depth of water to exercise safely in an aquatic environment.

FACILITIES AND EQUIPMENT

When considering an existing facility or when planning to build one, certain characteristics of the pool should be taken into consideration. The pool should not be smaller than 10 × 12 ft. It can be in-ground or above ground as long as access for the patient is well planned. Both a shallow area (2.5 ft) and a deep area (5+ ft) should be present to allow standing exercise and swimming or non-standing exercise.[7] The pool bottom should be flat and the depth gradations clearly marked. Water temperature will vary depending on the patient that is served. For the athlete, recommended pool temperature should be 26°C to 28°C (79°F to 82°F) but may depend on the available facility.[45] The water temperature suggested by the Arthritis Foundation for their programs is 29°C to 31°C (85°F to 89°F). Traditional chemicals

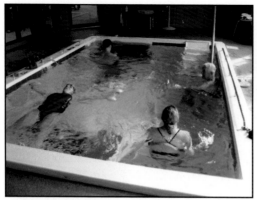

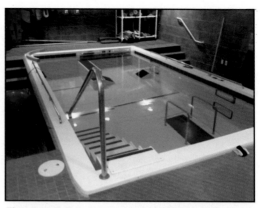

Figure 15-7. The SwimEx pool. This pool's even, controllable water flow allows for the application of individualized prescriptive exercise and therapeutic programs. As many as three patients can be treated simultaneously.

Figure 15-8. SwimEx custom pool with treadmill.

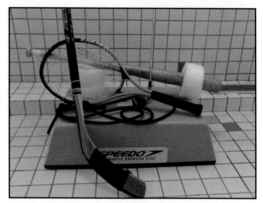

Figure 15-9. Custom pool equipment.

that have been used for pool treatment are chlorine and bromine, but additional options exist, including saltwater system pools.

Depending on the type of condition, the patient's perception of the water temperature may differ.

Some prefabricated pools come with an in-water treadmill or current-producing device (Figures 15-7 and 15-8). These devices can be beneficial but are not essential to treatment. An aquatic program will benefit from a variety of equipment that allows increasing levels of resistance and assistance, and also motivates the patient. Catalog companies and sporting goods stores are good resources for obtaining equipment. There are many styles and variations of equipment available: the athletic trainer needs to select equipment depending on the needs of the program. Creative use of actual sport equipment (baseball bats, tennis racquets, golf clubs, etc; Figures 15-9 to 15-12) is helpful to incorporate sport specific activities that challenge the athlete. Use of mask and snorkel will allow options for prone activities/swimming (Figures 15-13 and 15-14). Instruction in the proper use of the mask and snorkel is essential for the patient's comfort and safety. Equipment aids for aquatic therapy or so-called pool toys are limited in their use only by the imagination of the athletic trainer. What is important is to stimulate the patient's interest in therapy and to keep in mind what goals are to be accomplished.

The clothing of the athletic trainer is an important consideration. Secondary to the close

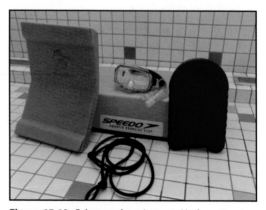

Figure 15-10. Other pool equipment. Underwater step, mask and snorkel, kickboard, tubing, and various sports equipment.

proximity of the athletic trainer to the patient with some treatments, wearing swimwear that covers portions of the lower extremities and upper trunk/upper extremities is an important aspect of professionalism in the aquatic

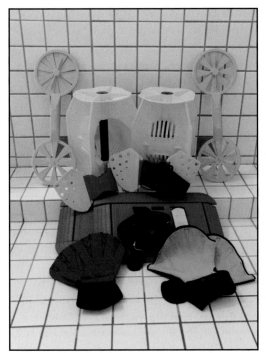

Figure 15-11. Equipment used for resistance or floatation.

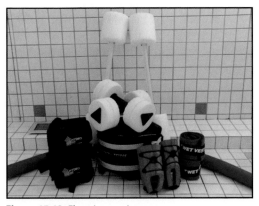

Figure 15-12. Flotation equipment.

environment. Footwear is another important consideration for the athletic trainer as well as the patient. Proper aquatic footwear provides stability, traction, prevents injuries, and maintains good foot position.

WATER SAFETY

A number of patients referred for aquatic therapy are uncomfortable in the water because of minimal experience in an aquatic environment. Swimming ability is not necessary to

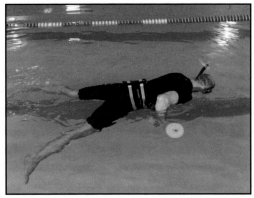

Figure 15-13. Prone kayak movement using mask and snorkel. Challenges the upper extremities and promotes stabilization of the trunk.

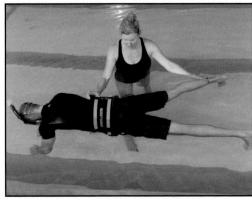

Figure 15-14. Prone hip abduction/adduction with manual resistance by athletic trainer. Note use of mask and snorkel, allowing the patient to maintain proper trunk and head/neck position.

participate in an aquatic exercise program, but instruction of water safety skills will allow for a satisfying experience for the patient. Patients may need an exercise bar or flotation noodle to assist with balance during ambulation in water, initially. When adding supine or prone activities into the patient's program, it is important to instruct the individual how to assume that position and return to upright position. This initial act will decrease fear and stress for the patient and also decrease stress to injured area.

AQUATIC TECHNIQUES

Aquatic techniques and activities can be designed to begin as active assisted movements and progress to strengthening, eccentric control, and functionally specific activities. Activities are selected based on several factors:

- Type of injury/surgery/condition
- Treatment protocols, if appropriate
- Results/muscle imbalances found in evaluation
- Goals/expected return to activities as stated by the patient

Aquatic programs are designed similarly to land-based programs, with the following components:

- Warm-up
- Mobility activities
- Strengthening activities
- Balance or neuromuscular response activities
- Endurance/cardiovascular activities, including possibilities for cross-training
- Sport or functionally specific activities
- Cool down/stretching

With these general considerations in mind, the following sections provide examples of aquatic exercises for the upper extremity, trunk, and lower extremity in a three-phase rehabilitation progression. What has been omitted from the four-phase rehabilitation scheme used throughout this textbook, in the current discussion, is the initial pain control phase. It is assumed that by the time the patient arrives for aquatic therapy, the patient has undergone previous treatment to manage acute injuries and painful conditions. Subsequently, the patient is ready to begin phases two through four of the four-phase approach.

Upper Extremity

The goal of rehabilitation is to restore function by restoring motion and synchrony of movement of all joints of the upper extremity. As listed above, the evaluation of upper extremity is important and identification of dysfunctional movements will assist in designing an effective program. Aquatic therapy may be used for treatment of the shoulder complex, elbow, wrist, and hand as one of the interventions to accomplish goals along with a land-based program. The following sections describe a rehabilitation progression for shoulder complex dysfunction.

Initial Level

The patient can be started at chest-deep water to allow for support of the scapulothoracic area. Walking forward, backward, and sideways will allow for warm-up, working on natural arm swing, and restoration of normal scapulothoracic motions, rotation, and rhythm. Initiation of activities to work on glenohumeral motions begins at the wall (patient with back against the wall); having the patient in neck- or shoulder-deep water gives the patient physical cues as to posture and quality of movement. The primary goal during the early phase is for the athletic trainer and patient to be aware of the amount of movement available without compensatory shoulder elevation (for example in the presence of an injury to the rotator cuff). The other options for positions during early treatment are supine and prone. The patient will need flotation equipment for cervical, lumbar, and lower-extremity support to have good positioning when in supine.

Supine activities include stretching, mobilization, and ROM. Stabilizing the scapula with one hand, the athletic trainer can work on glenohumeral motion with the patient (Figures 15-15 and 15-16). The patient can initiate gentle active movement in shoulder abduction and extension.

Prone activity can be performed depending on the patient's comfort in water and willingness to use a mask and snorkel. Flotation support around the pelvis allows the patient to concentrate on movement of the upper extremities without worrying about flotation of the trunk and legs. The patient is able to perform pendulum-type movements, proprioceptive neuromuscular facilitation (PNF) diagonals, and straight-plane movement patterns (flexion/extension and horizontal abduction/adduction) in their pain-free range. For the patient not comfortable with the prone position, an alternative position is the pendulum position in the standing position with the trunk flexed.

Deep-water activity can be integrated for conditioning/endurance building in early stages of upper-extremity rehabilitation. It is

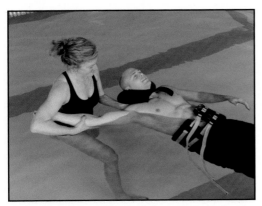

Figure 15-15. Range of motion with scapular stabilization.

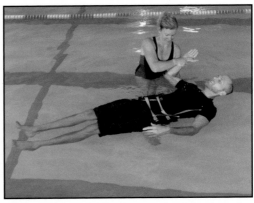

Figure 15-16. Internal and external rotation in supine. Note appropriate floatation support for the athlete.

important for the patient to perform pain-free range when performing endurance-type activities.

Intermediate Level

The program can be progressed to challenge strength by using equipment to resist motion through pain-free range. Increasing the surface area of the extremity or increasing the length of the lever arm will increase the difficulty of the activity. As the patient progresses into this phase, the limitations of the standing position become apparent. The athlete can work to the 90-degree angle but not overhead without exiting the water. It is important for the patient to maintain a neutral position of the spine and pelvic area to avoid injury and substitution patterns when performing strengthening activities while standing.

The patient will be able to progress with scapular stabilization from standing to supine and prone positions. Supine and prone positioning can allow for more functional movement patterns and core stabilization by the scapular muscles. Recall that prone activities such as alternate shoulder flexion, the "kayaking" type motion (Figure 15-13), PNF diagonal patterns, and horizontal shoulder abduction/adduction can all be performed using various types of equipment or manual resistance provided by the athletic trainer while in prone. Resistance to each of these motions could be added during this phase of rehab.

Supine positioning allows for work on shoulder internal and external rotation where resistance or speed can be added (Figure 15-16), as well as shoulder extension against resistance (Figure 15-17) in varying degrees of abduction. Internal and external rotation can be performed against resistance in standing. The land-based program and aquatic program should be coordinated to ensure continued improvement of strength, endurance, and function. The goal of treatment in the intermediate-level activities is development of strength and eccentric control throughout increasing ranges of motion.

Final Level

The goal of this level of treatment is high-level functional strengthening and training. Equally important is the transition from the aquatic environment to the land environment. Using sport equipment in treatment, if applicable, will keep an athlete motivated and working toward the goal of returning to sport (Figure 15-18). Increasing the resistance by using elastic or flotation attachments will keep it challenging (Figure 15-19). As in the intermediate level, the patient needs to be involved in a strengthening and training program on land.

Clinical Decision-Making Exercise 15-4

A 17-year-old high school baseball pitcher has undergone an ulnar collateral ligament repair of his dominant (right) elbow that used an autogenous graft. According to the postoperative protocol, resistive exercises at the elbow must be avoided for the next 4 weeks and a motion-limiting elbow brace must be worn during all activities for 5 weeks after surgery. How might aquatic exercises be used for this patient after the fifth week? Are there any precautions that must be observed?

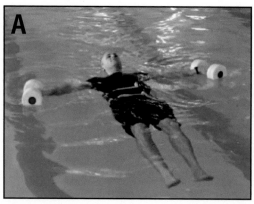
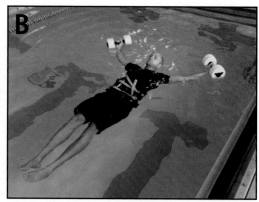

Figure 15-17. Supine shoulder extension at 2 different abduction angles, for scapular stabilization. (A) Middle trapezius; (B) lower trapezius.

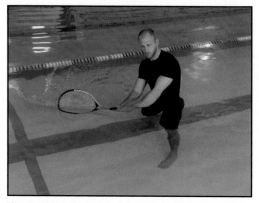
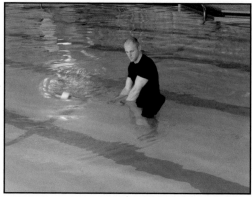

Figure 15-18. Example of sport-specific training in the aquatic environment. Useful for upper-extremity, core, and lower-extremity training.

Figure 15-19. Sport-specific training using buoyancy cuffs around a bat for resistance.

Spine Dysfunction

The unloading capability of water allows the patient ease of movement and some potential relief of symptoms. The patients will need to be shown how to obtain and maintain the neutral spine position in the water even if they have been instructed on land. The neutral spine position is the basis of treatment in land and water and will progress in level of difficulty. Activities of the trunk, upper extremities, and lower extremities all challenge trunk stability, strength, total body balance, and neuromuscular control. Directional movement preferences for relief of symptoms, such as extension- or flexion-biased exercises, can be integrated into the program. Pregnant patients who experience back pain often benefit from exercising in an aquatic environment secondary to the unloading forces on the lower back.

Initial Level

Using forward/backward/sideways walking is common for a warm-up activity in patients with spine dysfunction. It is an opportunity for the patient to become aware of postural dysfunctions and practice with changing alignment. Kim et al[31] studied aquatic backward locomotion exercise and reported that a training program emphasizing backward walking is as effective as a progressive resistive exercise training program using equipment with increasing lumbar extension after discectomy surgery. Backward ambulation has been shown to activate paraspinal muscles, the vastus medialis, and tibialis anterior more than forward walking.[35] Initially, the patient can start with a speed and length of stride that does not cause discomfort, and then can progress to normal walking speed so as to allow for return to function.

Initial instruction regarding the neutral spine position is the basis for treatment. The patient stands in a partial squat position with the back against the wall to offer feedback and allow him or her to monitor his or her response. There are a variety of ways to instruct the patient to contract the transversus abdominis muscle. It is important for the patient to have the awareness of maintaining a light transversus abdominis muscle contraction and keeping the lower-extremity muscles relaxed or "soft" during activities. Working on the endurance and prolonged hold of abdominal stabilization without increasing spinal discomfort is a goal for the initial level. Upper- and lower-extremity activities can be added so as to progressively challenge the patient's ability to stabilize without increasing symptoms. Initially begin with activities without additional equipment, while manipulating the speed of movement through controlled ranges of motion to challenge the ability to maintain the desired position.

Use of deep-water activities can be initiated early in rehabilitation. The patient should maintain a vertical position while performing small controlled movements of the upper and lower extremities. The Burdenko approach to aquatic activities uses deep-water activities before activities in shallow water. If dealing with radicular (sciatica) type symptoms, a trial of deep-water traction can be done. Flotation support of the upper body and trunk and placement of light weights on the ankles allows for gentle distraction of the lumbar spine. The patient can hang using the flotation devices placed on the upper body/trunk, and perform small pedaling motions as if bicycling/walking.[36]

Working on normalizing the gait pattern and developing the ability to weight bear equally on the lower extremities in any depth of water comfortable to the patient is important early in the therapeutic progression. Incorporation of activities to help centralize the symptoms are important, as well as encouraging the patient to perform only activities that maintain or diminish symptoms during the session. Gentle stretching and rotation movements can be performed within the pain-free motion to increase pelvic and lumbar spine mobility.

Intermediate Level

At this level, the patient is allowed to progress away from the wall, and the extremities or equipment is used to challenge his or her ability to stabilize. Stability can be initially challenged by moving the arms through the water to induce perturbation to the trunk (Figure 15-20). This can be made more challenging by increasing the speed of the upper-extremity movements or adding something to the hands such as webbed water gloves or floatation dumbbells. A kickboard can be used to mimic pushing, pulling, and lifting motions (Figures 15-21 and 15-22). Equipment that resists upper-extremity or lower-extremity movements in a single-leg stance or lunge position challenges the patient's balance, as well as stabilization using the abdominal and pelvic muscles (Figure 15-23). There is benefit to having the patient work on both bilateral and single-leg activities such as squats/calf raises that translate to some of the functional activities such as sit to stand and stair climbing. The patient's ability to stabilize can be further challenged using deep-water activities that require maintaining a vertical position while bringing knees to chest and progressing to tucking and rolling type movement (Figure 15-24). Activities can be created to work on diagonal and rotational motions of the spine and trunk, while maintaining the neutral position.

Activities in a supine position are effective for increasing trunk mobility and then progressing to work on trunk stability using Bad Ragaz techniques[21] (Figures 15-25 and 15-26). Activities in prone position provide an excellent method to challenge the patient's ability to maintain the neutral spine position, and the patient may need flotation equipment to accomplish that goal. The use of the mask and snorkel will allow for proper positioning of the spine while performing the activities (Figures 15-13 and 15-14). It is important to monitor and teach the patient the neutral spine position with each new position that is introduced in the treatment program. Activities can be simplified or progressed in difficulty according to patients' level of function or their ability to maintain the neutral spine position.

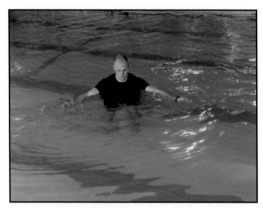

Figure 15-20. Anterior posterior trunk stabilization with upper extremity horizontal abduction/adduction. Note flexed knees and wide base of support.

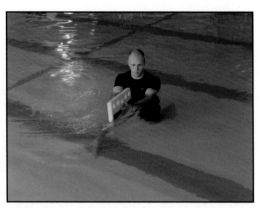

Figure 15-22. Trunk stabilization against oblique/diagonal forces, split stance.

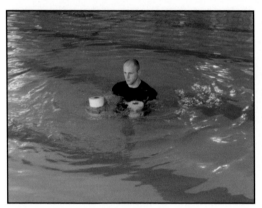

Figure 15-21. Trunk stabilization against anterior/posterior forces, split stance.

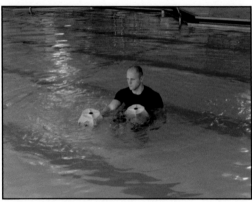

Figure 15-23. Challenging lower-extremity neuromuscular control and balance, as well as trunk control, in single-limb stance using upper-extremity resistance.

Final Level

Depending on the patient's needs and functional goals related to return to a desired level of activity, the program could be modified and progressed. For the patient returning to a demanding occupation, development of a program of lifting/pushing/pulling or other needs described by the patient can complement a work-conditioning program. For the patient returning to a sport, the athletic trainer and athlete can work together to develop specific challenging activities. The athletic trainer needs to be creative with the use of aquatic equipment and should use equipment specific to the athlete's sport to challenge the athlete to a higher level of trunk stabilization. It is important to integrate movement patterns that are opposite of the ones the athlete normally performs in the athlete's sport to challenge body symmetry during function. For example, if a gymnast or ice skater predominantly turns or rotates in one direction, have him or her practice turns in the opposite direction. The aquatic environment provides the athlete an alternate environment in which to train, that should be encouraged for the serious athlete to attempt to avoid overuse type of conditions that can occur. Especially important in this phase is the reintegration of the patient back into treatment and training on land, as the water environment does not allow the athlete to prepare for the exact speeds and forces experienced on land.

Lower-Extremity Injuries

Aquatic therapy is a common modality for rehabilitation of many injuries of the lower extremity because of the properties of unloading and hydrostatic pressure. At an early phase

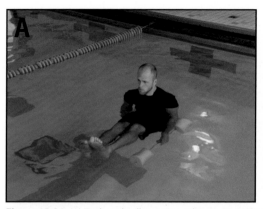
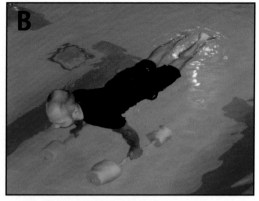

Figure 15-24. (A) Tuck-and-roll exercise, pike position; (B) tuck-and-roll exercise, tuck position.

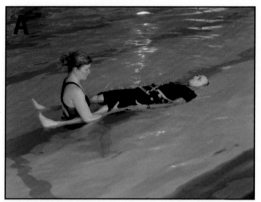
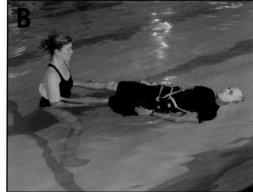

Figure 15-25. Bad Ragaz technique for trunk stabilization. (A) Note short lever arm with the athletic trainer contacting the LE's above the knee to protect the knee joint; (B) contact below the knees (if indicated) increases the trunk and LE stability demands.

of healing, the patient may need to use a flotation belt, vest, exercise bars, noodles, and various other buoyancy devices to provide support, depending on pain and how long he or she has been non-weight-bearing. The aquatic environment allows for limited weight bearing and restoration of gait by calculating the percentage of weight bearing allowed and weight of patient and then placing the patient in an appropriate depth of water, as discussed previously.

Initial Level

The expected goals of this phase of rehabilitation are the return of normal motion and early strengthening of affected muscles. The restoration of normal and functional gait pattern is also desired. Performing backward and sideways walking adds a functional dimension to the program in addition to traditional forward walking. ROM activities may involve

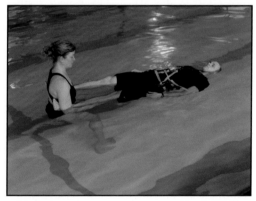

Figure 15-26. Bad Ragaz technique for oblique trunk stabilization.

active motions of the hip, knee, and ankle. Using cuffs, noodles, or kickboards under the foot will assist with increasing motion, due to the buoyancy offered by such equipment.

Exercises for strengthening noninvolved joints such as the hips or ankles can be performed with the patient who has had a knee injury. However, it is important to remember that resistance (manual or with devices) may need to be placed above the injured knee to decrease torque placed upon the knee. It is important to integrate conditioning and balance activities within this initial level (Figure 15-27). Standing activities should be performed with attention paid to maintaining the spine in a neutral position, as well as to challenging balance and neuromuscular control of the involved lower extremity (Figure 15-23).

Deep-water activities allow for conditioning and cross-training opportunities (Figure 15-28). The patient may initially need assistance with flotation devices, but can progress by decreasing the amount of flotation when able. For the patient who must be non-weight-bearing secondary to an injury or surgery, the deep water allows for a workout along with maintaining strength in uninvolved joints. Activities can involve running, bicycling, scissoring, or cross-country skiing motions, and also incorporate sport specific activities of the lower extremities, trunk, and upper extremities. The athletic trainer can also incorporate activities performed in the supine position. The patients need to be supported with flotation equipment that allow them to float evenly and without great effort to stay afloat. The athletic trainer can stabilize at the feet and have the patient work on active hip and knee flexion and extension to work on increasing ROM at the affected joint (Figure 15-29). Resistance of hip abduction and adduction can also be performed in a supine position. Again, attention must be paid to the location of applied force. Resistance placed upon the uninvolved leg movement will also allow for strengthening of the injured extremity. It should be noted that the athletic trainer must teach the patient how to safely return to the standing/vertical position from the supine or prone position especially with the use of equipment applied to lower extremities.

Intermediate Level

Depending on the injury, surgery, or condition, the patient can be progressed to the intermediate level when appropriate. The activities can be progressed by use of weights or

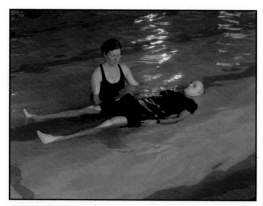

Figure 15-27. Supine hip abduction/adduction. Note the athletic trainer's hand placement above the knee to protect the knee ligaments.

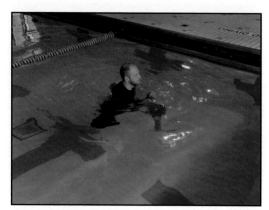

Figure 15-28. Deep-water running.

flotation cuffs to increase difficulty. As in the initial level, resistance may need to be placed more proximally in the presence of knee ligament injuries or surgeries. Performing circuits of straight-plane and diagonal patterns with both lower extremities can be progressed by performing with upper-extremity support on the wall and progressing to no support. The involved lower extremity can be challenged by using specific motions that mimic running (Figure 15-30). The patient can stand on an uneven surface, such as a noodle or cuff, to challenge balance and stabilization. Eccentric, closed chain activities can be performed in the shallow water with the patient standing on a noodle or kickboard for single-leg reverse squats, and using a noodle, kickboard, or bar for bilateral reverse-squat motions in deep-water (Figure 15-31) and progressing to a single-leg reverse squat. Bilateral lower-extremity

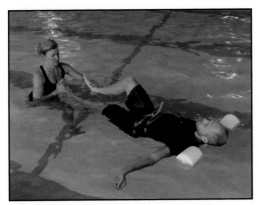

Figure 15-29. Supine alternating hip and knee flexion and extension, using Bad Ragaz technique. Hand contact by the athletic trainer gives the patient cues for movement.

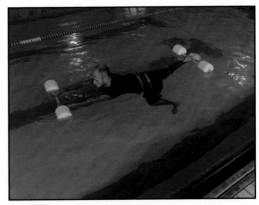

Figure 15-30. Supported single-lower-extremity running movement. Note the appropriate support of the patient with buoyancy belts and upper-extremity bell and lower-extremity bell under the stationary lower extremity. Also challenges trunk stabilization.

strength, endurance, and coordination can be challenged by kicking with a kickboard, using a flutter kick. This is also excellent for developing core control and aerobic endurance.

Performing deep-water tether running or sprinting forward and backward for increasing periods of time will allow for overall conditioning. The patient can progress to running in shallower water depending upon the condition of injury or surgery (Figure 15-32).

Supine activities can be continued with emphasis on strengthening and stabilization of the trunk, pelvis, and lower extremities. Placement of the athletic trainer's resistance will depend on the patient's strength, ability to stabilize, and how much time has elapsed since surgery or injury. Increasing the number of repetitions and/or speed of movement will provide more resistance and work on fatiguing muscle groups of the lower extremity. The prone position provides increased challenges to the patient to perform hip abduction and adduction along with hip and knee flexion and extension. As mentioned previously, the patient can use mask and snorkel or floatation equipment to help with positioning while in the prone position.

Sport-specific activities can be integrated into the program for the athlete. While practicing movement patterns needed for sport, the patient can start at chest depth and progress to shallow water. As with spine rehabilitation, there is benefit from practicing opposite movement patterns such as turns and jumps. The

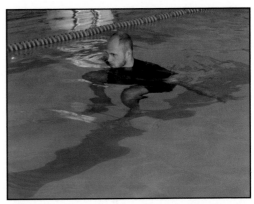

Figure 15-31. Reverse squat, bilateral, using flotation dumbell beneath the feet. Can be used for balance and neuromuscular coordination, as well as range of motion.

aquatic environment will allow for early initiation of a structured jumping and landing program. Some adaptations and proper instruction to the patient will provide similar positive effects as those seen in land-based programs.[40] Progression to the land-based jump/land program is recommended when appropriate.

Clinical Decision-Making Exercise 15-5

A 20-year-old female collegiate basketball player was injured and sustained a left ACL tear. She had a surgical repair using the hamstring graft. How soon can she begin with activities in the aquatic environment, and what would be the goals of early intervention?

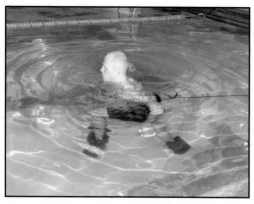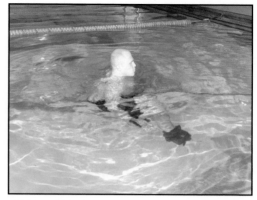

Figure 15-32. Deep water running against tubing resistance. (A) Forward; (B) backward.

Final Level

In the final level, the patient is involved with a high-level strengthening and training program. The aquatic program can and should be used to complement the land program. The athlete can continue to practice sport-specific activities and drills in varying levels of water. Decreasing the use of flotation equipment can increase the difficulty with deep-water activities. Using buoyancy cuffs on the ankles without using a flotation belt will challenge the athlete's ability to stabilize and perform running in deep water. Endurance training in an aquatic environment is a good alternative for the healthy athlete's conditioning programs and may help to prevent injuries. As with the upper extremity, this phase also requires integration of aquatic- and land-based exercises to successfully transition the athlete to full participation in sport on land.

SPECIAL TECHNIQUES

Bad Ragaz Ring Method

The Bad Ragaz technique originated in the thermal pools of Bad Ragaz, Switzerland, in the 1930s, and continued to evolve throughout the years. As a method, it focuses on muscle reeducation, strengthening, spinal traction/elongation, relaxation, and tone inhibition.[17] The properties of water—including buoyancy, turbulence, hydrostatic pressure, and surface tension—provide dynamic environmental forces during activities. The use of upper-extremity and lower-extremity PNF patterns add a 3-dimensional aspect to this method. Movement of the patient's body through the water provides the resistance.[11] The turbulent drag produced from movement is in direct relation to the patient's speed of movement. The athletic trainer provides the movement when the patient works on isometric (stabilization) patterns; however, the athletic trainer is in the stable/fixed position when the patient is performing isokinetic or isotonic activities[21] (Figures 15-26, 15-27, and 15-29). Stretching and lengthening responses can be obtained with passive or relaxed response from the patient; the athletic trainer needs to support and stabilize body segments to obtain desired response.

Awareness of body mechanics and prevention of injury are important to the athletic trainer when performing resistive Bad Ragaz–type activities. The athletic trainer should stand in waist-deep water, not deeper than the level of T8-T10,[21] and wear aqua shoes for traction and stability. The athletic trainer should stand with one foot in front of the other, with knees slightly bent, and legs shoulder-width apart, to compensate for the long lever arm force of the patient.

Burdenko Method

The Burdenko method uses motion as the principal healing intervention. According to Burdenko,[6] the components of dynamic healing include patterns of movement, injury assessment, and rehabilitation exercises that occur with the patient in a standing position; the psychology of the injured patient benefits from pain-free movement, and blood flow and neural stimulation being enhanced by activity.[6] Six essential qualities are necessary for perfecting and maintaining the art of movement: balance, coordination, flexibility, endurance, speed, and strength. Burdenko advocates the presentation of these qualities in exercise activities in the previously stated order. The activities are designed to challenge the center of buoyancy and center of gravity. Treatments/activities are initiated in deep water and incorporate shallow-water activities as patient succeeds by demonstrating control of movement while maintaining neutral vertical position. Integration of land exercise along with the aquatic activity addresses functional movement patterns. For further information on this technique, see "Suggested Readings" at the end of the chapter.

Halliwick Method

The Halliwick method is commonly used to teach individuals with physical disabilities to swim and to learn balance control in water. Developed by James McMillan, the Halliwick method or concept is based on a "Ten Point Programme."[9] This method is frequently used with the pediatric population, but portions of the technique can be used to improve and restore an adult patient's balance. Use of turbulent forces can assist in developing strategies for maintaining balance or challenge the patient to maintain a stable posture during a change in the direction of force. For example, the patient maintains a single-leg stance while the athletic trainer or another person runs around the patient offering turbulent perturbations (Figure 15-33). More information on the Halliwick technique is also available in the "Suggested Readings" section at the end of the chapter.

This exercise demonstrates the use of the principle of turbulence, generated in the Halliwick technique to challenge the stability of the patient.

Ai Chi

Ai chi is an Eastern-based treatment approach combining Tai Chi, Zen Shiatsu,

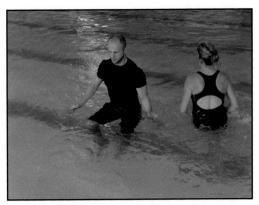

Figure 15-33. Balance and neuromuscular control restoration technique for trunk and single lower extremity.

Watsu, and Qi Gong in the water. Benefits of this approach include promoting relaxation by the use of diaphragmatic breathing that stimulates the parasympathetic nervous system, core strengthening, and increased flexibility. Performed in shoulder-depth water, it progresses from deep breathing to total-body movements through a characteristic sequence of postures.[42]

Clinical Decision-Making Exercise 15-6

A 12-year-old girl involved in high-level gymnastics has complaints of low back pain with 5- to 6-hour training sessions 5 to 6 days per week. She is diagnosed with grade 1 spondylolisthesis at L4-L5. What is a key principle or position that she needs to be taught, and how can aquatic activities complement your land program?

CONCLUSION

Aquatic rehabilitation is not typically the exclusive intervention option for most patients. The aquatic environment offers many positive psychological and physiologic effects during the early rehabilitation phase of injury.[37,54] However, in subsequent phases of rehabilitation, it is typical to use combinations of land- and water-based interventions to achieve rehabilitation goals. Because humans function in a "gravity environment," the transition from water to land is necessary for full rehabilitation for most patients. Some patients use the aquatic environment for continued strengthening and conditioning programs secondary to a painful response to land-based activities. Examples of this include those patients with pain that occurs with compressive forces at joints (such as cases of disc dysfunction, spinal stenosis, and osteoarthritis), as well as chronic neuromuscular conditions such as multiple sclerosis.

This chapter provides information regarding indications and benefits as well as contraindications and precautions to use of the aquatic environment for rehabilitation. Suggestions and exercises are offered to help the athletic trainer to incorporate aquatic exercise into a rehabilitation program. Using the principles provided and the examples of activities, athletic trainers can use their judgment, skill, and especially their creativity to develop an exercise program to meet their patient's goals. The old English proverb says, "We never know the worth of water 'til the well is dry." The worth and value of aquatic therapy as an intervention cannot be fully understood and appreciated until experienced and additional research is completed.

Summary

1. The buoyant force counteracts the force of gravity as it assists motion toward the water's surface and resists motion away from the surface.

2. Because of differences in the specific gravity of the body, the head and chest tend to float higher in the water than the heavier, denser extremities, making compensation with floatation devices necessary.

3. The three forces that oppose movement in the water are the cohesive force, the bow force, and the drag force.

4. Aquatic therapy allows for fine gradations of exercise, increased control over the percentage of weight bearing, increased ROM and strength in weak patients, and decreased pain and increased confidence in functional movements.

5. Pool size and depth, water temperature, and specific pool equipment vary depending on the clientele being treated and the resources available to the athletic trainer.

6. Application of the principle of buoyancy allows for progression of exercises.

7. Upper- and lower-extremity activities both require and provide a challenge to trunk and core stability.

8. The special techniques exclusive to the aquatic environment can be used to complement traditional land-based therapeutic interventions.

9. Aquatic therapy can help stimulate interest, motivation, and exercise compliance in pediatric, geriatric, neurological, and athletic patients.

10. The aquatic environment is an excellent medium to facilitate speedy functional return to work, activities of daily living, and sport.

11. It is typical to use a combination of land- and water-based therapeutic exercise protocols to achieve rehabilitation goals.

References

1. Arrigo C, ed. Aquatic rehabilitation. *Sports Med Update*. 1992;7(2).

2. Arrigo C, Fuller CS, Wilk KE. Aquatic rehabilitation following ACL-PTG reconstruction. *Sports Med Update*. 1992;7(2):22-27.

3. Asahina M, Asahina MK, Yamanaka Y, Mitsui K, Kitahara A, Murata A. Cardiovascular response during aquatic exercise in patients with osteoarthritis. *Am J Phys Med Rehabil*. 2010;89(9):731-735.

4. Bolton F, Goodwin D. *Pool Exercises*. Edinburgh, UK: Churchill-Livingstone; 1974.

5. Broach E, Groff D, Yaffe R, Dattilo J, Gast D. Effects of aquatic therapy on adults with multiple sclerosis. *Ann Ther Rec*. 1998;7:1-20.

6. Burdenko IN. *Sport-specific exercises after injuries — the Burdenko method*. Paper presented at the Aquatic Therapy Symposium 2002, August 22-25, Orlando, FL, 2002.

7. Butts NK, Tucker M, Greening C. Physiologic responses to maximal treadmill and deep water running in men and women. *Am J Sports Med*. 1991;19(6):612-614.

8. Campion MR. *Adult Hydrotherapy: A Practical Approach.* Oxford, UK: Heinemann Medical; 1990.

9. Cunningham J. Halliwick method. In: Ruoti RG, Morris DM, Cole AJ, eds. *Aquatic Rehabilitation.* Philadelphia, PA: Lippincott-Raven; 1997:305-331.

10. Cureton KJ. Physiologic responses to water exercise. In: Ruoti RG, Morris DM, Cole AJ, eds. *Aquatic Rehabilitation.* Philadelphia, PA: Lippincott-Raven; 1997:39-56.

11. Davis BC. A technique of re-education in the treatment pool. *Physiotherapy.* 1967;53(2):37-59.

12. Dioffenbach L. Aquatic therapy services. *Clin Manage.* 1991;11(1):14-19.

13. Dougherty NJ. Risk management in aquatics. *JOPERD.* 1990;(May/June):46-48.

14. Duffield NH. *Exercise in Water.* London, UK: Bailliere Tindall; 1976.

15. Edlich RF, Towler MA, Goitz RJ, et al. Bioengineering principles of hydrotherapy. *J Burn Care Rehabil.* 1987;8(6):580-584.

16. Ekdahl C, Jarnlo GB, Andersson SI. Standing balance in healthy subjects: use of quantitative test-battery on force platform. *Scand J Rehabil Med.* 1989;21:187-95.

17. Ekdahl C, Andersson SI. Standing balance in rheumatoid arthritis: a comparative study with healthy subjects. *Scand J Rheumatol.* 1989;18:33-42.

18. Eyestone ED, Fellingham G, George J, Fisher G. Effect of water running and cycling on maximum oxygen consumption and 2 mile run performance. *Am J Sports Med.* 1993;21(1):41-44.

19. Fawcett CW. Principles of aquatic rehab: a new look at hydrotherapy. *Sports Med Update.* 1992;7(2):6-9.

20. Fontana HDB, Haupenthal A, Ruschel C, Hubert M, Ridehalgh C, Roesler H. Effect of gender, cadence, and water immersion on ground reaction forces during stationary running. *J Orthop Sports Phys Ther.* 2012;42(5):437-443.

21. Garrett G. Bad Ragaz ring method. In: Ruoti RG, Morris DM, Cole AJ, eds. *Aquatic Rehabilitation.* Philadelphia, PA: Lippincott-Raven; 1997:289-292.

22. Geigle P, Daddona K, Finken K, et al. The effects of a supplemental aquatic physical therapy program on balance and girth for NCAA division III athletes with a grade I or II lateral ankle sprain. *J Aquatic Phys Ther.* 2001;9(1):13-20.

23. Genuario SE, Vegso JJ. The use of a swimming pool in the rehabilitation and reconditioning of athletic injuries. *Contemp Orthop.* 1990;20(4):381-387.

24. Golland A. Basic hydrotherapy. *Physiotherapy.* 1961;67(9):258-262, 1961.

25. Hall J, Phil M, Swinkels A, Briddon J. Does aquatic exercise relieve pain in adults with neurologic or musculoskeletal disease? A systematic review and meta-analysis of randomized controlled trials. *Arch Phys Med Rehabil.* 2008;89:873-883.

26. Haralson KM. Therapeutic pool programs. *Clin Manage.* 1985;5(2):10-13.

27. Harrison R, Bulstrode S. Percentage weight bearing during partial immersion in the hydrotherapy pool. *Physiother Theory Pract.* 1987;3:60-63.

28. Hertler L, Provost-Craig M, Sestili D, Hove A, Fees M. Water running and the maintenance of maximal oxygen consumption and leg strength in runners. *Med Sci Sports Exerc.* 1992;24(5):S23.

29. Hurley R, Turner C. Neurology and aquatic therapy. *Clin Manage.* 1991;11(1):26-27.

30. Irion JM. Aquatic therapy. In: Bandy WD, Sanders B, eds. *Therapeutic Exercise: Techniques for Intervention.* Baltimore, MD: Lippincott, Williams & Wilkins; 2001: 295-332.

31. Kim Y, Park J, Shim J. Effects of aquatic backward locomotion exercise and progressive resistance exercise on lumbar extension strength in patients who have undergone lumbar discectomy. *Arch Phys Med Rehabil.* 2010;91:208-214.

32. Kolb ME. Principles of underwater exercise. *Phys Ther Rev.* 1957;27(6):361-364.

33. Koszuta LE. From sweats to swimsuits: is water exercise the wave of the future? *Phys Sportsmed.* 1989;17(4):203-206.

34. Levin S. Aquatic therapy. *Phys Sportsmed.* 1991;19(10): 119-126.

35. Masumota K, Takasugi S, Hotta N, Fujishima K, Iwamato Y. A comparison of muscle activity and heart rate response during backward and forward walking on an underwater treadmill. *Gait Posture.* 2007;25:222-228.

36. McNamara C, Thein L. Aquatic rehabilitation of musculoskeletal conditions of the spine. In: Ruoti RG, Morris DM, Cole AJ, eds. *Aquatic Rehabilitation.* Philadelphia, PA: Lippincott-Raven; 1997:85-98.

37. McWaters JG. For faster recovery just add water. *Sports Med Update.* 1992;7(2):4-5.

38. Meyer RI. Practice settings for kinesiotherapy-aquatics. *Clin Kinesiol.* 1990;44(1):12-13.

39. Michaud TL, Brennean DK, Wilder RP, Sherman NW. Aquarun training and changes in treadmill running maximal oxygen consumption. *Med Sci Sports Exerc.* 1992;24(5):S23.

40. Miller MG. Berry DC, Gilders R, Bullard S. Recommendations for implementing an aquatic plyometric program. *Strength Cond J.* 2001;23(6):28-35.

41. Moor FB, Peterson SC, Manueall EM, et al. *Manual of Hydrotherapy and Massage.* Mountain View, CA: Pacific Press; 1964.

42. Morris DM. Aquatic rehabilitation for the treatment of neurologic disorders. In: Cole AJ, Becker BE, eds. *Comprehensive Aquatic Therapy.* Philadelphia, PA: Butterworth-Heinemann; 2004.

43. Morris D. Aquatic therapy to improve balance dysfunction in older adults. *Top Geriatr Rehabil.* 2010;26(2):104-119.

44. Nolte-Heuritsch I. *Aqua Rhythmics: Exercises for the Swimming Pool.* New York, NY: Sterling; 1979.

45. Petersen TM. Pediatric aquatic therapy. In: Cole AJ, Becker BE, eds. *Comprehensive Aquatic Therapy.* Philadelphia, PA: Butterworth-Heinemann; 2004.

46. Pöyhönen T, Kyröläinen H, Keskinen KL, Hautala A, Savolainen J, Mälkiä, E. Electromyographic and kinematic analysis of therapeutic knee exercises under water. *Clin Biomech (Bristol, Avon)*. 2001;16:496-504.

47. Pöyhönen TK, Keskinen L, Hautala A, Mälkiä E. Determination of hydrodynamic drag forces and drag coefficients on human leg/foot model during knee exercise. *Clin Biomech (Bristol, Avon)*. 2000;15:256-260.

48. Robertson JM, Brewster EA, Factora KI. Comparison of heart rates during water running in deep and shallow water at the same rating of perceived exertion. *J Aquatic Phys Ther*. 2001;9(1):21-26.

49. Simmons V, Hansen PD. Effectiveness of water exercise on postural mobility in the well elderly: an experimental study on balance enhancement. *J Gerontol*. 1996;51A(5):M233-M238.

50. Sova R. *Aquatic Activities Handbook*. Boston, MA: Jones & Bartlett; 1993.

51. Speer K, Cavanaugh JT, Warren RF, Day L, Wickiewicz TL. A role for hydrotherapy in shoulder rehabilitation. *Am J Sports Med*. 1993;21(6):850-853.

52. Suomi R, Koceja D. Postural sway characteristics in women with lower extremity arthritis before and after an aquatic exercise intervention. *Arch Phys Med Rehabil*. 2000;81:780-785.

53. Svendenhag J, Seger J. Running on land and in water: comparative exercise physiology. *Med Sci Sports Exerc*. 1992;24(10):1155-1160.

54. Thein JM, Thein BL. Aquatic-based rehabilitation and training for the elite athlete. *J Orthop Sports Phys Ther*. 1998;27(1):32-41.

55. Town GP, Bradley SS. Maximal metabolic responses of deep and shallow water running in trained runners. *Med Sci Sports Exerc*. 1991;23(2):238-241.

56. Triggs M. Orthopedic aquatic therapy. *Clin Manage*. 1991;11(1): 30-31.

57. Wilder RP, Brennan D, Schotte D. A standard measure for exercise prescription and aqua running. *Am J Sports Med*. 1993;21(1):45-48.

58. Wilder R, Brennan D. Aqua running. In: Cole AJ, Becker BE, eds. *Comprehensive Aquatic Therapy*. Philadelphia, PA: Butterworth-Heinemann; 2004.

SOLUTIONS TO CLINICAL DECISION-MAKING EXERCISES

15-1   This individual can begin initial activities when active assistive motion is allowed. Activities in this phase might include shoulder elevation (flexion and abduction) while standing in shoulder-deep water using the assistance of buoyancy. He will be able to benefit from strengthening and stabilization activities when he progresses to being able to do resistive activities.

15-2   It is important in this example to honor the prescribed weight-bearing restrictions imposed after surgery. The aquatic environment is an excellent choice for implementation of early rehabilitation after sufficient incisional healing or adequate coverage with a moisture-proof dressing. This environment is ideal for maintaining or improving ROM and strength without full weight bearing. Also, the aquatic environment offers the possibility of gradual weight-bearing progression and restoration of balance, neuromuscular control, and function.

15-3   The athletic trainer should recommend an alternate environment for maintenance of aerobic function. The aquatic environment is ideal for cross-training applications that decrease or eliminate weight bearing in the lower extremities. Excellent choices might include deep-water running and sport-specific lower-extremity strengthening in a diminished weight-bearing application (chest-deep water).

15-4   Initially the aquatic environment is ideal for developing ROM for elbow flexion and extension. It can also be used for light resistance training for elbow and shoulder musculature, being very cautious about valgus forces that might occur at the elbow due to drag forces that could occur during upper-extremity adduction and internal rotation motions against water resistance. Exercises could be progressed appropriately to include exercise directed at development of endurance, power, and sport-specific movements (pitching).

15-5   She could begin as soon as incisions are healed, or sooner if a moisture-barrier dressing is used. Goals would be:

- To control and decrease swelling because of the property of hydrostatic pressure;

- To restore gait pattern in an unloaded environment;
- To normalize motion in the left knee;
- To normalize neuromuscular control;
- To initiate and maintain her conditioning level with deep-water activities.

Awareness of graft vulnerability occurring at 4 to 8 weeks after surgery must be integrated into the program.

15-6 She needs to be taught neutral position and core strengthening. Activities that are specific to gymnastics and the events she participates in can be practiced and challenged in the aquatic environment. Integrating activities using opposite movement patterns can assist in developing core stabilization.

Suggested Readings

Berger MA, deGroot G, Hollander AP. Hydrodynamic drag and lift forces on human hand/arm models. *J Biomech.* 1995;28(2):125-133.

Brody LT, Geigle PR. *Aquatic Therapy for Rehabilitation and Training.* Champaign, IL: Human Kinetics; 2009.

Burdenko J, Connors E. *The Ultimate Power of Resistance.* Igor Publishing; 1999 [available only through mail order]. Burdenko Water & Sports Therapy Institute. Newton, MA; 1998.

Campion MR. *Adult Hydrotherapy: A Practical Approach.* Oxford, UK: Heinemann Medical; 1990.

Cassady SL, Nielsen DH. Cardiorespiratory responses of healthy subjects to calisthenics performed on land versus in water. *Phys Ther.* 1992;72(7):532-538.

Christie JL, Sheldahl LM, Tristani FE. Cardiovascular regulation during head-out water immersion exercise. *J Appl Physiol.* 1990;69(2):657-664.

Frangolias DD, Rhodes EC. Maximal and ventilatory threshold responses to treadmill and water immersion running. *Med Sci Sports Exerc.* 1995;27(7):1007-1013.

Green JH, Cable NT, Elms N. Heart rate and oxygen consumption during walking on land and in deep water. *J Sports Med Phys Fitness.* 1990;30(1):49-52.

Martin J. The Halliwick method. *Physiotherapy.* 1981;67: 288-291.

Sova R. *Aquatic Activities Handbook.* Boston, MA: Jones & Bartlett; 1993.

Please see videos on the accompanying website at

www.healio.com/books/sportsmedvideos

CHAPTER 16

Functional Progressions and Functional Testing in Rehabilitation

Michael McGee, EdD, LAT, ATC

After completion of this chapter, the athletic training student should be able to do the following:

- Develop the concept of a functional progression.
- Identify the goals of a functional progression.
- Recognize how and when functional progressions should be used in the rehabilitation process.
- Describe the physical benefits associated with a functional progression.
- Identify and describe the psychological benefits associated with a functional progression.
- Generalize the disadvantages associated with a functional progression.
- Incorporate the components of a functional progression.
- Develop a functional progression for a patient.
- Analyze various functional tests.
- Design a functional test for a patient.

In the athletic community, injuries and subsequent disability frequently occur. Disabilities can be described as restrictive influences that "disease and injury exert upon neuromotor performances."[19] Thus, to reduce the lasting effects of injury, the athletic trainer should direct rehabilitation toward improving neuromuscular coordination and agility, and not simply toward increasing strength and endurance. If rehabilitation is directed toward regaining range of motion (ROM), flexibility, strength, and endurance, and perhaps primarily toward increasing neuromuscular coordination and agility, a full return to activity is possible. However, if the

Prentice WE, ed.
Rehabilitation Techniques for Sports Medicine and Athletic Training (pp 415-441).
© 2015 SLACK Incorporated.

program simply provides a means for reducing signs and symptoms associated with the injury, the patient will not return to a safe and effective level of activity.[36] As a result, rehabilitation of athletic injuries needs to focus on return to preinjury activity levels.[29] Function refers to patterns of motion that use multiple joints acting with various axes and in multiple planes.[22] Traditional rehabilitation techniques, although vital to the return of function, often stress single joints in single planes of motion. To complement traditional rehabilitation, the athletic trainer can use functional rehabilitation techniques. Functional rehabilitation, along with traditional methods, will ready the patient for activity and competition more successfully than if either method is employed alone.[21]

THE ROLE OF FUNCTIONAL PROGRESSIONS IN REHABILITATION

Athletic trainers must adapt rehabilitation to the sports-specific demands of each individual sport and playing position. But rehabilitation programs in a clinical setting cannot predict the ability of the injured part to endure the demands of full competition on the playing field. For example, the complex factors surrounding a solid tackle in competition play cannot be produced in the clinical setting. The role of the functional progression is to improve and complete the clinical rehabilitation process.[39] A functional progression is a succession of activities that simulate actual motor and sport skills, enabling the patient to acquire or reacquire the skills needed to perform athletic endeavors safely and effectively.[9,13,21] The athletic trainer takes the activities involved in a given sport and breaks them down into individual components. In this way, the patient concentrates on individual parts of the game or activity in a controlled environment before combining them together in an uncontrolled environment as would exist during full competition. The functional progression places stresses and forces on each body system in a well-planned, positive, and progressive fashion, ultimately improving the patient's overall ability to meet the demands of daily activities as well as sport competition. The

functional progression is essential in the rehabilitation process because tissues not placed under performance-level stresses do not adapt to the sudden return of such stresses with the resumption of full activity. Thus, the functional progression is integrated into the normal rehabilitation scheme, as one component of exercise therapy, rather than replacing traditional rehabilitation altogether.[10]

BENEFITS OF USING FUNCTIONAL PROGRESSIONS

Using a functional progression in a rehabilitation program will help the patient and the athletic trainer reach the goals of the entire program. The goals of the functional progression generally include a restoration of (1) joint ROM, (2) strength, (3) proprioception, (4) agility, and (5) confidence. Achieving these goals allows the patient to reach the desired level of activity safely and effectively.[28] Functional progressions provide both physical and psychological benefits to the injured patient. The physical benefits include improvements in muscular strength and endurance, mobility and flexibility, cardiorespiratory endurance, and neuromuscular coordination, along with an increase in the functional stability of an injured joint. Psychologically, the progression can reduce the feelings of anxiety, apprehension, and deprivation commonly observed in the injured patient.[9,13,21]

Improving Functional Stability

Functional stability is provided by (1) passive restraints on the ligaments, (2) joint geometry, (3) active restraints generated by muscles, and (4) joint compressive forces that occur with activity and force the joint together.[27] Stability is maintained by the neuromuscular control mechanisms involved in proprioception and kinesthesia (as discussed in Chapter 5). Functional stability cannot always be determined by examining the patient in the clinic. Therefore, the functional progression can be used to evaluate functional stability both objectively and subjectively. Can the patient complete all tasks with no adverse effects? Does the patient appear to perform at the same level, or close to the same level, as prior to injury? Performance during a functional task can be evaluated for improvement, and functional testing can be incorporated to provide an objective measure of ability.[10] The patient can also give important feedback regarding function, pain, and stability while performing the functional tasks.

Muscular Strength

Increased strength is a physical benefit of the functional progression. Strength is the ability of the muscle to produce tension or apply force maximally against resistance. This occurs statically or dynamically, in relation to the imposed demands. Strength increases are possible if the load imposed on a muscle exceeds that muscle's anatomic capabilities during exercise. This is commonly referred to as the overload principle and is possible due to increased efficiency in motor unit recruitment and muscle fiber hypertrophy.[23] To see these improvements, the muscle must be worked to the point of fatigue with either high or low resistance. The functional progression will develop strength using the SAID (Specific Adaptation to Imposed Demands) principle. The muscles involved will be strengthened dynamically, under stresses similar to those encountered in competition.

Endurance

Muscular and cardiorespiratory endurance can both be enhanced with a functional progression. Endurance is necessary for long-duration activity, whether in daily living or in the repeated motor functions found with sport participation. The functional progression will enhance muscular endurance through the repetition of the individual activities and their combination into one general activity. The progression provides an environment for improving muscular strength and endurance without using more than one program. Cardiorespiratory endurance can be improved through the repetition of movements involved in the progression in the same way as regular fitness levels improve with continuous exercise.

Flexibility

With injury, tissues will shorten or tighten in response to immobilization. This can inhibit proper function. With a functional progression, the injured area is stressed within a controlled range. This stress should be significant enough to allow the tissue to elongate and return to proper length. This improved mobility and flexibility is crucial to the patient. Strength and endurance do not mean much if the injured body part cannot move through a full ROM. Tissues also become stronger with consistent stresses, so tissues other than muscle can also be improved with the functional progression.[23]

Muscle Relaxation

Relaxation involves the concerted effort to reduce muscle tension. The functional progression can teach an individual to recognize this tension and eventually control or remove it by consciously relaxing the muscles after exercise. The total body relaxation that can ensue relaxes the injured area, helping to relieve the muscle guarding that can inhibit the joint's full ROM.[23]

Motor Skills

Coordination, agility, and motor skills are complex aspects of normal function defined as appropriate contractions at the most opportune time and with the appropriate intensity.[23] A patient needs coordination, agility, and motor skills to transform strength, flexibility, and endurance into full-speed performance. This is especially important for an injured patient. If the patient does not regain or improve his or her coordination and agility, performance is hampered and can in itself lead to further injury. Repetition and practice are important to learning motor skills. Regular motions that are consciously controlled develop into automatic reactions via motor learning. This is possible due to the constant repetition and reinforcement of a particular skill.[19] To acquire these "automatic reactions," one needs an intact and functional neuromuscular system. Because this system is disturbed by injury, decreases in performance will occur, increasing the potential for injury. The functional progression can be used to minimize the loss of normal neuro-muscular control by providing exercises that stress proprioception, motor-skill integration, and proper timing. The functional progression is indicated for improvement in agility and skill because of the constant repetition of sport specific motor skills, use of sensory cues, and progressive increases in activity levels. Proprioception can be enhanced by stimulating the intra-articular and intramuscular mechano-receptors. These are all components of, or general principles for, enhancing neuromuscular coordination.[19] The practice variations used with functional progressions allow the patient to relearn the various aspects of their sport that they might encounter in competition. Rehabilitative exercise programs must stress neuromuscular coordination and agility. Increases in strength, endurance, and flexibility are unquestionably necessary for a safe and effective return to play, but without the neuromuscular coordination to integrate these aspects into proper function, little performance enhancement can occur. For this reason, functional progressions should become an integral part of the long-term rehabilitation stage so that injured patients can maximize their ability to return to competition at their pre-injury level.

PSYCHOLOGICAL AND SOCIAL CONSIDERATIONS

Functional progressions can also provide psychological benefits to the patient. Anxiety, apprehension, and feelings of deprivation are all common emotions found with injuries. The functional progression can aid the rehabilitation process and facilitate the return to play by diminishing these emotions. Chapter 4 discusses the psychological aspects of the rehabilitative process in more detail. This chapter will focus on the specific contributions of the functional progression.

Anxiety

Uncertainty about the future is a reason many patients give for their feelings of anxiety. Patients experience this insecurity because they have only a vague understanding of the severity of their injury and the length of time it will take for them to fully recover.[1] The progression can lessen anxiety because the patient is gradually placed into more demanding situations that allow the patient to experience success and not be concerned as much with failure in the future.

Deprivation

The patient might experience feelings of deprivation after losing direct contact with his team and coaches for an extended time. The functional progression can limit such feelings of deprivation, because the patient can exercise during regular team practice times at the practice site. By engaging in an activity that can be completed during practice, the patient remains close in proximity and socially feels little loss in team cohesion.[1]

Apprehension

Apprehension is often listed as an obstacle to performance and many times serves as a precursor to reinjury.[1] Functional progressions enable patients to adapt to the imposed demands of their sports in a controlled environment, helping to restore confidence, thus decreasing apprehension. Each success builds on past success, allowing the patient to feel in control as they return to full activity. Figure 16-1 provides a list of the physical and psychological benefits of functional progressions.

COMPONENTS OF A FUNCTIONAL PROGRESSION

Functional progressions can begin early post-injury. In general, the early focus of phase 1 in the progression is on restoration of joint ROM, muscular strength, and muscle endurance. The next phase of the progression focuses on incorporating proprioception and agility exercises into the program. These two phases can be two separate phases or, as is often the case, they may overlap. By including proprioception and agility exercises into the program, the injured area is positively stressed to improve the neurovascular, neurosensory, and kinetic functions.[28]

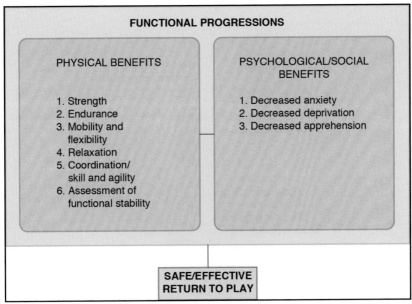

Figure 16-1. Physical and psychological benefits of using functional progressions.

The functional progression should allow for planned sequential activities that challenge the patient while allowing for success. The success will give the patient confidence in his or her ability to complete tasks and motivate the patient to attain the next goal. Neglecting to plan and use a simple progression can lead to reinjury, pain, effusion, tendinitis, or a plateau in performance. To plan appropriately, each decision for a patient should be based on individual results and performance rather than solely on time factors.[28]

Several factors must be addressed to provide a safe and effective return to play with the use of functional progressions. First, what are the physician's expectations for the patient's return to activity? Second, what are the patient's expectations for his or her return to activity? Third, what is the total disability of the patient? And fourth, what are the parameters of physical fitness for this patient? Keeping the total well-being of the injured patient in perspective is a significant factor.[9]

Activity Considerations

Exercise can be viewed from two perspectives. From one perspective, exercise is a single activity involving simple motor skills. From the second perspective, exercise involves the training and conditioning effect of repetitive activity.[19] It is well accepted that preinjury status can be regained only if appropriate activities of sufficient intensity are used to train and condition the patient. To provide the patient with these activities, four principles must be observed. First, the individuality of the patient, the sport, and the injury must be addressed. Second, the activities should be positive, not negative; no increased signs and symptoms should occur. Third, an orderly progressive program should be used. And fourth, the program should be varied to avoid monotony.[23] Steps to minimize monotony include the following:

1. Vary exercise techniques used

2. Alter the program at regular intervals

3. Maintain fitness base to avoid reinjury with return to play

4. Set achievable goals, reevaluate, and modify regularly

5. Use clinical, home, and on-field programs to vary the activity[19]

Patients are continually exposed to situations that make reinjury likely, so every effort should be made to understand and incorporate the inherent demands of the sport into the rehabilitation program. The athletic trainer can emphasize the importance of sport-specific

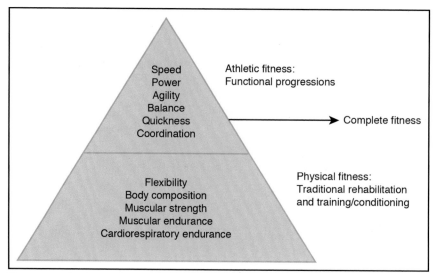

Figure 16-2. Combining components of physical fitness with components of athletic fitness in functional progressions.

activities to enhance the patient's return to activity, rather than simply concentrating on traditional rehabilitation methods involving only weight machines and analgesics.

The components of fitness are listed in Figure 16-2. There are two distinct components in this model. The physical fitness items used in more traditional rehabilitation programs should be merged with the athletic fitness items of functional progressions to maximize the patient's chance to regain preinjury fitness levels.

The components of a functional progression should aim to incorporate all the factors listed in Figure 16-2 under athletic fitness items.

DESIGNING A FUNCTIONAL PROGRESSION

Athletic trainers should consider all aspects of a patient's situation when designing a functional progression. There is no "cookbook" method that meets the needs of all patients. Athletic trainers should use their creativity when it comes to developing progressions for the patient. As previously mentioned, functional progressions may start early in the rehabilitation process and then culminate in a full return to participation. The following guidelines are suggestions for designing functional progressions that can meet the needs of various injury situations.

As with any rehabilitation program, the patient's current state should be evaluated first. This step may include a review of the patient's medical history, physician notes and/or rehabilitation protocols, a physical exam or injury evaluation, diagnostic testing, and functional testing. Once the status of the patient is established, planning for proper progression may occur. The planning will involve reviewing the expectations of the patient and the physician. What are the rehabilitation goals and parameters? At this point, the athletic trainer must determine whether the injury situation, the patient's goals, and the physician's expectations will work together. If not, the athletic trainer must work to bring the three together. The athletic trainer will also need to understand the demands of the sport and the position played by the patient. The patient, coaches, and other athletic trainers may serve as valuable resources for successful completion of this step.

A complete analysis of the demands that will be placed on the patient and the injured body part once return to play is achieved must be completed. All of the tasks involved in the activity should be ranked on a continuum from simple to difficult. Simple tasks may involve isolated joints, assisted techniques, or low-impact activities, whereas difficult tasks often group simple tasks together into one activity and involve higher-impact activity-related skills. Primary concerns should include the intention of the activity, what activities should be included, and the order in which the activities should occur.[42] For example, if throwing a baseball is the purpose, the progression can be broken into an ordered sequence like the following:

1. Grip the ball
2. Stance
3. Backswing of the upper limb
4. Forward swing of the upper limb
5. Release of the ball
6. Follow-through

It is imperative that the athletic trainer assess the patient periodically throughout the progression prior to moving to the next level in the progression. Assessment of present functional status of the injury should serve as a guide to a safe progression.[23] The assessment should be based on traditional assessment methods, such as goniometry, along with knowledge of the healing process and the patient's response to activity, functional testing, and subjective evaluation. Aggressive activities that lead to pain, effusion, or patient anxiety can be replaced with less-aggressive activities. Achieving a certain skill level in a functional progression occurs when the skill can be completed at functional speed with high repetitions and no associated increase in pain or effusion or decrease in ROM. The athletic trainer and the patient should realize, however, that setbacks will occur and are common. Sometimes it takes two steps forward and one step back to achieve the needed level of improvement.

Full Return to Play

Deciding whether a patient is ready to return to play at full participation is a difficult task. The decision requires a complete evaluation of the patient's condition, including objective observations and a subjective evaluation. The athletic trainer should feel that the patient is ready both physically and mentally before allowing a return to play.[12] Return to activity should not be attempted too soon, to avoid added stress to the injury, which can slow healing and result in a long, painful recovery or reinjury.[11] The following are criteria for allowing a full return to activity:

1. Physician's release
2. Free of pain
3. No swelling
4. Normal ROM
5. Normal strength (in reference to contralateral limb)
6. Appropriate functional testing completed with no adverse reactions

FUNCTIONAL TESTING

Functional testing involves having the patient perform certain tasks appropriate to his or her stage in the rehabilitation process to isolate and address specific deficits. As a result the athletic trainer is able to determine the patient's current functional level and set functional goals.[31] According to Harter, functional testing is an indirect measure of muscular strength and power. Function is "quantified" using maximal performance of an activity.[18] Harter describes three purposes of functional testing as follows:

1. Determine risk of injury due to limb asymmetry
2. Provide objective measure of progress during a treatment or rehabilitation program
3. Measure the ability of the individual to tolerate forces[18]

Functional testing can provide the athletic trainer with objective data for review. Traditional rehabilitation programs and improvements in strength and ROM do not always correlate with functional ability.[20] Functional testing should have a better correlation with functional ability.

When contemplating the use of a functional test or battery of tests, the athletic trainer must evaluate the test(s) chosen. Validity and reliability must be considered. A test should measure what it intends to measure (validity) and should consistently provide similar results (reliability) regardless of the evaluator. Other factors must be considered before releasing a patient to full activity. These include a subjective evaluation of the injury, performance on functional tests, presence or absence of signs and symptoms, other recognized clinical tests (isokinetic testing, special tests, etc), and the physician's approval. Functional testing should attempt to look at unilateral function and bilateral function in an attempt to determine whether the patient is compensating with the uninjured limb. Other considerations should include the stage of healing for the patient, appropriate rest time, and self-evaluation.[31]

Functional testing might be limited if the athletic trainer does not have normative values or preinjury baseline values for comparison. Obviously, a patient who cannot complete the test(s) is not ready for a return to play. However, what happens to the patient who can complete the test(s) but has no preinjury data available for comparison? The athletic trainer has to make a subjective decision based on the test results. If the normative data or preinjury data are available, the athletic trainer can make an objective decision. If a soccer player is able to complete a sprint test with a mean of 20 seconds but her preinjury time was 16 seconds, then she is only 85% functional. Without the preinjury data, the athletic trainer might be unable to determine the patient's functional level. Of course, the athletic trainer can always compare to the mean functional level of the uninjured team members to aid in the decision making. Other methods that will aid in objective decision making include limb symmetry and error scores. Limb symmetry can include strength, ROM, and other traditional measurements; however, in this case, limb symmetry refers to the functional ability of the limbs. For example, a single-leg hop that compares the ipsilateral limb with the contralateral limb uses the following formula

(ipsilateral limb/contralateral limb) × 100
= limb symmetry percentage

An 85% or better goal is the recognized standard for limb symmetry scores.[12,31] Error scores typically calculate the number of times an error is made during the testing time frame. Bernier describes an error test with the Stork Stand for the ankle. During the 20-second time frame, the number of errors is recorded

and compared to the score for the contralateral limb.[6]

Functional testing should be an easy task for athletic trainers and should be equally simple for patients to understand. Cost efficiency, time demands, and space demands are important concepts when considering the tests to use.

> **Clinical Decision-Making Exercise 16-1**
> A soccer midfielder is recovering from a grade 2 MCL sprain and has been cleared for sport-specific training. What types of activities could you use for this patient?

EXAMPLES OF FUNCTIONAL PROGRESSIONS AND TESTING

The Upper Extremity

Functional activities that will enhance the healing and performance of the upper extremity might include PNF patterns, swimming motions, closed kinetic chain activities, and using pulley machines or rubber tubing to simulate sport activity.[12] Functional rehabilitation for the shoulder joint needs to focus on proprioception and neuromuscular control. Myers and Lephart report that four "facets of functional rehabilitation must be addressed: awareness of proprioception, dynamic stabilization restoration, preparatory and reactive muscle facilitation, and replication of functional activities."[32] Activities that promote awareness of proprioception are described as activities that promote restoration of interrupted afferent pathways while facilitating compensatory afferent pathways. This improvement in afferent pathways will result in a return of kinesthesia and joint position sense at an early stage in the rehabilitation process. Dynamic stabilization involves training the muscular and tendinous structures to work together as "force-couples." The muscles of the glenohumeral joint along with the scapular stabilizers work together using co-contraction as a way of providing stability to the upper extremity. Preparatory and reactive muscle facilitation involves stressing the upper extremity with unexpected forces. These activities will allow the patient to improve both muscle stiffness and muscle reflex action. Finally, functional activities that mimic actual sport or activity participation should be included.[32]

Numerous activities can promote joint position sense. Isokinetic exercise, proprioception testing devices, goniometry, and electromagnetic motion analysis are all reported by Myers and Lephart[32] as potential means for achieving this goal. Patients can practice reproducing joint positions with visual cues and progress to using no external cues. Activities can be passive, where the patient attempts to recognize certain joint positions when passively moved by the athletic trainer; or active in nature, where the patient attempts to actively reproduce a specific position. The patient can also attempt to reproduce specific motion paths in an attempt to increase the functional component of the activity. All activities need to stress the joint at both the end ROM and midrange of motion. The end ROM will stress the capsuloligamentous afferents; the midrange motion will stress the musculotendinous mechanoreceptors. Attention to full ROM will maximize the functional training for complete joint position sense.[32]

Kinesthesia training can use activities similar to those for joint position sense. To stress kinesthetic awareness, the athletic trainer needs to remove external visual and auditory cues. During motion, the patient is instructed to signal when they first notice joint motion. The athletic trainer notes what degree of error occurs before the patient senses the motion.[32]

Dynamic stability stresses the training of the force couples provided by the scapular stabilizers and the muscles of the glenohumeral joint. Closed kinetic chain activities are believed to enhance coactivation of these force couples. Common examples of activities would include push-ups and variations on the push-up, slide board activities, weight-shifting activities, and press-ups.[32]

The athletic trainer can improve the patient's muscle preparation and reaction skills by incorporating rhythmic stabilization activities into the program along with the closed kinetic chain activities previously discussed. Rhythmic stabilization helps the patient prepare for motion, thus improving muscle stiffness, while also training for muscle reaction. Simple rhythmic stabilization activities are discussed in Chapter 14. Plyometric training is an excellent alternative activity to include for training the muscle for reaction and preparation. Finally, functional activities that stress sport specific skills should be included in the progression. PNF patterns can be used as an early alternative to sport specific activity to simulate the sport motions with less stress.[32]

King advocates that upper-extremity rehabilitation should focus on the glenohumeral joint, the scapulothoracic articulation,[22] and the core. An effort should be made to coordinate the rehabilitation process and incorporate activities that stress glenohumeral improvements along with scapular and core stability. The quadruped position allows the patient to work the muscles that connect the trunk and scapula in both a concentric and an eccentric manner.[22] This idea is consistent with Myers and Lephart's plan for improving dynamic stability and muscle readiness. King suggests using activities that use a quadruped position with stable and unstable surfaces along with movement patterns.[22]

Although many sport-specific skills for the upper extremity are completed in the open kinetic chain, closed kinetic chain activities are important for proper function. Athletic trainers should work to incorporate these activities into the rehabilitation process as a part of the functional progression. Open kinetic chain sport-specific activities are important as well.[8] A functional progression for the throwing shoulder should include the following steps. First, the patient must be instructed in and complete a proper warm-up. During the warm-up, the patient should practice the throwing motion at a slow velocity and with low stress. The activity can then progress through increasingly difficult stages as indicated in Table 16-1 and in more detail in Chapter 17. Table 16-2 provides an example of a functional progression for

Table 16-1 Upper-Extremity Progression for Throwing

1. Functional activity can begin early with assisted PNF techniques
2. Rubber tubing exercises simulating PNF patterns and/or sport motions
3. Swimming
4. Push-ups
5. Sport drills:

Interval throwing program

45 ft phase

Step 1:	1. Warm-up throwing	Step 2:	1. Warm-up throwing
	2. 25 throws		2. 25 throws
	3. Rest 10 minutes		3. 15 minute rest
	4. Warm-up throwing		4. Warm-up throwing
	5. 25 throws		5. 25 throws
			6. Rest 10 minutes
			7. Warm-up throwing
			8. 25 throws

Repeat steps 1 and 2 for 60, 90, 120, 150, and 180 feet, until full throwing from the mound or respective position is achieved. See Chapter 19 for a more detailed program.

Table 16-2 Interval Golf Rehabilitation Program

	Day 1	Day 2	Day 3
Week 1	5 min chipping/putting 5 min rest 5 min chipping	5 min chipping/putting 5 min rest 5 min chipping 5 min rest 5 min chipping	5 min chipping/putting 5 min rest 5 min chipping 5 min rest 5 min chipping
Week 2	10 min chipping 10 min rest 10 min short iron	10 min chipping 10 min rest 10 min short iron 10 min rest 10 min short iron	10 min short iron 10 min rest 10 min short iron 10 min rest 10 min short iron
Week 3	10 min short iron 10 min rest 10 min long iron 10 min rest 10 min long iron	10 min short iron 10 min rest 10 min long iron 10 min rest 10 min long iron	10 min short iron 10 min rest 10 min long iron 10 min rest 10 min long iron
Week 4	Repeat week 3, day 2	Play 9 holes	Play 18 holes

hitting a golf ball, and Table 16-3 provides a program for return to hitting a tennis ball. Any upper-extremity injury can benefit from one of these programs or can be exercised in similar fashion using any sport equipment needed for that sport.[34]

Clinical Decision-Making Exercise 16-2

A volleyball player has chronic impingement syndrome due to poor scapular stabilization. What types of functional activities would help this patient?

Table 16-3 Interval Tennis Program

	Day 1	Day 2	Day 3
Week 1	12 FH 8 BH 10 min rest 13 FH 7 BH	15 FH 8 BH 10 min rest 15 FH 7 BH	15 FH 10 BH 10 min rest 15 FH 10 BH
Week 2	25 FH 15 BH 10 min rest 25 FH 15 BH	30 FH 20 BH 10 min rest 30 FH 20 BH	30 FH 25 BH 10 min rest 30 FH 15 BH 10 OH
Week 3	30 FH 25 BH 10 OH 10 min rest 30 FH 25 BH 10 OH	30 FH 25 BH 15 OH 10 min rest 30 FH 25 BH 15 OH	30 FH 30 BH 15 OH 10 min rest 30 FH 15 BH 10 min rest 30 FH 30 BH 15 OH
Week 4	30 FH 30 BH 10 OH 10 min rest Play 3 games 10 FH 10 BH 5 OH	30 FH 30 BH 10 OH 10 min rest Play set 10 FH 10 BH 5 OH	30 FH 30 BH 10 OH 10 min rest Play 1.5 sets 10 FH 10 BH 3 OH
FH = Forehand BH = Backhand OH = Overhead			

The shoulder joint serves as a template for upper-extremity rehabilitation and functional progressions. Many of the activities for the shoulder are equally effective for rehabilitation of the elbow, wrist, and hand. Other activities that can be used for upper-extremity rehabilitation may focus more on the elbow or wrist/hand. An excellent example of functional elbow rehabilitation can be found with Uhl, Gould, and Geick's work with a football lineman.[41] The progression started with simulated lineman drills for the upper extremity in the pool. The patient then progressed to proprioception and endurance work using a basketball bounced against a wall and progressed to a medicine ball thrown against a plyoback.[35] There are many ways to functionally test a patient. The most common and often the simplest ways include timed performance. For the upper extremity, a throwing velocity test is often used. This can be accomplished two ways, depending on the athletic trainer's budget and the availability of complex testing tools. The first way includeds the following:

1. Test velocity in a controlled environment, preferably indoors to decrease effects of the weather.

2. Set up a standard pitching distance (60 feet, 6 inches).

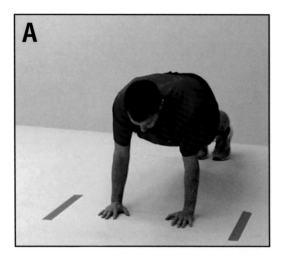

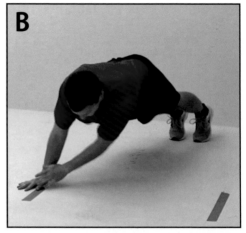

Figure 16-3. Closed kinetic chain upper-extremity stability test (CKC UE ST).

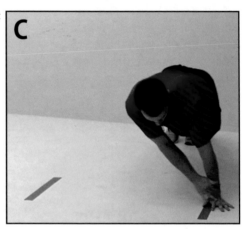

3. Have the patient use a windup motion.

4. Measure a maximum of five throws—measured in miles per hour with a calibrated Magnum X ban radar gun (CMI Corporation, Owensburg, KY) placed 36 inches high and to the right of the catcher.

5. Compute the mean of the five throws and compare to the pretest value.

Many athletic trainers do not have access to such equipment. A second way to test the upper extremity using velocity would be to use a similar setup but minus the radar gun. In this situation, the athletic trainer needs a stopwatch to time the flight of the ball. The athletic trainer begins timing as the patient releases the ball and stops when the catcher receives the ball. Again, a mean of five throws should be computed to help decrease testing error. The

first method will be the most accurate, but the second method can be used as an effective testing tool.

Other upper-extremity tests are possible. The closed kinetic chain upper-extremity stability test (CKC UE ST) can be used for an objective measure of upper extremity readiness for sport. In the CKC UE ST, the athletic trainer sets up a course using two strips of athletic tape placed on the ground parallel to each other 36 inches apart (Figure 16-3). The patient assumes a push-up position with hands on the appropriate tape strips. The patient then has 15 seconds to alternately reach across and touch the opposite tape strip. The patient should complete three trials with a maximal effort. The mean value is calculated as the patient's score. A standard 1-to-3 work-to-rest ratio is used allowing the patient to rest for 45 seconds in between each trial. Assessment of the score can be the total number of touches, the number of touches divided by body weight to normalize the data, or determining a power score by multiplying the mean score by 68% of the patient's body weight (weight of arms, head, and trunk) then dividing by 15 seconds. Goldbeck and Davies found that the CKC UE ST has a test–retest reliability of 0.922 and a coefficient of stability of 0.859, indicating that the test is a reliable evaluation tool.[15]

Uhl et al used sport-specific testing to determine the readiness for return of the football lineman.[41] The patient completed up-down drills, drive-blocking on a dummy (5 × 4 yards), blocking drill with a butt roll to both the right and the left, and finally a snap-pass protection drill against an opponent. Both athletic trainer and patient satisfaction and no report of pain indicated successful completion.[41] This is a great example of how the athletic training staff used sport-specific tasks to determine the functional level of the patient.

To functionally test the upper extremity, the key concept is to focus on the sport demand for the patient. Careful attention should focus on the skill involved with the sport. Does the patient perform a primarily open kinetic chain skill, or is the skill performed in a closed kinetic chain? A gymnast might need more closed kinetic chain testing than a tennis player. Similarly, the athletic trainer will not test a volleyball player using a pitching test. The athletic trainer will have to consult with the coach and determine what the patient needs to do, and from this devise a test battery. For the volleyball player, a serving test would obviously be better than the pitching test.

Clinical Decision-Making Exercise 16-3

A gymnast has a recurrent anterior dislocation of the glenohumeral joint. She has excellent muscular strength in both the glenohumeral muscles and the scapular muscles. She has had no problem regaining full ROM. She is extremely worried that the shoulder will dislocate again. Because strength and ROM are normal for this patient, what type of rehabilitation activities should the patient concentrate on to help improve her dynamic stability?

The Lower Extremity

The lower extremity follows the same basic pattern, with different exercises. The activities used should provide functional stress to the injured limb. An example of a functional progression for the lower extremity is found in Table 16-4. The lower extremity can be tested in many ways: sprint times, agility run times, jumping or hopping heights/distances, co-contraction tests, carioca runs, and shuttle runs.[16,33,38,40] The following are brief introductions to a variety of these tests.

Functional Activities

Functional activities can begin early in the rehabilitation process, almost immediately following injury. They can include both non-, partial-, and full-weight-bearing activities to regain proprioception, neuromuscular control, and balance. The patient should perform these activities in multiple planes of motion on both stable and unstable surfaces with eyes open then closed to provide an optimal challenge.[3,6,10] These exercises could include balancing on a BAPS board or Bosu Balance Trainer (Figure 16-4). The athletic trainer can also incorporate sport skills into balance exercises (see Chapter 7). As balance and neuromuscular control improve walking normally, then on heels, toes, and side shuffling laterally (Figure 16-5) can be incorporated. Both neuromuscular control and strength can be enhanced by multi-planar lunges (Figure 16-6); and forward and lateral step-ups (Figure 16-7).

Jogging

Jogging begins in a straight line, followed by jogging the curves on a track and then progressing to directional changes such as running "Ss" and "Zs" (Figures 16-8 and 16-9).

Sprint Tests

Jogging activities are replaced by sprinting actives that begin with sets of 10 straight line sprints of 10, 20, and 40 yards that are timed at each distance. During the sprinting phase it is important to introduce at speed running that involves more explosive acceleration and immediate deceleration (Figure 16-10). The sprint phase should also include both forward

TABLE 16-4 Lower-Extremity Functional Progression

1. Functional activity can begin early in the rehabilitation process with:
   - Assisted proprioceptive neuromuscular facilitation (PNF) techniques
   - Cycling
   - Non-weight-bearing (NWB) BAPS board or Bosu Balance exercises
   - Partial-weight-bearing (PWB) BAPS board or Bosu Balance exercises
   - Full-weight-bearing (FWB) BAPS board or Bosu Balance exercise (Figure 16-4)
   - Walking normal; heel; toe; sidestep/shuffle; slides (Figure 16-5)

2. Lunges:
   - Sagittal, frontal and transverse planes (Figure 16-6)
   - 90 degree pivot with weight or increased speed
   - 180 degree pivot with weight or increased speed

3. Step-ups:
   - Forward step-up, 50% to 75% max speed (Figure 16-7A)
   - Lateral step-up, 50% to 75% max speed (Figure 16-7B)

4. Jogging:
   - Straight-away on track; jog in turns (goal = 2 miles)
   - Complete oval of track (goal = 2 to 4 miles)
   - 100 yd "S" course 75% to 100% max speed with gradual increase in number of curves (Figure 16-8)
   - 100 yd–"8" course 75% to 100% max speed with gradual decrease in size of "8" to fit 5 × 10 yd (Figure 16-12)
   - 100 yd "Z" course 75% to 100% max speed with gradual increase in number of "Zs" (Figure 16-9)
   - Sidestep/shuffle slides

5. Sprints:
   - 10 yd × 10
   - 20 yd × 10
   - 40 yd × 10
   - Acceleration/deceleration; 50 yd × 10 (Figure 16-10)
   - "W" sprints × 10 (Figure 16-11)

6. Box runs:
   - 10 yd clockwise/counterclockwise × 10 (Figure 16-13)
   - Barrow Zig Zag Test (Figure 16-14)

7. Shuttle Runs -"suicides" (Figure 16-14)

8. Carioca: (Figure 16-16)
   - 30 yd × 5 right lead-off; 30 yd × 5 left lead-off

9. Jumping: (Figure 16-17)
   - Rope
   - Lines
   - Boxes, balls, etc

10. Hopping: (Figure 16-18)
    - Two feet
    - One foot
    - Alternate

11. Vertical jump using a vertec (Figure 16-19)

12. Co-contraction semicircular test (Figure 16-20)

13. Cutting, jumping, hopping on command

14. Sport drills used for preseason or in-season practice

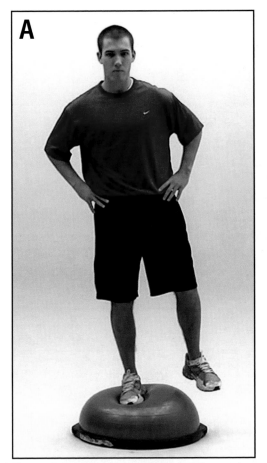

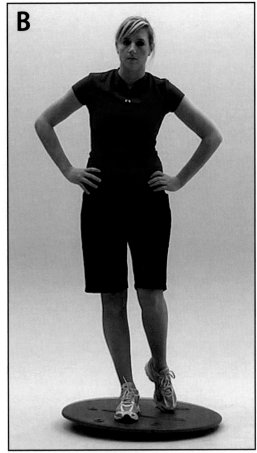

Figure 16-4. Balance exercises. (A) Bosu Balance trainer exercise; (B) BAPS board exercise.

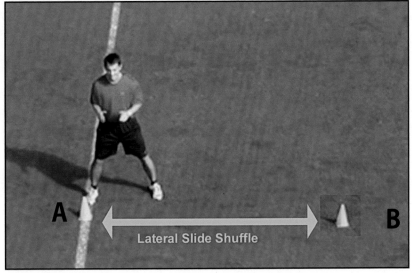

Figure 16-5. Shuffle slides. (A) Starting position; (B) finish position.

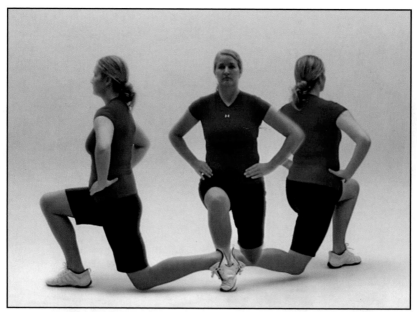

Figure 16-6. Multiplanar lunges can be done in the sagittal, frontal, and transverse planes.

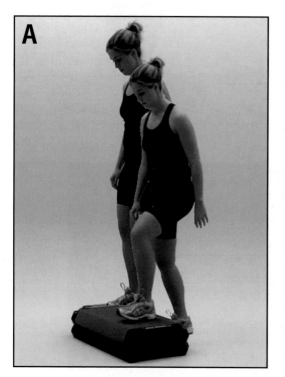

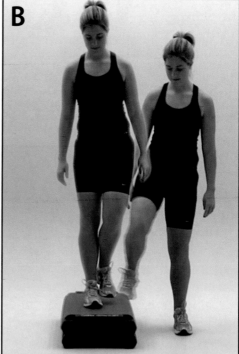

Figure 16-7. Step-ups. The patient steps (A) forward; or (B) laterally onto a step.

and backward sprints as in "W" sprints (Figure 16-11).

Agility Tests

Agility tests incorporate changes of direction, acceleration/deceleration, and quick starts and stops. For example, a simple figure 8 can be

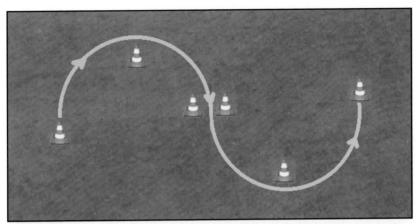

Figure 16-8. S course. The patient runs a set distance in a curving S pattern rather than straight ahead.

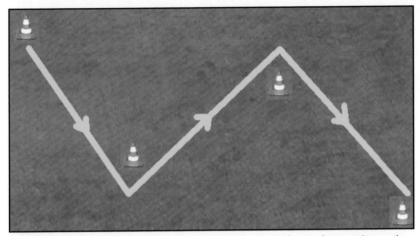

Figure 16-9. Z course. The patient runs a zigzag course to emphasize sharp cutting motions and quick, controlled directional changes.

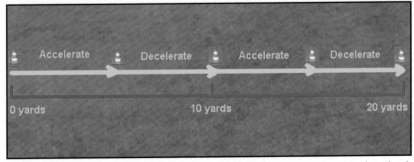

Figure 16-10. Acceleration/deceleration. The patient accelerates to a maximum, then decelerates almost to a stop, then repeats this within a relatively short distance.

set up with cones and the patient is instructed to travel the cones as fast as possible while being timed for performance (Figure 16-12). Gross et al described a figure 8 course that was 5 by 10 meters.[17] Each person in their study was instructed to complete three trips around the figure 8 while being timed. Two trials were conducted, and the best time was recorded.[17]

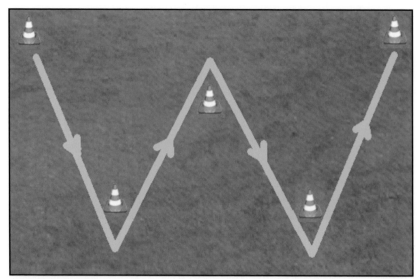

Figure 16-11. W sprints. The patient sprints forward to the first marker, then backpedals to the second, then sprints forward to the third, and so on.

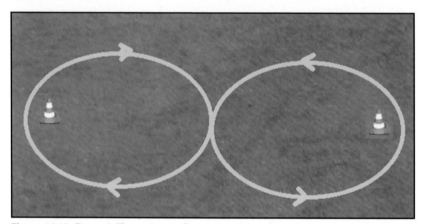

Figure 16-12. Figure 8. The patient walks, jogs, or runs a figure 8 pattern around cones or markers.

Anderson and Foreman point out that no standard in the literature dictates testing procedures for the figure 8.[4] A standard procedure should be developed by each athletic trainer or each institution to ensure the validity and reliability of the test.

Box shuttle runs are also beneficial as agility runs, because they emphasize pivoting and change of direction (Figure 16-13). The patient is instructed to travel around four cones arranged in a box formation. The time to complete the box is recorded. Shuttle runs require the patient to complete four 20-foot sprints for a total of 80 feet, incorporating three direction changes. It is common to take three trials, and the mean should be calculated.[24,25,26,30] Again, variations are prominent, with single laps vs multiple laps and the use of multiple movements (run, carioca, backpedal, etc). The Barrow Zigzag Run is a variation of the box run using five cones. The four cones of the box are set as usual, and the fifth cone is set in the center of the box. The box course is 16 feet by 10 feet. The patient travels around the cones as shown in Figure 16-14.

Nussbaum reports that the use of sprinting, cutting maneuvers, figure 8 runs, and backpedaling drills are all excellent means for assessing the functional performance of the lower extremity.[35] It is beneficial to use agility runs

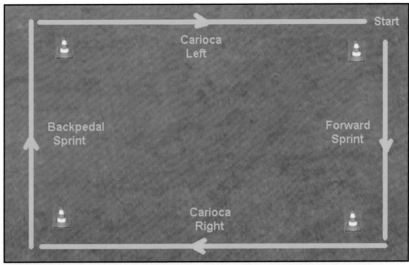

Figure 16-13. Box runs. Running both clockwise and counterclockwise, the patient runs around four markers set in a box shape, concentrating on abrupt directional changes at each corner.

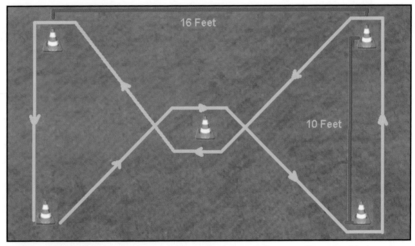

Figure 16-14. Barrow Zigzag Run test. The patient essentially runs a figure 8 with sharp turns at the corners. 16 ft × 10 ft Stop Start.

because the level of difficulty can be changed. Early in the rehabilitation process, large figure 8s that are more circular in shape can be used to provide functional data with low stress to the injury. As the injury heals, the figure 8 can be made tighter to provide greater stress to the injured body part.

Another common shuttle run is the line drill, sometimes called "suicide sprints" or "death warmed over" (Figure 16-15). The course is set with markers at various distances from the starting line. The patient is instructed to sprint and touch the first marker and then return to the starting position. The patient then continues the course, touching each marker and returning to the starting position. A total time is recorded.[4] This test is very flexible and can be used on basketball, volleyball, or tennis courts, as well as football, soccer, or other playing fields.

Carioca Runs

Carioca runs can be timed to measure improvement in function (Figure 16-16). The carioca run involves a lateral grapevine or crossover step over a total distance of 80 feet. First, choose which direction to face and maintain the stance. The patient will then carioca

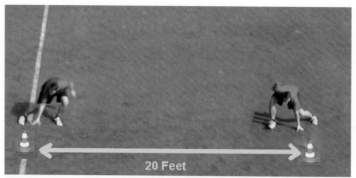

Figure 16-15. Shuttle runs involve four 20-foot sprints between cones.

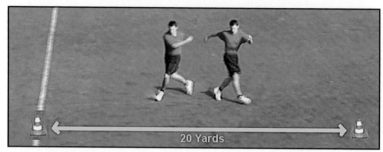

Figure 16-16. Carioca. The patient sidesteps onto the right foot, then steps across with the left foot in front of the right, then steps back onto the right foot, then the left foot steps across in back of the right, then back onto the right, and so on.

Figure 16-17. Timed exercise. The patient jumps side to side over a ball or other obstacle in a timed exercise.

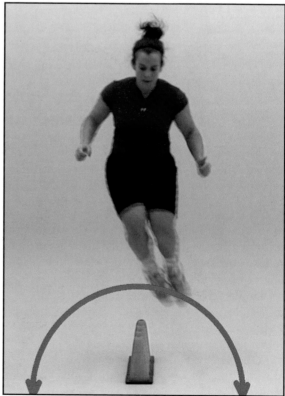

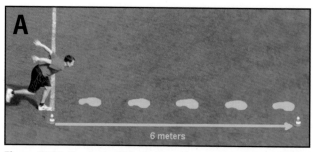
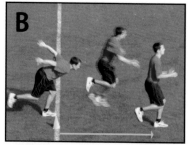

Figure 16-18. Hop tests. (A) In the timed hop test, time required to cover a 6-meter distance is measured in seconds; (B) the single hop for distance test measures the distance covered in a single hop. Both tests use a percentage of the injured leg compared to the uninjured leg.

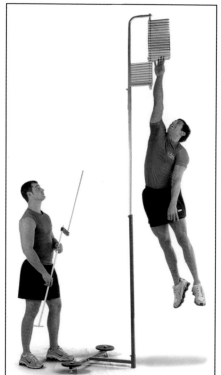

Figure 16-19. The Vertec can be used to measure vertical jump height

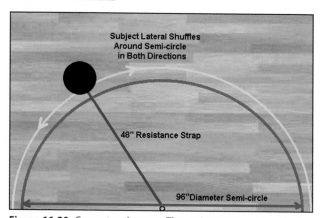

Figure 16-20. Co-contraction test. The patient moves in a side-step or shuffle fashion around the periphery of a semicircle, using surgical tubing for resistance.

40 feet, change direction without turning around, and return to the starting position. The time to complete the 80-foot course is recorded. Three trials should be used and the mean time calculated.[24,25,26]

Hopping Tests

Hopping tests are also found in the literature (Figure 16-18). Booher et al. and Worrell et al. report that hopping tests might not be sensitive enough to evaluate the functional abilities of patients.[7,44] However, hopping tests are noted in the literature and are used for clinical determination of function.[16] A variety of hop tests to determine lower-extremity limb symmetry have been used.[4,29,27] The more common hopping tests are the single-leg hop for distance, the timed hop test, the triple hop for distance, and the crossover hop for distance. The single-leg hop for distance requires the patient to attempt to hop as far as possible while landing on the same limb.[5] The timed hopping test measures the amount of time it takes the patient to hop a distance of 6 meters. The triple hop for distance measures the distance traveled by the patient with three consecutive hops. And finally, the crossover hop for distance measures the distance traveled using three consecutive hops while crossing over a strip 15 centimeters wide.[2,5,6,7,14,16,20,29]

Vertical Jump

The vertical jump test can also be used to evaluate the lower extremity.[5] A Vertec can be used to measure vertical jump height (Figure 16-19). If a Vertec is not available, the patient chalks the fingertips and jumps to touch a piece of paper (of a different color than the chalk). Three to five jumps should be attempted and the mean height recorded (measured from fingertips standing to the chalk mark).[4,7,39] Variations in the test also exist. Anderson and Foreman mention alterations that include "bilateral vs single-leg jump, countermovement vs static squat start, approach steps vs stationary start, and use of the upper extremities for propulsion vs restricted use of the upper extremities."[4] Many, more expensive testing devices are available that measure time differentials, force, and height.

Co-contraction Semicircular Test

The co-contraction semicircular test involves securing the patient in a 48-inch resistance strap (TheraBand) that is attached to the wall 60 inches above the floor (Figure 16-20). The strap is then stretched to twice its recoil length and the patient completes five 180-degree semicircles, with a radius of 96 inches, around a tape line. The patient is instructed to use a forward-facing lateral shuffle step. If the patient starts on the left, she or he will travel around the semicircle until reaching the right boundary. This semicircle counts as one repetition. The patient must complete five repetitions in the shortest amount of time possible. Three trials can be used, and the mean time is calculated. This test is designed to provide a dynamic pivot shift for the ACL-insufficient knee.[6,24,25,26,29]

Subjective Evaluation

Subjective evaluations of performance have been correlated with functional performance testing to determine predictive capabilities. Wilk et al found strong correlations between subjective scores and knee extension peak torques, knee extension acceleration, and functional testing; however, no significant relationship was noted with hamstring function.[43] This is in contrast to Shelbourne's research, which showed a poor relationship between subjective evaluation, functional tests, and knee strength. Shelbourne concluded that knee strength was a good measure of ability.[37] Subjective questionnaires or numeric scales might or might not be beneficial in the functional assessment of patients, based on the correlations. A low subjective score might indicate that the patient is apprehensive, which should serve as a warning sign of psychological unreadiness to return to play. The athletic trainer should determine whether subjective evaluation is useful with respect to the given patient. Obviously, budget considerations and availability of equipment will determine the types of tests the athletic trainer can use, but simple timed sprints can indicate improved performance just as well as the more complicated tests that involve expensive equipment.[3,24,25,26]

Table 16-5 CFPI Mean Index and Performance Test Means

	Males Means/standard deviation	Females Means/standard deviation
CFPI	31.551/2.867	36.402/3.489
Carioca	7.812/1.188	8.899/1.124
Co-contraction test	11.188/1.391	13.218/1.736
One-legged hop test	4.953/0.53	5.746/0.63
Shuttle run	7.596/0.654	8.539/0.69

> **Clinical Decision-Making Exercise 16-4**
>
> What type of functional testing could you use for a football receiver who has sustained a second-degree acromioclavicular sprain? What criteria for a return to play would you use?

CAROLINA FUNCTIONAL PERFORMANCE INDEX

The CFPI has been developed to help the athletic trainer evaluate lower-extremity functional performance.[29] The CFPI evaluates the patient's existing functional performance capability. McGee and Futtrell evaluated 200 collegiate athletes and non-athletes using a battery of tests that included the co-contraction test, carioca test, shuttle run test, and one-legged timed hopping test. Table 16-5 shows the mean and standard deviation for each of these tests for males and for females. From this series of tests, a normative CFPI index was determined for males and females that can be used in accurately assessing functional performance based on the results of only two of the tests—the carioca test and the co-contraction test.[29]

Using stepwise regression techniques, the following prediction equations were established:

Males: $1.09(x_1) + 1.415(x_2) + 8.305 = CFPI$
Females: $1.26(x_1) + 1.303(x_2) + 8.158 = CFPI$
(Where x_1 = co-contraction score in seconds, and x_2 = carioca score in seconds)

The athletic trainer can test any individual using these two tests (co-contraction and carioca) and determine their individual CFPI. The CFPI value for that individual can be compared to the mean normative CFPI indices of 31.551 for males and 36.402 for females. If baseline preinjury testing was done, then the preinjury CFPI can be compared to the postinjury CFPI to determine how the patient is progressing in their rehabilitation program. The CFPI provides a reliable objective criteria for functional performance testing.

APPLYING FUNCTIONAL PROGRESSIONS TO A SPECIFIC SPORT CASE

The following is an example of how a functional progression may be applied to a specific sport-related injury:

Subject: 20-year-old female soccer player.

History: Sustained anterior cruciate ligament (ACL) rupture of left knee while performing a cutting motion in practice. ACL reconstruction using an intra-articular patellar tendon graft was performed.

Rehabilitation for the first 2 months was conducted both at home and in a clinical setting. Emphasis of program concentrated on increasing range of motion (ROM) and decreasing pain and swelling, with some minor considerations to improving strength.

At 2 months postsurgery, the rehabilitation protocol consisted of emphasizing general physical fitness, strengthening via traditional rehabilitation means and strength testing, as well as improving ROM. At about 3 months postsurgery, a functional progression was initiated. The progression included the following activities an average of three times per week:

- Walking
- PNF techniques—using lower extremity D1, D2 patterns
- Jogging on track with walking of curves
- Jogging full track
- Running on track with jogging of curves
- Running full track

This progression occupied the majority of the next 2 months, coupled with traditional rehabilitation techniques to increase strength and maintain ROM. At 4 months, the progression intensified to a 5-day-a-week program including the following:

- Running for fitness—2 to 3 miles three times per week
- Lunges—90 degree, pivot, 180 degree
- Sprints—W, triangle, 6 second, 20 yd, 40 yd, 120 yd
- Acceleration/deceleration runs
- Shuffle slides progressing to shuffle run
- Carioca
- Ball work—Turn/stop the pass; turn/mark opponent; mark/steal/shoot the ball; two-touch and shoot; one touch and shoot; volley and shoot; passing; pass/knock/move; coerver drills; light drill work at practice; one-on-one; scrimmage (begin with short period, progress to full game); full active participation

Clinical Decision-Making Exercise 16-5

A patient had surgery 2 weeks ago for an ACL rupture. Acute inflammation is controlled, and he is clear to begin the next phase of rehabilitation. The physician prefers an accelerated protocol for the patient. What types of functional activities could you suggest for the patient?

Clinical Decision-Making Exercise 16-6

A male patient has a CFPI of 42.00 following an ACL reconstruction. At what percentage of the norm is the patient? What decision would you make about his return to play? What type of activities may help this patient improve his score?

CONCLUSION

Once the patient can safely and effectively perform all specific tasks leading up to the motor skill, they can return to activity. For example, a patient might progress from cycling, to walking, to jogging, to running, before returning to sprinting activities and competition in a 4×400 relay.

The athletic trainer must note that these are only examples. No one program will benefit every patient and every condition. Athletic trainers should use these activities, along with others they develop, to help maximize the patient's recovery. By providing patients with every option available in rehabilitation, the athletic trainer can return the patient to participation at preinjury status. The preinjury status achieved with the functional progression not only can return the patient to competition, but also can ensure a safer, more effective return to play.

Summary

1. Complete rehabilitation should strive to improve neuromuscular coordination and agility, strength, endurance, and flexibility.

2. The role of the functional progressions is to improve and complete the traditional rehabilitation process by providing sport-specific exercise.

3. The functional progression is a sequence of activities that simulate sport activity. The progression will begin easy and progress to full sport participation.

4. Each sport activity can be divided into smaller components, allowing the patient to progress from easy to difficult.

5. Functional progressions are highly effective exercise therapy techniques that should be incorporated in the long-term rehabilitation stage.

6. Functional progressions allow for improvements in strength, endurance, mobility/flexibility, relaxation, coordination/agility/skill, and assessment of functional stability.

7. Functional progression can benefit the patient psychologically and socially by decreasing the patient's feelings of anxiety, deprivation, and apprehension.

8. Components of a functional progression that should be addressed include development, choice of activity, implementation, and termination.

9. Many functional tests exist and should be administered when deciding whether to return a patient to competition.

References

1. Abrahamson E, Hyland V. 2010. Progressive systematic functional rehabilitation, In Comfort, P. *Sports Rehabilitation and Injury Prevention*. New York, John Wiley & Sons.

2. Adams D. Logerstedt D. 2012. Current concepts for anterior cruciate ligament reconstruction: A criterion-based rehabilitation progression. *Journal of Orthopedic and Sports Physical Therapy*; 42(7):601-614.

3. Anderson M. 1991. The relationships among isometric, isotonic, and isokinetic concentric and eccentric quadriceps and hamstring force and three components of athletic performance. *Journal of Orthopaedic and Sports Physical Therapy*; 14(3):114-120.

4. Anderson MA, and Foreman TL. 1996. Return to competition: Functional rehabilitation. In *Athletic injuries and rehabilitation*, edited by JE Zachazewski, DJ Magee, and WS Quillen. Philadelphia: W. B. Saunders.

5. Augustsson J, Thomeé R. 2006. Single-leg hop testing following fatiguing exercise: Reliability and biomechanical analysis. *Scandinavian Journal of Medicine & Science in Sports*; 16(2):111, 2006.

6. Bernier J, Sieracki NK, and Levy S. 2000. Functional rehabilitation of the ankle. *Athletic Therapy Today*; 5(2): 38–44.

7. Booher LD, KM Hench, TW Worrell, and J Stikeleather. 1993. Reliability of three single leg hop tests. *Journal of Sport Rehabilitation*; 2:165–70.

8. Brummit R, Dale R. 2008. Functional rehabilitation and exercise prescription for golfers. *Athletic Therapy Today*; 13(2):37-41.

9. Cates W, Cavanaugh J. 2009. *Advances in Rehabilitation and Performance Testing*, New York, Elsevier.

10. Clanton T, Matheny L. 2012. Return to play in athletes following ankle injuries. *Sports Health: A Multidisciplinary Approach*; 4(6):471-474

11. Davies G, and J Matheson. 2007. Functional testing as the basis for ankle rehabilitation progression. In *The unstable ankle*, Nyska M, ed. Champaign, IL, Human Kinetics.

12. Drouin J, and B Riemann. 2004. Lower extremity functional performance testing, Part 2. *Athletic Therapy Today*; 9(3):49.

13. Ellenbecker T, DeCarlo M. 2009. *Effective Functional Progressions in Sport Rehabilitation*, Champaign, IL, Human Kinetics.

14. Fitzgerald G, Lephart S. 2001. Hop tests as predictors of dynamic knee stability. *Journal of Orthopaedic and Sports Physical Therapy*; 31(10): 588–97.

15. Goldbeck TG, and GJ Davies. 2000. Test-retest reliability of the closed kinetic chain upper extremity stability test: A clinical field test. *Journal of Sport Rehabilitation*; 9(1): 35–45.

16. Grindem H, Logerstedt D. 2011. Single-legged hop tests as predictors of self-reported knee function in nonoperatively treated individuals with anterior cruciate ligament injury. *Am J Sports Med*; 39:2347–2354.

17. Gross MT, JR Everts, and SE Roberson. 1994. Effect of DonJoy ankle ligament protector and Aircast Sport-Stirrup orthoses on functional performance. *Journal of Orthopaedic and Sports Physical Therapy*; 19(3): 150–56.

18. Harter R. 1996. Clinical rationale for closed kinetic chain activities in functional testing and rehabilitation of ankle pathologies. *Journal of Sport Rehabilitation*; 5(1): 13–24.

19. Jokl E. 1964. *The scope of exercise in rehabilitation*. Lexington, MA, Charles C. Thomas.

20. Keskula DR, JB Duncan, and VL Davis. 1996. Functional outcome measures for knee dysfunction assessment. *Journal of Athletic Training*; 31(2): 105–10.

21. Kibler B, and Chandler J. 2008. Functional rehabilitation and return to training and competition. In Frontera W, *The Encyclopedia of Sports Medicine: An IOC Medical Commission Publication*. Oxford, United Kingdom, Blackwell Science Ltd.

22. King MA. 2000. Functional stability for the upper quarter. *Athletic Therapy Today*; 15(2):16–21.

23. Kisner C, and L Colby. 2012. *Therapeutic exercise foundations and techniques*. Philadelphia: F. A. Davis.

24. Lephart S. 1992. Relationship between selected physical characteristics and functional capacity in the anterior cruciate ligament-insufficient patient. *Journal of Orthopaedic and Sports Physical Therapy*; 16(4):164–81.

25. Lephart SM, and T Henry. 1995. Functional rehabilitation for the upper and lower extremity. *Orthopedic Clinics of North America*; 26(3):579–92.

26. Lephart S, D Perrin, K Minger, et al. 1991. Functional performance tests for the anterior cruciate ligament insufficient patient. *Journal of Athletic Training*; 26:44–50.

27. Logerstedt D, and Lynch A. 2013. Symmetry restoration and functional recovery before and after ACL reconstruction. *Knee Surg Spots Traumatol Arthrosc*; 21:859-868.

28. MacLean C, and J Taunton. 2001. Functional rehabilitation for the PCL-deficient knee. *Athletic Therapy Today*; 6(6):32–8.

29. McGee MR, and MD Futtrell. 1993. *Functional testing of patients and non-patients using the Carolina Functional Performance Index.* Unpublished master's thesis, University of North Carolina, Chapel Hill.

30. Mellion M. 2002. *Sports Medicine Secrets*, Philadelphia, Hanley & Belfus.

31. Mullin MJ. 2000. Functional rehabilitation of the knee. *Athletic Therapy Today*; 5(2):28-35.

32. Myers JB, and SM Lephart. 2000. The role of the sensorimotor system in the athletic shoulder. *Journal of Athletic Training*; 35(3):35–63.

33. Narducci E, Waltz A, Gorski K, et al. 2011. The clinical utility of functional performance tests within one year post ACL reconstruction. *Int J Sports Phys Ther*. 6(4):333–342.

34. Negrete R, and Hanney W. 2010. Reliability, minimal detectable change and normative values for tests of uppextremity function and power. *Journal of Strength and Conditioning*; 24(12):3318-3325.

35. Nussbaum ED, TM Hosea, SD Sieler, BR Incremona, and DE Kessler. 2001. Prospective evaluation of syndesmotic ankle sprains without diastasis. *American Journal of Sports Medicine*; 29(1): 31–35.

36. Reiman M, Manske R. 2009. *Functional Testing in Human Performance.* Champaign, IL, Human Kinetics.

37. Shellbourne D. 1987. Functional ability in athletes with anterior cruciate deficiency. *American Journal of Sports Medicine*; 15:628.

38. Souissi S, and Wong D. 2011. Improving functional performance and muscle power 4-6 months after ACL surgery. *Journal of Sports Science and Medicine*; 10:655-664

39. Tegner Y, J Lysholm, M Lysholm, et al. 1986. A performance test to monitor rehabilitation and evaluate anterior cruciate ligament injuries. *American Journal of Sports Medicine*; 14:156–159.

40. Tibone JM, MS Antich, GS Fanton, et al. 1986. Functional analysis of anterior cruciate ligament instability. *American Journal of Sports Medicine*; 13:34–39.

41. Uhl TL, M Gould, and JH Geick. 2000. Rehabilitation after posterolateral dislocation of the elbow in a collegiate football player: A case report. *Journal of Athletic Training*; 35(1):108–110.

42. Voight M, and Tippett S. 1995. *Functional Progressions for Sport Rehabilitation.* Champaign, IL, Human Kinetics.

43. Wilk KE, WT Romaniello, SM Soscia, and CA Arrigo. 1994. The relationship between subjective knee scores, isokinetic testing, and functional testing in the ACL-reconstructed knee. *Journal of Orthopaedic and Sports Physical Therapy*; 20(2): 60–71.

44. Worrell, TW, LD Booher, and KM Hench. 1994. Closed kinetic chain assessment following inversion ankle sprain. *Journal of Sport Rehabilitation*; 3(3):197–203.

SOLUTIONS TO CLINICAL DECISION-MAKING EXERCISES

16-1 Agility runs would be the most beneficial for this patient to allow for improvement in speed and direction change.

16-2 Closed kinetic chain activities that stress coactivation of the core, scapular stabilizers, and rotator cuff muscles would help the patient correct the strength deficits with the scapular stabilizers. Once improvements are noted with the CKC activities, sport-specific open kinetic chain activities would be indicated.

16-3 The patient is probably deficient in her proprioception and kinesthetic awareness. Upper-extremity CKC activities, rhythmic stabilization, and PNF diagonal patterns may benefit this patient.

16-4 Sport-specific and position-specific testing would be indicated. Open and closed kinetic chain testing would be necessary to evaluate all aspects of the patient's position. Criteria for return: no pain, full ROM, bilaterally equal strength, successful completion of functional test, self-evaluation, and physician's release.

16-5 Although it is early in the rehabilitation process, functional activities could begin. Closed kinetic chain activities such as mini-squats could be initiated safely. Gait training and functional activities in the pool could also benefit the patient in this stage.

16-6 The patient is at about 75% of function. Based on this score, the patient would continue his rehabilitation program and not return to full participation. Agility training, along with continuation of his strengthening program, will help the patient reach his goals.

Please see videos on the accompanying website at

www.healio.com/books/sportsmedvideos

SECTION IV

Rehabilitation Techniques for Specific Injuries

CHAPTER 17

Rehabilitation of Shoulder Injuries

Joseph B. Myers, PhD, ATC
Terri Jo Rucinski, MA, PT, ATC
William E. Prentice, PhD, PT, ATC, FNATA
Rob Schneider, PT, MS, LAT, ATC

After completion of this chapter, the athletic trainer should be able to do the following:

- Review the functional anatomy and biomechanics associated with normal function of the shoulder joint complex.

- Differentiate the various rehabilitative strengthening techniques for the shoulder, including both open and closed kinetic chain isotonic, plyometric, isokinetic, and proprioceptive neuromuscular facilitation exercises.

- Compare the various techniques for regaining range of motion, including stretching exercises and joint mobilization.

- Administer exercises that may be used to reestablish neuromuscular control.

- Relate biomechanical principles to the rehabilitation of various shoulder injuries/pathologies.

- Discuss criteria for progression of the rehabilitation program for different shoulder injuries/pathologies.

- Describe and explain the rationale for various treatment techniques in the management of shoulder injuries.

FUNCTIONAL ANATOMY AND BIOMECHANICS

The anatomy of the shoulder joint complex allows for tremendous range of motion (ROM). This wide ROM of the shoulder complex proximal permits precise positioning of the hand distally, to allow both gross and skilled movements. However, the high degree of mobility requires some compromise in stability, which, in turn, increases the vulnerability

Prentice WE, ed.
Rehabilitation Techniques for Sports Medicine and Athletic Training (pp 445-516).
© 2015 SLACK Incorporated.

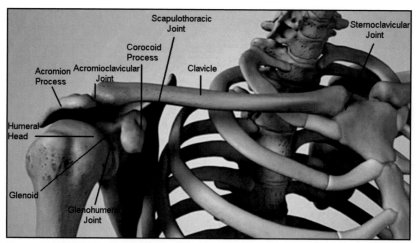

Figure 17-1. Skeletal anatomy of the shoulder complex.

of the shoulder joint to injury, particularly in dynamic overhead athletic activities.[5]

The shoulder girdle complex is composed of 3 bones—the scapula, the clavicle, and the humerus—that are connected either to one another or to the axial skeleton or trunk via the glenohumeral joint, the acromioclavicular joint, the sternoclavicular joint, and the scapulothoracic joint (Figure 17-1). Dynamic movement and stabilization of the shoulder complex require integrated function of all four articulations if normal motion is to occur.

Sternoclavicular Joint

The clavicle articulates with the manubrium of the sternum to form the sternoclavicular joint, the only direct skeletal connection between the upper extremity and the trunk. The sternal articulating surface is larger than the sternum, causing the clavicle to rise much higher than the sternum. A fibrocartilaginous disk is interposed between the two articulating surfaces. It functions as a shock absorber against the medial forces and also helps to prevent any displacement upward. The articular disk is placed so that the clavicle moves on the disk, and the disk, in turn, moves separately on the sternum. The clavicle is permitted to move up and down, forward and backward, in combination, and in rotation.

The sternoclavicular joint is extremely weak because of its bony arrangement, but it is held securely by strong ligaments that tend to pull

the sternal end of the clavicle downward and toward the sternum, in effect anchoring it. The main ligaments are the anterior sternoclavicular, which prevents upward displacement of the clavicle; the posterior sternoclavicular, which also prevents upward displacement of the clavicle; the interclavicular, which prevents lateral displacement of the clavicle; and the costoclavicular, which prevents lateral and upward displacement of the clavicle.[3]

It should also be noted that for the scapula to abduct and upward rotate throughout 180 degrees of humeral abduction, clavicular movement must occur at both the sternoclavicular and acromioclavicular joints. The clavicle must elevate about 40 degrees to allow upward scapular rotation.[93]

Acromioclavicular Joint

The acromioclavicular joint is a gliding articulation of the lateral end of the clavicle with the acromion process. This is a rather weak joint. A fibrocartilaginous disk separates the two articulating surfaces. A thin, fibrous capsule surrounds the joint.

The acromioclavicular ligament consists of anterior, posterior, superior, and inferior portions. In addition to the acromioclavicular ligament, the coracoclavicular ligament joins the coracoid process and the clavicle and helps to maintain the position of the clavicle relative to the acromion. The coracoclavicular ligament is further divided into the trapezoid ligament, which prevents overriding of the clavicle on the acromion, and the conoid ligament, which limits upward movement of the clavicle on the acromion. As the arm moves into an elevated position, there is a posterior rotation of the clavicle on its long axis that permits the scapula to continue rotating, thus allowing full elevation. The clavicle must rotate about 50 degrees for full elevation to occur, otherwise elevation would be limited to about 110 degrees.[93]

Coracoacromial Arch

The coracoacromial ligament connects the coracoid to the acromion. This ligament, along with the acromion and the coracoid, forms the coracoacromial arch over the glenohumeral joint. In the subacromial space between the coracoacromial arch superiorly and the humeral head inferiorly lies the supraspinatus tendon, the long head of the biceps tendon, and the subacromial bursa. Each of these structures is subject to irritation and inflammation resulting either from excessive humeral head translation or from impingement during repeated overhead activities. In asymptomatic individuals, the optimal subacromial space appears to be about 9 to 10 mm.[94]

Glenohumeral Joint

The glenohumeral joint is an enarthrodial, or ball-and-socket, synovial joint in which the round head of the humerus articulates with the shallow glenoid cavity of the scapula. The cavity is deepened slightly by a fibrocartilaginous rim called the glenoid labrum. The humeral head is larger than the glenoid, and at any point during elevation, only 25% to 30% of the humeral head is in contact with the glenoid.[47] The glenohumeral joint is maintained by both static and dynamic restraints. Position is maintained statically by the glenoid labrum and the capsular ligaments, and dynamically by the deltoid and rotator cuff muscles.

Surrounding the articulation is a loose, articular capsule that is attached to the labrum. This capsule is strongly reinforced by the superior, middle, and inferior glenohumeral ligaments and by the tough coracohumeral ligament, which attaches to the coracoid process and to the greater tuberosity of the humerus.[87]

The long tendon of the biceps muscle passes superiorly across the head of the humerus and then through the bicipital groove. In the anatomical position, the long head of the biceps moves in close relationship with the humerus. The transverse humeral functional anatomy and biomechanics ligament maintains the long head of the biceps tendon within the bicipital groove by passing over it from the lesser and the greater tuberosities, converting the bicipital groove into a canal.

Scapulothoracic Joint

The scapulothoracic joint is not a true joint, but the movement of the scapula on the wall of the thoracic cage is critical to shoulder joint motion.[92] The scapula is capable of 5 degrees of freedom movement, including three rotations (orientations) and two translations (positions).[54,76] Rotation of the scapula can occur around its three orthogonal axes, with upward/downward rotation occurring around an anteroposterior axis, internal/external rotation occurring around a superoinferior axis, and anterior/posterior tipping occurring around a mediolateral axis. In addition to rotating, the scapula can translate superoinferiorly (scapular elevation and depression), and anteroposteriorly on the thorax. Because anterior/posterior translation is limited by the rib cage, protraction/retraction results from the anterior/posterior translation (Figure 17-2). During humeral elevation (flexion, scaption, or abduction), the scapula and humerus must move in a synchronous fashion to maintain glenohumeral joint congruency, length–tension relationships for the numerous muscles attaching on the scapula, and adequate subacromial space clearance. Commonly termed scapulohumeral rhythm, as the humerus elevates, the scapula synchronously upwardly rotates, posteriorly tips, externally rotates, elevates, and translates posteriorly (retracts). Alterations in these scapular movement patterns have been identified in individuals with varying degrees of rotator tendinopathy (subacromial impingement and rotator cuff tears),[35,69,71,79,103,122] pathologic internal impingement,[61] glenohumeral instability,[88] frozen shoulder,[37,101] and osteoarthritis,[37] as well as highly influenced by fatigue,[32,33,108,119] upper-quarter posture and

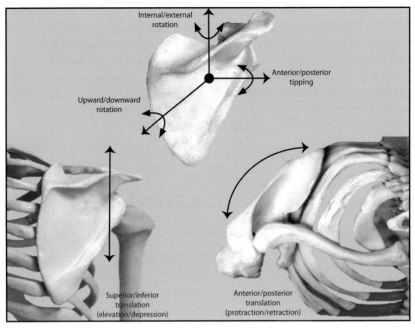

Figure 17-2. Scapular motions.

tightness,[11,12,13] and even history of participation in overhead athletics.[30,63,83,90]

Stability in the Shoulder Joint

Maintaining stability, while the four articulations of the shoulder complex collectively allow for a high degree of mobility, is critical in normal function of the shoulder joint. Instability is very often the cause of many of the specific injuries to the shoulder that are discussed later in this chapter. In the glenohumeral joint, the rounded humeral head articulates with a relatively flat glenoid on the scapula. During movement of the shoulder joint, it is essential to maintain the positioning of the humeral head relative to the glenoid. Likewise, it is also critical for the glenoid to adjust its position relative to the moving humeral head while simultaneously maintaining a stable base. The glenohumeral joint is inherently unstable, and stability depends on the coordinated and synchronous function of both static and dynamic stabilizers.[74]

Static Stabilizers

The primary static stabilizers of the glenohumeral joint are the glenohumeral ligaments, the posterior capsule, and the glenoid labrum.

The glenohumeral ligaments appear to produce a major restraint in shoulder flexion, extension, and rotation. The anterior glenohumeral ligament is tight when the shoulder is in extension, abduction, and/or external rotation. The posterior glenohumeral ligament is tight in flexion and external rotation. The inferior glenohumeral ligament is tight when the shoulder is abducted, extended, and/or externally rotated. The middle glenohumeral ligament is tight when in flexion and external rotation. Additionally, the middle glenohumeral ligament and the subscapularis tendon limit lateral rotation from 45 to 75 degrees of abduction and are important anterior stabilizers of the glenohumeral joint.[3] The inferior glenohumeral ligament is a primary check against both anterior and posterior dislocation of the humeral head and is the most important stabilizing structure of the shoulder in the overhead patient.[3]

The tendons of the rotator cuff muscles blend into the glenohumeral joint capsule at their insertions about the humeral head (Figure 17-3). As these muscles contract, tension is produced, dynamically tightening the capsule and helping to center the humeral head in the glenoid fossa. This creates both static and dynamic control of humeral head movement.

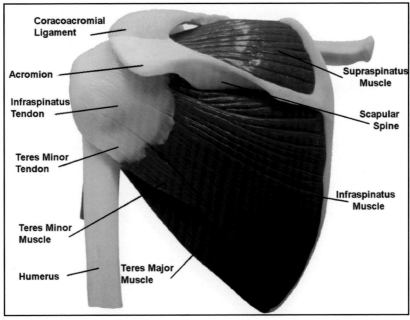

Figure 17-3. Shoulder complex ligaments and rotator cuff muscle and tendons–posterior view.

The posterior capsule is tight when the shoulder is in flexion, abduction, internal rotation, or any combination of these. The superior and middle segment of the posterior capsule has the greatest tension, while the shoulder is internally rotated.

The bones and articular surfaces within the shoulder are positioned to contribute to static stability. The glenoid labrum, which is tightly attached to the bottom half of the glenoid and loosely attached at the top, increases the glenoid depth about two times, enhancing glenohumeral stability.[66] The scapula faces 30 degrees anteriorly to the chest wall and is tilted upward 3 degrees to enable easier movement on the anterior frontal plane and movements above the shoulder.[4] The glenoid is tilted upward 5 degrees to help control inferior instability.[72]

The Dynamic Stabilizers of the Glenohumeral Joint

The muscles that cross the glenohumeral joint produce motion and function to establish dynamic stability to compensate for a bony and ligamentous arrangement that allows for a great deal of mobility. Movements at the glenohumeral joint include flexion, extension, abduction, adduction, horizontal adduction/abduction, circumduction, and humeral rotation.

The muscles acting on the glenohumeral joint may be classified into two groups. The first group consists of muscles that originate on the axial skeleton and attach to the humerus; these include the latissimus dorsi and the pectoralis major. The second group originates on the scapula and attaches to the humerus; these include the deltoid, the teres major, the coracobrachialis, the subscapularis, the supraspinatus, the infraspinatus, and the teres minor (Figures 17-3 and 17-4). These muscles constitute the short rotator muscles whose tendons insert into the articular capsule and serve as reinforcing structures. The biceps and triceps muscles attach on the glenoid and affect elbow motion.

The muscles of the rotator cuff, the subscapularis, infraspinatus, supraspinatus, and teres minor along with the long head of the biceps function to provide dynamic stability to control the position and prevent excessive displacement or translation of the humeral head relative to the position of the glenoid.[9,70,121]

Stabilization of the humeral head occurs through coactivation of the rotator cuff muscles. This creates a series of force couples that act to compress the humeral head into the

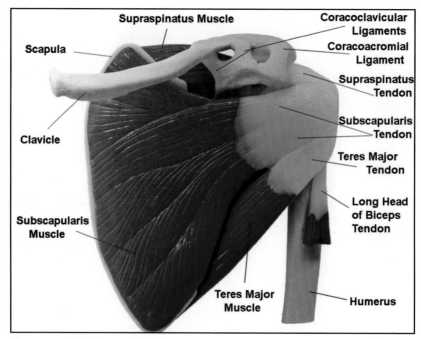

Figure 17-4. Shoulder complex ligaments and rotator cuff muscle and tendons–anterior view.

glenoid, minimizing humeral head translation. A force couple involves the action of two opposing forces acting in opposite directions to impose rotation about an axis. These force couples can establish dynamic equilibrium of the glenohumeral joint regardless of the position of the humerus. If an imbalance exists between the muscular components that create these force couples, abnormal glenohumeral mechanics occur.

In the frontal plane, a force couple exists between the subscapularis anteriorly and the infraspinatus and teres minor posteriorly. Coactivation of the infraspinatus, teres minor, and subscapularis muscles both depresses and compresses the humeral head during overhead movements.

In the coronal plane, there is a critical force couple between the deltoid and the inferior rotator cuff muscles. With the arm fully adducted, contraction of the deltoid produces a vertical force in a superior direction causing an upward translation of the humeral head relative to the glenoid. Coactivation of the inferior rotator cuff muscles produces both a compressive force and a downward translation of the humerus that counterbalances the force

of the deltoid, stabilizing the humeral head. The supraspinatus compresses the humeral head into the glenoid and, along with the deltoid, initiates abduction on this stable base. Dynamic stability is created by an increase in joint compression forces from contraction of the supraspinatus and by humeral head depression from contraction of the inferior rotator cuff muscles.[9,27,70,121]

The long head of the biceps tendon also contributes to dynamic stability by limiting superior translation of the humerus during elbow flexion and supination.

Scapular Stability and Mobility

Like the glenohumeral muscles, the scapular muscles play a critical role in normal function of the shoulder. The scapular muscles produce movement of the scapula on the thorax and help to dynamically position the glenoid relative to the moving humerus. They include the levator scapula and upper trapezius, which elevate the scapula; the middle trapezius and rhomboids, which retract the scapula; the lower trapezius, which retracts, upwardly rotates, and depresses the scapula; the pectoralis minor, which depresses the scapula; and the serratus anterior, which protracts and upwardly rotates the scapula (in combination with the upper and lower trapezius). Collectively, they function to maintain a consistent length–tension relationship with the glenohumeral muscles.[58,59,80]

The only attachment of the scapula to the thorax is through these muscles. The muscle stabilizers must fix the position of the scapula on the thorax, providing a stable base for the rotator cuff to perform its intended function on the humerus. It has been suggested that the serratus anterior moves the scapula while the other scapular muscles function to provide scapular stability.[58,59] The scapular muscles act isometrically, concentrically, or eccentrically, depending on the movement desired and whether the movement is speeding up or slowing down.[72]

Clinical Decision-Making Exercise 17-1

A varsity ice hockey player suffers a grade 1 acromioclavicular (AC) separation after being checked into the boards during a hockey game. The patient presents with the chief complaint of pain and the inability to abduct his affected arm. The physician was not able to see any widening of the AC joint with a weighted X-ray. The patient is referred to the athletic trainer for conservative management of his injury. What can the athletic trainer do to ensure that the patient's injury will heal and not lead to further dysfunction of the shoulder complex?

Plane of the Scapula

The concept of the plane of the scapula refers to the angle of the scapula in its resting position, usually 35 to 45 degrees anterior to the frontal plane toward the sagittal plane. When the limb is positioned in the plane of the scapula, the mechanical axis of the glenohumeral joint is in line with the mechanical axis of the scapula. The glenohumeral joint capsule is lax, and the deltoid and supraspinatus muscles are optimally positioned to elevate the humerus. Movement of the humerus in this plane is less restricted than in the frontal or sagittal planes because the glenohumeral capsule is not twisted.[39] Because the rotator cuff muscles originate on the scapula and attach to the humerus, repositioning the humerus into the plane of the scapula optimizes the length of those muscles, improving the length–tension relationship. This is likely to increase muscle force.[39] It has been recommended that many strengthening exercises for the shoulder joint complex be done in the scapular plane.[39,128,129]

REHABILITATION EXERCISES

Stretching Exercises

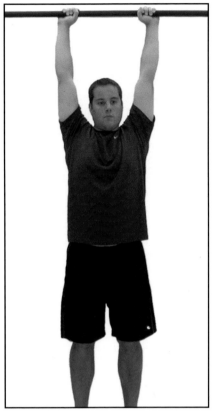

Figure 17-5. Static hanging: Hanging from a chinning bar is a good general stretch for the musculature in the shoulder complex.

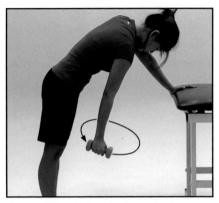

Figure 17-6. Codman's circumduction exercise: The patient holds a dumbbell in the hand and moves it in a circular pattern, reversing direction periodically. This technique is useful as a general stretch in the early stages of rehabilitation when motion above 90 degrees is restricted.

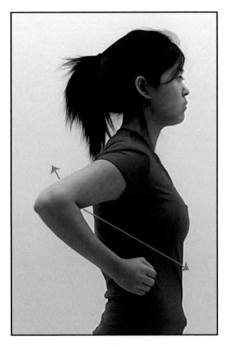

Figure 17-7. Sawing: The patient moves the arm forward and backward as if performing a sawing motion. This technique is useful as a general stretch in the early stages of rehabilitation when motion above 90 degrees is restricted.

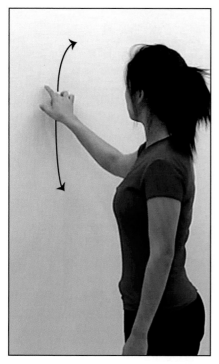

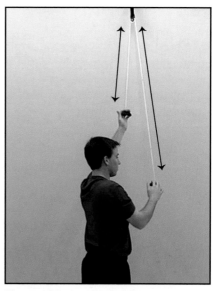

Figure 17-9. Rope and pulley exercise: This exercise may be used as an active-assistive exercise when trying to regain full overhead motion. ROM should be restricted to a pain-free arc.

Figure 17-8. Wall climbing: The patient uses the fingers to "walk" the hand up a wall. This technique is useful when attempting to regain full-range elevation. ROM should be restricted to a pain-free arc.

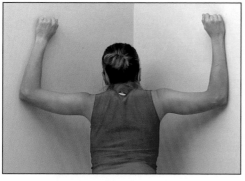

Figure 17-10. Wall/corner stretch: Used to stretch the pectoralis major and minor, anterior deltoid, and cora-cobrachialis, and the anterior joint capsule.

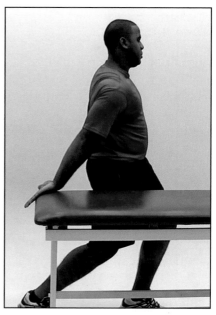

Figure 17-11. Shoulder flexors stretch standing: Used to stretch the anterior deltoid, coracobra-chialis, pectoralis major, and biceps muscles, and the anterior joint capsule.

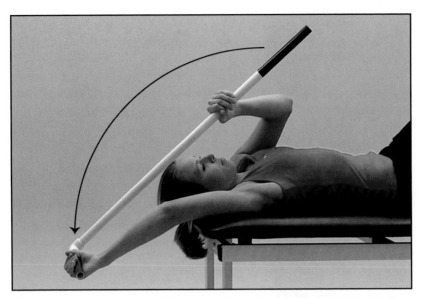

Figure 17-12. Shoulder extensor stretch using an L-bar: Used to stretch the latissimus dorsi, teres major and minor, posterior deltoid, and triceps muscles, and the inferior joint capsule.

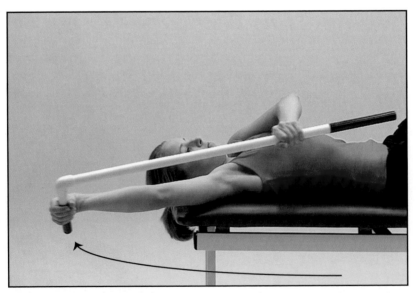

Figure 17-13. Shoulder adductors stretch using an L-bar: Used to stretch the latissimus dorsi, teres major and minor, pectoralis major and minor, posterior deltoid, and triceps muscles, and the inferior joint capsule.

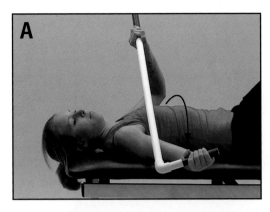

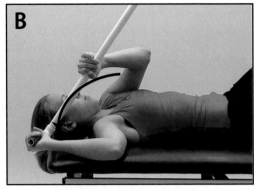

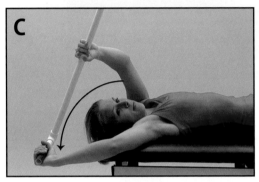

Figure 17-14. Shoulder medial rotators stretch using an L-bar. Used to stretch the subscapularis, pectoralis major, latissimus dorsi, teres major, and anterior deltoid muscles, and the anterior joint capsule. This stretch should be done at (A) 0 degrees; (B) 90 degrees; and (C) 135 degrees.

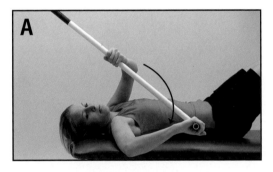

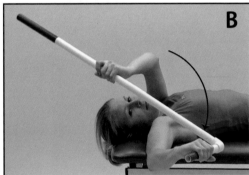

Figure 17-15. Shoulder external rotators stretch using an L-bar. Used to stretch the infraspinatus, teres minor, and posterior deltoid muscles, and the posterior joint capsule. This stretch should be done at (A) 90 degrees and (B) 135 degrees. (C) The Sleeper Stretch can also be used to stretch the external rotators.

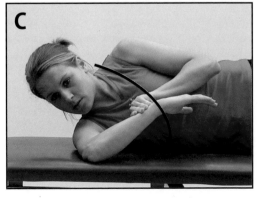

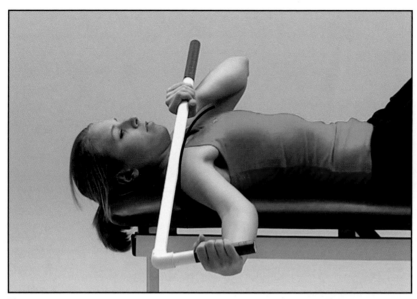

Figure 17-16. Horizontal adductors stretch using an L-bar. Used to stretch the pectoralis major, anterior deltoid, and long head of the biceps muscles, and the anterior joint capsule.

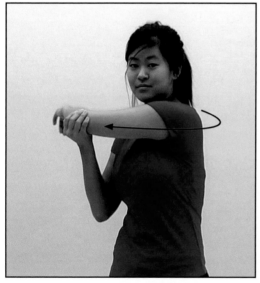

Figure 17-17. Horizontal abductors stretch. Used to stretch the posterior deltoid, infraspinatus, teres minor, rhomboids, and middle trapezius muscles, and the posterior capsule. This position might be uncomfortable for patients with shoulder impingement syndrome.

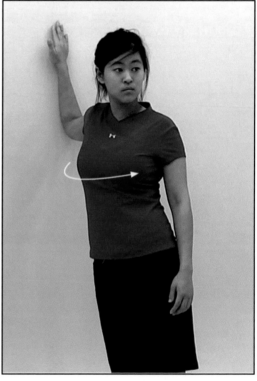

Figure 17-18. Anterior capsule stretch. Self-stretch using the wall.

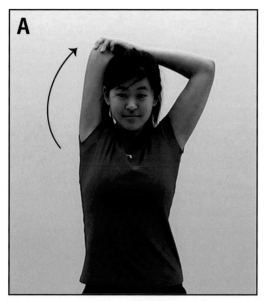

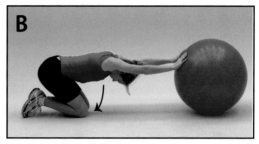

Figure 17-19. Inferior capsule stretch. (A) Self-stretch done with the arm in the fully elevated overhead position. This position might be uncomfortable for patients with shoulder impingement syndrome. (B) Inferior capsule stretch can also be done using a stability ball.

Strengthening Techniques

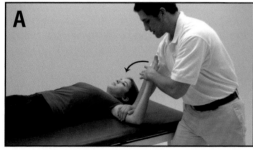

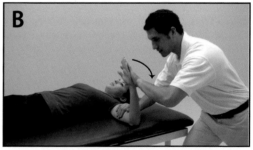

Figure 17-20. (A) Isometric medial rotation and (B) isometric lateral rotation are useful in the early stages of a shoulder rehabilitation program when full ROM isotonic exercise is likely to exacerbate a problem.

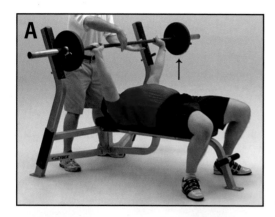

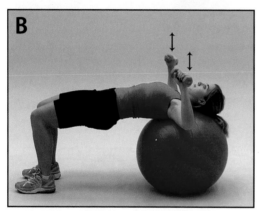

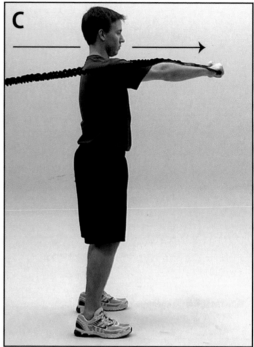

Figure 17-21. Chest press. Used to strengthen the pectoralis major, anterior deltoid, and triceps, and secondarily the coracobrachialis muscles. (A) Performing this exercise with the feet on the floor helps to isolate these muscles. (B) An alternate technique is to use dumbbells on an unstable surface such as a stability ball. (C) May also be done in a standing position using cable or tubing.

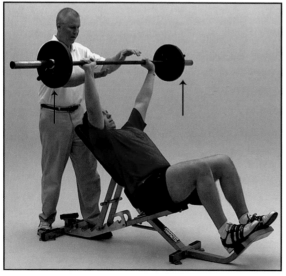

Figure 17-22. Incline bench press. Used to strengthen the pectoralis major (upper fibers), triceps, middle and anterior deltoid, and secondarily, the coracobrachialis, upper trapezius, and levator scapula muscles.

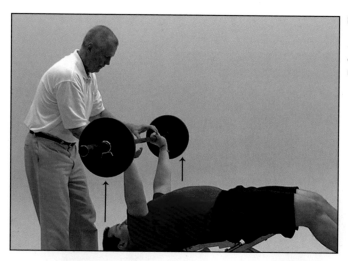

Figure 17-23. Decline bench press Used to strengthen the pectoralis major (lower fibers), triceps, anterior deltoid, coracobrachialis, and latissimus dorsi muscles.

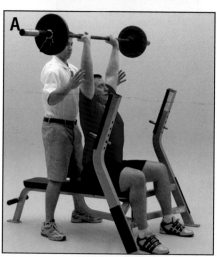

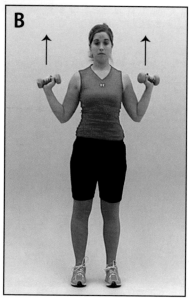

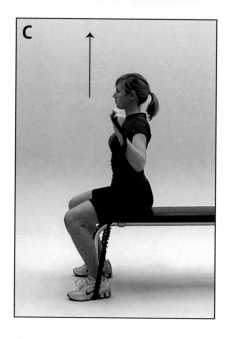

Figure 17-24. Military press. Used to strengthen the middle deltoid, upper trapezius, levator scapula, and triceps. (A) Performed in a seated position on a bench. (B) In a standing position using dumbbells. (C) In a seated position using cable or tubing.

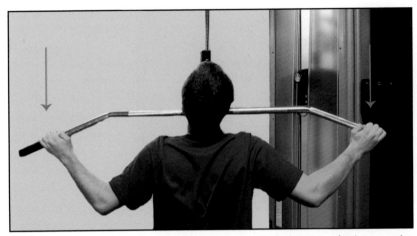

Figure 17-25. Lat pull-downs. Used to strengthen primarily the latissimus dorsi, teres major, and pectoralis minor, and secondarily the biceps muscles. This exercise should be done by pulling the bar down in front of the head. Pull-ups done on a chinning bar can also be used as an alternative strengthening technique.

Figure 17-26. Shoulder flexion. Used to strengthen primarily the anterior deltoid and coracobrachialis, and secondarily the middle deltoid, pectoralis major, and biceps brachii muscles. Note that the thumb should point upward.

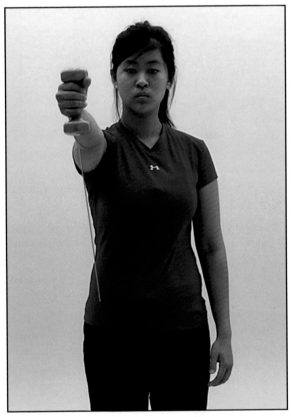

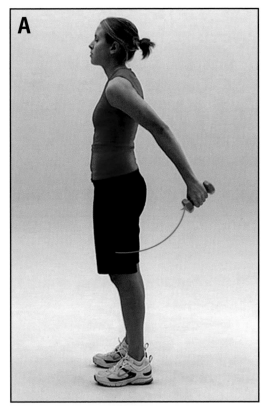
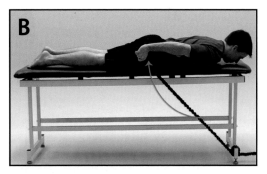
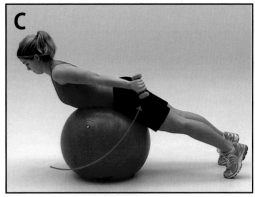

Figure 17-27. Shoulder extension. Used to strengthen primarily the latissimus dorsi, teres major, and posterior deltoid, and secondarily, the teres minor and the long head of the triceps muscles. Note that the thumb should point downward. May be done (A) standing using a dumbbell, (B) lying prone using cable or tubing, or (C) using dumbbells prone on a stability ball.

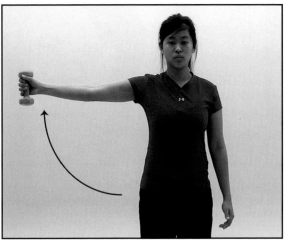

Figure 17-28. Shoulder abduction to 90 degrees. Used to strengthen primarily the middle deltoid and supraspinatus, and secondarily, the anterior and posterior deltoid and serratus anterior muscles.

Figure 17-29. Flys (shoulder horizontal adduction). Used to strengthen primarily the pectoralis major, and secondarily, the anterior deltoid. Note that the elbow may be slightly flexed. May be done in a supine position or standing with surgical tubing or wall pulleys behind.

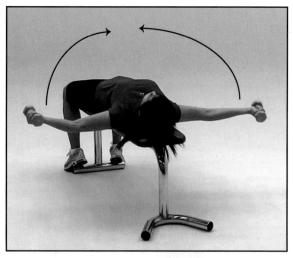

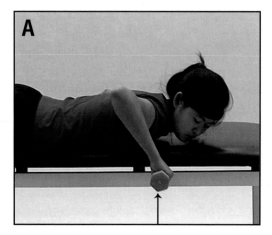

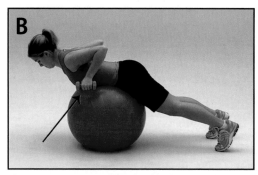

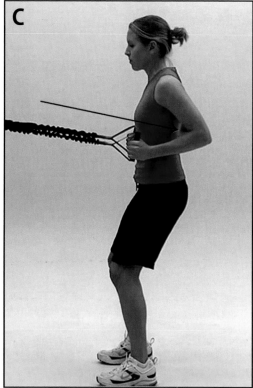

Figure 17-30. Reverse flys (shoulder horizontal abduction). Used to strengthen primarily the posterior deltoid, and secondarily, the infraspinatus, teres minor, rhomboids, and middle trapezius muscles. (A) May be done lying prone using dumbbells, (B) prone on a stability ball, and (C) standing using cables or tubing. Note that with the thumb pointed upward the middle trapezius is more active, and with the thumb pointed downward the rhomboids are more active.

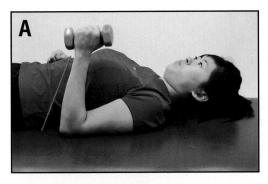

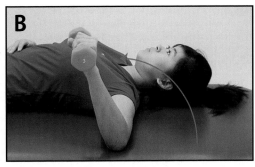

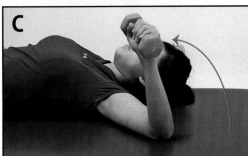

Figure 17-31. Shoulder medial rotation. Used to strengthen primarily the subscapularis, pectoralis major, latissimus dorsi, and teres major, and secondarily, the anterior deltoid. This exercise may be done isometrically or isotonically, either lying supine using a dumbbell or standing using tubing. Strengthening should be done with the arm fully adducted at 0 degrees, and also in 90 degrees and 135 degrees of abduction.

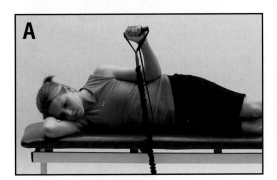

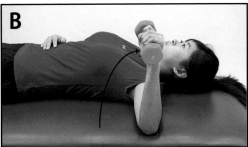

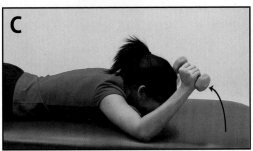

Figure 17-32. Shoulder lateral rotation. Used to strengthen primarily the infraspinatus and teres minor, and secondarily, the posterior deltoid muscles. This exercise may be done isometrically or isotonically, either lying prone using a dumbbell or standing using tubing. Strengthening should be done with the arm fully adducted at 0 degrees, and also in 90 degrees and 135 degrees of abduction.

Figure 17-33. Scaption. Used to strengthen primarily the supraspinatus in the plane of the scapula, and secondarily, the anterior and middle deltoid muscles. This exercise should be done standing with the arm horizontally adducted to 45 degrees.

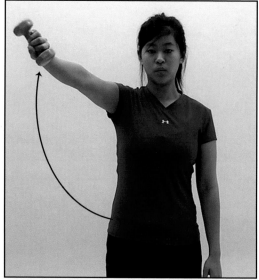

Figure 17-34. Alternative supraspinatus exercise. Used to strengthen primarily the supraspinatus, and secondarily, the posterior deltoid. In the prone position with the arm abducted to 100 degrees, the arm is horizontally abducted in extreme lateral rotation. Note that the thumb should point upward.

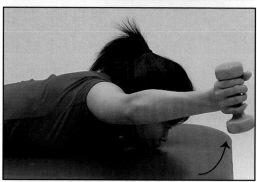

Figure 17-35. Shoulder shrugs. Used to strengthen primarily the upper trapezius and the levator scapula, and secondarily, the rhomboids.

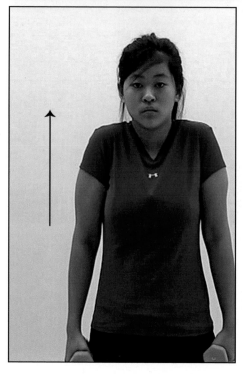

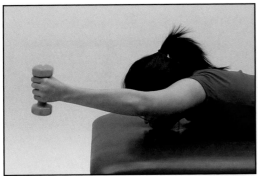

Figure 17-36. Superman. Used to strengthen primarily the inferior trapezius, and secondarily, the middle trapezius. May be done lying prone using either dumbbells or tubing.

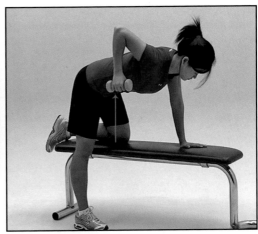

Figure 17-37. Bent-over rows. Used to strengthen primarily the middle trapezius and rhomboids. Done standing in a bent-over position with one knee supported on a bench.

Figure 17-38. Rhomboids exercise. Used to strengthen primarily the rhomboids, and secondarily, the inferior trapezius. Should be done lying prone with manual resistance applied at the elbow.

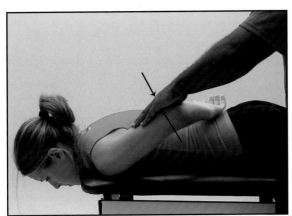

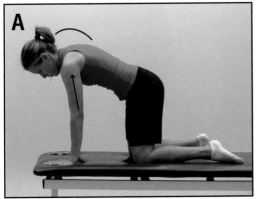

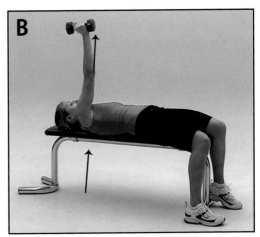

Figure 17-39. Push-ups with a plus. Used to strengthen the serratus anterior. There are several variations to this exercise, including (A) regular push-ups, and (B) weight-loaded push-ups with a plus.

Figure 17-40. Scapular strengthening using a Body Blade. Holding an oscillating Body Blade with both hands, the patient moves from a fully adducted position in front of the body to a fully elevated overhead position.

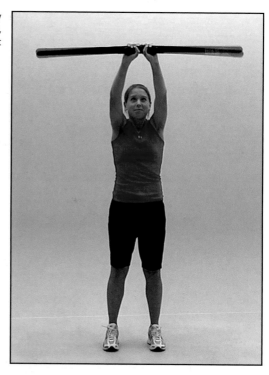

Closed Kinetic Chain Exercises

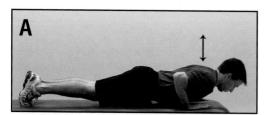

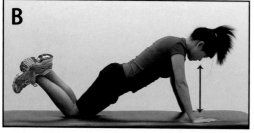

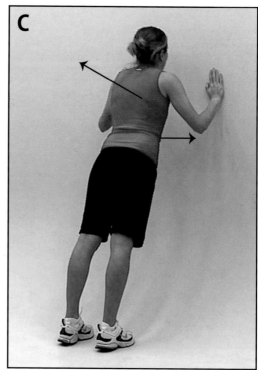

Figure 17-41. Push-ups. May be done with (A) weight supported on feet, or (B) modified to support weight on the knees. (C) Wall pushups.

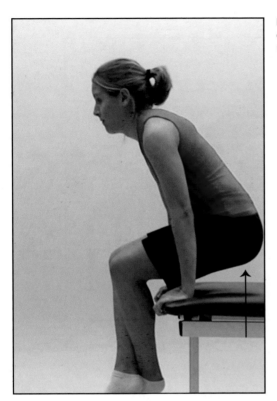

Figure 17-42. Seated push-up. Done sitting on the end of a table. Place hands on the table and lift weight upward off of the table isotonically.

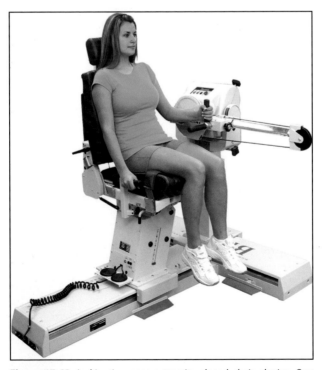

Figure 17-43. Isokinetic upper-extremity closed chain device. One of the only isokinetic closed kinetic chain exercise devices currently available. (Printed with permission from Biodex Medical Systems, Inc.)

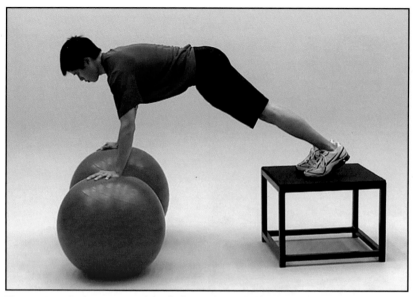

Figure 17-44. Push-ups on a stability ball. An advanced closed chain strengthening exercise that requires substantial upper body strength.

Plyometric Exercises

Figure 17-45. Cable or tubing. To strengthen the medial rotators, use a quick eccentric stretch of the medial rotators to facilitate a concentric contraction of those muscles.

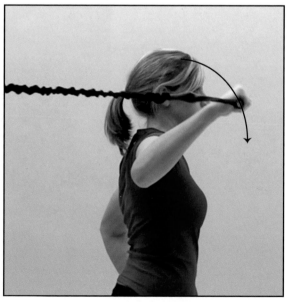

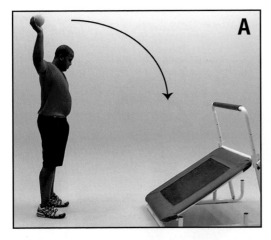

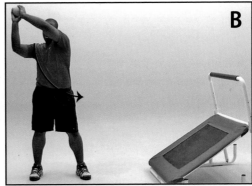

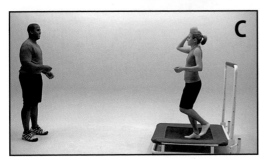

Figure 17-46. Plyoback. The patient should catch the ball, decelerate it, then immediately accelerate in the opposite direction. (A) Single-arm toss; (B) two-arm toss with trunk rotation; (C) standing single-leg and single-arm toss on unstable surface.

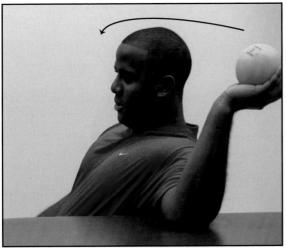

Figure 17-47. Seated single-arm weighted ball throw. The patient should be seated with the arm abducted to 90 degrees and the elbow supported on a table. The athletic trainer tosses the ball to the hand, creating an overload in lateral rotation that forces the patient to dynamically stabilize in that position.

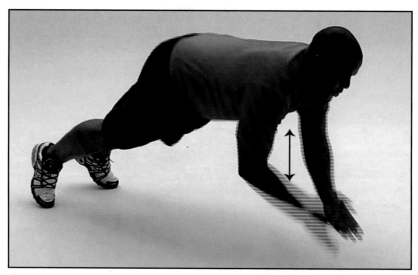

Figure 17-48. Push-ups with a clap. The patient pushes off the ground, claps his hands, and catches his weight as he decelerates.

Figure 17-49. Push-ups on boxes. When performing a plyometric pushup on boxes, the patient can stretch the anterior muscles, which facilitates a concentric contraction.

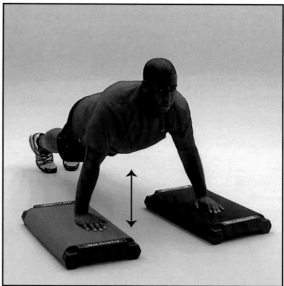

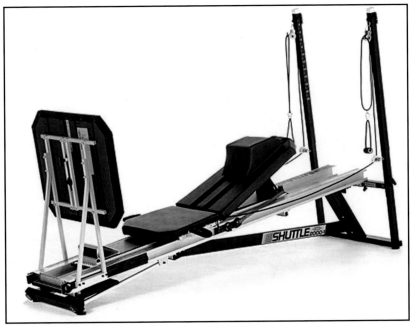

Figure 17-50. Shuttle 2000-1: The exercise machine can be used for plyometric exercises in either the upper or the lower extremity. (Printed with permission from Shuttle Systems.)

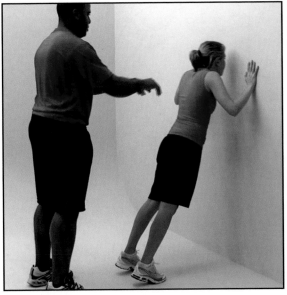

Figure 17-51. Push into wall. The athletic trainer stands behind the patient and pushes her toward the wall. The patient decelerates the forces and then pushes off the wall immediately.

Isokinetic Exercises

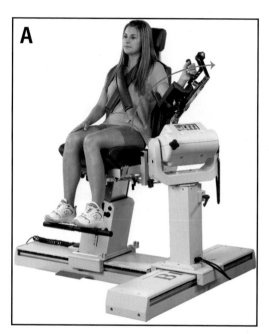

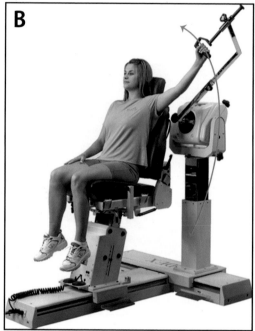

Figure 17-52. When using an isokinetic device for strengthening the shoulder, the patient should be set up such that strengthening can be done in a scapular plane. (A) Shoulder abduction/adduction; (B) internal and external rotation; and (C) diagonal 1 PNF pattern. (Printed with permission from Biodex Medical Systems.)

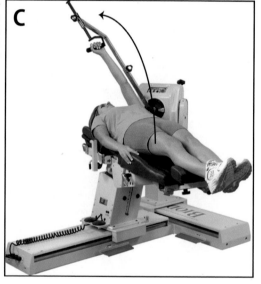

Strengthening Techniques

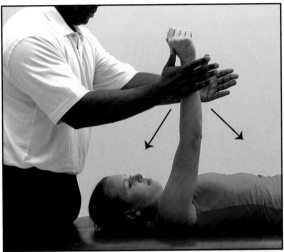

Figure 17-53. Rhythmic contraction. Using either a diagonal 1 (D1) or diagonal 2 (D2) pattern. The patient uses an isometric cocontraction to maintain a specific position within the ROM while the athletic trainer repeatedly changes the direction of passive pressure.

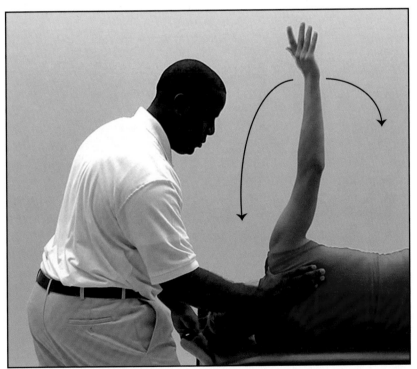

Figure 17-54. PNF technique for scapula. As the patient moves through either a D1 or a D2 pattern, the athletic trainer applies resistance at the appropriate scapular border.

Figure 17-55. The patient can use resistance from tubing through a PNF movement pattern.

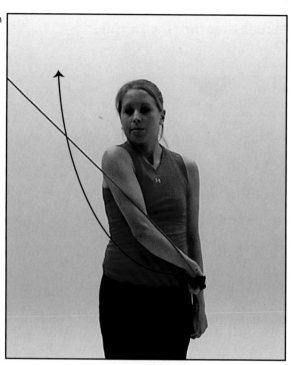

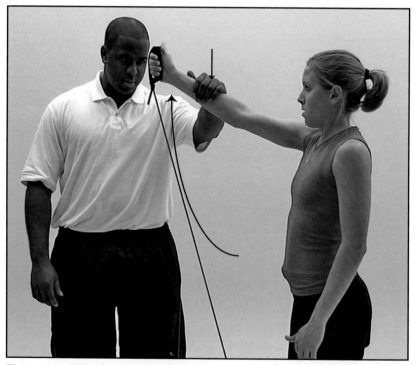

Figure 17-56. PNF using both manual resistance and surgical tubing rhythmic stabilization can be performed as the patient isometrically holds a specific position in the ROM with surgical tubing and force applied by the athletic trainer.

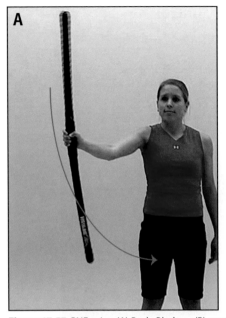

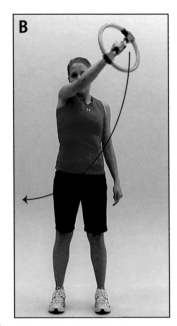

Figure 17-57. PNF using (A) Body Blade or (B) centrifugal ring blade.

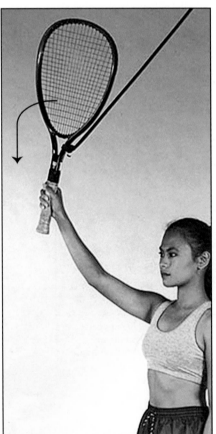

Figure 17-58. Surgical tubing may be attached to a tennis racket as the patient practices an overhead serve technique. This is useful as a functional progression technique.

Exercises to Reestablish Neuromuscular Control

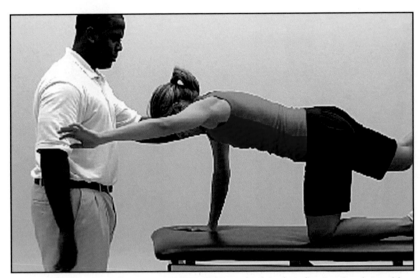

Figure 17-59. Weight shifting on a stable surface may be done kneeling in a 2-point position. The athletic trainer can apply random directional pressure to which the patient must respond to maintain a static position. In the 2- and 3-point positions, the arm that is supported in a closed kinetic chain is using shoulder force couples to maintain neuromuscular control.

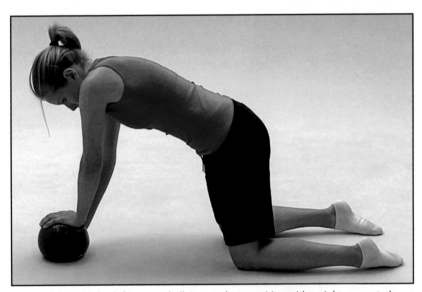

Figure 17-60. Weight shifting on a ball. In a push-up position with weight supported on a ball, the patient shifts weight from side to side and/or forward and backward. Weight shifting on an unstable surface facilitates cocontraction of the muscles involved in the force couples that collectively maintain dynamic stability

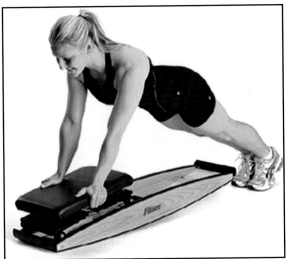

Figure 17-61. Weight shifting on a Fitter. In a kneeling position the patient shifts weight front to back using a Fitter. Weight shifting on an unstable surface facilitates cocontraction of the muscles involved in the force couples that collectively maintain dynamic stability. (Printed with permission from Fitter International, Inc.)

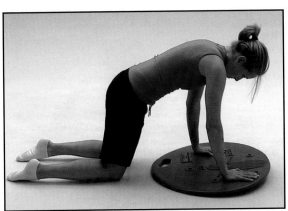

Figure 17-62. Weight shifting on a biomechanical ankle platform system (BAPS) board: In a kneeling position the patient shifts weight from side to side and/or backward and forward using a BAPS board. Weight shifting on an unstable surface facilitates cocontraction of the muscles involved in the force couples that collectively maintain dynamic stability.

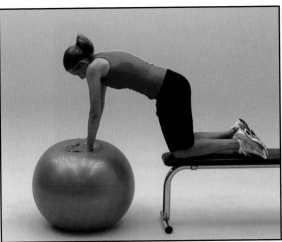

Figure 17-63. Weight shifting on a stability ball. With the feet supported on a bench, the patient shifts weight from side to side and/or backward and forward using a stability ball. Weight shifting on an unstable surface facilitates cocontraction of the muscles involved in the force couples that collectively maintain dynamic stability.

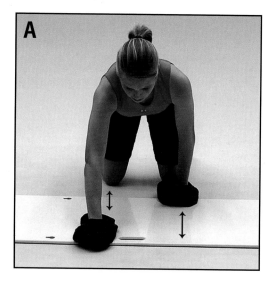

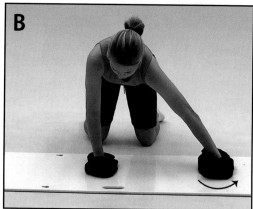

Figure 17-64. Slide board exercises. (A) Forward and backward motion, (B) wax-on/wax-off motion, (C) lateral motion. The patient shifts weight from side to side and/ or backward and forward using a slide board. Weight shifting on an unstable surface facilitates cocontraction of the muscles involved in the force couples that collectively maintain dynamic stability.

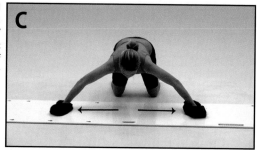

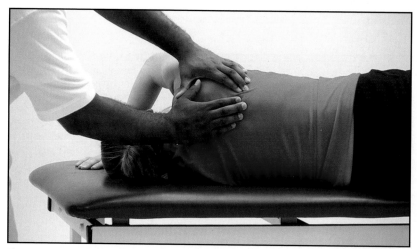

Figure 17-65. Scapular neuromuscular control exercises. The patient's hand is placed on the table, creating a closed kinetic chain, and the athletic trainer applies pressure to the scapula in a random direction. The patient moves the scapula isotonically into the direction of resistance.

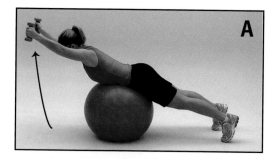

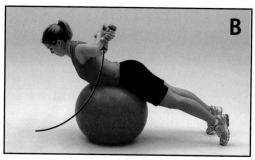

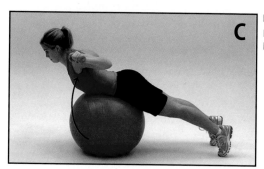

Figure 17-66. Stability ball exercises. The patient lies in a prone position on the stability ball and maintains a stable position and performs (A) Ys, (B) Ts, and (C) Ws.

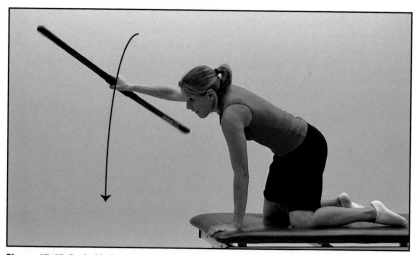

Figure 17-67. Body Blade exercises. The patient is in a 3-point kneeling position holding an oscillating Body Blade in one hand while working on neuromuscular control in the weight-bearing shoulder.

REHABILITATION TECHNIQUES FOR SPECIFIC INJURIES

Sternoclavicular Joint Sprains

Pathomechanics

Sternoclavicular (SC) joint sprains are not commonly seen as athletic injuries. Although they are rare, the joint's complexity and integral interaction with the other joints of the shoulder complex warrant discussion. The SC joint has multiple axes of rotation and articulates with the manubrium with an interposed fibrocartilaginous disc. Pathology of this joint can include injury to the fibrocartilage and sprains of the sternoclavicular ligaments and/or the costoclavicular ligaments.[49]

As stated earlier, the SC joint is extremely weak because of its bony arrangement. It is held in place by its strong ligaments that tend to pull the sternal end of the clavicle downward and toward the sternum. A sprain of these ligaments often results in either a subluxing SC joint or a dislocated SC joint. This can be significant because the joint plays an integral role in scapular motion through the clavicle's articulation with the scapula. Combined movements at the acromioclavicular and SC joints have been reported to account for up to 60 degrees of upward scapular rotation inherent in glenohumeral abduction.[3]

When this joint incurs an injury, a resultant inflammatory process occurs. The inflammatory process can cause an increase in the joint capsule pressure, as well as a stiffening of the joint due to the collagen tissue being produced for the healing tissues. The pathogenesis of this inflammatory process can cause an altering of the joint mechanics and an increase in pain felt at the joint. This often results adversely on the shoulder complex.[106]

Injury Mechanism

After motor vehicle accidents, the most common source of injuries to the SC joint is sports participation.[89] The SC joint can be injured by direct or indirect forces, resulting in sprains, dislocations, or physical injuries.[49] Direct force injuries are usually the result of a blow to the anteromedial aspect of the clavicle and produce a posterior dislocation.[49] Indirect force injuries can occur in many different sporting events, usually when the patient falls and lands with an outstretched arm in either a flexed and adducted position or extended and adducted position of the upper extremity. The flexed position causes an anterior lateral compression force to the adducted arm, producing a posterior dislocation. The extended position causes a posterior lateral compression force to the adducted arm, leading to an anterior dislocation. Lesser forces can also lead to varying degrees of sprains to the SC joint. Additionally, there have been reports of repetitive microtrauma to this joint in sports such as golf, gymnastics, and rowing.[95,106]

In golf, an example of mechanism of injury occurs during the backswing.[74] For a right-handed golfer, the SC joint is subject to medially directed forces on the left at the top of the backswing and on the right at the end of the backswing. When the right arm is abducted and fully coiled at the end of the backswing and the beginning of the downswing, there is a posterior retraction of the shoulder complex, resulting in an anterior SC joint stress. As a result of the repetitive nature of golf, this can cause repetitive microtrauma leading to irritation of the joint. Over time the joint may become hypermobile relative to its normal stable condition, allowing for degeneration of the soft tissue and fibrocartilaginous disc. This often results in a painful syndrome affecting the mechanics of the joint and muscular control of the shoulder complex.[95] Similar examples are found in gymnastics and rowing.

Rehabilitation Concerns

In addressing the rehabilitation of a patient with a SC joint injury, it is important to address the function of the joint on shoulder complex movement. The SC joint acts as the sole passive attachment of the shoulder complex to the axial skeleton. As noted earlier in the chapter, the clavicle must elevate about 40 degrees to allow upward scapular rotation.[93]

In most cases, the primary problem reported by the injured patient is discomfort associated with end-range movement of the shoulder complex. It is important to identify the cause of the pain (ie, ligamentous instability, disc degeneration, or ligamentous trauma).

In cases where there is ligamentous instability as well as disc degeneration, the rehabilitation should focus on strengthening the muscles attached to the clavicle in a range that does not put further stress on the joint. Muscles such as the pectoralis minor, sternal fibers of the pectoralis major, and upper trapezius are strengthened to help control the motion of the clavicle during motion of the shoulder complex. Exercises include incline bench press, shoulder shrugs, and the seated press-up, in a limited range of motion (ROM) (Figures 17-22, 17-35, and 17-42). In addition to addressing the dynamic supports of the SC joint, the athletic trainer should employ the appropriate modalities necessary to control pain and the inflammatory process. It is also noteworthy, in cases where dislocation or subluxation has occurred, to consider the structures in close proximity to the SC joint. In the case of a posterior dislocation, signs of circulatory vessel compromise nerve tissue impingement, and difficulty swallowing may be seen. It is important to avoid these symptoms and communicate with the patient's physician regarding any lasting symptoms.[106]

When dealing with ligamentous trauma that lacks instability, the athletic trainer should also address the associated pain with the appropriate modalities and use exercises that strengthen muscle with clavicular attachments. In all of the above scenarios, it is important to address the role of the SC joint on shoulder complex movement. A full evaluation of the shoulder complex should be performed to address issues related to scapular elevation. Exercises such as Superman, bent-over row, rhomboids, and push-ups with a plus should be included to help control upward rotation of the scapula (Figures 17-36 through 17-39). Appropriate progression should be followed while addressing the healing stages for the appropriate tissues.

Rehabilitation Progression

In the initial stages of rehabilitation, the primary goal is to minimize pain and inflammation associated with shoulder complex motion.

The athletic trainer should limit activities to midrange exercises and incorporate the use of therapeutic modalities along with the use of NSAID intervention from the physician. Ultrasound is often useful for increasing blood flow and facilitating the process of healing. Occasionally a shoulder sling or figure 8 strap can help minimize stress at the joint. During this phase of the rehabilitation progression, the therapist should identify the sport-specific needs of the patient to tailor the later phases of rehabilitation to the patient's demands. The patient should also continue to work on exercises that maintain cardiorespiratory fitness.

When the pain and inflammation have been controlled, the patient should gradually engage in a controlled increase of stress to the tissues of the joint. This is a good time to begin low-grade joint mobilizations resistance exercises for the muscles attaching to the clavicle. Exercises in this phase are best done in the midrange to minimize pain. As the patient's tolerance increases, the resistance and ROM can be increased. During this phase, it is also important to address any limitations there might be in the patient's ROM. Emphasis should be placed on restoring the normal mechanics of the shoulder complex during shoulder movements.

As the patient begins to enter the pain-free stages of the progression, the athletic trainer should gradually incorporate sport-specific demands into the exercise program. Examples of this are proprioceptive neuromuscular facilitation (PNF) with rubber tubing for the golfer (Figures 17-55 and 17-56); push-ups on a stability ball for the gymnast (Figure 17-44); and rowing machine for the rower.

Criteria for Returning to Full Activity

The patient may return to full activity when (a) the rehabilitation program has been progressed to the appropriate time and stress for the specific demands of the patient's sport; (b) the patient shows improved strength in the muscles used to protect the SC joint when compared to the uninjured side; and (c) the patient no longer has associated pain with movements of the shoulder complex that will inevitably occur with the demands of the sport.

Table 17-1 Acromioclavicular Sprain Classification

Type I
• Sprain of the AC ligaments
• AC ligament intact
• Coracoclavicular ligament, deltoid and trapezius muscles intact
Type II
• AC joint disrupted with tearing of the AC ligament
• Coracoclavicular ligament sprained
• Deltoid and trapezius muscles intact
Type III
• AC ligament disrupted
• AC joint displaced and the shoulder complex displaced inferiorly
• Coracoclavicular ligament disrupted with a coracoclavicular interspace 25% to 100% greater than the normal shoulder
• Deltoid and trapezius muscles usually detached from distal end of the clavicle
Type IV
• AC ligaments disrupted with the AC joint displaced and the clavicle anatomically displaced posteriorly through the trapezius muscle
• Coracoclavicular ligaments disrupted with wider interspace
• Deltoid and trapezius muscles detached
Type V
• AC and coracoclavicular ligaments disrupted
• AC joint dislocated and gross displacement between the clavicle and the scapula
• Deltoid and trapezius muscles detached from distal end of the clavicle
Type VI
• AC and coracoclavicular ligaments disrupted
• Distal clavicle inferior to the acromion or the coracoid process
• Deltoid and trapezius muscles detached from distal end of the clavicle

Acromioclavicular Joint Sprains

Pathomechanics

The acromioclavicular (AC) joint is composed of a bony articulation between the clavicle and the scapula. The soft tissues included in the joint are the hyaline cartilage coating the ends of the bony articulations, a fibrocartilaginous disc between the two bones, the AC ligaments, and the costoclavicular ligaments. There have been two conflicting papers regarding the motion available at the joint. Codman reported little movement at the joint, whereas Inman

reported exactly the opposite.[22,48] Multiple authors have reported degenerative changes at the AC joint by age 40 years in the average healthy adult.[29,102]

The AC joint provides the bridge between the clavicle and the scapula. When an injury occurs to the joint, all soft tissue should be considered in the rehabilitation process. An elaborate grading system has been reported to categorize injuries based on the soft tissue that is involved in the injury (Table 17-1).[99] Through evaluation by X-ray, the patient's injury should be categorized to provide the athletic trainer with a guideline for rehabilitation.

Injury Mechanism

Type I or type II AC joint sprains are most commonly seen in athletics as a result of a direct fall on the point of the shoulder with the arm at the side in an adducted position or falling on an outstretched arm. The injury mechanism for type III and type IV sprains usually involves a direct impact that forces the acromion process downward, backward, and inward while the clavicle is pushed down against the rib cage. The impact can produce a number of injuries such as (a) fracture of the clavicle; (b) AC joint sprain; (c) AC and coracoclavicular joint sprain; or (d) a combination of the previous injury with concomitant muscle tearing of the deltoid and trapezius at their clavicular attachments.[3] Another possible mechanism for injury to the AC joint is repetitive compression of the joint often seen in weight lifting.[106]

Rehabilitation Concerns

Management of AC injuries is dependent on the type of injury.[40] Age, level of play, and the demand on the patient can also factor into the management of this injury. Most physicians prefer to handle type I and type II injuries conservatively, but some authors suggest that type I and type II injuries can cause further problems to the patient later in life.[6,26] These injuries might require surgical excision of the distal 2 cm of the clavicle. The athletic trainer should consider when developing a treatment plan (a) the stability of the AC joint; (b) the amount of time the patient was immobilized; (c) pain, as a guide for the type of exercises being used; and (d) the soft tissue that was involved in the injury. Rehabilitation of these injuries should focus on strengthening the deltoid and trapezius muscles. Additional strengthening of the clavicular fibers of the pectoralis major should also be done. Other muscles that help restore the proper mechanics to the shoulder complex should also be strengthened.

Type I

Treatment for the type I injury consists of ice to relieve pain and a sling to support the extremity for several days. The amount of time in the sling usually depends on the patient's ability to tolerate pain and begin carrying their involved extremity with the appropriate posture. The athletic trainer can have the patient begin active assisted ROM immediately and then incorporate isometric exercises to the muscles with clavicular attachments. This will help restore the appropriate carrying posture for the involved upper extremity. When the patient is able to remove the sling, the athletic trainer should increase the exercise program to incorporate progressive resistance exercise (PRE) for the muscles with clavicular attachments and add exercises to encourage appropriate scapular motion. This will help prevent related shoulder discomfort due to poor glenohumeral mechanics after return to activity.

Type II

The treatment for type II injuries is also nonsurgical. Because this type of injury to the AC joint involves complete disruption of the AC ligaments, immobilization plays a greater role in the treatment of these patients. There is no consensus as to the duration of immobilization. Some authors recommend 7 to 14 days; others suggest using a sling that not only supports the upper extremity but depresses the clavicle.[1,106] This debate is fueled by disagreements regarding the time it takes the body to produce collagen and bridge the gap left from the injury. It has been reported that tissue mobilized too early shows a greater amount of type III collagen than the stronger type I collagen.[53] The time needed to heal the soft tissues involved in this injury must be considered prior to beginning exercises that stress the injury. Heavy lifting and contact sports should be avoided for 8 to 12 weeks.

Type III

Many authors recommend a nonoperative approach for this type of injury, most agreeing that a sling is adequate for allowing the patient to rest comfortably.[3] Use of this nonoperative technique is reported to have limited success. Cox reported improved results without support of the arm in 62% of his patients, whereas only 25% had relief after 3 to 6 weeks of immobilization and a sling.[26]

Operative management of this type of injury can be summarized with the following options:

1. Stabilization of clavicle to coracoid with a screw.

2. Resection of distal clavicle.

3. Transarticular AC fixation with pins.

4. Use of coracoclavicular ligament as a substitute AC ligament.

Taft et al found superior results with coracoclavicular fixation. They found that patients with AC fixation had a higher rate of post-traumatic arthritis than those managed with a coracoclavicular screw.[112]

Type IV, V, and VI

Types IV, V, and VI injuries require open reduction and internal fixation. Operative procedures are designed to attempt realignment of the clavicle to the scapula. The immobilization for this type of injury is longer and therefore the rehabilitation time is longer. After immobilization, the concerns are similar to those previously discussed.

Rehabilitation Progression

Early in the rehabilitation progression, the athletic trainer should be concerned with application of cold therapy and pressure for the first 24 to 48 hours to control local hemorrhage. Fitting the patient for a sling is also important to control the patient's pain. Time in the sling depends on the severity of the injury. After the patient has been seen by a physician for differential diagnosis, the rehabilitation progression should be tailored to the type of sprain according to the diagnosis.

Types I, II, and III sprains should be handled similarly at first, with the time of progression accelerated with less-severe sprains. Exercises should begin with encouraging the patient to use the involved extremity for activities of daily living and gentle ROM exercises. Return of normal ROM in the patient's shoulder is the first objective goal. The patient can also begin isometric exercises to maintain or restore muscle function in the shoulder. These exercises can be started while the patient is in the sling. Once the sling is removed, pendulum exercises can be started to encourage movement. In type III sprains, the athletic trainer should hold off doing passive ROM exercises in the end ranges of shoulder elevation for the first 7 days. The patient should have full passive ROM by 2 to

3 weeks. Once the patient has full active ROM, a program of progressive resistive exercises should begin. Strengthening of the deltoid and upper trapezius muscles should be emphasized. The athletic trainer should evaluate the patient's shoulder mechanics to identify problems with neuromuscular control and address specific deficiencies as noted. As the patient regains strength in the involved extremity, sport-specific exercises should be incorporated into the rehabilitation program. Gradual return to activity should be supervised by the patient's coach and athletic trainer.

In the case of types IV, V, and VI AC sprains, a postsurgical progression should be followed. The athletic trainer should design a program that is broken down into four phases of rehabilitation with the goal of returning the patient to activity as quickly as possible.[3] Contact with the physician is important to determine the time frame in which each phase may begin. Common surgeries for this injury include open reduction with pin or screw fixation and/or acromioplasty.

The early stage of rehabilitation should be designed with the goal of reestablishing pain-free ROM, preventing muscle atrophy, and decreasing pain and inflammation. ROM exercises may include Codman's exercises (Figure 17-6), rope and pulley exercises (Figure 17-9), L-bar exercises (Figures 17-12 to 17-16), and self-capsular stretches (Figures 17-17 and 17-19). Strengthening exercises in this phase may include isometrics in all of the cardinal planes and isometrics for medial and lateral rotation of the glenohumeral joint at 0 degrees of elevation (Figure 17-20).

As rehabilitation progresses, the athletic trainer has the goal of regaining and improving muscle strength, normalizing arthrokinematics, and improving neuromuscular control of the shoulder complex. Prior to advancing to this phase, the patient should have full ROM, minimal pain and tenderness, and a 4/5 manual muscle test for internal rotation, external rotation, and flexion. Initiation of isotonic PRE should begin. Shoulder medial and lateral rotation (Figures 17-31 and 17-32), shoulder flexion and abduction to 90 degrees (Figures 17-26 and 17-28), scaption (Figure 17-33), bicep curls, and triceps extensions should be included. Additionally, a program of scapular-stabilizing exercises should begin. Exercises should include Superman exercises (Figure 17-36), rhomboids exercises (Figure 17-38), shoulder shrugs (Figure 17-35), and seated push-ups (Figure 17-42). To help normalize arthrokinematics of the shoulder complex, joint mobilization techniques should be used for the glenohumeral, AC, SC, and scapulothoracic joints (Figures 13-10 to 13-20). To complete this phase the patient should begin neuromuscular control exercises (Figures 17-59 to 17-67), trunk exercises, and a low-impact aerobic exercise program.

During the advanced strengthening phase of rehabilitation, the goals should be to improve strength, power, and endurance of muscles as well as to improve neuromuscular control of the shoulder complex, and prepare the patient to return to sport-specific activities. Prior to advancing to this phase, the therapist should use the criteria of full pain-free ROM, no pain or tenderness, and strength of 70% compared to the uninvolved shoulder. The emphasis in this phase is on high-speed strengthening, eccentric exercises, and multiplanar motions. The patient should advance to surgical tubing exercises (Figure 17-45), plyometric exercises (Figures 17-46 to 17-51), PNF diagonal strengthening (Figures 17-53 to 17-58), and isokinetic strengthening exercises (Figure 17-52).

When the patient is ready to return to activity, the athletic trainer should progressively increase activities that prepare the patient for a fully functional return. An interval program of sport-specific activities should be started. Exercises from stage III should be continued. The patient should progressively increase the time of participation in sport-specific activities as tolerated. For contact and collision sport patients, the AC joint should be protected.

Criteria for Returning to Full Activity

Prior to returning to full activity the patient should have full ROM and no pain or tenderness. Isokinetic strength testing should meet the demands of the patient's sport, and the patient should have successfully completed the final phase of the rehabilitation progression.

Clavicle Fractures

Pathomechanics

Clavicle fractures are one of the most common fractures in sports. The clavicle acts as a strut connecting the upper extremity to the trunk of the body.[31] Forces acting on the clavicle are most likely to cause a fracture of the bone medial to the attachment of the coracoclavicular ligaments.[4] Intact AC and coracoclavicular ligaments help keep fractures nondisplaced and stabilized.

Injury Mechanism

In athletics, the mechanism for injury often depends on the sport played. The mechanism can be direct or indirect. Fractures can result from a fall on an outstretched arm, a fall or blow to the point of the shoulder, or less commonly a direct blow as in stick sports like lacrosse and hockey.[95]

Rehabilitation Concerns

Early identification of the fracture is an important factor in rehabilitation. If stabilization occurs early, with minimal damage and irritation to the surrounding structures, the likelihood of an uncomplicated return to sports is increased. Other factors influencing the likelihood of complications are injuries to the AC, coracoclavicular, and SC ligaments. Treatment for clavicle fractures includes approximation of the fracture and immobilization for 6 to 8 weeks. Most commonly a figure 8 wrap is used, with the involved arm in a sling.

When designing a rehabilitation program for a patient who has sustained a clavicle fracture, the athletic trainer should consider the function of the clavicle. The clavicle acts as a strut offering shoulder girdle stability and allowing the upper extremity to move more freely about the thorax by positioning the extremity away from the body axis.[42] Mobility of the clavicle is therefore very important to normal shoulder mechanics. Joint mobilization techniques are started immediately after the immobilization period to restore normal arthrokinematics. The clavicle also serves as an insertion point for the deltoid, upper trapezius, and pectoralis major muscles, providing stability and aiding in neuromuscular control of the shoulder complex. It is important to address these muscles with the appropriate exercises to restore normal shoulder mechanics.

Rehabilitation Progression

For the first 6 to 8 weeks, the patient is immobilized in the figure 8 brace and sling. If good approximation and healing of the fracture is occurring at 6 weeks, the patient may begin gentle isometric exercises for the upper extremity. Use of the involved extremity below 90 degrees of elevation should be encouraged to prevent muscle atrophy and excessive loss of glenohumeral ROM. After the immobilization period, the patient should begin a program to regain full active and passive ROM. Joint mobilization techniques are used to restore normal arthrokinematics (Figures 13-10 to 13-12). The patient may continue to wear the sling for the next 3 to 4 weeks while regaining the ability to carry the arm in an appropriate posture without the figure 8 brace. The patient should begin a strengthening program using progressive resistance as ROM improves. Once full ROM is achieved, the patient should begin resisted diagonal PNF exercises and continue to increase the strength of the shoulder complex muscle, including the periscapular muscles, to enable normal neuromuscular control of the shoulder.

Criteria for Return

The patient may return to activity when the fracture is clinically united, full active and passive ROM is achieved, and the patient has the strength and neuromuscular control to meet the demands of his or her sport.

Glenohumeral Dislocations/ Instabilities (Surgical vs Nonsurgical Rehabilitation)

Pathomechanics

Dislocations of the glenohumeral joint involve the temporary displacement of the humeral head from its normal position in the glenoid labral fossa. From a biomechanical perspective, the resultant force vector is directed outside the arc of contact in the glenoid fossa, creating a dislocating moment of the humeral head by pivoting about the labral rim.

Shoulder dislocations account for up to 50% of all dislocations. The inherent instability of the shoulder joint necessary for the extreme mobility of this joint makes the glenohumeral joint susceptible to dislocation. The most common kind of dislocation is that occurring anteriorly. Posterior dislocations account for only 1% to 4.3% of all shoulder dislocations. Inferior dislocations are extremely rare. Of dislocations caused by direct trauma, 85% to 90% are recurring.[104]

In an anterior glenohumeral dislocation, the head of the humerus is forced out of its anterior capsule in an anterior direction past the glenoid labrum and then downward to rest under the coracoid process. The pathology that ensues is extensive, with torn capsular and ligamentous tissue, possibly tendinous avulsion of the rotator cuff muscles, and profuse hemorrhage. A tear or detachment of the glenoid labrum might also be present. Healing is usually slow, and the detached labrum and capsule can produce a permanent anterior defect on the glenoid labrum called a Bankart lesion. Another defect that can occur with anterior dislocation can be found on the posterior lateral aspect of the humeral head called a Hill-Sachs lesion. This is caused by compressive forces between the humeral head and the glenoid rim while the humeral head rests in the dislocated position. Additional complications can arise if the head of the humerus comes into contact with and injures the brachial nerves and vessels. Rotator cuff tears can also arise as a result of the dislocation. The bicipital tendon might also sublux from its canal as the result of a rupture of the transverse ligament.[104]

Posterior dislocations can also result in significant soft-tissue damage. Tears of the posterior glenoid labrum are common in posterior dislocation. A fracture of the lesser tubercle can occur if the subscapularis tendon avulses its attachment.

Glenohumeral dislocations are usually very disabling. The patient assumes an obvious disabled posture and the deformity itself is obvious. A positive sulcus sign is usually present at the time of the dislocation, and the deformity can be easily recognized on an X-ray. As detailed previously, the damage can be extensive to the soft tissue.

Injury Mechanism

When discussing the mechanism of injury for dislocations of the glenohumeral joint, it is necessary to categorize the injury as traumatic or atraumatic, and anterior or posterior. An anterior dislocation of the glenohumeral joint can result from direct impact on the posterior or posterolateral aspect of the shoulder. The most common mechanism is forced abduction, external rotation, and extension that forces the humeral head out of the glenoid cavity.[73] An arm tackle in football or rugby or abnormal forces created in executing a throw can produce a sequence of events resulting in dislocation. The injury mechanism for a posterior glenohumeral dislocation is usually forced adduction and internal rotation of the shoulder or a fall on an extended and internally rotated arm.

The two mechanisms described for anterior dislocation can be categorized as traumatic or atraumatic. The following acronyms have been described to summarize the two mechanisms.[56]

Traumatic	Atraumatic
Unidirectional	Multidirectional
Bankart lesion	Bilateral involvement
Surgery required	Rehabilitation effective
	Inferior capsular shift recommended

The AMBRI group can be characterized by subluxation or dislocation episodes without trauma, resulting in a stretched capsuloligamentous complex that lacks end-range stabilizing ability. Several authors report a high rate of recurrence for dislocations, especially those in the TUBS category.[100]

Rehabilitation Concerns

Management of shoulder dislocation depends on a number of factors that need to be identified. Mechanism, chronology, and direction of instability all need to be considered in the development of a conservatively managed rehabilitation program. No single rehabilitation program is an absolute solution for success in the treatment of a shoulder dislocation. The athletic trainer should thoroughly evaluate the injury and discuss those objective findings with the team physician. The initial concern in rehabilitation focuses on maintaining appropriate reduction of the glenohumeral joint. The patient is immobilized in a reduced position for a time, depending on the type of management used in the reduction (surgical vs nonsurgical). For the purpose of this section, the discussion will continue with conservative management in mind. The principles of rehabilitation, however, remain constant regardless of whether the physician's management is surgical or nonsurgical. Surgical rehabilitation should be based on the healing time of tissue affected by the surgery. The limitations of motion in the early stages of rehabilitation should also be based on surgical fixation. It is extremely important that the athletic trainer and physician communicate prior to the start of rehabilitation. After the immobilization period, the rehabilitation program should be focused on restoring the appropriate axis of rotation for the glenohumeral joint, optimizing the stabilizing muscle's length–tension relationship, and restoring proper neuromuscular control to the shoulder complex. In the uninjured shoulder complex with intact capsuloligamentous structures, the glenohumeral joint maintains a tight axis of rotation within the glenoid fossa. This is accomplished dynamically with complex neuromuscular control of the periscapular muscles, rotator cuff muscles, and intact passive structures of the joint. Because the extent of damage in this type of injury is variable, the exercises employed to restore these normal mechanics should also vary.[99] As the athletic trainer helps the patient regain full ROM, a safe zone of positioning should be followed. Starting in the plane of the scapula is safe because the axis of rotation for forces acting on the joint fall in the center of this plane. The least-provocative position is somewhere between 20 and 55 degrees of scapular plane abduction. Keeping the humerus below 55 degrees prevents subacromial impingement, while avoiding full adduction minimizes excessive tension across the supraspinatus/coracohumeral and/or capsuloligamentous complex. As ROM improves, the therapist should progress the exercise program into positions outside the safe zone, accommodating the demands that the patient will need to meet. Specific strengthening exercises should be given to address the muscles of the shoulder complex responsible for maintaining the axis of rotation, such as the

Table 17-2 Exercise Modification Per Direction of Instability

Direction of Instability	Position to Avoid	Exercises to Be Modified or Avoided
Anterior	Combined position of external rotation and abduction	Fly, pull-down, push-up, bench press, military press
Posterior	Combined position of internal rotation, horizontal adduction, and flexion	Fly, push-up, bench press, weight-bearing exercises
Inferior	Full elevation, dependent arm	Shrugs, elbow curls, military press

supraspinatus and rotator cuff muscles. The periscapular muscles should also be addressed to provide the rotator cuff muscles with their optimal length–tension relationship for more efficient usage. In the later stages of rehabilitation, neuromuscular control exercises are incorporated with sport-specific exercises to prepare the patient for return to activity.[56]

Rehabilitation Progression

The first step in a successful rehabilitation program is the removal of the patient from activities that may put the patient at risk for reinjury to the glenohumeral joint. A reasonable time frame for return to activity is about 12 weeks, with unrestricted activity coming closer to 20 weeks. This is variable, depending on the extent of soft-tissue damage and the type of intervention chosen by the patient and physician. Some exercises previously used by the patient might produce undesired forces on noncontractile tissues and need to be modified to be performed safely. Push-ups, pull-downs, and the bench press are performed with the hands in close and avoiding the last 10 to 20 degrees of shoulder extension. Pull-downs and military presses are performed with wide bars and machines are kept in front rather than behind the head. Supine fly exercises are limited to 30 degrees in the coronal plane while maintaining glenohumeral internal rotation. Table 17-2 provides further modifications dependent on directional instability.[3]

During phase 1, the patient is immobilized in a sling. This lasts for up to 3 weeks with first-time dislocations. The goal of this phase is to limit the inflammatory process, decrease pain, and retard muscle atrophy. Passive ROM

exercises can be initiated along with low-grade joint mobilization techniques to encourage relaxation of the shoulder musculature. Isometric exercises are also started. The patient begins with submaximal contractions and increases to maximal contractions for as long as 8 seconds. The protective phase is a good time to initiate a scapulothoracic exercise program, avoiding elevated positions of the upper extremity that put stability at risk. Patients should begin an aerobic training regimen with the lower extremity, such as stationary biking.

Phase 2 begins after the patient has been removed from the sling. This phase lasts from 3 to 8 weeks post injury and focuses on full return of active ROM. The program begins with the use of an L-bar performing active assistive ROM (Figures 17-12 to 17-16). Manual therapy techniques can also begin using PNF techniques to help reestablish neuromuscular control (see Figures 12-3 to 12-10). Exercises with the hands on the ground can help begin strengthening the scapular stabilizers more aggressively. These exercises should begin on a stable surface like a table, progressing the amount of weight bearing by advancing from the table to the ground (Figure 17-59). Advancing to a less stable surface like a biomechanical ankle platform system (BAPS) board (Figure 17-62) or stability ball (Figure 17-63) will also help reestablish neuromuscular control.

At 6 to 12 weeks, the athletic trainer should gradually enter phase 3 of the rehabilitation progression. The goal of this phase is to restore normal strength and neuromuscular control. Prophylactic stretching is done, as full ROM should already be present. Scapular and rotator cuff exercises should focus on strength and endurance. Weight-bearing exercises should be made more challenging by adding motion to the demands of the stabilization. Scapular exercises should be performed in the weight room with guidance from the athletic trainer to meet the challenge of the patient's strength. Weight shifting on a fitter (Figure 17-61) and push-ups on a stability ball (Figure 17-44) for endurance are started. Strengthening exercises progress from PRE to plyometric. Rotator cuff exercises using surgical tubing with emphasis on eccentrics are added.[2] Progression to multi-angle exercises and sport specific positioning is started. The Body Blade is a good rehabilitation tool for this phase (Figure 17-67), progressing from static to dynamic stabilization and single-position to multiplanar dynamic exercises.

Phase 4 is the functional progression. Patients are gradually returned to their sport with interval training and progressive activity increasing the demands on endurance and stability. This can last as long as 20 weeks, depending on the patient's shoulder strength, lack of pain, and ability to protect the involved shoulder. The physician should be consulted prior to full return to activity.

Criteria for Return to Activity

At 20 to 26 weeks, the patient should be ready for return to activity. This decision should be based on (a) full pain-free ROM, (b) normal shoulder strength, (c) pain-free sport specific activities, and (d) ability to protect the patient's shoulder from reinjury. Some athletic trainers and physicians like the patient to use a protective shoulder harness during participation.

Clinical Decision-Making Exercise 17-2

A 40-year-old wrestling coach suffered an antero-inferior dislocation of his glenohumeral joint while attempting to take down an opponent. The joint needed to be relocated under anesthesia. X-rays showed no injury to the humeral head, and an MRI was negative for any other structural involvement. The physician's diagnosis was an acute dislocation. What can the athletic trainer recommend to the coach to prevent another dislocation?

Multidirectional Instabilities of the Glenohumeral Joint

Pathomechanics

Multidirectional instabilities are an inherent risk of the glenohumeral joint. The shoulder has the greatest ROM of all the joints in the human body. The bony restraints are minimal, and the forces that can be generated in over-head motions of throwing and other athletic activities far exceed the strength of the static restraints of the joint. Attenuation of force is multifactorial, with time, distance, and speed determining forces applied to the joint. Thus, stability of the joint must be evaluated based on the patient's ability to dynamically control all of these factors to have a stable joint. In cases of multidirectional instability, there are two categories for pathology: atraumatic and traumatic. The atraumatic category includes patients who have congenitally loose joints or who have increased the demands on their shoulder prior to having developed the muscular maturity to meet these demands. When forces are generated at the glenohumeral joint that the stabilizing muscles are unable to handle (this occurs most commonly during the deceleration phase of throwing), the humeral head tends to translate anteriorly and inferiorly into the capsuloligamentous structures.[123] Over time, repetitive microtrauma causes these structures to stretch. Lephart et al described the essential importance of tension in the anterior capsule of the glenohumeral joint as a protective mechanism against excessive strain in these capsuloligamentous structures.[65] They theorized that the loss of this protective reflex joint stabilization can increase the potential for continuing shoulder injury. Proprioceptive deficits have been identified in individuals with multidirectional instability[4] and even generalized laxity.[10] Increased translation of the humeral head also increases the demand on the posterior structures of the glenohumeral joint, leading to repetitive microtrauma and breakdown of those soft tissues.[123] In this type of instability, there will usually be some inferior laxity, leading to a positive sulcus sign. Although the anterior glenoid labrum is usually intact during the early stages of this instability, splitting and partial detachment can develop.[3]

The patient usually has some pain and clicking when the arm is held by the side. Any symptoms and signs associated with anterior or posterior recurrent instability may be present.

Injury Mechanism

It is generally believed that the cause of multidirectional instability is excessive joint volume with laxity of the capsuloligamentous complex. In the patient, this laxity might be an inherent condition that becomes more pronounced with the superimposed trauma of sport. This type of instability might also occur as a result of extensive capsulolabral trauma in patients who do not appear to have laxity of other joints.[95]

Rehabilitation Concerns

The rehabilitation concerns for multidirectional instability are similar to those already discussed in relation to shoulder instabilities. The complexity of this program is increased because of the addition of inferior instability. The success of the program is often determined by the patient's tissue status and compliance.[109] Additionally, this program emphasizes the anterior and posterior musculature. These muscles working together are referred to as force couples and are believed to be essential stabilizers of the joint.[16] The rehabilitation program should also address the neuromuscular control of these muscles to promote dynamic stability.[43] Compliance is often an extremely important factor in maintaining good results with this type of instability. The patient must continue to do the exercise program even after symptoms have subsided. If the patient is not compliant, subluxation usually recurs. For cases where conservative treatment is not successful, Neer recommended an inferior capsular shift surgical procedure that has proven successful in restoring joint stability when used in conjunction with a rehabilitation program.[85]

Surgical management of multidirectional instability remains controversial.[36] Arthroscopic thermal capsulorrhaphy, when performed alone, has fallen out of favor as the surgery of choice as a result of high failure rates and complications.[25,45,96] The role that the rotator interval plays with regard to instability has come to the forefront. Although the integrity of the rotator interval and its relationship to shoulder stability is agreed upon,[18,25,96] the closure of the rotator interval in unstable shoulders remains an orthopedic dilemma. Although the dilemma is ongoing as to whether this closure is performed arthroscopically or via an open incision, or in combination with thermal techniques, there are several factors that can be agreed upon. The first is that the redundant capsule needs to be imbricated, the labrum, reverse Bankart, or reverse bony Bankart need to be repaired, and the rotator interval needs to be closed.[10,12] Wilk et al[131] suggest a postoperative rehabilitation program that is based on six factors: (1) type of instability; (2) patient's inflammatory response to surgery; (3) concomitant surgical procedures; (4) precautions following surgery; (5) gradual rate of progression; and (6) team approach to treatment. These factors determine the type and aggressiveness of the program. First, it must be determined whether the instability is congenital or acquired. Congenital instabilities should be treated more conservatively. Second, some patients respond to surgery with excessive scarring and proliferation of collagen ground tissue. Progression should be adjusted weekly based on assessing capsular end feel. The third factor takes into account any other procedures performed at the time of surgery. Precautions should be followed based on the tissue healing time of the other procedures. Surgical precautions also should be communicated to the athletic trainer based on the tissues involved; passive ROM (PROM) after surgery should be cautious. The authors suggest conservative PROM progression for the first 8 weeks post surgery. The gradual progression (factor 5) contrasts to one that moves faster and then slows down. The speed of progression should be based on a weekly scheduled assessment of capsular end feel and progress. The sixth factor ensures a successful rehabilitation outcome by open and continuous communication between the patient, surgeon, and athletic trainer.[131]

Rehabilitation Progression

The rehabilitation program should begin with reestablishing muscle tone and proper scapulothoracic posture. This helps provide a steady base with appropriate length–tension relationships for the anterior and posterior muscles of the shoulder complex acting

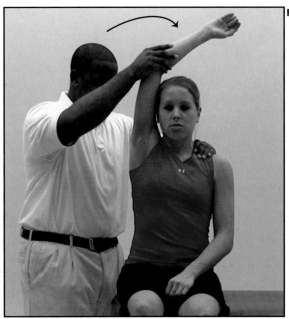

Figure 17-68. Neer impingement test.

as force couples. Strengthening of the rotator cuff muscles in the plane of the scapula should progress to higher resistance, starting at 0 degrees of shoulder elevation. As the patient becomes asymptomatic, the athletic trainer should incorporate an emphasis on neuromuscular control exercises like PNF, rhythmic stabilization, and weight-bearing activity to establish coactivation at the glenohumeral joint.[28] Sport-specific training can then be added, first in the rehabilitation setting and then in the competitive setting. For successful results, the patient might have to continue a program of maintenance for neuromuscular control for as long as they wish to be asymptomatic.

Shoulder Impingement

Pathomechanics

Shoulder impingement syndrome was first identified by Dr. Charles Neer[85] who observed that impingement involves a mechanical compression of the supraspinatus tendon, the subacromial bursa, and the long head of the biceps tendon, all of which are located under the coracoacromial arch. This syndrome has been described as a continuum during which repetitive compression eventually leads to irritation and inflammation that progresses to fibrosis and eventually to rupture of the rotator cuff.

Neer has identified three stages of shoulder impingement:

Stage I

- Seen in patients aged younger than 25 years with report of repetitive overhead activity

- Localized hemorrhage and edema with tenderness at supraspinatus insertion and anterior acromion

- Painful arc between 60 and 119 degrees; increased with resistance at 90 degrees

- Muscle tests revealing weakness secondary to pain

- Positive Neer or Hawkins-Kennedy impingement signs (Figures 17-68 and 17-69)

- Normal radiographs, typically

- Reversible; usually resolving with rest, activity modification, and rehabilitation program

Stage II

- Seen in patients age 25 to 40 years with report of repetitive overhead activity

- Many of the same clinical findings as in stage I

- Severity of symptoms worse than stage I, progressing to pain with activity and night pain

Figure 17-69. Hawkins-Kennedy impingement test.

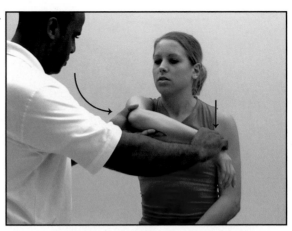

- More soft-tissue crepitus or catching at 100 degrees

- Restriction in PROM as a result of fibrosis

- Possibly radiographs showing osteophytes under acromion, degenerative AC joint changes

- No longer reversible with rest; possibly helped by a long-term rehabilitation program

Stage III

- Seen in patients aged older than 40 years with history of chronic tendinitis and prolonged pain

- Many of the same clinical findings as stage II

- Tear in rotator cuff usually less than 1 cm

- More limitation in active and passive ROM

- Possibly a prominent capsular laxity with multidirectional instability seen on radiograph

- Atrophy of infraspinatus and supraspinatus caused by disuse

- Treatment typically surgical following a failed conservative approach

Neer's impingement theory was based primarily on the treatment of older, nonathletic patients. The older population will likely exhibit what has been referred to as "outside" or "outlet" impingement.[8,85] In outside impingement there is contact of the rotator cuff with the coracoacromial ligament or the acromion with fraying, abrasion, inflammation, fibrosis, and degeneration of the superior surface of the cuff within the subacromial space. There might also be evidence of degenerative processes, including spurring, decreased joint space due to fibrotic changes, and decreased vascularity.

Internal or "nonoutlet" impingement is more likely to occur in the younger overhead patient. With internal impingement, the subacromial space appears relatively normal. With humeral elevation and internal rotation, the rotator cuff is compressed between the posterior superior glenoid labrum (or glenoid rim) and the humeral head. Although this compression is a normal biomechanical phenomenon, it can become pathologic in overhead patients because of the repetitive nature of overhead sports. The result is inflammation on the undersurface of the rotator cuff tendon, posterior superior tears in the glenoid labrum, and lesions in the posterior humeral head (Bankart lesion).

The mechanical impingement syndrome, as originally proposed by Neer, has been referred to as primary impingement. Jobe and Kvnite have proposed that an unstable shoulder permits excessive translation of the humeral head in an anterior and superior direction, resulting in what has been termed secondary impingement.[50] Based on the relationship of shoulder instability to shoulder impingement, Jobe and Kvnite have proposed an alternative system of classification:[50]

Group IA

- Found in recreational patients aged older than 35 years with pure mechanical impingement and no instability;

- Positive impingement signs
- Lesions on the superior surface of the rotator cuff, possibly with subacromial spurring
- Possibly some arthritic changes in the glenohumeral joint

Group IB

- Found in recreational patients aged older than 35 years who demonstrate instability with impingement secondary to mechanical trauma
- Positive impingement signs
- Lesions found on the undersurface of the rotator cuff, superior glenoid, and humeral head

Group II

- Found in young overhead patients (aged younger than 35 years) who demonstrate instability and impingement secondary to repetitive microtrauma
- Positive impingement signs with excessive anterior translation of humeral head
- Lesions on the posterior superior glenoid rim, posterior humeral head, or anterior inferior capsule
- Lesions on the undersurface of the rotator cuff

Group III

- Found in young overhead patients (aged younger than 35 years)
- Positive impingement signs with atraumatic multidirectional, usually bilateral, humeral instabilities
- Demonstrated generalized laxity in all joints
- Humeral head lesions as in group II but less severe

Group IV

- Found in young overhead patients (aged younger than 35 years) with anterior instability resulting from a traumatic event but without impingement
- Posterior defect in the humeral head
- Damage in the posterior glenoid labrum

It has also been proposed that wear of the rotator cuff is a result of intrinsic tendon pathology, including tendinopathy and partial or small complete tears with age-related thinning, degeneration, and weakening. This permits superior migration of the humeral head, leading to secondary impingement, thus creating a cycle that can ultimately lead to full-thickness tears.[120]

A "critical zone" of vascular insufficiency has been proposed to exist in the tendon of the supraspinatus, which is found at about 1 cm proximal to its distal insertion on the humerus. It has been hypothesized that when the humerus is adducted and internally rotated, a "wringing out" of the blood supply occurs in this tendon. Should this occur repetitively, such as in the recovery phase on a swimming stroke, ultimately irritation and inflammation may lead to partial or complete rotator cuff tears.[97]

It is likely that some as yet unidentified combination of mechanical, traumatic, degenerative, and vascular processes collectively lead to pathology in the rotator cuff.

Injury Mechanism

Shoulder impingement syndrome occurs when there is compromise of the subacromial space under the coracoacromial arch. When the dynamic and static stabilizers of the shoulder complex for one reason or another fail to maintain this subacromial space, the soft-tissue structures are compressed, leading to irritation and inflammation.[44] In athletes, impingement most often occurs in repetitive overhead activities such as throwing, swimming, serving a tennis ball, spiking a volleyball, or during handstands in gymnastics. There is ongoing disagreement regarding the specific mechanisms that cause shoulder impingement syndrome. It has been proposed that mechanical impingement can result from either structural or functional causes. Structural causes can be attributed to existing congenital abnormalities or to degenerative changes under the coracoacromial arch and might include the following:

- An abnormally shaped acromion (Figure 17-70). Patients with a type III or hook-shaped acromion are about 70% more likely to exhibit signs of impingement than those with a flat or slightly curved acromion.[7]

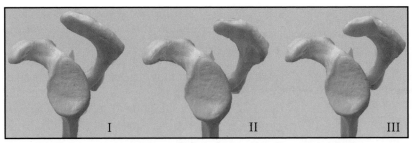

Figure 17-70. Acromion shapes. Type I, flat; type II, curved; and type III, hooked.

- Inherent capsular laxity compromises the ability of the glenohumeral joint capsule to act as both a static and a dynamic stabilizer.[50]

- Ongoing or recurring tendinitis or subacromial bursitis causes a loss of space under the coracoacromial arch, which can potentially lead to irritation of other, uninflamed structures, setting up a vicious degenerative cycle.[106]

- Laxity in the anterior capsule due to recurrent subluxation or dislocation can allow an anterior migration of the humeral head, which can cause impingement under the coracoid process.[126]

- Postural malalignments, such as a forward head, round shoulders, and an increased kyphotic curve that cause the scapular glenoid to be positioned such that the space under the coracoacromial arch is decreased, can also contribute to impingement.

Functional causes include adaptive changes that occur with repetitive overhead activities, altering the normal biomechanical function of the shoulder complex. These include the following:

- Failure of the rotator cuff to dynamically stabilize the humeral head relative to the glenoid, producing excessive translation and instability. The inferior rotator cuff muscles (infraspinatus, teres minor, subscapularis) should act collectively to both depress and compress the humeral head. In the overhead or throwing patient, the internal rotators must be capable of producing humeral rotation on the order of 7000 degrees per second.[117] The subscapularis tends to be stronger than the infraspinatus and teres minor, creating a strength imbalance in the existing force couple in the transverse plane. This imbalance produces excessive anterior translation of the humeral head. Furthermore, weakness in the inferior rotator cuff muscles creates an imbalance in the existing force couple with the deltoid in the coronal plane. Myers et al demonstrated that patients with subacromial impingement demonstrated decreased inferior cuff muscle coactivation while excessive activation of the middle deltoid is present.[82] The deltoid potentially produces excessive superior translation of the humeral head, decreasing subacromial space. Weakness in the supraspinatus, which normally functions to compress the humeral head into the glenoid, allows for excessive superior translation of the humeral head.[74]

- Because the tendons of the rotator cuff blend into the joint capsule, we rely on tension created in the capsule by contraction of the rotator cuff to both statically and dynamically center the humeral head relative to the glenoid. Tightness in the posterior and inferior portions of the glenohumeral joint capsule causes an anterosuperior migration of the humeral head, again decreasing the subacromial space. In the overhead patient, ROM in internal rotation is usually limited by tightness of both the muscles that externally rotate and the posterior capsule. There tends to be excessive external rotation, primarily due to laxity in the anterior joint capsule.[14]

- The scapular muscles function to dynamically position the glenoid relative to the humeral head, maintaining a normal length–tension relationship with the rotator cuff. As the humerus moves into elevation, the scapula should also move so that the glenoid is able to adjust regardless of the position of the elevating humerus. Weakness in the serratus anterior, which elevates, upward rotates, and abducts the scapula, or weakness in the levator scapula or upper trapezius, which elevate the scapula, will compromise positioning of the glenoid during humeral elevation, interfering with normal scapulohumeral rhythm.[23] Altered scapular movement patterns commonly identified in patients with subacromial impingement includes decreased upward rotation, external rotation, and posterior tipping, all of which have the potential to compromise subacromial space height, contributing to impingement.[23,35,69,71,122]

- It is critical for the scapula to maintain a stable base on which the highly mobile humerus can move. Weakness in the rhomboids and/or middle trapezius, which function eccentrically to decelerate the scapula in high-velocity throwing motions, can contribute to scapular hypermobility. Likewise, weakness in the inferior trapezius creates an imbalance in the force couple with the upper trapezius and levator scapula, contributing to scapular hypermobility.[23]

- An injury that affects normal arthrokinematic motion at either the SC joint or the AC joint can also contribute to shoulder impingement. Any limitation in posterior superior clavicular rotation and/or clavicular elevation will prevent normal upward rotation of the scapula during humeral elevation, compromising the subacromial space.

Rehabilitation Concerns

Management of shoulder impingement involves gradually restoring normal biomechanics to the shoulder joint to maintain space under the coracoacromial arch during overhead activities.[55,114] The athletic trainer should address the pathomechanics and the adaptive changes that most often occur with overhead activities.

Overhead activities that involve humeral elevation (full abduction or forward flexion) or a position of humeral flexion, horizontal adduction, and internal rotation are likely to increase the pain.[68] The patient complains of diffuse pain around the acromion or glenohumeral joint. Palpation of the subacromial space increases the pain.

Exercises should concentrate on strengthening the dynamic stabilizers, the rotator cuff muscles that act to both compress and depress the humeral head relative to the glenoid (Figures 17-31 and 17-32).[51,81,114] The inferior rotator cuff muscles in particular should be strengthened to recreate a balance in the force couple with the deltoid in the coronal plane. The supraspinatus should be strengthened to assist in compression of the humeral head into the glenoid (Figures 17-33 and 17-34).[113] The external rotators, the infraspinatus and teres minor, are generally weaker concentrically but stronger eccentrically than the internal rotators and should be strengthened to recreate a balance in the force couple with the subscapularis in the transverse plane.

The external rotators and the posterior portion of the joint capsule are tight and tend to limit internal rotation and should be stretched (Figures 17-15, 17-17, and 17-19). Both horizontal adduction and sleeper stretches have been demonstrated effective to stretch the posterior shoulder.[62,75] There is excessive external rotation because of laxity in the anterior portion of the joint capsule, and stretching should be avoided. There might be some tightness in both the inferior and the posterior portions of the joint capsule; this can be decreased by using posterior and inferior glenohumeral joint mobilizations (Figures 13-13, 13-14, 13-16, and 13-17).

Strengthening of the muscles that abduct, elevate, and upwardly rotate the scapula (these include the serratus anterior, upper trapezius, and levator scapula) should also be incorporated (Figures 17-35, 17-39, and 17-40). The middle trapezius and rhomboids should be strengthened eccentrically to help decelerate the scapula during throwing activities (Figures 17-37 and 17-38). The inferior trapezius should also be strengthened to recreate a balance in the force couple with the upper trapezius, facilitating scapular upward rotation and stability (Figure 17-36).

Anterior, posterior, inferior, and superior joint mobilizations at both the SC and the AC joint should be done to assure normal arthrokinematic motion at these joints (Figures 13-10 to 13-12).

Strengthening of the lower-extremity and trunk muscles to provide core stability is essential for reducing the stresses and strains placed on the shoulder and arm, and this is also important for the overhead patient (Figure 17-40).

Rehabilitation Progression

In the early stages of a rehabilitation program, the primary goal of the athletic trainer is to minimize the pain associated with the impingement syndrome. This can be accomplished by using some combination of activity modification, therapeutic modalities, and appropriate use of NSAIDs.

Initially, the athletic trainer should have a coach evaluate the patient's technique in performing the overhead activity to rule out faulty performance techniques. Once existing performance techniques have been corrected, the athletic trainer must make some decision about limiting the activity that caused the problem in the first place. Activity limitation, however, does not mean immobilization. Instead, a baseline of tolerable activity should be established. The key is to initially control the frequency and the level of the load on the rotator cuff and then to gradually and systematically increase the level and the frequency of that activity. It might be necessary to initially restrict activity, avoiding any exercise that places the shoulder in the impingement position, to give the inflammation a chance to subside. During this period of restricted activity, the patient should continue to engage in exercises to maintain cardiorespiratory fitness. Working on an upper-extremity ergometer will help to improve both cardiorespiratory fitness and muscular endurance in the shoulder complex.

Therapeutic modalities such as electrical stimulating currents and/or heat and cold therapy may be used to modulate pain. Ultrasound and the diathermies are most useful for elevating tissue temperatures, increasing blood flow, and facilitating the process of healing. NSAIDs prescribed by the team physician are useful not only as analgesics, but also for their long-lasting anti-inflammatory capabilities.

Once pain and inflammation have been controlled, exercises should concentrate on strengthening the dynamic stabilizers of the glenohumeral joint, stretching the inferior and posterior portions of the joint capsule and external rotators, strengthening the scapular muscles that collectively produce normal scapulohumeral rhythm, and maintaining normal arthrokinematic motions of the AC and SC joints.

REHABILITATION PLAN

ARTHROSCOPIC ANTERIOR CAPSULOLABRAL REPAIR OF THE SHOULDER COMPLEX

Injury situation A 27-year-old male baseball player returns to the throwing rotation of his baseball club after having elbow surgery five months earlier. Three weeks after returning, he starts complaining of posterior shoulder pain. After three months of using ice and NSAID therapy, he begins to have difficulty with his velocity and control of his pitches, and is now also experiencing anterior shoulder pain near the bicipital groove. The patient is diagnosed by an orthopedist with posterior impingement secondary to multidirectional instability of the glenohumeral joint. An MRI revealed an additional lesion of the superior labral attachment, and some degenerative tearing of the rotator cuff.

Signs and symptoms The patient complains of posterior cuff pain whenever he externally rotates. He has 165 degrees of external rotation and 35 degrees of internal rotation. Horizontal adduction of the humerus is only 15 degrees. Tenderness is present along the posterior glenohumeral joint line. He also has a positive O'Brien test for superior labral pathology (SLAP lesion), apprehension sign, and relocation test. The patient is evaluated for other factors that have stressed the throwing motion. Evaluation revealed an extremely tight hip flexibility pattern: bilateral hip flexion of 70 degrees, hip internal rotation of 15 degrees bilaterally, and hip external rotation of 50 degrees bilaterally.

Management plan The patient underwent arthroscopic anterior capsulolabral repair of the shoulder to address his instability and was rehabilitated with the goal of returning to play in 8 to 12 months.

PHASE ONE Protection Phase

GOALS: Allow soft-tissue healing, diminish pain and inflammation, initiate protected motion, and retard muscle atrophy.

Estimated length of time (ELT): Day 1 to Week 6 For the first 2 to 3 weeks the patient uses a sling, full time for 7 to 10 days, sleeping with it for the full 2 weeks, and then gradual weaning of the sling. Exercises include hand and wrist ROM and active cervical spine ROM. During this phase, cryotherapy is used before and after treatments. Passive and active assisted ROM for the glenohumeral joint is cautiously performed in a restricted ROM. Shoulder rotation is done in 20 degrees of abduction; external rotation (ER) is to 30 degrees and internal rotation (IR) is allowed to 25 or 30 degrees for the first 3 weeks, advancing to 50 degrees by week 6. Passive forward elevation (PFE) is progressed to 90 degrees for the first 3 weeks, advancing to 135 degrees by 6 weeks. Active assisted forward elevation (AFE) can be progressed between weeks 3 and 6 to 115 degrees. Moist heat can be used prior to therapy after 10 days. Passive ROM is performed by the athletic trainer and active-assisted ROM by the patient.

During this phase, ROM is progressed based on the end feel the athletic trainer gets when evaluating the patient. With a hard end feel, the athletic trainer may choose to be more aggressive, making sure not to surpass the ROM guidelines. A soft end feel dictates a slower progression. ROM is not the main focus of this phase; healing of the repaired tissue is the prime goal. The minimally invasive nature of arthroscopy leads to less pain and inflammation. Therefore, it is important to stress to the patient the importance of protection. Educating the patient to minimize load to less than 5 pounds and limiting repetitive activities is very important. ROM of the patient's hips is also addressed during this phase. Aggressive stretching and core stability exercises may be started to maintain an increased state of flexibility of the pitcher's total rotational capabilities.

Shoulder strengthening begins early in this phase with rhythmic stabilization, scapular stabilizing exercises, isometric exercises for the rotator cuff muscles, and PNF control exercises in a restricted ROM. Although scapular stabilizing exercises are begun, protraction should not begin until the end of this phase. Protraction has been shown to stress the anterior and inferior portions of the joint capsule. Scapula elevation and retraction are allowed.[125] By the end of this phase, the patient should have met all ROM goals set and they should be pain free within these guidelines. Advancement to the second phase should not occur unless these goals are met.

PHASE TWO Intermediate Phase

GOALS: Restore full ROM, restore functional ROM, normalize arthrokinematics, improve dynamic stability, and improve muscular strength.

Estimated length of time (ELT): Weeks 7 to 12 During this phase, the patient's ROM will ultimately be progressed to fully functional by 12 weeks: at week 9, PFE to 155 degrees, 75 degrees of ER at 90 degrees of abduction, 50 to 65 degrees of ER at 20 degrees of abduction, and 60 to 65 degrees of IR. Active forward elevation should progress to 145 degrees. Aggressive stretching may be used during this phase if the goal is not met by 9 weeks. This may include joint mobilization and capsular stretching techniques. From week 9 to week 12, the athletic trainer begins to gradually progress ROM exercises to a position functional for this pitcher.

In this phase, strengthening exercises include PRE in all planes of shoulder motion and IR- and ER-resisted exercises. Exercises begin in the scapular plane and work their way to more functional planes. Incremental stresses are added to the anterior capsule working toward the 90/90 position. Resistance progresses from isotonic to gentle plyometrics. Gentle plyometrics are defined as two-handed, low-load activity like the pushup. Rhythmic stabilization drills continue to be progressed with increasing difficulty. Aggressive strengthening may be initiated if ROM goals are achieved. Strengthening should emphasize high repetitions (30 to 50 reps) and low resistance (1 to 3 pounds). Weight room activities, including push-ups, dumbbell press (without allowing the arm to drop below the body), and latissimus pull-downs in front of body, bicep, and triceps exercises with arm at the side may begin. Exercises should be performed asymptomatically. If symptoms of pain or instability occur, a thorough evaluation of the patient should be performed and the program adjusted accordingly.

PHASE THREE Advanced Activity and Strengthening

GOALS: Improve strength, power, and endurance; enhance neuromuscular control; functional activities.

Estimated length of time (ELT): Weeks 12 to 24 The criteria for progression to this phase should be: Active range of motion (AROM) goals met without pain or substitution patterns and appropriate scapular posture and dynamic control present during exercises. The patient should maintain established ROM and should continue stretching exercises. Throwing-specific exercises are initiated, including throwing a ball into the plyoback.

During this phase, additional lifting exercises are added to begin building power and strength. Full dumbbell incline and bench press are added. Shoulder raises to 90 degrees in the sagittal and frontal planes, overhead dumbbell press, pectoralis major flys, and dead lifts can be worked in. Lifting exercises that put the bar behind the head and dips should still be avoided.

At week 16, the athletic trainer will initiate a formal interval-throwing program. Each step is performed at least two times on separate days prior to advancing. Throwing should be performed without pain or any increasing symptoms. If symptoms appear, the patient will be regressed to the previous step and remain there until symptom-free.

PHASE FOUR Return to Full Activity

GOALS: Complete elimination of pain and full return to activity.

Estimated length of time (ELT): Weeks 24 to 36 Usually by week 24 the patient will begin throwing off the pitcher's mound. In this phase, the number of throws, intensity, and type of pitch are progressed gradually to increase the stress at the glenohumeral joint. By 6 to 7 months the patient will progress to game-type situations and return to competition. The patient will begin by limiting his pitch count and progressing if he can maintain his pain- and symptom-free status. Full return may take as long as 9 to 12 months.

Criteria for Returning to Competitive Pitching

1. Full functional ROM
2. No pain or tenderness
3. Satisfactory muscular strength
4. Satisfactory clinical exam

DISCUSSION QUESTIONS

1. What other factors may affect the pitcher's ability to generate velocity of the baseball when he throws the ball?
2. Can the athletic trainer truly simulate the demands of pitching during the rehabilitation process?

3. Should the patient be allowed to take NSAIDs during the rehabilitation progression?
4. What muscles generate the greatest amounts of torque during the patient's throwing motion?
5. What other areas of the thrower's body should be targeted for strengthening, to ensure that he will recover his delivery speed and power?

Strengthening exercises are done to establish neuromuscular control of the humerus and the scapula (Figures 17-59 through 17-67). Strengthening exercises should progress from isometric pain-free contractions to isotonic full-range pain-free contractions. Humeral control exercises should be used to strengthen the rotator cuff to restrict migration of the humeral head and to regain voluntary control of the humeral head positioning through rotator cuff stabilization.[127] Scapular control exercises should be used to maintain a normal relationship between the glenohumeral and scapulothoracic joints.[58,59,68]

Closed kinetic chain exercises for the shoulder should be primarily eccentric. They tend to compress the joint, providing stability, and are perhaps best used for establishing scapular stability and control.

Gradually, the duration and intensity of the exercise may be progressed within individual patient tolerance limitations, using increased pain or stiffness as a guide for progression, eventually progressing to full-range overhead activities.

Criteria for Returning to Full Activity

The patient may return to full activity when (a) the gradual program used to increase the duration and intensity of the workout has allowed the patient to complete a normal workout without pain; (b) the patient exhibits improved strength in the appropriate rotator cuff and the scapular muscles; (c) there is no longer a positive impingement sign, drop arm test, or empty can test; and (d) the patient can discontinue use of anti-inflammatory medications without a return of pain. After return to play, or even as a prophylactic measure prior to injury athletes (especially those who participate in overhead sports) benefit from participation in an injury prevention program. Although the literature is currently void of scientifically validated injury prevention programs for the overhead patient, the literature and clinical experience do support the inclusion of overhead athletic specific resistance tubing exercises,[84,110,111] shoulder flexibility,[62,75] and upper quarter posture exercises[60] for purposes of injury prevention.

Rotator Cuff Tears and Tendinopathies

Pathomechanics

Rotator cuff injury has often been described as a continuum starting with impingement of the tendon that, through repetitive compression, eventually leads to irritation and inflammation and eventually fibrosis of the rotator cuff tendon. This idea began with the work of Codman in 1934 when he identified a critical zone near the insertion of the supraspinatus tendon.[78] Since then many researchers in sports medicine have studied this area and expanded the information base, leading to the identification of other causative factors.[51,91] Neer is also credited with developing a system of classification for rotator cuff disease. This system seemed to be appropriate until sports medicine professionals began dealing with overhead patients as a separate entity due to the acceleration of repetitive stresses applied to the shoulder. Disease in the overhead patient usually results from failure from one or both of these chronic stresses: repetitive tension or compression of the tissue. We now regard rotator cuff injury in athletics as an accumulation of microtrauma to both the static and the dynamic stabilizers of the shoulder complex. Meister and Andrews classified these causative traumas based on the pathophysiology of events leading to rotator cuff failure. Their five categories of classification for modes of failure are primary compressive, secondary compressive, primary tensile overload, secondary tensile overload, and macrotraumatic.[78]

Injury Mechanism

Rotator cuff tendinopathy is a gradation of tendon failure, so it is important to identify the causative factors. The following classification system helps group injury mechanisms to better aid the athletic trainer in developing a rehabilitation plan.

Primary compressive disease results from direct compression of the cuff tissue. This occurs when something interferes with the gliding of the cuff tendon in the already tight subacromial space. A predisposing factor in this category is a type III hooked acromion process, a common factor seen in younger patients with rotator cuff disease. Other factors in younger patients include a congenitally thick coracoacromial ligament and the presence of an osacromiale. In younger patients, a primary impingement without one of these associated factors is rare. In middle-aged athletes/patients, degenerative spurring on the undersurface of the acromion process can cause irritation of the tendon and eventually lead to complete tearing of the tendon. These individuals are often seen because they experience pain during such activities as tennis and golf.

Secondary compressive disease is a primary result of glenohumeral instability. The high forces generated by the overhead patient can cause chronic repetitive trauma to the glenoid labrum and capsuloligamentous structures, leading to subtle instability. Patients with inherent multidirectional instability, such as swimmers, are also at risk. The additional volume created in the glenohumeral capsule allows for extraneous movement of the humeral head, leading to compressive forces in the subacromial space.

Primary tensile overload can also cause tendon irritation and failure. The rotator cuff resists horizontal adduction, internal rotation, and anterior translation of the humeral head, as well as the distraction forces found in the deceleration phase of throwing and overhead sports. The repetitive high forces generated by eccentric activity in the rotator cuff while attempting to maintain a central axis of rotation can cause microtrauma to the tendon and eventually lead to tendon failure. This type of mechanism is not associated with previous instability of the joint. Causes for this mechanism often are found when evaluating the patient's mechanics and taking a complete history during the evaluation. The athletic trainer might find that the throwing patient had a history of injury to another area of the body where the muscles are used in the deceleration phase of overhead motion (eg, the right-handed pitcher who sprained his left ankle).

Secondary tensile disease is often a result of primary tensile overload. In this case, the repetitive irritation and weakening of the rotator cuff allows for subtle instability. In contrast to secondary compressive disease of the tendon, the rotator cuff tendon experiences greater distractive and tensile forces because the humeral head is allowed to translate anteriorly. Over time, the increased tensile force causes failure of the tendon.

Macrotraumatic failure occurs as a direct result of one distinct traumatic event. The mechanism for this is often a fall on an outstretched arm. This is rarely seen in patients with normal, healthy rotator cuff tendons. For this to occur, forces generated by the fall must be greater than the tensile strength of the tendon. Because the tensile strength of bone is less than that of young healthy tendon, it is rare to see this in a young patient. It is more common to see a longitudinal tear in the tendon with an avulsion of the greater tubercle.

Rehabilitation Concerns

When designing a rehabilitation program for rotator cuff tendinopathy, the basic concerns remain the same regardless of the extent to which the tendon is damaged. Instead, rehabilitation should be based on why and how the tendon has been damaged. Once the cause of the tendinopathy is identified and secondary factors are known, a comprehensive program can be designed. If a comprehensive rehabilitation program does not relieve the painful shoulder, surgical repair of the tendon and alteration of the glenohumeral joint are performed. Surgical rehabilitation is similar to the nonsurgical plan, with the time of progression altered based on tissue healing and tendon histology.

Conservative Management

Stage I of the rehabilitation process is focused on reducing inflammation and removing the patient from the activity that caused pain. Pain should not be a part of the rehabilitation process. The athletic trainer may employ therapeutic modalities to aid in patient comfort. A course of NSAIDs is usually followed during this stage of rehabilitation. ROM exercises begin, avoiding further irritation of the tendon. Attention is paid to restoring appropriate arthrokinematics to the shoulder complex. If the injury is a result of a compressive disease to the tendon, capsular stretching may be done (Figures 17-17 and 17-19). Active strengthening of the glenohumeral joint should begin, concentrating on the force couples acting around the joint. Beginning with isometric exercises for the medial and lateral rotators of the joint (Figure 17-20), and progressing to isotonic exercises if the patient does not experience pain (Figures 17-31 and 17-32). A towel roll under the patient's arm can help initiate coactivation of the shoulder muscles, increasing joint stability. Exercises might need to be altered to limit translational forces of the humeral head. Strengthening of the supraspinatus may begin if 90 degrees of elevation in the scapular plane is available (Figures 17-33 and 17-34). Aggressive pain-free strengthening of the periscapular muscles should also start, as the restoration of normal scapular control will be essential to removal of abnormal stresses of the rotator cuff tendon in later stages. The athletic trainer might want to begin with manual resistance, progressing to free-weight exercises (Figures 17-35 to 17-39).

In stage II, the healing process progresses and ROM will need to be restored. The athletic trainer might need to be more aggressive in stretching techniques, addressing capsular tightness as it develops. The prone-on-elbows position is a good technique for self-mobilization. This position should be avoided if compressive disease was part of the irritation. If pain continues to be absent, strengthening gets increasingly aggressive. Isokinetic exercises at speeds greater than 200 degrees per second for shoulder medial and lateral rotation may begin (Figure 17-52).[41]

Aggressive neuromuscular control exercises are started in this stage: quick reversals during PNF diagonal patterns, starting with manual resistance from the athletic trainer and advancing to resistance applied by surgical tubing (Figures 17-55 and 17-56). A Body Blade may also be used for rhythmic stabilization (Figure 17-57). The exercise program should now progress to free weights, and eccentric exercises of the rotator cuff should be emphasized to meet the demands of the shoulder in overhead activities. Strengthening of the deltoid and upper trapezius muscles can begin above 90 degrees of elevation. Exercises include the military press (Figure 17-24), shoulder flexion (Figure 17-26), and reverse flys (Figure 17-30). Push-ups can also be added. It might be necessary to restrict ROM so the body does not go below the elbow, to prevent excessive translation of the glenohumeral joint. Combining this exercise with serratus anterior strengthening in a modified push-up with a plus is recommended (Figure 17-39).

In the later part of this stage, exercises should progress to plyometric strengthening.[132] Surgical tubing is used to allow the patient to exercise in 90 degrees of elevation with the elbow bent to 90 degrees (Figure 17-45). Plyoball exercises are initiated (Figures 17-46 and 17-47). The weight and distance of the exercises can be altered to increase demands. The Shuttle 2000-1 is an excellent exercise to increase eccentric strength in a plyometric fashion (Figure 17-50).

Stage III of the rehabilitation focuses on sport-specific activities. With throwing and overhead patients, an interval overhead program begins. Total body conditioning, return of strength, and increased endurance are the emphasis. The patient should remain pain-free as sport-specific activities are advanced and a gradual return to sport is achieved.

Clinical Decision-Making Exercise 17-4

A 20-year-old baseball pitcher is complaining of posterior shoulder pain. He is unable to go fully into his cocking motion of his throw without pain. Upon further evaluation, the athletic trainer finds that the infraspinatus and supraspinatus are weak and painful. The patient is referred to a physician for evaluation. The physician refers the patient with anterior instability and secondary impingement. The patient has tissue breakdown occurring on the undersurface of the rotator cuff tendons. In what order should the athletic trainer address the patient's problems?

Postsurgical Management

If conservative management is insufficient, surgical repair is often indicated. Postsurgical outcomes for patients having had a rotator cuff repair can be quite good.[15,19,21,24,46,77,98,105,116,130] The type of repair done depends on the classification of the injury. Subacromial decompression has been described by Neer as a method to stimulate tissue healing and increase the subacromial space.[85] Additional procedures may be done as open repairs of the tendon along with a capsular tightening procedure. One example is a modified Bankart procedure and capsulolabral reconstruction.[49] Surgical repairs can be done both open or closed. Closed arthroscopic rotator cuff repairs are becoming more common. The arthroscopic cuff repair addresses the deficiency of the rotator cuff by repairing the tear through the use of sutures and/or suture anchors. The arthroscopic technique spares the atrophy of the deltoid muscles and limits the presence of adhesions. Patients tend to show a much more rapid recovery of function with this repair.[38,67,115]

Stage I usually begins with some form of immobilization. This does not mean complete lack of movement. Instead it refers to restricting positions based on the surgical repair. In open repairs, flexion and abduction might be restricted for as long as 4 weeks. When the repair addresses the capsulolabral complex, the patient might spend up to 2 weeks in an airplane splint (Figure 17-71). Some surgeons have adopted a delayed start to mobilization and rehabilitation because of a few studies that have shown improved healing rates without associated stiffness.[57] During this phase, load across the repaired tendon should be minimized. ROM should be passive and in a safe range. During weeks 0 to 4 post operation, the ROM in forward elevation should be kept below 125 degrees and external rotation (ER) should be at 20 degrees of abduction and less than 45 degrees. During weeks 4 to 6 post operation, forward elevation can advance to 145 degrees and ER to 60 degrees. The patient may also advance to abduction at 90 degrees to begin external rotation ROM up to 45 degrees.

Pain control and prevention of muscle atrophy are addressed in this stage. Shoulder shrugs, isometrics, and joint mobilization for pain control can be done. Later in this stage, active assistive exercises with the L-bar and multiangle isometrics are done in the pain-free ROM, usually best done in supine position during this phase.

Stage II collagen and elastin components have begun to stabilize. Healing tissue should have a decreased level of elastin and an increased level of collagen by now.[106,131] Regaining full ROM and increasing the stress to healing tissue for better collagen alignment is important in this stage. Achieving full passive ROM during this phase is important. Normalizing the quality of AROM and beginning to work on strength and endurance are also important goals. This phase often is defined by weeks 6 to 10 postoperative.

Active and active assisted ROM exercises are added, progressing from no resistance to resistance with light free weights. If a primary repair has been done to the tendon, resisted supraspinatus exercises should be avoided until 10 weeks. Internal rotation and external rotation stretches are introduced at 70 to 90 degrees of abduction. A full scapula strengthening program should be introduced. The restoration of normal arthrokinematics and scapulothoracic rhythm is addressed with exercises emphasizing neuromuscular control. Postural control and endurance should be addressed. The patient can use a mirror to judge progress. The patient may also begin a core exercise program and cardiovascular exercises at this time.

Stage III collagen and elastin components are nearing maturation.[99,131] By week 14, the tissue should be considered mature. Typically, this stage is defined as weeks 10 to 16 post operation. Goals during this stage are full AROM,

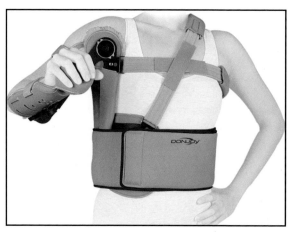

Figure 17-71. Airplane splint (Reprinted with permission from DonJoy.)

maintaining full PROM, gradual restoration of strength, power, and endurance, and optimal neuromuscular control. Closed chain exercise progression may be progressed. A balanced rotator cuff strengthening program should be followed, advancing out of the scapular plane and into the functional position for the patient.

Stage IV is typically defined by postoperative weeks 14 to 26 and begins the preparation for return to sports training. During this stage, strength training will be advanced to plyometric loading.

Criteria for Return to Activity

Return to full activity should be based on these criteria: (a) the patient has full AROM; (b) normal mechanics have been restored in the shoulder complex; (c) the patient has at least 90% strength in the involved shoulder compared to the uninvolved side; and, (d) there is no pain present during overhead activity.

Clinical Decision-Making Exercise 17-5

A 15-year-old female tennis player has been complaining of shoulder pain that stops her from completing her matches. The athletic trainer finds global scapular stabilizer weakness, as well as pain and weakness in her rotator cuff muscles. Her physician diagnoses shoulder impingement and rotator cuff tendinitis. An MRI revealed thickening of the supraspinatus and infraspinatus tendons. She is in the middle of her competitive tournament season and will begin her scholastic season in 3 months. What course should the athletic trainer recommend to ensure that her symptoms subside and she can compete successfully again?

Adhesive Capsulitis (Frozen Shoulder)

Pathomechanics

Adhesive capsulitis is characterized by the loss of motion at the glenohumeral joint. The cause of this arthrofibrosis is not well defined. One set of criteria used for diagnosis of a frozen shoulder was described by Jobe et al in 1996, and included: (a) decreased glenohumeral motion and loss of synchronous shoulder girdle motion; (b) restricted elevation (less than 135 degrees or 90 degrees, depending on the author); (c) external rotation 50% to 60% of normal; and (d) arthrogram findings of 5 to 10 mL volume with obliteration of the normal axillary fold.[52] Other authors have identified histologic changes in different areas surrounding the glenohumeral joint.[106] Travell and Simons explained that a reflex autonomic reaction could be the underlying cause, because of the presence of subscapularis trigger points.[118] The result is a chronic inflammation with fibrosis and rotator cuff muscles that are tight and inelastic.

Injury Mechanism

For the purposes of this chapter, we separate this diagnosis into two categories: primary vs secondary frozen shoulder. Adhesive capsulitis may be considered primary when it develops spontaneously; it is considered secondary when a known underlying condition (eg, a fractured humeral head) is present.

Primary frozen shoulder usually has an insidious onset. The patient often describes a sequence of painful restrictions in his or her shoulder, followed by a gradual stiffness with less pain. Factors that have been found to predispose a patient to idiopathic capsulitis include diabetes, hypothyroidism, and underlying cardiopulmonary involvement.[106] These factors were identified through epidemiologic studies and might have more to do with characteristic personalities of these patients. It is rare to see this type of frozen shoulder in the athletic population.

Secondary frozen shoulder is more commonly seen in the athletic population. It is associated with many different underlying diagnoses. Rockwood and Matsen listed eight categories of conditions that should be considered in the differential diagnosis of frozen shoulder: trauma, other soft-tissue disorders about the shoulder, joint disorders, bone disorders, cervical spine disorders, intrathoracic disorders, abdominal disorders, and psychogenic disorder (Table 17-3).[99]

Rehabilitation Concerns

The primary concern for rehabilitation is proper differential diagnosis. Attempting to progress the patient into the strength or functional activities portion of a rehabilitation program can lead to exacerbation of the motion restriction. The single best treatment for adhesive capsulitis is prevention.

Depending on the stage of pathology when intervention is started, the rehabilitation program time frame can be shortened. In all cases, the goals of rehabilitation are the same: first relieving the pain in the acute stages of the disorder, gradually restoring proper arthrokinematics, gradually restoring ROM, and strengthening the muscles of the shoulder complex.

Rehabilitation Progression

In the acute phase, Codman's exercises and low-grade joint mobilization techniques can be used to relieve pain. This may be accompanied by therapeutic modalities and passive stretching of the upper trapezius and levator scapulae muscles. The athletic trainer may also want to suggest that the patient sleep with a pillow under the involved arm to prevent internal rotation during sleep.

Table 17-3 Differential Diagnosis of Frozen Shoulder

Trauma
Fractures of the shoulder region
Fractures anywhere in the upper extremity
Misdiagnosed posterior shoulder dislocation
Hemarthrosis of shoulder secondary to trauma

Other Soft-Tissue Disorders about the Shoulder
Tendinitis of the rotator cuff
Tendinitis of the long head of biceps
Subacromial bursitis
Impingement
Suprascapular nerve impingement
Thoracic outlet syndrome

Joint Disorders
Degenerative arthritis of the AC joint
Degenerative arthritis of the glenohumeral joint
Septic arthritis
Other painful forms of arthritis

Bone Disorders
Avascular necrosis of the humeral head
Metastatic cancer
Paget disease
Primary bone tumor
Hyperparathyroidism

Cervical Spine Disorders
Cervical spondylosis
Cervical disc herniation
Infection

Intrathoracic Disorder
Diaphragmatic irritation
Pancoast tumor
Myocardial infarction

Abdominal Disorder
Gastric ulcer
Cholecystitis
Subphrenic abscess

Psychogenic

Adapted with permission from Rockwood CA, Matsen FA. *The Shoulder*. Philadelphia, PA: WB Saunders; 1990.

In the subacute phase, ROM is more aggressively addressed. Incorporating PNF techniques such as hold-relax can be helpful. Progressive demands should be placed on the patient with rhythmic stabilization techniques. Wall climbing (Figure 17-8) and wall/corner stretches (Figure 17-10) are also good additions to the rehabilitation program. As ROM returns, the program should start to address strengthening. Isometric exercises for the shoulder are often the best way to begin. Progressive strengthening will continue in the next phase.

The final phase of rehabilitation is a progressive strengthening of the shoulder complex. Exercises for maintenance of ROM continue, and a series of strengthening exercises should be added. The rehabilitation program should be tailored to meet the needs of the patient based on the differential diagnosis.

Criteria for Return to Activity

The patient may return to his or her previous level of activity once the proper physiologic and arthrokinematic motion has been restored to the glenohumeral joint. How long the patient went untreated and undiagnosed affects how long it takes to reach this point.

Thoracic Outlet Syndrome

Pathomechanics

Thoracic outlet syndrome is the compression of neurovascular structures within the thoracic outlet. The thoracic outlet is a cone-shaped passage, with the greater circumferential opening proximal to the spine and the narrow end passing into the distal extremity. On the proximal end, the cone is bordered anteriorly by the anterior scalene muscles, and posteriorly by the middle and posterior scalene muscles. Structures traveling through the thoracic outlet are the brachial plexus, subclavian artery and vein, and axillary vessels. The neurovascular structures pass distally under the clavicle and subclavius muscle. Beneath the neurovascular bundle is the first rib. At the narrow end of the cone, the bundle passes under the coracoid process of the scapula and into the upper extremity through the axilla. The distal end is bordered anteriorly by the pectoralis minor and posteriorly by the scapula.

Based on the anatomy of the thoracic outlet, there are several areas where neurovascular compression can occur. Therefore, pathology of the thoracic outlet syndrome is dependent on the structures being compressed.

Injury Mechanism

In 60% of the population affected by thoracic outlet syndrome, there is no report from the patient of an inciting episode.[64] Some of the theories presented by authors regarding the etiology of thoracic outlet syndrome include trauma, postural components, shortening of the pectoralis minor, shortening of the scalenes, and muscle hypertrophy.

There are four areas of vulnerability to compressive forces: the superior thoracic outlet, where the brachial plexus passes over the first rib; the scalene triangle, at the proximal end of the thoracic outlet, where there might be overlapping insertions of the anterior and middle scalenes onto the first rib; the costoclavicular interval, which is the space between the first rib and clavicle where the neurovascular bundle passes (the space can be narrowed by poor posture, inferior laxity of the glenohumeral joint, or an exostosis from a fracture of the clavicle); and under the coracoid process where the brachial plexus passes and is bordered anteriorly by the pectoralis minor.[106]

Rehabilitation Concerns

As described, thoracic outlet syndrome is an anatomy-based problem involving compressive forces applied to the neurovascular bundle. Conservative management of thoracic outlet syndrome is moderately successful, resulting in decreased symptoms 50% to 90% of the time. As the first course of treatment, rehabilitation should be based on encouraging the least provocative posture. Leffert advocated a detailed history and evaluation of the patient's activities and lifestyle to help identify where and when postural deficiency is occurring.[64]

Through a detailed history and evaluation of a patient's activity, the athletic trainer can identify the cause of compression in the thoracic outlet. The rehabilitation program should be tailored to encourage good posture throughout the patient's day. Therapeutic exercises should be used to strengthen postural muscles, such as the rhomboids (Figure 17-38), middle trapezius (Figure 17-37), and upper trapezius (Figure 17-35). Flexibility exercises are also used to increase the space in the thoracic outlet. Scalene stretches and wall/corner stretches (Figure 17-10) are used to decrease the incidence of muscle impinging on the neurovascular bundle. Proper breathing technique should also be reviewed with the patient. The scalene muscles act as accessory breathing muscles, and improper breathing technique can lead to tightening of these muscles.

Rehabilitation Progression

The rehabilitation process begins by detailed evaluation of the patient's activities and symptoms. First, the patient is removed from activities exacerbating the neurovascular symptoms until the patient can maintain a symptom-free posture. During this time, an erect posture is encouraged using stretching and strengthening exercises. Gradually encourage the patient to return to the his or her sport, for short periods, while maintaining a pain-free posture. The time of participation is increased at regular intervals if the patient remains free of pain. This helps build endurance of the postural muscles. Exercising on an upper-body ergometer, by pedaling backward, can help build endurance. As the patient returns to sports it may be necessary to alter strength-training methods that place the patient in a flexed posture.

Criteria for Return to Activity

If the patient responds to the rehabilitation program and can maintain a pain-free posture during the patient's sport specific activity, participation can be resumed. The patient should have no muscular weakness, neurovascular symptoms, or pain. If the patient fails to respond to therapy, and functionally significant pain and weakness persist, surgical intervention might be indicated. Surgical procedure depends on the anatomical basis for the patient's symptoms.

Clinical Decision-Making Exercise 17-6

A 19-year-old tennis player has been complaining of paresthesia in his dominant (right) arm for about 3 weeks. He does not remember doing anything that might have injured his shoulder but thinks this symptom started shortly after classes began this semester. When asked if anything in his normal routine had changed, he revealed that he had changed to a new racquet and was having to do a lot more work with a mouse on a computer. The patient was seen by a physician and diagnosed with thoracic outlet syndrome. The patient also reports symptoms occurring whenever he strikes a tennis ball with his forehand stroke. What can the athletic trainer recommend to help this patient recover?

Brachial Plexus Injuries (Stinger or Burner)

Pathomechanics

The brachial plexus begins at cervical roots C5 through C8 and thoracic root T1. The ventral rami of these roots are formed from a dorsal (sensory) and ventral (motor) root. The ventral rami join to form the brachial plexus. The ventral rami lie between the anterior and middle scalene muscles, where they run adjacent to the subclavian artery. The plexus continues distally passing over the first rib. It is deep to the sternocleidomastoid muscle in the neck.[86] Just caudal to the clavicle and subclavius muscle, the five ventral rami unite to form the three trunks of the plexus: superior, middle, and inferior. The superior trunk is composed of the C5 and C6 ventral roots. The middle trunk is formed by the C7 root, and the inferior trunk is formed by C8 and T1 ventral roots. After passing under the clavicle, the three trunks divide into three divisions that eventually contribute to the three cords of the brachial plexus.

The typical picture of a brachial plexus injury in sports is that of a traction injury. This syndrome is commonly referred to as burner or stinger syndrome. These injuries usually involve the C5 to C6 nerve roots. The patient will complain of a sharp, burning pain in the shoulder that radiates down the arm into the hand. Weakness in the muscles supplied by C5 and C6 (deltoid, biceps, supraspinatus, and infraspinatus) accompany the pain. Burning and pain are often transient, but weakness might last a few minutes or indefinitely.

Clancy et al classified brachial plexus injuries into three categories.[20] A grade I injury results in a transient loss of motor and sensory function that usually resolves completely within minutes. A grade II injury results in significant motor weakness and sensory loss that might last from 6 weeks to 4 months. Electromyography evaluation after 2 weeks will demonstrate abnormalities. Grade III lesions are characterized by motor and sensory loss for at least 1 year in duration.

Injury Mechanism

The structure of the brachial plexus is such that it winds its way through the musculoskeletal anatomy of the upper extremity as described. Clancy et al identified neck rotation, neck lateral flexion, shoulder abduction, shoulder external rotation, and simultaneous scapular and clavicular depression as potential mechanisms of injury.[20]

During neck rotation and lateral flexion to one side, the brachial plexus and the subclavius muscle on the opposite side are put on stretch and the clavicle is slightly elevated about its anteroposterior axis. If the arm is not elevated, the superior trunk of the plexus will assume the greatest amount of tension. If the shoulder is abducted and externally rotated, the brachial plexus migrates superiorly toward the coracoid process and the scapula retracts, putting the pectoralis minor on stretch. As the shoulder is moved into full abduction, a condition similar to a movable pulley is formed, where the coracoid process of the scapula acts as the pulley. In full abduction, most stress falls on the lower cords of the brachial plexus.[107] The addition of clavicular and scapula depression to the above scenarios would produce a downward force on the pulley system, bringing the brachial plexus into contact with the clavicle and the coracoid process. The portion of the plexus that receives the greatest amount of tensile stress depends on the position of the upper extremity during a collision.

Rehabilitation Concerns

Management of brachial plexus injuries begins with the gradual restoration of the patient's cervical ROM. Muscle tightness caused by the direct trauma, and by reflexive guarding that occurs because of pain, needs to be addressed. Gentle passive ROM exercises and stretching for the upper trapezius, levator scapulae, and scalene muscles should be done. The athletic trainer should be careful not to cause sensory symptoms.

Butler advocates using an early intervention with gentle mobilization of the neural tissues.[17] The goal of early mobilization is to prevent scarring between the nerve and the bed or within the connective tissue of the nerve itself as the nerve heals. He advocates low tensile loads to avoid the possibility of irritating a nerve lesion such as axonotmesis or neurotmesis. More chronic, repetitive injuries may use the neural tension test positions to do mobilizations with higher grades.

Strengthening of the involved muscles is also addressed in the rehabilitation program. Supraspinatus strengthening exercises, like scaption (Figure 17-33) and alternative supraspinatus exercises (Figure 17-34), should be performed. Other exercises for involved musculature are shoulder lateral rotation (Figure 17-32) for the infraspinatus, forward flexion and abduction to 90 degrees (Figures 17-26 and 17-28) to strengthen the deltoid, and bicep curls for elbow flexion.

The athletic trainer should also work closely with the patient's coach to evaluate the patient's technique and correct any alteration in form that might put the patient at risk for burners. Prior to return to activity, the patient's equipment should be inspected for proper fitting, and a cervical neck roll should be used to decrease the amount of lateral flexion that occurs during impact, as in tackling.

Rehabilitation Progression

The patient is removed from activity immediately after the injury. The rehabilitation progression should begin with the restoration of both AROM and PROM at the neck and shoulder. Neural tissue mobilizations using the upper limb tension testing positions should begin with the patient in the testing positions (Figure 8-4A and B).[17] For the median nerve, the testing position consists of shoulder depression, abduction, external rotation, and wrist and finger extension. For the radial nerve, the elbow is extended, the forearm pronated, the glenohumeral joint internally rotated, and the wrist, finger, and thumb flexed. The position for stretching the ulnar nerve consists of shoulder depression, wrist and finger extension, supination or pronation of the forearm, and elbow flexion. Mobilizations of distal joints, like the elbow and wrist, in large-grade movements should initiate the treatment phase. Progression should include grade 4 and grade 5 mobilizations in later phases of recovery.

As the patient regains ROM, strengthening of the neck and shoulder is incorporated into the rehabilitation program. Strengthening should progress from PRE-type strengthening with free weights to exercises that emphasize power and endurance. Functional progression begins with teaching proper technique for sport-specific demands that mimic the position of injury. The progressive return and proper technique are important to the rehabilitation program as they address the psychological component of preparing the patient for return to sport.

Criteria for Return to Activity

Patients are allowed to return to play when they have full, pain-free ROM, full strength, and no prior episodes in that context.[124] Additionally, football players should use a cervical neck roll. The patient's psychological readiness should also be considered prior to return to sport. Patients who are too protective of their neck and shoulder can expose themselves to further injury.

Myofascial Trigger Points

Pathology

Clinically, a trigger point (TP) is defined as a hyperirritable foci in muscle or fascia that is tender to palpation and may, upon compression, result in referred pain or tenderness in a characteristic "zone." This zone is distinct from myotomes, dermatomes, sclerotomes, or peripheral nerve distribution. TPs are identified via palpation of taut bands of muscle or discrete nodules or adhesions. Snapping of a taut band will usually initiate a local twitch response.[106]

Physiologically, the definition of a TP is not as clear. Muscles with myofascial TPs reveal no diagnostic abnormalities upon electromyographic examination. Routine laboratory tests show no abnormalities or significant changes attributable to TPs. Normal serum enzyme concentrations have been reported with a shift in the distribution of lactate dehydrogenaseisoenzymes. Skin temperature over active TPs might be higher in a 5- to 10-cm diameter.[118]

Travell and Simons classify TPs as follows:[118]

1. Active TPs. Symptomatic at rest with referral pain and tenderness upon direct compression. Associated weakness and contracture are often present.

2. Latent TPs. Pain is not present unless direct compression is applied. These might show up on clinical exam as stiffness and/or weakness in the region of tenderness.

3. Primary TPs. Located in specific muscles.

4. Associated TPs. Located within the referral zone of a primary TP's muscle or in a muscle that is functionally overloaded in compensation for a primary TP.

Pathology of a myofascial TP is identified with (a) a history of sudden onset during or shortly after an acute overload stress or chronic overload of the affected muscle; (b) characteristic patterns of pain in a muscle's referral zone; (c) weakness and restriction in the end ROM of the affected muscle; (d) a taut, palpable band in the affected muscle; (e) focal tenderness to direct compression in the band of taut muscle fibers; (f) a local twitch response elicited by snapping of the tender spot; and, (g) reproduction of the patient's pain through pressure on the tender spot.

Injury Mechanism

The most common mechanism for myofascial TPs in the shoulder region is acute muscle strain (Table 17-4). The damaged muscle tissue causes tearing of the sarcoplasmic reticulum and release of its stored calcium, with loss of the ability of that portion of the muscle to remove calcium ions. The chronic stress of sustained muscle contraction can cause continued muscle damage, repeating the above cycle of damage. The presence of the normal muscle adenosine triphosphate and excessive calcium initiate and

Table 17-4 Trigger Points of the Shoulder

Posterior Shoulder Pain
Deltoid
Levator scapulae
Supraspinatus
Subscapularis
Teres minor
Teres major
Serratus posterior superior
Triceps
Trapezius
Anterior Shoulder Pain
Infraspinatus
Deltoid
Scalene
Supraspinatus
Pectoralis major
Pectoralis minor
Biceps
Coracobrachialis
Source: Data from Travell and Simons.[118]

maintain a sustained muscle band contracture. This produces a region of the muscle with an uncontrolled metabolism, to which the body responds with local vasoconstriction. This region of increased metabolism and decreased local circulation, with muscle fibers passing through that area, causes muscle shortening independent of local motor unit action potentials. This taut band can be palpated in the muscle.

Rehabilitation Concerns

The principal mechanism of myofascial TPs is related to muscular overload and fatigue, so the primary concern is identification of the incriminating activity. The athletic trainer should take a detailed history of the patient's daily activity demands, as well as the changing demands of the patient's sport activities.

The cyclic nature of TPs requires interruption of the cycle for successful treatment. Interrupting the shortening of the muscle fibers and prevention of further breakdown of the muscle tissue components should be attempted using modified hold-relax techniques and post isometric stretching. Travell and Simons advocate a spray-and-stretch method, where vapocoolant spray is applied and passive stretching follows. Theoretically, when the muscle is placed in a stretched position and the skin receptors are cooled, a reflexive inhibition of the contracted muscle is facilitated, allowing for increased passive stretching.[118]

After a treatment session where PROM has been achieved, the muscle must be activated to stimulate normal actin and myosin cross bridging. Gentle AROM exercises or active assistive exercises with the L-bar might be a good activity to use as post treatment activity. Normal muscle activity and endurance must be encouraged after ROM is restored. A gradual progression of shoulder exercises with an endurance emphasis should be used.

Rehabilitation Progression

Treatment progression for TPs should begin with temporary removal from activities that overload the contracted tissue. The patient is then treated with myofascial stretching techniques, including positional release and Active Release Technique, to increase the length of the contracted tissue (see Chapter 8). Immediate use of the extended ROM should be emphasized. Strengthening exercises are added once the patient can maintain the normal muscle length without initiating the return of the contracted myofascial band. As strength and function of the involved muscles return, the patient may gradually return to the patient's sport.

Criteria for Return to Activity

The patient may return to activity in a relatively short time if the patient can demonstrate the ability to function without reinitiating the myofascial TPs and associated taut bands. Early return without meeting this criterion can lead to greater regionalization of the symptoms.

Summary

1. The high degree of mobility in the shoulder complex requires some compromise in stability, which, in turn, increases the vulnerability of the shoulder joint to injury, particularly in dynamic overhead athletic activities.

2. In rehabilitation of the SC joint, effort should be directed toward regaining normal clavicular motion that will allow the scapula to abduct and upward rotate throughout 180 degrees of humeral abduction. The clavicle must elevate about 40 degrees to allow upward scapular rotation.

3. AC joint sprains are most commonly seen in patients who experienced a direct fall on the point of the shoulder with the arm at the side in an adducted position or falling on an outstretched arm.

4. Management of AC injuries depends on the type of injury. Types I and II injuries are usually handled conservatively, focusing on strengthening of the deltoid, trapezius, and the clavicular fibers of the pectoralis major. Occasionally AC injuries require surgical excision of the distal portion of the clavicle.

5. Treatment for clavicle fractures includes approximation of the fracture and immobilization for 6 to 8 weeks, using a figure 8 wrap with the involved arm in a sling. Because mobility of the clavicle is important for normal shoulder mechanics, rehabilitation should focus on joint mobilization and strengthening of the deltoid, upper trapezius, and pectoralis major muscles.

6. Following a short immobilization period, rehabilitation for a dislocated shoulder should focus on restoring the appropriate axis of rotation for the glenohumeral joint, optimizing the stabilizing muscle's length–tension relationship, and restoring proper neuromuscular control of the shoulder complex. Similar rehabilitation strategies are applied in cases of multidirectional instabilities, which can occur as a result of recurrent dislocation.

7. Management of shoulder impingement involves gradually restoring normal biomechanics to the shoulder joint in an effort to maintain space under the coracoacromial arch during overhead activities. Techniques include strengthening of the rotator cuff muscles, strengthening of the muscles that abduct, elevate, and upwardly rotate the scapula, and stretching both the inferior and the posterior portions of the joint capsule and posterior rotator cuff musculature.

8. The basic concerns of a rehabilitation program for rotator cuff tendinopathy are based on why and how the tendon has been damaged. If a comprehensive rehabilitation program does not relieve the painful shoulder, surgical repair of the tendon and alteration of the glenohumeral joint are performed. Surgical rehabilitation is similar to the nonsurgical plan, with the time of progression altered, based on tissue healing and tendon histology.

9. In cases of adhesive capsulitis, the goals of rehabilitation are relieving the pain in the acute stages of the disorder, gradually restoring proper arthrokinematics, gradual restoration of ROM, and strengthening the muscles of the shoulder complex.

10. Rehabilitation for thoracic outlet syndrome should be directed toward encouraging the least-provocative posture combined with exercises to strengthen postural muscles (rhomboids, middle trapezius, upper trapezius) and stretching exercises for the scalenes to increase the space in the thoracic outlet to reduce muscle impingement on the neurovascular bundle.

11. Management of brachial plexus injuries includes the gradual restoration of cervical ROM, and stretching for the upper trapezius, levator scapulae, and scalene muscles.

12. After identifying the cause of myofascial TPs, rehabilitation may include a spray- and stretch method with passive

stretching, gentle active ROM exercises or active assistive exercises, encouraging normal muscle activity and endurance, and gradual improvement of muscle endurance.

References

1. Allman FL. Fractures and ligamentous injuries of the clavicle and its articulations. *J Bone Joint Surg Am.* 1967;49:774.

2. Anderson L, Rush R, Shearer L. The effects of a TheraBand exercise program on shoulder internal rotation strength. *Phys Ther Suppl.* 1992;72(6):540.

3. Andrews JR, Wilk EK, eds. *The Athlete's Shoulder.* New York, NY: Churchill Livingstone; 1994.

4. Barden JM, Balyk R, Raso VJ, Moreau M, Bagnall K. Dynamic upper limb proprioception in multidirectional shoulder instability. *Clin Orthop.* 2004;420:181-189.

5. Bateman JE. *The Shoulder and Neck.* Philadelphia, PA: WB Saunders; 1971.

6. Bergfeld JA, Andrish JT, Clancy GW. Evaluation of the acromioclavicular joint following first and second degree sprains. *Am J Sports Med.* 1978;6:153.

7. Bigliani L, Kimmel J, McCann P. Repair of rotator cuff tears in tennis players. *Am J Sports Med.* 1992;20(2):112-117.

8. Bigliani L, Morrison D, April E. The morphology of the acromion and its relation to rotator cuff tears. *Orthop Transcr.* 1986;10:216.

9. Blackburn T, McCloud W, White B. EMG analysis of posterior rotator cuff exercises. *Athl Train.* 1990;25(1):40-45.

10. Blasier RB, Carpenter JE, Huston LJ. Shoulder proprioception: effects of joint laxity, joint position, and direction of motion. *Orthop Rev.* 1994;23(1):45-50.

11. Borich MR, Bright JM, Lorello DJ, Cieminski CJ, Buisman T, Ludewig PM. Scapular angular positioning at end range internal rotation in cases of glenohumeral internal rotation deficit. *J Orthop Sports Phys Ther.* 2006;36(12):926-934.

12. Borstad JD. Resting position variables at the shoulder: evidence to support a posture-impairment association. *Phys Ther.* 2006;86(4):549-557.

13. Borstad JD, Ludewig MP. The effect of long versus short pectoralis minor resting length on scapular kinematics in healthy individuals. *J Orthop Sports Phys Ther.* 2005;35(4):227-238.

14. Brewster C, Moynes D. Rehabilitation of the shoulder following rotator cuff injury or surgery. *J Orthop Sports Phys Ther.* 1993;17(2):422-426.

15. Burkhart SS, Esch JC, Jolson RS. The rotator crescent and rotator cable: An anatomic description of the shoulder's "suspension bridge." *Arthroscopy.* 1993;9:611-616.

16. Burkhead W, Rockwood C. Treatment of instability of rotator cuff injuries in the overhead athlete. *J Bone Joint Surg Am.* 1992;74:890.

17. Butler D. *The Sensitive Nervous System.* Adelaide, Australia: Noigroup; 2000.

18. Caprise PA Jr, Sekiya JK. Open and arthroscopic treatment of multidirectional instability of the shoulder. *Arthroscopy.* 2006;22(10):1126-1131.

19. Carpenter JE, Thomopoulos S, Flanagan CL, DeBano CM, Soslowsky LJ. Rotator cuff defect healing: a biomechanical and histologic analysis in an animal model. *J Shoulder Elbow Surg.* 1998;7:599-605.

20. Clancy WG, Brand RI, Bergfeld AJ. Upper trunk brachial plexus injuries in contact sports. *Am J Sports Med.* 1977;5:209.

21. Clark JM, Harryman DT. Tendons, ligaments, and capsule of the rotator cuff: gross and microscopic anatomy. *J Bone Joint Surg Am.* 1992;74:713-725.

22. Codman EA. Ruptures of the supraspinatus tendon and other lesions in or about the subacromial bursa. In: Codman EA, ed. *The Shoulder.* Boston, MA: Thomas Todd; 1934.

23. Cools AM, Witvrouw EE, DeClercq GA, Voight LM. Scapular muscle recruitment pattern: EMG response of the trapezius muscle to the sudden shoulder movement before and after a fatiguing exercise. *J Orthop Sports Phys Ther.* 2002;32(5):221-229.

24. Cooper DE, O'Brien, SJ, Warren RF. Supporting layers of the glenohumeral joint: an anatomic study. *Clin Orthop.* 1993;(289):144-155.

25. Covey, Bahu AM, Ahmad C. Arthroscopic posterior/multidirectional instability. *Oper Tech Orthop.* 2008;18:33-45.

26. Cox JS. The fate of the acromioclavicular joint in athletic injuries. *Am J Sports Med.* 1981;9:50.

27. Culham E, Malcolm P. Functional anatomy of the shoulder complex. *J Orthop Sports Phys Ther.* 1993;18(1): 342-350.

28. Davies G, Dickoff-Hoffman S. Neuromuscular testing and rehabilitation of the shoulder complex. *J Orthop Sports Phys Ther.* 1993;18(2):449-458.

29. Depalma AF. *Surgery of the Shoulder.* 2nd ed. Philadelphia, PA: Lippincott; 1973.

30. Downar JM, Sauers EL. Clinical measures of shoulder mobility in the professional baseball player. *J Athl Train.* 2005;40(1):23-29.

31. Dvir Z, Berme N. The shoulder complex in elevation of the arm: a mechanism approach. *J Biomech.* 1978;11:219-225.

32. Ebaugh DD, McClure PW, Karduna AR. Effects of shoulder muscle fatigue caused by repetitive overhead activities on scapulothoracic and glenohumeral kinematics. *J Electromyogr Kinesiol.* 2006;16(3):224-235.

33. Ebaugh DD, McClure PW, Karduna AR. Scapulothoracic and glenohumeral kinematics following an external rotation fatigue protocol. *J Orthop Sports Phys Ther.* 2006;36(8):557-571.

34. Ellenbecker, T. 2006. *Shoulder Rehabilitation: Non-operative treatment.* New York, Thieme Publishers.

35. Endo K, Ikata T, Katoh S, Takeda Y. Radiographic assessment of scapular rotational tilt in chronic shoulder impingement syndrome. *J Orthop Sci.* 2001;6(1):3-10.

36. Favorito P, Langenderfer M, Colosimo A, Heidt R Jr, Carlonas R. Arthroscopic laser-assisted capsular shift in the treatment of patients with multidirectional shoulder instability. Am J Sports Med. 2002;30:322-328.

37. Fayad F, Roby-Brami A, Yazbeck C, et al. Three-dimensional scapular kinematics and scapulohumeral rhythm in patients with glenohumeral osteoarthritis or frozen shoulder. *J Biomech.* 2008;41(2):326-332.

38. Gerber C, Schneeberger AG, Beck M, Schlegel U. Mechanical strength of repairs of the rotator cuff. *J Bone Joint Surg Br.* 1994;76:371-380.

39. Greenfield B. Special considerations in shoulder exercises: plane of the scapula. In: Andrews J, Wilk K, eds. *The Athlete's Shoulder.* New York, NY: Churchill Livingstone; 1993.

40. Gryzlo SM. Bony disorders: clinical assessment and treatment. In: Jobe FW, ed. *Operative Techniques in Upper Extremity Sports Injuries.* St. Louis, MO: Mosby; 1996.

41. Hageman P, Mason D, Rydlund K. Effects of position and speed on concentric isokinetic testing of the shoulder rotators. *J Orthop Sports Phys Ther.* 1989;11:64-69.

42. Hart DL, Carmichael SW. Biomechanics of the shoulder. *J Orthop Sports Phys Ther.* 1985;6(4):229-234.

43. Hawkins R, Bell R. Dynamic EMG analysis of the shoulder muscles during rotational and scapular strengthening exercises. In: Post M, Morey B, Hawkins R, eds. *Surgery of the Shoulder.* St. Louis, MO: Mosby; 1990.

44. Hawkins R, Kennedy J. Impingement syndrome in athletes. *Am J Sports Med.* 1980;8:151.

45. Hawkins RJ, Krishnan SG, Karas SG, Noonan TJ, Horan MP. Electrothermal arthroscopic shoulder capsulorrhaphy: a minimum 2-year follow-up. *Am J Sports Med.* 2007;35(9):1484-1488.

46. Hirose K, Kondo S, Choi HR, Mishima S, Iwata H, Ishiguro N. Spontaneous healing process of a supra-spinatus tendon tear in rabbits. *Arch Orthop Trauma Surg.* 2004;124(9):647.

47. Howell S, Kraft T. The role of the supraspinatus and infraspinatus muscles in glenohumeral kinematics of anterior shoulder instability. *Clin Orthop.* 1991;263:128-134.

48. Inman VT, Saunders JB, Abbott CL. Observations on the function of the shoulder joint. *J Bone Joint Surg.* 1996;26:1.

49. Jobe FW, ed. *Operative Techniques in Upper Extremity Sports Injuries.* St. Louis, MO: Mosby; 1996.

50. Jobe FW, Kvitne RS, Giangarra CE. Shoulder pain in the overhand and throwing athletes. The relationship of anterior instability and rotator cuff impingement. *Orthop Rev.* 1989;18:963-975.

51. Jobe F, Moynes D. Delineation of diagnostic criteria and a rehabilitation program for rotator cuff injuries. *Am J Sports Med.* 1982;10(6):336-339.

52. Jobe FW, Schwab, Wilk KE, Andrews EJ. Rehabilitation of the shoulder. In: Brotzman SB, ed. *Clinical Orthopedics Rehabilitation.* St. Louis, MO: Mosby; 1996.

53. Kannus P, Josza L, Renstrom P, et al. The effects of training, immobilization and remobilization on musculoskeletal tissue: 2. Remobilization and prevention of immobilization atrophy. *Scand J Med Sci Sports.* 1992;2:164-176.

54. Karduna AR, McClure PW, Michener LA, Sennett B. Dynamic measurements of three-dimensional scapular kinematics: a validation study. *J Biomech Eng.* 2001;123(2):184-190.

55. Keirns M. Nonoperative treatment of shoulder impingement. In: Andrews J, Wilk K, eds. *The Athlete's Shoulder.* New York, NY: Churchill Livingstone; 2008:527-544.

56. Kelley MJ. Anatomic and biomechanical rationale for rehabilitation of the athlete's shoulder. *J Sport Rehabil.* 1995;4:122-154.

57. Kibler WB, McMullen J, Uhl T. Shoulder rehabilitation strategies, guidelines, and practice. *Orthop Clin North Am.* 2001;32:527-538.

58. Kibler WB. Role of the scapula in the overhead throwing motion. *Contemp Orthop.* 1998;22:525-532.

59. Kibler WB. The role of the scapula in athletic shoulder function. *Am J Sports Med.* 1998;26(2):325-337.

60. Kluemper M, Uhl TL, Hazelrigg H. Effect of stretching and strengthening shoulder muscles of forward shoulder posture in competitive swimmers. *J Sport Rehabil.* 2006;15:58-70.

61. Laudner KG, Myers JB, Pasquale MR, Bradley JP, Lephart SM. Scapular dysfunction in throwers with pathologic internal impingement. *J Orthop Sports Phys Ther.* 2006;36(7):485-494.

62. Laudner KG, Sipes RC, Wilson JT. The acute effects of sleeper stretches on shoulder range of motion. *J Athl Train.* 2008;43(4):359-363.

63. Laudner KG, Stanek JM, Meister K. Differences in scapular upward rotation between baseball pitchers and position players. *Am J Sports Med.* 2007;35(12):2091-2095.

64. Leffert RD. Neurological problems. In: Rockwood CA, Matsen FA, eds. *The Shoulder.* Philadelphia, PA: WB Saunders; 1990.

65. Lephart SM, Warner JP, Borsa PA, Fu HF. Proprioception of the shoulder joint in healthy, unstable, and surgically repaired shoulders. *J Shoulder Elbow Surg.* 1994;3(6):371-380.

66. Lew W, Lewis J, Craig E. Stabilization by capsule ligaments and labrum: stability at the extremes of motion. In: Masten F, Fu F, Hawkins R, eds. *The Shoulder: A Balance of Mobility and Stability.* Rosemont, IL: American Academy of Orthopedic Surgery; 1993.

67. Lewis CW, Schlegel TF, Hawkins RJ, James SP, Turner AS. The effect of immobilization on rotator cuff healing using modified Mason-Allen stitches: a biomechanical study in sheep. *Biomed Sci Instrum.* 2001;37:263-268.

68. Litchfield R, Hawkins R, Dillman C. Rehabilitation for the overhead athlete. *J Orthop Sports Phys Ther.* 1993;18(2):433-441.

69. Ludewig PM, Cook TM. Alterations in shoulder kinematics and associated muscle activity in people with symptoms of shoulder impingement. *Phys Ther.* 2000;80(3):276-291.

70. Ludewig PM, Cook MT. Translations of the humerus in persons with shoulder impingement syndromes. *J Orthop Sports Phys Ther.* 2002;32(6):248-259.

71. Lukasiewicz AC, McClure P, Michener L, Pratt N, Sennett B. Comparison of 3-dimensional scapular position and orientation between subjects with and without shoulder impingement. *J Orthop Sports Phys Ther.* 1999;29(10):574-583, discussion 584-576.

72. Magee D, Reid D. Shoulder injuries. In: Zachazewski J, Magee D, Quillen W, eds. *Athletic Injuries and Rehabilitation.* Philadelphia, PA: WB Saunders; 1995:509-542.

73. Matsen FA, Thomas SC, Rockwood AC. Glenohumeral instability. In: Rockwood CA, Matsen FA, eds. *The Shoulder.* Philadelphia, PA: WB Saunders; 1990.

74. McCarroll J. Golf. In: Pettrone FA, ed. *Athletic Injuries of the Shoulder.* New York, NY: McGraw-Hill; 1995.

75. McClure P, Balaicuis J, Heiland D, Broersma ME, Thorndike CK, Wood A. A randomized controlled comparison of stretching procedures for posterior shoulder tightness. *J Orthop Sports Phys Ther.* 2007;37(3):108-114.

76. McClure PW, Michener LA, Sennett BJ, Karduna AR. Direct 3-dimensional measurement of scapular kinematics during dynamic movements in vivo. *J Shoulder Elbow Surg.* 2001;10(3):269-277.

77. McGough RL, Debski RE, Taskiran E, Fu FH, Woo SL. Mechanical properties of the long head of the biceps tendon. *Knee Surg Sports Traumatol Arthrosc.* 1996;3:226-229.

78. Meister K, Andrews RJ. Classification and treatment of rotator cuff injuries in the overhead athlete. *J Orthop Sports Phys Ther.* 1993;18(2):413-421.

79. Mell AG, LaScalza S, Guffey P, et al. Effect of rotator cuff pathology on shoulder rhythm. *J Shoulder Elbow Surg.* 2005;14(1 Suppl S):58S-64S.

80. Moseley J, Jobe F, Pink M. EMG analysis of the scapular muscles during a shoulder rehabilitation program. *Am J Sports Med.* 1992;20:128-134.

81. Mulligan E. Conservative management of shoulder impingement syndrome. *Athl Train.* 1988;23(4):348-353.

82. Myers JB, Hwang JH, Pasquale MR, Blackburn JT, Lephart SM. Rotator cuff coactivation ratios in participants with subacromial impingement syndrome. *J Sci Med Sport.* 2009;12(6):603-608.

83. Myers JB, Laudner KG, Pasquale MR, Bradley JP, Lephart SM. Scapular position and orientation in throwing athletes. *Am J Sports Med.* 2005;33(2):263-271.

84. Myers JB, Pasquale MR, Laudner KG, Sell TC, Bradley JP, Lephart SM. On-the-field resistance tubing exercises for throwers: an electromyographic analysis. *J Athl Train.* 2005;40(1):15-22.

85. Neer C. Anterior acromioplasty for the chronic impingement syndrome in the shoulder: a preliminary report. *J Bone Joint Surg Am.* 1972;54:41.

86. Nicholas JA, Hershmann BE, eds. *The Upper Extremity in Sports Medicine.* St. Louis, MO: Mosby; 1990.

87. O'Brien S, Neeves M, Arnoczky A. The anatomy and histology of the inferior glenohumeral ligament complex of the shoulder. *Am J Sports Educ.* 1990;18:451.

88. Ogston JB, Ludewig PM. Differences in 3-dimensional shoulder kinematics between persons with multidirectional instability and asymptomatic controls. *Am J Sports Med.* 2007;35(8):1361-1370.

89. Omer GE. Osteotomy of the clavicle in surgical reduction of anterior sternoclavicular dislocations. *J Trauma.* 1967;7(4):584-590.

90. Oyama S, Myers JB, Wassinger CA, Ricci RD, Lephart SM. Asymmetric resting scapular posture in healthy overhead athletes. *J Athl Train.* 2008;43(6):565-570.

91. Ozaki J, Fujimoto S, Nakagawa Y. Tears of the rotator cuff of the shoulder associated with pathological changes in the acromion: a study of cadavers. *J Bone Joint Surg Am.* 1988;70:1224.

92. Paine R, Voight M. The role of the scapula. *J Orthop Sports Phys Ther.* 1993;18(1):386-391.

93. Peat M, Culham E. Functional anatomy of the shoulder complex. In: Andrews J, Wilk K, eds. *The Athlete's Shoulder.* New York, NY: Churchill Livingstone; 1993.

94. Petersson C, Redlund-Johnell I. The subacromial space in normal shoulder radiographs. *Acta Orthop Scand.* 1984;55:57.

95. Pettrone FA, ed. *Athletic Injuries of the Shoulder.* New York, NY: McGraw-Hill; 1995.

96. Provencher M, Saldua N. The rotator interval of the shoulder: anatomy, biomechanics, and repair techniques. *Oper Tech Orthop.* 2008;18:9-22.

97. Rathbun J, McNab I. The microvascular pattern of the rotator cuff . *J Bone Joint Surg Br.* 1970;52:540.

98. Reilly P, Amis AA, Wallace AL, Emery RJ. Supraspinatus tears: propagation and strain alteration. *J Shoulder Elbow Surg.* 2003;12:134-138.

99. Rockwood C, Matsen F. *The Shoulder.* Philadelphia, PA: WB Saunders; 1990.

100. Rowe CR. Prognosis in dislocation of the shoulder. *J Bone Joint Surg Am.* 1956;38:957.

101. Rundquist PJ, Anderson DD, Guanche CA, Ludewig PM. Shoulder kinematics in subjects with frozen shoulder. *Arch Phys Med Rehabil.* 2003;84(10):1473-1479.

102. Salter EG, Shelley BS, Nasca R. A morphological study of the acromioclavicular joint in humans [abstract]. *Anat Rec.* 1985;211:353.

103. Scibek JS, Mell AG, Downie BK, Carpenter JE, Hughes RE. Shoulder kinematics in patients with full-thickness rotator cuff tears after a subacromial injection. *J Shoulder Elbow Surg.* 2007;17(1):172-181.

104. Skyhar M, Warren R, Altcheck D. Instability of the shoulder. In: Nicholas A, Hershmann BE, eds. *The Upper Extremity in Sports Medicine.* St. Louis, MO: Mosby; 1990.

105. Soslowsky LJ, Thomopoulos S, Esmail A, et al. Rotator cuff tendinosis in an animal model: role of extrinsic and overuse factors. *Ann Biomed Eng.* 2002;30: 1057-1063.

106. Souza TA. *Sports Injuries of the Shoulder: Conservative Management.* New York, NY: Churchill Livingstone; 1994.

107. Stevens JH. The classic brachial plexus paralysis. In: Codman EA, ed. *The Shoulder.* Boston, MA: Thomas Todd; 1934:344-350.

108. Su KP, Johnson MP, Gracely EJ, Karduna AR. Scapular rotation in swimmers with and without impingement syndrome: practice effects. *Med Sci Sports Exerc.* 2004;36(7):1121-1123.

109. Sutter JS. Conservative treatment of shoulder instability. In: Andrews J, Wilk EK, eds. *The Athlete's Shoulder.* New York, NY: Churchill Livingstone; 1994.

110. Swanik KA, Lephart SM, Swanik CB, Lephart SP, Stone DA, Fu FH. The effects of shoulder plyometric training on proprioception and selected muscle performance characteristics. *J Shoulder Elbow Surg.* 2002;11(6):579-586.

111. Swanik KA, Swanik CB, Lephart SM, Huxel K. The effect of functional training on the incidence of shoulder pain and strength in intercollegiate swimmers. *J Sport Rehabil.* 2002;11(2):140-154.

112. Taft TN, Wilson FC, Ogelsby JW. Dislocation of the AC joint, an end result study. *J Bone Joint Surg Am.* 1987;69:1045.

113. Takeda Y, Kashiwaguchi S, Endo K, Matsuura T, Sasa T. The most effective exercise for strengthening the supraspinatus muscle. *Am J Sports Med.* 2002;30:374-381.

114. Thein L. Impingement syndrome and its conservative management. *J Orthop Sports Phys Ther.* 1989;11(5):183-191.

115. Thomopoulos S, Williams GR, Soslowsky LJ. Tendon to bone healing: differences in biomechanical, structural, and compositional properties due to a range of activity levels. *J Biomech Eng.* 2003;125:106-113.

116. Thompson WO, Debski RE, Boardman ND, et al. A biomechanical analysis of rotator cuff deficiency in a cadaveric model. *Am J Sports Med.* 1996;24:286-292.

117. Townsend H, Jobe F, Pink M. EMG analysis of the glenohumeral muscles during a baseball rehabilitation program. *Am J Sports Med.* 1991;19(3):264-272.

118. Travell JG, Simons GD. *Myofascial Pain and Dysfunction: The Trigger Point Manual.* Baltimore, MD: Williams & Wilkins; 1983.

119. Tsai NT, McClure PW, Karduna AR. Effects of muscle fatigue on 3-dimensional scapular kinematics. *Arch Phys Med Rehabil.* 2003;84(7):1000-1005.

120. Uthoff H, Loeher J, Sarkar K. The pathogenesis of rotator cuff tears. In: Takagishi N, ed. *The Shoulder.* Philadelphia, PA: Professional Post Graduate Services; 1987.

121. Von Eisenhart-Rothe R, Jager A, Englmeier K, Vogl TJ, Graichen H. Relevance of arm position and muscle activity in three-dimensional glenohumeral translation in patients with traumatic and atraumatic shoulder instability. *Am J Sports Med.* 2002;30:514-522.

122. Warner JJ, Micheli LJ, Arslanian LE, Kennedy J, Kennedy R. Scapulothoracic motion in normal shoulders and shoulders with glenohumeral instability and impingement syndrome: a study using moire topographic analysis. *Clin Orthop.* 1992;(285):191-199.

123. Warner J, Michili L, Arslanin L. Patterns of flexibility, laxity, and strength in normal shoulders and shoulders with instability and impingement. *Am J Sports Med.* 1990;17(4):366-375.

124. Warren RF. Neurological injuries in football. In: Jordan BD, Tsiaris P, Warren FR, eds. *Sports Neurology.* Rockville, MD: Aspen; 1989.

125. Weiser WM, Lee TQ, McMaster WC, McMahon PJ. Effects of simulated scapular protraction on anterior glenohumeral stability. *Am J Sports Med.* 1999;27(6):801-805.

126. Wilk K, Andrews J. Rehabilitation following subacromial decompression. *Orthopedics.* 1993;16(3):349-358.

127. Wilk K, Arrigo C. An integrated approach to upper extremity exercises. *Orthop Phys Ther Clin N Am.* 1992;9(2):337-360.

128. Wilk K, Arrigo C. Current concepts in the rehabilitation of the athletic shoulder. *J Orthop Sports Phys Ther.* 1993;18(1):365-378.

129. Wilk K, Arrigo C. Current concepts in rehabilitation of the shoulder. In: Andrews J, Wilk K, eds. *The Athlete's Shoulder.* New York, NY: Churchill Livingstone; 1993.

130. Wilk KE, Arrigo CA, Andrews JR. Current concepts: the stabilizing structures of the glenohumeral joint. *J Orthop Sports Phys Ther.* 1997;25:364-379.

131. Wilk KE, Reinhold MM, Dugas JR, Andrews JR. Rehabilitation following thermal-assisted capsular shrinkage of the glenohumeral joint: current concepts. *J Orthop Sports Phys Ther.* 2002;32(6):268-287.

132. Wilk K, Voight M, Kearns M. Stretch shortening drills for the upper extremity: theory and application. *J Orthop Sports Phys Ther.* 1993;17(5):225-239.

SOLUTIONS TO CLINICAL DECISION-MAKING EXERCISES

17-1 The patient is treated for pain using modalities like ice and electrical stimulation. He is told to wear a sling for a few days, until he can tolerate pain and begins to carry his arm in an appropriate manner. The athletic trainer begins the patient's rehabilitation with active-assisted ROM. He is then progressed to isometric exercises for muscles with clavicle attachments. When the appropriate carrying posture for the involved upper extremity is restored, the patient's exercises are progressed to incorporate scapular motion. This will help prevent related shoulder discomfort due to poor glenohumeral mechanics. A patient with this injury can usually return to play earlier if a pad is fitted for the involved upper extremity and there is no deficit in strength or ROM.

17-2 It is important to understand that 80% of first-time dislocations have subsequent dislocations and go on to need surgical correction. The coach should expect full recovery to take as long as 12 weeks. He will need to avoid combined positioning of external rotation and abduction. He must strengthen his rotator cuff muscles aggressively and restore neuromuscular control to the joint. The athletic trainer should emphasize that the joint must now rely on the dynamic stabilizers of the joint. The coach will need to maintain a level of healthy strength even after he has returned to his normal activities, because the dynamic stabilizers must maintain a level of proprioceptive awareness that is different from the passive structures.

17-3 The athletic trainer should explain to the patient that pain should not be part of the rehabilitation process. The swimmer should stop swimming and all other overhead activities. Therapeutic modalities may be used to aid in patient comfort. NSAIDs are usually taken during the early stages of the rehabilitation process. Exercises should begin by restoring the arthrokinematics of the shoulder complex. Active strengthening exercises are focused on restoring force couples acting around the joint. The patient should not be progressed until the athletic trainer is assured that exercises can be performed pain-free. Strength progression begins with isometrics, advancing to isotonic exercises and then to plyometric exercises. Force couples around the scapula should be aggressively strengthened prior to addressing those involving the rotator cuff. PNF exercises should follow a restored, force-couple driven, shoulder complex. Gradual movement of exercises to a more functional position should be achieved. Once the patient can do exercises in a functional ROM without pain, a return to swimming can be sought. The return should be gradual and deliberate. Increases should be based on pain-free activity. This should continue until the swimmer is back to her normal regimen.

17-4 It is important for the athletic trainer to address the underlying instability prior to addressing the pain caused by impingement. Stretching of the rotator cuff is also emphasized early to normalize the effects of the tight structures. Rotator cuff exercises should be done in a closed kinetic chain position to ensure maximum congruity of the glenohumeral joint. A progression of neuromuscular control exercises should also begin. Once the patient's pain subsides, a progression of neuromuscular control exercises should be emphasized. Exercise should then be advanced to include more challenging exercises outside of the safe zone. Modalities can be used to improve comfort and stimulate the healing process. The pitcher should also be evaluated and treated for any other areas of his body that may be predisposing him to compensate for a lack of ROM during the acceleration portion of his throwing motion.

17-5 The athletic trainer should first work to evaluate and correct any biomechanical weaknesses that might diminish the dynamic stability of the glenohumeral joint. The athletic trainer must limit the player's activities to eliminate overhead motions. No painful activity should be undertaken during the rehabilitation process. Once the strength deficits in the patient's muscles have been negated, the athletic trainer should gradually return the patient to practice activities. Return should be gradual, controlling the load on the rotator cuff muscles and systematically increasing the frequency of the activity. It may be necessary to avoid any actions that place the shoulder in an impingement position, to give the inflammation a chance to subside. It should be noted that during the rehabilitation process neuromuscular control should be addressed to help avoid impingement due to excessive movement of the humeral head. Pain and stiffness should be guides for the progression of activity. Anti-inflammatories should be used in the early stages of rehabilitation to better allow the patient to perform strengthening exercises. The patient should not return to full activity until there is no longer a positive impingement sign.

17-6   It is important for the athletic trainer to identify where the thoracic outlet is being impinged. It is equally important to identify the causative factors in the patient's symptoms. This patient has postural tendencies for scapular abduction and increased forces about the shoulder complex. Using a mouse on a computer encourages a protracted scapular posture with pectoralis minor hyperactivity. Increased forces cause hypertrophy of the anterior musculature and greater reaction forces that are leading to impingement of the thoracic outlet under the coracoid process. To remove the stress on the thoracic outlet, the athletic trainer must first remove the causative factors. The patient should be educated on a more optimal posture for using a mouse for long periods. The patient should have his racquet restrung. Removal of the patient from tennis activities is recommended until the patient can maintain a symptom-free posture. The athletic trainer should then focus on lengthening the pectoralis minor muscle and encouraging postural exercises for the scapular stabilizers. Exercises should focus on scapular adductors and upward rotators. Rehabilitation should progress to activities that gradually place the patient's shoulder complex in a more functional position. A return to hitting should be gradual, with adequate recovery time between sessions. The patient should increase his workouts at regular intervals as long as he remains pain-free. This will allow him to build endurance for this appropriate posture. He may return to full activity when he is symptom-free while hitting the number of forehands he would hit in a regular tennis match. If the patient fails to progress, he should be sent back to the referring physician to explore surgical options.

Please see videos on the accompanying website at

www.healio.com/books/sportsmedvideos

CHAPTER 18

Rehabilitation of Elbow Injuries

Pete Zulia, PT, SCS, ATC
William E. Prentice, PhD, PT, ATC, FNATA

After completion of this chapter, the athletic training student should be able to do the following:

- Discuss the functional anatomy and biomechanics associated with normal function of the elbow.

- Identify and discuss the various rehabilitative strengthening techniques for the elbow, including both open and closed kinetic chain isometric, isotonic, plyometric, and isokinetic exercises.

- Identify the various techniques for regaining range of motion, including stretching exercises and joint mobilizations.

- Identify the use of aquatic therapy in elbow rehabilitation.

- Discuss exercises that may be used to reestablish neuromuscular control.

- Discuss criteria for progression of the rehabilitation program for different elbow injuries.

FUNCTIONAL ANATOMY AND BIOMECHANICS

Anatomically, the elbow joint is three joints in one. The humeroulnar joint, the humeroradial joint, and the proximal radioulnar joint are the articulations that make up the elbow complex. The elbow allows for flexion, extension, pronation, and supination movement patterns about the joint complex. The bony limitations, ligamentous support, and muscular stability will help to protect it from vulnerability of overuse and resultant injury. In the athletic environment, the elbow complex can be subjected to forces that can result in various injuries ranging from overhead throwing injuries to blunt trauma.

The elbow complex is composed of three bones: the distal humerus, proximal ulna, and proximal radius. The articulations between these three bones dictate elbow movement patterns.[43] It is also important to mention that the

Prentice WE, ed.
Rehabilitation Techniques for Sports Medicine and Athletic Training (pp 517-546).
© 2015 SLACK Incorporated.

Figure 18-1. The elbow carrying angle is an abducted position of the elbow in the anatomical position. The normal carrying angle in females is 10 to 15 degrees and in males, 5 degrees.

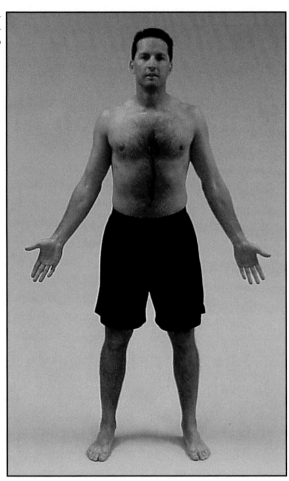

appropriate strength and function of the upper quarter (cervical spine to the hand) needs to be addressed when evaluating the elbow specifically. The elbow complex has an intricate articulation mechanically between the three separate joints of the upper quarter to allow for function to occur.

In the elbow, the joint capsule plays an important role. The capsule is continuous between the three articulations[29,31] and highly innervated. This is important for not only support of the complex, but also for proprioception of the joint. The capsule of the elbow functions as a neurological link between the shoulder and the hand. This has an effect on upper-quarter activity and is an obvious aspect of the rehabilitation process if injury does occur.

Humeroulnar Joint

The humeroulnar joint is the articulation between the distal humerus medially and the proximal ulna. The humerus has distinct features distally. The medial aspect has the medial epicondyle and an hourglass-shaped trochlea[19] located anteromedially on the distal humerus. The trochlea extends more distally than the lateral aspect of the humerus. The trochlea articulates with the trochlear notch of the proximal ulna.

Because of the more distal projection of the humerus medially, the elbow complex demonstrates a carrying angle that is an abducted position of the elbow in the anatomical position. The normal carrying angle (Figure 18-1) in females is 10 to 15 degrees and in males, 5 degrees.[3] When the elbow is in flexion, the ulna slides forward until the coronoid process of the ulna stops in the floor of the coronoid fossa of the humerus. In extension, the ulna will slide backward until the olecranon process of the ulna makes contact with the olecranon fossa of the humerus posteriorly.

Humeroradial Joint

The humeroradial joint is the articulation of the laterally distal humerus and the proximal radius. The lateral aspect of the humerus has the lateral epicondyle and the capitellum, which is located anteriolaterally on the distal humerus. With flexion, the radius is in contact with the radial fossa of the distal humerus, whereas in extension the radius and the humerus are not in contact.

Proximal Radioulnar Joint

The proximal radioulnar joint is the articulation between the radial notch of the proximal lateral aspect of the ulna, the radial head, and the capitellum of the distal humerus. The proximal and distal radioulnar joints are important for supination and pronation. When evaluating this motion, it is important to look at them as one, functionally. The proximal and distal aspects of this joint cannot function one without the other. Proximally, the radius articulates with the ulna by the support of the annular ligament, which attaches to the ulnar notch anteriorly and posteriorly. The ligament circles the radial head for support. The interosseous membrane is the connective tissue that functions to complete the interval between the two bones. When there is a fall on the outstretched arm, the interosseous membrane can transmit some forces off the radius, the main weight-bearing bone, to the ulna. This can help prevent the radial head from having forceful contact with the capitellum. Distally, the concave radius will articulate with the convex ulna. With supination and pronation, the radius will move on the ulna.

Ligamentous Support

The stability of the elbow first starts with the joint capsule that is continuous between all three articulations. The capsule is loose anteriorly and posteriorly to allow for movement in flexion and extension.[1] It is taut medially and laterally due to the added support of the collateral ligaments. The capsule is highly innervated for proprioception, as stated earlier.

The medial (ulnar) collateral ligament (MCL) is fan-shaped and has three aspects. The anterior aspect of the MCL is the primary stabilizer in the MCL from about 20 to 120 degrees of motion.[43] The posterior and the oblique aspect of the MCL add support and assist in stability to the MCL. The lateral elbow complex consists of four structures. The radial collateral ligament attachments are from the lateral epicondyle to the annular ligament. The lateral ulnar collateral ligament is the primary lateral stabilizer and passes over the annular ligament into the supinator tubercle. It reinforces the elbow laterally, and reinforces the humeroradial joint.[34,43] The assessory lateral collateral ligament passes from the tubercle of the supinator into the annular ligament. The annular ligament, as previously stated, is the main support of the radial head in the radial notch of the ulna. The interosseous membrane is a syndesmotic condition that connects the ulna and the radius in the forearm. This structure prevents the proximal displacement of the radius on the ulna.

The Dynamic Stabilizers of the Elbow Complex

The elbow flexors are the biceps brachii, brachialis, and brachioradialis muscles. The biceps brachii originate via two heads proximally at the shoulder: the long head from the supraglenoid tuberosity of the scapula and the short head from the coracoid process of the scapula. The insertion is from a common tendon at the radial tuberosity and lacertus fibrosis to origins of the forearm flexors. The biceps brachii function is flexion of the elbow and supination the forearm.[48] The brachialis originates from the lower two-thirds of the anterior humerus to the coronoid process and tuberosity of the ulna. It functions to flex the elbow. The brachioradialis, which originates from the lower two-thirds of the lateral humerus and attaches to the lateral styloid process of the distal radius, functions as an elbow flexor, semipronator, and semisupinator.

The elbow extensors are the triceps brachii and the anconeus muscles. The triceps brachii has a long, medial and lateral head origination. The long head originates at the infraglenoid tuberosity of the scapula, the lateral and medial heads to the posterior aspect of the humerus. The insertion is via the common tendon posteriorly at the olecranon. Through this insertion, along with the anconeus muscle that assists the triceps, extension of the elbow complex is accomplished.

The Elbow in the Upper Quarter

The elbow plays an important part in functional activity in the upper quarter. Anatomical position places the elbow in full extension and full supination. The elbow functions in flexion, extension, supination, and pronation movement patterns. The elbow allows for about 145 degrees of flexion and 90 degrees of both supination and pronation, although normals for range of motion (ROM) are individual for the involved and for the noninvolved joint.[26]

The capsule, as previously stated, is a proprioceptive link of the upper quarter to the hand. Functionally, the relationship between the hand and the shoulder needs the elbow for normal movement to occur. The connection between multijoint muscles that affect the elbow will work proximally and distally in the upper quarter as a whole.

The hand and wrist muscles add to the support of the capsule for stability. Function of the cervical spine and shoulder can also affect the elbow. Limitations in motion in either area can cause accommodations in the elbow complex. For example, for a patient who has a decrease in supination due to injury, an accommodation of the injury is an increase in adduction and external rotation at the shoulder and an increased valgus stress to the elbow to allow function to continue. This is why proper knowledge of biomechanics in the elbow complex and associated joints is essential for proper assessment of injury and rehabilitation.

REHABILITATION TECHNIQUES FOR THE ELBOW COMPLEX

Isotonic Open Kinetic Chain Strengthening Exercises

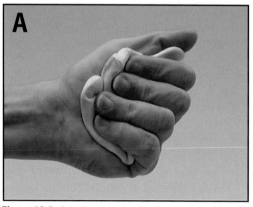 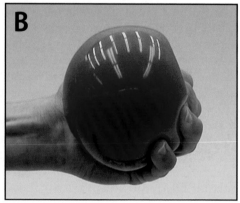

Figure 18-2. Gripping exercise. Used to strengthen the wrist flexors and the intrinsic muscles of the hand. (A) Putty; (B) ball.

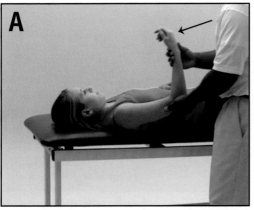
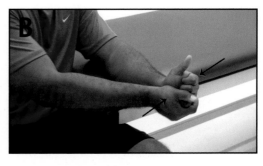

Figure 18-3. (A) Isometric wrist flexion and extension; (B) isometric wrist supination and pronation. The reeducation that the isometric contractions provide is a safe technique for the early stages of rehabilitation. Contractions can be performed in various angles prior to isotonic exercise.

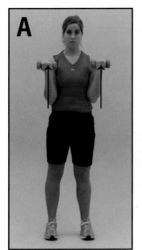
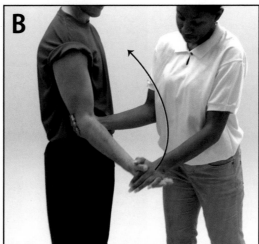
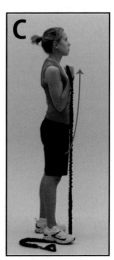

Figure 18-4. Isotonic elbow flexion. The biceps brachii, the brachialis, and the brachioradialis muscles are used when moving the elbow from full extension into full flexion. (A) Dumbell resistance; (B) manual resistance; (C) tension band or cable resistance.

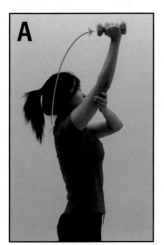
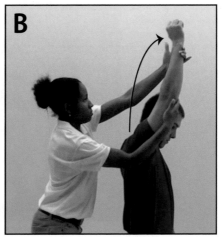
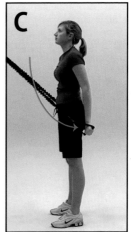

Figure 18-5. Isotonic elbow extension. The triceps muscle moves the arm from full flexion to full extension. (A) Dumbell resistance; (B) manual resistance; (C) tension band or cable resistance.

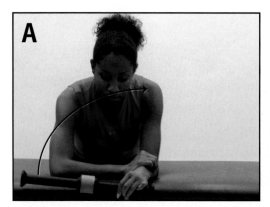
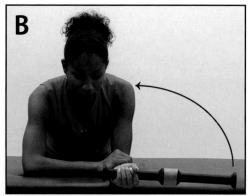

Figure 18-6. Isotonic wrist supination/pronation. The forearm is in a stable position on the table, and the elbow is in a 90-degree position. (A) Supinate the forearm while holding onto a weighted bar; (B) pronate the forearm while holding a weighted bar.

Figure 18-7. Concentric/eccentric flexion with the use of tension band for the benefits of maximum load on the muscle. A concentric contraction is done slowly, at first, then the speed is increased to mimic functional activity. An eccentric contraction is done by pulling the muscle into a shortened position, then allowing a lengthening contraction to take place by lowering the hand in control. Increased speed is introduced when proficiency is obtained.

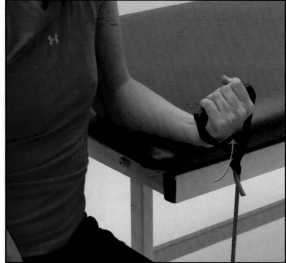

Figure 18-8. Concentric/eccentric extension with the use of a tension band for the benefits of maximum load on the muscle. A concentric contraction is done slowly at first, then the speed is increased to mimic functional activity. An eccentric contraction is done by pulling the muscle into a shortened position, then allowing a lengthening contraction to take place by lowering the hand in control. Increased speed is introduced when proficiency is obtained.

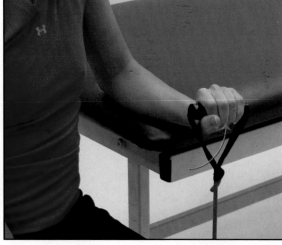

Closed Kinetic Chain Exercises

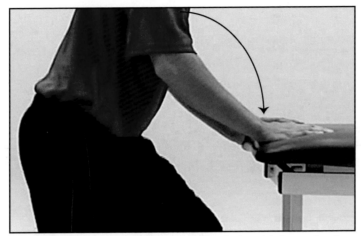

Figure 18-9. Closed kinetic chain static hold. The body weight is over the elbow in varying degrees for the purpose of bearing weight and initiating kinesthetic awareness in the elbow joint.

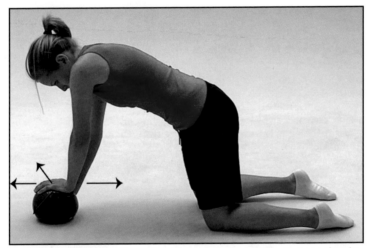

Figure 18-10. Plyoball ball exercises. This exercise is used for sport-specific rehabilitation in sports that require closed kinetic chain activity. There is stimulation of the joint receptors.

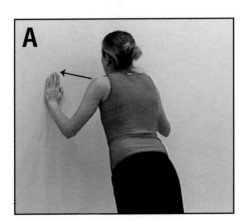

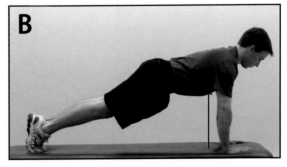

Figure 18-11. Push-ups. (A) Standing; (B) prone.

Plyometric Exercises

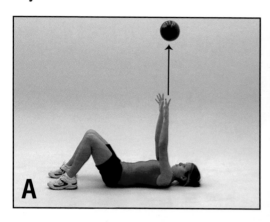
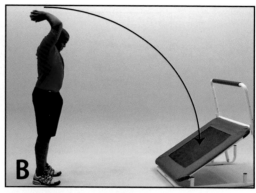
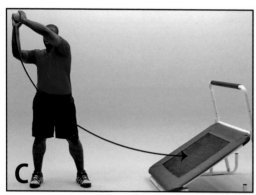
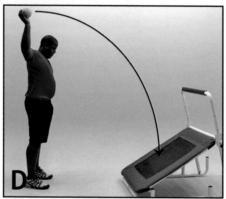

Figure 18-12. Plyometric exercise drills. Plyometric exercise has three phases: a quick eccentric load (stretch), a brief amortization phase, and a concentric contraction. (A) Elbow extension; (B) two-hand overhead toss; (C) two-hand side throws; (D) one-arm overhead throw.

Isokinetic Exercises

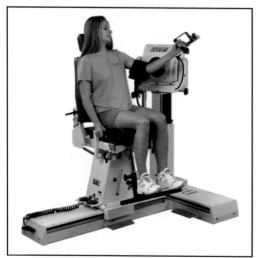
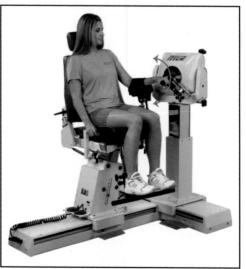

Figure 18-13. Isokinetic elbow flexion (hand positioned in supination). (Reprinted with permission from Biodex Medical Systems.)

Figure 18-14. Isokinetic wrist flexion/extension. (Reprinted with permission from Biodex Medical Systems.)

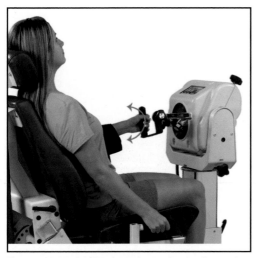

Figure 18-15. Isokinetic wrist supination/pronation. (Reprinted with permission from Biodex Medical Systems.)

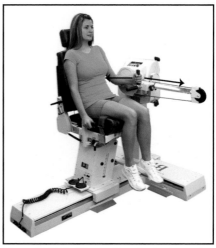

Figure 18-16. Isokinetic elbow flexion/extension with scapular retraction/protraction. (Reprinted with permission from Biodex Medical Systems.)

Stretching Exercises

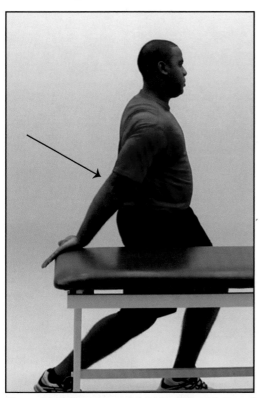

Figure 18-17. Stretching of the biceps brachii. Extend the elbow and pronate the wrist, bring the arm into extension.

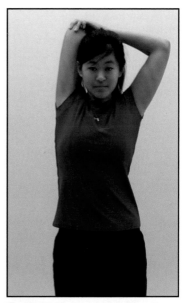

Figure 18-18. Stretching of the triceps. Flex arm with the elbow in flexion, passive force is applied by pulling the arm into flexion.

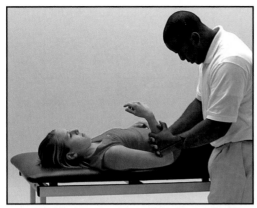

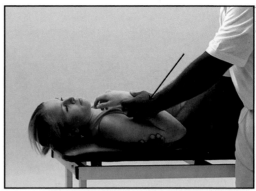

Figure 18-19. Passive distraction. The elbow is at 90 degrees while the patient is supine, and the arm is in the plane of the body, hands are clasped while a pull on the proximal radius and ulna is performed. Used to increase elasticity of the adhesed joint capsule to enhance ROM in all planes of motion.

Figure 18-20. Passive flexion. While the patient is supine and the arm is in the plane of the body, a push of the forearm toward the shoulder is performed to increase the angle of the elbow toward a straight position. Used to increase elasticity of the adhesed joint capsule to enhance ROM in all planes of motion.

Figure 18-21. Passive extension. While the patient is supine and the arm is in the plane of the body, a push of the forearm away from the shoulder is performed to decrease the angle of the elbow toward a straight position. Used to increase the elasticity of the adhesed joint capsule to enhance ROM in all planes of motion.

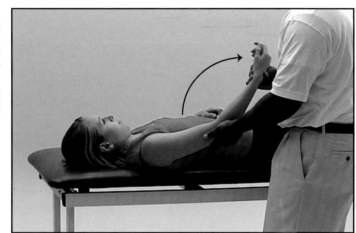

Figure 18-22. Long-duration, low-intensity passive ROM. Using a cuff weight at the wrist will increase ROM by stretching the joint capsule while the patient is supine and the arm is in anatomic position at the shoulder and the wrist.

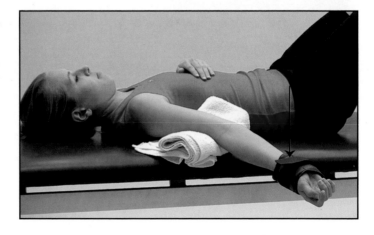

Exercises to Reestablish Neuromuscular Control

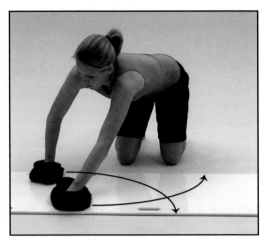

Figure 18-23. Slide board exercises. The closed kinetic chain patterns, as shown, incorporate joint awareness and movement for proprioceptive benefits. Stress to the patient the importance of developing the weight over the upper quarter while movement patterns are worked.

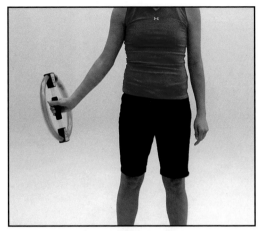

Figure 18-24. Proprioceptive oscillation. This is for kinesthetic/proprioceptive exercises for the elbow and the entire upper quarter. An upper-quarter exercise tool, there are three metal balls in the ring that move when the upper extremity generates the movement. This can be performed in various positions to mimic arm positioning in sport.

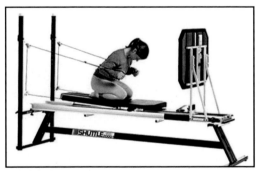

Figure 18-25. Kinesthetic training for timing. This device is used for the purpose of improving proprioception and timing with functional activity. The pulling of the handle causes the weight to move, and with the benefit of inertia, proprioceptive and kinesthetic awareness can improve. Printed with permission from Shuttle Systems.

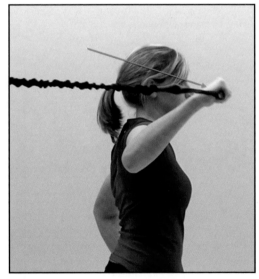

Figure 18-26. Surgical tubing exercises done in the scapular plane to mimic the throwing motion using internal and external rotation.

Bracing and Taping

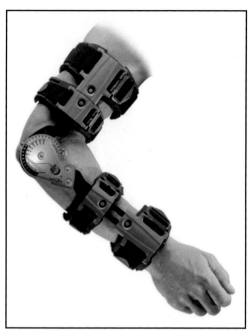

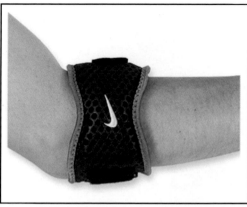

Figure 18-28. Elbow brace for lateral epicondylitis. This brace is used to decrease the tension of the extensor muscles at the elbow. The brace is applied over the extensor muscles just distal to the elbow joint.

Figure 18-27. Brace to protect the medial elbow structures. This brace is used when injury stress has occurred to the medial aspect of the elbow. The hinge design is developed for valgus and also varus stress, and can have limits on range of motion as well.

Figure 18-29. Elbow taping for hyperextension of the elbow uses a checkrein to limit extension in the joint.

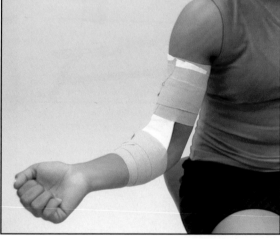

REHABILITATION TECHNIQUES FOR SPECIFIC INJURIES

Fractures of the Elbow

Pathomechanics

Fractures to the elbow proper will be specific to one or more bones in the elbow, with effects to the joint as a whole. The fractures seen in the humeral shaft and distal humerus, the radial head, and the proximal ulna will affect the function of the entire elbow complex, as well as the individual bones themselves.[44] Dislocations might accompany an elbow fracture, depending on the specific mechanism of injury. With elbow fractures, properly evaluating the neurovascular system is critical. The ulnar, radial, median, and musculocutaneous nerves pass the elbow in various positions anatomically. The brachial artery has various branches that provide the blood supply from the proximal elbow to the digits.

The radial, ulnar, and common interosseous arteries (and the collateral and recurrent arteries), specifically, provide the circulation off the brachial artery to the structures at and distal to the elbow.

Mechanism of Injury

The fracture of an elbow bone can have various injury mechanisms. The shaft of the humerus can fracture as a result of a direct force, as well as from a rotational component with the hand in a fixed position. There is also evidence that a direct blow can fracture the bones of the elbow, via a stick, helmet, or bat.[38] A rotational or twisting mechanism can also occur when pushing off on a fixed hand (eg, a gymnast on a vault)[11] and can cause the onset of immediate pain and loss of function. The increased load on the joint structures from a direct blow can increase the possibility of supracondylar fractures. Olecranon process fractures will occur with a fall directly on the tip of the elbow (eg, when a volleyball player falls on an elbow). A forearm fracture will often occur in the shafts of both the radius and ulna. A fracture of one of the forearm bones can result in a dislocation of the other bone.[8,41] Radial head fractures make up a third of all elbow fractures and a fourth of all elbow trauma.[44] They are more common in females than in males by a 2 to 1 ratio.[41] The mechanism of injury is an axial load being placed on a pronated arm. This can occur in skating falls and biking accidents when the posterolateral aspect of the radius is in contact with the capitellum.

This type of stress, in addition to the carrying angle, makes the medial collateral ligament susceptible to injury. A valgus stress can also injure the epiphyseal plate of an adolescent patient with an avulsion fracture as a possible result.

Rehabilitation Concerns

Undisplaced or minimally displaced fractures in adults and children are treated conservatively and require little or no immobilization. Cases managed using open reduction and internal fixation (ORIF) surgical procedures require only slightly longer periods of immobilization. The joint may be aspirated if the swelling is extremely painful. With the elbow flexed 90 degrees, a posterior plaster splint and sling are applied. Early motion is encouraged, and the splint is removed in 1 to 2 weeks, while a sling is continued for another 1 to 2 weeks as tolerated.

Displaced or comminuted radial head fractures in adults are usually treated by early surgery (within 24 to 48 hours) to minimize the likelihood of permanent restriction of joint motion, traumatic arthritis, soft-tissue calcification in the anterior elbow region, and myositis ossificans. Fractures in children with less than 15 to 30 degrees of angulation are treated as undisplaced fractures. Displaced fractures, or fractures angulated greater than 15 to 30 degrees, are treated by closed or open reduction.

Fractures of the olecranon can be either displaced or undisplaced. The extensor mechanism is intact in undisplaced fractures, and further displacement is unlikely. The undisplaced fracture is treated with a posterior plaster splint for 2 weeks, followed by a sling and progressive ROM exercises. Displaced fractures usually require open reduction and internal fixation to restore the bony alignment and repair the triceps insertion.

Regardless of the method of treatment, some loss of extension at the elbow is very likely; however, little functional impairment usually results.

Rehabilitation Progression

Immediately following the injury or with ORIF surgical procedures, the goal is to minimize pain and swelling by using cold, compression, and electrical stimulation. Active and passive ROM exercises (Figures 18-17 through 18-22) should begin immediately after injury. The goal should be to achieve 15 to 105 degrees of motion by the end of week 2. Within the first week, isometric elbow flexion and extension exercises (Figure 18-3A) and gentle isometric pronation/supination exercises (Figure 18-3B) should begin. Isotonic shoulder and wrist exercises should also be used and should continue to progress throughout the rehabilitation program. Joint mobilizations should begin during the second week in an attempt to minimize loss of extension (Figures 13-21 through 13-25).

Progressive lightweight (1 to 2 pound [lb]) isotonic elbow flexion exercises (Figure 18-4) and elbow extension exercises (Figure 18-5) can be incorporated during the third week and should continue for as long as 12 weeks. Active-assisted passive pronation/supination exercises (Figure 18-6) should begin at week 6, progressing as tolerated.

Beginning at week 7, eccentric elbow flexion and extension exercises (Figures 18-7 and 18-8) along with plyometric exercises can be used. Exercises designed to establish neuromuscular control, including closed kinetic chain activities, should also be used to help regain dynamic stability about the elbow joint (Figures 18-9 through 18-11, and 18-23 through 18-25). Functional training activities will also begin about this time and should progressively incorporate the stresses, strains, and forces that occur during normal activities. Isokinetic training for elbow flexion and extension can also begin at this time (Figures 18-13 to 18-16). Each of these exercises should continue in a progressive manner throughout the rehabilitative period.

Criteria for Return

Full return to activity is expected at about 12 weeks. The patient may return to full activity when specific criteria have been successfully completed. There should be clinical healing of the fracture site. ROM in flexion, extension, supination, and pronation should be within normal limits. Strength should be at least equal to the uninvolved elbow, and the patient should have no complaint of pain in the elbow while performing a progression of activities in normal conditions. The return to sport is progressed with the use of restrictions (eg, pitch counts in baseball), which can be helpful in objectively measuring activity and progression. The throwing progression for the elbow shows a gradual increase in activity in terms of time, repetitions, duration, and intensity (Table 18-1).

Clinical Decision-Making Exercise 18-1

A mountain biker fell off her bike while going downhill. As she fell, she tried to protect herself with an outstretched pronated arm. Afterward, she felt pain along the lateral side of the elbow with any movement in the arm. The biker had fractured the radial head. How should the athletic trainer manage this injury?

Osteochondritis Dissecans/ "Panner's Disease"

Pathomechanics

Osteochondritis dissecans and "Panner's disease" are injuries that affect the lateral aspect of the elbow. Osteochondritis dissecans is a condition that affects the central and/or lateral aspect of the capitellum or radial head in which an underlying osteochondral bone fragment becomes detached from the articular surface, forming a loose body in the joint. It can also be found in the knee and ankle joints.[45]

Osteochondritis dissecans is considered to be different from osteochondrosis but might represent different stages of the same disease.[41] With osteochondritis there is no inflammation. It is the most common cause of loose bodies in adolescents; and, although it is most often seen in pitchers, it can also be seen in gymnasts or basketball players aged between 12 and 15 years.[28,45] The primary cause is thought to be trauma due to a repetitive compressive force between the radial head and the capitellum at the radiocapitular joint with valgus forces that load the joint during throwing.[6]

Some confusion exists as to whether there is any difference between osteochondritis dissecans and Panner's disease. Although Panner's disease might just be a part of the spectrum of osteochondritis dissecans, it is probably better to limit the diagnosis of Panner's disease to children aged 10 years or younger at the time of onset.[42] Panner's disease is an osteochondrosis of the capitellum in which there is a localized avascular necrosis leading to loss of the subchondral bone of the capitellum that can cause softening and fissuring of articular surfaces of the radiocapitellar joint.[21] If loose bodies develop, Panner's disease will produce osteochondritis dissecans.[4]

Mechanism of Injury

Osteochondritis dissecans occurs due to compressive forces at the lateral aspect of the elbow. When the elbow is in the late cocking and acceleration phases of throwing motion, there is a valgus condition that causes a compressive force to the articular surface between the radial head and the capitellum.[21] The repetitive throwing motion causes vascular defects in the area. Panner's disease is an idiopathic condition that encompasses the entire capitellum.[19,45] In the young patient, throwing under guidance and with good technique is essential to preventing injuries.

Rehabilitation Concerns

Impaired motion and pain to the lateral aspect of the elbow are among the most common complaints. The caution is to avoid excessive and repetitive compression of the joint surfaces, which can lead to degenerative changes and the formation of loose bodies within the joint.[16,45]

Treatment of osteochondritis dissecans is variable. In some cases, lesions in the skeletally immature elbow will heal if properly managed. Treatment includes completely avoiding any throwing or impact-loading activities as seen in gymnastics. Pain, tenderness, contracture, and radiographic changes provide objective parameters to determine the activity of the disease. If there is formation of loose bodies or if healing has been incomplete (as is usually the case) and symptoms persist, surgical intervention is

necessary. Arthroscopic joint debridement and loose body removal has been advocated.[45]

Rehabilitation Progression

The functional progression after the injury has been diagnosed should be first and foremost pain-free. The injury is articular in nature, and a cautious rehabilitation program should be followed. ROM exercises should be full and pain-free (Figures 18-17 through 18-22). Strengthening exercises (Figures 18-4 through 18-6) will progress at the pain-free level and with restriction from increased pressure between the radius and the capitellum. The patient might have to decrease or modify the activity level to avoid the compressive nature in the joint. A slow, progressive program that gradually increases the load on the injured structure is essential.

Following arthroscopic debridement and removal of loose bodies, the goal is to minimize pain and swelling by using cold, electrical stimulation, and compression using a bulky dressing initially, followed by an elastic wrap. Active and passive ROM exercises (Figures 18-17 through 18-22) should begin immediately after surgery, as tolerated. The goal should be to achieve full ROM within 7 to 14 days after surgery, although the patient must continue to work on ROM throughout the rehabilitation period. Within the first 2 days, isometric elbow flexion and extension exercises (Figure 18-3A), and isometric pronation/supination exercises (Figure 18-3B) should begin. Isometric shoulder and wrist exercises should also be used and should continue to progress throughout the rehabilitation program.

Progressive lightweight (1 to 2 lb) isotonic elbow flexion exercises (Figure 18-4), elbow extension exercises (Figure 18-5), and pronation/supination exercises can be incorporated between days 3 and 7. Isotonic shoulder and wrist exercises should begin during this period and continue to progress throughout the rehabilitation program.

At 3 weeks, eccentric elbow flexion and extension exercises (Figures 18-7 and 18-8) can be used. Joint mobilizations should begin in an attempt to normalize joint arthrokinematics (see Figures 13-18 through 13-22). Beginning at week 5, in addition to continuing strengthening and ROM exercises, activities that progressively incorporate the stresses, strains, and forces that prepare the patient for gradual return to functional activities should begin. For throwing athletes, the interval throwing program can be initiated. Exercises designed to establish neuromuscular control, including closed kinetic chain activities, should also be used to help regain dynamic stability about the elbow joint (Figures 18-9 through 18-11, and 18-23 through 18-25).

Criteria for Return

The patient may return to full competitive activity when (1) full ROM in flexion, extension, supination, and pronation has been regained; (2) strength is at least equal to that in the uninvolved elbow; (3) there is no complaint of pain in the elbow while performing throwing or loading activities; and (4) the interval throwing program has been completed.

Realistically, the prognosis for full return to throwing or to loading activities, as in gymnastics and wrestling, especially at a competitive level, should be cautious. The athletic trainer should educate parents, coaches, and children about this problem so that early recognition and subsequent intervention and referral to medical personnel can reduce the likelihood of need for surgical intervention. Following an arthroscopic procedure, the patient might be able to return to full throwing activities in 7 to 8 weeks.

Clinical Decision-Making Exercise 18-2

A 9-year-old gymnast is experiencing increased pain at the lateral aspect of the elbow. Her symptoms started after an impact with the vault. She is experiencing difficulty and pain with motion in both flexion and extension, and she has not been able to compete. How should the athletic trainer manage this injury?

Ulnar Collateral Ligament Injuries

Pathomechanics

The medial complex of the elbow is susceptible to various injuries in the athletic population.[5] The repetitive stresses that are placed on the medial elbow increase the possibilities of injury. The ulnar collateral ligament, the medial aspect of the joint capsule, and the ulnar nerve can individually or collectively be stressed when valgus forces are applied to the elbow. The ulnar collateral ligament is composed of three bands: the anterior oblique ligament, which remains tight throughout full ROM; the posterior oblique ligament, which is tight during flexion and loose during extension; and the transverse oblique ligament, which remains tight throughout the range but provides little medial stability.[50] The anterior band of the ulnar collateral ligament has been demonstrated to be the primary structure resisting valgus stress at the elbow and is tight from 20 to 120 degrees of flexion. The osseous articulation of the elbow contributes little to medial stability with the arm in this position.[40]

The ulnar collateral ligament provides the primary resistance to valgus stresses that occur during the late cocking and early acceleration phases of throwing.[15] The moment during the throwing motion that places the most stress on the elbow is when the arm is fully cocked with maximal shoulder external rotation.[31,39] On examination the patient typically complains of pain along the medial aspect of the elbow. There is tenderness over the medial collateral ligament, usually at the distal insertion and occasionally in a more diffuse distribution. In some cases the patient might describe associated paresthesias in the distribution of the ulnar nerve with a positive Tinel's sign. When valgus stress is applied to the elbow at 20 to 30 degrees of flexion, local pain, tenderness, and end-point laxity are assessed. On standard X-ray, hypertrophy of the humeral condyle and posteromedial aspect of the olecranon, marginal osteophytes of the ulnohumeral or radiocapitellar joints, calcification within the medial collateral ligament, and/or loose bodies in the posterior compartment might be present.[13] The adolescent elbow has an increased injury potential due to ligament laxity, which can produce stress on the epiphyseal growth plate and an avulsion fracture of the medial epicondyle from the pull of the medial collateral ligament. This can occur in patients at or around the age of 13 years.[20]

Mechanism of Injury

The ulnar collateral ligament is most often injured as a result of a valgus force from the repetitive trauma of overhead throwing. It can also be injured during a forehand stroke in tennis, or in the trail arm during an improper golf swing. In the general population, acute injury to the ulnar collateral ligament rarely results in recurrent instability of the elbow. Stress of the medial complex can also result in ulnar nerve inflammation or impairment, or wrist flexor tendinitis.[33]

During the late cocking phase through the early acceleration phase of throwing, tremendously high, repetitive stresses are applied to the medial elbow joint, frequently resulting in ligament failure, tendinitis, or osseous changes. Injuries can vary in degree from an overuse flexor/pronator muscular strain to ligamentous sprains of the ulnar collateral ligament. These injuries can result in elbow flexion contractures or potentially increase the instability of the elbow in adolescents.

Rehabilitation Concerns

Most ulnar collateral ligament injuries can be managed without surgery.[17] Conservative treatment of patients with chronic ulnar collateral ligament injury should begin with rest and nonsteroidal anti-inflammatory medication. With resolution of symptoms, rehabilitation should be instituted with emphasis on strengthening. The athletic trainer along with the coach should analyze the athlete's throwing mechanics, which might include video assessment, to correct any existing faulty mechanics. If periods of rest and rehabilitation fail to result in a resolution of symptoms, surgical intervention might be necessary.

Operative management consists of repair or reconstruction. In the case of an acute rupture, surgical repair can be considered; however, the indications are extremely limited. The avulsed ligament should be without evidence of calcification, and if there is any question as to the quality of the tissue, reconstruction should be performed.

The ulnar collateral ligament is the primary stabilizer to valgus stress at the elbow, so reconstruction is vital to competitive throwing athletes who wish to return to their previous levels of performance. An autograft, using either the palmaris longus or extensor hallucis, is used to reconstruct the ulnar collateral ligament. The graft then simulates function of the ulnar collateral ligament, particularly the anterior oblique portion, providing the primary restraint to valgus stress during throwing. During this surgical procedure, the ulnar nerve is transposed medially and is held in place with fascial slings. Immediate postoperative precautions must be observed, especially in relation to the soft tissue of the fascial slings that stabilize the ulnar nerve.

Rehabilitation Progression

Following a requisite period of rest and rehabilitation techniques designed to reduce inflammation, the rehabilitation progression for ulnar collateral ligament injuries should concentrate primarily on strengthening of the flexor muscles, particularly the flexor carpi ulnaris and flexor digitorum superficialis, which can help prevent medial injury by providing additional support to medial elbow structures.[37] Strengthening exercises (Figures 18-2 through 18-8) should be done initially in the pain-free midrange of motion with a gradual increase of forces at the end ranges of motion. Exercises to increase both static and dynamic flexibility of the elbow without producing valgus stress should be incorporated (Figures 18-9 through 18-11). Support taping can also assist in the protection for return to activity (Figure 18-29).

Following a reconstruction of the ulnar collateral ligament, the initial goal is to decrease pain and swelling (using a compression dressing for 2 to 3 days) and to protect the healing reconstruction. The patient is placed in a 90-degree posterior splint for 1 week, during which time submaximal isometrics for the wrist musculature (Figure 18-2) and the elbow flexors and extensors (Figures 18-3A and B) are performed at multiple angles as long as all valgus stress is eliminated. Isometric shoulder exercises, except for external rotation, along with isometric biceps exercises should be used.

In the second week, the patient is placed into a ROM brace set at 30 to 100 degrees (Figure 18-27). ROM should be increased by 5 degrees of extension and 10 degrees of flexion each week, with full ROM at 6 to 7 weeks. In addition to the exercises used during the first week, wrist isometrics and elbow flexion and extension isometrics (Figure 18-3A) should begin.

At 4 weeks, progressive lightweight (1 to 2 lb) isotonic elbow flexion exercises (Figure 18-4), elbow extension exercises (Figure 18-5), and pronation/supination exercises (Figure 18-6) can be incorporated. Isotonic shoulder exercises (avoiding external rotation for 6 weeks) should begin during this period and continue to progress throughout the rehabilitation program. Passive elbow flexion and extension ROM exercises (Figures 18-20 and 18-21) may begin during this period.

At 6 weeks, isotonic strengthening exercises for the shoulder (now including external rotation), elbow, and wrist should continue to progress.

At 9 weeks, as strength continues to increase, more functional activities can be incorporated, including eccentric elbow flexion and extension exercises (Figures 18-7 and 18-8), PNF diagonal strengthening patterns (Figures 14-3 through 14-10), and plyometric exercises (Figure 18-12). Exercises designed to establish neuromuscular control, including closed kinetic chain activities, should also be used to help regain dynamic stability about the elbow joint (Figures 18-9 through 18-11, and 18-23 through 18-26).

Beginning at week 11, in addition to continuing strengthening and ROM exercises, activities that progressively incorporate the stresses, strains, and forces that prepare the patient for gradual return to throwing activities should begin. For throwing patients, the interval throwing program can be initiated at week 14 (Table 18-1).

Criteria for Full Return

Generally the throwing athlete can return to competitive levels at about 22 to 26 weeks post surgery. The patient may return to full competitive activity when (1) full ROM in flexion, extension, supination, and pronation has been regained; (2) strength is at least equal to that of the uninvolved elbow; (3) there is no complaint of pain in the elbow while performing throwing or loading activities; and (4) the interval throwing program has been completed.

Clinical Decision-Making Exercise 18-3

While sliding headfirst into third base, a baseball player caught his hand on the outer corner of the bag. As the third baseman grabbed the bag to come up to a standing position, she landed on the lateral aspect of the base runner's arm, causing increased force to the medial complex of the arm. There is increased pain and swelling to the medial aspect of the elbow, and the player complains of paresthesia along the medial aspect of the forearm. How should the athletic trainer manage this injury?

Nerve Entrapments

Pathomechanics and Injury Mechanism

The ulnar, median, and radial nerves are susceptible to injury and entrapment in the elbow. The ulnar nerve, which passes through the medial epicondylar groove, can be injured with medial stress to the elbow as previously described. The median nerve passing between the supracondylar process, and the medial epicondyle can become compressed. The radial nerve passes under the lateral head of the triceps and, if compressed, can cause weakness in the forearm extensors.[7] Whenever nerve compression conditions at the elbow are considered, the athletic trainer should also consider the possibility of compression lesions at other levels such as the cervical spine, brachial plexus, and wrist.

Ulnar Nerve Entrapment

Ulnar nerve compression can occur from a number of causes, including (1) direct trauma; (2) traction due to an increase of laxity in the medial complex, which causes a compressive force to be placed on the nerve resulting in a tension neuropathy; (3) compression due to a thickened retinaculum or a hypertrophied flexor carpi ulnaris muscle; (4) recurrent subluxation or dislocation; and (5) osseous degenerative changes.[12] In throwing patients, ulnar nerve irritation is most likely to develop secondary to mechanical factors that occur during the late cocking and early acceleration phases of the throwing motion. In these patients, ulnar neuritis often occurs along with medial instability and medial epicondylitis.[12]

The term cubital tunnel syndrome is used to identify a specific anatomic site for entrapment of the ulnar nerve. The ulnar nerve can be compromised by any swelling that occurs within the canal or with inflammatory changes that result in thickening of the fascial sheath.

The patient generally complains of medial elbow pain associated with numbness and tingling in the ulnar nerve distribution. Paresthesias may be present that radiate from the medial epicondyle distally along the ulnar aspect of the forearm into the fourth and fifth fingers. These sensory symptoms usually precede the development of motor deficits. There is tenderness at the cubital tunnel, which may include the medial epicondyle. Tinel's sign is generally present at the cubital tunnel. Subluxation of the ulnar nerve occurs in as many as 16% of patients with symptoms, particularly in those with a shallow medial epicondylar groove. Radiographs might show osteophytes on the humerus and olecranon, calcifications of the medial collateral ligament, and loose bodies.[12]

Median Nerve Entrapment

The median nerve can be compressed under the ligament of Struthers, within the pronator teres muscle, and under the superficial head of the flexor digitorum superficialis.[7] The compression can occur as a result of hypertrophy of the proximal forearm muscles, particularly the pronator teres muscle, that occurs with repetitive grip-related activity or pronation and extension of the forearm, as occurs in the racket sports and other grip/hold activities. The patient will usually describe aching pain and fatigue or weakness of the forearm muscles along with paresthesia in the distribution of the median nerve. Symptoms seem to worsen with repetitive pronation, as in practicing tennis serves. There is usually tenderness of the proximal pronator teres with a positive Tinel's sign. The patient might also complain of increased pain while sleeping.

Radial Nerve Entrapment

Entrapment of the radial nerve, specifically the posterior interosseous nerve, occurs within the radial tunnel and has been referred to as either radial tunnel syndrome in which there is pain with no motor weakness, or posterior interosseous nerve compression where there is motor weakness in the absence of pain.[12] The radial nerve innervates the brachioradialis as well as the extensor muscles of the proximal forearm. Radial nerve compression occurs in throwing mechanisms and overhead activities such as swimming and playing tennis. The patient typically complains of lateral elbow pain that is sometimes confused with lateral epicondylitis. There is tenderness distal to the lateral epicondyle over the supinator muscle. The pain is described as an ache that spreads into the extensor muscles and occasionally radiates distally to the wrist. Nocturnal pain might be present.

Rehabilitation Concerns

If rehabilitation begins early after onset of symptoms, treatment should include rest, avoiding activities that seem to exacerbate pain, use of anti-inflammatory medications, protective padding, and occasionally use of extension night splints. This should be followed by a rehabilitation program that concentrates on ROM exercises before return to sport. A concern that will arise and needs to be addressed with regard to nerve entrapments is that of decreased muscle function, which can lead to accommodative activity and possible muscle imbalance. If the patient remains symptomatic despite a conservative program, surgery is generally recommended. It should be noted that, although physical findings other than local tenderness might be minimal and electrodiagnostic tests are rarely positive, good-to-excellent results can be obtained by surgery. The surgical treatment options include decompression alone and subcutaneous, intramuscular, or submuscular transposition.

Rehabilitation Progression

Following a course of conservative care involving rest and anti-inflammatory medication, the rehabilitation program should concentrate on strengthening of the involved muscles to maintain a balance between agonist and antagonist muscles (Figures 18-2 through 18-8). In addition, maintaining ROM through aggressive stretching exercises will help to free up entrapped nerves (Figures 18-17 through 18-22). Massage techniques that can be used in the affected area can prevent the development of adhesions that would restrict injured nerves. Mobility of the nerve is critical in reducing nerve entrapment.

Following surgical decompression or transposition of an entrapped nerve, the initial goal is to decrease pain and swelling (using a compression dressing for 2 to 3 days). The patient is placed in a 90-degree posterior splint for 1 week, during which time gripping exercises (Figure 18-2), isometric shoulder exercises, and wrist ROM exercises are used. During weeks 2 and 3, the posterior splint ROM is limited to 30 to 90 degrees initially, progressing to 15 to 120 degrees. The splint may be removed for exercise. Isometric flexion and extension exercises (Figures 18-3A and B) are begun, and shoulder isometrics continue.

At 3 weeks, the splint can be discontinued. Progressive isotonic elbow flexion exercises (Figure 18-4), elbow extension exercises (Figure 18-5), and pronation/supination exercises (Figure 18-6) can be incorporated. Isotonic shoulder exercises should begin during this period and continue to progress throughout the rehabilitation program. Passive elbow flexion and extension ROM exercises (Figures 18-2 and 18-21) continue during this period with particular emphasis placed on regaining extension.

At 7 weeks, as strength continues to increase, more functional activities can be incorporated, including eccentric elbow flexion and extension exercises (Figures 18-7 and 18-8), PNF diagonal strengthening patterns (see Figures 14-3 through 14-10), and plyometric exercises (Figure 18-12). Exercises designed to establish neuromuscular control, including closed kinetic chain activities, should also be used to help regain dynamic stability about the elbow joint (Figures 18-9 through 18-11, and 18-23 through 18-26). For throwing patients, the interval throwing program can be initiated (Table 18-1).

Criteria for Return

The throwing athlete can return to competitive activity at about 12 weeks. The patient must be able to demonstrate full function of the elbow after nerve injury. ROM, strength, neuromuscular control, and functional activities must be comparable to preinjury levels. The patient must also appropriately demonstrate activities related to his or her sport, and perform these tasks without compensation or substitution of other structures. For example, a swimmer must demonstrate the proper mechanics in the elbow while performing the stroke with the involved extremity comparably to the uninvolved extremity. If it is not performed in a satisfactory manner, the rehabilitation will be continued until the stroke can be performed appropriately.

Elbow Dislocations

Pathomechanics

Generally elbow dislocations are classified as either anterior or posterior dislocations. Anterior dislocations and radial head dislocations are not common, occurring in only 1% to 2% of cases. There are several different types of posterior dislocations, which are defined by the position of the olecranon relative to the humerus: (1) posterior, (2) posterolateral (most common), (3) posteromedial (least common), or (4) lateral. Dislocations can be complete or perched. Compared with complete dislocations, perched dislocations have less ligament tearing, and thus they have a more rapid recovery and rehabilitation period.[2,50] In a complete dislocation there is rupture of the ulnar collateral ligament, a possibility that the anterior capsule will rupture, along with possible ruptures of the lateral collateral ligament, brachialis muscle, or wrist flexor/extensor tendons.[46] Fractures occur in 25% to 50% of patients with elbow dislocations, with a fracture of the radial head being most common. With rupture of the anterior oblique band of the ulnar collateral ligament, repair is sometimes necessary in patients if the injury occurs in the dominant arm.[22]

Injury Mechanism

Elbow dislocations most frequently occur as a result of elbow hyperextension from a fall on the outstretched or extended arm, although dislocation can occur in flexion.[30] The radius and ulna are most likely to dislocate posterior or posterolateral to the humerus. The olecranon process is forced into the olecranon fossa with such impact that the trochlea is levered over the coronoid process.[22] Flexion dislocation is often associated with radial head fractures.

If the dislocation is simple without associated fractures, reduction can result in a stable elbow if the forearm flexors, extensors, and annular ligament have maintained their continuity. In these cases, early motion is resumed and the ultimate prognosis is good. The injury will present with rapid swelling, severe pain at the elbow, and a deformity with the olecranon in posterior position, giving the appearance of a shortened forearm.[30]

Elbow dislocations that involve fractures of the bony stabilizing forces about the elbow, such as a radial head or capitular fracture/dislocation, creates a significant instability pattern that cannot completely be corrected on either the medial or the lateral side of the elbow alone for maximum functional return. These injuries must be treated surgically.

Rehabilitation Concerns

Following reduction of an elbow dislocation, the degree of stability present will determine the course of rehabilitation. If the elbow is stable, best results are obtained with a brief period of immobilization followed by rehabilitation that is focused on restoring early ROM within the limits of elbow stability. This is particularly true if the anterior band of the ulnar collateral ligament is stable.[47] Prolonged immobilization after dislocation has been closely associated with flexion contractures and more increased pain, with no decrease in instability. An unstable dislocation requires surgical repair of the ulnar collateral ligament and thus a longer period of immobilization.

Recurrent elbow dislocation is uncommon, occurring after only 1% to 2% of simple dislocations.[30] Recurrent instability is more likely if the initial dislocation involved a fracture or if the first incident took place during childhood.

An overly aggressive rehabilitation program is more likely to result in chronic instability, wheras being overly conservative can lead to a flexion contracture. Typically, flexion contracture is much more likely. It is not uncommon to have a flexion contracture of 30% at 10 weeks. After 2 years, a 10% flexion contracture is often still present.[2] Unfortunately, this flexion contracture does not improve with time. For the athlete, it is most desirable to regain full elbow extension. For nonathletes, it is more important

to ensure that the joint structure and ligaments are given sufficient time to heal, to decrease the risk for recurrent subluxation or dislocation.

Loss of motion, joint stiffness, and heterotopic ossification are more likely complications following dislocation.

Rehabilitation Progression

The rehabilitation progression is determined by whether the elbow is stable or unstable following reduction. If the elbow is stable, it should be immobilized in a posterior splint at 90 degrees of flexion for 3 to 4 days. During that period, gripping exercises (Figure 18-2) and isometric shoulder exercises are used. All exercises that place valgus stress on the elbow should be avoided. Therapeutic modalities should also be used to modulate pain and control swelling. On day 4 or 5, gentle active ROM elbow exercises (Figures 18-4 through 18-6) and gentle isometric elbow flexion and extension exercises (Figures 18-3A) can be done out of the splint. Passive stretching is absolutely avoided because of the tendency toward scarring of the traumatized soft tissue and the possibility of recurrent posterior dislocation. Shoulder and wrist isotonic exercises may be done in the splint. Gentle joint mobilizations can be used to regain normal joint arthrokinematics (see Figures 13-21 through 13-24).

At 10 days, the splint can be discontinued. Passive ROM exercises (Figures 18-20 through 18-21) can begin, progressing to stretching exercises (Figures 18-21 through 18-23). Progressive isotonic elbow flexion exercises (Figure 18-8), elbow extension exercises (Figure 18-5), and pronation/supination exercises (Figure 18-6) should continue and progress as tolerated. Isotonic shoulder exercises should continue to progress throughout the rehabilitation program. Eccentric elbow flexion and extension exercises (Figures 18-7 and 18-8), PNF diagonal strengthening patterns (see Figures 14-3 through 14-10), and plyometric exercises (Figure 18-12) may be incorporated as tolerated. Exercises designed to establish neuromuscular control, including closed kinetic chain activities, should also be used to help regain dynamic stability about the elbow joint (Figures 18-9 through 18-11 and 18-23 through 18-26). The patient should continue to wear the brace or use taping (Figure 18-29) to prevent elbow hyperextension and valgus stress during return to activities. For an unstable elbow, the goal during the first 3 to 4 weeks is to protect the healing soft tissue while decreasing pain and swelling. During this period, the protective brace should be set initially at 10 degrees less than the active ROM extension limit. Starting at week 1, a ROM brace preset at 30 to 90 degrees is implemented. Each week, motion in this brace is increased by 5 degrees of extension and 10 degrees of flexion. The brace can be discontinued when full ROM is achieved. During this period, gripping exercises (Figure 18-2) and wrist ROM exercises are used. All exercises that place valgus stress on the elbow should be avoided. Shoulder isometric exercises avoiding internal or external rotation may be used.

At 4 weeks, progressive lightweight (1 to 2 lb) isotonic elbow flexion exercises (Figure 18-4), elbow extension exercises (Figure 18-5), and pronation/supination exercises (Figure 18-6) may be incorporated. Isotonic shoulder exercises (avoiding internal and external rotation for 6 weeks) should begin during this period and continue to progress throughout the rehabilitation program. Passive elbow flexion and extension ROM exercises (Figures 18-20 and 18-21) may begin during this period.

At 6 weeks, isotonic strengthening exercises for the shoulder and external and internal rotation should begin and continue to progress.

At 9 weeks, as strength continues to increase, more functional activities can be incorporated, including eccentric elbow flexion and extension exercises (Figures 18-7 and 18-8), PNF diagonal strengthening patterns (see Figures 14-3 through 14-10), and plyometric exercises (Figure 18-12). Exercises designed to establish neuromuscular control, including closed kinetic chain activities, should also be used to help regain dynamic stability about the elbow joint (Figures 18-9 through 18-11 and 18-26 through 18-35). At 11 weeks, the patient can begin some sport activities as tolerated while continuing to progress the strengthening program. The protective brace should be worn whenever the patient is engaging in any type of sport activity.

Criteria for Full Return

The criteria for a return to full activity after an elbow dislocation are the same as for any return to full activity. The elbow must demonstrate full ROM, and the patient must demonstrate strength, endurance, and neuromuscular control skills appropriate to his or her sport without limiting performance. A functional progression must be demonstrated, and success in terms of the criteria of the rehabilitation protocol must be reached.

Clinical Decision-Making Exercise 18-4

An offensive tackle in football fell while finishing a block. His arm was fully extended, and he felt severe pain and had acute swelling to the elbow. He also noted deformity, with the elbow "stuck" in a flexed position. The elbow had dislocated. The team doctor performed a reduction on the field. The pain is not as severe post reduction. How should the athletic trainer manage this injury?

Medial and Lateral Epicondylitis

Pathomechanics and Injury Mechanism

The medial and the lateral epicondyles of the distal humerus are the tendon attachments of the wrist flexors and extensors.[37] The medial epicondyle serves as the attachment for the wrist flexors, and the wrist extensors attach to the lateral epicondyle.

Medial Epicondylitis

Medial epicondylitis (golfer's elbow, racquetball elbow, or swimmer's elbow in adults, and Little League elbow in adolescents) generally occurs as a result of repetitive microtrauma to the pronator teres and the flexor carpi radialis muscles during pronation and flexion of the wrist. The patient usually complains of pain on the medial aspect of the elbow, which is exacerbated when throwing a baseball, serving or hitting a forehand shot in racquetball, pulling during a swimming backstroke, or hitting a golf ball, in which case the trail arm is affected. There is tenderness at the medial epicondyle, and pain is exacerbated with resisted pronation, resisted volar flexion of the wrist, or passive extension of the wrist with the elbow extended.

REHABILITATION PLAN

MEDIAL ELBOW PAIN

Injury Situation A 23-year-old tennis player is complaining of increased pain to the medial aspect of the elbow. He has been experiencing pain primarily in overhand and forehand strokes. The pain has progressed over the past 4 weeks to now include periodic paresthesia from the medial joint down the medial aspect of the forearm to the fifth digit and one-half of the fourth digit. With cessation of activity, the pain subsides.

Signs and symptoms The patient's ROM is normal, although the end ranges of motion cause pain at the medial collateral ligament. Muscle testing shows strength to be normal throughout except for wrist flexion and ulnar deviation, which is 4/5 with a pain at the medial elbow. Palpation shows pain at the medial collateral ligament and a positive Tinel's sign at the ulnar nerve. There is pain and slight laxity to the medial collateral ligament with valgus testing.

Management plan Establish normal pain-free ROM and return to activity without pain or disability to the elbow.

PHASE ONE: Acute Inflammatory Stage

GOALS: Pain modulation and rehabilitate within healing constraints.

Estimated length of time (ELT): Day 1 to Day 7. The goal is to establish pain-free motion with a gradual and continual increase to full ROM with the use of modalities and passive, active-assistive, and active motion exercises. Stoppage of the activities that exacerbate symptoms is recommended in this time frame. Strengthening exercises that benefit strength and endurance can be done within the constraint of no pain before, during, or after exercise.

PHASE TWO: Fibroblastic-Repair Stage

GOALS: Increase the strength of the elbow flexors, extensors as well as the flexors, extensors, supinators, pronators, and ulnar and radial deviators of the wrist.

Estimated length of time (ELT): Day 8 to Week 3. Modalities such as electrical stimulation for muscle reeducation and pain modulation as well as ice are continued. A gradual progression of rehabilitation exercises (PRE) is begun. These exercises incorporate not only the elbow and wrist/hand, but also the shoulder for rotator cuff and scapular stabilization. Aquatic therapy can increase function with the benefits of buoyancy, and is also recommended for the elbow and upper extremity.

PHASE THREE: Maturation-Remodeling Stage

GOALS: Complete elimination of symptoms for return to sport.

Estimated length of time (ELT): Week 3 to Full Return. The patient can continue the PRE regimen and increase activity in the aquatic setting, with stroke mechanics in the water with a racquet to mimic all forces that will be used when back on the court. The patient should be accustomed to all strengthening and stretching exercises that will be continued after a pain-free return to play has been accomplished.

CRITERIA FOR RETURN TO PLAY

1. No pain with exercises.

2. Normal strength and flexibility in the elbow and upper quarter.

3. Successful completion of all functional progressions and return-to-sport activity without pain or dysfunction.

DISCUSSION QUESTIONS

1. What factors can increase the tension to the medial elbow in tennis?

2. What exercises in the aquatic setting can benefit this patient?

3. Describe the mechanics of the tennis swing that could be developed to decrease pressure to the medial elbow.

4. What modalities are to be used for this patient during and after the rehabilitation process?

5. Are there equipment modifications that can be addressed to help distribute pressure and tension away from the medial elbow?

Associated ulnar neuropathy at the elbow has been reported in 25% to 60% of patients with medial epicondylitis.[9]

Lateral Epicondylitis

Lateral epicondylitis (tennis elbow) occurs with repetitive microtrauma that results in either concentric or eccentric overload of the wrist extensors and supinators, most commonly the extensor carpi radialis brevis.[37] There is pain along the lateral aspect of the elbow, particularly at the origin of the extensor carpi radialis brevis. Pain increases with passive flexion of the wrist with the elbow extended, as it does with resisted wrist dorsiflexion. Pain with resisted wrist extension and full elbow extension indicates involvement of the extensor carpi radialis longus. Lateral epicondylitis usually results from repeated forceful wrist hyperextension, as often occurs in hitting a backhand stroke in tennis. For beginning tennis players, the backhand stroke is somewhat unnatural, and to get enough power to hit the ball over the net there is a tendency to use forced wrist hyperextension. In more advanced players, lateral epicondylitis can develop in a number of ways, including hitting a topspin backhand stroke using a "flick" of the wrist instead of a long follow-through; hitting a serve with the wrist in pronation and "snapping" the wrist to impart spin; using a racquet that is strung with too much tension (55 to 60 lb is recommended); using a grip size that is too small; and hitting a heavy, wet ball.[14,37] It must be emphasized that any activity that involves repeated forceful wrist extension can result in lateral epicondylitis.[14]

Rehabilitation Concerns

Medial and lateral epicondylitis, but particularly lateral epicondylitis, can be a lingering, limiting, frustrating, painful pathological conditions for both the patient and the sports therapist.[32] Perhaps the first step in treating these conditions is altering faulty performance mechanics to minimize the repetitive stress created by these activities. The stressful components of high-level activities can also be alleviated by altering the frequency, intensity, or duration of play.[35]

Two rehabilitation approaches may be taken in treating medial and lateral epicondylitis. The first approach involves using all of the normal measures to reduce inflammation and pain. Treatment may include several weeks of rest or at least restricted activity during which painful movements, like gripping activities that aggravate the condition, are avoided; using therapeutic modalities such as cryotherapy, electrical stimulating currents, ultrasound phonophoresis with hydrocortisone, or iontophoresis using dexamethasone, or extracorporal shockwave therapy;[25] and using nonsteroidal anti-inflammatory drugs. If pain persists, some physicians might recommend a steroid injection if they feel that the patient is incapable of progressing in the rehabilitation program. However, more than two or three steroid injections per year is inappropriate and probably harmful, because it can result in weakening of the surrounding normal tissues.

A second approach would be to realize that the patient has a chronic inflammation. For one reason or another the inflammatory phase of the healing process has not accomplished what it is supposed to and thus the inflammatory process is in effect "stuck." The goal in this approach is to "jump-start" the inflammatory process, using techniques that are likely to increase the inflammatory response, with the idea that increasing inflammation might allow healing to progress as normal to the fibroblastic and remodeling phases. To increase the inflammatory response, transverse friction massage can be used. This technique involves firm pressure massage over the point of maximum tenderness at the epicondyle in a direction perpendicular to the muscle fibers. The use of effleurage progressing to petrissage from origin to insertion of the extensor muscles is recommended. This massage will be painful for the patient, so it is recommended that a stretching of the wrist extensors followed by a 5-minute ice treatment be used prior to the massage to minimize pain. Transverse friction massage should be done for 5 to 7 minutes, every other day, using a maximum of five treatments. It is our experience that if the symptoms do not begin to resolve in 1 week to 10 days, it is unlikely that this approach will eliminate the problem.

It must also be emphasized that during this treatment period, all measures previously described to reduce inflammation should be avoided. Remember that the idea is to increase the inflammatory response. In those individuals who have persistent pain that does not resolve after 1 year of conservative treatment, surgery should be considered.

Clinical Decision-Making Exercise 18-5

A 12-year-old pitcher has been complaining of increased pain to the medial aspect of the elbow. He notes that his team was in an important tournament and he had been pitching more than he is used to in a week's time. The pain increases with any pronatory position associated with the snapping of the wrist into flexion at ball release. How should the athletic trainer manage this injury?

Rehabilitation Progression

Rehabilitation time frames will differ somewhat, depending on which of the two approaches is used in the early treatment of medial and lateral epicondylitis. Regardless of which technique is used, some submaximal exercise can begin during this period as long as it does not cause pain. If rest and anti-inflammatory measures are used, 2 or 3 weeks of restricted activity with very limited or no submaximal exercise might be necessary to control pain and inflammation. If the more aggressive approach using transverse friction massage is chosen, submaximal exercises can begin immediately within pain-free limits.

Exercise intensity should be based on patient tolerance but should adhere to an exercise progression. Throughout the rehabilitation process pain should always be a guide for progression. Each of the following exercises should continue

in a progressive manner throughout the rehabilitative period: gentle active and passive ROM exercises for both the elbow and wrist (Figures 18-17 through 18-22), gentle isometric elbow flexion and extension exercises (Figure 18-3A), gentle isometric pronation/supination exercises (Figure 18-3B), progressive isotonic elbow flexion exercises (Figure 18-4), elbow extension exercises (Figure 18-5), and pronation/supination exercises (Figure 18-6) beginning with light weight (1 to 2 lb). Lateral counterforce bracing should be used as a supplement to muscular strengthening exercises (Figure 18-28) with the patient gradually weaning from use as appropriate. Eccentric elbow flexion and extension exercises (Figures 18-7 and 18-8), along with plyometric exercises (Figure 18-12) and functional training activities should progressively incorporate the stresses, strains, and forces that occur during normal sport activities, gradually increasing the frequency, intensity, and duration of play.

Criteria for Full Return

Perhaps the biggest mistake made with epicondylitis is trying to progress too quickly in the exercise program and rushing full return to play. The athletic trainer should counsel the patient about doing too much too soon, cautioning that rapid increases in activity levels often exacerbate the condition. The involved muscles must regain appropriate strength, flexibility, and endurance with reduced inflammation and pain. Functional activity needs to progress slowly to prepare the patient for the return without restrictions.

AQUATIC THERAPY TECHNIQUES TO ASSIST IN THE REHABILITATION OF THE ELBOW

Aquatic therapy is very helpful in the rehabilitation of the elbow and the upper quarter as a whole. As described in Chapter 15, upward buoyancy counteracts the force of the earth's gravity. Therefore, activity performed in the water enhances achievement in comparison to land exercise.[27] Treatment techniques that traditionally are performed when the patient is

Table 18-1 Interval Throwing Program

45-Foot Phase	60-Foot Phase	90-Foot Phase
Step 1: A. Warm-up throwing B. 45 feet (25 throws) C. Rest 15 minutes D. Warm-up throwing E. 45 feet (25 throws)	Step 3: A. Warm-up throwing B. 60 feet (25 throws) C. Rest 15 minutes D. Warm-up throwing E. 60 feet (25 throws)	Step 5: A. Warm-up throwing B. 90 feet (25 throws) C. Rest 15 minutes D. Warm-up throwing E. 90 feet (25 throws)
Step 2: A. Warm-up throwing B. 45 feet (25 throws) C. Rest 10 minutes D. Warm-up throwing E. 45 feet (25 throws) F. Rest 10 minutes G. Warm-up throwing H. 45 feet (25 throws)	Step 4: A. Warm-up throwing B. 60 feet (25 throws) C. Rest 10 minutes D. Warm-up throwing E. 60 feet (25 throws) F. Rest 10 minutes G. Warm-up throwing H. 60 feet (25 throws)	Step 6: A. Warm-up throwing B. 90 feet (25 throws) C. Rest 10 minutes D. Warm-up throwing E. 90 feet (25 throws) F. Rest 10 minutes G. Warm-up throwing H. 90 feet (25 throws)
120-Foot Phase	**150-Foot Phase**	**180-Foot Phase**
Step 7: A. Warm-up throwing B. 120 feet (25 throws) C. Rest 15 minutes D. Warm-up throwing E. 120 feet (25 throws)	Step 9: A. Warm-up throwing B. 150 feet (25 throws) C. Rest 15 minutes D. Warm-up throwing E. 150 feet (25 throws)	Step 11: A. Warm-up throwing B. 180 feet (25 throws) C. Rest 15 minutes D. Warm-up throwing E. 180 feet (25 throws)
Step 8: A. Warm-up throwing B. 120 feet (25 throws) C. Rest 10 minutes D. Warm-up throwing E. 120 feet (25 throws) F. Rest 10 minutes G. Warm-up throwing H. 120 feet (25 throws)	Step 10: A. Warm-up throwing B. 150 feet (25 throws) C. Rest 10 minutes D. Warm-up throwing E. 150 feet (25 throws) F. Rest 10 minutes G. Warm-up throwing H. 150 feet (25 throws)	Step 12: A. Warm-up throwing B. 180 feet (25 throws) C. Rest 10 minutes D. Warm-up throwing E. 180 feet (25 throws) F. Rest 10 minutes G. Warm-up throwing H. 180 feet (25 throws)
		Step 13: A. Warm-up throwing B. 180 feet (25 throws) C. Rest 15 minutes D. Warm-up throwing E. 180 feet (25 throws) F. Rest 15 minutes G. Warm-up throwing H. 180 feet (25 throws)
		Step 14: Begin throwing off the mound or return to respective position

(continued)

Table 18-1 Interval Throwing Program (*continued*)

Interval Throwing Program—Phase 2	
Stage 1: Fastball only	**Stage 2: Fastball Only**
Step 1: Interval throwing 　　　15 throws off mound 50%	Step 9:　45 throws off mound 75% 　　　　15 throws in batting practice
Step 2: Interval throwing 　　　30 throws off mound 50%	Step 10: 45 throws off mound 75% 　　　　30 throws in batting practice
Step 3: Interval throwing 　　　45 throws off mound 50%	Step 11: 45 throws off mound 75% 　　　　45 throws in batting practice
Step 4: Interval throwing 　　　60 throws off mound 50%	**Stage 3**
Step 5: Interval throwing 　　　30 throws off mound 50%	Step 12: 30 throws off mound 75% 　　　　warm-up 　　　　15 throws off mound 50% 　　　　breaking balls 　　　　45–60 throws in batting practice (fastball only)
Step 6: 30 throws off mound 75% 　　　45 throws off mound 50%	
Step 7: 45 throws off mound 75% 　　　15 throws off mound 50%	Step 13: 30 throws off mound 75% 　　　　30 breaking balls 75% 　　　　30 throws in batting practice
Step 8: 60 throws off mound 50% 　　　15 throws off mound 50%	Step 14: 30 throws off mound 75 % 　　　　60 to 90 throws in batting practice 　　　　25% breaking balls
	Step 15: Simulated game: progressing by 15 throws per 　　　　workout
Note: Use interval throwing to 120-foot phase as a warm-up. All throwing off the mound should be done in the presence of the pitching coach to stress proper throwing mechanics. Use a speed gun to aid in effort control.	

in a supine, prone, or standing position can be done in the aquatic setting with less stress to the elbow, maximizing activity and benefiting the rehabilitation process (see Figures 15-15 through 15-23).

THROWING PROGRAM FOR RETURN TO SPORT

The patient progresses through a series of steps for return to her or his sport. For the throwing patient, the progression described in Table 18-1 is one of the final criteria for full return.[49,50] During this throwing progression, the patient is performing upper-quarter exercises that work on the cervical spine, the shoulder rotator cuff, and muscles that affect the glenohumeral joint, as well as exercises that work on the elbow, hand, and wrist. The proprioceptive and neuromuscular control effects stressed by this throwing program are critical in returning the patient to full activity. The throwing program is progressive in distance, repetition, duration, and intensity. It is imperative that the patient successfully complete the criteria at one level before progressing to the next.

Summary

1. The elbow joint is composed of the humeroulnar joint, humeroradial joint, and the proximal radioulnar joint. Motions in the elbow complex include flexion, extension, pronation, and supination.

2. Fractures in the elbow can occur from a direct blow or from falling on an outstretched hand. They may be treated by casting or in some cases by surgical reduction and fixation. Following surgical

fixation the patient might require 12 weeks for return.

3. Osteochondritis dissecans and Panner's disease are injuries that affect the lateral aspect of the elbow. Osteochondritis dissecans is associated with a loose body in the joint, whereas Panner's disease is an osteochondrosis of the capitellum. The prognosis for full return to throwing or loading activities should be cautious.

4. Injuries to the ulnar collateral ligament result from a valgus force from the repetitive trauma of overhead throwing, which occurs during the late cocking phase through the early acceleration phase of throwing. Reconstruction is vital to competitive throwing athletes, and rehabilitation can require as long as 22 to 26 weeks for full return.

5. In the case of entrapment of the ulnar, median, and radial nerves, mobility of the nerve is critical in reducing nerve entrapment. Rehabilitation should concentrate primarily on stretching to free up the nerve. If conservative treatment fails, surgical release might be indicated.

6. Elbow dislocations result from elbow hyperextension from a fall on an extended arm, with the radius and ulna dislocating posteriorly. The degree of stability present will determine the course of rehabilitation. If the elbow is stable, a brief period of immobilization is followed by rehabilitation. An unstable dislocation requires surgical repair and thus a longer period of immobilization.

7. Medial epicondylitis (golfer's elbow, racquetball elbow, swimmer's elbow, Little League elbow) results from repetitive microtrauma to flexor carpi radialis muscles during pronation and flexion of the wrist. Lateral epicondylitis (tennis elbow) occurs with concentric or eccentric overload of the wrist extensors and supinators, most commonly the extensor carpi radialis brevis.

References

1. An, K. N., and B. F. Morrey. 2009. Biomechanics of the elbow. In *The elbow and its disorders*, edited by B. F. Morrey. Philadelphia: W. B. Saunders.

2. Andrews, J. R., K. E. Wilk, and D. Groh. 2003. Elbow rehabilitation. In *Clinical orthopedic rehabilitation*, edited by B. Brotzman. St. Louis: Mosby.

3. Andrews, J. R., K. E. Wilk, Y. E. Satterwhite, and J. L. Tedder. 1993. Physical examination of the throwers elbow. *Journal of Orthopaedic and Sports Physical Therapy; 17*:296–304.

4. Andrich, J. 1995. Upper extremity injuries in the skeletally immature patient. In *The upper extremity in sports medicine*, edited by J. Nicholas and E. Hershman. St. Louis: Mosby.

5. Azar, F. M., and K. E. Wilk. 1996. Nonoperative treatment of the elbow in throwers. *Operative Techniques in Sports Medicine; 4*:91–99.

6. Bauer, M., K. Jonsson, P. O. Josefsson, and B. Linden. 1999. Osteochondritis dissecans of the elbow: A long-term follow-up study. *Clinical Orthopaedics and Related Research; 284*:156–160.

7. Bencardino, J. 2006. Entrapment Neuropathies of the Shoulder and Elbow in the Athlete. *Clinics in Sports Medicine; 25*(3):465.

8. Bruckner, J. D., A. H. Alexander, and D. M. Lichtman. 1996. Acute dislocations of the distal radioulnar joint. *Instructional Course Lectures; 45*:27–36.

9. Buettner, C., and D. Leaver-Dunn. 2000. Prevention and treatment of elbow injuries in adolescent pitchers. *Athletic Therapy Today; 5*(3):19.

10. Byron, P. 1997. Restoring function. *Journal of Hand Therapy; 10*(1):334–37.

11. Chehab, E., J. Toro, and D. Helfet. 2005. The management of fractures of the elbow joint in athletes. *International SportMed Journal; 6*(2):84.

12. Cordasco, F., and J. Parkes. 1995. Overuse injuries of the elbow. In *The upper extremity in sports medicine*, edited by J. Nicholas and E. Hershman. St. Louis: Mosby.

13. Davidson, P. A., M. Pink, J. Perry, and F.W. Jobe. 1995. Functional anatomy of the flexor pronator muscle group in relation to the medial collateral ligament of the elbow. *American Journal of Sports Medicine; 23*(2):245–250.

14. De Smedt, T. 2007. Lateral epicondylitis in tennis: Update on aetiology, biomechanics and treatment. *British Journal of Sports Medicine; 41*(11):816–819.

15. Dodson, C. 2006. Medial ulnar collateral ligament reconstruction of the elbow in throwing athletes. *American Journal of Sports Medicine; 34*(12):1926–1932.

16. Ferlic, D. C., and B. F. Morrey. 1993. Evaluation of the painful elbow: The problem elbow. In *The elbow and its disorders*, 2nd ed., edited by B. F. Morrey. Philadelphia: W. B. Saunders.

17. Field, L., and F. Savoie. 2000. Surgical treatment of ulnar collateral ligament injuries. *Athletic Therapy Today;* 5(3):25.

18. Fyfe, I., and W. D. Stanish. 1992. The use of eccentric training and stretching in the treatment and prevention of tendon injuries. *Clinics in Sports Medicine;* 3:601–624.

19. Guerra, J. J., and L. A. Timmerman. 1996. Clinical anatomy, histology, and pathomechanics of the elbow in sports. *Operative Techniques in Sports Medicine;* 4:69–76.

20. Harrelson, G. L. 2004. Elbow rehabilitation. In *Physical rehabilitation of the injured patient,* edited by J. Andrews and G. L. Harrelson. Philadelphia: W. B. Saunders.

21. Hennrikus, W. 2006. Elbow disorders in the young athlete. *Operative Techniques in Sports Medicine;* 14(3):165–172.

22. Kälicke, T. 2007. Dislocation of the elbow with fractures of the coronoid process and radial head. *Archives of Orthopaedic & Trauma Surgery* 127(10):925.

23. Kaminski, T., M. Powers, and B. Buckley. 2000. Differential assessment of elbow injuries. *Athletic Therapy Today;* 5(3):6.

24. Kao, J. T., M. Pink, F.W. Jobe, and J. Perry. 1995. Electromyographic analysis of the scapular muscles during a golfswing. *American Journal of Sports Medicine;* 23(1):19–23.

25. Kohia, M., J. Brackle, and K. Byrd. 2008. Effectiveness of physical therapy treatments on lateral epicondylitis. *Journal of Sport Rehabilitation;* 17(2):119.

26. Levangie, P. K., and C. C. Norkin. 2005. Function: Humeroulnar and humeroradial joints. In *Joint structure and function,* 2nd ed. Philadelphia: F. A. Davis.

27. Levin, S. 1991. Aquatic therapy. *Physician and Sports Medicine;* 19:119–126.

28. Levine, J. 2006. Arthroscopic management of osteochondritis dissecans of the elbow. *Operative Techniques in Sports Medicine;* 14(2):60–66.

29. Magee, D. J. 2008. *Elbow: Orthopedic physical assessment.* Philadelphia: W. B. Saunders.

30. Mehta, J. 2004. Elbow dislocations in adults and children. *Clinics in Sports Medicine;* 23(4):609–627.

31. Morrey, B. F. 2009. Anatomy of the elbow joint. In *The elbow and its disorders,* 2nd ed., edited by B. F. Morrey. Philadelphia: W. B. Saunders.

32. Murphy, K. 2006. Management of lateral epicondylitis in the athlete. *Operative Techniques in Sports Medicine* 14(2):67–77.

33. Nassab, P. 2006. Evaluation and treatment of medial ulnar collateral ligament injuries in the throwing athlete. *Sports Medicine & Arthroscopy Review;* 14(4):221–231.

34. Olsen, B. S., J. O. Sojbjerg, M. Dalstra, and O. Sneppen. 1996. Kinematics of the lateral ligamentous constraints of the elbow joint. *Journal of Shoulder and Elbow Surgery;* 5(5):333–341.

35. Plancher, K. D., J. Halbrecht, and G. M. Lourie. 1996. Medial and lateral epicondylitis in the patient. *Clinics in Sports Medicine;* 15(2):283–305.

36. Reinold, M., et al. 2000. Biomechanics and rehabilitation of elbow injuries during throwing. *Athletic Therapy Today;* 5(3):12.

37. Roetert, E. P., H. Brody, C. J. Dillman, J. L. Groppel, and J. M. Schultheis. 1995. The biomechanics of tennis elbow: An integrated approach. *Clinics in Sports Medicine;* 14(1):47–57.

38. Saliba, E. 1991. The upper arm, elbow, and forearm. In *AAOS athletic training and sports medicine,* 2nd ed., edited by L. Y. Hunter. Park Ridge, IL: AAOS.

39. Savoie, F. 2008. Primary repair of ulnar collateral ligament injuries of the elbow in young athletes. *American Journal of Sports Medicine;* 36(6):1066.

40. Shin, R., and D. Ring. 2007. The ulnar nerve in elbow trauma. *Journal of Bone & Joint Surgery;* 89(5):1108.

41. Sobel, J., and R. P. Nirschl. 1996. Elbow injuries. In *Athletic injuries and rehabilitation,* edited by J. Zachewski, D. Magee, and W. Quillen. Philadelphia: W. B. Saunders.

42. Stoane, J. M., M. R. Poplausky, J. O. Haller, and W. E. Berdon. 1995. Panner's disease: X-ray, MR imaging findings and review of the literature. *Computerized Medical Imaging and Graphics;* 19(6):473–476.

43. Stroyan, M., and K. E. Wilk. 1993. The functional anatomy of the elbow complex. *Journal of Orthopaedic and Sports Physical Therapy;* 17(6):279–288.

44. Struijs, P., and G. Smit. 2007. Radial head fractures: Effectiveness of conservative treatment versus surgical intervention. *Archives of Orthopaedic & Trauma Surgery;* 127(2):125.

45. Takahara, M. 2007. Classification, treatment, and outcome of osteochondritis dissecans of the humeral capitellum. *Journal of Bone & Joint Surgery, American Volume;* 89(6):1205.

46. Thomas, P. J., and R. C. Noellert. 1995. Brachial artery disruption after closed posterior dislocation of the elbow. *American Journal of Orthopedics;* 24(7):558–560.

47. Uhl, T. 2000. Uncomplicated elbow dislocation rehabilitation. *Athletic Therapy Today;* 5(3):31.

48. Warfel, J. H. 1993. Muscles of the arm. In *The extremities, muscles and motor points.* Philadelphia: Lea & Febiger.

49. Wilk, K. E. 1997. Personal communication with the author.

50. Wilk, K. E., C. Arrigo, and J. R. Andrews. 1993. Rehabilitation of the elbow in the throwing patient. *Journal of Orthopaedic and Sports Physical Therapy;* 17(6):305–317.

SOLUTIONS TO CLINICAL DECISION-MAKING EXERCISES

18-1 Axial loading injuries such as this will cause articular pain and potential epiphyseal plate pathology in the younger patient. The athletic trainer must work on the upper quarter as a whole by working on strength and function of the neck, shoulder, and wrist/hand. Techniques of functional progression and return-to-sport concepts must also be addressed.

18-2 Due to the complexities of this osteochondrotic condition, the athletic trainer should exercise extreme caution in the rehabilitation of this patient. The fact that there is an articular surface pathology associated with such a young patient requires pain-free activity initially that can be gradually progressed within pain-free limits.

18-3 With the instability noted to the medial complex as a whole, the athletic trainer must consider how this will affect other structures. The carrying angle increases medial stress anatomically, so increased laxity of the ligament and medial complex will increase pressure on the ulnar nerve. During rehabilitation, care must be taken not to increase paresthesia and weakness in the forearm.

18-4 The athletic trainer knows that the stability of the elbow after this injury will be the cornerstone of the rehabilitation progression. If there is stability, the increase in motion and loading with isometric, isotonic, and functional exercise can be progressive. If there is inherent instability due to a bony stabilizing force impairment, the rehabilitation will be more tenuous.

18-5 Skeletal immaturity and excessive activity are not compatible, so the athletic trainer must establish a pain-free rehabilitative progression. It is essential to increase the musculoskeletal balance in the upper extremity, develop a gradual increase in activity progression, such as pitch counts, and use a proper throwing progression.

Please see videos on the accompanying website at

www.healio.com/books/sportsmedvideos

CHAPTER 19

Rehabilitation of Wrist, Hand, and Finger Injuries

Anne Marie Schneider, OTR/L, CHT

After completion of this chapter, the athletic training student should be able to do the following:

- Discuss the functional anatomy and biomechanics associated with normal function of the wrist and hand.

- Discuss various rehabilitative strengthening techniques for the wrist and hand.

- Identify techniques for improving, including stretching exercises.

- Relate biomechanical and tissue healing principles to the rehabilitation of various wrist and hand injuries.

- Discuss criteria for progression of the rehabilitation program for different hand and wrist injuries.

- Describe and explain various splints for the hand and wrist and how they relate to protection and return to play.

- Describe and explain the rationale for various treatment techniques in the management of wrist and hand injuries.

FUNCTIONAL ANATOMY AND BIOMECHANICS

The hand is an intricate balance of muscles, tendons, and joints working in unison. Hands are almost always exposed and for that reason can be especially prone to injuries, especially during sport contact. Changing the mechanics can greatly alter the function and appearance of the hand.

The Wrist

The wrist is the connecting link between the hand and the forearm.[45] The wrist joint is composed of eight carpal bones and their articulations with the radius and ulna proximally, and the metacarpals distally. There is

Prentice WE, ed.
Rehabilitation Techniques for Sports Medicine and Athletic Training (pp 547-590).
© 2015 SLACK Incorporated.

an intricate relationship between the carpal bones. They are connected by ligaments to each other, and to the radius and ulna. The palmar ligaments from the proximal carpal row to the radius are strongest, followed by the dorsal ligaments (scaphoid-triquetrum, and distal radius to lunate and triquetrum), with intrinsic ligaments (scapholunate and lunotriquetral) being the weakest.[7] The carpal bones are arranged in two rows, proximal and distal, with the scaphoid acting as the functional link between the two.[45] The distal carpal row determines the position of the scaphoid and thus the lunate. With radial deviation, the distal row is displaced radially while the proximal row moves ulnarly. The distal portion of the scaphoid must shift to avoid the radial styloid. The scaphoid palmar flexes. This is reversed in ulnar deviation.[25] The total arc of motion for radial and ulnar deviation averages about 50 degrees, 15 degrees radially and 35 degrees ulnarly.[25] The uneven division is due to the buttressing effect of the radial styloid.[25]

Flexion and extension occur through synchronous movement of proximal and distal rows. The total excursion is equally distributed between the midcarpal and radiocarpal joints.[7] The arc of motion for flexion and extension is 121 degrees.[32]

There are no collateral ligaments in the wrist. Their presence would impede radial and ulnar deviation, allowing only flexion and extension. Cross sections through the wrist reveal that tendons of the extensor carpi ulnaris (ECU) at the ulnar aspect of the wrist, and the extensor pollicus brevis (EPB) and abductor pollicus longus (APL) on the radial side are in "collateral" position.[32] Electromyogram (EMG) studies show that ECU, EPB, and APL are active in wrist flexion and extension.[32] These muscles show only small displacement with flexion and extension so they are in an isometric position.[32] Their function can be described as an adjustable collateral system. The ECU shows activity in ulnar deviation and the APL and EPB in radial deviation.[32]

Stability of the ulnar side of the wrist is provided by the triangular fibrocartilage complex (TFCC).[45] This ligament arises from the radius and inserts into the base of the ulnar styloid, the ulnar carpus, and the base of the fifth metacarpal.[45] This ligament complex is the major stabilizer of the distal radioulnar joint (DRUJ) and is a load-bearing column between the distal ulna and ulnar carpus.[45] There are no muscular or tendinous insertions on any carpal bones except the flexor carpi ulnaris (FCU) into the pisiform.[45] Muscles that move the wrist and fingers cross the wrist and insert on the appropriate bones. There is a dorsal retinaculum (fascia) with six vertical septa that attach to the distal radius and partition the first five dorsal compartments.[32] These define fibroosseous tunnels that position and maintain extensor tendons and their synovial sheaths relative to the axis of wrist motion.[32] The sixth compartment that houses the ECU is a separate tunnel formed from infratendinous retinaculum. This allows unrestricted ulnar rotation during pronation and supination.[32] The retinaculum prevents bowstringing of the tendons during wrist extension.

Volarly, the long finger flexors, long thumb flexor, median nerve, and radial artery pass through the carpal tunnel. Bowstringing is prevented by the thick transverse carpal ligament.

The Hand

The metacarpal phalangeal (MCP) joints allow for multiplanar motion; however, the primary function is flexion and extension.[45] The metacarpal head has a convex shape that fits with a shallow concave proximal phalanx. The stability of the MCP joint is provided by its capsule, collateral ligaments, accessory collateral ligaments, volar plate, and musculotendinous units.[45] The collateral ligaments are laterally positioned and are dorsal to the axis of rotation. In extension the collateral ligament is lax, in flexion it is taut.[13] This is important to remember if immobilizing the MCP joint. If the joint is casted or splinted in extension, the lax collateral ligament will tighten, which will then prevent flexion once mobilization has begun. The accessory collateral ligament is volar to the axis of rotation and is taut in extension and lax in flexion.

The volar plate helps prevent hyperextension of the MCP joint. It forms the dorsal wall of the flexor tendon sheath and the A1 pulley.[45]

Several muscles cross the MCP joints. On the flexor surface the flexor digitorum superficialis

(FDS) and flexor digitorum profundus (FDP) are held close to the bones by pulleys. These pulleys prevent bowstringing during finger flexion. The FDS flexes the proximal interphalangeal (PIP) joint, and the FDP flexes the distal interphalangeal (DIP) joint. The interosseous muscles are lateral to the MCP joints and are responsible for abduction and adduction of the MCP joints. The lumbrical muscles are volar to the axis of rotation of the MCP joint, but then insert into the lateral bands and are dorsal to the PIP and DIP joints. Their function is MCP joint flexion and IP joint extension. (This is also the reason there can be IP extension with a radial nerve palsy.) Dorsally, the extensor mechanism crosses the MCP joint. The tendon is held centrally by the sagittal bands.

The Fingers

The IP joints are bicondylar hinge joints allowing flexion and extension. Collateral and accessory collateral ligaments stabilize the joints on the lateral aspect. The collateral ligament is taut in extension and lax in flexion. This is important when splinting the PIP joint. If it is not a contraindication to the injury (ie, PIP fracture dislocation), the joint should be splinted in full extension to help prevent flexion contractures.

On the flexor surface, the FDS bifurcates proximal to the PIP joint, allowing the FDP to become more superficial as it continues to insert on the distal phalanx, allowing DIP flexion. The FDS inserts on the middle phalanx for PIP flexion. Five annular pulleys and three cruciate pulleys between the MCP and DIP joints prevent bowstringing of the tendons and help provide nutrition to the tendons.

On the extensor surface, the common extensor tendon crosses the MCP joint then divides into three slips. The central slip inserts on the dorsal middle phalanx, allowing for PIP extension. The two lateral slips, called the lateral bands, get attachments from the lumbricals, travel dorsal and lateral to the PIP joint, rejoin after the PIP joint, and insert as the terminal extensor into the DIP joint. This is a delicately balanced system to extend the IP joints. Disruption of this system greatly alters the balance, and thus the dynamic function, of the hand.

REHABILITATION TECHNIQUES FOR SPECIFIC INJURIES

Distal Radius Fractures

Pathomechanics

Fractures of the distal radius can be described in many different ways, by several classification systems. For treatment, it is important to be able to describe the fracture and X-ray. Is the fracture intra-articular or extra-articular; displaced or nondisplaced; simple or comminuted; open or closed? Is the radius shortened? Is the ulna also fractured? Answers to these questions help guide treatment and expected outcomes.

Simple, extra-articular, nondisplaced fractures tend to heal without incident with immobilization, with full or nearly full motion expected following treatment.[1] As the fractures become more involved (intra-articular or comminuted), chances of full return of motion are decreased.

The normal anatomic radius is tilted volarly. If in a fracture the volar tilt becomes dorsal, motion will be affected. It can also lead to midcarpal instability, decreased strength, increased ulnar loading, and a dysfunctional DRUJ.[12]

The normal anatomic radius is longer than the ulna. If in a comminuted fracture the radius is shortened, this is the most disabling.[12] Radial shortening can lead to DRUJ problems, decreased mobility, and decreased power (strength). Articular displacement correction is critical. Radial shortening must be corrected via external fixation.

The external fixator will attach to the mid radius and to the second metacarpal shaft. Length may be restored and held with the traction bars of the external fixator. If the fixator was not in place and the fracture was not reduced, the weight and anatomy of the carpal bones and the force of the muscles would cause loss of reduction and shortening of the radius. The type of fracture, size of the fragments, and displacement determine initial treatment (cast vs fixator). Once reduced, the fractures must be closely monitored to be sure reduction is being maintained.

REHABILITATION TECHNIQUES

Strengthening Techniques

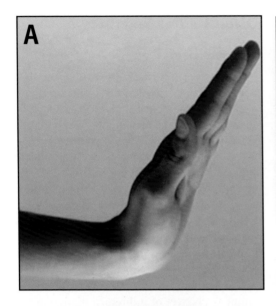
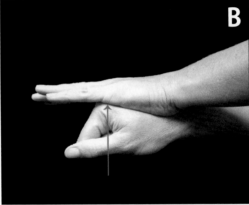
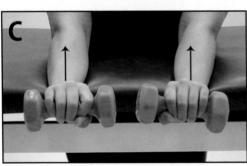
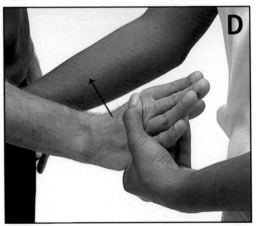

Figure 19-1. (A) Wrist extension should be done in pronation to work against gravity. This exercise encourages strength and motion of the common wrist extensor tendons (ECRL, ECRB, ECU). (B) Strengthening of wrist extensors can be initiated isometrically. (C) This position can be graded by adding weights. (D) Passive wrist extension helps regain motion in the wrist, which then needs to be maintained actively.

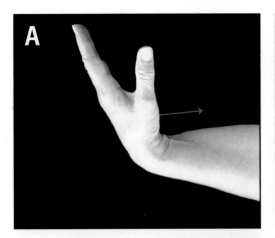
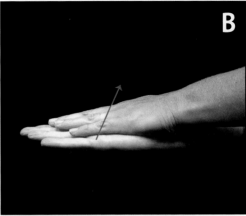
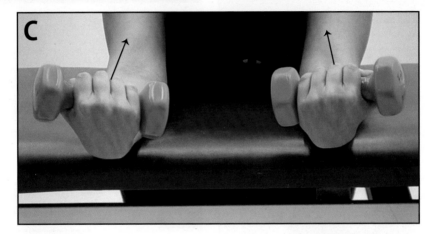
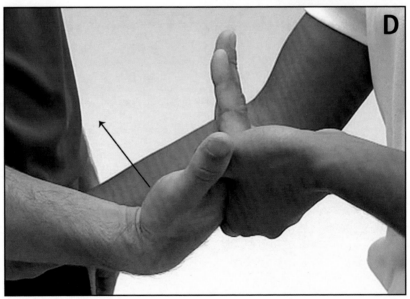

Figure 19-2. (A) Wrist flexion actively works on FCR and FCU. It may be done in pronation as gravity assists or in supination against gravity. (B) Strengthening of wrist flexors can begin isometrically. (C) Position may be graded by adding weights. (D) Passive wrist flexion should be done first by pulling out or distracting the wrist, then flexing.

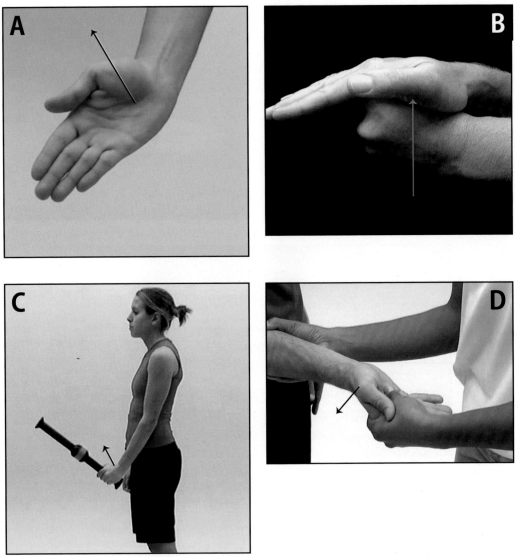

Figure 19-3. (A) Wrist radial deviation with neutral flexion and extension will exercise the FCR and ECRL. (B) Isometric wrist radial deviation. (C) It may be graded to include weights. (D) It may be manually resisted isotonically.

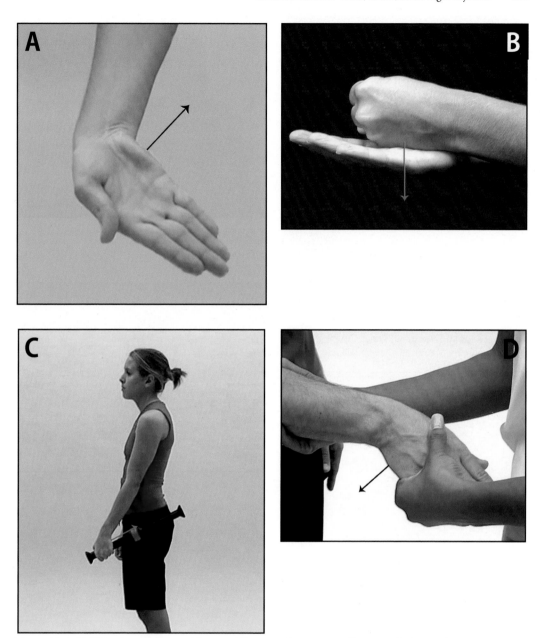

Figure 19-4. (A) Wrist ulnar deviation with neutral flexion and extension will exercise the ECU and FCU. (B) Isometric wrist ulnar deviation. (C) It may be graded to include weights. (D) It may be manually resisted isotonically.

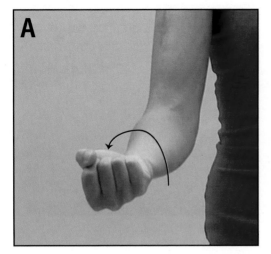

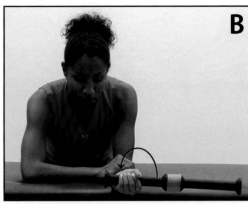

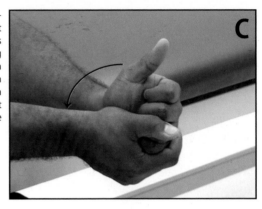

Figure 19-5. (A) Active supination exercises the supinator and the biceps. It should be done with elbow at 90 degrees of flexion with the humerus by the side. This eliminates shoulder rotation. (B) This can be graded using a hammer or weights for strengthening. The hammer with lever action being heavier on one end will also assist with passive motion. (C) Passive stretching should be done in the same position, with force applied proximal to the wrist applying pressure over the radius rather than torquing the wrist.

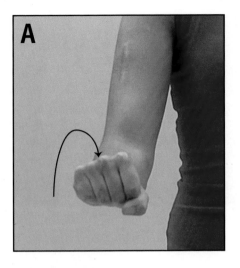

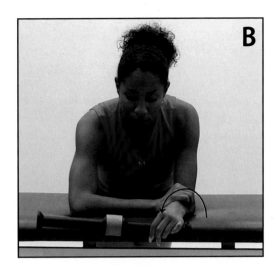

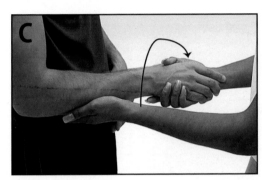

Figure 19-6. (A) Active pronation exercises the pronator. It should be done with elbow flexed to 90 degrees with the humerus by the side. This eliminates shoulder rotation. (B) This can be done with a hammer or weights for strengthening. (C) Passive stretching should be done in the same position with the pressure applied proximal to the wrist.

Figure 19-7. Thumb ROM is begun with opposition to each fingertip.

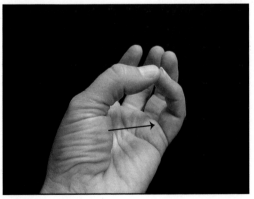

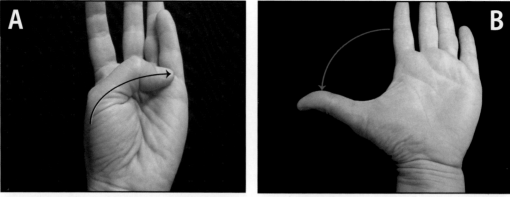

Figure 19-8. (A) Opposition can be progressed to composite flexion reaching for the base of the little finger. (B) Composite thumb extension.

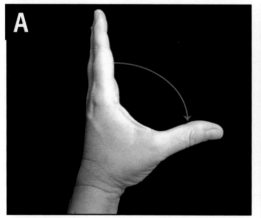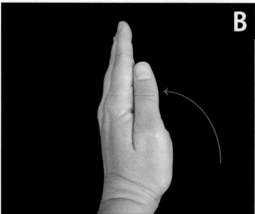

Figure 19-9. (A) Thumb abduction. (B) Thumb adduction.

Figure 19-10. Thumb retropulsion to test EPL function.

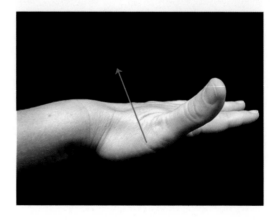

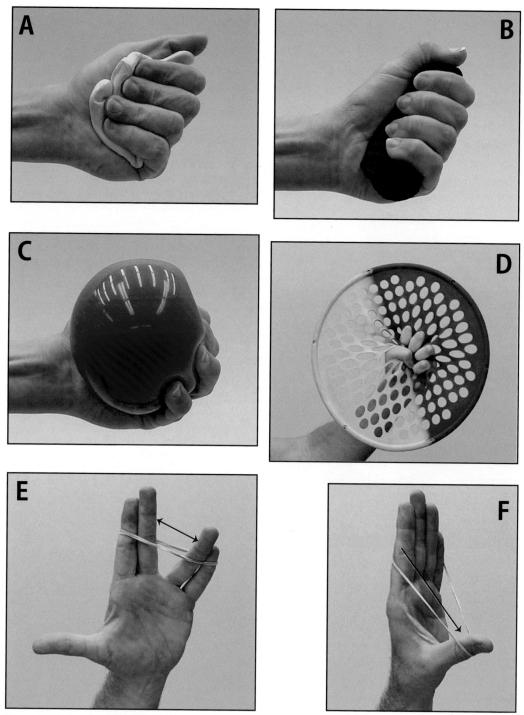

Figure 19-11. A variety of resistance devices are available for restoring hand grip function: (A) putty; (B) foam; (C) rubber ball; (D) power web; (E) rubber band finger abduction; (F) rubber band thumb abduction. *(continued)*

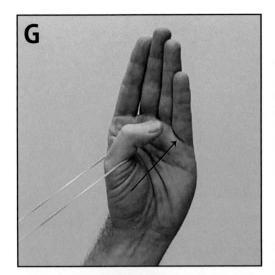

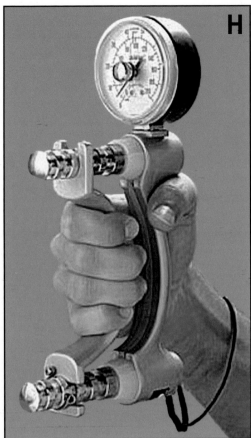

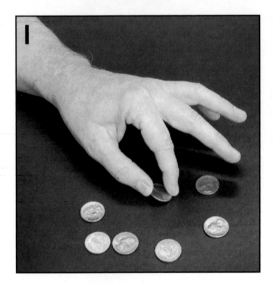

Figure 19-11. (*continued*) (G) Rubber band thumb opposition; (H) a grip dynamometer; (I) picking up coins.

Closed Kinetic Chain Exercises

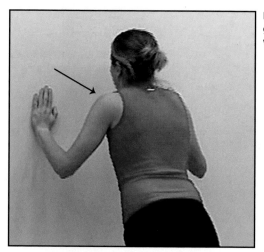

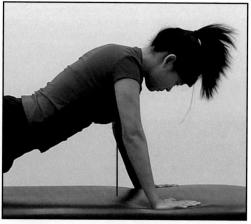

Figure 19-12. Wall push-ups encourage wrist motion and general upper-body strengthening. They also encourage weight-bearing and closed chain activities.

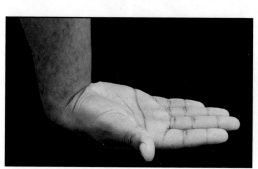

Figure 19-13. Push-ups can be progressed from the wall to a table or countertop. This encourages increased weight but not the full weight of floor push-ups.

Figure 19-14. Push-ups on the floor require full, or close to full, wrist motion and encourage full upper-body weight bearing on the wrist.

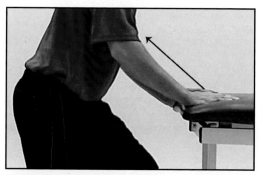

Figure 19-15. Stretching wrist extensor musculature is appropriate when tendinitis is present. The greatest stretch will occur with the elbow at full extension. If this stretch is too great, increase elbow flexion to a comfortable stretch point. Do not bounce at the end of a stretch.

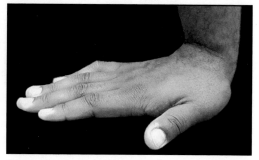

Figure 19-16. Stretching wrist flexor musculature is appropriate with flexor tendinitis. Again, the largest stretch will occur with full elbow extension. Modify elbow flexion as necessary. Stretching should not be painful.

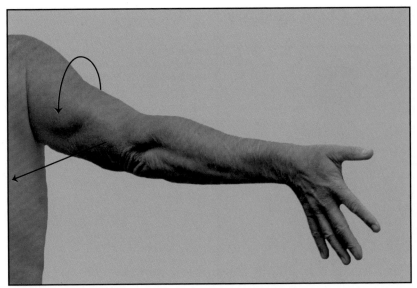

Figure 19-17. Butler describes median nerve gliding exercises to be done in the clinic. It is also important to teach athletes to stretch on their own. This is a median nerve glide that athletes can perform on their own against a wall. Start with arm at shoulder height, elbow extended, and wrist extension with palm against the wall. Rotate shoulder externally. Turn away from the wall to be perpendicular. The last step is to add lateral neck flexion. Stop at any point along this progression where numbness or burning is felt along the arm.

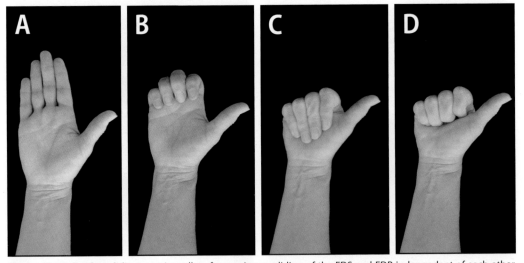

Figure 19-18. Tendon gliding exercises allow for maximum gliding of the FDS and FDP independent of each other. (A) Start with full composite finger extension, (B) move to hook fisting, which gives the maximum glide of the FDP, (C) return to extension, move to long fisting with MCP and PIP flexion and DIP extension for maximum FDS glide, (D) return to extension, then to composite flexion with full fisting.

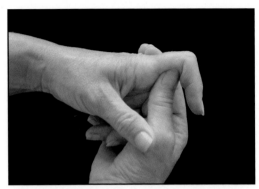

Figure 19-19. Blocked PIP exercises encourage FDS pull-through. Stabilizing the proximal phalanx then allows the flexion force to act at the PIP joint. It is most often used with tendon injuries or finger fractures.

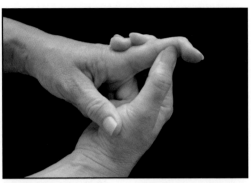

Figure 19-20. Blocked DIP exercises encourage FDP pull-through. Stabilizing the middle phalanx allows the flexion force to concentrate at the DIP joint. These are most often done with flexor tendon injuries, extensor tendon injuries, or finger fractures.

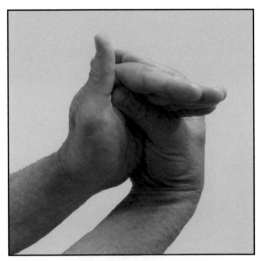

Figure 19-21. MCP flexion with IP extension exercises the intrinsic muscles of the hand. It may help with edema control and muscle pumping. This is most often done with distal radius fractures or MCP joint injuries. Performing IP extension with the MCP joints blocked in flexion concentrates the extension force at the IP joints. This is beneficial for IP joint injuries or tendon injuries.

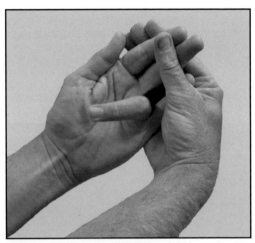

Figure 19-22. Isolated superficialis exercises are done for tendon gliding of the FDS. Noninvolved fingers should be held in full extension, allowing only the involved finger to flex. This is most helpful during flexor tendon lacerations.

Exercises to Reestablish Neuromuscular Control

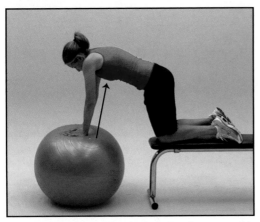

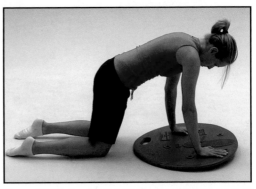

Figure 19-24. Kneeling on the floor and bearing weight on a BAPS board allows for weight bearing throughout the upper extremity, weight shifting, and balance activities.

Figure 19-23. Push-ups on the ball allow for an unstable surface, to encourage strengthening and upper extremity control. Overhead plyometric activities encourage endurance and strength of entire upper extremity.

Taping and Bracing Techniques

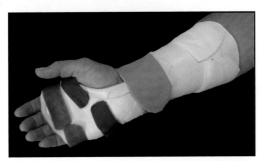

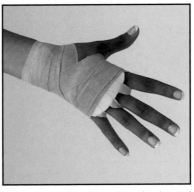

Figure 19-25. A wrist splint may be made dorsally, volarly, or circumferentially, depending on support needs and type of injury. These splints may be used for tendinitis, wrist fractures, wrist sprains, and carpal tunnel syndrome.

Figure 19-26. Wrist taping may be done when extra support is needed but hard plastic splinting is inappropriate.

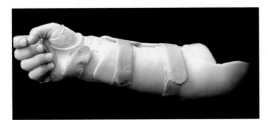

Figure 19-27. Circumferential wrist splint with separate elbow "sugartong" component to prevent supination and pronation.

Rehabilitation following a distal radius fracture is similar, regardless of method of fixation (cast, ORIF, or ex fix). Range of motion (ROM) and edema control of noninvolved joints are essential, so that when immobilization is discontinued rehabilitation can be concentrated on the wrist and forearm rather than also on the fingers, elbow, and shoulder.

Injury Mechanism

As is true of most wrist injuries, distal radius fractures occur from a fall on an outstretched hand. It might be a high-impact event but does not have to be.

Rehabilitation Concerns

Early and proper reduction and immobilization are of utmost importance. The fracture must be closely watched initially to be sure reduction is being maintained. Early ROM to noninvolved joints is imperative. This helps prevent muscle atrophy, aids in muscle pumping to decrease edema, and most importantly, maintains motion so treatment can focus on the wrist once the fracture is healed and fixation is removed.[1]

Other concerns include complications of carpal tunnel or reflex sympathetic dystrophy (RSD).[19] If present and first noted in the therapy clinic or athletic training room, referral should be made back to the physician as soon as possible. One other complication, which usually occurs late in a seemingly inconsequential nondisplaced distal radius fracture, is an extensor pollicus longus (EPL) rupture.[19] It is thought that this occurs from the EPL rubbing around the fracture site near Lister's tubercle. The patient would be unable to extend the thumb IP joint. The test for this is to put the injured hand flat on the table and try to lift the thumb off the table toward the ceiling. The term for this movement is *retropulsion* (Figure 19-10). This would need to be surgically repaired.

Rehabilitation Progression

Rehabilitation may be initiated while the wrist is immobilized. This should include shoulder ROM in all planes, elbow flexion and extension, and finger flexion and extension. Finger exercises should include isolated MCP flexion, composite flexion (full fist), and intrinsic minus fisting (MCP extension

with PIP flexion) (Figure 19-18). Coban or an Isotoner glove may be used for edema control if necessary.

If a fixator or pins are present, pin site care may be performed, depending on physician preference. Many physicians prefer hydrogen peroxide with a cotton applicator to remove the crusted areas from around the pins. A different applicator should be used on each pin, to prevent possible spread of infection. Some physicians allow patients to shower with the fixator in place (not soaking while bathing); other physicians prefer to cover the pin sites with a plastic bag to keep them dry.

Once immobilization is discontinued (at about 6 weeks for casting, 8 weeks with an external fixator, 2 weeks for ORIF with plate and screws), ROM to the wrist is begun. Active motion is begun immediately. Wrist flexion, extension, and radial and ulnar deviation are evaluated, then instructed. Wrist extension should be taught with finger (especially MCP) flexion (Figure 19-1). This isolates the wrist extensors and prevents "cheating" with the extensor digitorum communis (EDC). The importance of wrist extensor isolation is for hand function. If the EDC is used to extend the wrist, then flexing the fingers to grasp something will cause the wrist to also flex, because there is not enough wrist strength to keep the wrist extended. Tenodesis will extend the fingers, and the object will be dropped. Isolating wrist extension should be the emphasis of treatment on the first visit.

Passive ROM (PROM) may depend on physician preference. Many let PROM begin immediately, others prefer waiting 1 to 2 weeks (Figures 19-1 and 19-2) for passive stretching exercises. Forearm rotation (supination and pronation) must not be ignored. Active ROM (AROM) and PROM are both important. When stretching rotation passively, pressure should be applied at the distal radius, proximal to the wrist, not at the hand. This will help apply pressure where the limitations are and not put unnecessary torque across the carpus (Figures 19-5 and 19-6).

Active motion can be progressed to strengthening. Light weights, TheraBand, or tubing may be graded for all wrist and forearm motions. This can be in conjunction with or in a progression to closed chain weight-bearing activities. Start with wall push-ups, then progress to countertop or table, then to floor (Figures 19-12 through 19-14). Push-ups on a ball may be the next progression (Figure 19-23), along with kneeling on the floor and bearing weight on a BAPS board while shifting weight (Figure 19-24).

Using putty for grip strengthening can be started and upgraded to harder putty beginning about 1 to 2 weeks after immobilization. This also helps to strengthen the wrist musculature (Figure 19-11).

Plyometric exercises for the wrist and general upper-extremity strength are next. Activities are graded from a playground-type ball to a large gym ball to weighted balls. Activities can be done supine, against a wall, or, if available, using a rebounder. Specific return-to-sport exercises and activities must also be done.

Criteria for Return

Return to play depends on the sport and the severity of the fracture. If the fracture is nondisplaced, the patient usually may return to sport when it stops hurting (2 to 3 weeks, or sooner), with protection. There should be early signs of healing, no pain at rest, and no pain with a direct blow to the protection. If a nondisplaced fracture is treated by ORIF with plate and screw fixation, the patient might be able to return to play at about 3 weeks without protection if the sport is noncontact or with protection if a contact sport. At about 6 weeks, the patient may play without protection. The sport must be taken into consideration. An athlete in a high-contact sport might need protection longer than a patient in a noncontact sport. If the fracture was displaced, the patient is usually out of competition for about 6 weeks, then returns with protection for an additional 2 to 6 weeks (Figures 19-25 and 19-26). As with all injuries, return to sport depends on the sport, position played, and physician. The patient's strength must also be adequate for the position played, to prevent reinjury.

> **Clinical Decision-Making Exercise 19-1**
>
> A lacrosse player has had a blow to the dominant distal radial forearm with a stick. Radiographs are negative for fracture, but the player has localized edema (swelling), ecchymosis (bruising), localized pain, and "squeaking" with thumb motion. The physician has cleared him to play once the pain is gone and strength has returned. What can the athletic trainer do to help decrease inflammation and pain and increase ROM for return to play?

Wrist Sprain

Pathomechanics

The term *wrist sprain* is often seen when patients complain of pain and have a history of minor trauma. The diagnosis should be one of exclusion. Injuries that must be ruled out include scaphoid fracture, traumatic instability patterns, lunate fractures, dorsal chip fractures, other carpal fractures and injuries, and ligament tears.[12]

Injury Mechanism

The injury is usually a minor trauma, either a fall landing on an outstretched hand, a twisting motion, or some impact such as striking the ground with a club.

Rehabilitation Concerns

The primary concern is ruling out more serious injury. Once other diagnoses are ruled out, treatment is focused on edema control, pain control maintaining (or increasing) active and passive ROM to the wrist and other, noninvolved joints. If necessary, splint immobilization (Figure 19-25) may also be tried for pain relief. If activities increase pain, those activities should be examined to determine whether modifications can be made to decrease pain and increase activity level for return to sport.

Rehabilitation Progression

Following decrease in pain and edema, and return of ROM, strengthening should be performed to all wrist motions and, if necessary, to grip strength and entire arm. Refer to the section on distal radius fracture for specific exercises (Figures 19-1 through 19-14, 19-23, and 19-24). Joint mobilizations for the wrist can certainly help improve joint arthrokinematics and ROM (see Figures 13-26 to 13-30).

Criteria for Return

Patients may return to sport when comfortable. Taping the wrist (Figure 19-26) can help provide support and decrease pain. The patient should not return to play until all other serious conditions are ruled out.

Triangular Fibrocartilage Complex (TFCC)

Pathomechanics

The TFCC is the primary stabilizer of the radio-ulnar joint. It consists of dorsal and volar radio-ulnar ligaments, ulnar collateral ligament, meniscus homologue, articular disc, and extensor carpi ulnaris tendon sheath.[25] The TFCC functions as a cushion for the ulnar carpus and a major stabilizer of the distal radio-ulnar joint. The TFCC arises from the radius and inserts into the base of the ulna styloid. It flows distally (the ulnar collateral ligament), becomes thickened (the meniscus homologue), and inserts distally into the triquetrum, hamate, and base of the fifth metacarpal.[36] Blood supply to the TFCC is limited to the peripheral 15% to 20%. The central articular disc is relatively avascular.[45] Generally, the TFCC tears that occur traumatically are in the periphery and can be surgically repaired because of the blood supply. Most degenerative tears are central and are best treated by debridement.

Injury Mechanism

Injuries to wrist ligaments can occur after a collision on the field, a fall on an outstretched hand, a pileup on the field where the wrist is landed on and twisted, or hitting a bad shot in tennis or golf.[45]

Rehabilitation Concerns

The primary concern is correct diagnosis. The patient will usually present with ulnar-side wrist pain. There may have been an acute injury, or just pain from overuse. ROM should be evaluated actively and passively. Pain is usually present with extension, ulnar deviation, and forearm rotation.[45] Palpation to replicate pain should be performed. Start with the radial side of the wrist, away from the pain. Palpate the snuffbox for scaphoid pain, dorsally for scapholunate ligament pain, ulnar to that (just proximal to the third metacarpal) for lunate pain, then palpate over the ulna head, just distal to the ulna head, and on the ulnar border of the wrist. Joint mobilizations of the carpus on radius can be performed. This is followed by ulna on radius in neutral, then in supination, then in pronation. You are looking for reproduction of pain and excessive movement on any direction compared to the noninjured side. An arthrogram or wrist arthroscopy can confirm the diagnosis. If an acute injury not associated with significant separation from the radius or ulna, it can be treated by cast immobilization.[36] A peripheral tear of the radial or ulnar attachments should be repaired. There is good blood supply, and it has the potential to heal.[3,35] A central linear or flap tear can be arthroscopically debrided with good results.[39]

Rehabilitation Progressions

A patient who has had surgery for repair of the TFCC will be in a postoperative dressing for 10 days to 2 weeks. At that time, the sutures will be removed, and the patient will be placed into a protective splint. The author makes a circumferential wrist splint that immobilizes the wrist and goes two-thirds of the way up the forearm, leaving the fingers and thumb free. A second splint is then applied around the elbow and overlapping the wrist splint (Figure 19-27). This is to prevent supination and pronation. Some surgeons keep the arm immobilized for 4 weeks; others will allow active wrist flexion and extension (Figures 19-1 and 19-2) only during the first 4 weeks, preventing supination or pronation and radial and ulnar deviation. At 4 weeks, the elbow portion of the splint is removed, keeping the wrist splint applied (Figure 19-25). The patient may then begin active supination and pronation exercises (Figure 19-5 and 19-6) and continue with flexion and extension. At 8 weeks, splinting is usually discontinued and PROM exercises are started. Gentle strengthening begins between week 8 to week 10, with progression to weight bearing and plyometrics as tolerated (Figures 19-12 to 19-14, 19-23, and 19-24).

If the patient has been treated conservatively with a cast, once the cast is removed (at 6 to 8 weeks), begin AROM for 1 to 2 weeks, with progression to PROM, then strengthening. Many surgeons prefer to have AROM close to normal before beginning strengthening.

Criteria for Return

Return to sport with this injury, like many others, is dependent upon sport, position played, and ability to play in a splint or cast. As a general rule, the patient may begin conditioning activities (such as running) at 2 weeks, when the sutures are removed and the arm is placed in a long arm splint. At 8 weeks, he or she may begin weight lifting with the wrist taped for support. An athlete who plays a sport requiring stick work may begin stick skills at 10 weeks if this does not make the wrist more painful. Return to full activity usually occurs about 3 months after surgical repair, when the ligament is healed, the wrist is pain-free, and full ROM and strength have returned.

Scaphoid Fracture

Pathomechanics

Fractures of the scaphoid account for 60% of all carpal injuries.[31] The prognosis is related to the site of the fracture, obliquity, displacement, and promptness of diagnosis and treatment.[12] The blood supply of the scaphoid comes distal to proximal. Fracture through the waist of the proximal one-third of the scaphoid can result in delayed union or avascular necrosis secondary to poor blood supply. It can take 20 weeks for a proximal one-third fracture to heal, compared to 5 or 6 weeks at the scaphoid tuberosity.[12] Displacement of the fracture occurs at the time of injury and must be treated early using ORIF.

Ninety percent of scaphoid fractures heal without complications if treated early and properly.[31] If the fracture does go on to non-union, whether symptomatic or not, it should be treated. Not treating will lead to carpal instability and periscaphoid arthritis.[37] Diagnosis is made by X-ray. Patients will have wrist pain, especially in the anatomic snuffbox (Figure 19-28).

Injury Mechanism

Scaphoid fractures result from a fall on an outstretched hand. The radial styloid may impact against the scaphoid waist, causing a fracture.[7] The scaphoid fails in extension when the palmar surface experiences an excessive bending movement.[38] Because the scaphoid blocks wrist extension, it is at risk for injury.[12]

Rehabilitation Concerns

Of primary concern is proper diagnosis. If the patient has a history of falls on an outstretched hand and has pain in the anatomic snuffbox, but the initial X-ray is negative, they should be treated conservatively in a thumb spica cast for 2 weeks, then be X-rayed again.[20] If the X-ray is negative after 2 weeks, the cast may be removed and ROM begun. Another concern is scaphoid non-unions that can lead to carpal instability or periscaphoid arthritis. ROM of noninjured and noncasted joints must be maintained during prolonged periods of immobilization.

Rehabilitation Progressions

Treatment of the nondisplaced scaphoid is casting. Following casting, an additional 2 to 4 weeks of splinting (Figure 19-29) may be used, with the splint removed for the exercise program. AROM exercises of wrist flexion, wrist extension (with finger flexion to isolate wrist extensors), and radial and ulnar deviation are initiated following immobilization (Figures 19-1 through 19-4). Thumb flexion and extension, abduction and adduction, and opposition to each finger are also initiated (Figures 19-7 through 19-9). After about 2 weeks (sooner if cleared by the physician), PROM to the same motion is begun. Gentle strengthening with weights or putty may be started around the same time. Strengthening is progressed over the next several weeks to include weight-bearing activities, plyometrics, and general arm conditioning to return to sport-specific activity (Figures 19-12 through 19-14, 19-23, and 19-24).

Surgical repair rehabilitation follows the same progression as for nonsurgical rehabilitation. The time frame of immobilization might be less because of the repair of the scaphoid with rigid fixation.

Criteria for Return

Return to play depends on the sport, location and type of fracture, and type of immobilization. If the fracture is nondisplaced and treated in a cast, return to play in a padded cast might be at 2 or 3 weeks or sooner—when the arm stops hurting, there are early signs of healing,

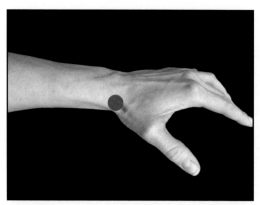

Figure 19-28. The dot indicates the anatomic snuffbox, under which the scaphoid is positioned. This area will be painful to palpation with scaphoid fracture or scapholunate ligament injury.

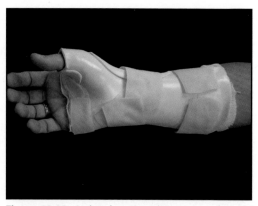

Figure 19-29. A thumb spica splint is circumferential and includes the thumb and wrist. It might or might not include the thumb IP joint. It is most commonly used for a scaphoid or thumb metacarpal fracture.

and there is no pain with a blow to the cast. The patient should continue to play with protection until the bone has healed and adequate strength has returned to help prevent reinjury, or new injury to a separate site. If the nondisplaced fracture has undergone ORIF or if the patient is participating in a noncontact sport, the patient may return, if cleared by the physician, in about 2 or 3 weeks without additional protection. An athlete in a contact sport should participate with protection. If the fracture is displaced and surgically repaired, time until return to play may be longer. The patient must wear a padded protective cast upon return to play. In all cases, close communication is essential for return to competition.

Lunate Dislocations

Pathomechanics

Stability of the carpus is dependent upon the maintenance of bony architecture interlaced with ligaments.[12] Most carpal dislocations are of the dorsal perilunate type. Many people believe that a lunate dislocation is the end of a perilunate dislocation.[12] The lunate dislocates palmarly with the loss of ligamentous stability.[26] It may be reduced, if seen early, by placing the wrist in extension and putting pressure on the lunate volarly (Figures 19-30 and 19-31). The wrist is then brought into flexion and immobilized. It is very common for reduction to be lost over time with this injury, so percutaneous pinning or ORIF is recommended.[12]

Median nerve compression is frequently caused by this injury. The palmarly displaced lunate puts pressure on the nerve. Symptoms might continue for several weeks following reduction of the lunate secondary to swelling and contusion of the nerve.[26]

Injury Mechanism

A violent hyperextension of the wrist is the injury mechanism.[7,12] A fall on the outstretched hand produces a translational compressive force when the lunate is caught between the capitate and the dorsal aspect of the distal radius articular surface.[12] If the lunate or scaphoid does not fracture, a periscaphoid or lunate dislocation can occur.

Rehabilitation Concerns

The primary concern is early surgical repair. Without surgical correction, complications include pain, weakness, wrist clicking, and bones slipping.[7] Carpal tunnel syndrome, if present, must be addressed at the time of surgery. ROM of noninvolved joints must be maintained during immobilization.

Rehabilitation Progressions

Progression is very similar to the rehabilitation of distal radius fractures and other wrist injuries. Following cast and pin removal (if applicable), AROM is begun. This is progressed to passive stretching and gentle strengthening. Strengthening becomes more aggressive with free weights, weight-bearing and plyometric activities. Motions that need to be addressed

REHABILITATION PLAN

ULNAR WRIST PAIN

Injury situation A 20-year-old college lacrosse player complains of pain in his nondominant (left) ulnar wrist. He has had this pain for several weeks, since he fell on his wrist while holding his lacrosse stick during practice, but he does not really know how he injured it. The pain has increased so much that he cannot control his stick to catch a ball or shoot.

Signs and symptoms The patient complains of pain in the wrist with gripping, forearm rotation, and trying to hold and shoot with his lacrosse stick. He has pain with end ROM for wrist extension, resisted wrist extension, and resisted supination. Palpation reveals pain in the ulnar side of the wrist. Joint mobilization of the radius on the ulna in neutral, supination, and pronation, and of the carpus on the radius shows minimal, if any, difference in joint mobility compared to the noninjured side, but is painful.

Management plan The goal is to decrease pain initially, regain ROM and strength, and determine whether a more serious injury has occurred.

Nonsurgical Plan

PHASE ONE: Acute Inflammatory Stage

GOALS: Decrease pain and begin ROM exercises
Estimated length of time (ELT): Day 1 to Day 14 Use ice for pain relief if swelling is present. Ice on the hand can be painful. Anti-inflammatory medications can help decrease edema and pain. Splinting the wrist when the patient is not involved in sport activity can provide pain relief as well. Begin AROM exercises in a pain-free range. If wrist taping provides sufficient support and pain relief, participation in sports may be allowed. If not, the patient may need to sit out practice for several days.

PHASE TWO: Fibroblastic-Repair Stage

GOALS: Increase ROM and strength; pain relief
Estimated length of time (ELT): Weeks 2 to 4 Ice, anti-inflammatory medications, and splinting may be continued. Continue with ROM exercises, adding supination and pronation. Strengthening may be started for the wrist and forearm if pain has decreased. Return to sport with taping if necessary. Fitness levels must be maintained if wrist pain continues and sport participation not possible.

PHASE THREE: Maturation-Remodeling Stage

GOALS: Complete elimination of pain and return to full activity.
Estimated length of time (ELT): Week 4 to Full Return Continue with ROM and strengthening. Return to activity as tolerated. Wean from splint. Wean from taping during activity.
Criteria for returning to competitive lacrosse
1. Pain is eliminated with ROM of wrist and forearm.
2. Full ROM in wrist and forearm.
3. Full return of strength in wrist, forearm, and grip.
If pain does not stop with ice, anti-inflammatory medications, and rest, the wrist might need further evaluation and prolonged immobilization. Prolonged ulnar-side wrist pain without relief might indicate a TRCC tear. The diagnosis can be confirmed with an arthrogram. An acute trauma can be surgically repaired. It is possible to delay repair until the end of the season if the patient is able to play without risk of further injury. Follow the plan above until surgery.

Surgical Plan

PHASE ONE: Acute Inflammatory Stage

GOALS: Protection of surgical repair

Estimated length of time (ELT): Day 10 post surgery to Week 4 The postoperative dressing is removed 10 days to 2 weeks after surgery. The sutures are removed, and the arm is placed in a circumferential wrist splint, with a sugartong component around the elbow to place the forearm in slight supination and prevent forearm rotation. AROM is begun for wrist flexion and extension only. No rotation or radial and ulnar deviation should be performed. (Check with the physician; some do not want any ROM activity for 4 weeks.) Conditioning, such as running, can begin at about 2 weeks, once the patient is comfortable in the protective splint.

PHASE TWO: Fibroblastic-Repair Stage

GOALS: Increasing ROM of the wrist and forearm, while protecting the surgical repair

Estimated length of time (ELT): Weeks 4 to 8 The elbow component of the splint is discontinued. Continue with the wrist splint. Continue with wrist ROM, beginning gentle PROM. Initiate forearm rotation actively. After about 2 weeks of AROM to rotation, begin PROM.

PHASE THREE: Maturation-Remodeling Stage

GOALS: Increasing ROM and strength, and return to sport activity.

Estimated length of time (ELT): Weeks 8 to 12 Initiate a strengthening program. Begin with isometrics, progress to weights, and then weight bearing. Weight lifting for return to sport can occur at 10 weeks, with the wrist taped for support if it is pain-free. Stick work can be initiated at that time as well. Return to competitive lacrosse occurs at about 12 weeks. Criteria for safe return are listed in nonsurgical plan.

DISCUSSION QUESTIONS

1. What other injuries could occur with a fall on a wrist?
2. What therapeutic modalities could help decrease pain?
3. If pain does not decrease with immobilization, modalities, and anti-inflammatory medications, should the athlete continue to play?
4. Explain why supination and pronation are not allowed initially.

for ROM and strengthening are flexion, extension, radial deviation, ulnar deviation, supination, and pronation (Figures 19-1 through 19-6, 19-12 through 19-14, 19-23, and 19-24).

Criteria for Return

The severity of this injury, and the need for ORIF secondary to frequent loss of reduction if not repaired, will keep this patient from competition for at least 8 weeks. Upon return at 8 weeks, the wrist may be taped for support and protection (Figure 19-26). The patient should not be favoring or protecting the hand during periods of noncompetition. Patients should have good ROM and strength prior to return to help prevent reinjury.

Hamate Fractures

Pathomechanics

Fractures of the hook of the hamate are more common than hamate body fractures.[34] The hook is the attachment for the pisohamate ligament, short flexor and opponens to the small finger, and the transverse carpal ligament.[45] Because of these attachments, if there is a hamate hook fracture there are deforming

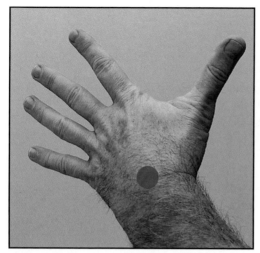

Figure 19-30. The dot indicates the position of the lunate and the location of pain with lunate or scapholunate ligament injuries.

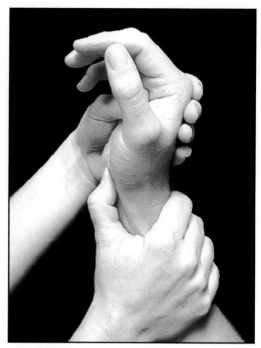

Figure 19-31. Hand placement to relocate a lunate.

forces on the fragment with intermittent tension. This makes it nearly impossible to align and immobilize the fracture, and as a result these often do not heal.[45] The hook can be palpated on the volar surface of the hand at the base of the hypothenar eminence deep and radial to the pisiform. The hamate is in close proximity to the ulnar nerve and artery on the ulnar side, and flexor tendons to the ring and small finger in the carpal canal on the radial side (Figure 19-32). There is a possibility of an ulnar neuropathy, tendinitis, or tendon rupture with this injury.[34]

Injury Mechanism

The suspected injury mechanism is a shearing force transmitted from the handle of a club to the hamate. It often occurs when striking an unexpected object (as when a golfer strikes a rock or tree root). It most frequently occurs in golfers but can occur in any stick sport, such as baseball or field hockey. There is also a possibility of a stress fracture from tension from ligament and muscle attachments, but this is rare.[7]

Rehabilitation Concerns

The first concern is diagnosis. Patients might have felt a snap or pop. They will have localized tenderness over the hamate hook, ulnar-side wrist pain, and weakness of grip that increases over time. A carpal tunnel view X-ray will confirm the diagnosis. The athletic trainer

must also be concerned and watch for signs of ulnar neuritis or neuropathy, and flexor tendon rupture.

Rehabilitation Progressions

Treatment has been described as casting an acute hamate hook fracture[34] or bone grafting a non-union.[40] However, as described previously, these fractures do not usually heal secondary to forces applied to the fracture fragment. Treatment for symptomatic hamate fractures is fragment excision.[34] Treatment following excision is edema control, scar massage (3 to 5 minutes, 5 times a day), and grip strengthening if necessary.

Criteria for Return

Acute injuries must be treated symptomatically. Tape or padding, if allowed, may be placed in the palm. Chronic fractures are also treated symptomatically, with pain being the limiting factor. It is not detrimental for the patient to continue to play with a fracture and have the fragment removed at the end of the season, as long as he or she is able to play with his or her symptoms. If the patient is unable to play, the injury should be surgically addressed.

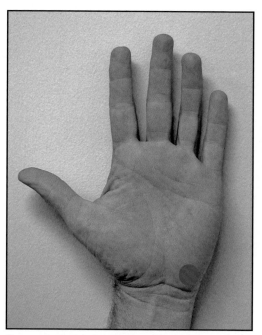

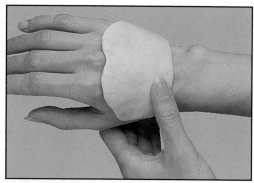

Figure 19-33. Otoform is used as a scar control pad. It comes in varying size containers. The needed amount of "putty" is taken from the jar, mixed with a catalyst, and applied directly to the scar area. Once it hardens, in 1 to 2 minutes, it can be rinsed and applied with Coban or a similar covering. It is usually worn 23 hours per day for scar control. It does need to be removed, as it does not breathe and skin can become macerated, or a rash can develop. It may also be worn during sport activity for additional protection to a sensitive area.

Figure 19-32. The dot indicates the point that will elicit pain with palpation (especially deep) for a hamate hook fracture. Some pain might also be referred to the ulnar wrist.

Once the fragment has been excised, the patient may return to sport as soon as he or she is comfortable. A small splint, padding, or scar control pad such as Topigel or Otoform (Figure 19-33) might be helpful initially for scar control and to decrease hypersensitivity around the incision area. Full return is expected.

Carpal Tunnel Syndrome

Pathomechanics

Carpal tunnel syndrome is compression of the median nerve at the level of the wrist. The carpal tunnel is made of the carpal bones dorsally and transverse carpal ligament volarly. Located in the carpal tunnel are the FDS and FDP tendons to all digits, FPL, median nerve, and median artery.[14] If tendons become inflamed, the space within the carpal tunnel is decreased and the nerve becomes compressed. Excessive wrist flexion or extension will also increase pressure in the carpal tunnel. Symptoms of classic carpal tunnel are numbness and tingling in the thumb through the radial half of the ring finger, pain or waking at night, and clumsiness or weakness in the hand.

Symptoms might increase with static positioning (eg, when driving or reading a newspaper).[14] Diagnosis is made by history, Phalen's test (Figure 19-34), Tinel's sign, nerve conduction studies, direct pressure over the carpal tunnel (Figure 19-35), and EMGs. Injection can help confirm diagnosis and may relieve symptoms.

Injury Mechanism

The incidence of carpal tunnel is extremely low in most patients,[24] but the injury is found in cyclists, throwers, and tennis players.[28] Pressure from resting on handlebars can cause symptoms. Sustained grip and the repetitive actions of throwers and racquet sports can also increase symptoms. Illnesses or injuries that have been associated with carpal tunnel include tenosynovitis from overuse or from rheumatoid arthritis, and external or internal pressure from conditions such as lipoma, diabetes, or pregnancy.[41] Acute carpal tunnel can occur following a fracture or other trauma, by either edema or a fracture fragment pressing on the median nerve.

Rehabilitation Concerns

Conservative treatment is tried first and consists of night splinting with the wrist in neutral position (Figure 19-25), anti-inflammatory medication, and relative rest from the aggravating source (if known). Occasionally

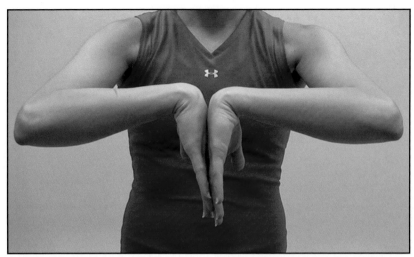

Figure 19-34. Phalen's test for carpal tunnel injury is extreme wrist flexion, which narrows the space in the carpal canal. The test is positive if there is numbness and tingling in the median nerve distribution within 60 seconds. Do not flex elbows or rest elbows on the table, as this can elicit ulnar nerve symptoms.

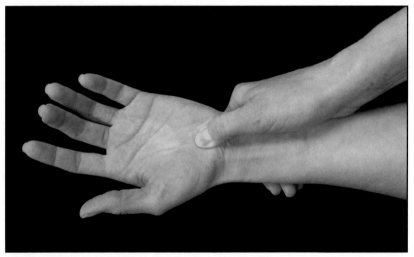

Figure 19-35. Firm pressure over the carpal tunnel can elicit numbness or tingling in the median nerve distribution. This alone is not indicative of carpal tunnel injury but provides more information.

physicians will recommend full-time wrist splinting. However, some prefer that wrist splints not be worn during the day, as this leads to muscle weakness and arm pain from distribution of forces to new areas. Injections may be done by the physician for symptom relief—this is also diagnostic. If the symptoms disappear with injection, the diagnosis is correct. Symptoms can recur. Nerve-gliding exercises[5,22] (Figure 19-17) and myofascial release might also help relieve symptoms. Activity

analysis and biomechanical analysis of activities that increase symptoms should be done to see if changes in technique will decrease symptoms. If conservative treatment fails, a carpal tunnel release may be performed. Rehabilitation following a release consists of wound care (if necessary), scar massage, and ROM exercises. Tendon-gliding exercises are done to improve ROM and isolation of tendons.[22] These exercises start with full-finger extension, then a hooked fist to maximize FDP pull-through in relation to FDS, then a long fist to maximize FDS pull-through, then a composite fist. Full extension should be performed between each position (Figure 19-18). Wrist ROM should also be performed (Figures 19-1 and 19-2).

Rehabilitation Progressions

Progression for carpal tunnel release includes grip strengthening. Exercises should begin slowly, to avoid increasing the symptoms. Wrist strengthening may also be performed. Strengthening is generally begun 2 to 4 weeks post surgery, after consultation with the physician. Upper-body conditioning should also be performed if necessary for return to sport.

Criteria for Return

Patients may continue to play with carpal tunnel. Activity should be examined, though, to see whether it could be altered to decrease symptoms. Activity level is based on symptoms. If conservative treatment fails and a release is performed, patients can typically return to sport once sutures are removed. Surgical release is rarely necessary in patients.

Ganglion Cysts

Pathomechanics

A ganglion cyst is the most common soft-tissue tumor in the hand.[4] It is a synovial cyst arising from the synovial lining of a tendon sheath or joint. The etiology is unclear. They are most common on the dorsal radial wrist but can also be volar (Figure 19-36). They originate deep in the joint and can be symptomatic before they appear at the surface. The usual origin is from the area of the scapholunate ligament.[4] Ganglion cysts are translucent, which can help confirm the diagnosis.

Treatment is aspiration of the cyst. Results of recurrence are variable. In adults, multiple aspirations are suggested, with success rates of 51% to 85%.[46] If multiple aspirations are not successful and cysts recur, they may be surgically excised.

Injury Mechanism

In the athletic population, it appears that ganglions most often form with repeated forceful hyperextension of the wrist, as would occur in weight lifters, shot putters, wrestlers, and gymnasts. Pain is the indication for treatment.

Rehabilitation Concerns

These patients do not need to be seen for rehabilitation once diagnosed and aspirated. The aspiration usually decreases pain and allows for full ROM. Following ganglion cyst excision, patients may need to be seen for ROM, passive stretching, strengthening, and scar control. ROM emphasis should be on wrist flexion and extension and finger flexion and extension (Figures 19-1, 19-2, and 19-18). Scar massage and desensitization may be done with lotion, rubbing on the scar, tapping on the scar, and performing vibration to the scar. Less noxious stimuli should be done first, with increasing difficulty being added to the program. Scar control pads such as Otoform (Figure 19-33) or Topigel sheeting may also be used, held in place with Coban.

Rehabilitation Progressions

Following excision and return of ROM, strengthening may be done as necessary for grip, wrist flexion and extension, and general upper-extremity return-to-play exercises.

Criteria for Return

Activity is limited by pain. Patients may participate with a ganglion if it is not symptomatic. If symptomatic, it may be aspirated with immediate return to activity. If it recurs, it may be aspirated again with no loss of playing time. If necessary, the ganglion may be excised at the end of the season. If excised, sport activity may begin once sutures are removed, at about 10 days. Full return is expected.

Boxer's Fracture

Pathomechanics

A boxer's fracture is a fracture of the fifth metacarpal neck. This is the most commonly fractured metacarpal.[16] It will frequently shorten and angulate on impact. There is a large amount of movement of the fifth metacarpal. For this reason, perfect anatomic reduction is not necessary. It should be noted, however, that excess angulation can lead to either an imbalance between the intrinsic and extrinsic

Figure 19-36. This is a dorsal wrist ganglion. These vary in size and shape and will transilluminate.

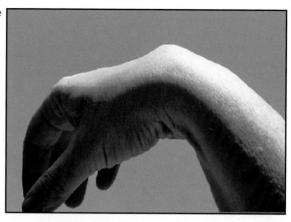

muscles of the hand, leading to clawing, or to a mass in the palm.[23]

Injury Mechanism

This injury occurs most frequently from contact against an object with a closed fist. The impact is usually through the fifth metacarpal head.

Rehabilitation Concerns

Of concern is skin integrity. The injuries frequently occur as a result of a fight, and pieces of tooth might be in an open wound. If the injury is closed, concern is for proper immobilization, edema control, and ROM of noninvolved joints—especially the IP joints of the small finger. Occasionally ORIF is required. Edema control is critical. AROM may be initiated 72 hours after the ORIF.[23]

Treatment is immobilization in a plaster gutter splint, or in a thermoplastic splint fabricated by a hand therapist (Figure 19-37). The latter is often preferred as it allows for skin hygiene, wrist ROM, and IP joint ROM. The splint immobilizes only the ring and small finger MCP joints. The splint is also easily remolded if necessary as edema decreases. Splinting is continued for about 4 weeks.

Rehabilitation Progression

During the time of immobilization, ROM to noninvolved joints is maintained by active and passive exercises. At about 4 weeks, the splint is discontinued, and ROM to MCP joints is begun. Buddy taping may be done to encourage ROM. Between 4 and 6, weeks gentle resistance may be performed, with vigorous activities at about 6 weeks.

Criteria for Return

A patient may return when there is a sign that the fracture is healing, it feels stable, and there is no pain with the fracture or movement. This is generally at 3 to 4 weeks with protection. Generally by 6 weeks, the patient may play with only buddy taping protection. This, as always, depends on the sport, the patient, and the physician.

DeQuervain's Tenosynovitis and Tendinitis

Pathomechanics

Tendinitis, most simply put, is inflammation of a tendon. It can occur on the dorsal wrist, volar wrist, or thumb. Symptoms are pain along the muscle, pain with resisted motions, and/or swelling. It is frequently caused by overuse. Injections can help relieve symptoms and confirm diagnosis.

DeQuervain's tenosynovitis is an inflammation in the first dorsal compartment; the abductor pollicus longus (APL) and extensor pollicus brevis (EPB) are affected.[2] The third dorsal compartment, the extensor pollicus longus (EPL), is usually not affected, and as such the IP joint of the thumb does not need to be included in any splint. The condition can be aggravated by excessive wrist radial and ulnar deviation, flexion and extension of the thumb, or abduction and adduction of the thumb,[17] Finklestein's test,[2] passive thumb flexion into the palm with passive wrist ulnar deviation, will be positive for pain (Figure 19-38). Always compare to the noninjured side, as this test can

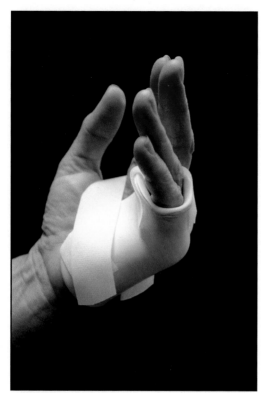

Figure 19-37. A boxer's fracture splint protects the ring and small finger proximal phalanxes and metacarpals, including the MCP joint. The splint may be modified for a different neck fracture (immobilizing the involved MCP joint). For a metacarpal shaft fracture possibly only the metacarpal will need to be in the splint, leaving the wrist and MCP joints free. For a metacarpal base fracture the splint might need to include the wrist, usually leaving the MCP joints free.

be uncomfortable normally. Resisted wrist flexion or extension will be positive for pain with wrist tendinitis.

Injury Mechanism

Tendinitis is usually caused by overuse. It can also be caused by weakness, poor body mechanics, or abnormal postures. DeQuervain's can be caused by repeated wrist radial and ulnar deviation. Less frequent causes include a direct blow to the radial styloid, acute strain as in lifting, or a ganglion in the first dorsal compartment.[17]

Rehabilitation Concerns

If a direct blow to the wrist or forearm or fall on outstretched hand has occurred, a fracture or ligament injury should be ruled out first. If no known injury has occurred, initial treatment is anti-inflammatory medication and rest from

aggravating activities. Modalities for edema reduction and pain control, such as ultrasound, iontophoresis, or ice, can be effective. Analysis of activity should be done to see if poor mechanics are aggravating symptoms. Look proximally to see if weak shoulder musculature or scapular stabilizers could be contributing to compensatory techniques and poor mechanics.

Splinting for wrist tendinitis includes the wrist only (Figure 19-25). Splinting for DeQuervain's includes the thumb MCP and CMC joints, and wrist, usually in a radial gutter fashion (Figure 19-39). Splinting is usually full-time except for hygiene for the first 2 to 3 weeks, then if symptoms are subsiding, wearing time is slowly decreased while activity is increased. If pain is persistent, splinting continues.

Rehabilitation Progressions

Stretching of the affected areas in a pain-free range (Figures 19-15 and 19-16) three times per day should begin immediately with rest (splinting) and anti-inflammatory medication. Once pain has decreased, strengthening of grip and wrist musculature may begin. Strengthening should begin isometrically, progressing to full ROM against gravity, and then light-weight eccentric exercises in the pain-free range (Figures 19-1 through 19-4). Progression to weight bearing and plyometrics may occur if there is no increase in symptoms (Figures 19-12 to 19-14, 19-23, and 19-24). If strengthening is begun too early, symptoms will be exacerbated. If tendinitis is a result of muscle imbalance, the weak muscle groups must be strengthened. If symptoms do not subside, and injections are helpful but do not cure the symptoms, a release of the first dorsal compartment, if DeQuervain's tenosynovitis, might need to be performed.

Criteria for Return

Pain and strength are limiting factors for return. Patients should have pain-free ROM to the affected part. Strength should be significant to prevent reinjury. The patient may participate prior to absence of pain if he or she is taped for support, use a splint for rest while he or she is not participating in sports, and if pain does not impair performance.

If a release is performed, it may be done at the end of the season if symptoms permit play.

If not, the patient can return when comfortable, as early as 10 days post surgery. Strength should be sufficient to prevent reinjury, aggravating forces should have been addressed, and support initially might be needed.

Clinical Decision-Making Exercise 19-2

A tennis player has been diagnosed by a physician with DeQuervain's tenosynovitis and wrist extensor tendinitis. She is in season and would like to continue to play. She has been referred to the athletic trainer for evaluation and rehabilitation for return to sport. What can the athletic trainer do to reduce the patient's symptoms?

Ulnar Collateral Ligament Sprain (Gamekeeper's Thumb)

Pathomechanics

The ulnar collateral ligament (UCL) injury to the MCP joint of the thumb is the most common ligament injury.[29,43] The injury can be classified as grade I or grade II, in which the majority of the ligament remains intact. Grade III is a complete disruption of the UCL, and surgical repair is recommended. Rupture occurs most often at the distal attachment of the ligament[15,21] (Figures 19-40 and 19-41).

The patient will complain of pain or tenderness on the ulnar side of the MCP joint. X-rays should be taken to rule out fracture. Following X-rays, MCP joint stability should be evaluated at full extension and at 30 degrees of flexion. These two positions will test the accessory collateral ligament and the proper collateral ligament, respectively. Angulation greater than 35 degrees or 15 degrees greater than the non-injured side indicates instability and surgery is recommended.[15]

If the ligament is completely torn, one must also worry about a Stener lesion. This is where the torn UCL protrudes beneath the adductor aponeurosis. This places the aponeurosis between the ligament and its insertion. If this occurs, reattachment will not occur spontaneously with casting or splinting, and surgery is needed.[29]

A more appropriate term for this injury in a patient would be *skier's thumb*. Initially,

Campbell described gamekeeper's injury as being due to chronic repeated stress on the UCL.[15] It was not an acute injury, as it most commonly is in sports.

Injury Mechanism

UCL injuries occur when a torsional load is applied to the thumb.[7] It frequently occurs in pole or stick sports (eg, skiing) where the thumb is abducted to hold the pole or stick and the patient falls and tries to catch herself on an outstretched hand, landing on an abducted thumb.[21,30,43] Defensive backs in football might also sustain this injury while abducting the thumb before making a tackle.[21]

Rehabilitation Concerns

Early diagnosis and treatment is important. An unstable thumb or Stener lesion, if not treated, will become chronically and painfully unstable with weak pinch and arthritis as sequelae.[15]

Treatment for incomplete (grade I or II) tears is immobilization in a thumb spica cast (Figure 19-29) for 3 weeks, with additional protective splinting for 2 weeks (Figure 19-42). AROM to flexion and extension may be performed following the first 3 weeks.

Treatment for complete tears (grade III, unstable MCP joint) should be surgical repair. Late reconstruction is not as successful as early surgery, so early operative treatment is recommended.[21] Postoperatively, a thumb spica cast or splint is worn for 3 weeks, with an additional 2 weeks of splinting except for exercise sessions of active flexion and extension.

Concerns during the initial 5 or 6 weeks post injury include protective immobilization, controlling edema, and maintaining motion in all noninvolved joints. An additional concern, once movement is begun, is to not place radial stress on the thumb to stretch the UCL.

Rehabilitation Progression

After protective splinting is discontinued (at about 5 to 6 weeks), exercises are upgraded from AROM of flexion and extension to active assistive and passive exercises. Care should be taken not to apply abduction stress to the MCP joint during the first 2 to 6 weeks following immobilization. Putty exercises for strength may be performed at about 8 weeks post injury.

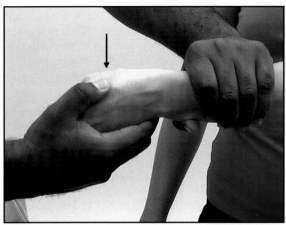

Figure 19-38. Finklestein's test will be positive for pain in DeQuervain's. Passive flexion of the thumb with wrist ulnar deviation is the provocative position. Always compare to the noninvolved side, as this test can be uncomfortable normally.

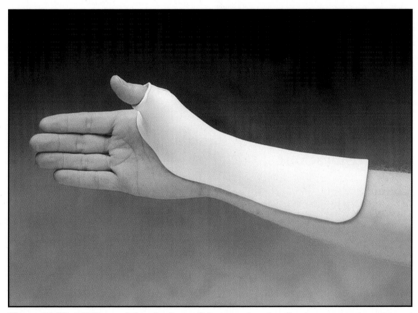

Figure 19-39. A DeQuervain's splint is a radial gutter thumb splint. It supports the wrist and thumb CMC and MCP joints. It is used to rest the thumb and wrist with DeQuervain's.

When measuring thumb ROM, always compare to the noninjured side. There is a large amount of variation in MCP and IP ROM from person to person.

Criteria for Return

Return-to-play decisions are made by the physician in conjunction with the sports medicine staff. Length of time to return to play is determined by the sport and position played, and whether the patient needs to use his or her thumb. For nonoperative treatment a cast or splint might provide adequate protection for return to play. Once the patient is medically cleared to play, a protective splint (Figure 19-42) or taping to prevent reinjury from extension and abduction (Figure 19-43) should be fabricated by a hand therapist or athletic trainer. Protective splinting during sports should continue for at least 8 weeks until pain and swelling subside and the patient has complete pain-free ROM.[21]

If surgical repair is performed, the patient will be out for a minimum of 2 weeks while the incision heals. After that, the position and sport determine the length of time until return. If the patient does not have to use his or her thumb, follow the protective splinting guidelines for nonoperative conditions. For either treatment where active thumb movement is necessary (eg, in the throwing hand of the quarterback), the patient will be out at least 4 to 6 weeks.[30] Strength should be sufficient and pain decreased to prevent reinjury.

Clinical Decision-Making Exercise 19-3

A basketball player's thumb was hyperextended when she caught a pass during practice. It began swelling immediately in the thenar area and MCP joint. She had pain and tenderness at the MCP joint. The athletic trainer referred her to the physician, who sent her back with the diagnosis of grade 2 UCL sprain. What can the athletic trainer do to decrease pain, provide stability, and return the patient to play?

Finger Joint Dislocations

Pathomechanics

Dislocation of the MCP joint is very infrequent. The force is dissipated by joint mobility.[42] These injuries can be a simple dorsal subluxation, in which the proximal phalanx rotates on the metacarpal head and locks the joint in 60 degrees of hyperextension, or an irreducible dorsal dislocation where the volar plate is interposed dorsally to the metacarpal head and prevents reduction. For a simple dislocation, after reduction some physicians splint the MCP joints in 50 degrees of flexion for 7 to 10 days.[42] Others buddy tape and allow full motion immediately. If the fracture is irreducible, it must be openly reduced with the volar plate retracted. The MCP joints are then splinted at 50 degrees or greater of flexion.

Dislocation of the PIP joint volarly is very rare and is usually a grade III irreducible fracture. It requires open reduction. Because it is very complex and rare in patients, it will not be covered in depth in this chapter.

Dorsal dislocations are much more common in sports. The patient might not even bring the injury to the attention of the athletic trainer, but might instead just pull the finger back into place independently. If a finger PIP is dorsally dislocated, immediate reduction (usually by physician) is preferred. If a physician is not present, and an experienced athletic trainer is not present, an X-ray should be taken prior to reduction to be sure there is no fracture. If there is no fracture, and the PIP joint is reduced and stable, the finger should be wrapped in Coban (Figure 19-44) for edema control and buddy taped to the adjacent finger. ROM is begun immediately (Figures 19-18 through 19-21). These injuries do not need to be splinted and should not be overtreated.

DIP joint dislocations are rarer than PIP dislocations.[10] Dorsal dislocations occur more frequently than volar. If the injury is closed, it is usually reducible. X-rays should be taken to rule out fracture. If the joint is reduced and there is no fracture, splint the DIP only in neutral for 1 to 2 weeks (Figure 19-48). If the DIP dislocation is open (and it frequently is) or is irreducible, it needs to be surgically addressed.[42] With all finger dislocations in a gloved patient, the glove must be removed to determine whether the injury is open or closed.

Injury Mechanism

The mechanism for all finger dislocations is a hyperextension force or a compressive load force.[7]

Rehabilitation Concerns

The initial concern is to rule out a fracture and relocate the injured joint. If the joint is not reducible, appropriate surgical intervention is needed. Once reduced, Coban (Figure 19-44) should be applied to decrease edema. Protective splinting or buddy taping is also applied. In PIP dorsal dislocations without fracture, immediate ROM is important to decrease stiffness. Complications of finger dislocations include pain, swelling, stiffness, or loss of reduction.

Rehabilitation Progressions

Simple dorsal subluxation of the MCP joints are reduced and splinted in 50 degrees of

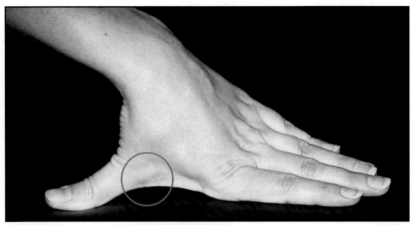

Figure 19-40. The ulnar collateral ligament provides support on the ulnar MCP joint. A fall on an abducted thumb can cause injury or rupture.

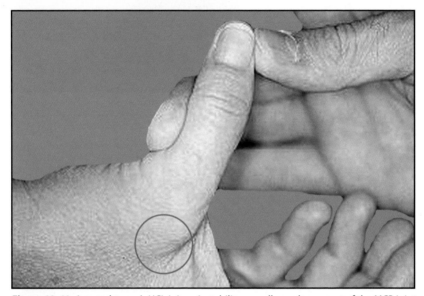

Figure 19-41. A gamekeeper's UCL injury. Instability as well as enlargement of the MCP joint is normal.

flexion for 7 to 10 days. Following splinting, AROM is begun. Because the joints are immobilized in flexion, the collateral ligaments remain taut and full MCP flexion should be maintained. Extension is not lost at the MCP joints with this injury. Progression is from full ROM to gentle strengthening to more aggressive strengthening.

If the MCP joint dislocation is irreducible, it will require open reduction. Pins may be placed holding MCP joints in flexion. If not, the hand needs to be splinted with MCP joints in flexion. Once motion is allowed, active flexion and extension are initiated. Stiffness can be a

problem, as can tendon adherence in the scar. Rehabilitation might be difficult and require consultation with a hand therapist for splinting to regain motion. ROM is progressed to activities of daily living (ADL), strengthening, and functional return to sport activities.

PIP dislocations without fractures, once reduced, need to be wrapped in Coban for edema control (Figure 19-44) and started on early motion. Exercises include composite flexion and extension, and blocked PIP and DIP flexion exercises (Figures 19-19 and 19-20). Buddy taping is often helpful to encourage ROM and provide protection. This is frequently

Figure 19-42. A gamekeeper's splint may also be called a hand-based thumb spica splint. It always includes the thumb MCP joint and may include the CMC or IP joint, depending on the injury or sport.

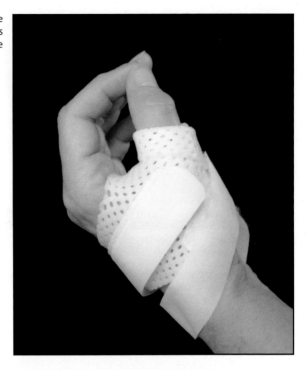

Figure 19-43. Thumb spica taping may be used when additional support is needed to the wrist and thumb. Tendinitis, gamekeeper's injuries, or healed fractures are some indications.

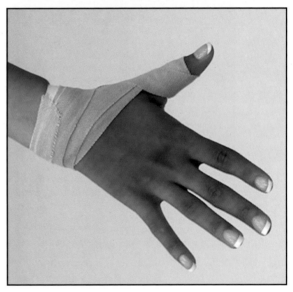

enough to maintain motion and strength. If stiffness does occur, a referral to a hand therapist may be necessary for dynamic splinting, serial casting, or an aggressive strength and motion program.

If the DIP is dislocated, closed, and easily reduced, it should be splinted in neutral to slight flexion for 1 to 2 weeks. AROM begins at 2 to 3 weeks, with protective splinting

continued between exercise sessions for 4 to 6 weeks.[55] At that time, putty for strengthening (Figure 19-11) and blocked DIP exercises (Figure 19-19) may begin.

Open or irreducible fractures require surgical wound care with debridement to prevent infection. These injuries are then treated like mallet fingers and progressed accordingly.[42]

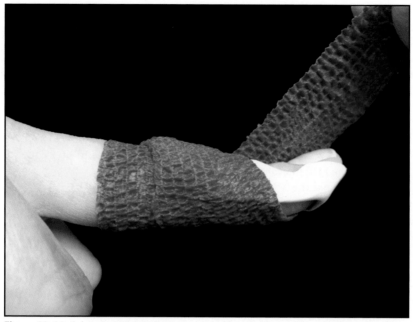

Figure 19-44. Coban is similar to Ace wrap in that it is elastic. It sticks to itself, so there is no need for clips. It comes in varying widths from 1 to 3 inches. One inch is perfect for fingers. Start wrapping from distal to proximal, pulling slightly but still leaving some wrinkles. Check circulation following application. Coban is perfect to help prevent swelling in finger injuries, especially PIP dislocations, immediately following injury.

Criteria for Return

Return to play for all finger joint dislocations is dependent upon the complexity of the dislocation and whether a fracture has occurred. If the MCP joints have a simple dislocation and are easily reduced, and remain reduced, the affected finger may be buddy taped, Coban wrapped for edema control, and protective-splinted for pain control if necessary, with return to sport immediately or within the first few days after injury. If it is a complex dislocation and surgery is necessary, the patient will be out a minimum of 2 to 3 weeks.

For PIP joint dorsal dislocations without fracture, once the joint is reduced and stable, the finger should be Coban wrapped and buddy taped. A dorsal Alumafoam splint is optional for pain control during sport activity. The patient may return to activity immediately. If the joint is not reducible, or there is a fracture, the length of time lost from sport will vary depending on the sport and severity of injury.

For DIP joint dislocations that are easily reduced, the patient may return immediately with Coban and splint. If the dislocation is open or irreducible, the patient can usually return once sutures are removed after surgery, at about 10 days, with protective splinting. The criteria for the DIP joint is very similar to criteria for mallet finger.

Clinical Decision-Making Exercise 19-4

A football player presents at the end of the season saying that 3 weeks ago he dislocated his finger during a game but pulled on it and "popped" it into place. He presents with swelling and redness at the PIP joint and passive extension to 30 degrees. He can flex the finger to the palm but is unable to make a tight fist. What should the athletic trainer address first and how?

Flexor Digitorum Profundus Avulsion (Jersey Finger)

Pathomechanics

Jersey finger is a rupture of the flexor digitorum profundus (FDP) tendon from its insertion on the distal phalanx. It most frequently occurs in the ring finger. It may be avulsed with or without bone. If avulsed with bone, depending on the size of the fragment, the tendon will usually not retract back into the palm, as it gets "caught" on the pulley system of the finger. If no bone, or only a very small fleck of bone, is avulsed, the tendon will retract back into the palm. This is the most common.[33] Each time the patient tries to flex his or her finger, the muscle is contracting but the insertion is not attached. This brings the insertion closer to its origin.

The way to isolate the FDP to evaluate function and integrity is to hold the MCP and PIP joints of the affected finger in full extension, then have the patient attempt to flex the DIP joint. If it flexes, it is intact. If it does not, it is ruptured (Figure 19-45).

If the tendon is ruptured, there are two options. The first is do nothing. If the tendon is not repaired, the patient will be unable to flex the DIP joint, might have decreased grip strength, and might have tenderness at the site of tendon retraction, but functionally should not have difficulty.[33,43] The second option is to have the tendon surgically repaired. If it is repaired, the patient should be informed that this is a labor-intensive operation and rehabilitation, there is a risk of scarring with poor tendon glide, and there is a risk of tendon rupture. The patient will not have full activity level for about 12 weeks after surgery. The repair should be done within 10 days of injury for the best results.

Injury Mechanism

Forceful hyperextension of the fingers while tightly gripping into flexion is the injury mechanism. It most frequently happens in football when a shirt is grabbed to try to make a tackle and the finger gets caught[33] (Figure 19-45).

Rehabilitation Concerns

This can be a very difficult injury to treat if surgically repaired. The surgery should be done by an experienced hand surgeon with rehabilitation by an experienced hand therapist.[8] Close communication between hand surgeon, hand therapist, and athletic training staff is a must. All protocols are guidelines and, as such, may need to be altered if complications such as infection, poor tendon glide, or excellent tendon glide occur. With this injury, unlike most others, the better a person is doing (ie, full active tendon glide) the more they are held back and protected. Good tendon glide is indicative of less scar, which means there is less scar holding the repaired tendon together, thus less tensile strength and increased chance of rupture. If a tendon is ruptured, it must be repaired again and the prognosis is poorer.

Proper patient education is a must. Instruction in what to expect, reasons for specific exercises, and consequences must be conveyed.

Rehabilitation Progressions

The following are guidelines. They are not all-inclusive, nor are they an indication that just anyone can treat this injury. For more specific information on the protocol, readers are encouraged to read and review the Roslyn Evans article on zone I flexor tendon rehabilitation.[11]

Between 2 and 5 days postoperative, the bulky dressing should be removed and a dorsal splint fabricated to hold the wrist in neutral, MCP joints in 30 degrees of flexion, and IP joints in full extension with the hood extending to the fingertips for protection (Figure 19-46). The affected DIP joint is splinted at 45 degrees of flexion with a second dorsal splint that extends from the PIP joint to the fingertip, held on with tape at the middle phalanx only. Exercises for the first 3 weeks are (1) passive DIP flexion; (2) full composite passive flexion, then extend MCP joints passively to a modified hook position; (3) hyperflexion of MCP joints with active extension of PIP joints to 0 degrees; and (4) strap or hold noninvolved fingers to the top of the splint. Position PIP joint in flexion passively then actively hold the joint in flexion (Figure 19-22). All exercises should be done with the splint on, at a frequency of 10 repetitions every waking hour. The patients should not use the injured hand for anything, extend the wrist or fingers with the splint off, or actively flex the fingers—all of these could cause tendon rupture. In addition, during the first weeks Coban (Figure 19-44) can be used for edema control and scar control. Scar massage may be performed in the splint. The dressing may be changed at home, but the DIP splint should remain in place at all times for 3 weeks.

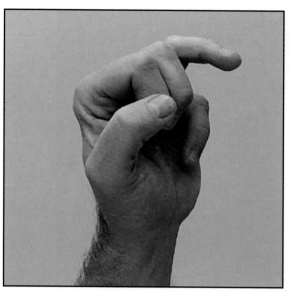

Figure 19-45. A jersey finger (FDP avulsion) injury is named for the injury mechanism—forced hyperextension with finger flexion, as in trying to grab a shirt during a tackle. The position of the DIP joint after injury will be extension or hyperextension.

Between 3 and 4 weeks post repair, the digital splint is discontinued, passive fist and hold is begun for composite flexion, and dorsal protective splinting is continued. Between 4 and 6 weeks, active hook fist and active composite fisting is begun, wrist ROM is begun, and gentle isolated profundus exercises are initiated (Figures 19-18 and 19-19). The splint may be discontinued if poor tendon glide is present.

At 6 to 8 weeks, the splint is discontinued, ADL may be done with the injured hand, and tendon-gliding exercises and blocked DIP exercises are continued. Light resistive exercises (putty) (Figure 19-11) may be initiated. Graded resistive exercises are begun if there is poor tendon glide. Be very careful during this time—it is a prime time for tendon ruptures. Patients are excited to be out of their splints and might overdo. Graded resistive exercises and dynamic splinting, if necessary, are initiated at 8 to 10 weeks.

Between 10 and 12 weeks, strengthening is begun. By 12 weeks, patients should be back with full tendon glide and good tendon strength to return to all normal activities. Activities and sports in which a sudden surprise force might pull on flexed fingers, such as rock climbing, windsurfing, water skiing, or dog walking, should not be done until 14 to 16 weeks postoperative.

Criteria for Return

Return to activity is dependent on sport and position played, and the decision must be made with physician, hand therapist, and athletic training staff involved. It will be 10 to 12 weeks before the patient can play without protection and with little risk of tendon reinjury. There are instances where a non-ball-handling patient may return sooner if cleared by the physician. In these cases, the patient's affected hand must be tightly taped into a fist and then casted with wrist in flexion, padded according to sport rules. Nothing hard should be placed in the patient's hand—if they squeeze against resistance, they might rupture. The patient and coaching staff must be made aware of the possibility of rupture with early return to sport.

Clinical Decision-Making Exercise 19-5

A football player makes a tackle and feels a pop in his ring finger. When he comes to the sideline, he is unable to flex his DIP joint actively. The team orthopedist diagnoses an FDP avulsion injury, or jersey finger. What can the athletic trainer do immediately on the field, and what information can be provided to the patient regarding treatment options?

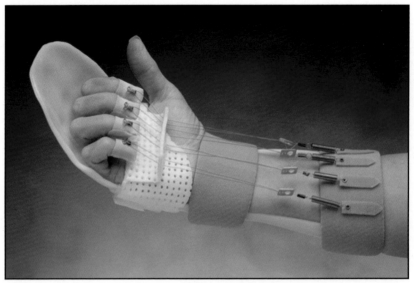

Figure 19-46. A flexor tendon splint—usually applied within 5 days post surgery—is dorsally based and includes the wrist in neutral to slight flexion, MCP joint flexion, and IP joint extension. Depending on the location of injury, the amount of flexion may be increased or decreased, and rubber band traction may be applied from fingernails to forearm strap.

Mallet Finger

Pathomechanics

A mallet finger is the avulsion of the terminal extensor tendon,[32] which is responsible for extension of the DIP joint. It can occur with or without fracture of bone. If there is a large fracture fragment, where the fracture fragment is displaced greater than 2 mm, or the DIP joint has volar subluxation on X-ray, the injury will require ORIF.

There is no other mechanism for extending the DIP joint. The presenting complaint is inability to extend the DIP joint (Figure 19-47).

Treatment is splinting the DIP joint in neutral to slight hyperextension (Figure 19-48) for 6 to 8 weeks with no flexion of the DIP joint.[9,27] If the DIP joint is flexed even once during that time, the 6 weeks starts again.

Injury Mechanism

Injury mechanism is forced flexion of the DIP joint while it is held in full extension.[27] It frequently happens when the end of the finger is struck by a ball.

Rehabilitation Concerns

Rehabilitation of the mallet finger is minimal. A splint may be custom made or prefabricated, such as a stack splint or Alumafoam. It should hold the DIP joint in neutral to slight hyperextension. Skin integrity needs to be monitored, and the splint modified or redesigned if breakdown occurs. ROM of noninvolved fingers and joints should be maintained. PIP flexion with the DIP splinted will not put tension on the injury and should be encouraged.

Rehabilitation Progressions

Once the tendon is healed, at about 6 to 8 weeks, splinting may be discontinued. If an extensor lag is present, splinting may be continued longer. Night splinting is often continued for 2 weeks after full-time splinting is discontinued. AROM to DIP joint following splint removal. No attempts to passively flex the finger to regain ROM should be attempted for 4 weeks. Blocked DIP flexion exercises are most important. Full ROM is usually gained through blocked exercises (Figures 19-19 and 19-20) and regular functional hand use.

Criteria for Return

Return to sports is permitted immediately with the DIP joint splinted in full extension. If the sport does not permit playing with the finger splint on, the patient will be out of competition for 8 weeks.

Clinical Decision-Making Exercise 19-6

A baseball player was fielding a ground ball when the ball popped up and jammed his fingertip. He continued to play. At the conclusion of the game, the ring finger has the DIP joint resting in 70 degrees of flexion. The finger is red over the dorsal DIP joint and swollen. What should the athletic trainer do?

Boutonniere Deformity

Pathomechanics

The posture of a finger with a boutonniere deformity is PIP joint flexion and DIP joint hyperextension (Figure 19-49). It is caused by interruption of the central slip and triangular ligament. Normally the central slip will initiate extension of flexed PIP joints. The lateral bands cannot initiate PIP joint extension but can maintain extension if passively positioned, because they are dorsal to the axis of motion. When the central slip is disrupted, the extensor muscle displaces proximally and shifts the lateral bands volarly. The FDS is unopposed without an intact central slip and will flex the PIP joint. As the length of time post injury increases, the lateral bands displace volarly and might become fixed to the joint capsule or collateral ligament. This makes passive correction very difficult. The DIP joint hyperextends because all the force to extend the PIP is transmitted to the DIP joint.[27]

Once a fixed deformity is present, it is much more difficult to treat. However, many patients do not seek immediate medical attention, feeling that the finger was "jammed" and will be fine in several days or weeks.

Treatment for the acute injury is uninterrupted splinting of the PIP joint in full extension for 6 weeks (Figure 19-50). The DIP joint is left free with motion encouraged. This will synergistically relax the extrinsic and intrinsic extensor tendon muscles and also exercises the oblique retinacular ligament.[32]

Following 6 weeks of immobilization, gentle careful flexion of the PIP joint is begun. Continue splinting for 2 to 4 weeks when not exercising. When full PIP joint extension can be maintained throughout the day, then night splinting only is appropriate. Length of treatment and splinting may be several months.

Injury Mechanism

Injury occurs when the extended finger is forcibly flexed, as when being hit by a ball or striking the finger on another player during a fall.[43]

Rehabilitation Concerns

Of primary concern is early and proper diagnosis and treatment. X-rays should be taken to rule out fracture or PIP joint dislocation. It is also very important to splint the PIP in full extension. If edema is present when initially splinted, as edema decreases the splint gets loose and full extension is no longer achieved. Passive flexion should not be performed to the PIP joint following removal of the splint. Blocked PIP ROM exercises are appropriate to isolate flexion (Figure 19-19). If diagnosis is made late and there is a fixed PIP flexion contracture, serial casting may be necessary to restore extension. Following return of full extension, the finger is then splinted for 8 weeks. One other factor to keep in mind is that initially a central slip injury does not present as a boutonniere, but rather a PIP flexor contracture. DIP hyperextension comes later.

Rehabilitation Progressions

The progression is increasing ROM following splint removal. Strengthening of grip may also be performed, if needed, at 10 to 12 weeks following acute injury (about 4 weeks following splinting).

Criteria for Return

The patient may return to activity when the finger is comfortable. The affected finger must be splinted at all times in full extension. If the sport does not allow for the finger to be splinted, the patient will be out about 8 weeks.

The author wishes to thank Dr. Wallace Andrew of Raleigh Orthopaedic Clinic for his support, knowledge, and willingness to answer my countless questions.

Figure 19-47. A mallet finger deformity with DIP flexion. There might or might not be redness dorsally.

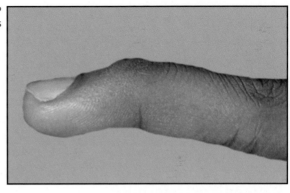

Figure 19-48. A mallet finger splint must hold the DIP in neutral to slight hyperextension. It may be dorsally based, volarly based, or circumferential. A stack-type splint is usually preferred since it rarely impedes PIP motion.

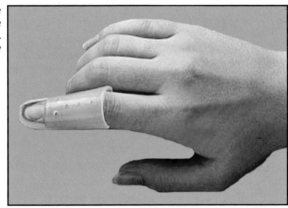

Figure 19-49. A boutonniere deformity might start as a PIP contracture. In time it will cause hyperextension of the DIP joint.

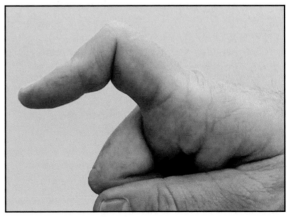

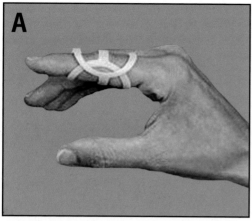
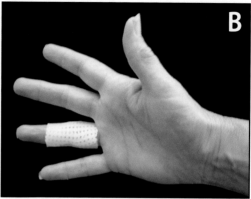

Figure 19-50. A boutonniere splint needs to immobilize the PIP joint in full extension, leaving the MCP and DIP joint free. (A) An oval 8 splint, (B) a splint made of two pieces of moldable thermoplastic that overlap and may be held in place with tape.

Summary

1. Flexor tendon injuries are very labor-intensive, significant injuries. An experienced hand surgeon and hand therapist must be involved in the care, and the patient must be made aware of what to expect.

2. The goal in the treatment of ulnar collateral ligament injuries (gamekeeper's thumb) is stability of the MCP joint. Patients will be stiff following immobilization—the athletic trainer should not passively push motion initially.

3. Early treatment of the boutonniere deformity is essential, as is proper splint position. The PIP joint should be fully extended with the DIP joint free.

4. The mallet finger must be splinted in full extension uninterrupted for 6 to 8 weeks. If the DIP joint is flexed, even once, any healing is disrupted and the 6 to 8 weeks begins again.

5. Dislocations of the MCP joints are very rare and are often complicated. Dorsal PIP dislocations without fracture are common and need early ROM and edema control. Splinting for comfort during competition is acceptable, but does not need to continue off-field unless the dislocation is unstable. DIP dislocations are frequently open and require surgery. They are treated like a mallet finger.

6. Boxer's fractures tend to heal without incident with full return of motion in 4 to 6 weeks. Splint immobilization should leave the PIP joint and wrist free to move.

7. Tendinitis and DeQuervain's tenosynovitis should be immobilized for 2 to 3 weeks with gentle pain-free ROM performed daily to maintain mobility. Activity should be increased as pain decreases.

8. Carpal tunnel syndrome is very rare in patients.

9. Ganglion cysts need to be treated only if symptomatic. Multiple aspirations may be performed during the season with excision postseason if necessary. There are usually few rehabilitation needs.

10. Wrist sprains are a diagnosis of exclusion. All other pathology must be ruled out prior to return to sport.

11. Lunate dislocations are serious injuries that require ORIF and possible lengthy rehabilitation.

12. Hamate hook fractures are not seen on regular X-ray views. A carpal tunnel view will confirm the diagnosis, and the fracture should be treated symptomatically.

13. Scaphoid fractures might not be seen on initial X-ray. If suspected, but the X-ray is negative, the patient should be treated as if a fracture is present, with X-rays

repeated in 2 weeks to confirm diagnosis. Early proper immobilization is important to the long-term outcome.

14. Distraction of the wrist while performing passive ROM after fracture can help increase motion and decrease pain during stretching.

References

1. Abramo, A. 2008. Evaluation of a treatment protocol in distal radius fractures. *Acta Orthopaedica* 79(3):376.

2. Baxter-Petralia, P., and V. Penney. 1992. Cumulative trauma. In *Concepts in hand rehabilitation*, edited by B. G. Stanley and S. M. Tribuzi. Philadelphia: F. A. Davis.

3. Bowers, W. H. 1998. The distal radio-ulnar joint. In *Operative hand surgery* 3rd ed., Green, D., and R. Hotchkiss. pp. 973–1019. New York: Churchill Livingstone.

4. Bush, D. C. 2002. Soft-tissue tumors of the hand. In *Rehabilitation of the hand and upper extremity* 5th ed., edited by Mackin, E. J. and A. D. Callahan. St. Louis: Mosby.

5. Butler, D. S. 1991. *Mobilization of the nervous system.* Melbourne: Churchill Livingstone.

6. Caditz, J. C., and A. M. Schneider. 1995. Modification of the digital serial plaster casting technique. *Journal of Hand Therapy* 8(3):215-216.

7. Cahalan, T. D., and W. P. Cooney. 1996. Biomechanics. In *Operative techniques in upper extremity sports injuries*, edited by Jobe, F. W., M. M. Pink, R. E. Glousman, R. S. Kvitne, and N. P. Zemel. St. Louis: Mosby.

8. Culp, R.W., and J. S. Taras. 2002. Primary care of flexor tendon injuries. In *Rehabilitation of the hand and upper extremity* 5th ed., edited by Mackin, E. J. and A. D. Callahan. St. Louis: Mosby.

9. Doyle, J. R. 1998. Extensor tendons: Acute injuries. In *Operative hand surgery* 4th ed., edited by Green, D. P. New York: Churchill Livingstone.

10. Dray, G. J., and R. G. Eaton. 1998. Dislocations and ligament injuries in the digits. In *Operative hand surgery* 4th ed., vol. 1, edited by Green, D. P. New York: Churchill Livingstone.

11. Evans, R. 1990. A study of the zone I flexor tendon injury and implications for treatment. *Journal of Hand Therapy* 3:133.

12. Frykman, G. K., and W. E. Kropp. 2002. Fractures and traumatic conditions of the wrist. In *Rehabilitation of the hand and upper extremity* 5th ed., edited by Mackin, E. J. and A. D. Callahan. St. Louis: Mosby.

13. Haugstvedt, J. 2004. Hand and Wrist Injuries. In *Clinical guide to sports injuries*, Bahr, R. ed. Champaign, IL: Human Kinetics.

14. Hunter, J. M., L. B. Davlin, and L. M. Fedus. 2002. Major neuropathies of the upper extremity: The median nerve. In *Rehabilitation of the hand and upper extremity* 5th ed., edited by Mackin, E. J. and A. D. Callahan. St. Louis: Mosby.

15. Husband, J. B., and S. A. McPherson. 1996. Bony skier's thumb injuries. *Clinical Orthopaedics and Related Research* 327:79–84.

16. Jupiter, J. B., and M. R. Belsky. 2002. Fractures and dislocations of the hand. In *Skeletal trauma*, edited by Browner, B. D., J. B. Jupiter, A. M. Levine, and P. G. Trafton. Philadelphia: W. B. Saunders.

17. Kirkpatrick, W. H., and S. Lisser. 2002. Soft-tissue conditions: Trigger fingers and DeQuervain's disease. In *Rehabilitation of the hand and upper extremity* 5th ed., edited by Mackin, E. J. and A. D. Callahan. St. Louis: Mosby.

18. Korman, J., R. Pearl, and V. R. Hentz. 1992. Efficacy of immobilization following aspiration of carpal and digital ganglion. *Journal of Hand Surgery* 17:1097.

19. Kozin, S. H., and M. B. Wood. 1993. Early soft tissue complications after fractures of the distal part of the radius. *Journal of Bone and Joint Surgery* 75A:144.

20. McCue, F. C. 1988. The elbow, wrist and hand. In *The injured patient* 2nd ed., edited by Kulund, D. Philadelphia: Lippincott.

21. McCue, F. C., and W. E. Nelson. 1993. Ulnar collateral ligament injuries of the thumb. *Physician and Sports Medicine* 21(9):67–80.

22. McKeon, J., and K. Yancosek. 2008. Neural gliding techniques for the treatment of carpal tunnel syndrome: A systematic review. *Journal of Sport Rehabilitation* 17(3):324.

23. Meyer, F. N., and R. L. Wilson. 2002. Management of nonarticular fractures of the hand. In *Rehabilitation of the hand and upper extremity* 5th ed., edited by Mackin, E. J. and A. D. Callahan. St. Louis: Mosby.

24. Mosher, F. J. 1986. Peripheral nerve injuries and entrapments of the forearm and wrist. In *American Academy of Orthopaedic Surgeons: Symposium on upper extremity injuries in patients*, edited by Pettrone, F. A. St. Louis: Mosby.

25. Palmer A. K., and F.W. Werner. Biomechanics of the distal radioulnar joint. In *Clinical orthopaedics and related research*, edited by Urist, M. R. Philadelphia: Lippincott.

26. Papadonikolakis, A. 2003. Transscaphoid Volar Lunate Dislocation. *Journal of Bone & Joint Surgery, American Volume* 85(9):1805.

27. Peterson, J., and L. Bancroft. 2006. Injuries of the fingers and thumb in the athlete. *Clinics in Sports Medicine* 25(3):527–542.

28. Pianka, G., and E. B. Hershman. 1990. Neurovascular injuries. In *Upper extremity in sports medicine*, edited by Nicholas, J. A. and E. B. Hershman. St. Louis: Mosby.

29. Rettig, A. 2003. Athletic injuries of the wrist and hand: Part I, Traumatic injuries of the wrist. *American Journal of Sports Medicine* 31(6):1038–1048.

30. Rettig, A. C. 1991. Current concepts in management of football injuries of the hand and wrist. *Journal of Hand Therapy* 4(2):42-50

31. Rizzo, M., and A. Shin. 2006. Treatment of acute scaphoid fractures in the athlete. *Current Sports Medicine Reports* 5(5):242.

32. Rosenthal, E. A. 2002. The extensor tendons: Anatomy and management. In *Rehabilitation of the hand and upper extremity* 5th ed., edited by Mackin, E. J. and A. D. Callahan. St. Louis: Mosby.

33. Shippert, B. A. 2007. Complex jersey finger: Case report and literature review. *Clinical Journal of Sport Medicine* 17(4):319–320.

34. Swan, M. 2003. Hook of hamate fractures. *New Zealand Journal of Sports Medicine* 31(3):76–77.

35. Thiru-Pathi, R. G., et al. 1986. Arterial anatomy of the triangular fibrocartilage of the wrist and its surgical significance. *Journal of Hand Surgery* 11(2):258–263.

36. Tracy, M. 2006. Arthroscopic management of triangular fibrocartilage tears in the athlete. *Operative Techniques in Sports Medicine* 14(2):95–100.

37. Vender, M. I. 1987. Degenerative changes in symptomatic scaphoid non-union. *Journal of Hand Surgery* 12A:514.

38. Viegas, S. F., et al. 1991. Simulated scaphoid proximal pole fracture. *Journal of Hand Surgery* 16A:485–500.

39. Warhold, L. G., and A. L. Osterman. 1992. Scaphoid fracture and non-union: Treatment by open reduction, bone graft and a Herbert screw. *Clinical Orthopaedics* 7:7–18.

40. Watson, H. K., and W. D. Rogers. 1989. Nonunion of the hook of the hamate: An argument for bone grafting the nonunion. *Journal of Hand Surgery* 14A:486–90.

41. Weinstein, S. M., and S. A. Herring. 1992. Nerve problems and compartment syndromes in the hand, wrist, and forearm. *Clinics in Sports Medicine* 11(1):161-188.

42. Wilson, R. L., and J. Hazen. 2002. Management of joint injuries and intraarticular fractures of the hand. In *Rehabilitation of the hand and upper extremity* 5th ed., edited by Mackin, E. J. and A. D. Callahan. St. Louis: Mosby.

43. Wright, H. H., and A. C. Rettig. 2002. Management of common sports injuries. In *Rehabilitation of the hand and upper extremity* 5th ed., edited by Mackin, E. J. and A. D. Callahan. St. Louis: Mosby.

44. Zemel, N. P. 1996. Anatomy and surgical approaches: Hand, wrist and forearm. In *Operative techniques in upper extremity sports injuries*, edited by Jobe, F. W., M. M. Pink, R. E. Glousman, R. S. Kvitne, and N. P. Zemel. St. Louis: Mosby.

45. Zemel, N. P. 1996. Fractures and ligament injuries of the wrist. In *Operative techniques in upper extremity sports injuries*, edited by Jobe, F. W., M. M. Pink, R. E. Glousman, R. S. Kvitne, and N. P. Zemel. St. Louis: Mosby.

46. Zubowicz, V. N., and C. H. Ishii. 1987. Management of ganglion cysts by simple aspiration. *Journal of Hand Surgery* 12:618.

SOLUTIONS TO CLINICAL DECISION MAKING EXERCISES

19-1 Oral anti-inflammatory medications and ice will be helpful initially to decrease pain and inflammation. Ultrasound or iontophoresis to the radial forearm may help with pain relief. ROM and wrist stretching should be done within pain limits as soon as possible following injury. A splint immobilizing the thumb and wrist (Figure 19-29) may be helpful for pain relief as well. If the patient can move his wrist without pain, but a blow to the area is painful, the area may be padded for return to play.

19-2 Splinting for immobilization between practice sessions can help decrease pain, as can oral anti-inflammatory medications and ultrasound or iontophoresis. Taping for support during play may help decrease pain. The practice schedule may need to be modified to decrease playing time during acute phase. Once the pain is decreasing, strength and body mechanics should be addressed. Ice following practice and play may also decrease symptoms.

19-3 Splinting for support should be initiated immediately to help provide stability and decrease chances of instability later. The splint should be worn full-time for about 4 weeks. If the patient is able to play in the splint, she may play. Be sure support is provided over the IP joint to prevent dislocation of that joint. Once the period of splinting is finished, taping the MCP joint during play and practice may provide support and pain relief. ROM exercises may be initiated if necessary; PROM is not done until 6 to 8 weeks post injury.

19-4 Extension should be addressed first. It is hardest to regain, as functionally it is not used much. Serial casting[10] will provide a sustained extension stretch, neutral warmth for pain relief, and immobilization to decrease edema. Because it may not be removed by the patient, compliance is better and results are quicker. Once extension is full, switch to a static splint, weaning out of it for flexion while maintaining extension.

19-5   Coban can be applied immediately to control swelling. Ice may be used, but ice can be uncomfortable in the hand. The athletic trainer needs to spend time with the patient, and with the parents, if appropriate, discussing options. The future needs of the patient should come before "I want to play" issues. If the tendon will be repaired, the best results will occur if it is repaired within 2 weeks of injury, and preferably within 5 to 7 days. If the tendon is repaired, the rehabilitation following surgery will last about 12 weeks. The patient will be in a splint full-time for 4 to 6 weeks following surgery. The patient will probably be in pain, and will usually be out of competition for 4 or more weeks, depending on the sport and position played. This is intensive rehabilitation, and the patient needs to be prepared for that. There is risk for re-rupture or infection. The patient who chooses not to have the tendon repaired will never again be able to actively flex the DIP joint. The athletic trainer can demonstrate this by bending all of his or her fingers except the DIP of the affected finger. Functionally, this is usually not a problem, but the patient's future plans need to be addressed. If the patient plans on medical school and surgery, or on playing an instrument, they should not choose to lose DIP flexion. The danger in not repairing the tendon is that if the joint hyperextends, if the patient pinches against it, the DIP will hyperextend. They will lose the stability of the joint. Functionally this may or may not be a problem. It is important to have close communication with all involved parties for this injury.

19-6   Referral for an X-ray should be made to be sure a more serious injury has not occurred. The most likely diagnosis is mallet finger. Treatment is full DIP extension by splinting. It is important to explain to the patient that he must keep his finger fully extended at all times. Flexing it once results in counting the 6 to 8 weeks again. The athletic trainer can make a splint and teach the patient how to remove the splint and reapply it safely. Once the 8 weeks of immobilization have passed, the athletic trainer can instruct the patient in AROM exercises and the importance of not pushing the DIP joint passively.

Please see videos on the accompanying website at

www.healio.com/books/sportsmedvideos

CHAPTER 20

Rehabilitation of Groin, Hip, and Thigh Injuries

Bernie DePalma, MEd, PT, ATC
Doug Halverson, MA, ATC, CSCS

After completion of this chapter, the athletic training student should be able to do the following:

- Understand the functional anatomy and biomechanics of the groin, hip, and thigh.

- Discuss athletic injuries to the groin, hip, and thigh and describe the biomechanical changes occurring during and after injury.

- Describe functional injury evaluation, using biomechanical changes to the groin, hip, and thigh.

- Recognize abnormal gait patterns as they relate to specific groin, hip, and thigh injuries and use this knowledge during the evaluation process and rehabilitation program.

- Explain the various rehabilitative techniques used for specific groin, hip, and thigh injuries, including open and closed kinetic chain strengthening exercises, stretching exercises, and plyometric, isokinetic, and PNF exercises.

- Discuss the role of functional evaluation in determining when to return a patient to competition, based on rehabilitation progression.

This chapter describes functional rehabilitation programs that follow groin, hip, and thigh injuries. The athletic trainer and patient, together, should develop the rehabilitation program with an emphasis on injury mechanism, the athletic trainer's functional and biomechanical evaluation, and clinical findings. Each exercise program should be presented to the patient in terms of short-term goals. One objective for the athletic trainer is to make the rehabilitation experience challenging for the patient while promoting adherence to the rehabilitation program.

Prentice WE, ed.
Rehabilitation Techniques for Sports Medicine and Athletic Training (pp 591-638).
© 2015 SLACK Incorporated.

Figure 20-1. Angle of torsion. With the femoral head and neck superimposed on the femoral condyles, you can see how the axis of the femoral head and neck and the axis of the femoral condyles intersect to create the angle of torsion.

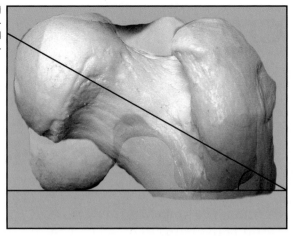

FUNCTIONAL ANATOMY AND BIOMECHANICS

The pelvis and hip are made up of the pelvic girdle and the articulation between the femoral head and the acetabulum. This articulation is considered a ball-in-socket joint with convex (femoral head) and concave (acetabulum) components connecting the lower extremity to the pelvic girdle.

The biomechanics of the hip joint can be affected by two natural bony alignments: the angle of inclination and femoral torsion. The angle of inclination is used to describe the position of the femoral head and neck with respect to the shaft of the femur.[9] An angle of inclination greater than 125 degrees, also known as coxa valga, creates a more superiorly directed femoral head and neck. This superior orientation decreases the shear forces across the femoral neck, decreases joint stability, and increases genu varum at the knee. The opposite can be found with an angle of inclination less than 125 degrees in which the femoral head and neck is more horizontally directed. This can only be assessed by measurement on X-ray.[24] Femoral torsion is the angle formed between the neck of the femur and the femoral condyles (Figure 20-1). An angle of torsion greater than 15 degrees is known as anteversion, which produces a more anteriorly directed femoral head and neck. It affects the lower extremity by decreasing hip joint stability, increasing femoral internal rotation, and producing a toe-in gait. Retroversion, or an angle less than 15 degrees, directs the femoral head and neck more posteriorly thereby increasing joint stability, femoral external rotation, and producing a toe-out gait.[24] This can be assessed clinically by using the Craig's test.[43] Changes in both these angles could cause changes in rotation of the femoral head within the acetabulum that predispose the patient to chronic injuries such as stress fractures and overuse hip injuries, as well as acute injuries, such as hip subluxation and labral tears.

The hip joint is a true ball-in-socket joint and has intrinsic stability not found in other joints. The acetabulum has a fibrocartilage rim known as the labrum which deepens the "socket" and helps stabilize the hip joint.[9] The hip joint is surrounded by three ligamentous structures that help to maintain the stability of an otherwise mobile joint. The iliofemoral ligament or Y ligament of Bigelow and pubofemoral ligament are positioned anteriorly and are taut in hip extension–external rotation and hip extension–abduction, respectively. The ischiofemoral ligament positioned posteriorly is taut in hip flexion and adduction. The ligamentum teres connects the femoral head to the acetabulum but is not considered a significant stabilizer.[12]

This intrinsic stability does not prevent the hip joint from retaining great mobility. During normal gait, the hip joint moves in all three planes: sagittal, frontal, and transverse. The pelvis itself moves in three directions: anteroposterior tilting, lateral tilting, and rotation. The iliopsoas muscle and other hip flexors, as

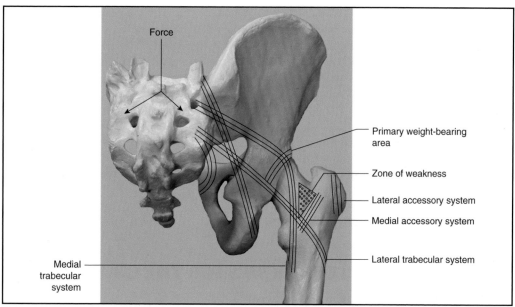

Figure 20-2. Forces transmitted through the hip and thigh cause pathomechanics that can result in injury.

well as extensors of the lumbar spine, perform anterior tilting in the sagittal plane and facilitate lumbar lordosis. The rectus abdominus, obliques, gluteus maximus, and hamstrings posteriorly tilt the pelvis and cause a decrease in lumbar lordosis. During lateral tilting in the frontal plane the hip joint acts as the center of rotation. Hip abduction or adduction is a result of pelvic lateral tilting. The hip abductors control lateral tilting by contracting isometrically or eccentrically.[9] Pelvic rotation occurs in the transverse plane, again using the hip joint as the axis of rotation. The gluteal muscles, external rotators, adductors, pectineus, and iliopsoas all act together to perform this movement in the transverse plane.[9] These movements of the pelvis are important when analyzing gait, doing injury evaluation, and teaching correct gait.

The forces transmitted up from the ground and through the hip joint show a very distinct pattern that can be used to understand the pathomechanics of certain injuries seen in the hip and thigh region. The forces transmitted through the femur are borne by the medial and lateral trabecular systems. The body's center of gravity and the medial angulation of the femur produce a three-point bending force on the femoral shaft in the frontal plane. This creates increased compressive forces along the medial

trabecular system and potential for increased tension forces along the lateral trabecular system (Figure 20-2). As the forces are transmitted proximally through the femur, a similar bending situation can be seen in the femoral neck. The medial and lateral trabecular systems intersect at the inferior aspect of the femoral neck through which the compressive forces are transmitted to the hip joint. This produces a condition where there is an area of weakness in the superior aspect of the femoral neck due to the relative increase in tensile load. Bone is better at resisting compressive forces that can be an important factor as the body attempts to absorb the increased loads that occur during activity. Forces at the hip joint are known to be 2 to 3 times body weight during level walking, 5 times body weight during running, greater than 7 times body weight with stair climbing, and over 8 times body weight during stumbling.[3,7,9,54]

The most frequently injured structures of the groin, hip, pelvis, and thigh are the muscles and tendons that perform the movements. The majority of these muscles originate on the pelvis or the proximal femur. The iliac crest serves as the attachment site for the abdominal muscles, the ilium serves as the attachment for the gluteals, and then the gluteals insert to the proximal femur. The pubis and pubic bone serve as the attachments for the adductors, as does the deep posterior abdominal muscle wall, and the iliopsoas inserts distally to the lesser trochanter of the proximal femur. Due to all the attachments in a small area, injury to these structures can be very disabling and difficult to distinguish.[9,33,35]

The quadriceps inserts by a common tendon to the proximal patella. The rectus femoris is the only quadriceps muscle that crosses the hip joint, which not only extends the knee but also flexes the hip. This is very important in differentiating hip flexor strains (eg, iliopsoas vs rectus femoris) and the ensuing treatment and rehabilitation programs.

The hamstrings all cross the knee joint posteriorly, and all except the short head of the biceps femoris cross the hip joint. These biarticular muscles produce forces dependent upon the position of both the knee joint and the hip joint. The positions of the hip and knee during movement and injury mechanism play a very important role and provide information to use when rehabilitating and preventing hamstring injuries.

REHABILITATION TECHNIQUES FOR THE GROIN, HIP, AND THIGH

Stretching Techniques, Strengthening Exercises

Figure 20-3. Lateral hip shifts on a stability ball.

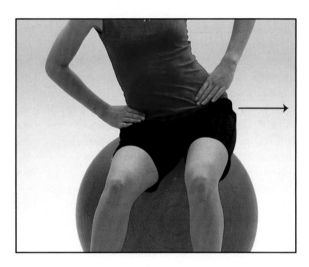

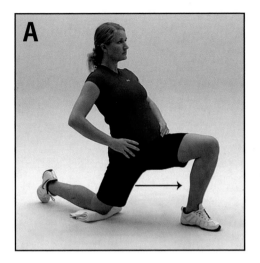

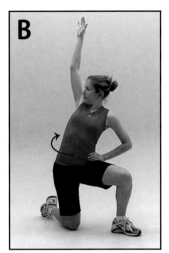

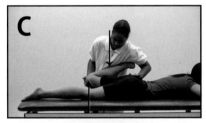

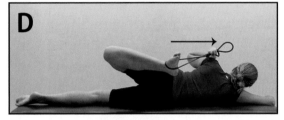

Figure 20-4. Hip flexor Stretches. (A) Kneeling hip flexor stretch, (B) with rotation, (C) prone manual stretch, (D) sidelying using tubing.

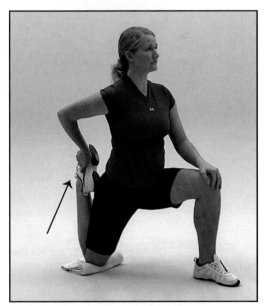

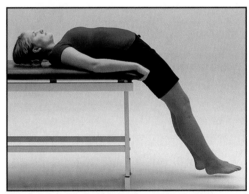

Figure 20-6. Hip flexors passive static stretch over end of table with hip extended.

Figure 20-5. Hip flexor stretch with knee flexed to isolate the rectus femoris.

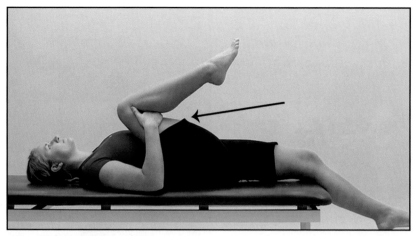

Figure 20-7. Supine gluteus maximus stretch.

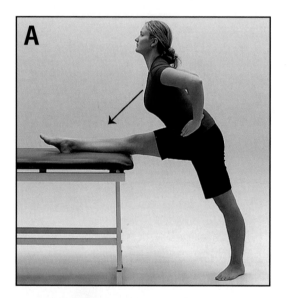

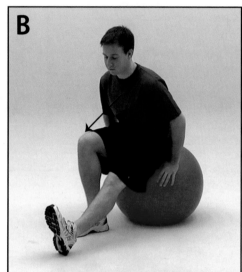

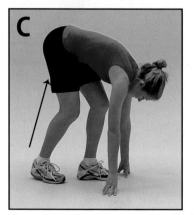

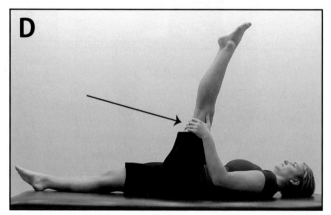

Figure 20-8. Hamstring stretches. (A) Standing ballet stretch (maintain lordotic curve), (B) on stability ball, (C) standing with trunk flexion, (D) supine.

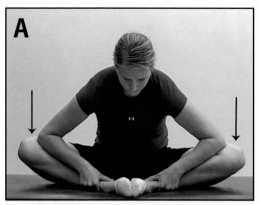

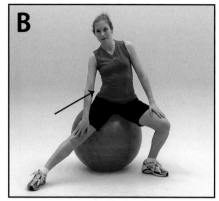

Figure 20-9. Seated hip adductor stretches. (A) Butterfly stretch, (B) seated on stability ball.

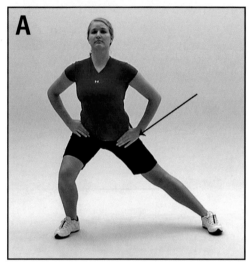

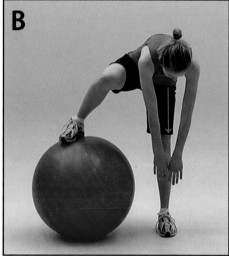

Figure 20-10. Standing hip adductor stretches. (A) Lunge stretch, (B) stability ball stretch.

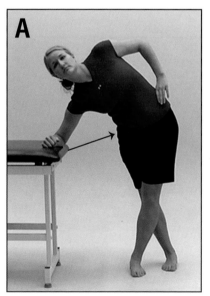

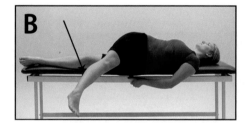

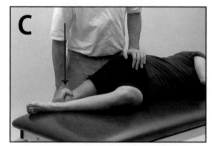

Figure 20-11. Hip adductor stretches. (A) Standing, (B) supine, (C) sidelying partner stretch.

Figure 20-12. Hip internal rotator stretch.

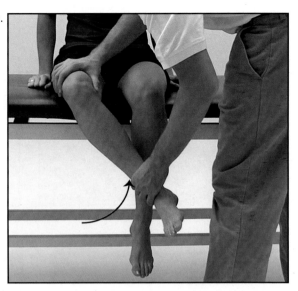

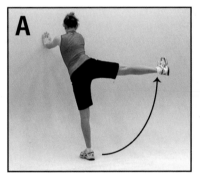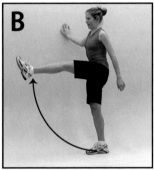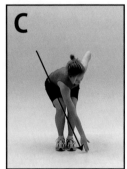

Figure 20-13. Dynamic stretching. (A) Hip adductors and abductors, (B) hip flexors and extensors, (C) hip extensors.

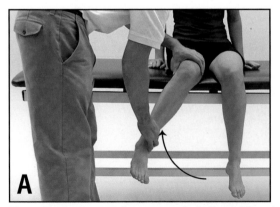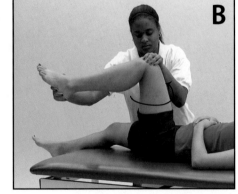

Figure 20-14. Hip external rotator stretch. (A) Sitting, (B) supine.

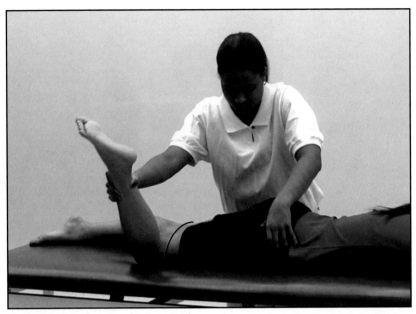

Figure 20-15. Piriformis evaluation stretch test.

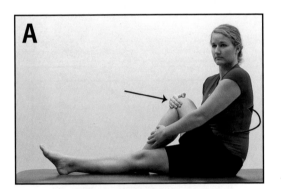

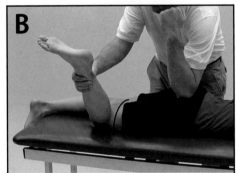

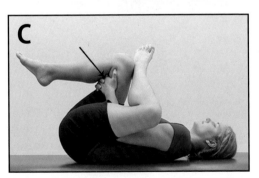

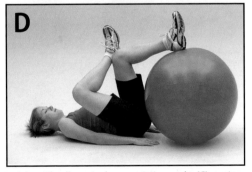

Figure 20-16. Piriformis stretches. (A) Sitting, (B) prone stretch with elbow in lesser sciatic notch, (C) supine, (D) supine using stability ball.

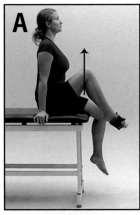

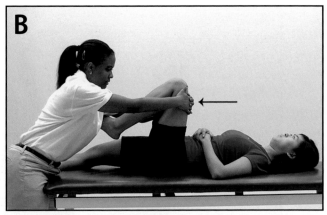

Figure 20-17. Pain-free hip flexion iliopsoas progressive resistive strengthening exercises. (A) Using cuff weights, (B) manually resisted.

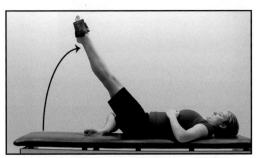

Figure 20-18. Weighted-cuff resisted straight leg raises (quadriceps and iliopsoas).

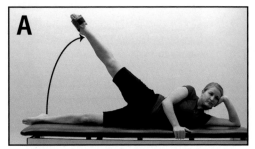

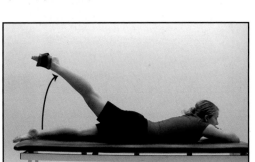

Figure 20-19. Weighted-cuff resisted hip extension (gluteus maximus and hamstring).

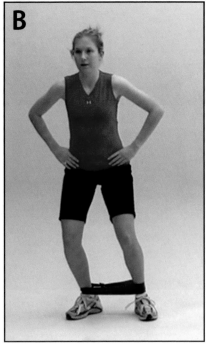

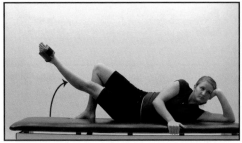

Figure 20-20. Weighted-cuff resisted hip adduction (adductor magnus, brevis, longus, pectineus, and gracilis).

Figure 20-21. (A) Weighted cuff resisted hip adduction. (B) Monster walks using Theraband resistance (gluteus medius, maximus, and tensor fascia latae).

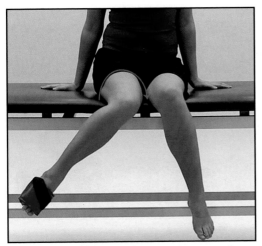

Figure 20-22. Weighted-cuff resisted hip internal rotation (gluteus minimus, tensor fascia latae, semitendinosus, and semimembranosus).

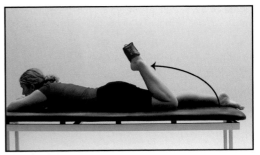

Figure 20-25. Weighted-cuff resisted prone hamstring single-leg strengthening exercises.

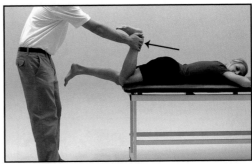

Figure 20-26. Manual resistance hamstring strengthening to fatigue. Patient lies prone with knee over the edge of treatment table. With the patient in full knee extension, resistance is applied to the back of the heels as the patient contracts concentrically to full knee flexion for a count of 5 seconds. After a 2-second pause at full flexion, resistance is applied into extension for a count of 5 as the patient contracts the hamstrings eccentrically.

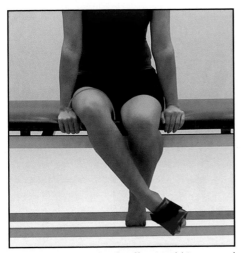

Figure 20-23. Weighted-cuff resisted hip external rotation (piriformis and gluteus maximus).

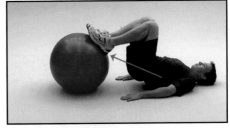

Figure 20-27. Hamstring strengthening exercise on stability ball. Patient moves stability ball away extending the hip.

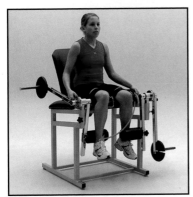

Figure 20-24. Seated hamstring progressive resistive strengthening exercises (maintain lordotic lumbar curve). Isotonics performed on the NK table.

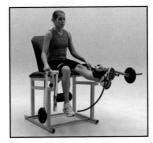

Figure 20-28. Seated single-leg resisted quadriceps extension on an NK table.

Figure 20-29. Seated quadriceps double-leg extension on a knee machine (Reprinted with permission from Body-Solid.)

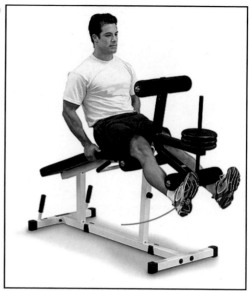

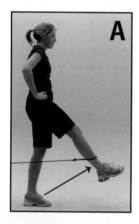

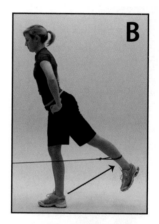

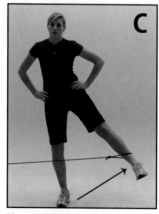

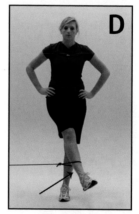

Figure 20-30. Multi-directional hip strengthening using cable or resistance band. (A) hip flexion (with knee extended iliopsoas, with knee flexed-rectus femoris), (B) hip extension (with knee extended semimembranosus, tendinosis, and gluteus maximus; with knee bent biceps femoris and gluteus maximus), (C) hip abduction (gluteus medius, tensor fascia lata), (D) hip adduction (adductor longus-magnus-brevis, pectineus, gracilis).

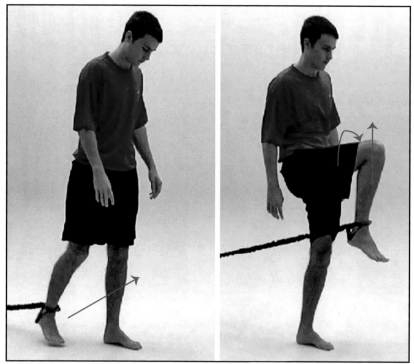

Figure 20-31. Tubing or cable resisted hip adduction, flexion, and internal rotation,

Closed Kinetic Chain Strengthening Exercises

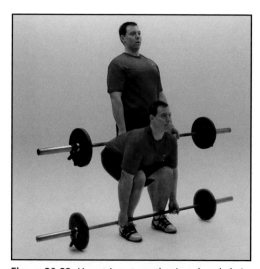

Figure 20-32. Hamstring-strengthening closed chain. Slightly flexed knee stiff-legged dead lifts. Rotate at the hip joint into flexion and keep back arched in lordotic curve until there is tightness in the hamstring muscles. Then use the hamstring muscles to extend the hip joint to the upright position.

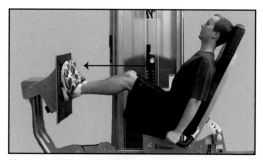

Figure 20-33. Leg press with feet high on the foot plate and shoulder-width apart to work the upper hamstring while keeping knees over the feet (not over the toes or in front of the toes). Seat setting should be close so that at the bottom of the motion the hips are lower than the knees (quadriceps, upper hamstrings, and gluteus maximus).

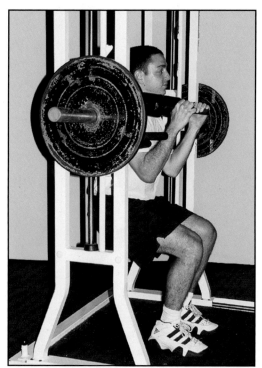

Figure 20-34. Smith press squats with feet placement forward of the patient's center of gravity and close (within 1 to 2 inches of each other); or hack squat (quadriceps, upper hamstrings, and gluteus maximus). The patient descends, keeping a lordotic curve in the low back, until the hip joints break parallel (lower than the knee joints).

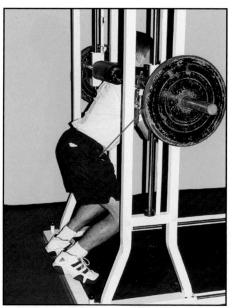

Figure 20-35. Smith press squats with feet behind the patient's center of gravity and hip in extension (as on a hip sled) (quadriceps, lower lateral hamstring, and gluteus maximus). The patient descends while keeping a lordotic curve in the low back.

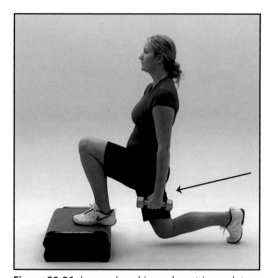

Figure 20-36. Lunges (quadriceps, hamstrings, gluteus maximus, groin muscles, and iliopsoas) stepping onto 4- to 6-inch step height. Once the foot hits the step, the patient should bend the back knee straight down toward the floor to work the upper hamstring of the front leg and the hip flexors of the back leg.

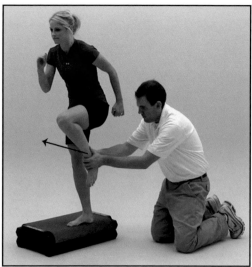

Figure 20-37. Standing running pattern, manual resistance. Resistance is applied to the back of the heel, resisting hip flexion and knee flexion to terminal position, then resisting hip extension and knee extension back down to starting position. The patient contracts as fast as possible through the entire range of running motion.

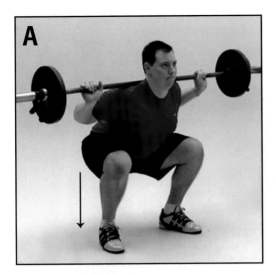

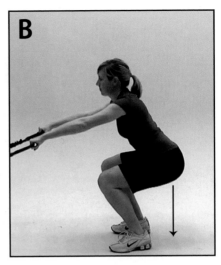

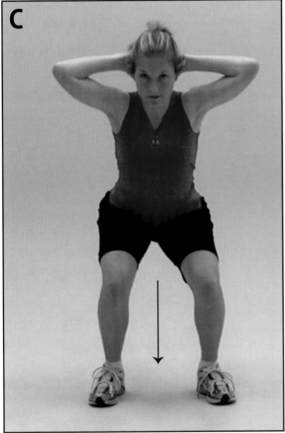

Figure 20-38. Squat exercises. (A) Using barbell, (B) using cable or tubing resistance, (C) prisoner squats.

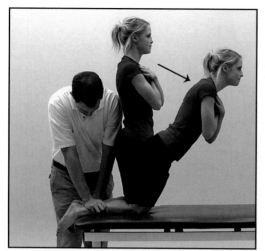

Figure 20-39. Hamstring leans—kneeling eccentric hamstring lowering exercises. With the patient kneeling on a treatment table and feet hanging over the end, the athletic trainer stabilizes the lower legs as the patient lowers the body, eccentrically contracting the hamstrings. The patient should maintain a lumbar lordotic curve and stay completely erect, avoiding any hip flexion.

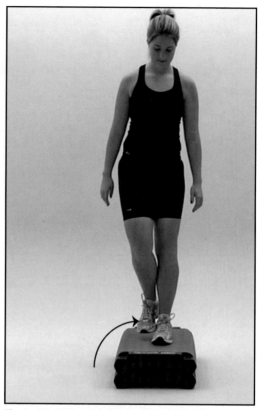

Figure 20-40. Lateral step-ups (quadriceps, hamstrings, gluteus maximus, gluteus medius, and tensor fascia latae) using repetitions and sets, or time, 2 to 3 days per week.

Isokinetic Exercises

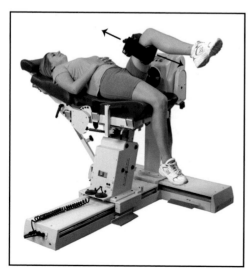

Figure 20-41. Seated isometric hip internal and external rotation strengthening. (Reprinted with permission from Biodex Medical Systems.)

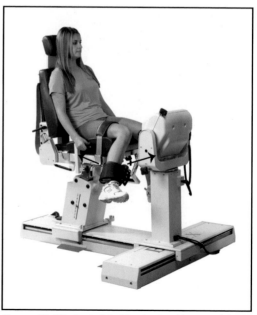

Figure 20-42. Seated isokinetic quadricep and hamstring strengthening. (Reprinted with permission from Biodex Medical Systems.)

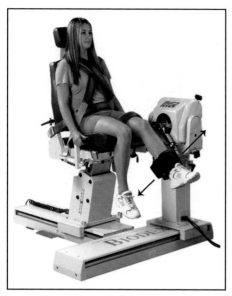

Figure 20-43. Supine isokinetic hip flexion and extension strengthening. (Reprinted with permission from Biodex Medical Systems.)

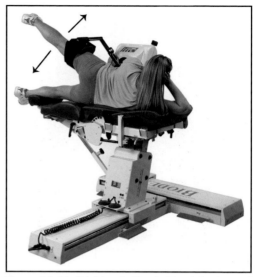

Figure 20-44. Sidelying isokinetic hip abduction and adduction. (Reprinted with permission from Biodex Medical Systems.)

Plyometric Exercises

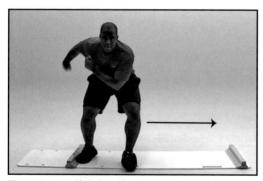

Figure 20-45. Slide board or Fitter, keeping knees bent and maintaining a squat position for the entire workout (increases hamstring activity).

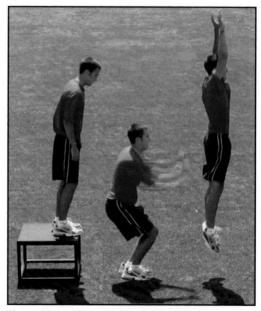

Figure 20-46. Plyometric jump-down exercises.

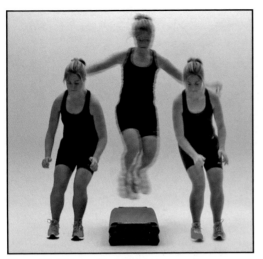

Figure 20-47. Lateral bounding.

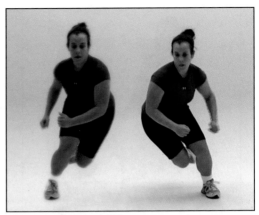

Figure 20-48. Lateral sliding.

REHABILITATION TECHNIQUES FOR ACUTE GROIN, HIP, AND THIGH INJURIES

Preferred treatment and rehabilitation of these injuries are broken down into phases. The early phase of rehabilitation consists of treatments using ice, compression, and modalities to reduce pain. Initiation of pain-free active range of motion (ROM) should begin as early as possible. Try to avoid any movement that causes pain, especially passive started too early. Oral anti-inflammatory medication is also beneficial in the early stages to reduce pain and inflammation and facilitate early ROM. After the acute phase, the athletic trainer should use modalities in combination with active ROM and active resistive pain-free strengthening exercises. The resistive exercises should include both open and closed kinetic chain, as well as concentric and eccentric contractions. Pain-free stretching is also started in this phase. The later phases of the rehabilitation allow the athletic trainer to progress the patient into plyometric activities, sport-specific functional training with agility, and ground/power-based activities. Keep in mind that the time sequences for programs and phases are approximations and should be adjusted depending upon the degree of injury, the sport, and the individual patient.

Iliac Crest Contusions (Hip Pointer)

Pathomechanics

A hip pointer can best be described as a subcutaneous contusion. In most cases, the contusion can cause separation or tearing of the origins or insertions of the muscles that attach to the prominent bony sites.[23] Usually the patient has no immediate concern, but within hours of the injury, bleeding, swelling, and pain can severely limit the patient's movement. In rare cases, a fracture of the crest may occur.[1] Care should also be taken to rule out more serious injuries such as the example of one patient who reported the signs and symptoms of a hip pointer on the field and later was determined to have a ruptured spleen.

Injury Mechanism

A hip pointer is usually caused by a direct blow to the iliac crest or the anterosuperior iliac spine. A common differential diagnosis that should be considered is a strain of the abdominal muscles at their attachment to the anterior and inferior iliac crest. This can be differentiated from a contusion by obtaining a good history of the mechanism of injury at the time it occurs. Muscle injuries typically result from a forceful eccentric contraction.[46]

Rehabilitation Concerns

An X-ray should be taken to rule out iliac crest fractures or avulsion fractures, especially in younger patients.[36] If the hip pointer is not treated early, within about 2 to 4 hours, the patient may experience severe pain and limited ROM of the trunk because of the muscle attachments involved.

As in most contusions, the hip pointer is graded. A patient with a grade 1 hip pointer might have both normal gait cycle and normal posture. The patient might complain of slight pain on palpation with little or no swelling. This patient might also present with full ROM of the trunk, especially when checking for lateral side bending to the opposite side of the injury.

A patient with a grade 2 hip pointer might have moderate to severe pain on palpation, noticeable swelling, and an abnormal gait cycle. The gait cycle might be changed because of a short swing-through phase on the affected side; the patient might take a short step and be reluctant to keep the foot off the ground. The patient's pelvis and therefore posture might be slightly tilted to the side of the injury. Active hip and trunk flexion might cause pain, especially if the anterosuperior iliac spine is involved because of the insertion of the sartorius muscle. ROM might be limited, especially lateral side bending to the opposite side of the injury and trunk rotation in both directions.

A patient with a grade 3 hip pointer might have severe pain on palpation, noticeable swelling, and possible discoloration. The patient's gait cycle could be abnormal, with very slow, deliberate ambulation and extremely short stride length and swing-through phase. The patient's posture might present a severe lateral tilt to the affected side. Trunk ROM could be limited in all directions. Active hip and trunk flexion might reproduce pain.

With all hip pointers, continue with ice, compression, and rest. Subcutaneous steroid injection has been known to decrease inflammation and enable early ROM exercises. Transcutaneous electrical nerve stimulation (TENS) may be helpful on the day of injury to decrease pain and allow early ROM exercises. To regain normal function and speed recovery, use ice massage with pain-free trunk ROM exercises at the same time. Concentrate on lateral hip shifts to the side opposite to the injury (Figure 20-3). Other modalities such as ultrasound and electric stimulation are beneficial for increasing ROM and functional movement. Pain-free active motion and active resistance ROM exercises are vital to the functional recovery process. Active motion helps promote healing and decreases the time the patient is prohibited from practice and competition. Exercises as shown in Figures 20-17 through 20-23, 20-30, and 20-31 should be used to progress the patient. Trunk-strengthening exercises may also be added.

Rehabilitation Progression

A grade 1 hip pointer usually does not prevent the patient from competing. A patient with a grade 2 hip pointer could miss 5 to 14 days, and a patient with a grade 3 hip pointer could miss 14 to 20 days of competition. A patient with a grade 2 or 3 hip pointer can progress to active resistive strengthening exercises, if pain-free, after the initial 2 days of ice, compression, and active ROM.

Criteria for Full Return

The patient is capable of returning to competition when full trunk ROM is obtained and the patient can perform all sport-specific activities, such as cutting and changing directions (see Figures 16-4 through 16-14). Compression should be maintained throughout the period, and on returning to competition the patient should wear a custom-made protective relief doughnut pad with a hard protective shell over the top.

Clinical Decision-Making Exercise 20-1

A college football athlete sustained a direct hit to his lateral abdominal and rib area. After trying to play through the pain, he reported severe pain and tenderness on, and slightly anterior to, the iliac crest. The team physician's evaluation shows a grade 2 hip pointer. The next day, the patient reports to the athletic trainer with severe pain, swelling, and posture tilted to the side of the injury. The patient walks very slowly and with a limp. What can the athletic trainer recommend to help with pain and ROM and eventually to get the patient to a full return to football?

Injury to the Anterosuperior Iliac Spine and Anteroinferior Iliac Spine

Pathomechanics

Pain at the site of the anterosuperior iliac spine might indicate contusion or apophysitis, an inflammatory response to overuse. Severe pain associated with disability requires an X-ray to rule out an avulsion fracture.[1]

As with the anterosuperior iliac spine, the anteroinferior iliac spine can also present with apophysitis or a contusion. An avulsion fracture should also be ruled out with severe pain. These injuries are seen more often in younger patients.[48]

Injury Mechanism

The anterosuperior iliac spine serves as an attachment for the sartorius, and the anteroinferior iliac spine serves as an attachment for the rectus femoris. In both cases a violent, forceful passive stretch of the hip into extension or a violent, forceful active contraction into flexion can cause injury to these sites.[52] Apophysitis or a contusion to these two sites may accompany a hip pointer to the iliac crest.

Rehabilitation Concerns and Progression

After ruling out an avulsion fracture, rehabilitation for these injuries should follow the same guidelines as for a hip pointer.

Posterosuperior Iliac Spine Contusion

Pathomechanics

Contusions to the posterosuperior iliac spine must be differentiated from vertebral fractures and more serious internal organ injuries.[1] Depending upon the patient's pain and ROM, an X-ray can be taken to rule out vertebral fractures, vertebral transverse process fractures, and fractures of the posterosuperior iliac spine. Unlike the ASIS and AIIS, other injuries to this area are not common because of the lack of muscle attachments.[28] Avulsion fractures are rare in this area, although a fracture of the posterosuperior iliac spine should be ruled out.

The injury can be painful but usually does not cause disability.

Injury Mechanism and Rehabilitation Concerns

A contusion to the posterosuperior iliac spine is usually caused by a direct blow or fall. A patient with a contusion might complain of pain on palpation and have swelling that is usually not extensive. The patient's gait cycle may look normal except in severe cases, when the patient may take short, choppy steps to avoid the pain associated with landing at heel strike. In severe cases, the patient's posture may show a slight forward flexion tilt of the trunk. This patient might show full active ROM of the trunk, with mild discomfort. In moderate to severe cases, up to 3 days of rest may be needed before return to competition.

Rehabilitation Progression and Criteria for Full Return

The same treatment can be followed that is used for hip pointers. Pain-free active and passive ROM exercises of the trunk and hip can be used in sets and repetitions, with stretches held for 20 to 30 seconds for each repetition. Guidelines for return to competition are the same as for a hip pointer, and protective padding is recommended.

Quadriceps Contusion

Pathomechanics

Because the quadriceps muscle is in the front of the thigh, a direct blow to the area that causes the muscle to compress against the femur can be very disabling.[1,45] A direct blow to the anterior portion of the muscle is usually more serious and disabling than a direct blow to the lateral quadriceps area because of the differences in muscle mass present in the two areas. Blood vessels that break cause bleeding in the area where muscle tissue has been damaged.[5] If not treated correctly or if treated too aggressively, a quadriceps contusion can lead to the formation of myositis ossificans (see the following section on myositis ossificans). At the time of injury, the patient may develop pain, loss of function to the quadriceps mechanism, and loss of knee flexion ROM. How relaxed the quadriceps were at the time of injury, and how forceful the blow was, determine the grade of injury.

Injury Mechanism

A patient with a grade 1 contusion may present a normal gait cycle, negative swelling, and only mild discomfort on palpation. The patient's active knee flexion ROM while lying prone should be within normal limits. Resistive knee extension while sitting and lying supine with the knee bent over the end of a table might not cause discomfort.

A patient with a grade 2 contusion may have a normal gait cycle, but before notifying the athletic trainer of the injury might attempt to continue to participate while the injury progressively becomes disabling. If the gait cycle is abnormal, the patient will splint the knee in extension and avoid knee flexion while bearing weight because the knee feels like it will give out. This patient might also externally rotate the extremity to use the hip adductors to pull the leg through during the swing-through phase. This move might be accompanied by hiking the hip at push-off, which causes tilting of the pelvis in the frontal plane. Swelling may be moderate to severe, with a noticeable defect and pain on palpation. While the patient is lying prone, active ROM in the knee may be limited, with possibly 30 to 45 degrees of motion lacking. Resistive knee extension while sitting and lying supine with the knee bent over the end of a table may be painful, and a noticeable weakness in the quadriceps mechanism may be evident. A grade 2 quadriceps contusion to the lateral thigh area is usually less painful because of the lack of muscle mass involved at the injury site. The patient might experience pain on palpation but not have disability. While the patient is lying prone, knee flexion, ROM will show a small limitation but should fall within normal limits. Resistive knee extension while the patient is sitting and lying supine with the knee bent over the end of a table may cause mild discomfort with good strength present.

A patient with a grade 3 contusion might herniate the muscle through the fascia to cause a marked defect, severe bleeding, and disability. The patient may not be able to ambulate without crutches. Pain, severe swelling, and a bulge of muscle tissue may be present on palpation.

When the patient is lying prone, knee flexion active ROM may be severely limited. Active resistive knee extension while the patient is sitting and lying supine with the knee bent over the end of a table might not be tolerated, and severe weakness may be present.

Rehabilitation Concerns and Progression

Initial injury management of quadriceps contusions involving knee flexion can significantly decrease a patient's total time lost.[2,44] Aronen et al found a dramatic improvement in time to return to play when the patient was initially treated with ice and immobilization of the knee at 120 degrees of flexion regardless of the severity of the injury. This immobilization lasted for 24 hours.[2]

A patient with a grade 1 quadriceps contusion should begin ice and 24-hour compression immediately. Twenty-four-hour compression should be continued until all signs and symptoms are absent. Gentle, pain-free quadriceps stretching exercises (Figures 20-4 and 20-5) may be performed on the first day. Quadriceps progressive resistive strengthening exercises may also be performed as soon as possible, usually on the second day, in the order given and pain-free (Figures 20-18, 20-28, 20-29) hip flexion with knee both extended and flexed (Figures 20-30A and B, 20-31 through 20-38, 20-40), and isokinetics (Figures 20-42 through 20-44). This patient's active ROM should be carefully monitored. If motion decreases, the injury should be updated to a grade 2 contusion and treated as such.

A patient with a grade 2 contusion should be treated very conservatively. Crutches should be used until a normal gait can be accomplished free of pain. Ice, 24-hour compression, and electrical muscle stimulation modalities may be started immediately to decrease swelling, inflammation, and pain and to promote ROM.[40] Compression should be applied at all times to counteract bleeding into the area. Pain-free quadriceps isometric exercises may be performed as soon as possible, usually within the first 3 days. Between days 3 and 5, ice is continued with pain-free active ROM, while the patient is sitting and lying prone. Active ROM lying supine with the knee bent over the end of a table can be added. Passive stretching is not used until the later phases of rehabilitation. Massage and heat modalities are also contraindicated in the early phases because of the possibility of promoting bleeding and eventually myositis ossificans. At about day 5, the patient may perform straight-leg raises without weights and then progress to weights, pain-free (Figure 20-18). As active ROM increases and approaches 95 to 100 degrees of knee flexion, swimming, aquatic therapy, and biking may be performed if the bicycle seat height is adjusted to the patient's available pain-free ROM. Between days 7 and 10, heat in the form of hot packs, ultrasound, or whirlpool may be used, as long as swelling is negative and the patient is approaching full active ROM while lying prone. Pain-free quadriceps progressive resistive strengthening exercises may be performed in the order given (Figures 20-18, 20-28, 20-29), hip flexion with knee both extended and flexed, (Figures 20-30A and B, 20-31 through 20-38, 20-40), and isokinetics (Figures 20-42 through 20-44). Ice or heat modalities, with active ROM, should be continued before all exercises as a warm-up. Pain-free quadriceps stretching exercises should not be rushed and can be started between 10 and 14 days (Figures 20-4, 20-5). Jogging, slide board (Figure 20-45), plyometrics (Figures 20-46 through 20-48), and sport specific functional drills (see Figures 16-4 through 16-14) may be used after the fourteenth day.

A patient with a grade 3 quadriceps contusion should use crutches, rest, ice, 24-hour compression, and electrical muscle stimulation modalities immediately to decrease pain, bleeding, and swelling and counteract atrophy.[40] After surgery has been ruled out, the patient may begin pain-free isometric quadriceps exercises between days 5 and 7. Ice and 24-hour compression should be continued from day 1 through day 7. Pain-free active ROM exercises may be performed while the patient is sitting and lying prone around day 7. Active ROM while lying supine with the knee bent over the end of a table can also be added. At about day 10, the patient may perform straight-leg raises without weights and then progress to weights by day 14 (Figure 20-18). Electrical muscle stimulation modalities may be very helpful in this phase to counteract muscle atrophy

and reeducate muscle contraction. Again, as active ROM increases and approaches 95 to 100 degrees of knee flexion, swimming, aquatic therapy, and biking may be performed if the bicycle seat height is adjusted to the patient's pain-free available ROM. After day 14, the patient may use heat in the form of hot packs or whirlpool, as long as the swelling has decreased and the patient has gained active ROM. At about the third week of rehabilitation, pain-free quadriceps progressive resistive strengthening exercises may be performed in the order presented (Figures 20-18, 20-28, 20-29), hip flexion with knee both extended and flexed (Figures 20-30A and B, 20-31 through 20-38, 20-40), and isokinetics (Figures 20-42, 20-43). Pain-free quadriceps stretching may also be performed (Figures 20-4, 20-5) if the patient is careful not to overstretch the quadriceps muscles. In general, the patient may be able to progress to jogging, slide board (Figure 20-45), plyometrics (Figures 20-46 to 20-48), and sport-specific functional drills (see Figures 16-4 through 16-14) around 3 weeks post injury. The rehabilitation timetables presented for grades 2 and 3 quadriceps contusions may be modified, depending upon the severity of the injury within its grade.

Criteria for Full Return

All patients need to achieve equal passive knee flexion and regain quadriceps tone, control (vastus medialis) and strength prior to being returned to play. They also need to pass functional testing of sports specific drills by the athletic trainer. Protective padding should always be used to protect the injured area after return to play and prevent the incidence of myositis ossificans.[2]

A patient with a grade 1 quadriceps contusion might not miss competition, but compression and protective padding should be worn until the patient is symptom-free.

A patient with a grade 2 quadriceps contusion might miss 3 to 20 days of participation, depending upon the severity of the injury. Compression and protective padding should be worn during all competition until the patient is symptom-free. A patient with a grade 2 quadriceps contusion to the lateral thigh area might not miss competition but should wear compression and protective padding during participation.

A patient with a grade 3 quadriceps contusion might miss 3 weeks to 3 months of competition time. Again, compression and protective padding should be worn during all competition until the patient is symptom-free. Grade 3 lateral quadriceps contusions are very rare due to the lack of muscle belly tissue. If a grade 3 lateral quadriceps contusion is diagnosed, a femoral contusion and possible fracture should be ruled out.

Myositis Ossificans

Pathomechanics and Injury Mechanism

With a severe direct blow or repetitive direct blows to the quadriceps muscles that cause muscle tissue damage, bleeding, and injury to the periosteum of the femur, ectopic bone production may occur.[1,27] Calcium formation will typically become visible on X-ray films between 3 to 6 weeks post injury. If the trauma was to the quadriceps muscles only and not the femur, a smaller bony mass may be seen on X-ray films.[1]

If quadriceps contusions and strains are properly treated and rehabilitated, myositis ossificans can be prevented. Myositis ossificans can be caused by trying to "play through" a grade 2 or 3 quadriceps contusion or strain and by early use of massage, active ROM into pain, passive stretching exercises into pain, ultrasound, and other heat modalities.[1]

Rehabilitation Concerns and Progression

After 1 year, surgical removal of the bony mass may be helpful. If the bony mass is removed too early, the trauma caused by the surgery can actually enhance the condition. After diagnosis by X-ray film, treatment and rehabilitation should follow the guidelines for a grade 2 or 3 quadriceps contusion or quadriceps strain (see treatment and rehabilitation for grade 2 and 3 quadriceps contusions and strains). The bony mass usually stabilizes after the sixth month.[23] If the mass does not cause disability, the patient should be closely monitored and follow the treatment and

rehabilitation programs outlined in grade 2 and 3 quadriceps contusions and strains. It has also been recommended that myositis be treated using acetic acid with iontophoresis.[56]

Quadriceps Muscle Strain

Pathomechanics

A strain to the large quadriceps muscles in the front of the thigh can be very disabling, especially when the rectus femoris muscle is involved due to its involvement at two joints.[19] The four quadriceps muscles share the same innervation and tendon of insertion. The rectus femoris is the only quadriceps muscle that crosses the hip joint, therefore it is considered a biarticular muscle. The quadriceps muscles are very similar to the hamstrings in that they produce a great deal of force and contract in a rapid fashion.[9] Most strains occur at the musculotendinous junctions. A strain shows acute pain, possibly after a workout has been completed, swelling to a specific area, and loss of knee flexion. If the rectus femoris is involved, knee flexion ROM lying prone (hip in extended position) will be severely limited and painful. Rectus femoris involvement is more disabling than a strain to any of the other quadriceps muscles.

Injury Mechanism

Muscle strains and contusion will present similar signs and symptoms but with no history of direct contact to the quadriceps area, the injury should be treated as a muscle strain. A quadriceps strain that involves the rectus femoris usually occurs because of a sudden, violent, forceful contraction of the hip and knee into flexion, with the hip initially extended. An overstretch of the quadriceps, with the hip in extension and the knee flexed, can also cause a quadriceps strain. Tight quadriceps, imbalance between quadriceps muscles, and leg length discrepancy can predispose someone to a quadriceps strain.[1]

A patient with a grade 1 quadriceps strain may complain of tightness in the front of the thigh. The patient may be ambulating with a normal gait cycle and present with a history of the thigh feeling fatigued and tight. Swelling might not be present, and the patient usually has very mild discomfort on palpation. With the patient sitting over the edge of a table, resistive knee extension might not produce discomfort. If the patient is lying supine with the knee flexed over the edge of a table, resistive knee extension may produce mild discomfort, if the rectus femoris is involved. With the patient lying prone, active knee flexion may produce a full pain-free ROM, with some tightness at extreme flexion.

A patient with a grade 2 quadriceps strain may have an abnormal gait cycle. The knee may be splinted in extension. The patient may present an externally rotated hip to use the adductors to pull the leg through and avoid hip extension, during the swing-through phase from push-off, especially when the rectus femoris is involved. In severe cases, it may also be accompanied by hiking the hip during the swing-through phase, which causes a tilting of the pelvis in the frontal plane. The patient may have felt a sudden twinge and pain down the length of the rectus femoris during activity.[9] Swelling may be noticeable, and palpation may produce pain. A defect in the muscle may also be evident in a grade 2 strain. Resistive knee extension, both when sitting and when lying supine, may reproduce pain. Lying supine and resisting knee extension may be more painful when the rectus femoris is involved. With the patient lying prone, active knee flexion ROM may present a noticeable decrease, in some cases a decrease up to 45 degrees. With a quadriceps strain, any decrease in knee flexion ROM should classify the injury as a grade 2 or 3 strain.

A patient with a grade 3 quadriceps strain may be unable to ambulate without the aid of crutches and will be in severe pain, with a noticeable defect in the quadriceps muscle. Palpation will usually not be tolerated, and swelling will be present almost immediately. The patient may not be able to extend the knee actively and against resistance. An isometric contraction will be painful and may produce a bulge or defect in the quadriceps muscle, especially if the rectus femoris is involved. With the patient lying prone, active knee flexion ROM may be severely limited and might not be tolerated.

Rehabilitation Concerns and Progression

A patient with a grade 1 quadriceps strain should start ice, compression, pain-free active ROM, and isometric quadriceps exercises immediately. Pain-free quadriceps progressive resistive strengthening exercises may be performed within the first 2 days, in the order given (Figures 20-18, 20-28 and 20-29), hip flexion with knee both extended and flexed (Figures 20-30A and B, 20-31 through 20-38, and 20-40), and isokinetics (Figures 20-41 through 20-44). The NK table (Figure 20-28) is used because of its ability to change the force on the quadriceps muscles by changing the lever arm, and therefore the torque and forces placed upon the injured muscle(s). It is very important that this patient be able to stretch pain-free and begin pain-free stretching as described in Figures 20-4 and 20-5. Compression should be used at all times until the patient is free of pain and no longer complaining of tightness.

A patient with a grade 2 quadriceps strain should begin ice, 24-hour compression, and crutches immediately for the first 3 to 5 days. Electrical muscle stimulation modalities may be used acutely to decrease swelling, inflammation, and pain and promote ROM.[26] At about day 3, or sooner if pain-free, the patient may perform quadriceps isometric exercises and pain-free quadriceps active ROM exercises, both sitting and lying prone. These active ROM exercises are then progressed to the supine position with the knee bent over the end of a table to allow more efficiency and ROM to the rectus femoris muscle, but with no resistance or weight. Ice used in conjunction with active ROM, as described above, is very helpful in regaining motion, and strengthening the quadriceps muscles without pain. Passive stretching exercises to the quadriceps muscles are not recommended in the rehabilitation program until later phases because a passive stretch might have been the cause of the strain. Twenty-four hour compression is continued until full pain-free ROM is achieved. A pain-free normal gait cycle is reviewed and emphasized, with and without crutches.

At about days 3 to 7, the patient may begin heat before exercise even though ice is still preferred if the patient has not obtained full pain-free ROM. During this phase of rehabilitation, pain-free progressive resistive exercises such as straight-leg raises may be implemented (Figure 20-18). Weights should be added as strength increases.

At about days 5 to 7 and within pain-free limits, this patient may begin the slide board (Figure 20-45), plyometrics (Figures 20-46 through 20-48), and sport-specific functional drills (see Figures 16-4 through 16-14).

Continue pain-free quadriceps progressive resistive strengthening exercises on days 7 through 14. The patient should be progressed, in the order given and pain-free, through the exercises shown in Figures 20-18, 20-28, and 20-29, hip flexion with knee both extended and flexed (Figures 20-30A and B, 20-31 to 20-38, 20-40), and isokinetics (Figures 20-41 through 20-44). Swimming and biking can also be performed as long as the patient avoids forceful kicking. The bike seat should be adjusted to accommodate a pain-free ROM. Pain-free passive quadriceps stretching exercises are not performed until days 7 to 14 (Figures 20-4, 20-5). All exercises should be pain-free.

A patient with a grade 3 quadriceps strain should be on crutches for 7 to 14 days or longer to allow for rest and normal gait before walking without crutches. Twenty-four hour compression, ice, and electrical muscle stimulation modalities should be used immediately. Quadriceps stretching exercises are not performed until later phases. Twenty-four-hour compression is maintained until the patient has full pain-free ROM. When pain-free, the patient may begin quadriceps isometric exercises. Gentle pain-free quadriceps active ROM exercises, while the patient is lying prone and/or sitting, should be performed if special attention is paid to avoiding an overstretch of the quadriceps muscles. Ice, in conjunction with active ROM while sitting over the end of a table, is very useful in regaining ROM. Heat (hot packs, whirlpool, or ultrasound) may be used if the patient is approaching full ROM and signs of acute inflammation have decreased. Pain-free straight-leg raises without weight may be performed. Weight may be added after days 10 to 14 (Figure 20-18).

Depending upon active ROM, swimming and biking may be added to the rehabilitation program. The bicycle seat height should be adjusted to accommodate the patient's available ROM. Also, depending upon active ROM, pain-free quadriceps active progressive resistive strengthening exercises may be performed after the third week, in the order given (Figures 20-18, 20-28, 20-29), hip flexion with knee both extended and flexed (Figures 20-30A and B, 20-31 to 20-38, 20-40), and isokinetics (Figures 20-41 through 20-44).

Depending on the severity of the injury, the patient should have full active ROM by the fourth week. Only when full active ROM is accomplished should quadriceps stretching exercises be added (Figures 20-4 and 20-5).

At about day 14 or later, and within pain-free limits, this patient may begin the slide board (Figure 20-45), plyometrics (Figures 20-46 through 20-48), and sport-specific functional drills (see Figures 16-4 through 16-14).

Criteria for Full Return

A patient with a grade 1 quadriceps strain might not miss competition but should be watched closely and started on a rehabilitation and strengthening program immediately.

A patient with a grade 2 quadriceps strain might miss 7 to 20 days of competition, depending upon the amount of active ROM present. The lack of ROM and the number of competition days missed are usually directly correlated.

A patient with a grade 3 quadriceps strain might miss 3 to 12 weeks of competition. In severe cases, surgery may be a consideration.

In all situations, the patient should not return to competition until plyometrics (Figures 20-46 through 20-48) and sport-specific functional drills (see Figures 16-4 through 16-14) are accomplished pain-free.

Clinical Decision-Making Exercise 20-2

A female volleyball athlete has been diagnosed with a grade 2 quadriceps strain after lunging for a ball. The athletic trainer has determined that the rectus femoris is involved and that the patient has lost 45 degrees of knee flexion while lying prone. What can the athletic trainer recommend to help this patient return to play?

Hamstring Strains

Pathomechanics

Hamstring strains are common, and the causes are numerous.[57] The ability of the hamstring muscles and quadriceps muscles to work together is very complex because the hamstrings cross two joints.[26] This produces forces and therefore stresses on the hamstrings dependent upon the positions of the hip and knee. Some dissection research has shown that there is consistent overlap of tendon vertically, over the course of the muscle, with the exception of the semitendinosus. With research showing the musculotendinous junction as the main injury site, anywhere along the muscle/tendon is susceptible to injury.[9]

The patient might report a "pop." Palpation is the easiest way to identify the site and extent of injury. Even though bleeding (ecchymosis) may be present, some people believe that this is not associated with the degree or severity of injury.[9] A patient with a grade 1 hamstring strain will complain of sore hamstring muscles, with some pain on palpation and possibly minimal swelling. A patient with a grade 2 hamstring strain may report having heard or felt a "pop" during the activity. At the first or second day, moderate ecchymosis may be observed. Palpation may produce moderate to severe pain, and even though a defect and noticeable swelling in the muscle belly may be evident, the grade 2 hamstring strain most likely occurs at the musculotendinous junction either mid to high semimembranosus/tendinosis or distal lateral biceps femoris. A patient with a grade 3 strain may report having heard or felt a "pop" during the activity. The athletic trainer may detect swelling and severe pain on palpation. A noticeable defect may be present, again at the musculotendinous junction as described above. After the first through third days, moderate to severe ecchymosis may be observed.

Injury Mechanism

A quick, explosive contraction that involves a "rapid activity" could lead to a strain of the hamstring muscles. Many theories try to explain the cause of hamstring strains. Imbalance with the quadriceps is one theory, according to which the hamstring muscles should have 60% to 70% of the quadriceps muscles' strength. Other possibilities are hamstring muscle fatigue, running posture and gait, leg-length discrepancy, decreased hamstring ROM, and an imbalance between the medial and lateral hamstring muscle.[1]

Another factor that plays a role in injury, as well as rehabilitation, is that the semitendinosus, semimembranosus, and long head of the biceps femoris are innervated from the tibial branch of the sciatic nerve, while the short head of the biceps femoris is innervated by the peroneal branch of the sciatic nerve. This innervation difference makes the short head a completely separate muscle—"a factor implicated in the etiology of hamstring muscle strains," as described by DeLee and Drez.[9]

Two phases of the running gait described by DeLee and Drez show that the biomechanics within the support phase and the recovery phase may predispose the patient to hamstring strains. During the support phase, foot strike, mid-support, and take-off occurs. During recovery phase, follow-through, forward swing, and foot descent occurs. The two portions of these two phases that are implicated in hamstring strains are the late-forward swing segment of the recovery phase and the take-off phase of the support phase. Electromyelogram (EMG) data show that the semimembranosus is very active during the late forward-swing segment and that the biceps femoris is inactive. At take-off of the support phase, the biceps femoris shows maximal activity.[9] This shows that the mid to high semimembranosus and semitendinosus strains may occur during the deceleration portion of the running cycle while the distal lateral biceps femoris strains are occurring at the take-off or push-off portion of the running cycle. The rehabilitation implications are connected to the position of the hip and knee while rehabilitating to isolate and identify the specific muscle and nerve innervation involved.[5] Using the correct biomechanical positions during rehabilitation, based on the EMG findings presented, will enhance rehabilitation and improve preventive programs.

Rehabilitation Concerns

A patient with a grade 1 hamstring strain may have a normal gait cycle. Hip flexion ROM is probably normal, with a tight feeling reported at the extreme range of hip flexion. Resistive knee flexion and hip extension with the knee extended are probably free of pain or possibly produce a tight feeling with good strength present.

A patient with a grade 2 hamstring strain usually ambulates with an abnormal gait cycle. The patient may lack heel strike and land during the foot-flat phase of the gait cycle. The swing-through phase may be limited because of the patient's unwillingness to flex the hip and knee. The patient may tend to ambulate with a flexed knee. Resistive knee flexion and hip extension with the knee extended may cause moderate to severe pain. The patient may also have a noticeable weakness on resistive knee flexion and hip extension with the knee extended and flexed. Resistive hip extension with the knee flexed also tests the strength of the gluteus maximus muscle. Passive hip flexion with the knee extended may also produce moderate to severe pain. The patient's ROM may be moderately to severely limited in hip flexion with the knee extended and moderately limited in hip flexion with the knee flexed.

A patient with a grade 3 hamstring strain may be unable to ambulate without the aid of crutches. The patient may have poor strength and be unable to resist knee flexion and hip extension with the knee extended. The patient may have fair strength upon resistive hip extension with the knee flexed because of the gluteus maximus muscle. Resisting these motions usually causes pain. Passive hip flexion, with the knee extended, might not be tolerated because of pain. Passive hip flexion, knee flexed, may be moderately to severely limited.

Because most hamstring injuries occur due to a "rapid activity" that involves an explosive concentric contraction during toe-off or a strong eccentric contraction during deceleration swing-through, it is our belief that the hamstring should be rehabilitated in a "rapid activity" fashion with high intensity and a high volume of exercises. After the initial treatment of ice, rest, compression, and active ROM, the following exercises, in the order given and with a load that doesn't produce pain, should be instituted. Alternating a single-joint open chain exercise with a multi-joint closed chain exercise, with 30 seconds rest between sets and actual exercises, has been shown to facilitate rapid healing and earlier return to activity, as well as present preventive advantages. (Again, all exercises are performed pain-free and in the order given.)

Depending on the degree of injury, the patient should warm up by using a stationary bike, Stairmaster, and/or aquatic therapy followed by pain-free stretching. It has been shown that the Stairmaster produces more hamstring activity than the bike and may be used in later stages to provide more hamstring isolation.[9] Stretching includes the exercises shown in Figure 20-8.

Grade 1 and 2 strains can expect to begin following the stretching program with pain-free strengthening about 3 to 5 days post-injury. The strengthening exercises are demonstrated in Figures 20-19, 20-24 through 20-27, and Figure 20-30E. The closed kinetic chain exercise shown in Figure 20-32 is also added as long as the patient keeps the stretch of the hamstring pain-free.

After a few days of performing those exercises, the following strengthening exercises may be added, in order, as long as they are performed pain-free: open chain (Figure 20-24), followed by closed chain (Figure 20-33) and then open chain (Figure 20-26) (if pain-free), followed by closed chain (Figure 20-34, feet in front for a mid-high strain, or Figure 20-35, feet in back for a lower/ lateral strain. The exercise in Figure 20-38 can be added at this time, combined with the exercise in Figure 20-32, as described previously.

Again, after a few more days the following strengthening exercises should be added, in order, as long as they are performed without pain: open chain (Figure 20-25, after single-leg concentric, follow with heavy negative repetitions/sets—two legs up, one leg down eccentrically, for 2 sets of 8 repetitions), followed by closed chain (Figures 20-32 and 20-36), and ending with Figure 20-39. Also at this time, PNF exercises shown in Figures 14-11 through 14-17 can be added.

After a week or so performing the preceding exercises, the following exercises can be added: Figure 20-37 (for both mid/high and lower/

lateral strains) and Figure 20-43 for mid/high strain or Figure 20-41 for low/lateral strain.

The time between adding new open and closed chain combinations depends on the degree of injury and whether the exercises are all performed pain-free. For example, with a moderate grade 2 hamstring strain, progression to all strengthening exercises described takes place in the first 3 to 10 days. With a more severe grade 2 hamstring strain, progressing to all the strengthening exercises described may take 2 weeks. For a grade 3 hamstring strain, the strengthening progression described works best after 3 to 4 weeks of healing has been allowed and all exercises can be accomplished pain-free. This program also works well prophylactically during the off-season; a modified version can be effective during the season.

Rehabilitation Progression

Each exercise done in the order given and sets, reps, and suggested rest periods should be progressed based on daily evaluation that involves pain, ROM, muscle strength from previous workout session, and how the patient subjectively feels. Days between strengthening workout sessions should be used for aerobic conditioning such as biking, Stairmaster, and aquatic therapy, as well as slide board activity (Figure 20-45) followed by stretching, as described above.

A pain-free normal gait cycle should be taught as soon as possible, and crutches should be used to accomplish a normal gait cycle. Ice, compression, and gentle, pain-free hamstring stretching exercises, making sure the patient maintains a lumbar lordotic curve to isolate the hamstring muscles, are performed on day 1. Electrical muscle stimulation modalities may be used to promote ROM and to decrease pain and spasm.[26] Active knee and hip ROM while lying prone may also be performed on days 1 through 3, if the patient can do so without pain. Hamstring isometric exercises are taught as soon as possible, again within pain-free limits. Starting pain-free active ROM, as soon as possible, is very important and usually decreases the length of time a patient misses competition. At about day 3, the patient may begin heat in the form of hot packs and whirlpool, combined with pain-free stretching exercises described earlier. If pain-free, the above strengthening program may be started between days 3 and 7. Hamstring injuries that appear to have a slower recovery than expected or experience recurrent injuries may be hindered by the presence of adverse neural tension. Turl et al found 57% of patients with a history of repetitive hamstring strains also had a positive slump sit test. These data suggested that adverse neural tension (ANT) may result from or be a contributing factor in the etiology of repetitive hamstring strains.[53] Treatment of adverse neural tension should be included in all hamstring rehab programs, for specifics, see the section regarding piriformis syndrome later in the chapter.

Criteria for Full Return

A patient with a grade 1 hamstring strain might not miss competition but should be watched closely for further injury. The rehabilitation program described should begin immediately to avoid further injury. A patient with a grade 2 hamstring strain could miss 5 to 20 days of competition. A patient with a grade 3 hamstring strain could miss 3 to 12 weeks of competition or more. In all situations the patient should not return to competition until plyometrics (Figures 20-45 through 20-48) and sport-specific functional drills (see Figures 16-4 through 16-14) are accomplished pain-free. Once you begin sport specific drills, it is advised to warm up the patient's core body temperature. This can be accomplished by using hamstring functional activities such as backpedals, side shuffles, carioca, plyometrics, and straight-ahead pain-free strides up to 100 yards in length.

Clinical Decision-Making Exercise 20-3

A football running back has suffered a grade 2 hamstring strain. His pain is in the middle upper aspect of the hamstring muscle. The team physician has referred the patient back to the athletic trainer for rehabilitation and return to play. What can the athletic trainer recommend for this patient to return to play at full speed?

Hamstring Tendinopathy

Pathomechanics

Another injury that occurs to the hamstring muscles is a strain (microtear) and/or inflammation of the hamstring tendons near their attachments to the tibia and fibula. Injury to the gastrocnemius muscle tendons in the same area must be ruled out.

Injury Mechanism

The patient might report pain but might not experience disability. A patient with a hamstring tendon strain or tendinitis may present a history of overuse and chronic pain for a few days with no specific mechanism of injury.

Rehabilitation Concerns, Rehabilitation Progression, and Criteria for Full Return

Palpation helps to isolate which tendon or tendons are involved and resistive knee flexion, with the tibia in internal and external rotation, aids in the evaluation. If resistive ankle plantar flexion with the knee in extension does not reproduce symptoms, gastrocnemius involvement may be ruled out. A patient who presents with this condition responds nicely to 1 to 2 days of rest with oral anti-inflammatory medication. Ice, massage, and ultrasound help decrease inflammation and pain. Gentle hamstring stretching exercises (Figures 20-7, 20-8) with the hip in internal and external rotation help to isolate the tendon or tendons involved, and PNF stretching (see Figures 14-11 through 14-17) should be performed on day 1. Hamstring progressive resistive strengthening exercises that isolate the hamstring muscles can be performed on day 1 (Figures 20-19, 20-24 to 20-27, 20-30E), along with eccentric hamstring leans (Figure 20-39), if they can be performed without pain.

Groin and Hip Flexor Strain

Pathomechanics

The number one cause of groin pain is a strain to the adductor muscles. A groin strain can occur to any muscle in the inner hip area. Whether it is to the sartoris, rectus femoris, the adductors, or the iliopsoas, the muscle and degree of injury must be determined and the injury treated accordingly.[8]

Discomfort may start as mild but develop into moderate to severe pain with disability if not treated correctly. A chronic strain can cause bleeding into the groin muscles, resulting in myositis ossificans (see the section on myositis ossificans). If a groin strain is treated acutely, myositis ossificans can be avoided.

Injury Mechanism and Rehabilitation Concerns

A groin strain can develop from overextending and externally rotating the hip or from forcefully contracting the muscles into flexion and internal rotation as involved in running, jumping, twisting, and kicking. Differential diagnosis and treatment may be difficult because of the number of muscles in the area.

With a grade 1 groin strain, the patient may complain of mild discomfort with no loss of function and full ROM and strength. Point tenderness may be minimal, with negative swelling. The gait cycle may be normal.

With a grade 2 groin strain, palpation may reproduce pain and show a minimal to moderate defect. Swelling might also be detected. This patient may show an abnormal gait cycle. Ambulation may be slow, and the stride length may be shortened on the affected side. The patient may tend to hike the hip and tilt the pelvis in the frontal plane rather than drive the knee through during the swing-through phase. ROM may be severely limited, and resistance could cause an increase in pain. When the iliopsoas is involved, the patient may experience severe pain after the initial injury. This is thought to be caused by spasm of the iliopsoas muscle, which tilts the pelvis in the frontal plane. The patient will walk with a flexed hip and knee and will be unable to extend the hip during the push-off phase of the gait cycle because the muscle spasm does not allow hip extension and active hip flexion during swing-through. This patient will also externally rotate the hip to use the hip adductors for the swing-through phase.

A patient with a grade 3 groin strain may need crutches to ambulate. A moderate to severe defect may be detected in the involved muscle or tendon. Point tenderness may be severe, with noticeable swelling. ROM is severely limited, especially if the iliopsoas is involved. The patient might splint the legs together and be apprehensive about allowing movement in abduction. Resistance might not be tolerated.

Differentiating a hip adductor strain from a hip flexor strain is the first step in treating this injury. Resistive adduction while lying supine with the knee in extension may significantly increase pain if the hip adductors are involved. Flexing the hip and knee and resisting hip adduction may also increase pain. If the injury is a pure hip adductor strain, the supine position with the knee extended may reproduce more discomfort than flexing the hip and knee. If resistive adduction with the hip and knee flexed produces more discomfort, the hip flexor may also be involved.

With the patient lying supine, more pain on resistive hip flexion with the knee in flexion tests for iliopsoas involvement. More pain on resistive hip flexion with the knee extended (straight leg raise) tests for rectus femoris involvement. After determining the muscle or muscle groups involved and the degree of the injury, treatment and rehabilitation is the next step.

Rehabilitation Progression and Criteria for Full Return

With a grade 1 strain, modalities and pain-free hip stretching exercises can begin immediately (Figures 20-4 through 20-6, 20-9, 20-10, 20-13). Pain-free progressive strengthening exercises may also be performed (Figures 20-17, 20-18, 20-20, 20-22, 20-23, 20-30A and B), progressing to flexion with knee straight, flexed, and adducted (Figures 20-31, 20-36, 20-37, 20-40), and PNF exercises (see Figures 14-11 through 14-17). Depending upon the severity of the injury, this patient need not miss competition time and can be progressed to the slide board (Figure 20-45), plyometrics (Figures 20-46 through 20-48), and sport-specific functional drills (see Figures 16-4 through 16-14) as soon as pain allows.

A patient with a grade 2 strain should be started immediately, with gentle, pain-free, active ROM exercises of the hip. When the iliopsoas is involved, it has been found that lying supine on a treatment table with the leg

and hip hanging over the end of the table, with the hip in a passively extended position, while applying ice for 15 to 20 minutes, can help eliminate muscle spasm and pain (Figure 20-6). Electrical muscle stimulation modalities can be very useful in the early stages to decrease inflammation, pain, and spasm and to promote ROM.[40] Isometrics should also be performed as soon as they can be managed without pain. If crutches are used, a normal gait cycle is taught. The patient can begin pain-free stretching as soon as possible (Figures 20-4 through 20-6, 20-9, 20-10, 20-13). As soon as pain allows, the patient can begin pain-free strengthening exercises (Figures 20-17, 20-18, 20-20, 20-22, 20-23, 20-29, 20-30A and B), flexion and adduction strengthening exercises (Figures 20-31, 20-36, 20-37, 20-40), and PNF (see Figures 14-14 through 14-20). After about 1 week, the patient can begin pain-free slide board exercises (Figure 20-45) and plyometrics (Figures 20-46 through 20-48), as well as sport-specific functional drills (see Figures 16-4 through 16-14). This patient may miss 3 to 14 days of competition, depending on the severity of injury. Hip adductor strains usually take longer to treat and rehabilitate than hip flexor strains of the same grade, especially if the muscle spasm involved with a hip flexor is eliminated as soon as possible. Treatment and rehabilitation should be modified accordingly.

A patient with a grade 3 strain should be iced, compressed, immobilized, and non-weight-bearing. Electrical muscle stimulation modalities are useful in the acute stage to decrease inflammation and pain and to promote ROM. Rest for 1 to 3 days is recommended, with compression at all times. If the iliopsoas is involved, passive stretching with ice (Figure 20-6) can be started after the third day.

If surgery is ruled out, the patient may perform pain-free isometric exercises between days 3 and 5. Slow, pain-free, active ROM exercises may also be performed between days 3 and 5. A normal gait cycle should be emphasized using crutches. Crutches should not be eliminated until the patient can ambulate with a normal, pain-free gait cycle. Between days 7 and 10, the patient may perform pain-free stretching exercises (Figures 20-4 through 20-6, 20-9, 20-10, 20-12) and can begin progressive resistive strengthening exercises without pain, progressing in weight and motion (Figures 20-17, 20-18, 20-20, 20-22, 20-23, 20-29, 20-30A and B), flexion and adduction (Figures 20-31, 20-36, 20-37, 20-40), and PNF (see Figures 14-11 through 14-17). The patient needs to achieve a good strength level, usually within 10 days after starting progressive resistive strengthening exercises, to perform pain-free slide board exercises (Figure 20-45) and plyometrics (Figures 20-46 through 20-48), as well as sport-specific functional activities (see Figures 16-4 through 16-14).

Treatment and rehabilitation timetables may be modified. The modifications should be based on the degree of injury within the grade presented. This patient could potentially miss 3 weeks to 3 months of competition.

Avulsion Fracture Femoral Trochanter

Pathomechanics and Injury Mechanism

Patients might suffer an isolated avulsion fracture of the femoral trochanters. When the greater trochanter is involved, the cause is usually a violent, forceful contraction of the hip abductor muscles. An avulsion fracture of the lesser trochanter occurs because of a violent, forceful contraction of the iliopsoas muscle.[41]

Palpation may produce pain and possibly a noticeable defect of the greater trochanter. Resistive movements and passive ROM of the hip may reproduce pain. X-rays must be taken to confirm the injury. Immobilization may be the treatment of choice for an incomplete avulsion fracture. With a complete avulsion fracture, internal fixation is usually required.

Rehabilitation Concerns, Progression, and Criteria for Full Return

During the initial immobilization period, as prescribed by the physician, the patient with a femoral avulsion fracture should perform isometric hip exercises on the first day of rehabilitation, with isometric quadriceps and hamstring exercises and ankle-strengthening exercises. Crutches should be used for the first 6 weeks or until a pain-free normal gait cycle can be accomplished. Full weight bearing can be achieved during the first 4 to 6 weeks per the physician's instructions. After 6 weeks, the patient may perform pain-free active ROM exercises, as well as pain-free stretching exercises (Figures 20-4 through 20-10, 20-16). When pain allows, the patient may add stretching (Figures 20-11 through 20-14, 20-16). The patient may also begin pain-free straight leg raise exercises (Figures 20-18 through 20-20), and progress to hip abduction and rotation (Figures 20-21 through 20-23). During about week 8, the patient may perform hip progressive resistive exercises in all four directions (Figure 20-30). Swimming can be added as soon as pain allows, and biking is performed when sufficient ROM is attained. The patient is then progressed to closed chain weight-bearing lifting activities (Figures 20-32 through 20-34, 20-36 through 20-38, 20-40). Jogging, plyometrics (Figures 20-46 through 20-48), slide board (Figure 20-45), and sport-specific functional drills (see Figures 16-4 through 16-14) can be started as soon as the patient is pain-free and has the necessary strength base.[31]

Avulsion Fracture Ischial Tuberosity

Pathomechanics

The ischial tuberosity is a common site of injury to the hamstring muscle group (the biceps femoris, semitendinosus, and semimembranosus). All three hamstring muscles originate from the ischial tuberosity. The most common ischial injury, as it relates to the hamstring group, is an avulsion fracture of the tuberosity.[4,39]

Injury Mechanism

This injury usually results from a violent, forceful flexion of the hip, with the knee in extension.[1] A less severe irritation of the hamstring origin at the ischial tuberosity may also develop.

Rehabilitation Concerns, Rehabilitation Progression, and Criteria for Full Return

A patient with a less severe injury or irritation of the hamstring origin at the ischial tuberosity may complain of discomfort on sitting for

REHABILITATION PLAN

FEMORAL STRESS FRACTURE

Injury situation An 18-year-old female cross-country athlete visits the athletic training room during the fourth week of cross-country practices her freshman year in college. She has been experiencing right thigh pain about mid-thigh since the end of the summer, and the pain has increased during the past 4 weeks. At first, it was present only toward the end of her running workouts and immediately after running. Lately, her pain has been a constant dull ache during the day and has increased during workouts to the point where she can no longer finish an entire workout. Her coach told her she probably has a quadriceps strain and she should go see the athletic trainer.

Signs and symptoms The patient is complaining of a constant dull ache to the anterior thigh about mid quadriceps that increases with activities such as walking around campus and cross-country workouts. During the last 6 weeks of her summer vacation (before reporting for her freshman year of college) she increased her mileage and started running 7 days per week in preparation for college competition. Upon reporting to campus, she began intensive workouts with the team, again increasing her mileage and continuing to train 7 days per week. There was no specific mechanism of injury. She didn't get hit, fall, or remember feeling thigh pain during a specific run/workout. The pain developed over time (during the last 6 weeks of the summer).

The patient is wearing older running shoes, which appear worn down, and she reports having more than 500 miles on them. She is currently wearing these shoes to train.

During palpation, the patient describes a low-grade pain about mid-thigh in an area 1 to 2 inches in length. There is no noticeable swelling or muscle defect. She shows full active and passive quadriceps and hip ROM when seated, lying supine, and lying prone. There is mild discomfort on resistive knee extension both seated and lying supine with the knee bent over the end of the table. The right hip shows a significant decrease in strength compared to the left hip in the movements of abduction, flexion, and extension. She shows mild tightness in her hamstrings equally bilateral. She also shows a slightly increased Q angle and does show excessive pronation upon weight bearing in her right foot but not in her left. She presents normal alignment with the subtalar joint in neutral non-weight-bearing. Also, to observation, her right quadriceps is slightly smaller and less defined than her left quadriceps. Her leg lengths are about the same.

Management plan The initial goal is to eliminate the cause of pain and refer the student-patient to the team physician. The main question is whether this patient has a femoral stress fracture or simply a low-grade quadriceps strain that needs rehabilitation and active rest. The team physician reports a negative X-ray but orders a bone scan, which is scheduled for 1 week from the date of the X-ray. The patient is also referred back to the athletic trainer for treatment and rehabilitation for a possible stress fracture.

PHASE ONE: Active Rest

GOALS: Protection

Estimated length of time (ELT): Days 1 to 14 Until the results of the bone scan are reported, the patient is treated as though she does have a stress fracture. Due to the patient's sport and history (the cumulative stress overload of running 7 days per week during the previous 10 weeks while wearing shoes with more than 500 miles on them), the patient is placed on a stress fracture cyclic rehabilitation program. During this phase, the bone scan results return positive for a right mid-shaft femoral stress fracture.

Based on bone physiology, a schedule is made that presents to the patient no running, jumping, or forced weight-bearing activities every third week after 2 weeks of stressing the bone in a pain-free "normal" manner. This cycle is repeated—2 weeks of "normal" pain-free activity followed by 1 week of either eliminating weight-bearing activities or at least cutting it back to half the "normal" activity level and possibly returning to crutches with partial weight bearing. This cycling of activities every third week promotes the resorptive process to slow down and the reparative process to catch up, enhancing new bone growth at the fracture site.

The following schedule is developed and the patient is instructed in a non-weight-bearing to partial-weight-bearing cardiovascular program.

1. Biking 30 to 40 minutes daily (5 days per week).
2. Aquatic therapy non-weight-bearing swimming, treading water, etc, 2 to 3 days per week.
3. Aquatic therapy with partial-weight-bearing chest-height water-walking 10 to 20 minutes, or to pain-free limits, 2 days per week.
4. Pain-free open chain quadriceps, hamstring, and hip-strengthening exercises, 2 or 3 days per week.

Ice and electrical stimulation are used to decrease discomfort. Crutches should be used for pain-free partial weight bearing. An orthotic that doesn't require posting, but provides a rigid arch support, should be constructed to correct the excessive pronation during weight bearing.

PHASE TWO: Reparative Phase

GOALS: Rest and Repair

Estimated length of time (ELT): Weeks 2 to 3 This phase of the rehabilitation program continues with modalities to decrease pain and maintain active ROM at the hip and knee. During the third week, the patient discontinues weight-bearing/partial-weight-bearing activities to provide rest from the stress and to allow the reparative process to work at a faster rate than the resorptive stress process.

1. This phase begins with returning the patient to crutches non-weight-bearing for 7 days.
2. Aquatic therapy with non-weight-bearing deep-water treading and swimming only (discontinue chest water-walking for 7 days).
3. Biking and open chain strengthening are continued.

PHASE THREE: Second 2-Week Cycle of Weightbearing Stress

GOALS: Gradually Progress Exercise

Estimated length of time (ELT): Weeks 4 to 5 This phase begins the second 2-week cycle of stressing the bone to promote bone formation after a 7-day period (phase 2) of the non-weight-bearing reparative process/cycle.

1. If fully pain-free, eliminate crutches (as long as the patient has a normal gait pain-free).
2. Continue biking.
3. Begin Stairmaster (weight-bearing) pain-free, 20 to 30 minutes for 2 to 3 days per week.
4. Aquatic therapy with waist-deep water-walking and possibly jogging if pain-free. Also can add carioca and backward walking, 15 to 20 minutes total time over 2 or 3 days per week.
5. Continue open chain strengthening and add closed-chain leg press and squats. Weight appropriate to complete 3 or 4 sets of 10 reps without pain, 2 days per week.

PHASE FOUR: Reparative Phase

GOALS: Rest and Repair

Estimated length of time (ELT): Week 6 This phase is a 7-day rest period to again allow the resorptive process to slow down and the reparative process to speed up, which continues to enhance new bone formation.

1. This phase begins with returning the patient to crutches for partial weight bearing (50% to 75%). The patient may not wish to return to crutches. The athletic trainer can win compliance by explaining the bone physiology and trying to get the patient to look long-term.

2. Weight bearing in the pool is eliminated. Deep-water treading and swimming are continued.
3. The Stairmaster is eliminated, the bike is continued.
4. Closed chain strengthening is eliminated and open chain is continued.

For cardiovascular conditioning, the time spent in aquatic therapy and on the bike can be increased accordingly.

PHASE FIVE: Return To Normal Activity

GOALS: Return to normal activity

Estimated length of time (ELT): Weeks 7 to 8 The third cycle of weight bearing is also called the return to "normal" activity phase. This is when the patient is tested for returning to a running program specific to cross-country (sport-specific).
1. This phase begins with the elimination of crutches again.
2. Closed-chain strengthening is started again.
3. Stairmaster is started again.
4. Aquatic therapy with weight bearing is started again. This is progressed to running in waist-deep water and possibly plyometrics in waist-deep water.
5. Dry-land running is started and progressed if pain-free, 3 or 4 days per week.

If, by the end of this 2-week phase, the patient has progressed pain-free with all activities, she can begin training with her team and return to competition when appropriate. At this time in the calendar/schedule, this patient may be starting the indoor track and field program and should be watched closely. If necessary, another week of a non- to partial-weight-bearing reparative cycle could be added (week 9).

If pain returns during phase 5, another 3-week cycle, phase 6 (2 weeks of weight bearing, followed by 1 week of non-weight bearing) should be added to the rehabilitation program, and the patient should continue in this manner until pain-free.

OTHER POINTS OF INTEREST

This patient should be asked about her nutritional habits (assessment) and menstrual cycle, as these can also contribute to stress fractures. If the patient continues to have problems with bone pain and repetitive stress fractures in the future, a bone density test should be conducted and the patient should be referred to a nutritionist and a gynecologist.

DISCUSSION QUESTIONS
1. Would medications and/or supplements help with this problem?
2. Would a running-gait biomechanical analysis help with diagnosis and prevention?
3. Should an External Bone Healing Stimulator be considered?
4. How many weeks of sport participation would you expect a cross-country patient to miss during this type of rehabilitation program?
5. How would you communicate the diagnosis/problem, rehabilitation program/process, and timetable to the patient and coach?

extended periods and discomfort on palpation. This patient may also complain of pain while walking up stairs or uphill. The patient may ambulate with a normal gait cycle. Also, the patient may be able to jog normally, but pain may be present with attempts at sprinting. Resistive knee flexion and resistive hip extension with the knee in an extended position may reproduce the pain. Passive hip flexion with the knee in extension may also cause discomfort.

After the initial treatment phase of ice and other modalities, the patient may begin gentle, pain-free hamstring stretching exercises (Figures 20-7 and 20-8). To isolate the hamstring muscle while stretching, the patient should maintain a lordotic curve in the lumbar back area while flexing at the trunk to stretch the hamstrings (Figure 20-8A). Pain-free hamstring muscle progressive resistive strengthening exercises may also be performed, as soon as possible, (Figures 20-19, 20-24 through 20-26, 20-37), closed chain extension exercises (Figures 20-32 through 20-40), and PNF exercises (see Figures 14-11 through 14-17). This patient might not miss competition time and can be progressed functionally as tolerated.

Rehabilitation Concerns

The more severe ischial tuberosity avulsion fracture presents a different clinical picture. Palpation may produce moderate to severe pain, and the patient may be in moderate to severe pain with a very abnormal gait cycle. The patient's gait cycle may lack a heel-strike phase and have a very short swing-through phase.[4] The patient may attempt to keep the injured extremity behind or below the body to avoid hip flexion during the gait cycle. Resistive knee flexion and hip extension with the knee in an extended or flexed position may reproduce the pain. Passive hip flexion with the knee extended and with the knee flexed may cause moderate to severe pain at the ischial tuberosity. X-rays might or might not show the injury.[46]

After week 3 and the initial acute phase of treatment with modalities, the patient may begin pain-free active ROM lying prone and supine. Pain-free hamstring stretching exercises (Figures 20-7 and 20-8) may also be performed. Regaining full ROM during the rehabilitation program is very important. Many patients never gain full hip flexion ROM after this injury.

Weeks 6 through 12 are devoted to pain-free hamstring progressive resistive strengthening exercises (Figures 20-19, 20-24 through 20-26, 20-30), closed chain extension exercises (Figures 20-32 through 20-34, 20-38, 20-40), isokinetics (Figures 20-41 through 20-44) and PNF exercises (see Figures 14-11 through 14-17). After 2 to 3 weeks the patient may progress to the exercises as shown in Figures 20-36, 20-37 and 20-39.

Rehabilitation Progression and Criteria for Full Return

Surgery is usually not necessary. Immobilization and limiting physical activity are usually enough to allow healing. Ice and limited physical activity that involves hip flexion and forceful hip extension and knee flexion for the first 3 weeks are usually all that is necessary. Crutches should be used until normal gait is taught. During weeks 6 to 12, the patient will begin activities such as swimming, biking, and jogging, but the patient should avoid forceful knee and hip flexion and forceful hip extension. After week 12 the patient, without pain, may progress to the slide board (Figure 20-45), plyometrics (Figures 20-46 through 20-48), and sport specific functional drills (see Figures 16-4, 16-7 through 16-14) and then progress to the exercises shown in Figures 16-5 and 16-6.

Fractures of the Inferior Ramus

Pathomechanics

Stress and avulsion fractures should be ruled out before treating the pubic area for injury. The extent of an avulsion fracture must be diagnosed by X-ray. In some cases, a palpable mass may be detected under the skin. Stress fractures may be diagnosed with the same symptoms as in osteitis pubis. With a stress fracture an X-ray might appear normal until the third or fourth week. Obtaining a good history can aid in diagnosing a stress fracture.

Injury Mechanism

Avulsion fracture of the inferior ramus is usually caused by a violent, forceful contraction of the hip adductor muscles or forceful passive movement into hip abduction, as in a split. Stress fractures can occur from overuse (see treatment for femoral stress fractures).

Rehabilitation Concerns, Progression, and Criteria for Full Return

Rest is the key in treating fractures of the inferior ramus. Hip stretching and strengthening exercises may be performed, as in pubic injuries, within a pain-free ROM. An avulsion fracture might keep a patient out of competition for up to 3 months. A patient with a stress fracture may miss 3 to 6 weeks of competition. Rest from the activities that cause muscle contraction forces at the inferior ramus should be avoided, and closed chain stabilization exercises as described in pubic symphysis injury rehabilitation should be used. Return to activity should be gradual and deliberate, and must be pain-free.

Traumatic Femoral Neck Fractures

Pathomechanics and Injury Mechanism

A femoral neck fracture is often associated with osteoporosis and is rarely seen in athletics.[18,50] However, a twisting motion combined with a fall can produce this fracture. Because the femoral neck fracture can disrupt the blood supply to the head of the femur, avascular necrosis is often seen later. This injury must receive proper initial treatment.

Rehabilitation Concerns, Progression, and Criteria for Full Return

After surgery or during immobilization, isometric hip exercises are started immediately. Patients, especially younger patients, are progressed slowly. A normal gait cycle should be taught to the patient as soon as possible. In some cases where osteoporosis has been known to be involved, exercise has been shown to increase bone density and reverse the rate of osteoporosis. Progress the patient with functional ROM and functional strength, aquatic therapy, and biking, if pain-free. Within 6 to 8 weeks, gentle active hip ROM exercises with no weight can be performed (Figures 20-17 through 20-23). Stretching exercises are performed at about week 8 (Figures 20-4 through 20-12) and progress to stretches for hip rotation and the piriformis (Figures 20-13, 20-14, 20-16). Progressive resistive muscle-strengthening exercises should be started after 2 to 4 weeks of active ROM and stretching exercises. At about week 12, weight can be added to the exercises shown in Figures 20-17 through 20-23, and the exercises shown in Figures 20-25, 20-28, and 20-30 can be added, along with closed chain exercises (Figures 20-32 through 20-34, 20-36 through 20-38, 20-40).

After the patient's strength level has reached the "norms," the patient may begin pain-free slide board (Figure 20-45), plyometrics (Figures 20-46 through 20-48), and sport-specific functional drills (see Figures 16-4, 16-7 through 16-14), and then progress to the exercises shown in Figures 16-5 and 16-6.

Acetabulum Labral Tear

Pathomechanics

Moul and Leslie present an excellent review of acetabulum labral tear and present a case history that is very familiar to the athletic trainer working with chronic hip, groin, and lower abdominal pain. Diagnosis of acetabulum labral tear is difficult, much like diagnosing "sports hernia." After months of treatment, including rest, for hip flexor/adductor strains, snapping hip syndrome, hip bursitis, and hip sprains and strains in general, the patient usually does not show improvement. Recently it has been shown that a relatively minor hip twist caused by direct blow, forceful cutting during changing directions, or a quick movement at the hip caused by a slip can cause a tear of the acetabular labrum. The patient may report hyperextending the hip with or without abduction. Previously, it was thought that a more serious hip dislocation had to occur to cause this injury.[36]

In 1999, Hase and Ueo described signs that help diagnose acetabulum labral tears. These include hip "catching" and "clicking," pain with internal rotation of the hip with it flexed at 90 degrees, axial compression of the hip joint with the hip flexed at 90 degrees and slightly adducted, and pain at the greater trochanter.[17]

The patient's gait might suggest a severe hip flexor strain, with the hip flexed and guarded. The patient might report groin and lower abdominal pain. At this point, the patient is usually treated for hip flexor/adductor strain and checked for possible hernia, which is always negative. As time passes, the patient will report and show signs of loss of hip ROM and strength, with either no change in pain or an increase in pain. At this point, the patient may report an audible "clicking" and/or "catching" with pain associated. If not performed previously, MRI may show a tear in the labrum. It is recommended that early intervention using diagnostic tools such as MRI, MRI arthrogram, and CT arthrogram scans may save time and pain. The question remains, how much time should pass before such diagnostic tools are ordered?

Rehabilitation Concerns, Progression, and Criteria for Full Return

Treatments of acetabulum labral tears have varied, with mixed results. Conservative treatment such as crutches, modalities, and nonsteroidal anti-inflammatory medications may have a positive effect acutely, but over time signs and symptoms usually return.

Injecting the capsular area outside the joint might result in improvement initially, but over time the patient will revert to preinjection status. The same has been reported with intra-articular injections.[6] The benefit of intra-articular injection is that it can help with differential diagnosis and ruling out snapping of the iliopsoas tendon over the iliopectineal eminence.[36]

It appears that the treatment of choice is to surgically remove or debride the labral tear arthroscopically. Hase and Ueo reported return to full pain-free activities (some in 6 weeks) in most patients (83%), compared to conservative treatment (13%).[17,36]

Rehabilitation after acetabulum labral tear arthroscopic resection follows this progression: Following an arthroscopic excision at the torn piece of labrum, beginning a day or two after surgery the patient is allowed to perform pain-free active ROM (without weight) as shown in Figures 20-17 through 20-23. At about day 5, the patient may begin adding weight to the exercises described in Figures 20-17 through 20-23 and also add the exercises shown in Figures 20-30A–E and 20-31. At about week 3, the patient can add pain-free stretching as shown in Figures 20-4, and 20-7 through 20-16. Also at week 3 or 4, if pain-free, the patient can add Figures 20-32 through 20-38, and 20-40. At about weeks 4 to 6, the patient can begin sport-specific functional training and return when all activities are pain-free.

Clinical Decision-Making Exercise 20-4

A male college soccer player has been receiving treatment for a groin strain for 6 weeks and has participated in his sport with pain. During the 6 weeks of treatment with modalities including ice, heat, electric stimulation, ultrasound, phonophoresis, oral anti-inflammatory medications, as well as modifying his run conditioning and practice schedule with the coach, the patient reported no change in symptoms. What can the athletic trainer recommend at this point to help this patient?

Hip Dislocation

Pathomechanics

Dislocation of the hip joint is extremely rare in athletics and takes a considerable amount of force because of the deep-seated ball-in-socket joint.[37,47] Fractures and avascular necrosis, which is a degenerative condition of the head of the femur caused by a disruption of blood supply during dislocation, should always be considered.[9,15,25] Dislocation should be treated as a medical emergency. The patient should be checked for distal pulses and sensation. The sciatic nerve should be examined to see if it has been crushed or severed.[1] Do this by checking sensation and foot and toe movements. If the sciatic nerve is damaged, knee, ankle, and toe weakness may be pronounced.

Injury Mechanism

A hip dislocation is generally a posterior dislocation that takes place with the knee and hip in a flexed position. The patient may be totally disabled, in severe pain, and usually unwilling to allow movement of the extremity. The trochanter may appear larger than normal with the extremity in internal rotation, flexed, and adducted.[42] X-ray studies should be performed before anesthetized reduction.[37]

Rehabilitation Concerns, Progression, and Criteria for Full Return

Two or three weeks (and in some cases, a longer period) of immobilization is initially needed. Rehabilitation of the thigh, knee, and ankle may be included at this time. Pain-free hip isometric exercises should be performed. Electrical muscle stimulation modalities may be used initially to promote muscle reeducation and retard muscle atrophy.[46] At about 3 to 6 weeks, pain-free active ROM exercises can be performed (Figures 20-17 through 20-23) with no resistance or weight. Crutch walking is progressed and performed until the patient can ambulate with a normal gait cycle and without pain. At about 6 weeks, the patient may perform gentle progressive resistive strengthening exercises with a weight cuff or weight boot. All six movements of the hip should be included in the progressive resistive strengthening exercises (hip flexion, abduction, extension, adduction, internal rotation, and external rotation) (Figures 20-17 through 20-23, and 20-30) and PNF exercises (see Figures 14-11 through 14-17). Pain-free stretching exercises should not be performed until 8 to 12 weeks (Figures 20-4, 20-5, 20-7 through 20-16). At about 12 weeks, the patient may begin closed chain exercises (Figures 20-32 through 20-40), as well as open chain exercises (Figure 20-31). At 16 to 20 weeks, the patient may progress to pain-free slide board (Figure 20-45), plyometric exercises (Figures 20-46 through 20-48), and sport-specific functional activities (see Figures 16-4, 16-7 through 16-14) and then progress to the functional exercises (see Figures 16-5 and 16-6). If pain returns, the patient must eliminate plyometrics and functional activities until they can be performed pain-free. This patient may return to competition in 6 to 12 months if there have been no delays and the patient is pain-free with all activity.

CHRONIC GROIN, HIP, AND THIGH INJURIES

Sciatica (Direct Trauma, Piriformis Syndrome, Neural Tension)

Pathomechanics

The sciatic nerve is a continuation of the sacral plexus as it passes through the greater sciatic notch and descends deeply through the back of the thigh.[34] Hip and buttock pain is often diagnosed as sciatic nerve irritation. Sciatica is a phrase used to describe any pain produced by irritation of the sciatic nerve, but there are many potential causes of this irritation. The sciatic nerve can be irritated by a low back problem, direct trauma, or trauma from surrounding structures such as the piriformis muscle, in which case sciatic nerve irritation is also called piriformis syndrome.[1,26] Piriformis syndrome is seen more in women than men, and the cause of this condition is typically due to a tight piriformis muscle as the nerve passes underneath the muscle or to an anatomical variation in which the nerve goes through the muscle. In about 15% of the population, the sciatic nerve passes through the piriformis muscle, separating it in two.[28]

Injury to the hamstring muscles can also cause sciatic nerve irritation, as can irritation from ischial bursitis. In a traumatic accident that causes posterior dislocation of the femoral head, the sciatic nerve might be crushed or severed and require surgery.[28]

Injury Mechanism

The most common cause of sciatic nerve irritation in athletics, especially contact sports, is a direct blow to the buttock. Because of the large muscle mass, this injury is not usually disabling when the sciatic nerve is not involved. When the sciatic nerve is involved, however, the patient may experience pain in the buttock, extending down the back of the thigh, possibly into the lateral calf and foot. Sciatic pain is usually a burning sensation.[46]

Rehabilitation Concerns

With sciatica, the athletic trainer must rule out disk disease before starting any exercise rehabilitation program. Stretching exercises that are indicated for sciatica, such as trunk and hip flexion, might be contraindicated for disk disease. To differentiate low back problems (disk disease) from piriformis syndrome as the cause of sciatica, determine whether the patient has low back pain with radiation into the extremity. An MRI is very useful for differentiating sciatica due to piriformis vs due to disk disease. Back pain is most likely midline, exacerbated by trunk flexion and relieved by rest. Coughing and straining may also increase back pain and possibly the radiation. Muscle weakness and sensory numbness may also be found in a patient with disk disease.[16] Patients with piriformis syndrome may have the same symptoms without the low back pain and without the low back pain being reproduced with coughing and straining. If, after treatment and rehabilitation, the patient still maintains neurological deficits, further evaluation to rule out disk disease is necessary.

In the case of piriformis syndrome, the patient might report a deep pain in the buttock without low back pain and possibly radiating pain in the back of the thigh, lateral calf, and foot, also indicating sciatica.[28] The athletic trainer's evaluation should include the low back, as well as the hip and thigh. The patient's gait cycle could include lack of heel strike, landing in the foot-flat phase, a shortening of the stride, and possible ambulation with a flexed knee to relieve the stretch on the sciatic nerve. The patient's posture, in severe cases, shows a flexed knee with the leg externally rotated. Palpation in the sciatic notch could also produce pain.

With the patient lying prone and the hip in a neutral position with the knee in flexion, active resistive external rotation and passive internal rotation of the hip might reproduce the pain (Figure 20-15).[28] Performed supine, straight leg raises performed passively or actively might also cause symptoms. With the patient supine and the knee in extension and relaxed, a decrease in passive internal rotation of the hip joint compared to the uninjured side may indicate piriformis tightness.

Another possible explanation for the irritation of the sciatic nerve would be Adverse Neural Tension (ANT). Gallant described this condition as the inability of the nervous system to move concurrently with changes in body position. This inability of the nerve to glide proximally and distally due to restrictions from the surrounding structures (ie, piriformis, hamstring muscles) would also produce radicular symptoms as hip flexion ROM increased. ANT could also present itself following direct trauma in which the nerve itself became inflamed or injured. This would most often be caused by swelling in the endoneural tube, which would increase the pressure around the nerve and produce similar radicular symptoms. ANT treatments usually involve neural mobilizations in which the nerve is moved

through large amplitude, mid-ranges of motion (grade 3) to help the nerve to regain its mobility independent of the surrounding structures. Neural mobilizations that are small amplitude, end-ROM (grade 4) can be used to help decrease the swelling found in the endoneural tube and improve radicular symptoms. Patients who are really symptomatic can be started with grade 1 and 2 mobilizations or even begin by mobilizing the opposite limb.[13,20,22,53]

> ### Clinical Decision-Making Exercise 20-5
>
> A female college soccer player reports to the athletic trainer with pain in the buttocks and burning down the back of the thigh to the lateral calf. After the athletic trainer obtains a history, the patient reports having fallen on her buttocks two days earlier in a game. The patient does not report having any back pain. After the patient is diagnosed with sciatica caused by the direct blow to the buttocks and the sciatic nerve, what can the athletic trainer recommend to help with the burning pain in the buttocks, thigh, and calf?

Rehabilitation Progression

Severe sciatica caused by piriformis syndrome can keep the patient out of competition for 2 to 3 weeks or longer. If the sciatic nerve is irritated and the patient complains of radiation into the extremity, the first 3 to 5 days should consist of rest and modalities to decrease the pain associated with sciatica.

After the acute pain has been controlled, the patient may perform pain-free stretching exercises for the low back and hamstring muscles, as long as disk disease has been ruled out. Stretching exercises (Figures 20-7, 20-8, 20-13, 20-16) can be used to treat piriformis syndrome. Piriformis strengthening may be accomplished through resistive external rotation of the hip (Figure 20-23).

Reviewing a normal gait cycle can also aid in gaining ROM if the patient has been ambulating with a flexed knee. The hamstrings, as well as the sciatic nerve, may have shortened in this case.

Criteria for Full Return

The patient should be capable of performing pain-free activity, such as running and cutting, without neurological symptoms, before returning to competition (see Figures 16-4 through 16-14). Participating with constant radiation into the extremity poses a risk for developing chronic problems. The best method of treatment is prevention by instituting a good flexibility program for all athletes.

Trochanteric Bursitis

Pathomechanics

The most commonly diagnosed hip bursitis is greater trochanteric bursitis. The greater trochanteric bursa lies between the gluteus maximus and the surface of the greater trochanter.[28,51] Bursitis and other disorders of the bursa are often mistaken for other injuries because of the location of numerous other structures around the bursa. The bursa is a structure that normally lies within the area of a joint and produces a fluid that lubricates the two surfaces between which it lies. It also may attach, very loosely, to the joint capsule, tendons, ligaments, and skin. Therefore, it is indirectly involved with other close structures.[18] The function of the bursa is to dissipate friction caused by two or more structures moving against one another. Bursitis associated with bleeding into the bursa is the most disabling form. With hemorrhagic bursitis, swelling and pain may limit motion.[38] The athletic trainer must also consider the possibility of an infected bursa. If it is suspected, the patient should be referred for a medical evaluation immediately.

Injury Mechanism

Bursitis in general is usually caused by direct trauma or overuse stress. One possible cause for trochanteric bursitis may be irritation caused by the iliotibial band at the insertion of the gluteus maximus.[28] Repetitive irritation such as running with one leg slightly adducted (as on the side of a road), can cause trochanteric bursitis on the adducted side.

Trochanteric bursitis caused by overuse is mostly seen in women runners who have an increased Q angle with or without a leg-length discrepancy.[1] Tight adductors can cause a runner's feet to cross over the midline, resulting in excessive tilting of the pelvis in the frontal plane, and consequently place an exceptional amount of force on the trochanteric bursa.[23]

Lateral heel wear in running shoes can also cause excessive hip adduction that may indirectly result in trochanteric bursitis. In contact sports, a direct blow may result in a hemorrhagic bursitis, which could be extremely painful to the patient.[18]

Rehabilitation Concerns

Traumatic trochanteric bursitis is more easily diagnosed than overuse trochanteric bursitis. Palpation produces pain over the lateral hip area and greater trochanter. In both cases the patient's gait cycle may be slightly abducted on the affected side to relieve pressure on the bursa. A patient's attempt to remove weight from the affected extremity may cause a shortened weight-bearing phase. The patient might report an increase in pain on activity, and active resistive hip abduction might also reproduce the pain.

A complete history must be taken to determine the cause of trochanteric bursitis. The patient's gait cycle, posture, flexibility, and running shoes should be examined. Oral anti-inflammatory medication usually helps decrease pain and inflammation initially. After the initial treatment of ice, compression, and other modalities, the patient can use various stretching exercises (Figures 20-4, 20-7 through 20-16).

Rehabilitation Progression

An orthotic evaluation should be performed to check for any malalignment that may have caused dysfunction, excessive adduction, or leg-length discrepancy. Progressive resistive strengthening exercises in hip abduction may be performed when the patient is free of pain. Also see treatment for all hip bursitis injuries.

Criteria for Full Return

This patient could miss 3 to 5 days of competition, depending on the severity of the bursitis. For contact sports, a protective pad should be worn upon return to competition after the patient can perform the sport-specific functional tests (see Figures 16-4 through 16-14).

Ischial Bursitis

Pathomechanics and Injury Mechanism

The ischial bursa lies between the ischial tuberosity and the gluteus maximus (also see Trochanteric Bursitis, Pathomechanics). Ischial bursitis is often seen in people who sit for long periods.[30] In athletes, ischial bursitis is more commonly caused by direct trauma, such as falling or a direct hit when the hip is in a flexed position that exposes the ischial area.

Rehabilitation Concerns

The patient might report trauma to the area. With the hip in a flexed position, palpation over the ischial tuberosity might reproduce the pain. The patient might experience pain on ambulation when the hip is flexed during the gait cycle. Also, stair climbing and uphill walking and running may reproduce pain.

Rehabilitation Progression

Treatment for ischial bursitis should include positioning the patient with the hip in a flexed position to expose the ischial area. After the initial phase of treatment with ice and anti-inflammatory medication, the patient may begin a pain-free stretching program (Figures 20-7 through 20-14, 20-16).

Criteria for Full Return

Depending on injury severity, this patient need not miss competition time. Avoiding direct trauma to the area usually allows healing within 3 to 5 days. For contact sports, a protective pad should be worn. Sport-specific functional testing and exercises should be performed as described above before the patient returns to competition.

Iliopectineal Bursitis

Pathomechanics and Injury Mechanism

Iliopectineal bursitis is often mistaken for a strain of the iliopsoas muscle and can be difficult to differentiate. Rarely seen in patients, iliopectineal bursitis could potentially be caused by a tight iliopsoas muscle. Osteoarthritis of the hip can also cause iliopectineal bursitis.[30]

Rehabilitation Concerns

Resistive hip flexion—sitting with the knee bent or lying supine with the knee extended—may reproduce the pain associated with iliopectineal bursitis. Also, passive hip extension with the knee extended may produce pain. Palpable pain in the inguinal area may also help in evaluating the patient. In some cases, the nearby femoral nerve may become inflamed and cause radiation into the front of the thigh and knee.[30] Osteoarthritis must be ruled out in evaluating iliopectineal bursitis.

Rehabilitation Progression

Oral anti-inflammatory medication may be helpful initially. A form of deep heat or ice massage may be used to aid in decreasing inflammation and pain. The iliopsoas tendon must be stretched (Figures 20-4 through 20-6), and hip flexion strengthening exercises are performed pain-free with the knee straight (Figures 20-18 and 20-30B).

Clinical Decision-Making Exercise 20-6

A female track athlete who competes in the long jump and short sprints has been diagnosed by the team physician with a grade 2 hip flexor strain to the deep iliopsoas muscle. The patient is in severe pain and ambulating very slowly with a flexed hip and knee. What can the athletic trainer recommend to decrease pain and improve her gait?

Snapping or Clicking Hip Syndrome

Pathomechanics and Injury Mechanism

Clinically, snapping hip syndrome is secondary to what could be a number of causes.[9] Excessive repetitive movement has been linked to snapping hip syndrome in dancers, gymnasts, hurdlers, and sprinters where a muscle imbalance develops.[1] The most common causes of the "snapping," when muscle is involved, is the iliotibial band over the greater trochanter resulting in trochanteric bursitis (see Trochanteric Bursitis) and the iliopsoas tendon over the iliopectineal eminence. Other extra-articular causes of the snapping are the iliofemoral ligaments over the femoral head, and the long head of the biceps femoris over the ischial tuberosity.[9] Extra-articular causes commonly occur when the hip is externally rotated and flexed. Other causes or anatomical structures that can predispose "snapping hip" are a narrow pelvic width, abnormal increases in abduction ROM, and lack of ROM into external rotation, or tight internal rotators.[1] Intra-articular causes are less likely but may consist of loose bodies, synovial chondromatosis, osteocartilaginous exostosis, acetabulum labral rim tear of fibrocartilage, and possibly subluxation of the hip joint itself.[9,36]

Rehabilitation Concerns, Progression, and Criteria for Full Return

Due to the extra-articular causes, the hip joint capsule, ligaments, and muscles become loosened and allow the hip to become unstable. The patient will complain of a snapping, and this snapping might be accompanied by severe pain and disability upon each snap.

The key to treating and rehabilitating the snapping hip syndrome is to decrease pain and inflammation with ice, anti-inflammatory medication, and other modalities such as ultrasound. This could significantly decrease the pain initially so that the patient can begin a stretching and strengthening program. The most important aspect of the evaluation process is to find the source of the imbalance (which muscles are tight and which are weak).

In the case of the iliopsoas muscle snapping over the iliopectineal eminence, the following stretches should be used (Figures 20-4 through 20-6). Strengthening should take into account the entire hip, especially the hip extensors and internal and external rotators (Figures 20-19, 20-22 and 20-23).

After pain has subsided and the patient can actively flex the hip pain-free, the patient can begin strengthening exercises for the hip flexor (Figures 20-17, 20-18, and 20-30), flexion with the knee straight. After the first 3 to 5 days, the patient can begin jogging and sport-specific functional drills (see Figures 16-4, 16-7 through 16-14) and progress to the exercises shown in Figures 16-5 and 16-6 if all are pain-free.

Sport Hernia/Groin Disruption

Pathomechanics

The syndrome of groin pain often includes the posterior abdominal wall. This syndrome has manifested itself over the past 10 years and has created much confusion when diagnosing, treating, and rehabilitating. Many of these patients will complain of groin pain and will show no improvement during a period of 4, 6, or even 12 months. All kinds of treatment and rehabilitation, including extended rest, tend not to produce positive results.

This non-descriptive groin pain has come under the umbrella *sports hernias*. The phrases groin disruption and athletic pubalgia have also been used interchangeably.[33,35] The anatomy and physiology involved are not fully understood because there hasn't been a detailed description with empirical evidence in the literature.[33] What is known is that a sports hernia is described as a weakening of the posterior inguinal wall with possibly an undetectable inguinal hernia due to the location behind the posterior wall.[35]

Injury Mechanism and Rehabilitation Concerns

Due to the many biomechanical movements that occur in sports, the pelvis is torqued in all its planes. The forces produced by the muscles that both stabilize and move the pelvis result in injury to the abdominal muscles, hip flexor, and adductor groups.[33] A patient with a sports hernia will usually present the same signs and symptoms as those who have osteitis pubis and adductor strains. The symptoms will simply last longer, even with conservative treatment. The patient will continuously present a gradual increase in symptoms over time with deep groin/pelvis pain. Pain may radiate into the lower abdominal area. A weakness of the abdominal muscles during pelvic and trunk stabilization may create a compartment syndrome-like injury caused when combined with repeated adduction of the hip. When symptoms persist, the patient usually responds extremely well to surgical repair.[33,35] The patient will usually have pain with resistive hip adduction and resisted sit-up. Some patients may describe a trunk hyperextension injury that may have occurred some time ago. The abdominal muscles and adductor site of insertion onto the pubic bone are the main sites of pain. Other injuries, such as osteitis pubis, tendinitis, bursitis, and adductor muscles strains, can contribute to the symptoms. Significant inflammation occurs where the adductors attach to the pubis and along the posterior aspect of the adductor insertion. The *pelvic floor repair* is described as the surgical reattachment of the abdominal muscles to the pubic bone. There are also numerous other components of this repair described in the literature. This procedure helps stabilize the anterior pelvis and has been shown to be very successful.[33]

X-rays, bone scans, and MRIs can be helpful in differential diagnosis, but they usually are not helpful in diagnosing sports hernias.[35]

Rehabilitation Progreession and Criteria for Full Return

After pelvic floor repair, the first 4 weeks and first phase of rehabilitation involves nothing more than rest with no activity or exercising. At about week 5, the patient can begin posterior pelvic tilts (Figure 24-23; hold 5 seconds for 3 sets of 10 repetitions), along with gentle pain-free stretching of the iliopsoas, hamstrings, groin, hip extensors, quadriceps, and trunk. (See the stretches in Figures 20-4 to 20-10, and trunk side bends shown in Figure 24-11). The patient may also at this time begin aquatic therapy involving simple walking forward, walking backward, and side walking.

At about week 8, the patient can add the strengthening exercises shown in Figures 20-15 to 20-21, all performed without weight. Aquatic therapy can be progressed to jogging and running forward, backward, and to the sides (carioca). At this time, the patient can also begin cardiovascular work on the Stairmaster, bike, and/or upper body ergometer. At about 10 weeks, the patient can begin stretching all muscles and add weight to the straight-leg raises begun previously. Abdominal crunches (Figure 24-24) can be added if pain-free. In the sport of ice hockey, the patient may begin light skating (pain-free) at this time. For dry land patients, progressive jogging can also be added at 10 weeks.

At 12 weeks, the patient can begin weightlifting exercises such as squats, power lifts, lunges, and plyometrics. The patient can progress the running program and add sport-specific drills.

From 3 months forward, the patient may be cleared for sport participation if all activities are pain-free.

Osteitis Pubis

Pathomechanics

Osteitis pubis is a condition described as pain located in the area of the pubic symphysis. Unless the patient reports being hit or experiencing some kind of direct trauma, pubic pain might be caused by osteitis pubis, fractures of the inferior ramus (stress fractures and avulsion fractures), or a groin strain.[1]

Because an overuse situation and rapid repetitive changes of direction predispose a patient to this injury, osteitis pubis is seen mostly in distance running, football, wrestling, and soccer. Constant movement of the symphysis in sports such as football and soccer produces inflammation and pain.

Injury Mechanism

Repetitive stress on the pubic symphysis, caused by the insertion of muscles into the area, creates a chronic inflammation.[1] Increased stress can also occur due to excessive motion. If the hip and/or sacroiliac joints have restricted motion, the stress of increased motion will be transferred to the pubic symphisis.[29,55] Direct trauma to the symphysis can also cause periostitis. Symptoms develop gradually, and might be mistaken for muscle strains. Exercises that aid muscle strains might cause more irritation to the symphysis; thus, early active exercises are contraindicated.[23]

Rehabilitation Concerns

Referral to a physician to rule out hernia problems, infection, and prostatitis may be helpful in evaluating osteitis pubis.[23] Changes in X-ray films can take 4 to 6 weeks to show. The patient should be treated symptomatically.

A patient with osteitis pubis may have pain in the groin area and might complain of an increase in pain with running, sit-ups, and squatting.[1] The patient might also complain of lower abdominal pain with radiation into the inner thigh. Differentiating osteitis pubis from a muscle strain is difficult.

Palpation over the pubic symphysis may reproduce pain. In severe cases, the patient may show a waddling gait because of the shear forces at the symphysis.[1] Rest is the main course of treatment, with modalities and anti-inflammatory medication to ease pain. As soon as pain permits, the patient should begin pain-free adductor stretching exercises, as shown in Figures 20-7 and 20-8, as well as stretches for the hip internal and external rotators.[55] Also, pain-free abdominal strengthening, low back strengthening, and open chain hip abductor, adductor, flexor, and extensor strengthening can be started (Figures 20-17 through 20-21). Because excessive movement that causes shear forces at the symphysis is the main cause of pain, stabilization exercises that concentrate on tightening the muscles around the pubic symphysis are recommended. The patient is asked to concentrate on tightening the buttock, groin, abdomen, and low back (the entire pelvic area) while performing a closed chain exercise such as the leg press (Figure 20-33) and lunges (Figure 20-36). This stabilization technique helps to control excessive movement at the pubic symphysis while the patient performs movements at other joints. These closed chain exercises may be started, for stabilization purposes, and might actually be pain-free before the start of open chain exercises.

Rehabilitation Progression and Criteria for Full Return

The lower body must be protected from shear forces to the symphysis area. Most patients will miss 3 to 5 days of competition. In severe cases, from 3 weeks up to 3 months and possibly 6 months of rest and treatment may be necessary. In severe cases, the patient should not participate until able to perform pain-free plyometric exercises (Figures 20-45 through 20-48). Sport-specific functional drills may be started as soon as the patient can perform them pain-free (see Figures 16-4 through 16-14).

Femoral Stress Fractures

Pathomechanics and Injury Mechanism

A stress fracture, often described as a partial or incomplete fracture of the femur, may be seen because of repetitive microtrauma or cumulative stress overload to a localized area of the bone.[10,58] Young patients are more likely to develop this injury. The patient may complain of pinpoint pain that increases during activity. The initial X-ray film is usually negative. Obtaining a good history is very important and should include activities, change in activities and surfaces, and running gait analysis.[58]

The basic biomechanics and biodynamics of normal bone are very important in understanding the mechanism by which femoral stress fractures occur and recover. A process of bone resorption, followed by new bone formation, in normal bone, is constantly occurring through turning over and remodeling by the dynamic organ itself.[54] This remodeling occurs in response to weight bearing and muscular contractions that cause increased stress on the bone. Responses by the bone to these loads allow the bone to become as strong as it has to be to withstand the stresses placed upon it during the required activity.[11,58] Because bone is a dynamic tissue, there is a cell system in place that carries out the process of constant bone breakdown and bone repair for the task at hand. There are two types of bone cells responsible for this dynamic procedure—osteoclasts, which resorb bone, and osteoblasts, which produce new bone to fill the areas that have been resorbed.[58] When stress is applied, the osteoblasts produce new bone at a rate comparable to the osteoclasts. When the stress is applied over time, as in overuse injuries, the osteoclasts work at a faster rate than the osteoblasts and a stress fracture occurs. Some studies have shown that this stress reaction occurs about the third week of a workout session.[14,42] This becomes very important when developing a rehabilitation program in reference to using the advantages of bone physiology within the rehabilitation program to facilitate new bone formation.

Rehabilitation Concerns, Progression, and Criteria for Full Return

As with all stress fractures, finding the cause is the first step in treatment and rehabilitation.[49] The patient may perform pain-free thigh strengthening and stretching exercises and progress as shown in the sections on hamstring and quadriceps rehabilitation programs.

The most important treatment for stress fractures is rest, especially from the sport or activity that caused the fracture. In a period of 6 to 12 weeks, most femoral stress fractures heal clinically if the specific cause is discontinued.[58] The resorptive process will slow down and the reparative process will catch up with simple rest from the activity that caused the problem. Rest should be "active." This allows the patient to exercise pain-free and helps prevent muscle atrophy and deconditioning. Except in special "problem" fractures, immobilization in a cast or brace is usually unnecessary. When there is excessive pain or motion of the part, casts or braces may be used. In noncompliant patients, a cast or some form of immobilization may be recommended. Non-weight-bearing or partial-weight-bearing with crutches is highly recommended as the process of ambulating with a normal gait, while using crutches, can facilitate bone formation at the fracture site.[32]

Until ordinary, "normal" activities are pain-free with no tenderness or edema over the fracture site and no abnormal gait patterns during ambulation, the patient is held back from sport activities. Pain-free rehabilitation should start immediately and continue throughout the recovery period with a slow progressive return to activity. Immediately discontinue all activity with recurrence of any symptoms.[58]

The first phase of the rehabilitation program begins when the stress fracture is diagnosed. This phase consists of modalities to decrease pain and swelling and to increase or maintain active ROM to the hip, knee, and ankle joints.[58] The second phase of rehabilitation begins as acute pain subsides. This phase consists of functional rehabilitation and conditioning in a progression of sport specific training. Keeping in mind bone physiology as described, the patient who has begun sport specific training is advised not to run, jump, or force activity during the third week after 2 weeks of vigorous "normal" exercise or rehabilitation and conditioning. This cycle is repeated—2 weeks of vigorous normal activity, followed by 1 week of either eliminating running and jumping or at least cutting it back to half the normal activity level. This cycling of activities every third week facilitates osteoblast function (bone formation) and new bone growth at the fracture site as the osteoblasts are able to keep pace with and actually work faster than the osteoclasts.

Rehabilitation and treatment should be an ongoing process as described above, with general physical conditioning as part of the "active rest" period. Aquatic exercise and conditioning, such as swimming, treading water, running in a swimming pool, biking, Stairmaster, and the slide board (Figure 20-45), should be started as soon as they are pain-free. These activities could come under the umbrella of "normal" exercise or rehabilitation and conditioning. Upper-body ergometers may also be used. A patient with a femoral stress fracture should also be evaluated for lower-extremity deformities and foot malalignments.[58] Orthotics can be very useful in treating a femoral stress fracture if a malalignment is found.

Summary

1. Injuries to the groin, hip, and thigh can be extremely disabling and often require a substantial amount of time for rehabilitation.

2. Hip pointers are contusions of the soft tissue in the area of the iliac crest and must be treated aggressively during the first 2 to 4 hours after injury.

3. Protection is the key to treatment and rehabilitation of quadriceps contusions and accompanying myositis ossificans.

4. Strains of the groin musculature, the hamstring, and the quadriceps muscles can require long periods of rehabilitation for the patient. Early return often exacerbates the problem.

5. The femur is subject to stress fractures, avulsion fractures of the lesser trochanter, and traumatic fractures of the femoral neck.

6. Hip dislocations are rare in patients and requires 6 to 12 months of rehabilitation or more before the patient can return to full activity.

7. Piriformis syndrome sciatica should be specifically differentiated from other problems that produce low back pain or radiating pain in the buttocks and leg. Rehabilitation programs are extremely variable for different conditions and can even be harmful if used inappropriately.

8. Trochanteric bursitis is relatively common in patients, as is ischial bursitis.

Treatment involves efforts directed at protection and reduction of inflammation in the affected area.

9. Snapping or clicking hip syndrome most often occurs when the iliotibial band snaps over the greater trochanter, causing trochanteric bursitis. Acetabulum labral tears should be ruled out.

10. Prolonged groin pain can include the posterior abdominal wall. This non-descriptive groin pain, called *sports hernia*, lasts over 4 to 6 months and responds well to surgery.

11. Osteitis pubis and fractures of the inferior ramus both produce pain at the pubic symphysis and are best treated with rest.

References

1. Arnheim, D.D., and W.E. Prentice. 2014. *Principles of athletic training.* 15th ed. New York: McGraw-Hill.

2. Aronen, J.G., et al. 2006. Quadriceps contusions: Clinical results of immediate immobilization in 120 degrees of knee flexion. *Clin J Sport Med* 16(5):383–387.

3. Bergmann, G., F. Graichen, and A. Rohlmann. 2004. Hip joint contact forces during stumbling. *Langenbecks Arch Surg* 389(1):53–59.

4. Berry, J.M. 1992. Fracture of the tuberosity of the ischium due to muscular action. *Journal of American Medical Association* 59:1450.

5. Brunet, M. and R. Hontas, eds. 1994. The thigh. In *Orthopaedic sports medicine*, Vol. 2, ed. J.C. DeLee and D. Drez. W. B. Saunders: Philadelphia.

6. Byrd, J.W.T. 1994. Labral lesions: An elusive source of hip pain: Case reports and literature review. *Arthroscopy*, 12:603–612.

7. Crowninshield, R.D., et al. 1978. A biomechanical investigation of the human hip. *J Biomech* 11(1–2):75–85.

8. Daniels, L. and C. Worthingham. 2007. *Muscle testing: Techniques of manual examination.* Philadelphia: W.B. Saunders.

9. DeLee, J.C. and D. Drez. 1994. *Orthopaedic sports medicine.* Vol. 2. Philadelphia: W. B. Saunders.

10. Devas, M.B. 1995. *Stress fractures.* New York: Longman.

11. Frost, H. 1964. *Laws of bone structures.* Springfield, IL: Charles C. Thomas.

12. Fuss, F.K. and A. Bacher. 1991. New aspects of the morphology and function of the human hip joint ligaments. *Am J Anat* 192(1)1–13.

13. Gallant, S. 1998. Assessing adverse neural tension in athletes. *Journal of Sport Rehabilitation* 7:128–139.

14. Gilbert, R.S., and H.A. Johnson. 1966. Stress fractures in military recruits: A review of 12 years' experiences. *Military Medicine* 131:716–721.

15. Gordon, E.J., 1981. Diagnosis and treatment of common hip disorders. *Medical Trauma Technology* 28(4):443.

16. Harvey, J. 1985. *Rehabilitation of the injured patient: Clinics in sports medicine.* Philadelphia: W. B. Saunders.

17. Hase, T. and T. Ueo. 1999. Acetabular labral tears: Arthroscopic diagnosis and treatment. *Arthroscopy* 15:138–141.

18. Hunter-Griffen, L., ed. 1987. *Overuse injuries: Clinics in sports medicine.* W. B. Saunders: Philadelphia.

19. Jaivin, J., and J. Fox. 1995. Thigh Injuries. In *The lower extremity and spine in sports medicine*, Nicholas, J., and E. Hershman, editors. Mosby: St. Louis.

20. Johnson, E.K., and C.M. Chiarello. 1997. The slump test: The effects of head and lower extremity position on knee extension. *J Orthop Sports Phys Ther* 26(6):310–317.

21. Kornberg, C., and P. Lew. 1989. The effect of stretching neural structures on grade one hamstring injuries. *J Orthop Sports Phys Ther* 10(12):481–487.

22. Kornberg, C., and T. McCarthy. 1992. The effect of neural stretching technique on sympathetic outflow to the lower limbs. *J Orthop Sports Phys Ther* 16(6):269–274.

23. Kuland, D.N. 1982. *The injured patient.* Philadelphia: Lippincott.

24. LeVangie, P., and L. Norkin. 2005. *Joint structure and function: A comprehensive analysis.* 4th ed. Philadelphia: F. A. Davis.

25. Lewinneck, G. 1980. The significance and comparison analysis of the epidemiology of hip fractures. *Clinical Orthopedics* 152:35.

26. Lewis, A. 1997. *Normal human locomotion.* Hamden, CT: Quinnipiac College.

27. Lipscomb, A.B. 1976. Treatment of myositis ossificans traumatic in patients. *Journal of Sports Medicine* 4:61.

28. Magee, D.J. 2007. *Orthopedic physical assessment.* Philadelphia: Elsevier Health Sciences

29. Major, N.M., and C.A. Helms. 1997. Pelvic stress injuries: the relationship between osteitis pubis (symphysis pubis stress injury) and sacroiliac abnormalities in patients. *Skeletal Radiol* 26(12):711–717.

30. Malone, T., et al. 1996. *Orthopedic and sports physical therapy.* St. Louis: Mosby.

31. Mbubaegbu, C.E., D. O'Doherty, and A. Shenolikar. 1998. Traumatic apophyseal avulsion of the greater trochanter: Case report and review of the literature. *Injury* 29(8):647–649.

32. Mendez, A., and R. Eyster. 1992. Displaced nonunion stress fracture of the femoral neck treated with internal fixation and bone graft. *American Journal of Sports Medicine* 20(2):220–223.

33. Meyers, W.C., et al. 2000. Management of severe lower abdominal or inguinal pain in high-performance patients. *American Journal of Sports Medicine* 28(1):2–8.

34. Moore, K.L. 1985. *Clinically oriented anatomy.* Baltimore: Williams & Wilkins.

35. Morelli, V., and V. Smith. 2001. Groin injuries in athletics. *Journal of the American Academy of Family Physicians* 2001(October).

36. Moul, J.L., and A. Leslie. 2001. Acetabulum labrum tear in a male collegiate soccer player: A case report. *NATA News from the Journal of Athletic Training* (October).

37. Nadkarni, J. 1991. Simultaneous anterior and posterior dislocation of the hip. *Journal of Postgraduate Education* 37(2):117–118.

38. Norkin, L., and P. LeVange. 1983. *Joint structure and function.* Philadelphia: F. A. Davis.

39. Orava, S., and U. Kujala. 1995. Rupture of the ischial origin of the hamstrings. *American Journal of Sports Medicine* 22(6):702–705.

40. Prentice, W.E. 2009. *Therapeutic Modalities in Sports Medicine and Athletic Training.* New York: McGraw-Hill.

41. Pruner, R., and C. Johnston. 1991. Avulsion fracture of the ischial tuberosity. *Pediatric Orthopedics* 13(3):357–358.

42. Romani, W.A., et al. 2007 Mechanisms and management of stress fractures in physically active persons. *J Athl Train* 37(3):306–314.

43. Ruwe, P.A., et al. 1992. Clinical determination of femoral anteversion: A comparison with established techniques. *J Bone Joint Surg Am* 74(6):820–830.

44. Ryan, J.B., et al. 1991. Quadriceps contusions: West Point update. *Am J Sports Med* 19(3):299–304.

45. Ryan, J., J. Wheeler, and W. Hopkinson. 1991. Quadriceps contusion: West Point Update. *American Journal of Sports Medicine* 19:299–303.

46. Sanders, B., and W. Nemeth. 1996. Hip and Thigh Injuries. In *Athletic injuries and Rehabilitation,* J. Zachazewski, D. Magee, and S. Quillen, eds. Philadelphia. W. B. Saunders:

47. Schlickewei, W., and B. Elsasser. 1993. Hip dislocation without fracture. *Injury* 24(1):27–31.

48. Sim, F., M. Rock, and S. Scott. 1995. Pelvis and hip injuries in patient: Anatomy and function. In *The lower extremity and spine in sports medicine,* J. Nicholas and E. Hershman, eds. Mosby: St. Louis.

49. Stanitski, C.L., J.H. McMaster, and P.E. Scranton. 1978. On the nature of stress fractures. *American Journal of Sports Medicine* 6:391–396.

50. Stevens, J. 1962. The incidence of osteoporosis in patients with femoral neck fractures. *Journal of Bone and Joint Surgery* 44:520.

51. Tinker, R. 1979. *Ramamurti's orthopaedics in primary care.* Baltimore: Williams & Wilkins.

52. Torg, J., J. Vegso, and P. Torg. 1987. *Rehabitation of athletic injuries: A guide to therapeutic exercise.* St. Louis: Mosby.

53. Turl, S.E., and K.P. George. 1998. Adverse neural tension: A factor in repetitive hamstring strain? *J Orthop Sports Phys Ther* 27(1):16–21.

54. Van den Bogert, A.J., L. Read, and B.M. Nigg. 1999. An analysis of hip joint loading during walking, running, and skiing. *Med Sci Sports Exerc* 31(1):131–142.

55. Verrall, G.M., et al. 2005. Hip joint range of motion reduction in sports-related chronic groin injury diagnosed as pubic bone stress injury. *J Sci Med Sport* 8(1):77–84.

56. Wieder, D. 1992. Treatment of traumatic myositis ossificans with acetic acid and iontophoresis. *Physical Therapy* 72:133–137.

57. Worrell, T. and D. Perrin. 1992. Hamstring muscle injury: The influence of strength, flexibility, warm up, and fatigue. *Journal of Orthopaedic and Sports Physical Therapy* 16:12–18.

58. Zelko, R.R. and B.F. DePalma. 1986. Stress fractures in patients: Diagnosis and treatment. Forum Medicus: Postgraduate Advances in Sports Medicine I–XI.

SOLUTIONS TO CLINICAL DECISION-MAKING EXERCISES

20-1 It is important to rule out a fracture and other internal organ injuries. The athletic trainer should refer the patient back to the team physician for a final diagnosis, possible oral anti-inflammatory medications, and/or injection. Pain management should begin with modalities such as ice and electric stimulation, as well as active ROM exercises (side bending). Ice and compression should be continued until full active ROM is accomplished and functional rehabilitation has begun. Upon return to football, the patient should wear protective padding.

20-2   The patient may be suffering from a severe spasm to the iliopsoas muscle. Having the patient lie supine on a treatment table with the leg and hip hanging over the end of the table with the hip in a passive extended stretch position may help eliminate or ease the spasm and acute pain. Pain management modalities (ice, electric stimulation, etc.) can be used with the passive stretching. Once pain has been managed, the patient should be directed in stretching and strengthening exercises, as well as a progression into running and jumping. The patient needs to know it could take 3 to 7 days or more before she will be able to begin running and jumping.

20-3   It is important for the athletic trainer to educate the patient as to which part of his hamstring has been injured biomechanically and how long it will take to rehabilitate. The athletic trainer should then communicate a clear timeline and progression of treatment and rehabilitation involving modalities, stretching, and strengthening, including open and closed chain strengthening exercises performed in a high-intensity manner. The patient should start modalities with 24-hour compression. A realistic functional rehabilitation timetable should be discussed with progression to full speed and return to sport. The patient should then be participating in a hamstring maintenance in-season program 1 or 2 days per week for injury prevention.

20-4   This patient should be referred to the team physician for follow-up to rule out abdominal pathologies, genitourinary abnormalities, hip disorders, and pelvic stress fractures. The team physician should then follow with diagnostic testing (X-ray, bone scan, MRI, etc). If all are negative, the athletic trainer should treat the injury as a chronic groin strain (and possibly osteitis pubis) and recommend a stretching and strengthening closed chain stabilization program. The team physician could also consider injection with anti-inflammatory medication. The athletic trainer should also recommend further modification of the patient's practice and conditioning program to the patient and coach.

20-5   It is important to perform a thorough low back, hip, and thigh evaluation to rule out disk injury, hip injury (eg, subluxation), and hamstring injury. Once those injuries are ruled out, the athletic trainer should provide pain management modalities for the first 3 to 5 days with rest. The athletic trainer should then progress the patient with pain-free stretching exercises and functional rehabilitation.

20-6   The patient should start modalities with 24-hour compression. As soon as the patient can tolerate it (around days 1 to 3), isometric quadriceps setting and pain-free active ROM lying supine with the knee bent over the end of a table, and lying prone should be started with ice. A clear progression of active ROM to pain-free passive stretching and strengthening with the hip in extension should be outlined for the patient. The goal should be full pain-free ROM with the hip extended and full functional rehabilitation to prepare the patient for sport participation.

Please see videos on the accompanying website at

www.healio.com/books/sportsmedvideos

CHAPTER 21

Rehabilitation of Knee Injuries

Darin A. Padua, PhD, ATC
Michelle C. Boling, PhD, LAT, ATC
William E. Prentice, PhD, PT, ATC, FNATA

After completion of this chapter, the athletic training student should be able to do the following:

- Review the functional anatomy and biomechanics associated with normal function of the knee joint.

- Assemble the various rehabilitative strengthening techniques for the knee, including both open and closed kinetic chain isotonic, plyometric, and isokinetic exercises.

- Identify the various techniques for regaining range of motion.

- Recognize exercises that may be used to reestablish neuromuscular control.

- Explain the rehabilitation progressions for various ligamentous and meniscal injuries.

- Discuss the role of jump-landing training in preventing knee injuries.

- Describe and explain the rationale for various treatment techniques in the management of injuries to the patellofemoral joint and the extensor mechanism.

FUNCTIONAL ANATOMY AND BIOMECHANICS

The knee is part of the kinetic chain and is directly affected by motions and forces occurring in and being transmitted from the foot, ankle, and lower leg. In turn, the knee must transmit forces to the thigh, hip, pelvis, and spine.[160] Abnormal forces that cannot be distributed must be absorbed by the tissues. In a closed kinetic chain (CKC), forces must be either transmitted to proximal segments or absorbed in a more distal joint. The inability of this closed system to dissipate these forces typically leads to a breakdown in some part of the system. Certainly, as part of the kinetic chain,

Prentice WE, ed.
Rehabilitation Techniques for Sports Medicine and Athletic Training (pp 639-709).
© 2015 SLACK Incorporated.

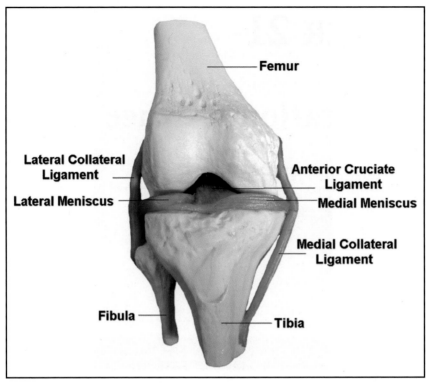

Figure 21-1. Anatomy of the knee, anterior view.

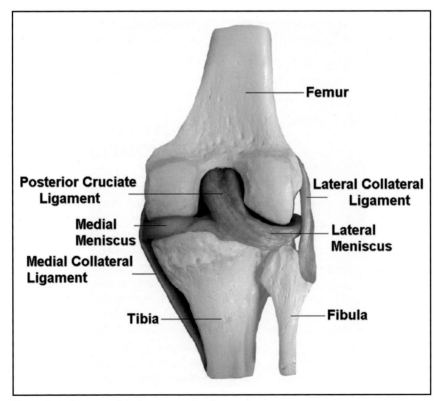

Figure 21-2. Anatomy of the knee, posterior view.

the knee joint is susceptible to injury resulting from absorption of these forces. The knee is commonly considered a hinge joint because its two principal movements are flexion and extension (Figures 21-1 and 21-2). However, the knee is capable of movement in six degrees of freedom—three rotations and three translations—thus the knee joint is truly not a hinge joint.[160] The stability of the knee joint depends primarily on the ligaments, the joint capsule, and muscles that surround the joint. The knee is designed primarily to provide stability in weight bearing and mobility in locomotion; however, it is especially unstable laterally and medially.

Movement between the tibia and the femur involves the physiological motions of flexion, extension, and rotation, as well as arthrokinematic motions including rolling and gliding. As the tibia extends on the femur, the tibia glides and rolls anteriorly. If the femur is extending on the tibia, gliding occurs in an anterior direction, whereas rolling occurs posteriorly. Axial rotation of the tibia relative to the femur is an important component of knee motion. In the "screw home" mechanism of the knee, as the knee extends, the tibia externally rotates. Rotation occurs because the medial femoral condyle is larger than the lateral femoral condyle. Thus, when weight bearing, the tibia must rotate externally to achieve full extension. The rotational component gives a great deal of stability to the knee in full extension. When weight bearing, the popliteus muscle must contract and externally rotate the femur to "unlock" the knee so that flexion can occur.

Collateral Ligaments

The medial collateral ligament (MCL) is divided into two parts, the stronger superficial portion and the thinner and weaker "deep" medial ligament or capsular ligament, with its accompanying attachment to the medial meniscus.[158] The superficial position of the MCL is separate from the deeper capsular ligament at the joint line. The posterior aspect of the ligament blends into the deep posterior capsular ligament and semimembranous muscle. Fibers of the semimembranous muscle go through the capsule and attach to the posterior aspect of the medial meniscus, pulling it backward during

knee flexion. The MCL functions as the primary static stabilizer against valgus stress. The MCL is taut at full extension and begins to relax between 15 to 20 degrees of flexion and comes under tension again at 60 to 70 degrees of flexion, although a portion of the ligament is taut throughout the range of motion (ROM).[8,82,158] Its major purpose is to prevent the knee from valgus and external rotating forces.

The medial collateral ligament was thought to be the principal stabilizer of the knee in a valgus position when combined with rotation. In the normal knee, valgus loading is greatest during the push-off phase of gait when the foot is planted and the tibia is externally rotated relative to the femur. It is now known that the anterior cruciate ligament (ACL) plays an equal or greater part in this function.[150] The lateral collateral ligament (LCL) is a round, fibrous cord about the size of a pencil. It is attached to the lateral epicondyle of the femur and to the head of the fibula. The LCL functions with the iliotibial band, the popliteous tendon, the arcuate ligament complex, and the biceps tendons to support the lateral aspect of the knee. The LCL is under constant tensile loading, and the thick, firm configuration of the ligament is well designed to withstand this constant stress.[82] The lateral collateral ligament is taut during knee extension but relaxed during flexion.

Clinical Decision-Making Exercise 21-1

A high school football player suffered an isolated grade 2 sprain of his MCL 3 days ago. At the emergency room, the X-ray result was negative and he was given a straight-leg immobilizer and crutches. He was instructed to begin walking after 1 week and return to play when the pain subsides. He has never before sustained a knee injury and is having difficulty regaining pain-free ROM. He has been referred to the athletic trainer in the local sports medicine clinic. What can the athletic trainer do to help increase ROM in the patient's injured leg?

Capsular Ligaments

The deep medial capsular ligament is divided into three parts: the anterior, medial, and posterior capsular ligaments. The anterior capsular ligament connects with the extensor mechanism and the medial meniscus through the coronary ligaments. It relaxes during knee extension and tightens during knee flexion. The primary purposes of the medial capsular ligaments are to attach the medial meniscus to the femur and to allow the tibia to move on the meniscus inferiorly. The posterior capsular ligament is called the posterior oblique ligament. It attaches to the posterior medial aspect of the meniscus and intersperses with the semimembranous muscle. Along with the MCL, the pes anserinus tendons, and the semimembranosus, the posterior oblique ligament reinforces the posteromedial joint capsule.

The arcuate ligament is formed by a thickening of the posteriorlateral capsule. Its posterior aspect attaches to the fascia of the popliteal muscle and the posterior horn of the lateral meniscus. This arcuate ligament and the iliotibial band, the popliteus, the biceps femoris, and the LCL reinforce the posteriorlateral joint capsule.

The iliotibial band becomes taut during both knee extension and flexion. The popliteal muscle stabilizes the knee during flexion and, when contracting, protects the lateral meniscus by pulling it posteriorly. The biceps femoris muscle also stabilizes the knee laterally by inserting into the fibular head, iliotibial band, and capsule.

Cruciate Ligaments

The ACL prevents the tibia from moving anteriorly during weight bearing, stabilizes the knee in full extension, and prevents hyperextension. It also stabilizes the tibia against excessive internal rotation and serves as a secondary restraint for valgus/varus stress with collateral ligament damage. The ACL works in conjunction with the thigh muscles, especially the hamstring muscle group, to stabilize the knee joint.

During extension, there is external rotation of the tibia during the last 15 degrees of the ACL unwinding. In full extension, the ACL is tightest, and it loosens during flexion. When the knee is fully extended, the posterolateral portion of the ACL is tight. In flexion, the posterolateral fibers loosen and the anteromedial fibers tighten.

Some portion of the posterior cruciate ligament is taut throughout the full ROM. As the femur glides on the tibia, the posterior cruciate ligament becomes taut and prevents further gliding. In general, the posterior cruciate ligament prevents excessive internal rotation. Hyperextension of the knee guides the knee in flexion and acts as a drag during the initial glide phase of flexion.

Menisci

The medial and lateral menisci function to improve the stability of the knee, increase shock absorption, and distribute weight over a larger surface area. The menisci help to stabilize the knee, specifically the medial meniscus, when the knee is flexed at 90 degrees. The menisci transmit one-half of the contact force in the medial compartment and an even higher percentage of the contact load in the lateral compartment.

During flexion the menisci move posteriorly, and during extension they move anteriorly, primarily due to attachments of the medial meniscus to the semimembranosus, and the lateral meniscus to the popliteus tendon. During internal rotation, the medial meniscus moves anteriorly relative to the medial tibial plateau, and the lateral meniscus moves posteriorly relative to the lateral tibial plateau. In internal rotation, the movements are reversed.

The Function of the Patella

Collectively, the quadriceps muscle group, the quadriceps tendon, the patella, and the patellar tendon, form the extensor mechanism. The patella aids the knee during extension by lengthening the lever arm of the quadriceps muscle. It distributes the compressive stresses on the femur by increasing the contact area between the patellar tendon and the femur.[128] It also protects the patellar tendon against friction. Tracking within this groove depends on the pull of the quadriceps muscle, patellar tendon, depth of the femoral condyles, and shape of the patella.

During full extension the patella lies slightly lateral and proximal to the trochlea. At 20 degrees of knee flexion, there is tibial rotation, and the patella moves into the trochlea. At

30 degrees the patella is most prominent. At 30 degrees and more, the patella moves deeper into the trochlea. At 90 degrees, the patella again becomes positioned laterally. When knee flexion is 135 degrees, the patella has moved laterally beyond the trochlea.[128]

Muscle Actions

For the knee to function properly, numerous muscles must work together in a highly complex and coordinated fashion. Knee movement requires various lower-extremity muscles to act as agonists, antagonists, synergists, stabilizers, and neutralizers, to act as force-couples to produce force, reduce force, and dynamically stabilize the knee.[29] Traditional rehabilitation has focused on uniplanar force production movements, yet athletic movement demands required multiplanar force with various muscular requirements. Following is a list of knee actions and the muscles that are involved in the agonist movement action, but athletic trainers also need to take into account the various muscle demands for proper movement production.

- Knee flexion is executed by the biceps femoris, semitendinous, semimembranous, gracilis, sartorius, gastrocnemius, popliteus, and plantaris muscles.

- Knee extension is executed by the quadriceps muscle of the thigh, consisting of three vasti—the vastus medialis, vastus lateralis, and vastus intermedius—and by the rectus femoris.

- External rotation of the tibia is controlled by the biceps femoris. The bony anatomy also produces external tibial rotation as the knee moves into extension.

- Internal rotation is accomplished by the popliteus, semitendinous, semimembranous, sartorius, and gracilis muscles. Rotation of the tibia is limited and can occur only when the knee is in a flexed position.

- The iliotibial band on the lateral side primarily functions as a dynamic lateral stabilizer and weak knee flexor.

REHABILITATION TECHNIQUES

Range of Motion Exercises

After injury to the knee, some loss of motion is likely. This loss can be caused by the effects of the injury, the trauma of surgery, or the effects of immobilization. Waiting for ligaments to heal completely is a luxury that cannot be afforded in an effective rehabilitation program. Ligaments do not heal completely for 18 to 24 months, yet periarticular tissue changes can begin within 4 to 6 weeks of immobilization.[80] This is marked histologically by a decrease in water content in collagen and by an increase in collagen crosslinkage.[80] The initiation of an early ROM program can minimize these harmful changes (Figures 21-3 through 21-17). Controlled movement should be initiated early in the recovery process and progress based on healing constraints and patient tolerance toward a normal range of about 0 to 130 degrees.

Pitfalls that can slow or prevent regaining normal ROM include imperfect surgical technique (improper placement of an anterior cruciate replacement), development of joint capsule or ligament contracture, and muscular resistance caused by pain.[55,80,90] The surgeon must address motion lost from technique, but the athletic trainer can successfully deal with motion lost from soft tissue contracture or muscular resistance.

To effectively alleviate lost motion, the cause of the limitation must be identified. An experienced athletic trainer can detect soft-tissue resistance to motion by the quality of the feel of the resistance at the end of the range. Muscular resistance, which restricts normal physiological movement, has a firm end feel and can best be treated by using proprioceptive neuromuscular facilitation (PNF) stretching techniques in combination with appropriate therapeutic modalities (heat, ice, electrical stimulation, etc).[131]

Strengthening Exercises

A primary goal in knee rehabilitation is the return of normal strength to the musculature

REHABILITATION EXERCISES

Stretching Techniques

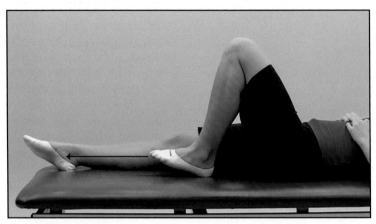

Figure 21-3. Active knee slides on table.

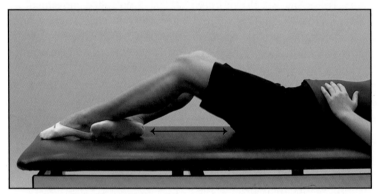

Figure 21-4. Active assistive knee slides use the good leg supporting the injured knee to regain flexion and extension.

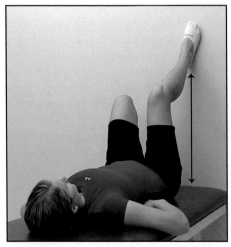

Figure 21-5. Wall slides are done to regain flexion and extension.

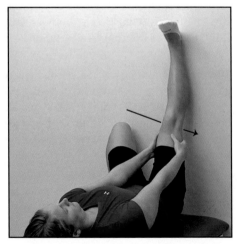

Figure 21-6. Active assistive knee slides on wall.

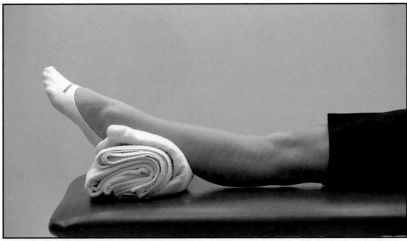

Figure 21-7. Knee extension with the foot supported on a rolled-up towel is used to regain knee extension.

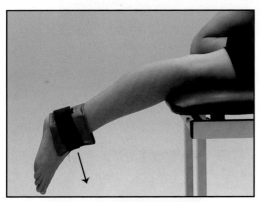

Figure 21-8. Knee extension in prone position with an ankle weight around the foot is used to regain extension.

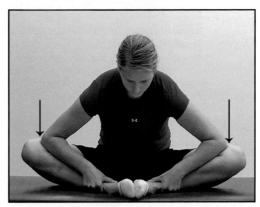

Figure 21-9. Groin stretch. Muscles: adductor magnus, longus, and brevis; pectineus; gracilis.

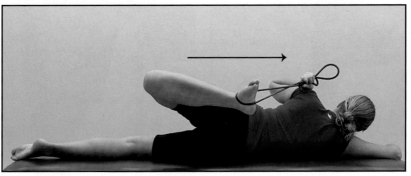

Figure 21-10. Side-lying knee extensor stretch using sport cord.

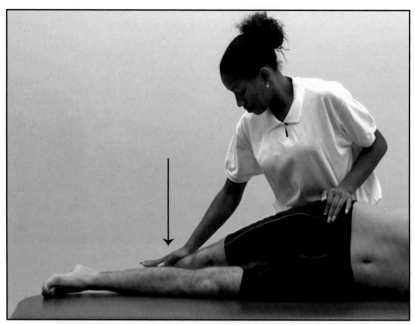

Figure 21-11. Iliotibial band stretch. The iliotibial band may be stretched in a variety of ways that use a scissoring position with extreme hip adduction. The major problem with these techniques is the lack of stabilization of the pelvis and therefore loss of stretch force transmission to the iliotibial band. To maximize the stretch, the pelvis must be manually stabilized to prevent lateral pelvic tilt. If the tensor fascia lata portion is tight, the hip should be flexed, abducted, extended, and adducted, in sequence, to position the tensor fascia lata fibers directly over the trochanter (rather than anterior to it) to produce maximal stretch.[9]

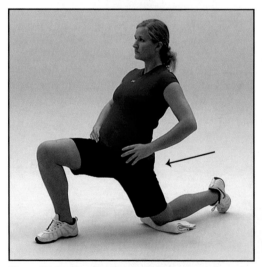

Figure 21-12. Kneeling thrusts. Muscles: rectus femoris.

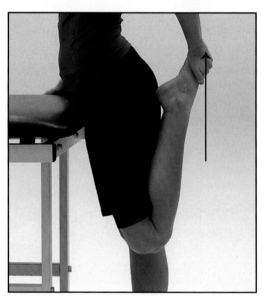

Figure 21-13. Standing knee extensors stretch. Muscles: quadriceps.

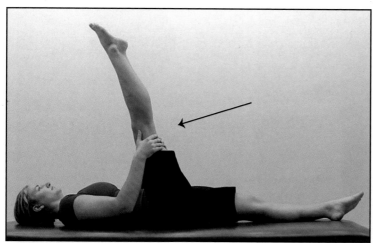

Figure 21-14. Knee flexor stretch. Muscles: hamstrings. Note: Externally rotated tibia stretches the semimembranous and semitendinous; internally rotated tibia stretches the biceps femoris.

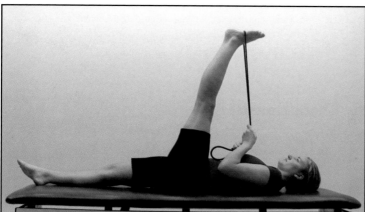

Figure 21-15. Knee flexor stretch using sport cord.

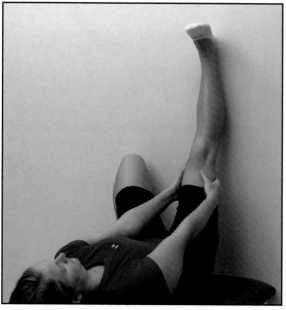

Figure 21-16. Knee flexor stretch against wall.

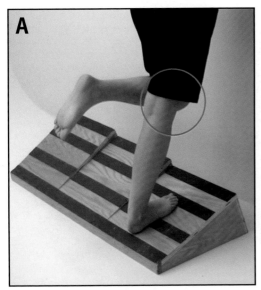 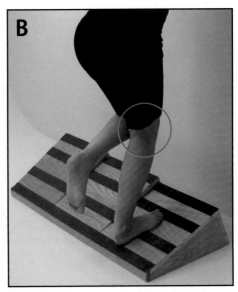

Figure 21-17. Ankle plantarflexors stretch. Muscles: (A) gastrocnemius, knee extended; (B), soleus, knee flexed.

Isotonic Open Kinetic Chain Exercises

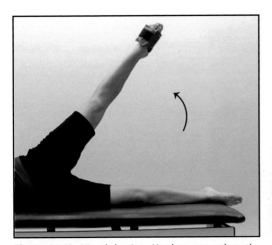 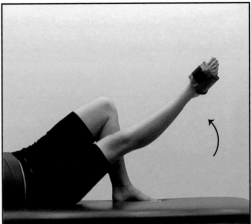

Figure 21-18. Hip abduction. Used to strengthen the gluteus medius and tensor fascia lata, which share a common tendon, the iliotibial band. The tensor fascia lata serves as a weak knee flexor and helps to provide stability laterally. Weight may be above knee as well.

Figure 21-19. Hip adduction. Used to strengthen the adductor magnus, longus, and brevis; pectineus, gracilis. The gracilis is the only one of the hip adductors to cross the knee joint. Weight placed above knee eliminates the gracilis.

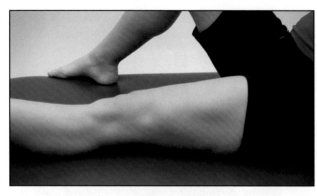

Figure 21-20. Quad sets are done isometrically with the knee in full extension to help the patient relearn how to contract the quadriceps following injury or surgery.

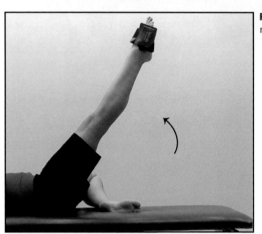

Figure 21-21. Straight leg raising is done early in the rehabilitation for active contraction of the quadriceps.

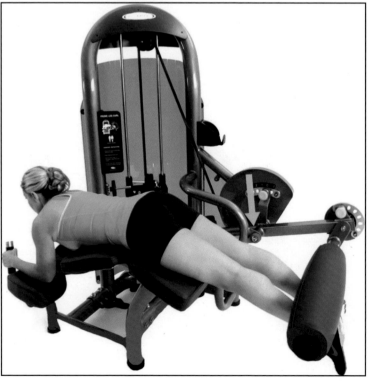

Figure 21-22. Knee flexion. Primary muscles: biceps femoris, semimembranous, semitendinous. Secondary muscles: gracilis, gastrocnemius, sartorius, popliteus. Note: Biceps femoris is best strengthened with tibia rotated externally; semimembranous and semitendinous muscles are best strengthened with tibia rotated internally. (Reprinted with permission from Matrix Fitness.)

Figure 21-23. Knee extension. Primary muscles: rectus femoris, vastus lateralis, vastus intermedialis, vastus medialis.

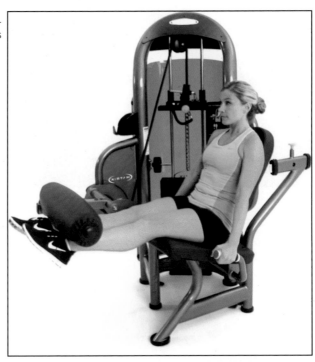

Closed Kinetic Chain Strengthening Exercises

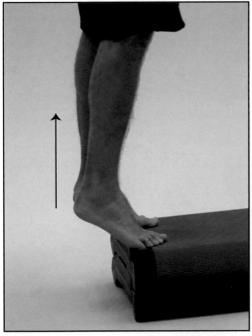

Figure 21-24. Ankle plantarflexion standing on box. Primary muscles: gastrocnemius and soleus.

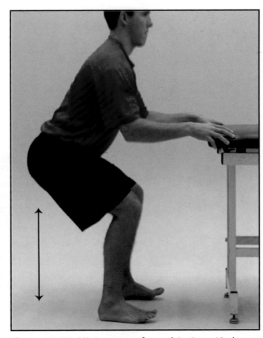

Figure 21-25. Minisquat performed in 0 to 40 degree range.

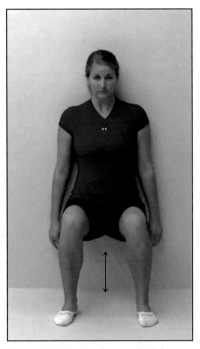

Figure 21-26. Standing wall slides are done to strengthen the quadriceps.

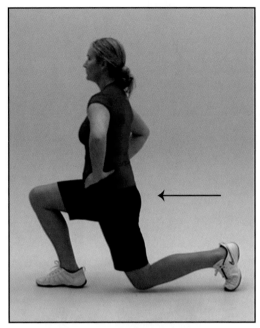

Figure 21-27. Lunges are done to strengthen quadriceps eccentrically.

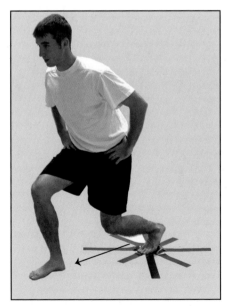

Figure 21-28. Lunges performed at different angles of the "clock face." Maintain a good squat position in each direction.

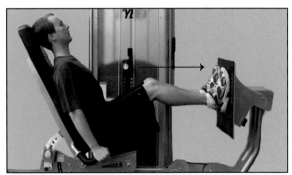

Figure 21-29. Leg-press exercise. The seat may be adjusted to whatever knee joint angle is appropriate. (Reprinted with permission from Reyes Fitness.)

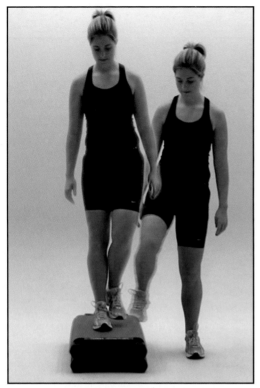

Figure 21-30. Lateral step-ups as well as forward step-ups may be done using different stepping heights. Retro step-downs should emphasize eccentric quadriceps control.

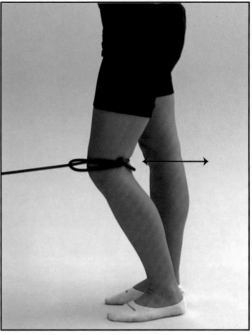

Figure 21-31. Terminal knee extensions using surgical tubing resistance for strengthening primarily the vastus medialis.

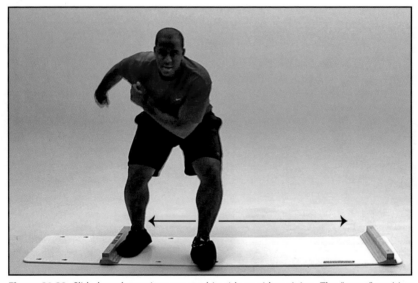

Figure 21-32. Slide board exercises are used in side-to-side training. The "squat" position should be emphasized.

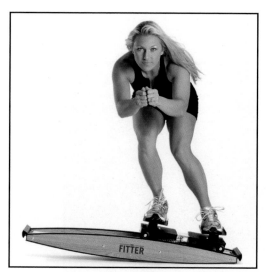

Figure 21-33. The Fitter is useful in side-to-side functional training. (Reprinted with permission from Fitter.)

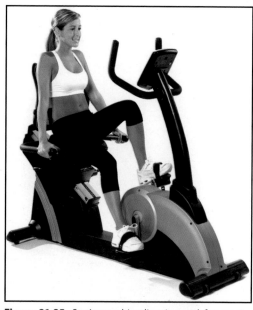

Figure 21-35. Stationary bicycling is good for regaining ROM, with seat adjusted to the appropriate height, and also for maintaining cardiorespiratory endurance. (Reprinted with permission from Smooth Fitness and Health.)

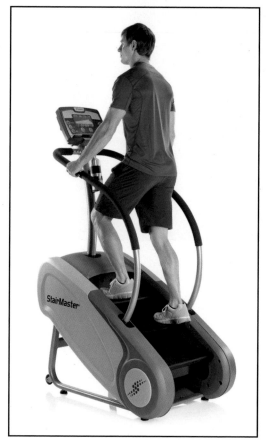

Figure 21-34. Stairmaster stepping machine allows the patient to maintain constant contact with the step. (Rerinted with permission from StairMaster.)

Plyometric Exercises

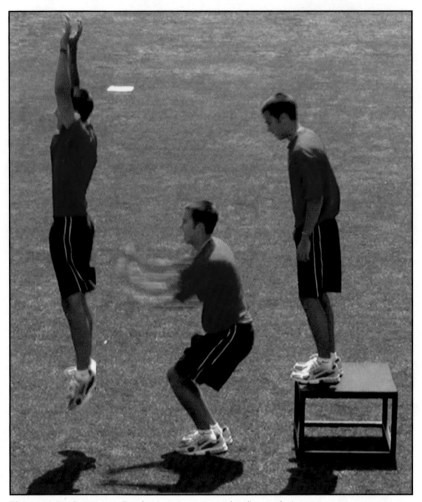

Figure 21-36. Box jumps. Emphasize proper jump-loading technique.

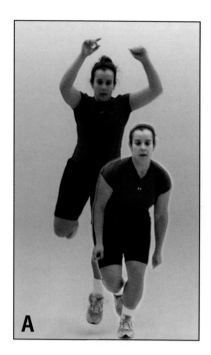

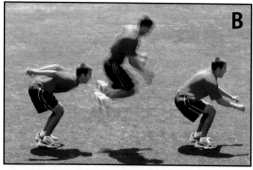

Figure 21-37. Jumping and bounding. (A) Single-leg; (B) double-leg bounding hops.

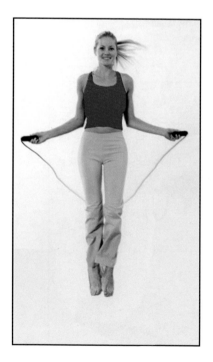

Figure 21-38. Rope skipping is a plyometric exercise that is also good for improving cardiorespiratory endurance.

Isokinetic Exercises

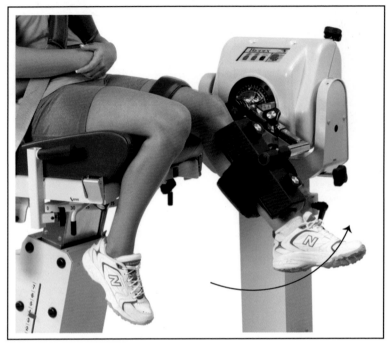

Figure 21-39. Knee extension set-up to strengthen the quadriceps. (Reprinted with permission from Biodex Medical Systems.)

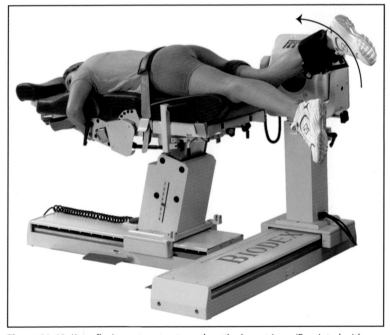

Figure 21-40. Knee flexion set-up to strengthen the hamstrings. (Reprinted with permission from Biodex Medical Systems.)

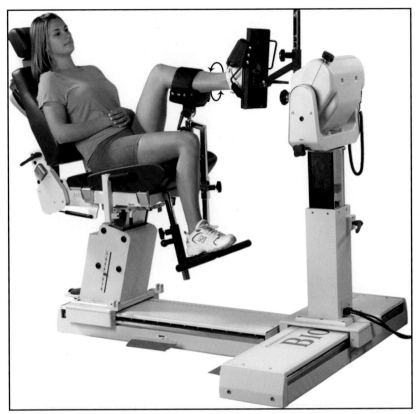

Figure 21-41. Tibial rotation is done with resistance at the ankle joint and is an extremely important, though often neglected, aspect of knee rehabilitation. (Reprinted with permission from Biodex Medical System.)

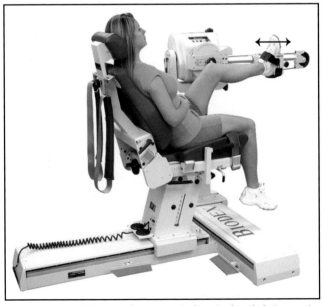

Figure 21-42. Biodex manufactures an isokinetic closed-chain exercise device. (Reprinted with permission from Biodex Medical Systems.)

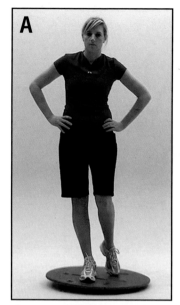

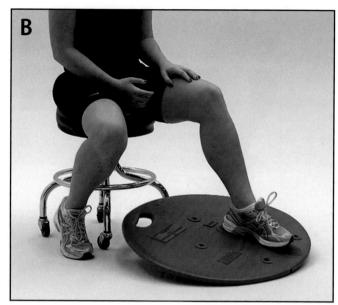

Figure 21-43. BAPS board exercise. (A) Standing; (B) sitting.

Exercises to Reestablish Neuromuscular Control

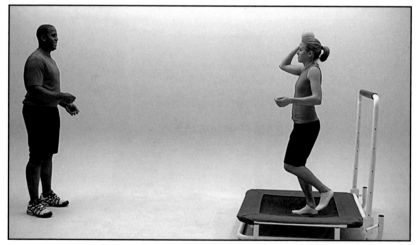

Figure 21-44. Minitramp provides an unstable base of support to which other functional plyometric activities may be added.

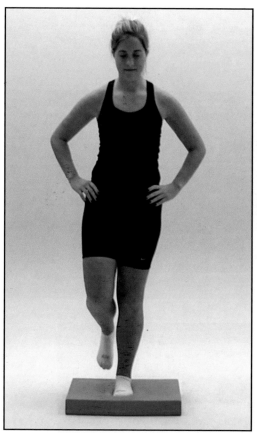

Figure 21-45. A foam pad is more cost-effective than a minitramp for providing an unstable surface.

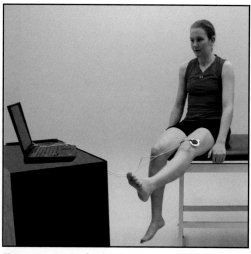

Figure 21-46. Biofeedback units can be used to help the patient learn how to fire a specific muscle or muscle group.

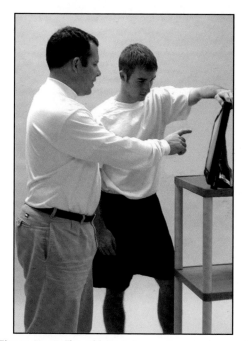

Figure 21-47. The athletic trainer can emphasize good technique with the aid of a video monitor.

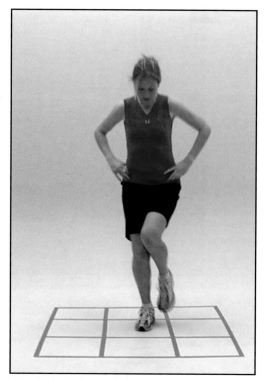

Figure 21-48. The single-leg Shark Skill Test is a useful exercise for functional neuromuscular training.

Figure 21-49. Speed and agility drills done on a high knee trainer or speed ladder are important components for functional activities prior to return to play. (Reprinted with permission from Perform Better, Cranston RI.)

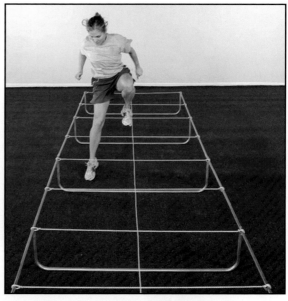

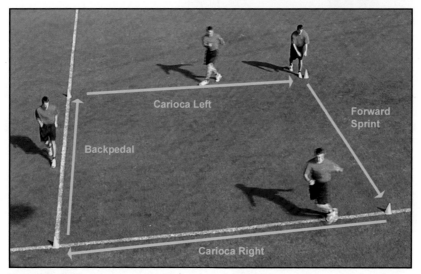

Figure 21-50. Running progression exercises demonstrating proper running technique should include directional changes and pivoting and cutting.

surrounding the knee. Along with the return of muscular strength, it is also important to improve muscular endurance and power.[135]

It is critically important to understand that strength will be gained only if the muscle is subjected to overload. However, it is also essential to remember that healing tissues can be further damaged by overloading the injured structure too aggressively. Especially during the early phases of rehabilitation, muscular overload needs to be carefully applied to protect the damaged structures. The recovering knee needs protection, and the high-resistance, low-repetition program designed to strengthen a healthy knee can compromise the integrity of the injured knee.[100] The strengthening phase of rehabilitation must be gently progressive and will generally progress from isometric to isotonic to isokinetic to plyometric to functional exercise.

For years, open kinetic chain exercises were the treatment of choice. However, more recently, closed kinetic chain exercises have been widely used and recommended in the rehabilitation of the injured knee. Closed kinetic chain exercises may be safely introduced early in the rehabilitation process for virtually all types of knee injury.[22,38,142,143,157] Closed kinetic chain activities may involve isometric, isotonic, plyometric, and even isokinetic techniques. For years, there has been debate over using open kinetic chain (OKC) vs closed kinetic chain (CKC) exercises for knee rehabilitation, especially with regard to ACL postsurgical rehabilitation.[47,146,156] Several biomechanical investigations have demonstrated that OKC exercises increase anterior tibial shear forces during isokinetic knee extension exercises, in contrast, CKC squat exercises decrease force production.[95] Research on knee muscle activity while performing OKC and CKC exercise experiments has shown that, overall, OKC exercises generate more rectus femoris activity and CKC exercises more vastus medialis and lateralis activity.[40] This suggests that OKC exercises may be better for patients with isolated rectus femoris weakness, and CKC exercise may be better for vasti musculature strengthening, particularly pathologies involving the patellofemoral joint. Tibiofemoral compressive forces also were reported to be greater in CKC exercises

than in OKC exercises, with the squat producing the most compressive force. Another biomechanical investigation[95] also supports these data and has shown that CKC exercises increase compressive forces and co-contraction, whereas OKC exercises at the same angles increase shear force and provide less co-contraction.

Current research has looked at both the force and the strain on the cruciate ligaments during common rehabilitation exercises. An investigation on ACL strain in vivo indicated increased ACL strain during CKC squat from 45 degrees to full extension. OKC knee extension demonstrated a similar pattern, producing ACL strain between 30 degrees and full extension.[12] Exercises producing the lowest ACL strain include mostly hamstring activity, quadriceps contraction at knee angles greater than 60 degrees, and isotonic knee flexion-extension angles between 35 and 90 degrees.[12] Patellofemoral force during isometric knee extension has been shown to be greatest near full extension. However, during dynamic OKC knee extension, maximum patellofemoral force occurs with 60 to 80 degrees of knee flexion.[40] This information suggests that dynamic knee extension exercises should be done at lower (0 to 60 degrees) or higher (80 to 90 degrees) knee ranges when patellofemoral stress is a primary concern.

CKC exercises may be best for preparing a patient for competition when dynamic stability and functional movement technique are vital to injury prevention. However, specific isolated contractions of certain muscles or muscle groups may demand the use of specific OKC muscle-strengthening exercises. Clinicians should take into consideration the most current biomechanical data to establish the appropriate exercise protocols for various knee ailments and stages of rehabilitation.

Clinical Decision-Making Exercise 21-2

A high school wrestler suffers from anterior knee pain. The patient has no history of previous knee problems and cannot recall any specific mechanism of injury. He complains of increased pain whenever pressure is applied to the tibial tubercle region and is having extreme difficulty finishing practice. How should the athletic trainer manage this condition?

Joint Mobilization Techniques

Joint capsule or ligamentous contractures have a leathery end feel and might not respond to conventional simple passive, active-assistive, and active motion exercises.[55] These contractures can limit the accessory motions of the joint, and until the accessory motions are restored, conventional exercises will not produce positive results. Accessory motions in the knee joint must occur between the patella and femur, the femur and tibia, and the tibia and fibula. Restriction in any or all of these accessory motions must be addressed early in the rehabilitation program.

Mobilization of a knee that is restricted by soft-tissue constraints may be accomplished by specifically applying graded oscillations to the restricted soft tissue as discussed in Chapter 13 (see Figures 13-55 through 13-61). In doing so, the athletic trainer is addressing a specific limiting structure rather than assaulting the entire joint with a "crank til you cry" technique. After the release of the soft-tissue contracture, accessory motion should improve, and so should physiological motion.

REHABILITATION TECHNIQUES FOR LIGAMENTOUS AND MENISCAL INJURIES

Medial Collateral Ligament Sprain

Pathomechanics

The MCL is the most commonly injured ligament in the knee.[113] About 65% of MCL sprains occur at the proximal insertion site on the femur. Individuals with proximal injuries tend to have more stiffness but less residual laxity than those with injuries nearer the tibial insertion. Tears of the medial meniscus are occasionally associated with grades 1 and 2 MCL sprains but almost never occur with grade 3 sprains.

Diagnosis of MCL sprains can usually be made by physical evaluation and do not generally require MRI. The grade of ligament injury is usually determined by the amount of joint laxity. In a grade 1 sprain, the MCL is tender due to microtears but has no increased laxity and there is a firm end point. A grade 2 sprain involves an incomplete tear with some increased laxity with valgus stress at 30 degrees of flexion and minimal laxity in full extension, yet there is still a firm end point. There is tenderness to palpation, hemorrhage, and pain on valgus stress test. A grade 3 sprain is a complete tear with significant laxity on valgus stress in full extension. No end point is evident, and pain is generally less than with grades 1 or 2. Significant laxity with valgus stress testing in full extension indicates injury to the medial joint capsule and to the cruciate ligaments.[75]

Injury Mechanism

An MCL sprain almost always occurs with contact from a laterally applied valgus force to the knee that is sufficient to exceed the strength of the ligament. This is especially true with grade 3 sprains. Very rarely, an MCL sprain can occur with noncontact and result in an isolated MCL tear. It has also been suggested that the majority of grade 2 sprains occur through indirect rotational forces associated with valgus movement of the knee.[142] The patient will usually explain that the knee was hit on the lateral side with the foot planted, and that there was immediate pain on the medial side of the knee that felt more like a "pulling" or "tearing" than a "pop." Swelling occurs immediately, and some ecchymosis likely will appear over the site of injury within 3 days.

Rehabilitation Concerns

Since the early 1990s, the treatment of MCL sprains has changed considerably. Typically grade 3 MCL sprains were treated surgically to repair the torn ligament and then immobilized for 6 weeks. However, several studies have demonstrated that treating patients with isolated MCL sprains nonoperatively with immobilization is as effective as treating them surgically, regardless of the grade of injury, the age of the patient, or the activity level.[74] This is especially true with isolated MCL tears where the ACL is intact.[2,152] Patients with a combined MCL-ACL injury will most likely have an ACL reconstruction without MCL repair, and this procedure appears to provide sufficient functional stability. Three conditions must be met for healing to occur at the MCL: (1) the ligament fibers must remain in continuity or within a well-vascularized soft-tissue bed; (2) there must be enough stress to stimulate and direct the healing process; and (3) there must be protection from harmful stresses.[158]

With grade 2 and 3 sprains, there will be some residual laxity because the ligament has been stretched, but this does not seem to have much effect on knee function. Patients with grade 1 and 2 sprains may be treated symptomatically and may be fully weight bearing as soon as tolerated. It is possible that a patient with a grade 1 and occasionally even a grade 2 sprain can continue to play. With grade 3 sprains, the patient should not be allowed to play and a rehabilitative brace should be worn for 4 to 6 weeks set from 0 to 90 degrees to control valgus stress (Figure 21-53).

Rehabilitation Progression

Initially, cold, compression, elevation, and electrical stimulation can be used to control swelling, inflammation, and pain. It may be necessary to have the patient on crutches initially, progressing to full weight bearing as soon as tolerated. The patient should use crutches until (1) full extension without an extension lag can be demonstrated; and (2) the patient can walk normally without gait deviation. For patient comfort, a knee immobilizer may be worn for a few days to a week following injury with grade 2 sprains requiring 7 to 14 days in either an immobilizer or a brace.

The patient with a grade 1 sprain can, on the second day following injury, begin quad sets (Figure 21-20) and straight leg raising (Figure 21-21). Early pain-free ROM exercises should be incorporated with grade 1 sprains, whereas grade 2 sprains may require 4 to 5 days for inflammation to subside. With grade 1 and 2 sprains, the patient may begin knee slides on a treatment table (Figure 21-3), wall slides (Figure 21-5), active assistive slides (Figure 21-4 and 21-6), or riding an exercise bike with the seat adjusted to the appropriate height to permit as much knee flexion as can be tolerated (Figure 21-35). As pain subsides and ROM improves, the patient may incorporate isotonic open chain flexion and extension

exercises (Figures 21-21 and 21-23), but the patient should concentrate on closed chain strengthening exercises, as tolerated, throughout the rehabilitation process (Figures 21-25 to 21-35). Functional PNF patterns stressing tibial rotation should be incorporated for strengthening, with resistance increasing as the patient becomes stronger (see Figures 14-14 through 14-21). As strength improves, the patient should engage in plyometric exercises (Figures 21-36 through 21-38) and functional activities to enhance the dynamic stability of the knee (see Chapter 16). With a grade 1, sprain the patient should be able to return to full activity in 3 to 5 weeks.

With a grade 3 sprain, the patient will be in a brace for 2 to 3 weeks with the brace locked from 0 to 45 degrees, and at 0 to 90 degrees for another 2 or 3 weeks, during which time isometric quad sets and SLR strengthening exercises may be performed as tolerated.[23] The patient should remain non-weight-bearing with crutches for 3 weeks. The strengthening program should progress as with grade 1 and 2 sprains, with return to activity at about 3 months.[23,149]

Criteria for Return

The patient may return to activity when (1) they have regained full ROM; (2) they have equal bilateral strength in knee flexion and extension; (3) there is no tenderness; and (4) they can successfully complete functional performance tests such as hopping, shuttle runs, carioca, and co-contraction tests.

Lateral Collateral Ligament Sprains

Pathomechanics

Fortunately, the lateral aspect of the knee is well supported by secondary stabilizers. Isolated injury to the LCL is rare in athletics, and when it does occur it is critical to rule out other ligamentous injuries.[142] Most LCL sprains in the athletic population result from a stress placed on the lateral aspect of the knee. Isolated sprain of the LCL is the least common of all knee ligament sprains.[113] LCL sprains result in disruption at the fibular head either with or without avulsion in about 75% of cases, with 20% occurring at the femur, and only 5% as mid-substance tears.[150] It is not uncommon to see associated injuries of the peroneal nerve, because the nerve courses around the head of the fibula. A complete disruption of the LCL often involves injury to the posterolateral joint capsule as well as the PCL and occasionally the ACL.[33,82,100]

The extent of laxity determines the severity of the injury. In a grade 1 sprain the LCL is tender due to microtears with some hemorrhage and tenderness to palpation. However, there is no increased laxity and there is a firm end point. A grade 2 sprain involves an incomplete tear with some increased laxity with varus stress at 30 degrees of flexion and minimal laxity in full extension, yet there is still a firm end point. There is tenderness to palpation, hemorrhage, and pain on a varus stress test. A grade 3 sprain is a complete tear with significant laxity on varus stress in 30 degrees of flexion and in full extension compared to the opposite knee. No end point is evident, and pain is generally less than with grades 1 or 2. Significant laxity with varus stress testing in full extension indicates injury to the posterolateral joint capsule, the PCL, and perhaps the ACL.

Injury Mechanism

An isolated LCL injury is almost always the result of a varus stress applied to the medial aspect of the knee. Occasionally a varus stress may occur during weight bearing when weight is shifted away from the side of injury, creating stress on the lateral structures.[79] Patients who sustain an LCL sprain will report that they heard or felt a "pop" and that there was immediate lateral pain. Swelling will be immediate and extra-articular with no joint effusion unless there is an associated menicus or capsular injury.

Rehabilitation Concerns

Patients with grade 1 and 2 sprains that exhibit stability to varus stress may be treated symptomatically and may be full weight bearing as soon as tolerated. For patient comfort a knee immobilizer may be worn for a few days to a week following injury. However, the use of a brace is not necessary. It is possible that a patient with a grade 1 and occasionally even a grade 2 sprain can continue to play. With grade

2 and 3 sprains, there will be some residual laxity, because the ligament has been stretched. Grade 3 sprains may be managed nonoperatively with bracing for 4 to 6 weeks limited to 0 to 90 degrees of motion. However, grade 3 MCL tears with associated ligamentous injuries that result in rotational instabilities are usually managed by surgical repair or reconstruction. This is certainly the case if the patient has chronic varus laxity and intends to continue participation in athletics, or if there is a displaced avulsion.

Rehabilitation Progression

The rehabilitation progression following LCL sprains should follow the same course as was previously described for MCL sprains. In the case of a grade 3 LCL sprain that involves multiple ligamentous injury with associated instability that is surgically repaired or reconstructed, the patient should be placed in a postoperative brace with partial weight bearing for 4 to 6 weeks. At 6 weeks, a rehabilitation program involving a carefully monitored, gradual, sport-specific functional progression should begin. In general, the patient may return to full activity at about 6 months.[79]

Criteria for Return

The patient may return to activity when (1) he or she has regained full ROM; (2) he or she has equal bilateral strength in knee flexion and extension; and (3) he or she can successfully complete functional performance tests such as hopping, shuttle runs, carioca, and co-contraction tests, as described in Chapter 16.

Anterior Cruciate Ligament Sprain

Pathomechanics

Injury to the ACL can significantly impair normal function of the knee complex. In simple terms, the ACL functions as a primary stabilizer to prevent anterior translation of the tibia on the fixed femur and posterior translation of the femur if the tibia is fixed as in a closed chain. Specific movement patterns directly influence the load and deformational forces on the ACL.[11,48,49,86,87,103] Anterior tibial shear force is the primary factor that contributes to increased ACL loading. Knee flexion angle greatly influences ACL loading as quadriceps contractions at low knee flexion angles (0 to 30 degrees) can generate significant anterior tibial shear forces that facilitate high levels of ACL loading.[6,12,34,37] Isolated knee valgus and tibial rotation also causes ACL loading, but the magnitude of ACL loading is smaller in comparison to isolated anterior tibial shear force.[103] However, when knee valgus and tibial rotation are applied in combination with each other or with anterior tibial shear force, the amount of ACL load is greatly magnified.[11,86,87,103]

The risk for ACL injury is greatest in younger individuals (eg, high school and college ages).[94] More ACL reconstruction procedures are performed for high school and college-age persons than for all other age groups combined.[139,165] The rate of ACL injury is typically greater in females than males, with most research indicating that recreational and competitive female athletes injure their ACL two to five times more than their male counterparts.[4,5,14,39,53,59,94,98,112] However, because males have greater exposure to sports and recreational activities than females, the absolute number of ACL injuries in males is greater than the absolute number in females in every age group except at age 15 years.[166] This apparent contradiction is, in fact, an established feature of the epidemiology of ACL injury.[2] Males account for the majority of injuries in the general population, but, when stratified by physical activity (ie, examining specific sports), females are consistently observed to be at higher risk.[4,5,14,39,53,59,94,98,112]

Tears of the ACL occur in the mid-substance of the ligament about 75% of the time, with 20% of the tears at the femur and 5% at the tibia.[54] As with MCL and LCL sprains, the severity of the injury is indicated by the degree of laxity or instability. A grade 1 sprain of the ACL results in partial microtears with some hemorrhage, but there is no increased laxity and there is a firm end point. A grade 2 sprain involves an incomplete tear with hemorrhage, some loss of function, and increased anterior translation, yet there is still a firm end point. A grade 2 sprain is painful, and pain increases with Lachman's and anterior drawer stress tests.

A grade 3 sprain is a complete tear with significant laxity with Lachman's and anterior drawer stress tests. There is also rotational instability as indicated by a positive pivot shift. No end point is evident. The patient will most often report feeling and hearing a "pop" and a feeling that the knee "gave out." There is significant pain initially, but pain decreases substantially within several minutes. With a complete ACL tear, insignificant hemarthrosis occurs within 1 to 2 hours.

The term *anterior cruciate deficient knee* refers to a grade 3 sprain in which there is a complete tear of the ACL. It is generally accepted that a torn ACL will not heal.[146] An ACL-deficient knee will exhibit rotational instability that may eventually cause functional disability in the patient. Additionally, rotational instability can lead to tears of the meniscus and subsequent degenerative changes in the joint.

Injury Mechanism

The ACL can be injured in several different ways, but non-contact injury mechanisms are most common. There has been considerable discussion on the specific mechanisms that are responsible for injury to the ACL.[56] To date there is no agreement on one single injury mechanism. However, there is agreement that the ACL may be injured either by direct contact or by a non-contact mechanism. Non-contact mechanisms are about 80% more likely to cause an ACL injury.[64]

It has become clear that a non-contact injury involves a combination of multiple plane forces collectively acting on the knee joint.[18,143] Most typically, the athlete is decelerating from a jump or forward running.[41,64,122] The foot contacts the ground with the heel, or in a flat-foot position, with little plantar flexion. Weight bearing creates an axial force with the knee near full extension and abducted or in knee valgus.[18] The axial and valgus forces in combination with a contraction of the quadriceps group, produces both an anterior shear and an internal rotation subluxation of the lateral tibia on the femur.[142] This position imposes a substantial strain on the ACL thus increasing its risk for injury. It should be added that while internal rotation creates greater loading forces on the ACL, external rotation has also produced tears of the ACL.[142]

Most recently it has become apparent the position of the hips also has a substantial impact on the incidence of ACL injury.[43] It appears that if the hip is adducted relative to the pelvis, the chances of ACL injury are significantly increased. Additionally, in ACL injuries the pelvis on the opposite (non-weight-bearing) side drops into a Trendelenberg position thus further increasing hip adduction on the weight bearing side and forcing the knee into a more varus position increasing the chance of ACL injury even further.[43]

In a contact injury, the athlete is decelerating and usually changing directions. The foot is planted on the ground with the knee abducted. There is contact from another athlete most often from lateral and posterior direction that forces the knee into a valgus and internally rotated position with anterior shear. Once again, in this position, the ACL is at risk for injury. A tear of the ACL and MCL, and possibly a detachment of the medial meniscus, was originally described by O'Donohue as the "unhappy triad."[117]

ACL Injury Risk Factors

Numerous risk factors for ACL injury have been presented in the literature.[4,59,60,71,78,88] Motivated by concern for the high incidence of anterior cruciate ligament injuries occurring in 15- to 25-year-old patients, the International Olympic Committee put forth a consensus statement in 2008 highlighting what is currently known regarding the increased incidence of noncontact ACL injuries in female athletes. The consensus of the Hunt Valley Conference was that ACL risk factors are multifactorial, with four distinct areas of risk factors: external, internal, hormonal, and biomechanical.

External Risk Factors

The external risk factors include type of competition (game vs practice), footwear and playing surface, protective equipment, and meteorological conditions. At present, there is no evidence to indicate that these factors influence noncontact ACL injury risk, but additional research is needed in this area.

Internal Risk Factors

The internal risk factors include anatomical factors. The conference decided that there was a great amount of information on femoral intercondylar notch size, ACL size, and lower-extremity anatomic alignment (eg, Q-angle, pronation, and tibial torsion) as they related to ACL injury. However, because of the difficulty of obtaining valid and reliable measurements, no consensus on their role in ACL injury could be reached.

Hormonal Risk Factors

A systematic review of literature investigated the effects of menstrual cycle phase on noncontact ACL injury risk.[65] The majority of studies showed an effect of the first half, or preovulatory phase, of the menstrual cycle for increased risk for sustaining noncontact ACL injuries. Clinically, these findings suggest that females may be more predisposed to noncontact ACL injuries during the preovulatory phase of the menstrual cycle.[65]

Biomechanical Risk Factors

The knee is only one part of the kinetic chain; therefore, the roles of the trunk, hip, and ankle may have importance to ACL injury risk. The conference agreed that common biomechanical factors in many ACL injuries include impact on the foot rather than the toes during landing or when changing directions while running, awkward body movements, and biomechanical perturbations prior to injury. The common at-risk situation for noncontact ACL injuries appears to be deceleration, which occurs when the patient pivots, changes direction, or lands from a jump. The group also noted that neuromuscular factors (eg, joint stiffness, muscle activation latencies, muscle recruitment patterns) are important contributors to the increased risk for ACL injuries in females and appear to be the most important reason for the differing ACL injury rates between males and females. The final factor stated was that strong quadriceps activation during eccentric contraction was considered to be a major factor in ACL injury.

ACL Injury Prevention Programs: Prehabilitation

Although current literature is mixed, the highest quality data support the efficacy of exercise-based injury prevention programs. In early 2006, Padua and Marshall published a systematic literature review that indicated there was moderate evidence supporting the efficacy of generalized exercise programs to decrease ACL and lower extremity injuries.[123] Nine papers met eligibility criteria,[25,62,64,85,99,114,119,144,155] though only three studies had sample sizes sufficient to draw a strong conclusion.[99,114,119] Each of these three studies showed exercise-based injury prevention programs to be effective. However, later in 2006 the results of a fourth large cohort study were published by Pfeiffer that showed no effect from an injury prevention training program.[127] A fifth injury prevention trial by Steffen was published in early 2008.[147] Each of these studies and a recent study by Gilchrist will be examined below. These five studies constitute the current evidence base for exercise-based injury-prevention programs.

In 2005, Mandelbaum et al investigated the effects of a plyometric-agility training program, PEP (Prevent injury, Enhance Performance), on ACL injury incidence. In a non-randomized cohort study involving 5,703 female soccer players ages 14 to 18 years, Mandelbaum demonstrated a dramatic 88% (Year 1) and 74% (Year 2) decrease in noncontact ACL injury in the intervention (n = 1885) vs the control (n = 3818) group.[99] The training program took about 20 minutes to complete and was to be performed prior to each soccer practice and game. The main weaknesses of this study were that patients were not randomly assigned to groups and compliance with the exercise program was not monitored. Despite these limitations, this research provides evidence to indicate that a preventive exercise intervention reduces the risk for injury in adolescents participating in soccer.

Additional research on exercise-based interventions has been performed in team handball players. Myklebust et al performed a non-randomized, phased-intervention cohort study using physical therapists to supervise and monitor compliance in female handball.[114] There was no overall difference in the incidence of ACL injuries between the control (n = 1705) and balance training groups (n = 942). However, elite division players who completed 15 sessions of balance training showed decreased ACL injury risk. Again in team handball, Olsen et al conducted a cluster-randomized, controlled

trial in adolescent male and female patients who performed a 20-minute injury-prevention program.[119] Over the course of one season, the intervention group (n = 958) experienced significantly fewer lower extremity injuries than the control group (n = 879). Compliance was not monitored. Although Myklebust and Olsen present evidence that exercise-based injury-prevention programs can reduce injury in handball patients, these results require generalization to sporting activities that are more common to U.S. and international patients (such as soccer and basketball).

A recent investigation by Gilchrist et al followed up the positive results of Mandelbaum and Olsen. Female soccer teams at 61 U.S. universities were randomized to receive training in the 20-minute PEP program or no program. Compliance was monitored by unannounced spot checks. Though Gilchrist's primary results have not yet been published, the work is cited in a recent review article as showing a 78% reduction in ACL injury rate.[52] This study contains many commendable features including randomization, compliance monitoring, and standardized exercise teaching methods. However, the study was performed in a relatively elite population served by a highly organized support staff of trainers and coaches. It is unclear if an injury-prevention program would have the same effect or even be feasible in a less structured setting, like a community youth soccer league. Intervening in younger, community-level patients is critical since there are many more patients and ACL injuries at the community level than on collegiate teams.

In contrast to the positive results of the above studies, Pfeiffer et al reported no effect on non-contact ACL injury rate from a 2-year, nonrandomized trial.[127] High school, female basketball, soccer, and volleyball patients (n = 577) performed a 20-minute program twice weekly. The control group consisted of 862 female patients from schools that did not wish to participate in the trial. Pfeifer reports three noncontact ACL injuries in each of the groups (total noncontact ACL injuries = 6) over 2 years—an injury rate substantially lower than previously reported data. This likely indicates incomplete injury surveillance, a serious threat to study validity in large trials of multiple teams. Exercise instruction and compliance with the program were not monitored. Finally, Pfeiffer's groups were not randomized. This null result may be the result of bias. Potentially, the teams that were more willing to adopt the intervention were more sensitized to the issue of sports injury, and thus were also better at reporting injuries to the researchers, thereby masking any potential intervention effect. Use of a randomized design, monitoring of intervention compliance, and validation of injury endpoints would have improved this study.

Also reporting negative results are Steffen, et al[147] Using a cluster-randomized design,[59] Norwegian youth soccer teams were given a 20-minute exercise-based injury prevention program while 54 teams were instructed to continue their usual warm-up pattern. No difference in ACL injury or all lower extremity injury rates were found. Compliance with the training routine was monitored and proved to be poor. Only 14 of the 59 teams in the intervention arm performed at least 20 sessions of the injury prevention exercises over a 7-month season.

Although there is conflicting evidence, the best designed studies support the beneficial effect of exercise-based injury prevention programs. However, many critical questions remain unanswered, prohibiting wide spread implementation of these programs.

Rehabilitation Concerns

After the diagnosis of injury to the ACL, the patient, the physician, the athletic trainer, and the patient's family are faced with various treatment options. The conservative approach is to allow the acute phase of the injury to pass and to then implement a vigorous rehabilitation program. If it becomes apparent that normal function cannot be recovered with rehabilitation, and if the knee remains unstable even with normal strengthening and hamstring retraining, then reconstructive surgery is considered. For a sedentary individual, this approach may be acceptable, but most patients prefer a more aggressive approach.

The older and more sedentary the individual, the less appropriate a reconstruction. This individual may not have the inclination or the time for an extensive rehabilitation program and may not be greatly inconvenienced by

some degree of knee instability. Conversely, the ideal patient is a young, motivated, and skilled patient who is willing to make the personal sacrifices necessary to successfully complete the rehabilitation process. Wilk and Andrews state that any active individual with a goal of returning to stressful pivoting activities should undergo surgical ACL reconstruction.[158] Thus, successful surgical repair/reconstruction of the ACL-deficient knee largely depends upon patient selection.[80] The following would be indications for deciding to surgically repair/reconstruct the injured knee:

- The ACL-injured individual is highly athletic
- The injured person is unwilling to change their active lifestyle
- There is rotational instability and a feeling of the knee "giving way" in normal activities
- There is injury to other ligaments and/or the menisci
- There are recurrent effusions
- There is failure at rehabilitation and instability after 6 months of intensive rehabilitation[80]
- Surgery is necessary to prevent the early onset of degenerative changes within the knee[82]

In the case of a partially torn ligament, the medical community is split on a treatment approach. Some feel that a partially damaged ACL is incompetent, and the knee should be viewed as if the ligament were completely gone. Others prefer a prolonged initial period of immobilization and limited motion, hoping that the ligament will heal and remain functional. Decisions to treat a patient nonoperatively should be based on the individual's preinjury status and willingness to engage only in activities such as jogging, swimming, or cycling that will not place the knee at high risk.[115] This is clearly a case where the patient may wisely seek several opinions before choosing the treatment course.

The most widely accepted opinion seems to be that when more than one major ligament is disrupted and there is functional disability, surgery is indicated. The surgical approach to ACL pathology is either repair or reconstruction. With a surgical repair, the damaged ligament is sutured if the tear is in the midsubstance of the ligament, or the bony fragment is reattached in the case of an avulsion injury. However, it is generally felt that direct repair of an isolated ACL tear will tend to have a poor result.[1] In the case of suturing, the repair may be augmented with an internal splint or an extra-articular reconstruction, which seems to be more successful than a direct repair.[137]

Surgical reconstruction is performed using either an extra-articular or an intra-articular technique. An extra-articular reconstruction involves taking a structure that lies outside of the joint capsule and moving it so that it can affect the mechanics of the knee in a manner that mimics normal ACL function. The iliotibial band is the most commonly used structure. This procedure is effective in reducing the pivot shift phenomena that is found in anterolateral rotational instability but cannot match the normal biomechanics of the ACL.[80,100] Isolated extra-articular reconstructions can be effective in patients with mild to moderate instability. Also it may be the treatment of choice in patients who cannot afford the commitment of time and resources for an intra-articular reconstruction.[80] The rehabilitation after an extra-articular reconstruction is aggressive and permits an earlier return to functional activities, but as an isolated procedure it is not recommended for high-level patients.

Intra-articular reconstruction involves placing a structure within the knee that will roughly follow the course of the ACL and will functionally replace the ACL. Techniques for reconstructive surgery for the ACL continue to evolve and the choice of a particular technique is most often based on the surgeon's preference and expertise. Currently there appear to be at least four primary surgical techniques that use autografts for reconstructing a torn ACL.

A bone-patellar tendon-bone graft uses the central one-third of the patellar tendon. Since the mid 1980s it has been the "gold standard" choice for the majority of surgeons because of an excellent surgical outcome success rate of 90% to 95%.[38,43,80,135,157]

A hamstring tendon graft uses the tendons of either the semitendinosus, the gracilis, or both.[81] As graft fixation techniques and hardware have improved, so has the popularity of this technique. Although it is generally considered to be a more technically difficult surgery, it requires a smaller incision, and there is less anterior pain and quadriceps atrophy than with a patellar tendon graft. However a hamstring tendon graft technique involves soft tissue to bone healing, which occurs at a significantly slower rate than bone to bone healing following a patellar tendon graft. Currently, there does not appear to be any strong evidence to suggest that either technique is superior in terms of outcomes.

A third, less widely used technique, uses a graft from the quadriceps tendon just above the patella that has bone on one end and soft tissue on the other. There seems to be less chance of patellar tendinitis and kneeling pain associated with quadriceps tendon grafts. They are often used for revision ACL surgeries.

Allografts can use patellar, hamstring or Achilles tendons and are used more often in revisions when an autograft has already be used. But most surgeons prefer to use an autograft for an initial reconstruction. Allografts take longer to heal than autografts, but recovery from surgery is quicker because of less pain and tissue healing from not having to harvest the patient's own tissue. The main problems with allografts are disease transmission and rejection of the tissue. It has been demonstrated that at 6 months post surgery, allografts show a prolonged inflammatory response and a more significant decrease in their structural properties.[81] Rehabilitation following an allograft reconstruction should be less aggressive than with an autograft reconstruction.[79]

Procedures that use synthetic replacements have generally not produced favorable results.

Surgical technique is crucial to a successful outcome. Improper placement of the tendon graft by only a few millimeters can prevent the return of normal motion.

In cases where there is reconstruction of the ACL along with a repair of a torn meniscus, the time required for rehabilitation will be slightly longer. This will be discussed in detail in the section on meniscal injury.

Rehabilitation Progression

Nonoperative Rehabilitation

If the ACL-deficient knee is to be treated nonoperatively, it is critical to rule out any other existing problems (torn meniscus, loose bodies, etc) and correct those problems before proceeding with rehabilitation.[115] Initial treatment should involve controlling swelling, pain, and inflammation through the use of cold, compression, and electrical stimulation. If necessary, the knee can be placed in an immobilizer for the first few days for comfort and minimal protection, with the patient ambulating on crutches until they regain full extension and can walk without an extension lag. The patient can begin immediately following injury with quad sets (Figure 21-20) and straight leg-raising (Figure 21-21) to regain motor control and minimize atrophy. Early pain-free ROM exercises using knee slides on a treatment table (Figure 21-3), wall slides (Figure 21-5), active assistive slides (Figures 21-4 and 21-6), or riding an exercise bike with the seat adjusted to the appropriate height to permit as much knee flexion as can be tolerated (Figure 21-35).

As pain subsides and ROM improves, the patient may incorporate isotonic open chain flexion and extension exercises (Figures 21-22 and 21-23). With open chain strengthening exercises, it has been recommended that extension be restricted initially to 0 to 45 degrees for as long as 8 to 12 weeks (6 to 9 weeks being a minimum) to minimize stress on the ACL.[115] Strengthening exercises should be emphasized for both the hamstrings and the gastrocnemius muscles (Figure 21-24), which act to translate the tibia posteriorly, minimizing anterior translation. Closed chain strengthening exercises (Figures 21-25 through 21-35) are thought to be safer because they minimize anterior translation of the tibia. Closed chain exercises are used to regain neuromuscular control by enhancing dynamic stabilization through co-contraction of the hamstrings and quadriceps (Figures 21-43 through 21-46). Closed chain exercises also minimize the possibility of developing patellofemoral pain. A goal of these strengthening exercises should be to achieve a quadriceps/hamstring strength ratio of 1 to 1.

It is important to incorporate PNF strengthening patterns that stress tibial rotation (see Figures 14-14 through 14-21). These manually resisted PNF patterns are essentially the only way to concentrate on strengthening the rotational component of knee motion, which is essential to normal function of the knee. Unfortunately many of the more widely known and used rehabilitation protocols fail to address this critical rotational component.

Perturbation training may be particularly important for those with an ACL-deficient knee. Perturbation training is a type of neuromuscular exercise focused on improving knee stability and involves the manipulation of an unstable support surface while the patient maintains his or her balance.[72] The inclusion of perturbation training should be performed in combination with the other types of exercises described above to facilitate strength, cardiorespiratory endurance, and agility.

Perturbation training includes three conditions: rollerboard, rockerboard, and rollerboard with block. The use of verbal cues such as "keep your knee soft," "keep your trunk still," and "relax between perturbations" are commonly employed during perturbation training to direct patients on successful completion of the tasks and further enhance neuromuscular control. The perturbation training program should be progressive in nature. Hurd et al describe the phasic and progressive nature of perturbation training as follows.[72] During the early phase of training, the patient should be exposed to perturbations in all directions. The patient is provided minimal verbal cues as they explore to develop the appropriate neuromuscular response patterns to the perturbations without creating a rigid co-contraction of knee musculature. During the middle phase, the addition of light sport-specific activity can be employed during perturbation training. During this phase, the patient should develop improved accuracy in using appropriate neuromuscular responses to the applied perturbation intensity, direction, and speed. In the final or late phase of perturbation training, the difficulty of perturbations is enhanced by using sport-specific stances. Focus should be on obtaining accurate, selective muscular responses to the applied

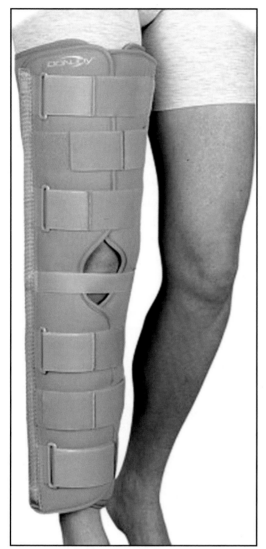

Figure 21-51. A knee immobilizer can be used for comfort following injury. (Reprinted with permission from DonJoy.)

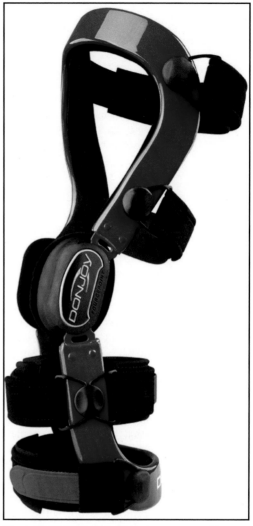

Figure 21-52. A functional knee brace can provide some protection to the injured knee. (Reprinted with permission from Bledsoe.)

perturbations in any of the applied directions and of any intensity magnitude or speed.

The use of functional knee braces for a patient with either a partial ACL tear or an ACL-deficient knee is controversial (Figure 21-52). These braces have not been shown to control translation, especially at functional loads.[15,131] However, there may be some benefit in terms of increased joint position sense, through stimulation of cutaneous sensory receptors, that may enhance both conscious and subconscious awareness of the existing injury.[93]

It is incumbent on the athletic trainer to counsel the patient with regard to the precautions that must be exercised when engaging in physical activity with an ACL-deficient knee. Nonoperative treatment is appropriate for an individual who does not plan on engaging in the types of activities that can potentially create stresses that can further damage the supporting structures of that joint. If the patient is not willing to make lifestyle changes relative to those activities, then surgical intervention may be a better treatment alternative.

Surgical Reconstruction

There is great debate as to the course of rehabilitation following ACL reconstruction. Traditionally, rehabilitation has been conservative, and there are a great number of physicians and athletic trainers who maintain this basic traditional philosophy.[35,126] However, in recent years, the trend has been to become more aggressive in rehabilitation of the reconstructed ACL, primarily as a result of the reports of success by Shelbourne and Nitz.[141] This has been referred to as an accelerated protocol. They have demonstrated that this program returning the patient to normal function early results in fewer patellofemoral problems, and reduces the number of surgeries to obtain extension, all without compromising stability.[143] The accelerated rehabilitation protocol is not without its detractors. Some clinicians feel that it places too much stress on vulnerable tissues and that there are not sufficient scientific data to justify the protocol.[43,116,125,157]

There is now such a variety of accelerated and nonaccelerated programs that the difference between "traditional" and "accelerated" has been blurred. Depending on the injury, many factors—such as type of patient, time of athletic season—have been driving the rehabilitation process to a greater extent than science-based outcomes. More studies need to be conducted to better predict the ideal rehabilitation protocol, yet individual differences may never allow for a single protocol to be used for all patients.

The traditional protocol emphasizes the following:

- Slow progression to regain flexion and extension
- Partial- or non-weight bearing postoperatively
- Closed chain exercises at 3 to 4 weeks postoperatively
- Return to activity at 6 to 9 months[35,43,157]

The accelerated protocol emphasizes the following:

- Immediate motion, including full extension
- Immediate weight bearing within tolerance
- Early closed chain exercise for strengthening and neuromuscular control
- Return to activity at 2 months and to competition at 5 to 6 months[143]

Preoperative period. Regardless of the various recommended time frames for rehabilitation, the rehabilitative process begins immediately following injury in what has been referred to as the preoperative phase. There is general agreement that surgical reconstruction be delayed until pain, swelling, and inflammation have subsided and ROM, quadriceps muscle control, and a normal gait pattern have been regained during this preoperative phase. This appears to occur at about 2 to 3 weeks post injury.[61] It also appears that delaying surgery decreases the incidence of postoperative arthrofibrosis.[139]

Postoperative period. Perhaps the single most important rehabilitation consideration postoperatively has to do with the initial strength of the graft and how the graft heals and matures. It has been demonstrated that the tensile strength of a 10 mm central third patellar tendon graft is about 107% of the normal ACL initially, and it has been predicted that the strength is at 57% at 3 months, 56% at 6 months, and 87% at 9 months.[18] Stress on the graft should be minimized during the period of graft necrosis (6 weeks), revascularization (8 to 16 weeks), and remodeling (16 weeks).[157] Assuming that the surgical technique for reconstruction is technically sound, the graft is at its strongest immediately following surgery, so rehabilitation can be very aggressive early in the process. Also it appears that an aggressive rehabilitation program minimizes complications and maximizes restoration of function following ACL reconstruction.[79]

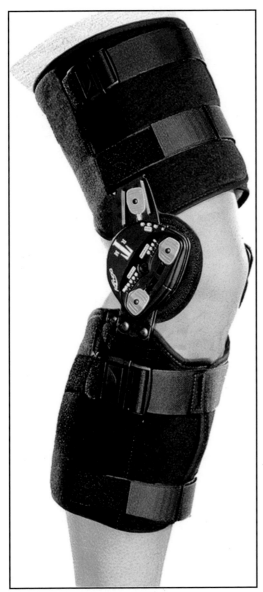

Figure 21-53. In a rehabilitative brace the range of movement can be restricted and changed whenever appropriate. (Reprinted with permission from DonJoy.)

A two-part systematic literature review focused on randomized controlled trials in ACL reconstruction rehabilitation has been published and helps to summarize the evidence in this area.[163,164]

Controlling swelling. Immediately following surgery, the goal is to minimize pain and swelling by using cold, compression, and electrical stimulation. A Cryo-cuff is widely used for this purpose. Significant swelling can initially inhibit firing of the quadriceps.

Bracing. The patient is placed in a rehabilitative brace and most often locked in either full extension,[100] or 0 to 90 degrees passive with 40 to 90 degrees active ROM, for the first 2 weeks (Figure 21-53). The brace will be worn for 4 to 6 weeks, or until knee flexion exceeds the limits of the brace, and may be removed for exercise and for bathing. Shelbourne and Nitz recommend that a knee immobilizer be used for the first 2 weeks but that at the end of the first week the patient be fitted for a functional brace, which should be worn for protection throughout the rehabilitation process.[143] No studies have shown adverse outcomes when wearing a brace. However, only one study has shown a potentially clinically meaningful finding by reporting improved knee extension following locking the brace in full extension during the first postoperative week.[110] Based on this body of evidence there does not appear to be a general consensus as to the value of wearing a functional brace during return to activity. This decision should be made on an individual basis.

Weight bearing. Generally the patient is placed on crutches either with 50% weight bearing,[125] or progressed to full weight bearing as tolerated[143] for the first 2 weeks. The patient can get off the crutches when there is minimal swelling, no extension lag, and sufficient quadriceps strength to allow for nearly normal gait. This may take anywhere from 2 to 6 weeks. In a study comparing immediate weight bearing as tolerated vs a 2-week delay, it was shown that no deleterious effects were observed for knee stability or function and the development of anterior knee pain might be less by facilitating earlier recruitment of the vastus medialis oblique when weight bearing early.

Range of motion. ROM exercises can begin immediately. Some clinicians advocate the judicious use of continuous passive motion (CPM) machines that may be applied immediately after surgery (Figure 21-54),[105,116,118,136] whereas others prefer that the patient engage in active ROM exercises as soon as possible (Figures 21-3 through 21-8). Based on the findings of the systematic literature review there does not appear to be a major benefit for CPM, except for possible decreases in pain.[163] Thus, future research is needed to investigate this area to justify the costs associated with CPM.

In their accelerated rehabilitation program, Shelbourne and Nitz emphasize the importance of early restoration of full knee extension.[141] Full extension can be achieved using knee extension on a rolled-up towel (Figure 21-7) or prone leg hangs (Figure 21-8). Exercises to maintain full extension should be emphasized throughout the rehabilitation process. Active knee extension should be limited to 60 to 90 degrees to minimize anterior tibial translation, whereas knee flexion should reach 90 degrees by the end of the second week. Full flexion (135 degrees) should be achieved at 5 to 6 weeks. Once knee flexion reaches 100 to 110 degrees, the patient may begin stationary cycling to help with regaining ROM (Figure 23-35).

During the second week, the athletic trainer should teach the patient self-mobilization techniques for the patella (see Figure 13-58). Restriction of patellar motion can interfere with regaining both flexion and extension. The grade of mobilization used should be based on the degree of inflammation, and should avoid creating additional pain and swelling.[131]

Strengthening. Initially, strengthening exercises should avoid placing high levels of stress on the graft. Quad sets (Figure 21-20) and straight leg raises (Figure 21-21) using co-contraction of the hamstrings should begin immediately to prevent shutdown of the quadriceps. Progressive resistive exercise can begin during the second week for hamstrings (Figure 21-21), hip adductors (Figure 21-19), hip abductors (Figure 21-18), and gastrocnemius muscles (Figure 21-24). Strengthening exercises for all of these muscle groups, particularly emphasizing strengthening of the hamstrings, should continue throughout rehabilitation.

The rationale and biomechanical advantages for using closed kinetic chain strengthening exercises in the rehabilitation of various knee injuries was discussed in detail in Chapter 12. In relation to ACL reconstruction rehabilitation, the use of closed kinetic chain exercises seems promising when considering that closed kinetic chain exercises may achieve the following: (1) promote normal muscle activation and co-activation; (2) maintain and promote muscle strength and endurance; (3) provide sensory feedback; (4) increase quadriceps activation

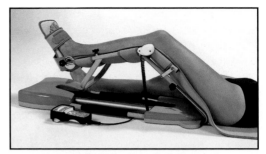

Figure 21-54. A CPM device may be used to help regain ROM.

without increasing ACL strain on reconstructed limb; (5) provide benefit of functional specificity of training; and (6) induce stronger contractions within the hamstring muscles, which may promote knee joint stability.[58]

When using the different closed kinetic chain exercises, it is essential to emphasize co-contraction of the hamstrings, both to stabilize the knee and to provide a posterior translational force to counteract the anterior shear force created by the quadriceps during knee extension. Once flexion reaches 90 degrees, which should generally be in 1 to 2 weeks, the patient can begin closed kinetic chain mini squats in the 40- to 90-degree range (Figure 21-25), lateral step-ups (Figure 21-30), standing wall slides (Figure 21-26) or leg presses (Figure 21-29).

Open kinetic chain quadriceps strengthening exercises should be completely avoided in the early stages of rehabilitation, due to the anterior shear forces, which are greatest from 30 degrees of flexion to full extension. However, at some point in the later stages of rehabilitation, open kinetic chain quadriceps strengthening exercises may be safely incorporated (Figure 21-23).

It should be reemphasized that the graft is at its weakest between weeks 8 to 14, during the period of revascularization. Therefore caution should be exercised relative to strengthening exercises during this period. The accelerated program has recommended that isokinetic testing begin at about 2 months. Other programs recommend that testing be delayed until 4 or 5 months. This should be done only using an antishear device with a 20-degree terminal extension block.[60,99] Isokinetic strengthening exercises may be safely incorporated at about 4 months (Figures 21-39 to 21-42). PNF strengthening patterns that stress tibial rotation may also be used. These manually resisted PNF patterns are essentially the only way to concentrate on strengthening the rotational component of knee motion, which is essential to normal function of the knee. Because the PNF patterns are done in an open kinetic chain, they should involve only active contraction through the functional movement pattern. Progressively resisted patterns can be used beginning at about 5 months (see Figures 14-14 through 14-21).

Reestablishing neuromuscular control. Along with the early controlled weight-bearing and closed chain exercises that act to stimulate muscle and joint mechanoreceptors, seated BAPS board exercises to reestablish balance and neuromuscular control should also begin early in the rehabilitation process (Figure 21-43B). Balance training using a standing BAPS board (Figure 21-43A), and lateral shifting for strengthening and agility using the Fitter (Figure 21-33), may be incorporated at 6 weeks.

Cardiorespiratory endurance. Cycling on an upper-extremity ergometer may begin during the first week. Cycling on a stationary bike can begin as early as possible when the patient achieves about 100 to 110 degrees of flexion (Figure 21-35). Walking with full weight bearing on a treadmill can usually begin at about 3 weeks, using forward walking initially then progressing to retro walking. Swimming is considered to be a safe activity at 4 to 5 weeks. Stair climbing (Figure 21-34) or cross-country skiing can begin as early as week 6 or 7. Recommendations for progressing to jogging/running are as early as 4 months in the accelerated program but are more often closer to 6 months.

Functional training. Functional training should progressively incorporate the stresses, strains, and forces that occur during normal running, jumping, and pivoting activities in a controlled environment (Figures 21-49 and 21-50).[23,41] Exercises such as single- and double-leg hopping, carioca, shuttle runs, vertical jumping, rope skipping, and co-contraction activities, most of which were described in Chapter 16, should be incorporated. In the more traditional programs these activities may begin at about 4 months, although in the accelerated program they may begin as early as 5 or 6 weeks.

Movement Technique Assessment. Throughout the rehabilitation process the athletic trainer should be evaluating movement technique to discern if any compensations or problems exist. One current theory attributes increased risk for ACL injury to the biomechanical technique patterns used by individuals when running, pivoting, and jump-landing.[89,121] Prior to return to play and throughout the rehabilitation process, motion analysis of the injured patient's movements should be monitored (Figure 21-47). It has been shown that video replay feedback can help teach the patient proper jump-landing technique and reduce possible deleterious forces.[108,122,130] Performance tests are vital to assess the injured patient's ability to regain movement times, but analysis of how the performance was conducted is also vital in preventing reinjury or compensatory problems. If poor technique previously existed or poor compensatory techniques have been developed, then the predisposition for injury remains and the athletic trainer has missed a critical final step of the rehabilitation process. The following movement tasks may be used to systematically evaluate for the presence of movement impairments: double leg squats, single leg squats, and jump-landings.[9,67] The clinician should look for the presence of the following movement impairments: decreased knee flexion, decreased hip flexion, increased knee valgus, inability to maintain toes straight (toe-out or toe-in), and poor trunk control (lateral trunk flexion, increased trunk flexion).

Criteria for Return

Physicians typically have varying criteria for full return of the patient following injury to the anterior cruciate. Perhaps the greatest variability exists in the recommended time frames for full return. Among the more widely used protocols are the following recommendations:

- Shelbourne and Nitz — 4 to 6 months
- Andrews and Wilk — 5 to 6 months
- Fu and Irrgang — 6 to 9 months
- Campbell Clinic — 6 to 12 months
- Paulos and Stern — 9 months

- Kerlan and Jobe — 9 months

In general the following criteria appear to be the most widely accepted: (1) no joint effusion; (2) full ROM; (3) isokinetic testing indicates that strength of the quadriceps and hamstrings are at 85% to 100% of the uninvolved leg; (4) satisfactory ligament stability testing using a KT-1000 arthrometer;[2] (5) successful progression from walking to running; and (6) successful performance during functional testing (hop tests, agility runs, etc).

Posterior Cruciate Ligament Sprains

Pathomechanics

Isolated tears of the posterior cruciate ligament (PCL) are not common but certainly do occur in athletes. It is more likely that the PCL is injured concurrently with the ACL, MCL, LCL, or menisci. The PCL is the strongest ligament in the knee and functions with the ACL to control the rolling and gliding of the tibiofemoral joint and has been called the primary stabilizer of the knee. More specifically, the PCL prevents 85% to 90% of the posterior translational force of the tibia on the femur. This is evident in the PCL-deficient knee when, upon descending an incline, the force of gravity works to increase the anterior glide of the femur on the tibia; without the PCL the femur will sublux on the tibia from midstance to toe-off, where the quadriceps are less effective in controlling the anterior motion of the femur on the tibia.[101,102]

The majority (70%) of PCL tears occur on the tibia, whereas 15% occur on the femur and 15% are midsubstance tears.[106] In the PCL-deficient knee, there is an increased likelihood of meniscus lesions and chondral defects, most often involving the medial side.[51]

The extent of laxity determines the severity of the injury. In a grade 1 sprain, the PCL is tender due to microtears with some hemorrhage and tenderness to palpation. However, there is no increased laxity and there is a firm end point. A grade 2 sprain involves an incomplete tear with some increased laxity in a positive posterior drawer test, yet there is still a firm end point. There is tenderness to palpation, hemorrhage, and pain on posterior drawer test. A grade 3 sprain is a complete tear with significant posterior laxity in posterior drawer, posterior sag, and reverse pivot shift tests when compared to the opposite knee. No end point is evident, and pain is generally less than with grades 1 or 2.

Injury Mechanism

In athletics, the most common mechanism of injury to the PCL is with the knee in a position of forced hyperflexion with the foot plantar flexed. The PCL can also be injured when the tibia is forced posteriorly on the fixed femur or the femur is forced anteriorly on the fixed tibia.[100] It is also possible to injure the PCL when the knee is hyperflexed and a downward force is applied to the thigh.

Forced hyperextension will usually result in injury to both the PCL and the ACL. If an anteromedial force is applied to a hyperextended knee, the posterolateral joint capsule may also be injured. If enough valgus or varus force is applied to the fully extended knee to rupture either collateral ligament, it is possible that the PCL may also be torn. The patient will indicate that they felt and heard a "pop" but will often feel that the injury was minor and that they can return to activity immediately. There will be mild to moderate swelling within 2 to 6 hours.

Rehabilitation Concerns

Perhaps the greatest concern in rehabilitating a patient with an injured PCL is the fact that the arthrokinematics of the joint are altered, and this change can eventually lead to degeneration of both the medial compartment and the patellofemoral joint.[79]

The decision as to whether the PCL-deficient knee is best treated nonoperatively or surgically is controversial. This is primarily due to the relative lack of data-based information in the literature regarding the normal history of PCL tears. Many patients with an isolated PCL tear do not seem to exhibit functional performance limitations and can continue to compete athletically, while others occasionally are limited in performing normal daily activities.[51] Parolie and Bergfeld reported a more than 80% success rate with nonoperative treatment.[124] On the other hand, Clancy reported a high incidence of femoral condylar articular injury involving degenerative changes that may eventually result in arthritis in patients 4 years after PCL injury. Thus surgical reconstruction has been advocated[28,102] It is generally believed that the surgical treatment of PCL tears is technically difficult. Surgery to reconstruct a PCL-deficient knee is most often indicated with avulsion injuries. Reconstructive procedures using the semitendinous tendon, the tendon of the medial gastrocnemius, the Achilles tendon, the patellar tendon, or synthetic material to replace the lost PCL have been recommended.[79] Both autografts and allografts have been used.

Rehabilitation Progression

Nonoperative Rehabilitation

If the PCL-deficient knee is to be treated nonoperatively, initial treatment should involve controlling swelling, pain, and inflammation through the use of cold, compression, and electrical stimulation. If necessary, the knee can be placed in an immobilizer for the first few days for comfort and minimal protection, with the patient ambulating on crutches until he or she regains full extension and can walk without an extension lag. Because there is often little functional limitation, the patient may progress rapidly through the rehabilitative process, the rate of progression limited only by pain and swelling.

The patient can begin immediately following injury with quad sets (Figure 21-20) and straight leg raising (Figure 21-21) to regain motor control and minimize atrophy. Early pain-free ROM exercises can begin using knee slides on a treatment table (Figure 21-3), wall slides (Figure 21-5), active assistive slides (Figure 21-4 and 21-6), or riding an exercise bike with the seat adjusted to the appropriate height to permit as much knee flexion as can be tolerated (Figure 21-35). Hamstring exercises should be avoided initially to minimize posterior laxity.

Nonoperative rehabilitation should focus primarily on quadriceps strengthening. As pain subsides and ROM improves, the patient may incorporate isotonic open chain extension exercises (Figure 21-23). With open chain quadriceps strengthening exercises, it has been recommended that extension be restricted initially in the 45 to 20 degrees range to avoid developing patellofemoral pain.[73] It has also been recommended that quadriceps strength

in the PCL-deficient knee be greater than 100% of the uninjured knee, particularly in patients attempting to fully return to sport activity.[124]

Open chain hamstring strengthening exercises using knee flexion that increase posterior translation of the tibia should be avoided. Posterior tibial translation can be minimized by strengthening the hamstrings using open chain hip extension with the knee fully extended (Figure 20-30E). Closed chain exercises (Figures 21-25 through 21-35) that use a co-contraction of the quadriceps to reduce posterior tibial translation and also to minimize the possibility of developing patellofemoral pain may safely be used to strengthen the hamstrings.

The use of functional knee braces for a patient with a PCL-deficient knee is generally not recommended, because functional braces are designed primarily for ACL-deficient knees. However, there may be some benefit in terms of increased joint position sense, through stimulation of cutaneous sensory receptors, that may enhance both conscious and subconscious awareness of the existing injury.[93]

Because of the tendency toward progressive degeneration of the medial aspect of the knee with a PCL-deficient knee, it is incumbent on the athletic trainer to counsel the patient to avoid repetitive activities that produce pain or swelling.

Clinical Decision-Making Exercise 21-4

A high school football kicker suffered an isolated grade 2 sprain of his PCL in his nonkicking leg. The team physician has decided to allow the player to return to play once pain-free ROM and strength are regained. The patient has regained complete use of the leg, except he feels unstable when planting to kick. What should the athletic trainer do to increase stability in the injured leg during the kicking maneuver?

Surgical Rehabilitation

The time frame for the maturation and healing process for a PCL graft has not been documented in the literature, as it has been for ACL grafts. The course of rehabilitation following surgical reconstruction of the PCL is not well defined, and recommended rehabilitation protocols are difficult to find. Clancy has perhaps the largest study of operative PCL reconstructions using a patellar tendon graft.[28]

Immediately following surgery, the goal is to minimize pain and swelling by using cold, compression, and electrical stimulation. A Cryo-cuff may be used to accomplish this. The patient is placed in a rehabilitative brace and locked in 0 degrees of extension at all times for the first week (Figure 21-53). During the second week, the brace may be unlocked for ambulation and passive ROM exercises. The brace will be worn for 4 to 6 weeks until the patient can achieve 90 to 100 degrees of flexion. Generally the patient is placed on crutches with full weight bearing as soon as possible, but he or she should stay on crutches for 4 to 6 weeks until he or she can achieve full extension.

Quad sets (Figure 21-20) and straight leg raises (Figure 21-21) done in the brace can begin at 2 to 4 weeks. Resisted exercise can begin during the second week for hip adductors (Figure 21-19) and hip abductors (Figure 21-18). After surgical reconstruction of the PCL, it is important to limit hamstring function to reduce the posterior translational forces.[101] Strengthening exercises for the hamstrings should be avoided initially because they tend to place stress on the graft. At 4 to 6 weeks, closed chain exercises from 0 to 45 degrees of flexion are initiated. Resisted terminal knee extensions in a closed chain should also be used (Figure 21-31).

Along with the early controlled weight-bearing and closed chain exercises begun at about 6 weeks that act to stimulate muscle and joint mechanoreceptors, seated BAPS board exercises to reestablish balance and neuromuscular control should also begin early in the rehabilitation process (Figure 21-43B).

Cycling on a stationary bike can begin at 6 weeks when the patient achieves about 100 to 110 degrees of flexion (Figure 21-35). Walking with full weight bearing on a treadmill can begin when the patient has no extension lag and has sufficient quadriceps strength to allow for nearly normal gait. Progressing to jogging/running is generally not recommended until 9 months. Functional training should progressively incorporate the stresses, strains, and forces that occur during normal running, jumping, and pivoting activities in a controlled environment (see Chapter 16).

Criteria for Return

In general the following criteria for return appear to be the most widely accepted: (1) there is no joint effusion; (2) there is full ROM; (3) isokinetic testing indicates that strength of the quadriceps is greater than 100% of the uninvolved leg; (4) the patient has made successful progression from walking to running; and (5) the patient has successful performance during functional testing (hop tests, agility runs, etc).

Meniscal Injury

Pathomechanics

The menisci aid in joint lubrication, help distribute weight-bearing forces, help increase joint congruency (which aids in stability), act as a secondary restraint in checking tibiofemoral motion, and act as a shock absorber.[24,96]

The medial meniscus has a much higher incidence of injury than the lateral meniscus. The higher number of medial meniscal lesions may be attributed to the coronary ligaments that attach the meniscus peripherally to the tibia and also to the capsular ligament. The lateral meniscus does not attach to the capsular ligament and is more mobile during knee movement. Because of the attachment to the medial structures, the medial meniscus is prone to disruption from valgus and torsional forces.

A meniscus tear can result in immediate joint-line pain localized to either the medial or the lateral side of the knee. Effusion develops gradually over 48 to 72 hours, although a tear at the periphery might produce a more acute hemarthrosis. Initially pain is described as a "giving-way" feeling, but the knee may be "locked" near full extension due to displacement of the meniscus. A knee that is locked at 10 to 30 degrees of flexion may indicate a tear of the medial meniscus, whereas a knee that is locked at 70 degrees or more may indicate a tear of the posterior portion of the lateral meniscus.[32] A positive McMurray's test usually indicates a tear in the posterior horn of the meniscus. The knee that is locked by a displaced meniscus may require unlocking with the patient under anesthesia so that a detailed examination can be conducted. If discomfort, disability, and locking of the knee continue, arthroscopic surgery may be required to remove a portion of the meniscus. If the knee is not locked but shows indications of a tear, the physician might initially obtain an MRI. A diagnostic arthroscopic examination may also be performed. Diagnosis of meniscal injuries should be made immediately after the injury has occurred and before muscle guarding and swelling obscure the normal shape of the knee.

Injury Mechanism

The most common mechanism of meniscal injury is weight bearing combined with internal or external rotation while extending or flexing the knee.[26] A valgus or varus force sufficient to cause disruption of the MCL or LCL also might produce an ACL tear as well as a meniscus tear. A large number of medial meniscus lesions are the outcome of a sudden, strong, internal rotation of the femur with a partially flexed knee while the foot is firmly planted, as would occur in a cutting motion. As a result of the force of this action, the medial meniscus is detached and pinched between the femoral condyles.

Meniscal lesions can be longitudinal, oblique, or transverse. Stretching of the anterior and posterior horns of the meniscus can produce a vertical-longitudinal or "bucket handle" tear. A longitudinal tear can also result from forcefully extending the knee from a flexed position while the femur is internally rotated. During extension the medial meniscus is suddenly pulled back, causing the tear. In contrast, the lateral meniscus can sustain an oblique tear by a forceful knee extension with the femur externally rotated.

Rehabilitation Concerns

Quite often in the athletic population, the choice is to initially treat meniscus tears conservatively, taking a "wait and see" approach. Occasionally the patient will be able to complete the competitive season by simply dealing with the associated symptoms of a torn meniscus, with the idea that the problem will be taken care of surgically at the end of the season. In some individuals the symptoms may resolve so that there is no longer a need for surgery.

The problem is that once a meniscal tear occurs, the ruptured edges harden and can eventually atrophy. On occasion, portions of the meniscus may become detached and wedge themselves between the articulating surfaces of the tibia and femur, imposing a chronic locking, "catching," or "giving way" of the joint. Chronic meniscal lesions can also display recurrent swelling and obvious muscle atrophy around the knee. The patient might complain of an inability to perform a full squat or to change direction quickly when running without pain, a sense of the knee collapsing, or a "popping" sensation. Displaced meniscal tears can eventually lead to serious articular degeneration with major impairment and disability. Such symptoms and signs usually warrant surgical intervention.

Three surgical treatment choices are possible for the patient with a damaged meniscus: partial meniscectomy, meniscal repair, and meniscal transplantation. It was not too long ago that the accepted surgical treatment for a torn meniscus involved total removal of the damaged meniscus. However, total meniscectomy has been shown to cause premature degenerative arthritis. With the advent of arthroscopic surgery, the need for total meniscectomy has been virtually eliminated. In surgical management of meniscal tears, every effort should be made to minimize loss of any portion of the meniscus.

The location of the meniscal tear often dictates whether the surgical treatment will involve a partial meniscectomy or a meniscal repair. Tears that occur within the inner third of the meniscus will have to be resected because they are unlikely to heal, even with surgical repair, due to avascularity. Tears in the middle third of the meniscus and, particularly in the outer third, may heal well following surgical repair because they have a good vascular supply. Partial meniscectomy of a torn meniscus is much more common than meniscal repair.

Rehabilitation Progressions

Nonoperative Management

If a consensus decision is made by the physician, the patient, and the athletic trainer to treat a meniscus tear nonoperatively, the patient may return to full activity as soon as the initial signs and symptoms resolve. Rehabilitation efforts should be directed primarily at minimizing pain and controlling swelling in addition to getting the patient back to functional activities as soon as possible. Generally the patient may require 3 to 5 days of limited activity to allow for resolution of symptoms.

Partial Menisectomy

Postsurgical management for a partial menisectomy that is not accompanied by degenerative change or injury to other ligaments initially involves controlling swelling, pain, and inflammation through the use of cold, compression, and electrical stimulation. The patient should ambulate on crutches for 1 to 3 days, progressing to full weight bearing as soon as tolerated until regaining full extension and walking without a limp or an extension lag. Early pain-free ROM exercises using knee slides on a treatment table (Figure 21-3), wall slides (Figure 21-5), active assistive slides (Figure 21-4 and 21-6), and stationary cycling (Figure 21-35) can begin immediately along with quad sets (Figure 21-20) and straight leg raising (Figure 21-21), which are used to regain motor control and minimize atrophy. As pain subsides and ROM improves, the patient may incorporate isotonic open and closed chain exercises (Figures 21-21). Functional activity training may begin as soon as the patient feels ready. It is not uncommon in the athletic population for functional activity training to begin within 3 to 6 days after a partial menisectomy, although it is more likely that full return will require about 2 weeks.

Meniscal Repair

The repair of a damaged meniscus involves the use of absorbable sutures, vascular access channels drilled from vascular to nonvascular areas, and the insertion of a fibrin clot.[26] Rehabilitation after arthroscopic surgery for a partial menisectomy with no associated capsular damage is rapid, and the likelihood of complications is minimal.

Rehabilitation after either meniscal repair or menicus transplant requires that joint motion be limited and thus is more prolonged than for a partial menisectomy. For the patient it is essential that some type of cardiorespiratory endurance conditioning be incorporated throughout the period of immobilization. Because of the limitation of the rehabilitative brace, use of an upper-extremity ergometer is perhaps the most effective way to maintain endurance.

The patient is placed in a rehabilitative brace locked in full extension for the first 2 weeks, both for protection and to prevent flexion contractures (Figure 21-53). During this period, there is partial weight bearing on crutches. Submaximal isometric quad sets (Figure 21-20) are performed in the brace along with hip abduction and adduction strengthening exercises (Figures 21-18 and 21-19).

For weeks 2 to 4, motion in the brace is limited to 20 to 90 degrees of flexion, and for weeks 4 to 6, motion is limited in the 0 to 90 degrees range. Hip exercises and isometric quad sets should continue. ROM exercises using knee slides (Figure 21-3), wall slides (Figure 21-5), and active assistive slides (Figures 21-4 and 21-6), should all be done in the brace within the protected range. Partial weight bearing on crutches should progress to full weight bearing after 6 weeks.

At 6 weeks the brace can be removed and the knee rehabilitation progressions described above may be incorporated, as tolerated by the patient, to regain full ROM and normal muscle strength. Generally the patient can return to full activity at about 3 months.

If a patient has had an ACL reconstruction in addition to a meniscal repair, the healing constraints associated with meniscal repair must be taken into consideration in the rehabilitation plan.[149] ROM exercises, strengthening exercises, and weight bearing all have some mechanical impact on the meniscus. If the rehabilitation protocols for other ligament injuries are more aggressive or accelerated, the guidelines for meniscus repair healing must be incorporated into the treatment plan.

Meniscal Transplant

Meniscal transplants using either allografts or synthetic material have been recommended.[50,148] Although reports of the efficacy of these procedures have been inconsistent,[32] generally the preference seems to be an allograft using bone plugs and suturing to the capsule at the periphery of the graft.[50] Meniscal transplants are markedly less common than either menisectomy or repair.

It is recommended that following transplantation, a rehabilitative brace be locked in full extension for 6 weeks. The brace may be unlocked during this period to allow passive ROM exercises in the 0 to 90 degrees range. Isometric quad sets and hip exercises are performed throughout this 6-week period. Also only partial weight bearing on crutches is allowed.

At 6 weeks the brace is unlocked, and there should be progression to full weight bearing. Use of the brace may be discontinued at 8 weeks or whenever the patient can achieve full extension, flexion to 100 degrees, and a normal gait.[79] At that point, progressive strengthening, ROM, and functional training techniques as described previously can be incorporated when appropriate. Full return is expected in 9 to 12 months.

Criteria for Return

Time frames required for full return following nonoperative management, partial menisectomy, meniscal repair, and meniscal transplant were discussed previously. Generally, with meniscus injury, the patient may return to activity when (1) swelling does not occur with activity; (2) full ROM has been regained; (3) there is equal bilateral strength in knee flexion and extension; and (4) the patient can successfully complete functional performance tests such as hopping, shuttle runs, carioca, and cocontraction tests.

REHABILITATION TECHNIQUES FOR PATELLOFEMORAL AND EXTENSOR MECHANISM INJURIES

Complaints of pain and disability associated with the patellofemoral joint and the extensor mechanism are exceedingly common among the athletic population. The terminology used to describe this anterior knee pain has been a source of some confusion and thus requires some clarification. At one time, it was not uncommon for every patient who walked into a sports medicine clinic complaining of anterior knee pain to be diagnosed as having chondromalacia patella. However, there can be many other causes of anterior knee pain, and chondromalacia patella is only one of these causes. The term patellofemoral arthralgia is a catchall term used to describe anterior knee pain. Chondromalacia patella, along with patellofemoral stress syndrome, patellar tendinitis, patellar bursitis, chronic patellar subluxation, acute patellar dislocation, and a synovial plica, are all conditions that can cause anterior knee pain. The treatment and rehabilitation of patients complaining of anterior knee pain can be very frustrating for the athletic trainer. The more conservative approach to treatment of patellofemoral pain described below should be used initially. If this approach fails, surgical intervention may be required.

Patellofemoral Stress Syndrome

Pathomechanics

Patients presenting with patellofemoral pain typically exhibit relatively common symptoms.[46] They complain of nonspecific pain in the anterior portion of the knee. It is difficult to place one finger on a specific spot and be certain that the pain is there. Pain seems to be increased when either ascending or descending stairs or when moving from a squatting to a standing position. Patients also complain of pain when sitting for long periods—this has occasionally been referred to as the "moviegoer's sign." Reports of the knee "giving away" are likely, although typically no instability is associated with this problem. When evaluating the pathomechanics of the patellofemoral joint, the athletic trainer must assess static alignment, dynamic alignment, and patellar orientation.

Static Alignment

Static stabilizers of the patellofemoral joint act to maintain the appropriate alignment of the patella when no motion is occurring (Figure 21-55). The superior static stabilizers are the quadriceps muscles (vastus lateralis, vastus intermedius, vastus medialis, rectus femoris). Laterally, static stabilizers include the lateral retinaculum, vastus lateralis, and iliotibial band. Medially, the medial retinaculum and the vastus medialis are the static stabilizers.

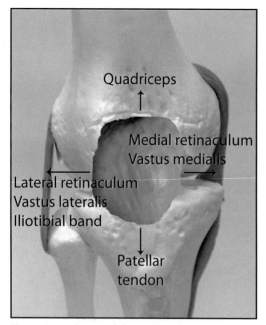

Figure 21-55. Static and dynamic patellar stabilizers.

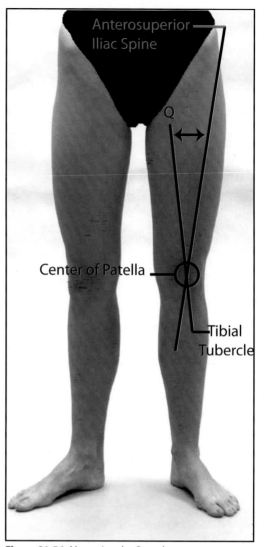

Figure 21-56. Measuring the Q-angle.

Inferiorly, the patellar tendon stabilizes the patella.

Dynamic Alignment

Dynamic alignment of the patella must be assessed during functional activities. It is critical to look at the tracking of the patella from an anterior view during normal gait. Muscle control should be observed while the patient engages in other functional activities, including stepping, bilateral squats, or one-legged squats.

A number of different anatomical factors can affect dynamic alignment. It is essential to understand that both static and dynamic structures must create a balance of forces about the knee. Any change in this balance might produce improper tracking of the patella and patellofemoral pain.

Increased Q-angle. The Q-angle (Figure 21-56) is formed by drawing a line from the anterosuperior iliac spine to the center of the patella. A second line drawn from the tibial tubercle to the center of the patella that intersects the first line forms the Q-angle. A normal Q-angle falls between 10 to 12 degrees in the male and 15 to 17 degrees in the female. Q-angle can be increased by lateral displacement of the tibial tubercle, external tibial torsion, or femoral neck anteversion. The Q-angle

is a static measurement and might have no direct correlation with patellofemoral pain.[45] However, dynamically this increased Q-angle may increase the lateral valgus vector force, thus encouraging lateral tracking, resulting in patellofemoral pain[63] (Figure 21-57).

Dynamic Q-angle may be affected by abnormal biomechanics occurring at the hip and knee.[69] Increased hip adduction and hip internal rotation during functional activities can lead to increased knee valgus, thus increasing the valgus force vector on the patella. This increased hip adduction and internal rotation may be due to weakness of the hip abductors and hip external rotators; therefore, it is

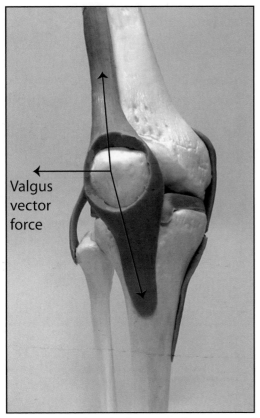

Figure 21-57. A lateral valgus vector force is created when the quadriceps is contracted.

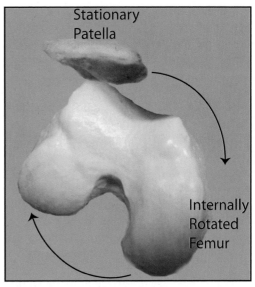

Figure 21-58. Femoral internal rotation during dynamic weight-bearing activities can affect patellar positioning. The femor can rotate without associated patellar movement.

imperative to evaluate the hip musculature in individuals with patellofemoral pain.

Femoral rotation. Femoral rotation during dynamic tasks has been reported to play a role in patellar malalignment. With the use of MRI, researchers have determined that the femur can rotate under the patella during weight-bearing stance.[129,151] Therefore, an increase in femoral rotation during dynamic activities may cause the patella to be laterally positioned, leading to improper tracking of the patella and patellofemoral pain (Figure 21-58).

A-angle. The A-angle (Figure 21-59) measures the patellar orientation to the tibial tubercle. It is created by the intersection of lines drawn bisecting the patella longitudinally and from the tibial tubercle to the apex of the inferior pole of the patella. An angle of 35 degrees or greater has been correlated with patellofemoral pathomechanics, resulting in patellofemoral pain.[7]

Iliotibial band. The distal portion of the iliotibial band interdigitates with both the deep transverse retinaculum and the superficial oblique retinaculum. As the knee moves into flexion, the iliotibial band moves posteriorly, causing the patella to tilt and track laterally.[46]

Vastus medialis oblique insufficiency. The vastus medialis oblique (VMO) functions as an active and dynamic stabilizer of the patella. Anatomically it arises from the tendon of the adductor magnus.[21] Normally, the VMO is tonically active electromyographically throughout the ROM. In individuals with patellofemoral pain, it is phasically active, and it tends to lose fatigue-resistant capabilities.[134] The VMO is innervated by a separate branch of the femoral nerve; therefore, it can be activated as a single motor unit.[8] In normal individuals the VMO to vastus lateralis (VL) ratio has been shown to be 1 to 1.[133] However, in individuals who complain of patellofemoral pain the VMO to VL ratio is less than 1 to 1.

Vastus lateralis. The vastus lateralis interdigitates with fibers of the superficial lateral retinaculum. Again, if this retinaculum is tight or if a muscle imbalance exists between the vastus lateralis and the vastus medialis with the lateralis being more active, lateral tilt or tracking of the patella may occur dynamically.[45]

Excessive pronation. Excessive pronation may result from existing structural deformities in the foot. With over pronation there is excessive subtalar eversion and adduction with an obligatory internal rotation of the tibia, increased internal rotation of the femur, and thus an increased lateral valgus vector force at the knee that encourages lateral tracking.[55] Various structural deformities in the feet that can cause knee pain should be corrected biomechanically according to techniques recommended in Chapter 23.

Tight hamstring muscles. Tight hamstring muscles cause an increase in knee flexion. When the heel strikes the ground, there must be increased dorsiflexion at the talocrural joint. Excessive subtalar joint motion may occur to allow for necessary dorsiflexion. As stated previously this produces excessive pronation with concomitant increased internal tibial rotation and a resultant increase in the lateral valgus vector force.

Tight gastrocnemius muscle. A tight gastrocnemius muscle will not allow for the 10 degrees of dorsiflexion necessary for normal gait. Once again this produces excessive subtalar motion, increased internal tibial rotation, and increased lateral valgus vector force.[55]

Patella alta and baja. In patella alta, the ratio of patellar tendon length to the height of the patella is greater than the normal 1 to 1 ratio. In patella alta the length of the patellar tendon is 20% greater than the height of the patella. This creates a situation where greater flexion is necessary before the patella assumes a stable position within the trochlear groove, and thus there is an increased tendency toward lateral subluxation.[76]

Patella baja is a condition in which the patella lies inferior to the normal position and may also restrict knee flexion ROM. Knee injuries (eg, patellar tendon rupture, ACL reconstructions using quadriceps tendon) may cause a patella baja condition. Aggressive joint mobilization and soft-tissue manipulation is important to prevent these conditions from occurring post injury. Strengthening exercises are also necessary to establish increased patellar stabilization during ROM.

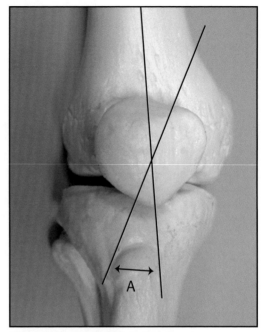

Figure 21-59. Measurement of the A-angle.

Patellar Orientation

Patellar orientation is the positioning of the patella relative to the tibia. Assessment should be done with the patient in supine position. Four components should be assessed when looking at patellar orientation: glide, tilt, rotation, and anteroposterior tilt.

Glide component. This component assesses the lateral or medial deviation of the patella relative to the trochlear groove of the femur. Glide should be assessed both statically and dynamically. Figure 21-60 provides an example of a positive medial glide.

Tilt component. Tilt is determined by comparing the height of the medial patellar border with the lateral patellar border. Figure 21-61 shows an example of a positive lateral tilt.

Rotation component. Rotation is identified by assessing the deviation of the longitudinal axis (a line drawn from superior pole to inferior pole) of the patella relative to the femur. The point of reference is the inferior pole. If the inferior pole is more lateral than the superior pole, a positive external rotation exists (Figure 21-62).

Anteroposterior tilt component. This must be assessed laterally to determine if a line drawn from the inferior patellar pole to the superior

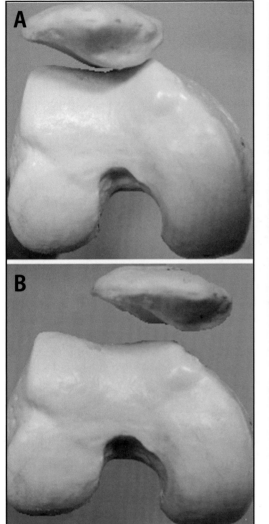

Figure 21-60. Glide component. (A) Normal positioning; (B) positive medial glide component.

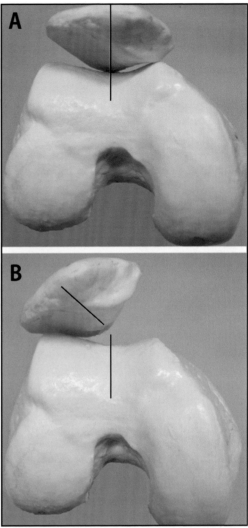

Figure 21-61. Tilt component. (A) Normal positioning; (B) positive lateral tilt component.

patellar pole is parallel to the long axis of the femur. If the inferior pole is posterior to the superior pole, the patient has a positive antero-posterior tilt component (Figure 21-63).

Rehabilitation Concerns

Traditionally, rehabilitation techniques for patients complaining of patellofemoral pain tended to concentrate on avoiding those activities that exacerbated pain (for example, squatting or stair climbing), occasional immobilization, and strengthening of the quadriceps group using open kinetic chain exercises. The current treatment approach has a new direction and focus that includes strengthening of both the quadriceps and also the hip musculature (see Chapter 20), through closed kinetic chain exercise regaining optimal patellar positioning and tracking, and regaining neuromuscular control to improve lower limb mechanics.

Strengthening Techniques

Earlier in this chapter, closed kinetic chain exercises were recommended for strengthening in the rehabilitation of ligamentous knee injuries. These same exercises are also useful in the rehabilitation of patellofemoral pain, not because anterior shear is reduced but because of how they affect patellofemoral joint reaction force (PFJRF).

REHABILITATION PLAN

ISOLATED GRADE 2 MCL INJURY IN COLLEGIATE FOOTBALL PLAYER

Injury situation: A 20-year-old collegiate football offensive lineman sustained an isolated grade 2 MCL sprain 2 days ago. He has been experiencing localized pain along the medial aspect of the knee and has been unable to ambulate without the aid of crutches. He wishes to participate in the homecoming game in 4 weeks.

Signs and symptoms: The patient complains of pain in the medial aspect of the knee when he attempts to bear weight. Pain is increased during the valgus stress test, and a soft end point is felt. During palpation there is noticeable pain on the superior border of the MCL; this increases when the knee is passively flexed and extended. There is moderate discoloration and swelling along the medial aspect of the knee extending down into the lower extremity.

Management plan The goal is to reduce pain initially and increase pain-free ROM.

PHASE ONE: Acute Inflammatory Stage

GOALS: Modulate pain and begin appropriate ROM exercises.

Estimated length of time (ELT): Day 1 to Day 4 Ice and electrical stimulation are applied to decrease pain. Anti-inflammatory medications can help reduce the amount of swelling; also apply a compression wrap. The patient is restricted from practice for a few weeks and instructed to perform rehabilitation in the athletic training room during the morning rehabilitation hours. He is fitted with a protective knee brace and he is instructed to increase bearing weight while crutch walking. ROM exercises—wall slides, prone hangs, and table glides—are begun. Quadriceps strengthening begins with isometric exercises using quad setting, short arc motions, and complete ROM exercises as tolerated. Leg abduction exercises and positions that increase valgus stress should be avoided. Hamstring and gastrocnemius/soleus flexibility should be emphasized.

PHASE TWO: Fibroblastic-Repair Stage

GOALS: Increase leg strength and improve flexibility.

Estimated length of time (ELT): Days 5 to 14 Ice and electrical stimulation may be continued as needed. Crutch walking should be eliminated, and the protective knee brace may be discontinued except when the patient is performing dynamic active exercises. Aggressive quadriceps/hamstring stretching exercises should be used as tolerated. Isometric and isotonic strengthening exercises should concentrate on the entire lower-extremity chain and include dynamic motions as tolerated. Controlled closed kinetic chain exercises, particularly mini squats and step-ups, should be recommended and performed as tolerated. Aquatic exercise (walk, jog, and swim) should be emphasized as tolerated, while avoiding increased valgus stress on the knee. Functional activities that emphasize core stability (thigh, trunk, and hip musculature) should begin once the patient is able to do them without pain. Fitness levels must be maintained, by using either an upper-extremity bicycle ergometer or aquatic exercise.

PHASE THREE: Maturation-Remodeling Stage

GOALS: Complete elimination of pain and full return to activity.

Estimated length of time (ELT): Day 15 to full return The patient should be gradually weaned from wearing the protective brace while rehabilitating, but encouraged to wear a medial supportive brace during football activities. The patient should be observed and monitored closely prior to full return to play to evaluate any biomechanical deformities in technique that may be a result of the injury. Videotape replay may be useful for analyzing technique and gait prior to and after return to practice and should be evaluated by the athletic trainer for possible compensations that may lead to additional problems. The patient must continue his strengthening and flexibility routine and incorporate functional tasks specific to his sport and position to increase strength, speed, power, and agility.

CRITERIA FOR RETURNING TO COMPETITIVE FOOTBALL

1. Pain, inflammation, and discoloration are eliminated in the lower extremity during all movement tasks.
2. Lower-extremity strength is good, especially in the quadriceps.
3. Core stability (thigh, trunk, and hip musculature) strength is good.
4. Biomechanical movement techniques are good.
5. The patient feels ready to return to play and has regained confidence in the injured knee.

DISCUSSION QUESTIONS

1. What other anatomic structures can potentially be disturbed if return to play activity is resumed too early?
2. What is the estimated total healing time for partially torn medial collateral ligament tissue?
3. Describe the characteristics of the protective knee brace used during football activities.
4. Explain the possible biomechanical movement strategies that may be used as compensation techniques for the injured knee.
5. Describe the potential sport/position demands imposed on this football offensive lineman and functional exercises that may be used during the rehabilitation process.

More traditional rehabilitation techniques focused on reducing the compressive forces of the patella against the femur and reducing PFJRF. PFJRF increases when the angle between the patellar tendon and the quadriceps tendon decreases (Figure 21-64). PFJRF also increases when the quadriceps tension increases to resist the flexion moment created by the lever arms. PFJRF can be minimized by maximizing the area of surface contact of the patella on the femur. As the knee moves into greater degrees of flexion, the area of surface contact increases, distributing the forces associated with increased compression over a larger area (Figure 21-65), minimizing the compressive forces per unit area.[54]

Rehabilitation techniques involving closed kinetic chain exercises try to maximize the area of surface contact. With closed kinetic chain exercises, as the angle of knee flexion decreases, the flexion moment acting on the knee increases. This requires greater quadriceps and patellar tendon tension to counteract the effects of the increased flexion moment arm, resulting in an increase in PFJRF as flexion increases. However, the force is distributed over a larger patellofemoral contact area, minimizing the increase in contact stress per unit area. Therefore it appears that closed kinetic chain exercises may be better tolerated by the patellofemoral joint than open kinetic chain exercises.

Regaining Optimal Patellar Positioning and Tracking

This second goal in our current treatment approach is based on the work of an Australian physiotherapist, Jenny McConnell.[52,107] This goal can be accomplished by stretching the tight lateral structures, correcting patellar orientation, and improving the timing and force of the VMO contraction.

Stretching

Successfully stretching the tight lateral structures involves a combination of both active and passive stretching techniques. Active stretching techniques include mobilization techniques as discussed in Chapter 13. Specific techniques should involve medial patellar glides and medial patellar tilts along the longitudinal axis of the patella (see Figure 13-58). Passive stretch is accomplished through a long-duration stretch created by the use of very specific

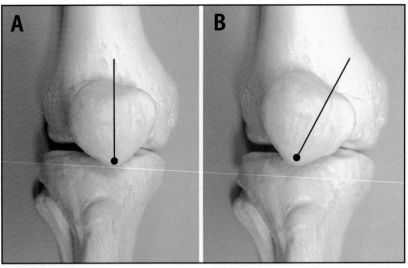

Figure 21-62. Rotation component. (A) Normal. (B) Positive external rotation.

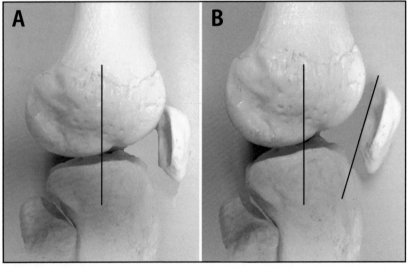

Figure 21-63. Anteroposterior tilt component (lateral view). (A) Normal; (B) positive inferior anteroposterior tilt.

taping techniques to alter patellar alignment and orientation.

Correcting Patellar Orientation

After a thorough assessment of patellofemoral mechanics as described earlier, the athletic trainer should have the patient perform an activity that produces patellofemoral pain, such as step-ups or double- or single-leg squats to establish a baseline for comparison.

Closed kinetic chain exercises were discussed in detail in Chapter 12. In the case of patellofemoral rehabilitation, closed kinetic chain exercises that strengthen both the hip and knee musculature have been shown to decrease pain and increase strength.[20,104,153] Ireland has shown that women with patellofemoral pain are more likely to demonstrate weakness in hip abduction and external rotation.[78] Mini squats from 0 to 40 degrees (Figure 21-25), leg press from 0 to 60 degrees (Figure 21-29), lateral step-ups using an 8-inch step (Figure 21-30), a stepping machine (Figure 21-34), a stationary bike (Figure 21-35), slide board exercises (Figure 21-32), and a Fitter (Figure 21-33) are all examples of closed kinetic chain strengthening

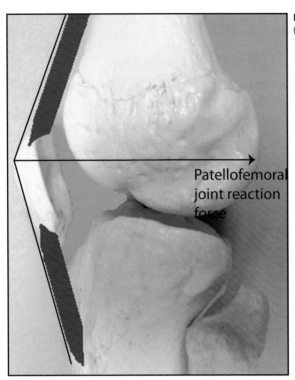

Figure 21-64. Patellofemoral joint reaction forces (PFJRF).

Patellofemoral joint reaction force

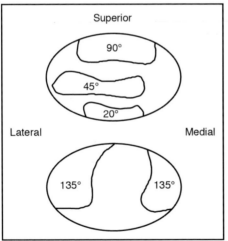

Figure 21-65. Compression force and contact stress. Even though compression forces increase with increasing knee flexion, the amount of contact stress per unit area decreases.

Superior

90°

45°

20°

Lateral   Medial

135°   135°

exercises that may be used in patellofemoral rehabilitation.

It should be stressed that not all individuals who complain of patellofemoral pain exhibit a positive patellar orientation component. In patients who do, patellofemoral orientation can be corrected to some degree by using tape. Correction of patellar positioning and tracking is accomplished by using passive taping of the patella in a more biomechanically correct position. In addition to correcting the orientation of the patella, the tape provides a prolonged stretch to the soft tissue structures that affect patellar movement.

Taping should be done using two separate types of highly adhesive tape available from several different manufacturers. A base layer using white tape is applied directly to the skin from the lateral femoral condyle to just posterior to the medial femoral condyle, making

REHABILITATION PLAN

PATELLOFEMORAL PAIN IN A HIGH SCHOOL VOLLEYBALL PLAYER

Injury situation: A 16-year-old high school female volleyball player complains of pain in her left anterior knee. She has been experiencing this pain for several weeks. At first, pain was present only during and immediately after practice, but lately her knee seems to ache all the time. Her pain has increased to the point where she now has difficulty completing a practice session.

Signs and symptoms: The patient complains of pain in the anterior aspect of the knee while walking, running, ascending and descending stairs, or squatting. Pain is increased during the patellar grind test. During palpation there may be pain on the inferior border of the patella or when the patella is compressed within the femoral groove while the knee is passively flexed and extended. She has tightness of the hamstrings, an increased Q-angle, excessive pronation in her left foot, and weakness in her vastus medialis obliques (VMO).

Management Plan The goal is to reduce pain initially and then identify and correct faulty biomechanics that may collectively contribute to her anterior knee pain.

PHASE ONE: Acute Inflammatory Stage

GOALS: Modulate pain and begin appropriate strengthening exercises
Estimated length of time (ELT): Day 1 to Day 4 Use ice and electrical stimulation to decrease pain. If there appears to be inflammation, anti-inflammatory medications may be helpful. McConnell taping should be used to try to correct any patellar malalignment that may exist. The patient may need to be restricted from practice for a few days; at least reduce the amount of lower-extremity activity, which may be exacerbating her condition. An orthotic insert should be constructed to correct any excessive pronation during gait. Quadriceps strengthening should begin with isometric exercises using quad setting, short arc motions, and complete ROM exercises from 90 degrees of flexion to full extension. None of the isometric exercises should increase her pain level; if they do, they should be eliminated and pain-free exercises should be incorporated.

PHASE TWO: Fibroblastic-Repair Stage

GOALS: Increase VMO strength and improve hamstring flexibility
Estimated length of time (ELT): Days 5 to 14 Ice and electrical stimulation may be continued. McConnell taping technique should also be continued with day-to-day reassessment of its effectiveness. Biofeedback may help the patient learn to contract the VMO better. The effectiveness of the orthotic should be reassessed, and appropriate correction adjustments should be made. Aggressive hamstring-stretching exercises should be used. Quadriceps strengthening should concentrate on VMO activation and progress from isometrics to full-range isotonics as soon as full ROM-resisted exercise no longer causes pain. Closed kinetic chain exercises, particularly mini squats and step-ups, should be recommended. The patient may resume practice, but activities that seem to increase pain should be modified or replaced with alternative activities. Functional activities that emphasize core stability (thigh, trunk, and hip musculature) should be emphasized once pain-free activities are conducted. Fitness levels must be maintained using stationary cycling, aquatic exercises, or other nonballistic types of aerobic exercise that do not increase knee pain.

PHASE THREE: Maturation-Remodeling Stage

GOALS: Complete elimination of pain and full return to activity
Estimated length of time (ELT): Week 3 to Full Return The patient should be gradually weaned from McConnell taping. It may be helpful for the patient to wear a neoprene sleeve during activity for joint warming and psychological support. The patient should be observed and monitored

closely prior to full return to play, to evaluate any biomechanical deformities in technique that may contribute to her knee pain. Videotape replay may be useful for gait analysis consisting of walking, running, pivoting, and jump-landing activities. The patient must continue her strengthening and flexibility routine, taking into consideration any practice or game demands that may impose too much of an overload. The patient should now be fully accustomed to the orthotic insert. It may be necessary to continue to use alternative fitness activities that reduce the strain on her knee during the season and possibly indefinitely.

CRITERIA FOR RETURNING TO COMPETITIVE BASKETBALL

1. Pain is eliminated in squatting and in ascending or descending stairs.
2. There is good hamstring flexibility.
3. Quadriceps strength is good, especially the VMO.
4. Core stability (thigh, trunk, and hip musculature) strength is good.
5. Biomechanical gait techniques are good.
6. The patient feels ready to return to play and has regained confidence in the injured knee.

DISCUSSION QUESTIONS

1. What other factors can potentially contribute to patellofemoral pain?
2. What therapeutic modalities might potentially be used to control pain?
3. Describe the characteristics of the orthotic that might be used to correct excessive pronation.
4. Will medications help in managing this problem?
5. Explain the McConnell taping technique that would likely be used to correct this problem.

certain that the patella is completely covered by the base layer (Figure 21-66). This tape is used as a base to which the other tape is adhered to correct patellar alignment.

The glide component should always be corrected first, followed by the component found to be the most excessive. If no positive glide exists, begin with the most pronounced component found. The glide component should always be corrected with the knee in full extension. To correct a positive lateral glide, attach the tape one thumb's breadth from the lateral patellar border, push the patella medially, gather the soft tissue over the medial condyle, push toward the condyle, and adhere to the medial condyle (Figure 21-67).

The tilt component should be corrected with the knee flexed 30 to 45 degrees. To correct a positive lateral tilt, from the middle of the patella pull medially to lift the lateral border. Again, gather the skin underneath, and adhere to the medial condyle (Figure 21-68).

The rotational component is corrected in 30 to 40 degrees of flexion. To correct a positive external rotation, from the middle of the inferior border pull upward and medially while rotating the superior pole externally (Figure 21-69).

To correct a positive anteroposterior superior tilt, place the knee in full extension. Adhere a 6-inch strip of tape over the lower half of the patella, and press directly posterior, adhering with equal pressure on both sides (Figure 21-70).

One piece of tape can be used to correct two components simultaneously. For example, when correcting a lateral glide along with an anteroposterior inferior tilt, follow the same taping procedure for the glide component except that the tape should be applied to the upper half of the patella.

After this taping procedure, the athletic trainer should reassess the activity that caused the patient's pain. In many cases the patient will indicate improvement almost immediately. If not, the order of the taping or the way the patella is taped may have to be changed considerably. The tape should be worn 24 hours a day initially, and the athletic trainer should instruct the patient in how to adjust and tighten the tape as necessary.

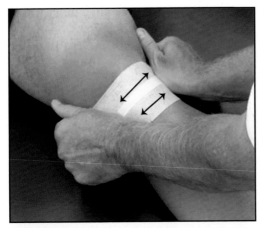

Figure 21-66. Application of base tape.

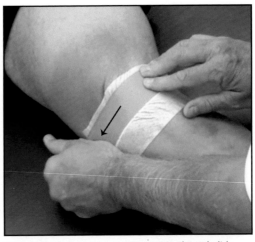

Figure 21-67. Taping to correct positive lateral glide.

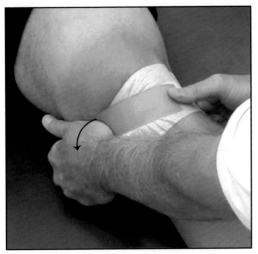

Figure 21-68. Taping to correct positive lateral tilt.

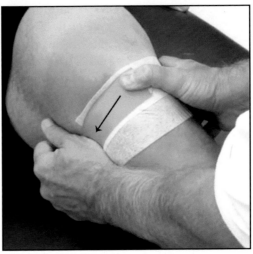

Figure 21-69. Taping to correct positive external rotation.

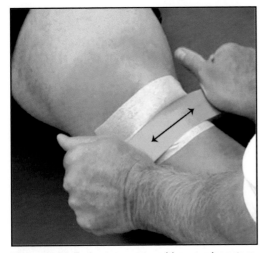

Figure 21-70. Taping to correct positive superior antero-posterior tilt.

It is important to understand that taping changes the forces acting on the patella and thus the kinematics of the knee joint. Taping essentially attempts to decrease the lateral pull on the patella. When combined with an increase in the force and timing of the VMO contraction, this will result in alteration of the balance of forces on the patella. Interestingly, a study by Bockrath et al demonstrated that patellar taping reduced pain in patients with anterior knee pain, but radiographic studies before and after taping revealed no change in patellofemoral congruency or patellar rotational angles. Hence the reduction in pain was not associated with positional change of the patella.[17]

Reestablishing Neuromuscular Control

Establishing neuromuscular control involves improving the timing and force of VMO contraction. It is perhaps most important for the athletic trainer to emphasize the quality rather than the quantity of the contraction. This means that training the VMO should concentrate more on motor skill acquisition than on strengthening activities. Strengthening should occur concomitantly with improvement in motor skill.

As mentioned previously, the VMO-to-VL strength ratio should be 1 to 1. In patients who have a VMO-to-VL ratio of less than 1 to 1 with patellofemoral pain, training efforts should focus on selectively strengthening the VMO. Isolating and training the VMO selectively requires concentration on the part of the patient. Techniques of facilitation, such as manually stroking or taping the VMO or the use of biofeedback, are recommended. The use of a dual-channel biofeedback unit capable of monitoring both VMO and VL electromyographic activity can help the patient gain neuromuscular control over both the force of contraction and timing for the firing of the VMO.

The VMO is a tonic muscle that acts to stabilize the patella both statically and dynamically, so it should be active throughout the ROM. Training goals should be directed toward increasing the force of the VMO contraction both concentrically and eccentrically throughout the ROM. Because the VMO arises from the adductor magnus tendon, adduction exercises may be used to facilitate VMO contraction. The VMO should be trained to respond to a new length–tension relationship between the agonist (VMO) and the antagonist (VL).

Several sources have indicated that the VMO has a separate nerve supply from the rest of the quadriceps, although this is in our opinion somewhat debatable.[7,21,42] Nevertheless, assuming this is the case, the patient should be taught to fire the VMO before the VL. Neuromuscular control of the VMO firing should help the patient maintain appropriate patellar alignment.

VMO exercises should concentrate on controlling the firing of the VMO. Exercises should be performed slowly and with concentration to selectively activate muscles. The athletic trainer should address concentric and eccentric control in a variety of functional tasks and positions. Mini squats, step-ups or step-downs, and leg presses are good exercises for establishing concentric and eccentric control. Training on a BAPS board DynaDisc or Bosu Balance Trainer (see Figures 7-16 and 21-43) is useful for proprioceptive training. It is extremely important to concentrate on VMO control during gait-training activities.

Criteria for Return

Taping should continue throughout the VMO training period. Again, tape should initially be worn 24 hours a day. The patient may be weaned from tape progressively when he or she demonstrates VMO control. Examples of functional criteria for weaning include when the patient can keep the VMO activated for 5 minutes during a walking gait and when the patient can fire the VMO either before or simultaneously with the VL consistently in step-downs for 1 minute. At this point, tape may be left off every third day for 1 week, then every second day for 1 week, then worn only during activity, and finally worn only if pain is present. Taping can be eliminated altogether when the patient can perform step downs for 5 minutes with appropriate timing and when she or he can sustain a quarter to a half squat for 1 minute without VMO loss.

Chondromalacia Patella

Pathomechanics and Injury Mechanism

Chondromalacia patella can occur either as a consequence of patellofemoral stress syndrome or from a direct impact to the patella. It is a softening and deterioration of the articular cartilage on the back of the patella that has been described as undergoing three stages: swelling and softening of the articular cartilage, fissuring of the softened articular cartilage, and deformation of the surface of the articular cartilage caused by fragmentation.[24]

The exact cause of chondromalacia is unknown. As indicated previously, abnormal patellar tracking could be a major etiological factor. However, individuals with normal tracking have acquired chondromalacia, and some individuals with abnormal tracking are free of it.[19]

The patient may experience pain in the anterior aspect of the knee while walking, running, ascending and descending stairs, or squatting. There may be recurrent swelling around the kneecap and a grating sensation when flexing and extending the knee. There may also be crepitation and pain during a patellar grind test. During palpation there may be pain on the inferior border of the patella or when the patella is compressed within the femoral groove while the knee is passively flexed and extended. Degenerative arthritis occurs on the lateral facet of the patella, which makes contact with the femur when the patient performs a full squat.[19] Degeneration first occurs in the deeper portions of the articular cartilage, followed by blistering and fissuring that stems from the subchondral bone and appears on the surface of the patella.[19,24]

Rehabilitation Concerns

Chondromalacia patella is initially treated conservatively using the same rehabilitation plan as was described for patellofemoral stress syndrome.[106] If conservative measures fail to help, surgery may be the only alternative. Some of the following surgical measures have been recommended[19]: realignment procedures such as lateral release of the retinaculum; moving the insertion of the vastus medialis muscle forward; shaving and smoothing the irregular surfaces of the patella and/or femoral condyle; in cases of degenerative arthritis, removing the lesion through drilling; elevating the tibial tubercle; or, as a last resort, completely removing the patella.

Rehabilitation Progression

Chondromalacia patella is a degenerative process that unfortunately does not tend to get better or resolve with time. There are times when the knee is painful and other times when it feels alright. Perhaps the key to managing chondromalacia is to maintain strength of the quadriceps muscle group and in particular the VMO. Closed chain exercises are recommended because they tend to decrease the patellofemoral joint reaction forces. The patient must be consistent in these strengthening efforts.

Irritating activities that tend to exacerbate pain, such as stair climbing, squatting, and long periods of sitting, should be avoided. Isometric exercises or closed chain isotonics performed through a pain-free arc to strengthen the quadriceps and hamstring muscles should be routinely done. The use of oral anti-inflammatory agents and small doses of aspirin may help to modulate pain. Wearing a neoprene knee sleeve helps certain patients but does absolutely nothing for others. Use of an orthotic device to correct pronation and reduce tibial torsion is helpful in many instances.

Criteria for Return

As long as the patient can tolerate the pain and discomfort that occurs with chondromalacia patella, he or she can continue to train and compete. Again, the key is essentially to "play games" with this condition, training normally when there is no pain and backing off when the knee is painful.

Clinical Decision-Making Exercise 21-5

A triathlete has been complaining of knee pain for several months. She has no previous history of a knee injury, but her training regimen is intense, involving 3 hours of training each day. A physician diagnosed her with chondromalacia patella. She has been referred to the athletic trainer for evaluation and rehabilitation. What can the athletic trainer do to help reduce the patient's symptoms and signs?

Acute Patellar Subluxation or Dislocation

Pathomechanics

The patella, as it tracks superiorly and inferiorly in the femoral groove, can be subject to direct trauma or degenerative changes, leading to chronic pain and disability.[70] Of major importance are those conditions that stem from abnormal patellar tracking within the femoral groove. Improper patellar tracking leading to patellar subluxation or dislocation can result from a number of biomechanical factors, including femoral anteversion with increased internal femoral rotation, genu valgum with a concomitant increase in the Q-angle, a shallow femoral groove, flat lateral femoral condyles, patella alta, weakness of the vastus medialis muscle relative to the vastus lateralis, ligamentous laxity with genu recurvatum, excessive external rotation of the tibia, pronated feet, a tight lateral retinaculum, and a patella with a positive lateral tilt. Each of these factors was discussed in detail earlier in this chapter.

Injury Mechanism

When the patient plants the foot, decelerates, and simultaneously cuts in an opposite direction from the weight-bearing foot, the thigh rotates internally while the lower leg rotates externally, causing a forced knee valgus. The quadriceps muscle attempts to pull in a straight line and as a result pulls the patella laterally, creating a force that can sublux the patella. As a rule, displacement takes place laterally, with the patella shifting over the lateral condyle.

A chronically subluxing patella places abnormal stress on the patellofemoral joint and the medial restraints. The knee may be swollen and painful. Pain is a result of swelling but also results because the medial capsular tissue has been stretched and torn. Because of the associated swelling the knee is restricted in flexion and extension. There may also be a palpable tenderness over the adductor tubercle where the medial retinaculum (patellar femoral ligament) attaches.

Acute patellar dislocation most often occurs when the foot is planted and there is contact with another athlete on the medial surface of the patella, forcing it to dislocate laterally. The patient reports a painful "giving way" episode. The patient experiences a complete loss of knee function, pain, and swelling, with the patella remaining in an abnormal lateral position. A physician should immediately reduce the dislocation by applying mild pressure on the patella with the knee extended as much as possible. If a time has elapsed before reduction, a general anesthetic may have to be used. After aspiration of the joint hematoma, ice is applied, and the joint is immobilized. A first-time patellar dislocation is sometimes associated with loose bodies from a chondral or osteochondral fracture as well as articular cartilage lesions. Thus some physicians advocate arthroscopic examination following patellar dislocation.[138]

Rehabilitation Progression

Chronic Patellar Subluxation

Rehabilitation for a chronically subluxing patella should focus on addressing each of the potential biomechanical factors that either individually or collectively contribute to the pathomechanics. It is important to regain a balance in strength of all musculature associated with the knee joint. Postural malalignments must be corrected as much as possible. Shoe orthotic devices may be used to reduce foot pronation and tibial internal rotation, and subsequently to reduce stress to the patellofemoral joint.

Particular attention should be given to strengthening the quadriceps through closed kinetic chain exercises; strengthening the hip abductors (Figure 21-18), hip adductors (Figure 21-19), and gastrocnemius (Figure 21-24); stretching the tight lateral structures using a combination of patellar mobilization glides (see Figure 13-58) and medial patellar tilts along the longitudinal axis of the patella as well as stretching for the iliotibial band (Figure 21-11) and biceps femoris (Figures 21-10 and 21-14); correcting patellar orientation; and establishing neuromuscular control by improving the timing and force of the VMO contraction.

If the patient does not respond to extensive efforts by the athletic trainer to correct the pathomechanics and subluxation remains a recurrent problem, surgical intervention may be necessary. However, a surgical release of the lateral retinacular ligaments does not appear to be a particularly effective procedure and should be done only after failure of more conservative treatment.

Acute Patellar Dislocation

In the case of acute patellar dislocation, following reduction, the knee should be placed in an immobilizer immediately, and it is recommended that it remain in place for 3 to 6 weeks with the patient ambulating on crutches until regaining full extension and walking without an extension lag. The patient can begin immediately following the dislocation with isometric quad sets (Figure 21-20) and straight leg raising (Figure 21-21), always paying close attention to achieving a good contraction of the VMO. Early pain-free ROM exercises including knee slides on a treatment table (Figures 21-3), wall slides (Figures 21-5 and 21-6), or active assistive slides (Figures 21-4 and 21-6) can be used.

As pain subsides and ROM improves, the patient should incorporate closed chain strengthening exercises (Figures 21-25 through 21-35) to minimize stress on the patellofemoral joint. Strengthening should be directed toward increasing the force of the VMO contraction both concentrically and eccentrically throughout the ROM. Neuromuscular control of the VMO firing should help the patient maintain appropriate patellar alignment. It is also important to concentrate on VMO control during gait-training activities.

After 3 to 6 weeks when immobilization is discontinued, the patient should wear a neoprene knee sleeve with a lateral horseshoe-shaped felt pad that helps the patella track medially (Figure 21-71). This support should be worn while running or performing in sports.

Criteria for Return

The patient should have good quadriceps strength and should be able to demonstrate VMO control during functional activities. Examples of functional criteria include when the patient can keep the VMO activated for 5 minutes during a walking gait and when the patient can fire the VMO either before or simultaneously with the vastus lateralis consistently in step-downs for 1 minute. The patient should be able to perform step-downs for 5 minutes with appropriate timing and sustain a quarter to a half squat for 1 minute without VMO loss.

Patellar Tendinitis (Jumper's Knee)

Pathomechanics and Injury Mechanism

Jumper's knee occurs when chronic inflammation develops in the patellar tendon either at the superior patellar pole (usually referred to as quadriceps tendinitis), the tibial tubercle, or most commonly at the distal pole of the patella (patellar tendinitis). It usually develops in athletes involved in activities that require

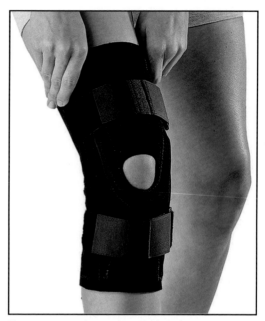

Figure 21-71. A brace that can help limit patellar dislocation and/or subluxation should have a felt horseshoe applied laterally. (Reprinted with permission from DonJoy.)

repetitive jumping; hence the name. Point tenderness on the posterior aspect of the inferior pole of the patella is the hallmark of patellar tendinitis. This condition is felt to be related to the shock-absorbing function (an eccentric contraction) that the quadriceps provides upon landing from a jump. Initially the patient complains of a dull aching pain after jumping or running following repetitive jumping activities. Pain usually disappears with rest but returns with activity. Pain becomes progressively worse until the patient is unable to continue. There are also reports of difficulty in stair climbing and an occasional feeling of "giving way."

Rehabilitation Concerns

Because jumper's knee involves a chronic inflammation, rehabilitation strategies may take one of two courses. The athletic trainer may choose to use traditional techniques designed to reduce the inflammation, which include rest, anti-inflammatory medication, ice, and ultrasound. Another, more aggressive approach would be to use a transverse friction massage technique designed to exacerbate the acute inflammation so that the healing process is no longer "stuck" in the inflammatory response phase and can move on to the fibroblastic-repair phase. The technique involves a 5- to 7-minute friction massage at the inferior pole of the patella in a direction perpendicular to the direction of the tendon fibers, performed every other day for about 1 week. During this treatment, all other medicative or modality efforts to reduce inflammation should be eliminated. It is our experience that if pain is not decreased after 4 or 5 treatments it is unlikely that this technique will resolve the problem.

Ruptures of the patellar tendon are rare in young patients but increase in incidence with age. A sudden powerful contraction of the quadriceps muscle with the weight of the body applied to the affected leg can cause a rupture of the patellar tendon.[160] The rupture may occur to the quadriceps tendon or to the patellar tendon. Usually rupture does not occur unless there has been a prolonged period of inflammation of the patellar tendon that has weakened the tendon. Seldom does a rupture occur in the middle of the tendon; usually the tendon is torn from its attachment. The quadriceps tendon ruptures from the superior pole of the patella, whereas the patellar tendon ruptures from the inferior pole of the patella. A rupture of the patellar tendon usually requires surgical repair.

Rehabilitation Progression

Regardless of which of the two treatment approaches is used, once the problem begins to resolve, the patient should engage in a thorough warm-up prior to activity. Initially, jumping and running activities should be restricted. Strengthening of the quadriceps is critical during rehabilitation. Success has been reported using eccentric strengthening exercises for both the quadriceps and the ankle dorsiflexors.[30,82,111] Curwin and Stanish have theorized that a graded program of eccentric stress will stimulate the tendon to heal.[31] They feel that rest does not stimulate healing, while low- to moderate-level eccentric exercise will. Their program consists of five parts: warm-up, stretching, eccentric squatting, stretching, and ice.[10,30] The eccentric squats, called drop squats, are performed with the patient moving slowly from standing to a squat position and return. To increase stress, the speed of the drop is increased until a mild level of pain is experienced (Figure 21-72A). The goal is to perform 3 sets of 10 repetitions at a speed that causes mild pain during the last set. The presence of mild pain is indicative of the mild stress. Several studies suggest standing on a 25-degree decline board while performing eccentric training of the quadriceps (Figure 21-72B).[136] Evidence suggest patellar tendon strain is significantly greater, stop angles of the ankle and hip joints are significantly smaller, and EMG amplitudes of the knee extensor muscles are significantly greater during exercise on the decline board compared with standard squats.

Jensen and DiFabio have suggested treating patellar tendinitis with a program of isokinetic eccentric quadriceps training[83] (Figure 21-39). The program begins with 6 sets of 5 repetitions at 30 degrees per second 3 times per week, progressing over an 8-week period to 4 sets of 5 repetitions each at 30, 50, and 70 degrees per second.[83] Vigorous quadriceps and hamstring stretching precede and follow each workout (Figures 21-13 and 21-14).

The use of a tenodesis strap or a brace worn about the patellar tendon has also been recommended for patellar tendinitis (Figure 21-73). It appears that the effectiveness of this strap in reducing pain varies from one patient to another.

Injection of cortisone into the tendon to reduce inflammation is not recommended because it will tend to weaken the tendon and can predispose the patient to patellar tendon rupture.

One vital piece of the rehabilitation process that has often been ignored is the jump-landing technique used by the injured patient.[31,108,121] Patellar tendinitis often arises in individuals who jump a lot during sport activities (eg, volleyball, basketball, and soccer), yet the analysis of the jump–landing technique is overlooked. Muscular strength, flexibility, and neuromuscular control are often assessed properly, but the contribution of movement technique assessment is the final piece of the puzzle. A patient who has sufficient muscular and neuromuscular contributions to joint stability can get joint overload and injury from poor jump–landing technique. The use of instructional feedback such as videotape replay and verbal cues has been shown to reduce the forces associated with jump-landing, thus possibly reducing the risk

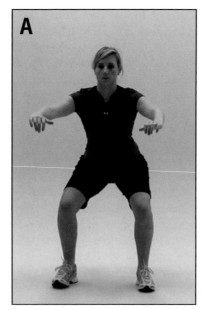 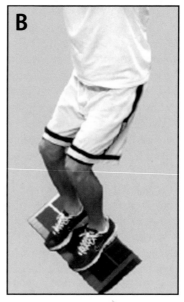

Figure 21-72. Drop squats are performed with the patient moving slowly from standing to a squat position and return. (A) Drop squats; (B) standing on 25 degree board.

of jump-landing injuries.[108,122,130] Instruction in proper landing technique must be sport and position specific and should include a combination of videotape replay from the athletic trainer (Figure 21-47) to provide specific feedback (eg, land with two feet, feet shoulder-width apart, and bend to absorb impact) and verbal cues (eg, soft knees, load hips, quiet sound, and toe-to-heel landing).[66,109,121,122,130] Improving soft-tissue structures surrounding the injured joint is necessary, but poor jump–landing technique will constantly exacerbate the tendinitis problem.

Criteria for Return

The patient may return to full activity when pain has subsided to the point where he or she is capable of performing jumping and running activities without increased swelling or exacerbation of pain. There should be normal strength in the quadriceps bilaterally.

Clinical Decision-Making Exercise 21-6

A high school volleyball player has been complaining of patellar tendon pain for 2 weeks following the start of preseason practice. She complains of sharp shooting pain in the inferior pole of the patellar tendon region during jumping activities, with increased pain during the plyometric conditioning program conducted at the end of each practice. She has tried to continue playing, but now she is noticeably limping. The coach has told her to discontinue practice and see the athletic trainer. How should the athletic trainer manage this condition?

Bursitis

Pathophysiology

Bursitis in the knee can be acute, chronic, or recurrent. Although any one of the numerous knee bursae can become inflamed, anteriorly the prepatellar, deep infrapatellar, and

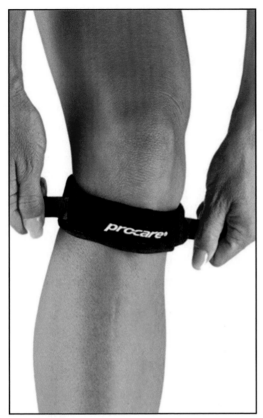

Figure 21-73. A tenodesis strap can be used to help control patellar tendinitis. (Reprinted with permission from DonJoy.)

suprapatellar bursae have the highest incidence of irritation in sports. The pathophysiological reaction that occurs with bursitis follows the normal course of the inflammatory response as described in Chapter 2.

Swelling patterns can often help differentiate bursitis from other conditions in the injured knee. With bursitis, swelling is localized to the bursa. For example, prepatellar bursitis results in localized swelling above the knee that is ballottable. In the more severe cases, it may seem to extend over the lower portion of the vastus medialis. Swelling is not intra-articular, and there may be some redness and increased temperature. In acute prepatellar bursitis, the ROM of the knee is not restricted except in the last degrees of flexion when pain-producing pressure is felt in the bursa, whereas a true hemarthrosis or synovitis of the knee joint most frequently shows a more significant limitation of terminal flexion and extension of the joint.[19]

Injuries to the ligaments of the knee and also fractures of the patella may occur along with acute prepatellar bursitis. Patellar fractures can occur from a direct blow to the patella with the knee held in flexion. A violent contraction of the quadriceps mechanism can also produce transverse patellar fractures, which should be ruled out with radiographs. Infection of the infrapatellar bursa can be similarly difficult to diagnose because of its deep location. It is a rare condition and requires aspiration for diagnosis.

Swelling posteriorly in the popliteal fossa does not necessarily indicate bursitis but could instead be a sign of Baker's cyst. A Baker's cyst is connected to the joint, which swells because of a problem in the joint and not due to bursitis. A Baker's cyst is often asymptomatic, causing little or no discomfort or disability.

Injury Mechanism

The cause of prepatellar bursitis can involve either a single trauma, as would occur in falling on a flexed knee, or it can result from repetitive crawling or kneeling on the knee, as would occur in wrestling. Acute or posttraumatic inflammation is not uncommon. The prepatellar bursa is more likely to become inflamed from continued kneeling, whereas the deep infrapatellar becomes irritated from repetitive stress to the patellar tendon, as is the case in jumper's knee.

Rehabilitation Concerns and Progression

Acute prepatellar bursitis should be treated conservatively, and rehabilitation should begin with ice, compression, anti-inflammatory medication, and possibly a brief period of immobilization in a knee splint. If necessary, the patient should walk on crutches until he or she has regained quadriceps control and can ambulate without a limp. The compression wrap should be applied from the foot upward to the middle of the thigh in a manner that maintains constant pressure on the bursa. The leg should be elevated as much as possible. The patient should begin with quad sets (Figure 21-20) and straight leg raising (Figure 21-21), both to maintain function of the quadriceps and to use active muscle contractions to help facilitate resorption of fluid. On the second day, the patient may begin ROM exercises doing knee slides on a treatment table (Figure 21-3), wall slides (Figure 21-5), or active assistive slides (Figures 21-4 and 21-6). The compression wrap should be left in place until there is no evidence of fluid reaccumulation.

Occasionally, a physician may choose to aspirate the bursa to relieve the pressure and speed up the recovery period. If so, it is essential to take necessary precautions to prevent contamination and subsequent infection. If infection does occur, it should be treated with antibiotics.

In cases of chronic bursitis, the techniques for controlling swelling listed above should be used. A compression wrap needs to be worn constantly. Unfortunately, there will generally not be complete resolution. Chronic bursitis becomes a recurrent problem with thickening of the bursa and reaccumulation of fluid. In these cases, injection with a corticosteroid or surgical excision of the bursa may be necessary.

Criteria for Return

The patient may return to full activity when there is no reaccumulation of fluid following their exercises, when there is full ROM, and when there is normal quadriceps control.

Iliotibial Band Friction Syndrome

Pathomechanics

The iliotibial band is a tendinous extension of the fascia covering the gluteus maximus and tensor fasciae latae muscles proximally. It attaches distally at Gerdy's tubercle on the proximal portion of the lateral tibial. As the patient flexes and extends the knee, the tendon glides anteriorly and posteriorly over the lateral femoral condyle. This repetitive motion, as typically occurs in runners, may produce irritation and inflammation of the tendon.

Iliotibial band friction syndrome involves localized pain about 2 cm above the joint line over the lateral femoral condyle when the knee is in 30 degrees of flexion. Pain appears to radiate toward the lateral joint line and down toward the proximal tibia, becoming increasingly severe as the patient continues to run. Eventually it becomes so symptomatic that the activity must be discontinued.

The patient has tenderness, crepitus, and an area of swelling over the lateral condyle. In some instances patients with iliotibial band friction syndrome also have a history of trochanteric bursitis and pain along the iliac crest at the origin at the tensor fasciae latae. Leg length discrepancies, contractures of the tensor fasciae latae and gluteus maximus, tightness of the hamstrings and quadriceps, genu varum, excessive pronation leading to increased internal tibial torsion, and a tight heel cord can individually or collectively increase the tension of the iliotibial band across the femoral condyle. Ober's test to detect tightness in this muscle group will be positive.

Injury Mechanism

As is the case in many injuries associated with running, there is often a history of poor training techniques that may include running on irregular surfaces (such as on the side of the road), downhill running, or running long distances without gradually building up to that level. Symptoms frequently develop in patients who do not have an adequate stretching program.

Rehabilitation Concerns and Progression

Initial treatment for iliotibial band friction syndrome is directed at reducing the local inflammatory reaction by using rest, ice, ultrasound, and oral anti-inflammatory medications.[44] Rehabilitation should focus on correcting the underlying biomechanical factors that may cause the problem. If Ober's test is positive, stretching exercises to correct this static contracture should be used (Figure 21-11).[44] Some patients also have hip flexion contractures with a positive Thomas test and require stretching of the iliopsoas and the anterior capsule, as well as the tensor fasciae latae. Myofascial release stretching as shown in Figure 8-8A also helps reduce pain and increase motion. Exercises to improve hip abductor strength and integrated movement patterns should also be incorporated.[44]

During normal gait, pronation leads to an obligatory internal rotation of the tibia. Orthotics may help reduce this pronation and relieve symptoms at the knee. Generally 4 to 6 weeks of conservative treatment is required to control the symptoms of iliotibial band syndrome. Although conservative treatment is usually effective in controlling symptoms, occasionally cases of iliotibial band syndrome do not respond and require surgical treatment. As was the case with patellar tendinitis, transverse friction massage used to increase the inflammatory response appears to be effective in treating iliotibial band friction syndrome. A 5- to 7-minute friction massage to the iliotibial band over the lateral femoral condyle in a direction perpendicular to the direction of the tendon fibers should be done every other day for about 1 week. During this treatment, all other medicative or modality efforts to reduce inflammation should be eliminated.

Criteria for Return

When the local tenderness over the lateral epicondyle has subsided, the patient may resume running but should avoid prolonged workouts and running on hills and irregular surfaces. If it is necessary to run on the side of the road, it is essential that the patient alternate sides of the road during workouts. Shortening the stride and applying ice after running may also be beneficial.

Patellar Plica

Pathomechanics

A plica is a fold in the synovial lining of the knee that is a remnant from the embryological development within the knee. The most common synovial fold is the infrapatellar plica, which originates from the infrapatellar fat pad and extends superiorly in a fanlike manner. The second most common synovial fold is the suprapatellar plica, located in the suprapatellar pouch. The least common, but most subject to injury, is the mediopatellar plica, which is band-like, begins on the medial wall of the knee joint, and extends downward to insert into the synovial tissue that covers the infrapatellar fat pad.[16] The mediopatellar plica can bowstring across the anteromedial femoral condyle, impinging between the articular cartilage and the medial facet of the patella with increasing flexion. A plica is often associated with a torn meniscus, patellar malalignment, or osteoarthritis. Because most synovial plicae are pliable, most are asymptomatic; however, the mediopatellar plica may be thick, nonyielding, and fibrotic, causing a number of symptoms.

Injury Mechanism

The patient may or may not have a history of knee injury. If symptoms are preceded by trauma, it is usually one of blunt force such as falling on the knee or of twisting with the foot planted, either of which can lead to inflammation and hemorrhage. Inflammation leads to fibrosis and thickening with a loss of extensibility.

As the knee passes 15 to 20 degrees of flexion, a snap may be felt or heard. Internal and external tibial rotation can also produce this snapping. The mediopatellar plica can snap over the medial femoral condyle, contributing to the development of chondromalacia.[16] A major complaint is recurrent episodes of painful pseudo-locking of the knee when sitting for a period. Such characteristics of locking and snapping could be misinterpreted as a torn meniscus. The patient complains of pain while ascending or descending stairs or when squatting. Unlike meniscal injuries, there is little or no swelling and no ligamentous laxity.

Rehabilitation Concerns and Progression

Initially, a plica should be treated conservatively to control inflammation with rest, anti-inflammatory agents, and local heat. If the plica is associated with improper patellar tracking, the pathomechanics should be corrected as previously discussed. If conservative treatment is unsuccessful, the plica may be surgically excised, usually with good results.[36]

Criteria for Return

The patient can return to full activity when she or he can perform normal functional activities with minimal or no pain and without a recurrence of swelling.

Osgood-Schlatter Disease

Pathomechanics and Injury Mechanism

Two conditions common to the immature adolescent's knee are Osgood-Schlatter disease and Larsen-Johansson disease. Osgood-Schlatter disease is characterized by pain and swelling over the tibial tuberosity that increases with activity and decreases with rest. Traditionally Osgood-Schlatter disease was described as either a partial avulsion of the tibial tubercle or an avascular necrosis of the same. Current thinking views it more as an apophysitis characterized by pain at the attachment of the patellar tendon at the tibial tubercle with associated extensor mechanism problems. The most commonly accepted cause of Osgood-Schlatter disease is repeated stress of the patellar tendon at the apophysis of the tibial tubercle. Complete avulsion of the patellar tendon is an uncommon complication of Osgood-Schlatter disease.

This condition first appears in adolescents and usually resolves when the patient reaches the age of 18 or 19 years. The only remnant is an enlarged tibial tubercle. Repeated irritation causes swelling, hemorrhage, and gradual degeneration of the apophysis as a result of impaired circulation. The patient complains of severe pain when kneeling, jumping, and running. There is point tenderness over the anterior proximal tibial tubercle.

Larsen-Johansson disease, although much less common, is similar to Osgood-Schlatter disease, but it occurs at the inferior pole of the patella. As with Osgood-Schlatter disease, the cause is believed to be excessive repeated strain on the patellar tendon. Swelling, pain, and point tenderness characterize Larsen-Johansson disease. Later, degeneration can be noted during X-ray examination.

Rehabilitation Concerns and Progression

Management is usually conservative and includes the following: Stressful activities are decreased until the apophyseal union occurs, usually within 6 months to 1 year; ice is applied to the knee before and after activities; isometric strengthening of quadriceps and hamstring muscles is performed; and severe cases may require a cylindrical cast. Treatment is symptomatic with emphasis on icing, quadriceps strengthening, hamstring stretching, and activity modification. Only in extreme cases is immobilization necessary.

Summary

1. To be effective in a knee rehabilitation program, the athletic trainer must have a good understanding of the functional anatomy and biomechanics of knee joint motion.

2. Techniques of strengthening involving closed kinetic chain, isometric, isotonic, isokinetic, and plyometric exercises are recommended after injury to the knee because of their safety and because they are more functional than open chain exercises.

3. ROM may be restricted either by lack of physiological motion, which may be corrected by stretching, or by lack of accessory motions, which may be corrected by patellar mobilization techniques. Constant passive motion may be used postoperatively to assist the patient in regaining ROM.

4. PCL, MCL, and LCL injuries are generally treated nonoperatively, and the patient is progressed back into activity rapidly within his or her limitations.

5. The current surgical procedure of choice for ACL reconstruction uses an intra-articular patellar tendon graft.

6. Recent trends in rehabilitation after ACL reconstruction are toward an aggressive, accelerated program that emphasizes immediate motion, immediate weight bearing, early closed chain strengthening exercises, early return to activity, and jump–landing training.

7. The current trend in treating meniscal tears is to surgically repair the defect if possible or perform a partial meniscectomy arthroscopically. Repaired menisci should be immobilized non-weight-bearing for 4 to 6 weeks.

8. It is critical to assess the mechanics of the patellofemoral joint in terms of static alignment, dynamic alignment, and patellar orientation to determine what specifically is causing pain.

9. Rehabilitation of patellofemoral pain concentrates on strengthening the quadriceps through closed kinetic chain exercises, regaining optimal patellar positioning and tracking, and regaining neuromuscular control to improve lower-limb mechanics.

References

1. Anderson, A., R. Snyder, and C. Federspiel. 1992. Instrumented evaluation of knee laxity: A comparison of five arthrometers. *Am J Sport Med* 20:135–140.

2. Anderson, C., and J. Gillquist. 1992. Treatment of acute isolated and combined ruptures of the ACL: A long-term followup study. *Am J Sport Med* 20:7–12.

3. Arendt, E., and R. Dick. 1995. Knee injury patterns among men and women in collegiate basketball and soccer. NCAA data and review of literature. *Am J Sport Med* 23(6):694–701.

4. Arendt, E.A., J. Agel, and R. Dick. 1999. Anterior cruciate ligament injury patterns among collegiate men and women. *J Ath Train* 34(2):86–92.

5. Arendt, E. 1997. Anterior cruciate ligament injuries in women. *Sport Medicine and Arthroscopy Review,* 5(2):149–155

6. Arms, S., M. Pope, R. Johnson, R. Fischer, I. Arvidsson, and E. Eriksson. 1984. The biomechanics of anterior cruciate ligament rehabilitation and reconstruction. *Am J Sports Med* 12:8–18.

7. Arno, S. 1990. The A-angle: A quantitative measurement of patellar alignment and realignment. *Journal of Orthopaedic and Sports Physical Therapy* 12[C]:237–242.

8. Aronson, P, et al. 2010. Tibiofemoral joint positioning for the valgus stress test. *Journal of Athletic Training* 45(4):357-393.

9. Bell, D.R., D.A. Padua, and M.A. Clark. 2008. Muscle strength and flexibility characteristics of people displaying excessive medial knee displacement. *Arch Phys Med Rehabil* 89:1323–1328.

10. Bennet, J., and W. Stauber. 1986. Evaluation and treatment of anterior knee pain using eccentric exercise. *Medicine and Science in Sports and Exercise* 18(5):526-530.

11. Berns, G.,M. Hull, and H. Patterson H. 1992. Strain in the anteromedial bundle of the anterior cruciate ligament under combination loading. *J Orthop Res* 10:167–176.

12. Beynnon, B.D., B.C. Fleming, R.J. Johnson, C.E. Nichols, P.A. Renstrom, and M.H. Pope. 1995. Anterior cruciate ligament strain behavior during rehabilitation exercises in vivo. *Am J Sports Med* 23(1):24–34.

13. Beynnon, B. D., and B. C. Fleming. 1998. Anterior cruciate ligament strain in-vivo: A review of previous work. *Journal of Biomechanics* 31:519–525.

14. Bjordal, J.M., F. Arnly, B. Hannestad, and T. Strand. 1997. Epidemiology of anterior cruciate ligament injuries in soccer. *Am J Sports Med* 25:341–345.

15. Black, K., and W. Raasch. 1995. Knee braces in sports. In *The lower extremity and spine in sports medicine,* edited by Nicholas, J. and E. Hershman. St. Louis: Mosby.

16. Blackburn, T. 1982. An introduction to the plica. *Journal of Orthopaedic and Sports Physical Therapy* 3:171.

17. Bockrath, K. 1993. *Effect of patellar taping on patellar position and perceived pain.* Poster presentation. APTA Combined Sections, San Antonio.

18. Boden, B. 2010. Non-contact ACL ligament injury: Mechanism and risk factors, *Journal of the Amercian Academy of Orthopedic Surgeons* 18(9):520-527.

19. Boland, A., and M. Hulstyn. 1995. Soft tissue injuries of the knee. In *The lower extremity and spine in sports medicine,* edited by Nicholas, J. and E. Hershman. St. Louis: Mosby.

20. Boling, M.C., L.A. Bolgla, C.G. Mattacola, T.L. Uhl, and R.G. Hosey. 2006. Outcomes of a weight-bearing rehabilitation program for patients diagnosed with patellofemoral pain syndrome. *Arch Phys Med Rehabil* 87:1428-435.

21. Bose, K., R. Kanagasuntheram, and M. Osman. 1980. Vastus medialis oblique: An anatomic and physiologic study. *Orthopaedics* 3:880–883.

22. Brewster, C., D. Moynes, and F. Jobe. 1983. Rehabilitation for the anterior cruciate reconstruction. *Journal of Orthopaedic and Sports Physical Therapy* 5:121–126.

23. Brotzman, B., and P. Head. 1996. The knee. In *Clinical orthopedic rehabilitation,* edited by Brotzman, B. St. Louis: Mosby.

24. Calliet, R. 1983. *Knee pain and disability.* Philadelphia: F. A. Davis.

25. Caraffa, A., G. Cerulli, M. Projetti, G. Aisa, and A. Rizzo. 1996. Prevention of anterior cruciate ligament injuries in soccer. A prospective controlled study of proprioceptive training. *Knee Surg Sports Traumatol, Arthroscopy* 4:19–21.

26. Cavenaugh, J. 1991. Rehabilitation following meniscal surgery. In *Knee ligament rehabilitation,* edited by Engle, R. New York: Churchill Livingstone.

27. Clancy, W., D. Nelson, and B. Reider. 1982. Anterior cruciate ligament reconstruction using one third of the patellar ligament augmented by extra-articular tendon transfers. *Journal of Bone and Joint Surgery* 62A:352.

28. Clancy, W., R. Narechania, and T. Rosenberg. 1981. Anterior and posterior cruciate ligament reconstruction in rhesus monkeys. *Journal of Bone and Joint Surgery* 63A:1270–1284.

29. Clark, M. 2000. *Integrated training for the new millennium.* Thousand Oaks, CA: National Academy of Sports Medicine.

30. Coleman, J., M. Adrian, and H. Yamamoto. 1984. *The teaching of the mechanics of jump landing.* Paper presented at the Second National Symposium on Teaching Kinesiology and Biomechanics in Sports, Colorado Springs, 12–14 January AAHPER.

31. Curwin, S., and W.D. Stanish. 1984. *Tendinitis: Its etiology and treatment.* New York: Collamore Press.

32. DeHaven, K., and R. Bronstein. 1995. Injuries to the meniscii in the knee. In *The lower extremity and spine in sports medicine,* edited by Nicholas, J. and E. Hershman. St. Louis: Mosby.

33. DeLee, J., M. Riley, and C. Rockwood. 1983. Acute straight lateral instability of the knee. *American Journal of Sports Medicine* 11:404–411.

34. DeMorat, G., P. Weinhold, J.T. Blackburn, S. Chudik, and W.E. Garrett. 2004. Aggressive quadriceps loading can induce noncontact anterior cruciate ligament injury. *Am J Sports Med* 32:477–483.

35. DePalma, B., and R. Zelko. 1986. Knee rehabilitation following anterior cruciate injury or surgery. *Athletic Training* 21(3):200–206.

36. Dorchak, J. 1991. Arthroscopic treatment of symptomatic synovial plica of the knee. *American Journal of Sports Medicine* 19:503.

37. Draganich, L.F., R.J. Jaeger, and A.R. Kralj. 1989. Coactivation of the hamstrings and quadriceps during extension of the knee. *J Bone Jt Surg* 71(7):1075–1081.

38. Engle, R., and D. Giesen. 1991. ACL reconstruction rehabilitation. In *Knee ligament rehabilitation,* edited by Engle, R. New York: Churchill Livingstone.

39. Engstrom, B., C. Johansson, and H. Tornkvist. 1991. Soccer injuries among elite female players. *Am J Sport Med* 19(4):372–375.

40. Escamilla, R. F., G. S. Fleisig, and N. Zheng, et al. 1998. Biomechanics of the knee during closed kinetic chain and open kinetic chain exercises. *Medicine and Science in Sports and Exercise* 30:556–569.

41. Fagenbaum R. 2003. Jump landing strategies in male and female college athletes and the implications of such strategies for anterior crucial ligament injuries, *Am J Sports Med* 31(2):233.

42. Ficat, P., and D. Hungerford. 1977. *Disorders of the patellofemoral joint.* Baltimore: Williams & Wilkins.

43. Frank B., Bell, D.R., Norcross, M.F., Blackburn, J.T., Goerger, B.M., Padua, D.A. 2013. Trunk and hip biomechanics influence anterior cruciate loading mechanisms in physically active patients, *American Journal of Sports Medicine,* doi: 10.1177/0363546513496625

44. Fredricson, M., Weir, A. 2006. Practical management of iliotibial band friction syndrome in runners. *Clinical Journal of Sports Medicine* 16(3):261-268.

45. Fulkerson, J. 1989. Evaluation of peripatellar soft tissues and retinaculum in patients with patellofemoral pain. *Clinics in Sports Medicine* 8(2):197–202.

46. Fulkerson, J., and D. Hungerford. 1990. *Disorders of the patellofemoral joint.* Baltimore: Williams & Wilkins.

47. Fulkerson, J., and E. Arendt. 2000. Anterior knee pain in females. *Clinical Orthopaedics* 372:69–73.

48. Fung, D.T., R.W. Hendrix, J.L. Koh, and L.Q. Zhang. 2002. ACL impingement prediction based on MRI scans of individual knees. *Clin Orthop Relat Res* 460:210–218.

49. Fung, D.T., and L. Zhang. 2003. Modeling of ACL impingement against the intercondylar notch. *Clin Biomech* 18:933–941.

50. Garret, J., and R. Stevensen. 1991. Meniscal transplantation in the human knee: A preliminary report. *Arthroscopy* 7:57–62.

51. Geissler, W., and T. Whipple. 1993. Intraarticular abnormalities in association with PCL injuries. *American Journal of Sports Medicine* 21:846–849.

52. Gilchrist, J., B. Mandelbaum, and H. Melancon. 2008. Randomized Controlled Trial to Prevent Noncontact Anterior Cruciate Ligament Injury in Female Collegiate Soccer Players [Preview]. *American Journal of Sports Medicine* 36(8):1476.

53. Gomez, E., J.C. DeLee, and W.C. Farney. 1996. Incidence of injury in Texas girls' high school basketball. *American Journal of Sports Medicine* 24(5):684–687.

54. Goodfellow, J., D. Hungerford, and C. Woods. 1976. Patellofemoral mechanics and pathology: II. Chondromalacia patella. *Journal of Bone and Joint Surgery* 58[B]:287.

55. Gould, J., and G. Davies. 1990. *Orthopaedic and sports physical therapy.* St Louis: Mosby.

56. Griffin L, Albohm M, Arendt E. 2006. Understanding and preventing noncontact anterior cruciate ligament injuries: a review of the Hunt Valley II meeting, *American Journal of Sports Medicine* 34(9):1513.

57. Griffis, N.D., S.W. Vequist, K.M. Yearout, et al. Injury prevention of the anterior cruciate ligament, Presented at the 15th Annual Meeting of the American Orthopaedic Society for Sports Medicine, Traverse City, Michigan. (20 June, 1989).

58. Grodski, M., and R. Marks. 2008. Exercises following anterior cruciate ligament reconstructive surgery: Biomechanical considerations and efficacy of current approaches. *Res Sports Med* 16:75–96.

59. Gwinn, D.E., J.H. Wilckens, E.R. McDevitt, G. Ross, and T. Kao. 2000. The relative incidence of anterior cruciate ligament injury in men and women at the United States naval academy. *Am J Sports Med* 28(1):98–102.

60. Harmon, K., and M. Ireland. 2000. Gender differences in noncontact anterior cruciate ligament injuries. *Clinics in Sports Medicine* 19:287–302.

61. Harner, C., J. Irrgang, and L. Paul. 1992. Loss of motion after ACL reconstruction. *American Journal of Sports Medicine* 20:99–106.

62. Heidt, R.S., L.M. Sweeterman, Jr., R.L. Carlonas, J.A. Traub, and F.X. Tekulve. 2000. Avoidance of soccer injuries with preseason conditioning. *Am J Sports Med* 28(5):659–662.

63. Henning, C.E., and N.D. Griffis. 1990. *Injury prevention of the anterior cruciate ligament* [Videotape]. Mid-American Center for Sports Medicine.

64. Hewett T, Ford K, Myer G. 2006. Anterior cruciate ligament injuries in female athletes, parts 1 and 2: a meta-analysis of neuromuscular interventions aimed at injury prevention, *American Journal of Sports Medicine* 34(3):490.

65. Hewett, T.E. 2000. Neuromuscular and hormonal factors associated with knee injuries in female patients: Strategies for intervention. *Sports Medicine* 29(5):313–327.

66. Hewett, T.E., A.L. Stroupe, T.A. Nance, and F.R. Noyes. 1996. Plyometric training in female patients: Decreased impact forces and increased hamstring torques. *American Journal of Sports Medicine* 24(6):765–73.

67. Hirth, C.J. 2007. Clinical movement analysis to identify muscle imbalances and guide exercise. *Ath Ther Today* 4:10–14.

68. Hodges, P.W., and J. McConnell. 2002. Physical therapy, alters recruitment of the vasti in patellofemoral pain syndrome. *Med Sci Sports Exerc* 34:1879–1885.

69. Host, J., R. Craig, and R. Lehman. 1995. Patellofemoral dysfunction in tennis players: A dynamic problem. *Clin Sports Med* 14:177–203.

70. Hughston, J., W. Walsh, and G. Puddu. 1984. *Patellar subluxation and dislocation*. Philadelphia: W. B. Saunders.

71. Hungerford, D., and M. Barry. 1979. Biomechanics of the patellofemoral joint. *Clinical Orthopedics* 144:9–15.

72. Hurd, W., M. Axe, and L. Snyder-Mackler. 2009. Management of the patient with anterior cruciate ligament deficiency. *Sports Health* 1:39–46.

73. Huston, L., M. Greenfield, and E. Wojtys. 2000. Anterior cruciate ligament injuries in the female patient: Potential risk factors. *Clinical Orthopaedics* 372:50–63.

74. Indelicato, P., J. Hermansdorfer, and M. Huegel. 1990. Nonoperative management of incomplete tears of the MCL of the knee in intercollegiate football players. *Clinical Orthopedics* 256:174–77.

75. Inoue, M. 1987. Treatment of MCL injury: The importance of the ACL ligament on varus-valgus knee laxity. *American Journal of Sports Medicine* 15:15.

76. Insall, J. 1979. Chondromalacia patella: Patellar malalignment syndromes. *Orthopedic Clinics of North America* 10:117–1125.

77. Ireland, M.L. 1999. Anterior cruciate ligament injury in female patients: Epidemiology. *J Ath Train* 34(2):150–154.

78. Ireland, M. et al. 2003. Hip strength in females with and without patellofemoral pain. *Journal of Orthopaedic and Sports Physical Therapy* 33(11):671–676.

79. Irrgang, J., M. Safran, and F. Fu. 1995. The knee: Ligamentous and meniscal injuries. In *Athletic injuries and rehabilitation*, edited by Zachazewski, J. D. Magee, and W. Quillen. Philadelphia: W. B. Saunders.

80. Jackson, D., and D. Drez. 1987. *The anterior cruciate deficient knee*. St Louis: Mosby.

81. Jackson, D., E. Grood, and J. Goldstein. 1993. A comparison of patellar tendon autograft and allograft used for ACL reconstruction in the goat model. *American Journal of Sports Medicine* 21:176–181.

82. Jenkins, D. 1985. *Ligament injuries and their treatment*. Rockville, MD: Aspen.

83. Jensen, J., and R. DiFabio. 1989. Evaluation of eccentric exercise in the treatment of patellar tendinitis. *Physical Therapy* 69(3):211–216.

84. Johnson, D. 1982. Controlling anterior shear during isokinetic knee exercise. *Journal of Orthopaedic and Sports Physical Therapy* 4(1):27.

85. Junge, A., D. Rosch, L. Peterson, T. Graf-Baumann, and J. Dvorak. 2002. Prevention of soccer injuries: A prospective intervention study in youth amateur players. *Am J Sports Med* 30(5):652–659.

86. Kanamori, A., S.L. Woo, C.B. Ma, et al. 2000. The forces in the anterior cruciate ligament and knee kinematics during a simulated pivot shift test: A human cadaveric study using robotic technology. *Arthroscopy* 16(6):633–639.

87. Kanamori, A., J. Zeminski, T.W. Rudy, G. Li, F.H. Fu, and S.L. Woo. 2002. The effect of axial tibial torque on the function of the anterior cruciate ligament: A biomechanical study of a simulated pivot shift test. *Arthroscopy* 18(4):394–398.

88. Kirkendall, D., and W. Garrett. 2000. The anterior cruciate ligament enigma: Injury mechanisms and prevention. *Clinical Orthopaedics* 372:64–68.

89. Kirkendall, D., and W. Garrett. 2001. Motor learning and sports injury: A role in anterior cruciate ligament injury. In *Women's health in sports and exercise: American Academy of Orthopaedic Surgeons symposium*, edited by Garrett, W. et al. Rosemont, IL: American Academy of Orthopaedic Surgeons.

90. Kramer, P. 1983. Patellar malalignment syndrome: Rationale to reduce lateral pressure. *Journal of Orthopaedic and Sports Physical Therapy* 8(6):301.

91. Krosshaug, T., A. Nakamae, and B.P. Boden, et al. 2007. Mechanisms of anterior cruciate ligament injury in basketball: Video analysis of 39 cases. *Am J Sports Med* 35(3):359–367.

92. LaPrade, R., and Q. Burnett. 1994. Femoral intercondylar notch stenosis and correlation to anterior cruciate ligament injuries: A prospective study. *American Journal of Sports Medicine* 21:198–202.

93. Lephart, S., M. Kocher, and F. Fu. 1992. Proprioception following anterior cruciate ligament reconstruction. *Journal of Sport Rehabilitation* 1:188–196.

94. Lindenfeld, T.N., D.J. Schmitt, M.P. Hendy, R.E. Mangine, and F.R. Noyes. 1994. Incidence of injury in indoor soccer. *Am J Sports Med* 21(3):364–371.

95. Lutz, G. S., R. A. Palmitier, K. N. An, and Y. S. Chao. 1993. Comparison of tibiofemoral joint forces during open kinetic chain and closed kinetic chain exercises. *Journal of Bone and Joint Surgery* 75A:732–739.

96. Lutz, G., and R. Warren. 1995. Meniscal injuries. In *Rehabilitation of the injured knee*, edited by Griffin, L. St. Louis: Mosby.

97. Malone, T.R., W.T. Hardaker, and W.E. Garrett. 1993. Relationship of gender to anterior cruciate ligament injuries in intercollegiate basketball players. *J South Orthop Assoc* 2(1):36–39.

98. Malone, T. 1992. *Relationship of gender in ACL injuries of NCAA Division I basketball players*. Paper presented at Specialty Day Meeting of the AOSSM, Washington, DC, February.

99. Mandelbaum, B.R., H.J. Silvers, and D.S. et al. 2005. Effectiveness of a neuromuscular and proprioception training program in preventing anterior cruciate ligament injuries in female patients: A 2-year follow-up. *Am J Sports Med* 33(7):1003–1110.

100. Mangine, R. 1988. *Physical therapy of the knee*. New York: Churchill Livingstone.

101. Mangine, R., and M. Eifert-Mangine. 1991. Postoperative PCL reconstruction rehabilitation. In *Knee ligament rehabilitation*, edited by Engle, R. New York: Churchill Livingstone.

102. Mansmann, K. 1991. PCL reconstruction. In *Knee ligament rehabilitation*, edited by Engle, R. New York: Churchill Livingstone.

103. Markolf, K., D. Burchfield, M. Shapiro, M. Shepard, G. Finerman, and J. Slauterbeck. 1995. Combined knee loading states that generate high anterior cruciate ligament forces. *J Orthop Res* 13:930–935.

104. Mascal, C.L., R. Landel, and C. Powers. 2003. Management of patellofemoral pain targeting hip, pelvis, and trunk muscle function: 2 case reports. *J Orthop Sports Phys Ther* 33:647–660.

105. McCarthy, M., C. Yates, and J. Anderson, et al. 1993. The effects of immediate CPM on pain during the inflammatory phase of soft tissue healing following ACL reconstruction. *Journal of Orthopaedic and Sports Physical Therapy* 17(2):96–101.

106. McConnell, J. 1986. The management of chondromalacia patella: A long-term solution. *Australian Journal of Physiotherapy* 32(4):215–223.

107. McConnell, J., and J. Fulkerson. 1995. The knee: Patellofemoral and soft tissue injuries. In *Athletic injuries and rehabilitation*, edited by Zachazewski, J. D. Magee, and W. Quillen. Philadelphia: W. B. Saunders.

108. McNair, P., and R. Marshall. 1994. Landing characteristics in subjects with normal and anterior cruciate ligament deficient knee joints. *Archives of Physical Medicine and Rehabilitation* 75:584–589.

109. McNair, P., H. Prapavessis, and K. Callender. 2000. Decreasing landing forces: Effect of instruction. *British Journal of Sports Medicine* 34:293–296.

110. Melegati, G., D. Tornese, M. Bandi, P. Volpi, H. Schonhuber, and M. Denti. 2003. The role of the rehabilitation brace in restoring knee extension after anterior cruciate ligament reconstruction: A prospective controlled study. *Knee Surg Sports Traumatol Arthrosc* 9:102–108.

111. Mellion, M., ed. 1987. *Office management of sports injury and athletic problems*. Philadelphia: Hanley & Belfus.

112. Messina, D.F., W.C. Farney, and J.C. DeLee. 1999. The incidence of injury in Texas high school basketball: A prospective study among male and female patients. *Am J Sport Med* 27(3):294–299.

113. Miyasaka, D. R. Danieal, and M. Stone. 1991. The incidence of knee ligament injuries in the population. *American Journal of Knee Surgery* 4:3–8.

114. Mykelbust, G., L. Engebretsen, I.H. Braekken, A. Skjolberg, O. Olsen, and R. Barh. 2003. Prevention of anterior cruciate ligament injuries in female team handball players: A prospective study over three seasons. *Clin J Sport Med* 13:71–78.

115. Nichols, C., and R. Johnson. 1991. Cruciate ligament injuries: Non-operative treatment. In *Ligament and extensor mechanism injuries of the knee*, edited by Scott, N. St. Louis: Mosby.

116. Noyes, F., R. Mangine, and S. Barber. 1987. Early knee motion after open and arthroscopic anterior cruciate ligament reconstruction. *American Journal of Sports Medicine* 15:149.

117. O'Donohue, D. 1970. *Treatment of injuries to patients*. Philadelphia: W. B. Saunders.

118. O'Driscoll, S., F. Keely, and R. Salter. 1986. The chondrogenic potential of free resurfacing of major full-thickness defects in joint surfaces under the influence of continuous passive motion: An experimental investigation in the rabbit. *Journal of Bone and Joint Surgery* 68A:1017.

119. Olsen, O.E., G. Mykelbust, L. Engebretsen, I. Holme, and R. Bahr. 2005. Exercises to prevent lower limb injuries in youth sports: Clulster randomised controlled trial. *Br J Sports Med* 330:449.

120. Olsen, O.E., G. Myklebust, L. Engebretsen, and R. Bahr. 2004. Injury mechanisms for anterior cruciate ligament injuries in team handball: A systematic video analysis. *Am J Sports Med* 32(4):1002–1012.

121. Onate, J. A. 2001. *Noncontact knee injury prevention plan (NC-LEIPP)*. Workshop presented at the National Athletic Trainers' Association 52nd Annual Meeting, Los Angeles, June.

122. Onate, J. A., K. M. Guskiewicz, and R. J. Sullivan. 2001. Augmented feedback reduces jump-landing forces. *Journal of Orthopaedic and Sports Physical Therapy* 31(9): 511–517.

123. Padua, D.A., and S.W. Marshall. 2006. Evidence supporting ACL Injury Prevention Exercise Programs: A review of the literature. *Athletic Therapy Today* 11:11–25.

124. Parolie, J., and J. Bergfeld. 1986. Long-term results of nonoperative treatment of PCL injuries in the patient. *American Journal of Sports Medicine* 14:35–38.

125. Paulos, L., and J. Stern. 1993. Rehabilitation after anterior cruciate ligament surgery, In *The anterior cruciate ligament*, edited by Jackson, D. New York: Raven Press.

126. Paulos, L., F. Noyes, and E. Grood. 1981. Knee rehabilitation after anterior cruciate ligament reconstruction and repair. *American Journal of Sports Medicine* 9:140–149.

127. Pfeiffer, R.P., K.G. Shea, D. Roberts, S. Grandstrand, and L. Bond. 2006. Lack of effect of a knee ligament injury prevention program on the incidence of noncontact anterior cruciate ligament injury. *J Bone Joint Surg* 88(8):1769–1774.

128. Pittman, M., and V. Frankel. 1995. Biomechanics of the knee in athletics. In *The lower extremity and spine in sports medicine*, edited by Nicholas, J. and E. Hershman. St. Louis: Mosby.

129. Powers, C.M., S.R. Ward, M. Fredericson, M. Guillet, and F.G. Shellock. 2003. Patellofemoral kinematics during weightbearing and non-weight-bearing knee extension in persons with lateral subluxation of the patella: A preliminary study. *J Orthop Sports Phys Ther* 33:677–685.

130. Prapavessis, H., and P. McNair. 1999. Effects of instruction in jumping technique and experience jumping on ground reaction forces. *Journal of Orthopaedic and Sports Physical Therapy* 29:352–356.

131. Prentice, W. 1988. A manual resistance technique for strengthening tibial rotation. *Athletic Training* 23(3):230–233.

132. Prentice, W., and T. Toriscelli. 1988. The effects of lateral knee stabilizing braces on running speed and agility. *Athletic Training* 23(3): 230.

133. Quillen, W., and J. Gieck. 1988. Manual therapy: Mobilization of the motion restricted knee. *Athletic Training* 23(2):123–130.

134. Reynold, L., T. Levin, and J. Medoiros et al. 1983. EMG activity of the vastus medialis oblique and the vastus lateralis and their role in patellar alignment. *American Journal of Physical Medicine and Rehabilitation* 62(2):61–71.

135. Richardson, C. 1985. *The role of the knee musculature in high speed oscillating movements of the knee.* MTAA 4th Biennial Conference Proceedings. Brisbane, Australia.

136. Rutland, M, et al. 2010. Evidence-supported rehabilitation of patellar tendinopathy. *North American Journal of Sports Physical Therapy* 5(3):166–178.

137. Salter, R. 1983. Clinical applications for basic research on continuous passive motion for disorders and injuries of synovial joints: A preliminary report of a feasibility study. *Journal of Orthopaedic Research* 3:325.

138. Sgaglione, N., R. Warren, and T. Wickiewicz. 1990. Primary repair with semitendinosis augmentation of acute ACL injuries. *American Journal of Sports Medicine* 18:64–73.

139. Shea, K.G., R.P. Pfeiffer, J.H. Wang, M. Curtin, and P.J. Apel. 2004. Anterior cruciate ligament injury in pediatric and adolescent soccer players: An analysis of insurance data. *J Pediatr Ortho* 24(6):623–628.

140. Shea, K., and J. Fulkerson. 1995. Patellofemoral joint injuries. In *Rehabilitation of the knee*, edited by Griffin, L. St. Louis: Mosby.

141. Shelbourne, K., and P. Nitz. 1992. Accelerated rehabilitation after ACL reconstruction. *Journal of Orthopaedic and Sports Physical Therapy* 15(6):256–264.

142. Shimokochi, Y: Mechanisms of non-contact ACL injury, *J Ath Train* 43(4):396-408, 2008.

143. Schultz, S et al. 2012. ACL Research Retreat VI: An update on ACL injury risk and prevention. *J Ath Train* 43(4):396-408.

144. Soderman, K., S. Werner, T. Pietila, B. Engstrom, and H. Alfredson. 2000. Balance board training: Prevention of traumatic injuries of the lower extremities in female soccer players? A prospective randomized intervention study. *Knee Surg Sports Traumatol, Arthroscopy* 8:356–363.

145. Sommerlath, K., J. Lysholm, and J. Gillquist. 1991. The long-term course of treatment of acute ACL ruptures: A 9 to 16 year followup. *American Journal of Sports Medicine* 19:156–162.

146. Souryal, T., T. Freeman, and J. Evans. 1993. Intercondylar notch size and ACL injuries in patients: A prospective study. *American Journal of Sports Medicine* 21:535–539.

147. Steffen, K., G. Myklebust, and O.E. Olsen, 2009. Preventing injuries in female youth football–A cluster-randomized controlled trial. *Scan J Med Sci Sports*; 18(5):605-614.

148. Steinkamp, L.A., M.F. Dillingham, M.D. Markel, et al. 1993. Biomechanical considerations in patellofemoral joint rehabilitation. *American Journal of Sports Medicine* 21:438-44.

149. Stone, K., and T. Rosenberg. 1993. Surgical technique of meniscal transplantation. *Arthroscopy* 9:234-237.

150. Sweitzer, R., D. Sweitzer, and A. Sarantini. 1991. Rehabilitation for ligament and extensor mechanism injuries. In *Ligament and extensor mechanism injuries of the knee*, edited by Scott, N. St. Louis: Mosby.

151. Tennant, S., A. Williams, V. Vedi, C. Kinmont, W. Gedroyc, and D.M. Hunt. 2001. Patello-femoral tracking in the weight-bearing knee: A study of asymptomatic volunteers utilising dynamic magnetic resonance imaging: A preliminary report. *Knee Surg Sports Traumatol Arthrosc* 9(3):155–162.

152. Tria, A., and K. Klein. 1991. *An illustrated guide to the knee.* New York: Churchill Livingstone.

153. Tyler, T.F., M.P. McHugh, G.W. Gleim, and S.J. Nicholas. 1998. The effect of immediate weightbearing after anterior cruciate ligament reconstruction. *Clin Orthop* 357:141–148.

154. Tyler, T.F., S.J. Nicholas, M.J. Mullaney, and M.P. McHugh. 2006. The role of hip muscle function in the treatment of patellofemoral pain syndrome. *Am J Sports Med* 34: 630–636.

155. Wedderkopp, N., M. Kaltoft, B. Lundgaard, M. Rosendahl, and K. Froberg. 1999. Prevention of injuries in young female European team handball: A prospective intervention study. *Scan J Med Sci Sports* 9(1):41–47.

156. Weiss, J., S. Woo, and K. Ohland. 1991. Evaluation of a new injury model to study MCL healing: Primary repair vs. non-operative treatment. *Journal of Orthopedic Research* 9:516–528.

157. Wilk, K.E., R.F. Escamilla, and G.S. Fleisig, et al. 1996. A comparison of tibiofemoral joint forces and electromyographic activity during open and closed kinetic chain exercises. *American Journal of Sports Medicine* 24:518–27.

158. Wilk, K., and J. Andrews. 1992. Current concepts in treatment of ACL disruption. *Journal of Orthopaedic and Sports Physical Therapy* 15(6):279–93.

159. Wilk, K., and W. Clancey. 1991. Medial collateral ligament injuries: Diagnosis, treatment, and rehabilitation. In *Knee ligament rehabilitation*, edited by Engle, R. New York: Churchill Livingstone.

160. Woo, S. L., R. E. Debaski, J. D., Withrow, and M. A. Janaushek. 1999. Biomechanics of knee ligaments. *American Journal of Sports Medicine* 27(4):533–543.

161. Woodall, W., and J. Welsh. 1991. A biomechanical basis for rehabilitation programs involving the knee joint. *Journal of Orthopaedic and Sports Physical Therapy* 11(11):535.

162. Wright, R.W., and G.B. Fetzer. 2007. Bracing after ACL reconstruction: A systematic review. *Clin Orthop* 465:162–168.

163. Wright, R.W., E. Preston, and B.C. Fleming. 2008. A systematic review of anterior cruciate ligament reconstruction rehabilitation. Part I: Continuous passive motion, early weight bearing, postoperative bracing, and home-based rehabilitation. *J Knee Surg* 21:214–217.

164. Wright, R.W., E. Preston, and B.C. Fleming. 2008. A systematic review of anterior cruciate ligament reconstruction rehabilitation. Part 2: Open versus closed kinetic chain exercises, neuromuscular electrical stimulation, accelerated rehabilitation, and miscellaneous topics. *J Knee Surg* 21:217–222.

165. Yu, B., D.T. Kirkendall, T.N. Taft, and W. Garrett, Jr. 2002. Lower extremity motor control-related and other risk factors for noncontact anterior cruciate ligament injuries. *American Orthopaedic Society for Sports Medicine Instructional Course Lectures* 51:315–324.

166. Zarins, B., and D. Fish. 1995. Knee ligament injury. In *The lower extremity and spine in sports medicine*, edited by Nicholas, J. and E. Hershman. St. Louis: Mosby.

SOLUTIONS TO CLINICAL DECISION-MAKING EXERCISES

21-1 The athletic trainer should recommend that the patient remove the straight-leg immobilizer and begin crutch walking while bearing weight on the injured leg as tolerated. ROM exercises that emphasize pain-free movement should be instituted. Stationary bicycling for ROM purposes can be initiated as tolerated. Isometric strengthening exercises should avoid increased MCL pain and leg abduction movements that place the knee in a valgus position causing strain on the MCL.

21-2 The athletic trainer should recommend that the patient reduce competition for a few days to allow for the reduction of inflammation. The patient should start ice treatments following physical activity and initiate strengthening and stretching of the quadriceps and hamstring musculature. A protective kneepad will help alleviate contact pressure when the patient returns to play, and the patient should continue with ice, stretching, and strengthening exercises following return to activity. The athletic trainer should continue to monitor signs and symptoms, to avoid escalation of knee problems that may require casting or surgical intervention.

21-3 It is important to understand that once a ligament has been sprained, the inherent stability provided to the joint by that ligament has been lost and will never be totally regained. Thus, the patient must rely on the other structures that surround the joint, the muscles and their tendons, to help provide stability. It is essential for the patient to work hard on strengthening exercises for all of the muscle groups that play a role in the function of the knee joint.

21-4 The athletic trainer should continue with ROM and strengthening activities of the quadriceps and surrounding musculature. The athletic trainer should start introducing dynamic stability exercises (eg, low-level plyometrics, single-leg static and dynamic exercises, and proprioception training) that mimic the planting aspect of the kicking maneuver. A prophylactic knee brace may also aid in stability and should not impair the patient because it is the non-kicking leg.

21-5 The athletic trainer should recommend shortening the training sessions; in particular, the running phase of training should be limited. Isometric exercises that are pain-free to strengthen the quadriceps and hamstring muscles can be used initially, progressing to closed chain strengthening exercises. Oral anti-inflammatory agents and small doses of aspirin may help control swelling and reduce pain. Pain might also be reduced by wearing a neoprene sleeve and an orthotic device that corrects pronation and reduces tibial torsion.

21-6 Following an initial evaluation that indicates infrapatellar tendinitis, acute care for the patient should be application of ice. Rehabilitation should consist of flexibility and strengthening exercises for the quadriceps and hamstring musculature, while not causing increased patellar tendon pain. A jump–landing video analysis probably will reveal poor landing technique, with the knees in full extension and a hard landing sound that indicates increased landing forces. A tendinosis strap may be recommended, but strengthening and proper jump–landing technique should be emphasized. The athletic trainer should discuss with the coach reducing plyometric exercises to two or three times per week and beginning each session with a review of proper jump–landing technique.

Please see videos on the accompanying website at

www.healio.com/books/sportsmedvideos

CHAPTER 22

Rehabilitation of Lower-Leg Injuries

Christopher J. Hirth, MSPT, PT, ATC

After completion of this chapter, the athletic training student should be able to do the following:

- Discuss the functional anatomy and biomechanics of the lower leg during open chain and weight-bearing activities such as walking and running.

- Identify the various techniques for regaining range of motion, including stretching exercises and joint mobilizations.

- Discuss the various rehabilitative strengthening techniques, including open and closed chain isotonic exercise, balance/proprioceptive exercises, and isokinetic exercise for dysfunction of the lower leg.

- Identify common causes of various lower-leg injuries and provide a rationale for treatment of these injuries.

- Discuss criteria for progression of the rehabilitation program for various lower-leg injuries.

- Describe and explain the rationale for various treatment techniques in the management of lower-leg injuries.

FUNCTIONAL ANATOMY AND BIOMECHANICS

The lower leg consists of the tibia and fibula and four muscular compartments that either originate on or traverse various points along these bones. Distally the tibia and fibula articulate with the talus to form the talocrural joint. Because of the close approximation of the talus within the mortise, movement of the leg will be dictated by the foot, especially upon ground contact. This becomes important when examining the effects of repetitive stresses placed upon the leg with excessive compensatory pronation secondary to various structural lower-extremity malalignments.[78,79] Proximally the tibia articulates with the femur to form the

Prentice WE, ed.
Rehabilitation Techniques for Sports Medicine and Athletic Training (pp 711-747).
© 2015 SLACK Incorporated.

tibiofemoral joint, as well as serving as an attachment site for the patellar tendon, the distal soft-tissue component of the extensor mechanism. The lower leg serves to transmit ground reaction forces to the knee as well as rotatory forces proximally along the lower extremity that may be a source of pain, especially with athletic activities.[56]

Compartments of the Lower Leg

All muscles work in a functionally integrated fashion in which they eccentrically decelerate, isometrically stabilize, and concentrically accelerate during movement.[50] The muscular components of the lower leg are divided anatomically into four compartments. In an open kinetic chain position, these muscle groups are responsible for movements of the foot, primarily in a single plane. When the foot is in contact with the ground, these muscle–tendon units work both concentrically and eccentrically to absorb ground reaction forces, control excessive movements of the foot and ankle to adapt to the terrain, and, ideally, provide a stable base to propel the limb forward during walking and running.

The anterior compartment is primarily responsible for dorsiflexion of the foot in an open kinetic chain position. Functionally these muscles are active in the early and midstance phase of gait, with increased eccentric muscle activity directly after heel strike to control plantarflexion of the foot and pronation of the forefoot.[21] Electromyographic (EMG) studies have noted that the tibialis anterior is active in more than 85% of the gait cycle during running.[54]

The deep posterior compartment is made up of the tibialis posterior and the long toe flexors and is responsible for inversion of the foot and ankle in an open kinetic chain. These muscles help control pronation at the subtalar joint and internal rotation of the lower leg.[21,54] Along with the soleus, the tibialis posterior will help decelerate the forward momentum of the tibia during the midstance phase of gait.

The lateral compartment is made up of the peroneus longus and brevis, which are responsible for eversion of the foot in an open kinetic chain. Functionally, the peroneus longus plantarflexes the first ray at heel off, while the peroneus brevis counteracts the supinating forces of the tibialis posterior to provide osseous stability of the subtalar and midtarsal joints during the propulsive phase of gait. This is a prime example of muscles working synergistically to isometrically stabilize during movement. EMG studies of running report an increase in peroneus brevis activity when the pace of running is increased.[54]

The superficial posterior compartment is made up of the gastrocnemius and soleus muscles, which in open kinetic chain position are responsible primarily for plantarflexion of the foot. Functionally these muscles are responsible for acting eccentrically, controlling pronation of the subtalar joint and internal rotation of the leg in the midstance phase of gait and acting concentrically during the push-off phase of gait.[21,54]

REHABILITATION TECHNIQUES FOR SPECIFIC INJURIES

Tibial and Fibular Fractures

Pathomechanics

The tibia and fibula constitute the bony components of the lower leg and are primarily responsible for weight bearing and muscle attachment. The tibia is the most commonly fractured long bone in the body, and fractures are usually the result of either direct trauma to the area or indirect trauma such as a combination rotatory/compressive force. Fractures of the fibula are usually seen in combination with a tibial fracture or as a result of direct trauma to the area. Tibial fractures will present with immediate pain, swelling, and possible deformity and can be open or closed in nature. Fibular fractures alone are usually closed and present with pain on palpation and with ambulation. These fractures should be treated with immediate medical referral and most likely a period of immobilization and restricted weight bearing for weeks to possibly months, depending on the severity and involvement of the injury. Surgery such as open reduction with

REHABILITATION TECHNIQUES FOR THE LOWER LEG

Strengthening Techniques

Isotonic Open Kinetic Chain Exercises

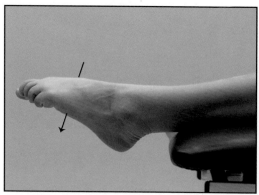

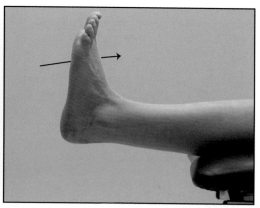

Figure 22-1. Active range of motion ankle plantarflexion. Used to activate the primary and secondary ankle plantarflexor muscle–tendon units after a period of immobilization or disuse. This exercise can be performed in a supportive medium such as a whirlpool.

Figure 22-2. Active range of motion ankle dorsiflexion. Used to activate the tibialis anterior, extensor hallucis longus, and extensor digitorum longus muscle–tendon units after a period of immobilization or disuse.

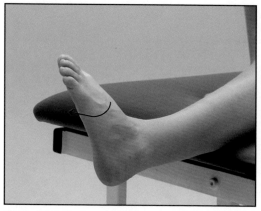

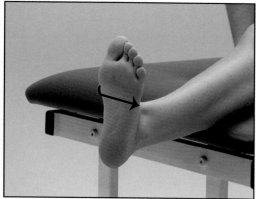

Figure 22-3. Active range of motion ankle inversion. Used to activate the tibialis posterior, flexor hallucis longus, and flexor digitorum longus muscle–tendon units after a period of immobilization or disuse.

Figure 22-4. Active range of motion ankle eversion. Used to activate the peroneus longus and brevis muscle–tendon units after a period of immobilization or disuse.

Figure 22-5. Resistive range of motion ankle plantarflexion with rubber tubing. Used to strengthen the gastrocnemius, soleus, and secondary ankle plantarflexors, including the peroneals, flexor hallucis longus, flexor digitorum longus, and tibialis posterior, in an open chain. This exercise will also place a controlled concentric and eccentric load on the Achilles tendon.

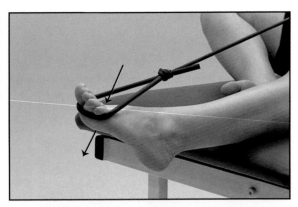

Figure 22-6. Resistive range of motion ankle dorsiflexion with rubber tubing. Used to isolate and strengthen the ankle dorsiflexors, including the tibialis anterior, extensor hallucis longus, and extensor digitorum longus, in an open chain.

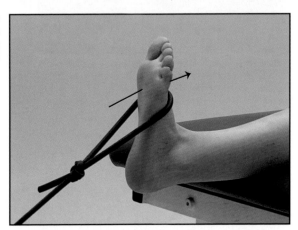

Figure 22-7. Resistive range of motion ankle inversion with rubber tubing. Used to isolate and strengthen the ankle inverters, including the tibialis posterior, flexor hallucis longus, and flexor digitorum longus, in an open chain.

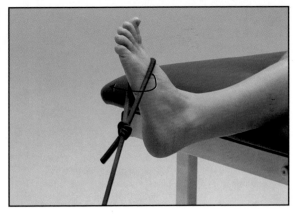

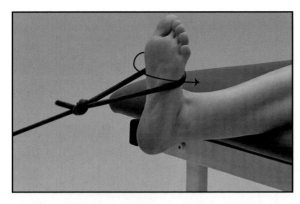

Figure 22-8. Resistive range of motion ankle eversion with rubber tubing. Used to isolate and strengthen the ankle everters, including the peroneus longus and peroneus brevis, in an open chain.

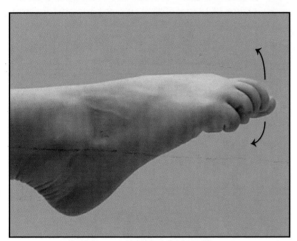

Figure 22-9. Active range of motion toe flexion/extension. Used to activate the long toe flexors, extensors, and foot intrinsic musculature. This exercise will also help to improve the tendon-gliding ability of the extensor hallucis longus, extensor digitorum longus, flexor hallucis longus, and flexor digitorum longus tendons after a period of immobilization.

Closed Kinetic Chain Strengthening Exercises

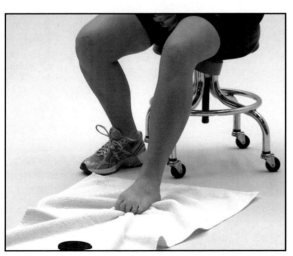

Figure 22-10. Towel-gathering exercise. Used to strengthen the foot intrinsics and long toe flexor and extensor muscle–tendon units. A weight can be placed on the end of the towel to require more force production by the muscle–tendon unit as range of motion and strength improve.

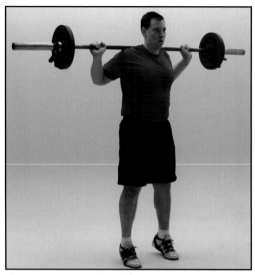

Figure 22-11. Heel raises. Used to strengthen the gastrocnemius musculature and will directly load the Achilles tendon.

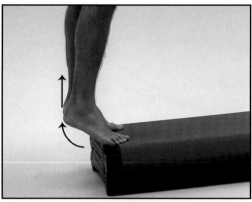

Figure 22-12. Two-legged heel raise. Used to strengthen the gastrocnemius when the knee is extended and the soleus when the knees are flexed. The flexor hallucis longus, flexor digitorum longus, tibialis posterior, and peroneals will also be activated during this activity. The patient can modify concentric and eccentric activity depending on the type and severity of the condition. For example, if an eccentric load is not desired on the involved side, the patient can raise up on both feet and lower down on the uninvolved side until eccentric loading is tolerated on the involved side.

Figure 22-13. One-legged heel raise. Used to strengthen the gastrocnemius and soleus muscles when the knee is extended and flexed, respectively. This can be used as a progression from the two-legged heel raise.

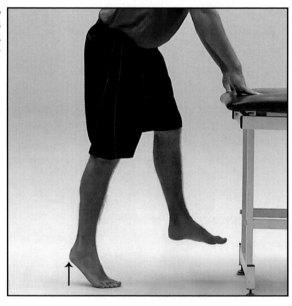

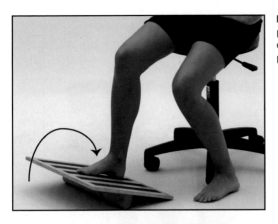

Figure 22-14. Seated closed chain ankle dorsiflexion/plantarflexion active ROM. Used to activate the ankle dorsiflexor/plantarflexor musculature in a closed chain position.

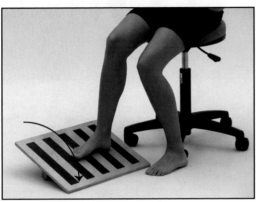

Figure 22-15. Seated closed chain ankle inversion/eversion active ROM. Used to activate the ankle inverter/everter musculature in a closed chain position.

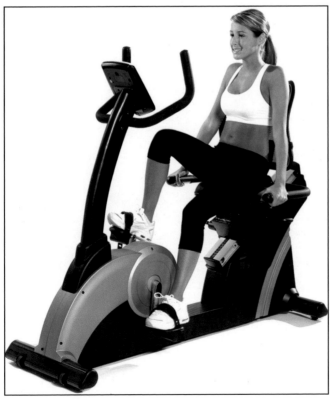

Figure 22-16. Stationary cycle. Used to reduce impact of weight-bearing forces on the lower extremity while also maintaining cardiovascular fitness levels. (Reprinted with permission from Smooth Fitness.)

Figure 22-17. Stair-stepping machine. Used to progressively load the lower extremity in a closed chain as well as maintain and improve cardiovascular fitness. (Reprinted with permission from Stairmaster, Inc.)

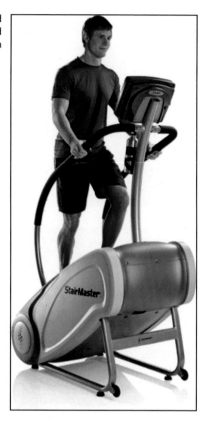

Stretching Exercises

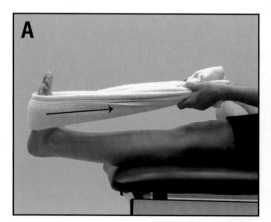

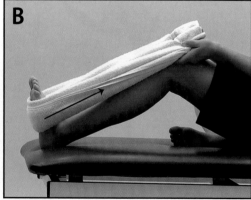

Figure 22-18. Ankle plantarflexors towel stretch. (A) Used to stretch the gastrocnemius when the knee is extended; and (B) the soleus when the knee is flexed. The Achilles tendon will be stretched with both positions. The patient can hold the stretch for 20 to 30 seconds.

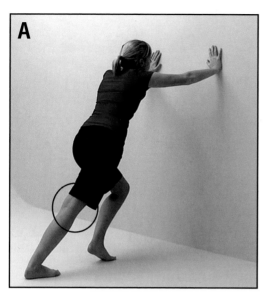

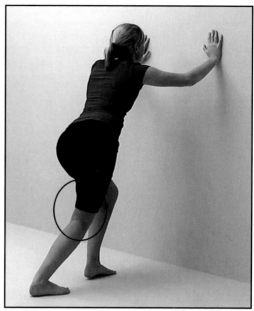

Figure 22-19. (A) Standing gastrocnemius stretch. Used to stretch the gastrocnemius muscle. The Achilles tendon will also be stretched. (B) Standing soleus stretch. Used to stretch the soleus muscle. The Achilles tendon will also be stretched.

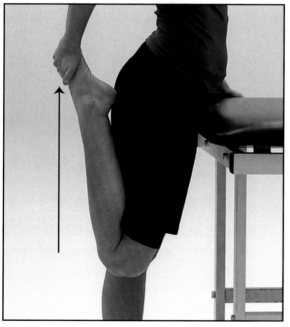

Figure 22-20. Standing ankle dorsiflexor stretch. Used to stretch the extensor hallucis longus, extensor digitorum longus, tibialis anterior, and anterior ankle capsule.

Figure 22-21. Standing ankle dorsiflexor stretch. Used to stretch the extensor hallucis longus, extensor digitorum longus, tibialis anterior, and anterior ankle capsule. This is an aggressive stretch that can be used in the later stages of rehabilitation to gain end ROM ankle dorsiflexion.

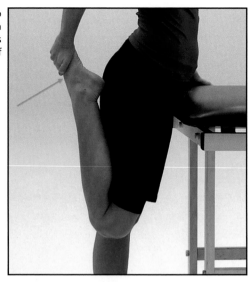

Exercises to Reestablish Neuromuscular Control

Figure 22-22. Standing double-leg balance on Bosu Balance Trainer. Used to activate the lower-leg musculature and improve balance and proprioception in the lower extremity.

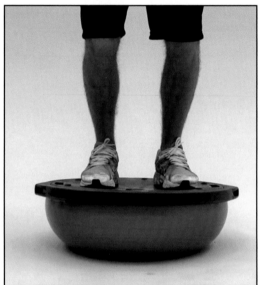

Figure 22-23. Standing single-leg balance board activity. Used to activate the lower-leg musculature and improve balance and proprioception in the involved extremity.

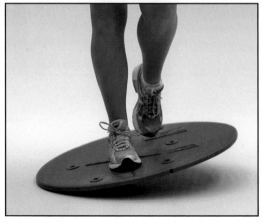

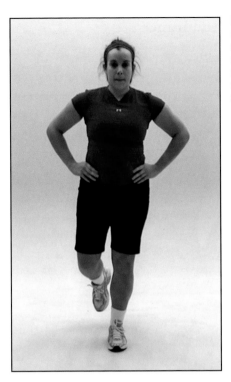

Figure 22-24. Static single-leg standing balance progression. Used to improve balance and proprioception of the lower extremity. This activity can be made more difficult with the following progression: (A) single-leg stand, eyes open; (B) single-leg stand, eyes closed; (C) single-leg stand, eyes open, toes extended so only the heel and metatarsal heads are in contact with the ground; (D) single-leg stand, eyes closed, toes extended.

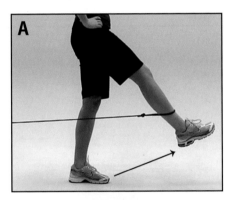

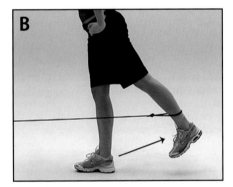

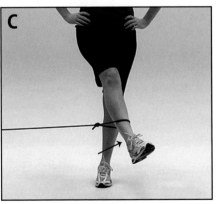

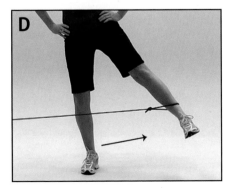

Figure 22-25. Single-leg standing rubber-tubing kicks. Used to improve muscle activation of the lower leg to maintain single-leg standing on the involved extremity while kicking against the resistance of the rubber tubing. (A) Extension; (B) flexion; (C) adduction; (D) abduction.

Exercises to Improve Cardiorespiratory Endurance

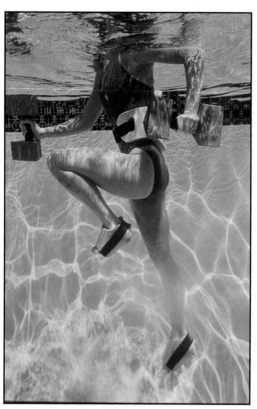

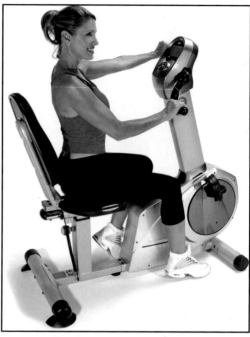

Figure 22-27. Upper-body ergometer. Used to maintain cardiovascular fitness when lower-extremity ergometer is contraindicated or too difficult for the patient to use. (Reprinted with permission from Stamina Products.)

Figure 22-26. Pool running with flotation device. Used to reduce impact weight-bearing forces on the lower extremity while maintaining cardiovascular fitness level and running form.

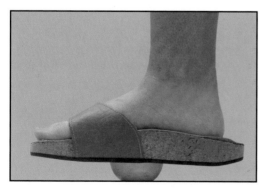

Figure 22-28. Exercise sandals (OPTP, Minneapolis, MN). Wooden sandals with a rubber hemisphere located centrally on the plantar surface.

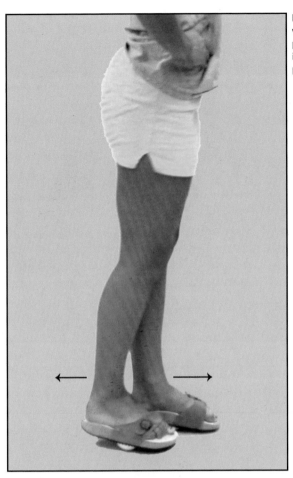

Figure 22-29. Exercise sandal forward and backward walking. Used to enhance balance and proprioception and increase muscle activity in the foot intrinsics, lower-leg musculature, and gluteals. The patient takes small steps forward and backward.

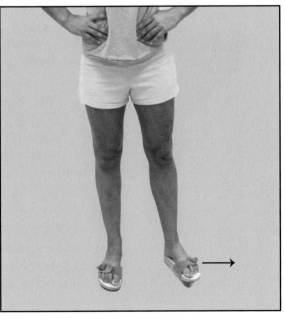

Figure 22-30. Exercise sandals sidestepping. Used to enhance balance and proprioception in the frontal plane. Increases muscle activity of the lower-leg musculature and foot intrinsics. The patient moves directly to the left or right along a straight line with the toes pointed forward.

Figure 22-31. Exercise sandals butt kicks. Used to promote balance and proprioception along with increased muscle activity of the foot intrinsics, lower-leg musculature, and gluteals. This exercise enhances single-leg stance in the exercise sandals.

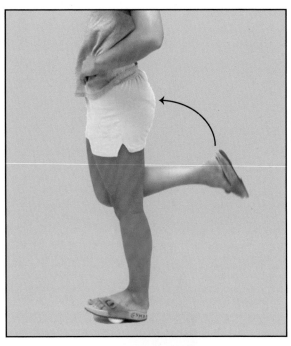

Figure 22-32. Exercise sandals high knees. Used to enhance balance and proprioception and muscle activity of the foot intrinsics, lower-leg musculature, and especially the gluteals. The patient should maintain an upright posture and avoid trunk flexion with hip flexion. This exercise promotes single-leg stance progression for a short time.

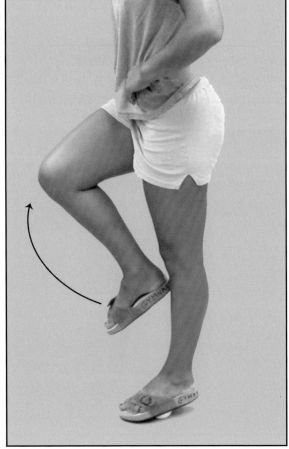

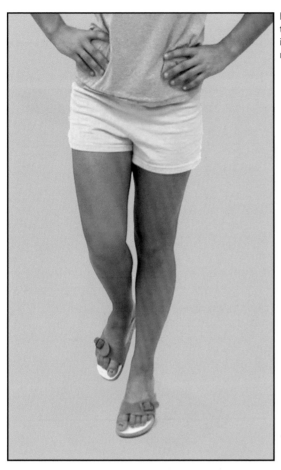

Figure 22-33. Exercise sandals single-leg stance. Used to enhance balance, proprioception, and muscle activity in the entire lower extremity. This exercise is the most demanding in the exercise sandal progression.

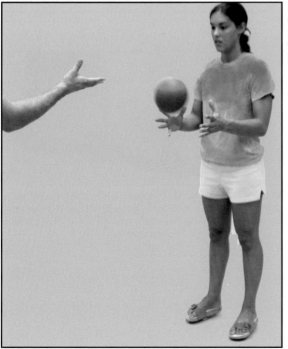

Figure 22-34. Exercise sandal ball catch. Used to enhance balance, proprioception, and lower-leg muscle activity. The patient focuses on catching and throwing the ball to the athletic trainer while moving laterally to the left or right.

Figure 22-35. Achilles tendon eccentric muscle loading. Used to enhance gastrocnemius (knee straight) and soleus (knee bent) strength and Achilles tendon tensile strength. The patient uses the uninvolved side to elevate onto the patient's toes and then places all weight on toes of the involved side to eccentrically lower. Initially, the patient lowers to the step and then progresses below the level of the step. Extra weight can be added via a backpack.

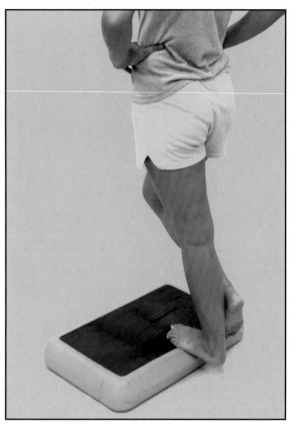

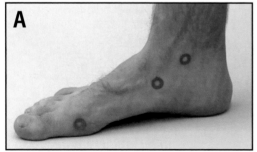 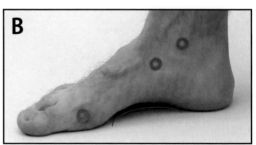

Figure 22-36. Short foot concept. Used to enhance and strengthen the foot intrinsic muscles. The patient is instructed to shorten the foot from front to back while keeping the toes straight. The metatarsal heads should stay in contact with the ground. The athletic trainer can palpate the foot intrinsics and will notice a raised longitudinal arch with a flexible foot type. The shortened foot should be maintained at all times while in the exercise sandals.

internal fixation of the bone, usually of the tibia, is common.

Injury Mechanism

The two mechanisms of a traumatic lower-leg fracture are either a direct insult to the bone or indirectly through a combined rotatory/compressive force. Direct impact to the long bone, such as from a projectile object or the top of a ski boot, can produce enough damaging force to fracture a bone. Indirect trauma from a combination of rotatory and compressive forces can be manifested in sports when an athlete's foot is planted and the proximal segments are rotated with a large compressive force. An example of this could be a football running back attempting to gain more yardage while an opposing player is trying to tackle him from above the waist and applying a superincumbent compressive load. If the patient's foot is planted and immovable and the lower extremity is rotated, the superincumbent weight of the defender may be enough to cause a fracture in the tibia. A fibular fracture may accompany the tibial fracture.

Rehabilitation Concerns

Tibial and fibular fractures are usually immobilized and placed on a restricted weight-bearing status for a time to facilitate fracture healing. Immobilization and restricted weight bearing of a bone, its proximal and distal joints, and surrounding musculature will lead to functional deficits once the fracture is healed. Depending on the severity of the fracture, there also may be postsurgical considerations such as an incision and hardware within the bone. Complications following immobilization include joint stiffness of any joints immobilized, muscle atrophy of the lower leg and possibly the proximal thigh and hip musculature, as well as an abnormal gait pattern. Bullock-Saxton demonstrated changes in gluteus maximus EMG muscle activation after a severe ankle sprain.[13] Proximal hip muscle weakness is magnified by the immobility and non-weight-bearing action that accompanies lower-leg fractures. It is important that the athletic trainer perform a comprehensive evaluation of the patient to determine all potential rehabilitation problems, including range of motion (ROM), joint mobility, muscle flexibility, strength and endurance of the entire involved lower extremity, balance, proprioception, and gait. The athletic trainer must also determine the functional demands that will be placed on the patient upon return to competition and set up short- and long-term goals accordingly. Upon cast removal it is important to address ROM deficits. This can be managed with passive, then active, ROM exercises in a supportive medium such as a warm whirlpool (Figures 22-1 to 22-4, 22-9, 22-14 through 22-17). Joint stiffness can be addressed via joint mobilization to any joint that was immobilized (see Figures 13-61 to 13-68). It is possible to have posttraumatic edema in the foot and ankle after cast removal that can be reduced with massage. Strengthening exercises can help facilitate muscle firing, strength, and endurance (Figures 22-5 to 22-8 and 22-10 to 22-17). Balance and proprioception can be improved with single-leg standing activities and balance board activities (Figures 22-22 to 22-25). Cardiovascular endurance can be addressed with pool activities including swimming and pool running with a flotation device, stationary cycling, and the use of an upper-body ergometer (Figures 22-16, 22-26 and 22-27). A stair stepper is also an excellent way to address cardiovascular needs as well as lower-extremity strength, endurance, and weight bearing (Figure 22-17).

Once the patient demonstrates proficiency in static balance activities on various balance modalities, more dynamic neuromuscular control activities can be introduced. Exercise sandals (OPTP, Minneapolis, MN) can be incorporated into rehabilitation as a closed kinetic chain functional exercise that places increased proprioceptive demands on the patient. The exercise sandals are wooden sandals with a rubber hemisphere located centrally on the plantar surface (Figure 22-28). The patient can be progressed into the exercise sandals once he or she demonstrates proficiency in barefoot single-leg stance. Prior to using the exercise sandals the patient is instructed in the short-foot concept—a shortening of the foot in an anteroposterior direction while the long toe flexors are relaxed, thus activating the short toe flexors and foot the intrinsics (Figure 22-36).[37] Clinically, the short foot appears to enhance the longitudinal and transverse arches of the foot. Once the patient can perform the short-foot concept in the sandals, the he or she is progressed to walking in place and forward walking with short steps (Figure 22-29). The patient is instructed to assume a good upright posture while training in the sandals. Initially, the patient may be limited to 30 to 60 seconds while acclimating to the proprioceptive demands. Once the patient appears safe with walking in place and small-step forward walking, the patient can follow a rehabilitation progression (Table 22-1 and Figures 22-30 to 22-34).

Table 22-1 Exercise Sandal Progression

1. Walking in place
2. Forward/backward walking—small steps
3. Sidestepping
4. Butt kicks
5. High knees
6. Single-leg stance—10 to 15 seconds
7. Ball catch—sidestepping
8. Sport-specific activity
   - Each activity can be performed for 30 to 60 seconds with rest between each activity.
   - All exercises should be performed with short-foot and good standing posture except where sport-specific activity dictates otherwise.

The exercise sandals offer an excellent means of facilitating lower-extremity musculature that can be affected by tibial and fibular fractures. Bullock-Saxton et al noted increased gluteal muscle activity with exercise sandal training after 1 week.[14] Myers et al also demonstrated increased gluteal activity, especially with high-knees marching in the exercise sandals.[48] Blackburn et al have shown increased activity in the lower-leg musculature, specifically the tibialis anterior and peroneus longus, while performing the exercise sandal progression activities.[11] The lower-leg musculature is usually weakened and atrophied from being so close to the trauma. The exercise sandals offer an excellent means of increasing muscle activation of the lower-leg musculature in a functional weight-bearing manner.

Rehabilitation Progression

Management of a post-immobilization fracture requires good communication with the physician to determine progression of weight-bearing status, any assistive devices to be used during the rehabilitation process, such as a walker boot, and any other pertinent information that can influence the rehabilitation process. It is important to address ROM deficits immediately with active ROM (AROM), passive stretching, and skilled joint mobilization. Isometric strengthening can be initiated and progressed to isotonic exercises once ROM has been normalized. After weight-bearing status is determined, gait training to normalize walking should be initiated. Assistive devices should be used as needed. Strengthening of the involved lower extremity can be incorporated into the rehabilitation process, especially for the hip and thigh musculature. It is important for the therapist to identify and address this hip muscular weakness early on in rehabilitation through open and closed chain strengthening. Balance and proprioceptive exercises can begin once there is full pain-free weight-bearing on the involved lower extremity.

As ROM, strength, and walking gait are normalized, the patient can be progressed to a walking/jogging progression and a sport-related functional progression. It must be realized that the rate of rehabilitation progression will depend on the severity of the fracture, any surgical involvement, and length of immobilization. The average healing time for uncomplicated nondisplaced tibial fractures is 10 to 13 weeks; for displaced, open, or comminuted tibial fracture, it is 16 to 26 weeks.[67]

Fibular fractures may be immobilized for 4 to 6 weeks. Again, an open line of communication with the physician is required to facilitate a safe rehabilitation progression for the patient.

Criteria for Full Return

The following criteria should be met prior to the return to full activity: (a) full ROM and strength, compared to the uninvolved side; (b) normalized walking, jogging, and running gait; (c) ability to hop for endurance and 90%

hop for distance compared to the uninvolved side, without complaints of pain or observable compensation; and (d) successful completion of a sport-specific functional test.

Clinical Decision-Making Exercise 22-1

A patient presents to the athletic training clinic 8 weeks after tibial fracture. An X-ray reveals excellent bony healing. The cast was removed today, and the physician would like him to begin rehabilitation. The evaluation reveals moderate atrophy of the lower leg and quadriceps musculature, along with severe restriction in foot and ankle joint ROM. Gait abnormalities are also present. Muscle testing reveals significant weakness throughout the entire lower extremity. What rehabilitation exercises could this patient start with to address some of his orthopedic problems?

Tibial and Fibular Stress Fractures

Pathomechanics

Stress fractures of the tibia and fibula are common in sports. Studies indicate that stress fractures of the tibia occur at a higher rate than those of the fibula.[7,8,45] Stress fractures in the lower leg are usually the result of the bone's inability to adapt to the repetitive loading response during training and conditioning of the athlete. The bone attempts to adapt to the applied loads initially through osteoclastic activity, which breaks down the bone. Osteoblastic activity, or the laying down of new bone, will soon follow.[53,77] If the applied loads are not reduced during this process, structural irregularities will develop within the bone, which will further reduce the bone's ability to absorb stress and will eventually lead to a stress fracture.[8,27]

Repetitive loading of the lower leg with a weight-bearing activity such as running is usually the cause of tibial and fibular stress fractures. Romani reports that repetitive mechanical loading seen with the initiation of a stressful activity may cause an ischemia to the affected bone.[58] He reports that repetitive loading may lead to temporary oxygen debt of the bone, which signals the remodeling process

to begin.[58] Also, microdamage to the capillaries further restricts blood flow, leading to more ischemia, which again triggers the remodeling process—leading to a weakened bone and a setup for a stress fracture.[58]

Stress fractures in the tibial shaft mainly occur in the mid anterior aspect and the posteromedial aspect.[7,45,55,77] Anterior tibial stress fractures usually present in patients involved in repetitive jumping activities with localized pain directly over the mid anterior tibia. The patient will complain of pain with activity that is relieved with rest. The pain can affect activities of daily living (ADL) if activity is not modified. Vibration testing using a tuning fork will reproduce the symptoms, as will hopping on the involved extremity. A triple-phase technetium-99 bone scan can confirm the diagnosis faster than an X-ray, as it can take a minimum of 3 weeks to demonstrate radiographic changes.[53,55,77] Posteromedial tibial pain usually occurs over the distal one-third of the bone with a gradual onset of symptoms.

Focal point tenderness on the bone will help differentiate a stress fracture from medial tibial stress syndrome (MTSS), which is located in the same area but is more diffuse upon palpation. The procedures listed above will be positive and will implicate the stress fracture as the source of pain. Fibular stress fractures usually occur in the distal one-third of the bone with the same symptomatology as for tibial stress fractures. Although less common, stress fractures of the proximal fibula are noted in the literature.[45,73,88]

Injury Mechanism

Anterior tibial stress fractures are prevalent in patients involved with jumping. Several authors have noted that the tibia will bow anteriorly with the convexity on the anterior aspect.[18,53,56,77] This places the anterior aspect of the tibia under tension that is less than ideal for bone healing, which prefers compressive forces. Repetitive jumping will place greater tension on this area, which has minimal musculotendinous support and blood supply. Other biomechanical factors may be involved, including excessive compensatory pronation at the subtalar joint to accommodate lower-extremity structural alignments such as forefoot varus, tibial varum, and femoral anteversion. This excessive pronation might not affect the leg during ADL or with moderate activity, but might become a factor with increases in training intensity, duration, and frequency, even with sufficient recovery time.[30,77] Increased training may affect the surrounding muscle–tendon unit's ability to absorb the impact of each applied load, which places more stress on the bone. Stress fractures of the distal posteromedial tibia will also arise from the same problems as listed above, with the exception of repetitive jumping. Excessive compensatory pronation may play a greater role with this type of injury. This hyperpronation can be accentuated when running on a crowned road; such is the case of the uphill leg.[60] Also, running on a track with a small radius and tight curves will tend to increase pronatory stresses on the leg that is closer to the inside of the track.[60] Excessive pronation may also play a role with fibular stress fractures. The repeated activity of the ankle everters and calf musculature pulling on the bone may be a source of this type of stress fracture.[53] Training errors of increased duration and intensity along with worn-out shoes will only accentuate these problems.[60] Other factors, including menstrual irregularities, diet, bone density, increased hip external rotation, tibial width, and calf girth, also have been identified as contributing to stress fractures.[8,29]

Rehabilitation Concerns

Immediate elimination of the offending activity is most important. The patient must be educated on the importance of this to prevent further damage to the bone. Many patients will express concerns about fitness level with loss of activity. Stationary cycling and running in the deep end of the pool with a flotation device can help maintain cardiovascular fitness (Figures 22-16 and 22-26). Eyestone et al demonstrated a small, but statistically significant, decrease in maximal aerobic capacity when water running was substituted for regular running.[23] This was also true with using a stationary bike.[23] These authors recommend that intensity, duration, and frequency be equivalent to regular training. Wilder et al note that water provides a resistance that is proportional to the effort exerted.[84] These authors found that cadence,

via a metronome, gave a quantitative external cue that with increased rate showed high correlation with heart rate.[84] Nonimpact activity in the pool or on the bike will help maintain fitness and allow proper bone healing. Proper footwear that matches the needs of the foot is also important. For example, a high arched or pes cavus foot type will require a shoe with good shock-absorbing qualities. A pes planus foot type or more pronated foot will require a shoe with good motion control characteristics. Recent evidence-based reviews indicate that shock-absorbing insoles can have a preventative effect with tibial stress fractures.[65] A detailed biomechanical exam of the lower extremity, both statically and dynamically, may reveal problems that require the use of a custom foot orthotic. Stretching and strengthening exercises can be incorporated in the rehabilitation process. The use of ice and electrical stimulation to control pain is also recommended.

The use of an Aircast with patients who have diagnosed stress fractures has produced positive results.[20] Dickson and Kichline speculate that the Aircast unloads the tibia and fibula enough to allow healing of the stress fracture with continued participation.[20] Swenson et al reported that patients with tibial stress fractures who used an Aircast returned to full unrestricted activity in 21 ± 2 days; patients who used a traditional regimen returned in 77 ± 7 days.[76] Fibular and posterior medial tibial stress fractures will usually heal without residual problems if the above mentioned concerns are addressed. Stress fractures of the mid anterior tibia can take much longer, and residual problems might exist months to years after the initial diagnosis, with attempts at increased activity.[18,22,55,56] Initial treatment may include a short-leg cast and non–weight-bearing for 6 to 8 weeks.

Batt et al noted that use of a pneumatic brace in those individuals allowed for return to unrestricted activity, an average of 12 months from presentation.[4] The proposed hypothesis for use of a pneumatic brace is that elevated osseous hydrostatic and venous blood pressure produces a positive piezoelectric effect that stimulates osteoblastic activity and facilitates fracture healing.[87] Rettig et al used rest from the offending activity as well as electrical stimulation in the form of a pulsed electromagnetic field for a period of 10 to 12 hours per day. The authors noted an average of 12.7 months from the onset of symptoms to return to full activity with this regimen.[56] They recommended using this program for 3 to 6 months before considering surgical intervention.[56] Chang and Harris noted good to excellent results with a surgical procedure involving intramedullary nailing of the tibia with individuals with delayed union of this type of stress fracture.[18] Surgical procedures involving bone grafting have also been recommended to improve healing of this type of stress fracture.

Rehabilitation Progression

After diagnosis of the stress fracture, the patient may be placed on crutches, depending on the amount of discomfort with ambulation. Ice and electrical stimulation can be used to reduce local inflammation and pain. The patient can immediately begin deep-water running with the same training parameters as his or her regular regimen if he or she is pain-free. Stretching exercises for the gastrocnemius–soleus musculature can be performed two to three times per day (Figure 22-19). Isotonic strengthening exercises with rubber tubing can begin as soon as tolerated on an every-other-day basis, with an increase in repetitions and sets as the athletic trainer sees fit (Figures 22-5 to 22-8).

Strengthening of the gastrocnemius can be done initially in an open chain and eventually be progressed to a closed chain (Figures 22-5, 22-12, and 22-13). The patient should wear supportive shoes during the day and avoid shoes with a heel, which can cause adaptive shortening of the gastrocnemius–soleus complex and increase strain on the healing bone. Custom foot orthotics can be fabricated for motion control to prevent excessive pronation for those patients who need it. Foot orthotics can also be fabricated for a high-arched foot to increase stress distribution throughout the plantar aspect of the whole foot vs the heel and the metatarsal heads. Shock-absorbing materials can augment these orthotics to help reduce ground reaction forces. The exercise sandal progression can also be introduced to help facilitate lower-leg muscle activity and strength (Figures 22-29 to 22-34 and 22-36).

As the symptoms subside during a period of 3 to 4 weeks and X-rays confirm that good callus formation is occurring, the patient may be progressed to a walking/jogging progression on a surface suitable to that patient's needs. The patient must demonstrate pain-free ambulation prior to initiating a walk/jog program. A quality track or grass surface may be the best choice to begin this progression. The patient may be instructed to jog for 1 minute, then walk for 30 seconds for 10 to 15 repetitions. This can be performed on an every-other-day basis with high-intensity/long-duration cardiovascular training occurring daily in the pool or on the bike. The patient should be reminded that the purpose of the walk/jog progression is to provide a gradual increase in stress to the healing bone in a controlled manner. If tolerated, the jogging time can be increased by 30 seconds every 2 to 3 training sessions until the patient is running 5 minutes without walking. The above progression is a guideline and can be modified based on individual needs.

Romani has developed a three-phase plan for stress fracture management.[58] Phase 1 focuses on decreasing pain and stress to the injured bone while also preventing deconditioning. Phase 2 focuses on increasing strength, balance, and conditioning, and normalizing function, without an increase in pain. After 2 weeks of pain-free exercise in phase 2, running and functional activities of phase 3 are introduced. Phase 3 has functional phases and rest phases. During the functional phase, weeks 1 and 2, running is progressed; in the third week, or rest phase, running is decreased. This is done to mimic the cyclic fashion of bone growth. During the first 2 weeks, as bone is resorbed, running will promote the formation of trabecular channels; in the third week, while the osteocytes and periosteum are maturing, the impact loading of running is removed.[58] This cyclic progression is continued over several weeks as the patient becomes able to perform sport-specific activities without pain.[58]

Criteria for Full Return

The patient can return to full activity when: (a) there is no tenderness to palpation of the affected bone and no pain of the affected area with repeated hopping; (b) plain films demonstrate good bone healing; (c) there has been successful progression of a graded return to running with no increase in symptoms; (d) gastrocnemius–soleus flexibility is within normal limits; (e) hyperpronation has been corrected or shock-absorption problems have been decreased with proper shoes and foot orthotics if indicated; and (f) all muscle strength and muscle length issues of the involved lower extremity have been addressed.

Clincial Decision-Making Exercise 22-2

A college freshman cross-country patient presents with localized posterior medial shin pain. She notes a gradual onset in the last 2 weeks with an increase in her training volume. She has been training primarily on concrete and asphalt, and also on trails wet from excessive rainfall. What advice can the athletic trainer give this patient to help her eliminate this problem?

Compartment Syndromes

Pathomechanics and Injury Mechanism

Compartment syndrome is a condition in which increased pressure within a fixed osseofascial compartment causes compression of muscular and neurovascular structures within the compartment. As compartment pressures increase, the venous outflow of fluid decreases and eventually stops, causing further fluid leakage from the capillaries into the compartment. Eventually arterial blood inflow also ceases secondary to rising intracompartmental pressures.[82] Compartment syndrome can be divided into three categories: acute compartment syndrome, acute exertional compartment syndrome, and chronic compartment syndrome. Acute compartment syndrome occurs secondary to direct trauma to the area and is a medical emergency.[38,74,82] The patient will complain of a deep-seated aching pain, tightness, and swelling of the involved compartment. Reproduction of the pain will occur with passive stretching of the involved muscles. Reduction in pedal pulses and sensory changes of the involved nerve can be present, but are not reliable signs.[82,86] Intracompartmental pressure measurements

will confirm the diagnosis. Emergency fasciotomy is the definitive treatment.

Acute exertional compartment syndrome occurs without any precipitating trauma. Cases have been cited in the literature in which acute compartment syndrome has evolved with minimal to moderate activity. If not diagnosed and treated properly, it can lead to poor functional outcomes for the patient.[24,86] Again, intracompartmental pressures will confirm the diagnosis, with emergency fasciotomy being the treatment of choice. Chronic compartment syndrome (CCS) is activity-related in that the symptoms arise rather consistently at a certain point in the activity. The patient complains of a sensation of pain, tightness, and swelling of the affected compartment that resolves upon stopping the activity. Studies indicate that the anterior and deep posterior compartments are usually involved.[6,57,64,75,85] Upon presentation of these symptoms, intracompartmental pressure measurements will further define the severity of the condition. Pedowitz et al developed modified criteria using a slit-catheter measurement of the intracompartmental pressures. These authors consider one or more of the following intramuscular pressure criteria as diagnostic of CCS: (A) preexercise pressure greater than 15 mm Hg; (B) a 1-minute postexercise pressure of 30 mm Hg; (C) a 5-minute postexercise pressure greater than 20 mm Hg.[51]

Rehabilitation Concerns

Management of CCS is initially conservative with activity modification, icing, and stretching of the anterior compartment and gastrocnemius–soleus complex (Figures 22-21 to 22-23). A lower-quarter structural exam along with gait analysis might reveal a structural variation that is causing excessive compensatory pronation and might benefit from the use of foot orthotics and proper footwear. However, these measures will not address the issue of increased compartment pressures with activity. Cycling has been shown to be an acceptable alternative in preventing increased anterior compartment pressures compared to running and can be used to maintain cardiovascular fitness.[2] If conservative measures fail, fasciotomy of the affected compartments has produced favorable results in a return to higher level of activity.[57,61,82,85] The patient should be counseled regarding the outcome expectations after fasciotomy for CCS. Howard reported a clinically significant improvement in 81% of the anterior/lateral releases and a 50% improvement in deep posterior compartment releases with CCS.[36] Slimmon et al noted that 58% of the patients responding to a long-term follow-up study for CCS fasciotomy reported exercising at a lower level than before the injury.[68] Micheli et al noted that female patients may be more prone to this condition and that for reasons unclear, they did not respond to the fasciotomy as well as their male counterparts.[46]

Rehabilitation Progression

Following fasciotomy for CCS, the immediate goals are to decrease postsurgical pain, swelling with RICE (rest, ice, compression, elevation), and assisted ambulation with the use of crutches. After suture removal and soft-tissue healing of the incision has progressed, AROM and flexibility exercises should be initiated (Figures 22-1 to 22-4, 22-18 to 22-21). Weight bearing will be progressed as ROM improves. Gait training should be incorporated to prevent abnormal movements in the gait pattern secondary to joint and soft-tissue stiffness or muscle guarding. AROM exercises should be progressed to open chain exercises with rubber tubing (Figures 22-5 to 22-8).

Closed kinetic chain activities can also be initiated to incorporate strength, balance, and proprioception that may have been affected by the surgical procedure (Figures 22-11 to 22-15 and 22-22 to 22-25). Lower-extremity structural variations that lead to excessive compensatory pronation during gait should be addressed with foot orthotics and proper footwear after walking gait has been normalized. These measures should help control excessive movements at the subtalar joint/lower leg and thus theoretically decrease muscular activity of the deep posterior compartment, which is highly active in controlling pronation during running.[54] Cardiovascular fitness can be maintained and improved with stationary cycling and running in the deep end of a pool with a flotation device (Figures 22-16 and 22-26). When ROM, strength, and walking gait have normalized, a walking/jogging progression can be initiated.

Criteria for Full Return

The patient may return to full activity when: (a) there is normalized ROM and strength of the involved lower leg; (b) there are no gait deviations with walking, jogging, and running; and (c) the patient has completed a progressive jogging/running program with no complaints of CCS symptoms. It should be noted that patients undergoing anterior compartment fasciotomy may not return to full activity for 8 to 12 weeks after surgery, and patients undergoing deep posterior compartment fasciotomy may not return until 3 to 4 months postsurgery.[40,61]

Clinical Decision-Making Exercise 22-3

A female lacrosse player has been diagnosed with anterior compartment syndrome. She presents to the athletic training clinic for recommendations on rehabilitation exercises and activity modification prior to attempts at surgery. Prior to being diagnosed, the patient had been running long distances on an urban, hilly course for conditioning. She has a history of lower-extremity musculoskeletal dysfunction, including decreased flexibility and excessive pronation. List and discuss recommendations the athletic trainer can give to this patient to alleviate the symptoms of anterior compartment syndrome.

Muscle Strains

Pathomechanics

The majority of muscle strains in the lower leg occur in the medial head of the gastrocnemius at the musculotendinous junction.[28] The injury is more common in middle-aged patients and occurs in activities requiring ballistic movement, such as tennis and basketball. The patient may feel or hear a pop, as if being kicked in the back of the leg. Depending on the severity of the strain, the athlete may be unable to walk secondary to decreased ankle dorsiflexion in a closed kinetic chain, which passively stretches the injured muscle and causes pain during the push-off phase of gait. Palpation will elicit tenderness at the site of the strain, and a palpable divot may be present, depending on the severity of the injury and how soon it is evaluated.

Injury Mechanism

Strains of the medial head of the gastrocnemius usually occur during sudden ballistic movements. A common scenario is the patient lunging with the knee extended and the ankle dorsiflexed. The ankle plantar flexes, in this case the medial head of the gastrocnemius, are activated to assist in push-off of the foot. The muscle is placed in an elongated position and activated in a very short period. This places the musculotendinous junction of the gastrocnemius under excessive tensile stress. The muscle–tendon junction, a transition area of one homogeneous tissue to another, is not able to endure the tensile loads nearly as well as the homogeneous tissue itself, and tearing of the tissue at the junction occurs.

Rehabilitation Concerns

The initial management of a gastrocnemius strain is ice, compression, and elevation. It is important for the patient to pay special attention to compression and elevation of the lower extremity to avoid edema in the foot and ankle that can further limit ROM and prolong the rehabilitation process. Gentle stretching of the muscle–tendon unit should be initiated early in the rehabilitation process (Figure 22-18). Ankle plantar flexor strengthening with rubber tubing can also be initiated when tolerated (Figure 22-5). Weight bearing may be limited to an as-tolerated status with crutches. The foot/ankle will prefer a plantar flexed position, and closed kinetic chain dorsiflexion of the foot and ankle, which is required during walking, will stress the muscle and cause pain. Pulsed ultrasound can be used early in the rehabilitation process and eventually progressed to continuous ultrasound for its thermal effects. A stationary cycle can be used for an active warm-up as well as cardiovascular fitness. A heel lift may be placed in each shoe to gradually increase dorsiflexion of the foot and ankle as the patient is progressed off crutches. Standing, stretching, and strengthening can be added as soft-tissue healing occurs and ROM and strength improve. Eventually the patient can be progressed to a walking/jogging program and sport-specific activity. It is important that the patient warm up and stretch properly before activity, to prevent reinjury.

Rehabilitation Progression

Early management of a medial head gastrocnemius strain focuses on reduction of pain and swelling with ice, compression, and elevation and modified weight bearing. The patient is encouraged to perform gentle towel stretching for the affected muscle group several times per day (Figure 22-18). AROM of the foot and ankle in all planes will also facilitate movement and act to stretch the muscle (Figures 22-1 to 22-4). With mild muscle strains, the patient may be off crutches and performing standing calf stretches and strengthening exercises by about 7 to 10 days with a normal gait pattern (Figures 22-12, 22-13, and 22-19). Moderate to severe strains may take 2 to 4 weeks before normalization of ROM and gait occur. This is usually because of the excessive edema in the foot and ankle. Strengthening can be progressed from open to closed chain activity as soft-tissue healing occurs (Figures 22-14, 22-15, and 22-22 through 22-25). As walking gait is normalized, the patient is encouraged to begin a graduated jogging program in which distance and speed are modulated throughout the progression. Most soft-tissue injuries demonstrate good healing by 14 to 21 days post injury. In the case of mild muscle strain, as the patient becomes more comfortable with jogging and running, plyometric activities can be added to the rehabilitation process. Plyometric activities should be introduced in a controlled fashion with at least 1 to 2 days of rest between activities to allow for muscle soreness to diminish. As the patient adapts to the plyometric exercises, sport-specific training should be added. Care should be taken to save sudden, ballistic activities for when the patient is warmed up and the gastrocnemius is well stretched.

Criteria for Full Return

The patient may return to full activity when the following criteria have been met: (a) full ROM of the foot and ankle; (b) gastrocnemius strength and endurance are equal to the uninvolved side; (c) ability to walk, jog, run, and hop on the involved extremity without any compensation; and (d) successful completion of a sport-specific functional progression with no residual calf symptoms.

Clinical Decision-Making Exercise 22-4

A male tennis player presents to the athletic training clinic with medial calf pain while playing tennis. He noted a sudden onset of pain while serving. List stretching and strengthening exercises in a progressive order that the athletic trainer could provide to the patient.

Medial Tibial Stress Syndrome

Pathomechanics

MTSS is a condition that involves increasing pain about the distal two-thirds of the posterior medial aspect of the tibia.[27,70] The soleus and tibialis posterior have been implicated as muscular forces that can stress the fascia and periosteum of the distal tibia during running activities.[2,26,64] In a cadaveric dissection study, Beck and Osternig implicated the soleus, and not the tibialis posterior, as the major contributor to MTSS.[5] Magnusson et al noted reduced bone mineral density at the site of MTSS, but could not ascertain whether this was the cause or the result.[42] Bhatt reported abnormal histologic appearance of bone and periosteum in longstanding MTSS.[10] Pain is usually diffuse about the distal medial tibia and the surrounding soft tissues and can arise secondary to a combination of training errors, excessive pronation, improper footwear, and poor conditioning level.[16,66] Initially, the area is diffusely tender and might hurt only after an intense workout. As the condition worsens, daily ambulation may be painful and morning pain and stiffness may be present. There is limited evidence in the literature that interventions used in rehabilitation are effective at preventing MTSS.[19,88] Rehabilitation of this condition must be comprehensive for each individual and address several factors, including musculoskeletal, training, and conditioning, as well as proper footwear and orthotics intervention.

Injury Mechanism

Many sources have linked excessive compensatory pronation as a primary cause of MTSS.[16,26,64,70,80] Bennett et al reported that a pronatory foot type was related to MTSS. The authors noted that the combination of a patient's sex and navicular drop test measures provided an accurate prediction for the development of MTSS in high school runners.[9] Subtalar joint pronation serves to dissipate ground reaction forces upon foot strike to reduce the impact to proximal structures. If pronation is excessive, or occurs too quickly, or at the wrong time in the stance phase of gait, greater tensile loads will be placed on the muscle–tendon units that assist in controlling this complex triplanar movement.[31,78] Lower extremity structural variations, such as a rear-foot and forefoot varus, can cause the subtalar joint to pronate excessively to get the medial aspect of the forefoot in contact with the ground for push-off.[70] The magnitude of these forces will increase during running, especially with a rear-foot striker. Sprinters may present with similar symptoms but with a different cause, that being overuse of the plantarflexors secondary to being on their toes during their event. Training surfaces including embankments and crowned roads can place increased tensile loads on the distal medial tibia, and modifications should be made whenever possible.

Rehabilitation Concerns

Management of this condition should include physician referral to rule out the possibility of stress fracture via the use of bone scan and plain films. Activity modification along with measures to maintain cardiovascular fitness should be set in place immediately.

Correction of abnormal pronation during walking and running can be addressed with antipronation taping and temporary orthotics to determine their effectiveness. Vicenzino et al reported that these measures were helpful in controlling excessive pronation.[83] If the above measures are helpful, a custom foot orthotic can be fabricated. Masse' Genova and Gross noted that foot orthotics significantly reduced maximum calcaneal eversion and calcaneal eversion at heel rise with abnormal pronators during treadmill walking.[44] Proper footwear, especially running shoes with motion-control features, can also be very helpful in dealing with MTSS. Although the above-mentioned measures provide passive support to address abnormal pronation, exercise sandals may provide a dynamic approach to managing excessive pronation issues. Michell et al noted a trend in reduced rear-foot eversion angles in

2-dimensional rear-foot kinematics during barefoot treadmill walking with abnormal pronators in patients who trained in the exercise sandals for 8 weeks.[47] The patients also demonstrated improved balance in a single-leg stance and subjectively noted improved foot function.[47] These improvements might be a result of increased muscle activity of the foot intrinsics via the short-foot concept and increased activity of the lower-leg musculature that may assist in controlling pronation. Also, the exercise sandals appear to place the foot in a more supinated position, which may enhance the cuboid pulley mechanism and its effects on the function of the first ray during the push-off phase of gait.[35] Ice massage to the affected area may help reduce localized pain and inflammation. A flexibility program for the gastrocnemius–soleus musculature should be initiated.

Clinical Decision-Making Exercise 22-5

A former athlete who is currently training for a 10K race presents to the athletic training clinic with "shin splints." She runs during her lunch hour in an urban area, and during the past 2 weeks she has doubled her mileage, which has not allowed her time to stretch after training. She notes that her running shoes are about 1 year old. What advice can the athletic trainer give to this individual?

Rehabilitation Progression

Running and jumping activities may need to be completely eliminated for the first 7 to 10 days after diagnosis. Pool workouts with a flotation device will help maintain cardiovascular fitness during the healing process. Gastrocnemius–soleus flexibility is improved with static stretching (Figure 22-19). Ice and electrical stimulation can be used to reduce inflammation and modulate pain in the early stages. As the condition improves, general strengthening of the ankle musculature with rubber tubing can be performed along with calf muscle strengthening (Figures 22-5 to 22-8, 22-12, and 22-13). These exercises may cause muscle fatigue but should not increase the patient's symptoms. The exercise sandal progression can be introduced to enhance dynamic pronation control at the foot and ankle (Table

22-1; Figures 22-29 to 22-34, and 22-36). An isokinetic strengthening program of the ankle inverters and everters can be used to improve strength and has been shown to reduce pronation during treadmill running (Figure 22-24).[25] As mentioned previously, it is imperative that all structural deviations that cause pronation be addressed with a foot orthotic or at least proper motion-control shoes. As pain to palpation of the distal tibia resolves, the patient should be progressed to a jogging/running program on grass with proper footwear. This may involve beginning with a 10- to 15-minute run and progressing by 10% every week. In the case of track athletes, a pool or bike workout can be implemented for 20 to 30 minutes after the run to produce a more demanding workout. The patient needs to be compliant with a gradual progression and should be educated to avoid doing too much, too soon, which could lead to a recurrence of the condition or possibly a stress fracture.

Criteria for Full Return

The patient may return to full activity when: (a) there is minimal to no pain to palpation of the affected area; (b) all causes of excessive pronation have been addressed with an orthotic and proper footwear; (c) there is sufficient gastrocnemius–soleus musculature flexibility; and (d) the patient has successfully completed a gradual running progression and a sport-specific functional progression without an increase in symptoms.

Clinical Decision-Making Exercise 22-6

A patient presents to the athletic training clinic from the physician with a referral to fabricate orthotics for abnormal pronation. List some possible structural causes of abnormal pronation the athletic trainer can look for during the evaluation.

Achilles Tendinopathy

Pathomechanics

Achilles tendinitis is an inflammatory condition that involves the Achilles tendon and/or its tendon sheath, the paratenon. Often there is excessive tensile stress placed on the tendon repetitively, as with running or jumping activities, that overloads the tendon, especially on its medial aspect.[49,63] This condition can be divided into Achilles paratenonitis or peritendinitis, which is an inflammation of the paratenon or tissue that surrounds the tendon, and tendinosis, in which areas of the tendon consist of mucinoid or fatty degeneration with disorganized collagen.[63] The patient often complains of generalized pain and stiffness about the Achilles tendon region that when localized is usually 2- to 6-cm proximal to the calcaneal insertion. Uphill running or hill workouts and interval training will usually aggravate the condition. There may be reduced gastrocnemius and soleus muscle flexibility in general that may worsen as the condition progresses and adaptive shortening occurs. Muscle testing of the above muscles may be within normal limits, but painful, and a true deficit may be observed when performing toe raises to fatigue as compared to the uninvolved extremity.

Injury Mechanism

Achilles tendinopathy will often present with a gradual onset over time. Initially the patient may ignore the symptoms, which may present at the beginning of activity and resolve as the activity progresses. Symptoms may progress to morning stiffness and discomfort with walking after periods of prolonged sitting. Repetitive weight-bearing activities, such as running, or early season conditioning in which the duration and intensity are increased too quickly with insufficient recovery time, will worsen the condition. Excessive compensatory pronation of the subtalar joint with concomitant internal rotation of the lower leg secondary to a forefoot varus, tibial varum, or femoral anteversion will increase the tensile load about the medial aspect of the Achilles tendon.[32,63] Decreased gastrocnemius–soleus complex flexibility can also increase subtalar joint pronation to compensate for the decreased closed kinetic chain dorsiflexion needed during the early and mid-stance phase of running. If the patient continues to train, the tendon will become further inflamed and the gastrocnemius–soleus musculature will become less efficient secondary to pain inhibition. The tendon may be warm and painful to palpation, as well as thickened, which may indicate the chronicity of the condition. Crepitus may be palpated with

AROM plantar and dorsiflexion and pain will be elicited with passive dorsiflexion.

Rehabilitation Concerns

Achilles tendinitis can be resistant to a quick resolution secondary to the slower healing response of tendinous tissue. It has also been noted that an area of hypovascularity exists within the tendon that may further impede the healing response. It is important to create a proper healing environment by reducing the offending activity and replacing it with an activity that will reduce strain on the tendon. Studies have shown that the Achilles tendon force during running approaches 6 to 8 times body weight.[63] Addressing structural faults that may lead to excessive pronation or supination should be done through proper footwear and foot orthotics, as well as flexibility exercises for the gastrocnemius–soleus complex. Soft-tissue manipulation of the gastrocnemius–soleus with a foam roller can be helpful prior to stretching. Modalities such as ice can help reduce pain and inflammation early on, and ultrasound can facilitate an increased blood flow to the tendon in the later stages of rehabilitation. Cross-friction massage may be used to break down adhesions that may have formed during the healing response and further improve the gliding ability of the paratenon. Strengthening of the gastrocnemius–soleus musculature must be progressed carefully so as not to cause a recurrence of the symptoms. Lastly a gradual progression must be made for a safe return to activity to avoid having the condition becoming chronic.

Rehabilitation Progression

Activity modification is necessary to allow the Achilles tendon to begin the healing process. Swimming, pool running with a flotation device, stationary cycling, and use of an upper-body ergometer are all possible alternative activities for cardiovascular maintenance (Figures 22-16, 22-26, and 22-27). It is important to reduce stresses on the Achilles tendon that may occur with daily ambulation. Proper footwear with a slight heel lift, such as a good running shoe, can reduce stress on the tendon during gait. Structural biomechanical abnormalities that manifest with excessive pronation or supination should be addressed with a custom foot orthotic. Placing a heel lift in the shoe or building it into the orthotic can reduce stress on the Achilles tendon initially, but should be gradually reduced so as not to cause an adaptive shortening of the muscle-tendon unit. Gentle pain-free stretching can be performed several times per day and can be done after an active or passive warm-up with exercise or modalities such as superficial heat or ultrasound (Figures 22-18 and 22-19). Open kinetic chain strengthening with rubber tubing can begin early in the rehabilitation process and should be progressed to closed kinetic chain strengthening in a concentric and eccentric fashion using the patient's body weight with modification of sets, repetitions, and speed of exercise to intensify the rehabilitation session (Figures 22-5, 22-12, and 22-13).

Good results have been reported with the use of eccentric training of the gastrocnemius–soleus musculature with chronic Achilles tendinosis.[1,52,59] Alfredson's protocol proposed a regimen of isolated eccentric loading of the Achilles tendon using body weight that involved a 12-week protocol of "heel drops" (Figure 22-35).[1] The protocol suggests three sets of fifteen reps done twice each day with the knee straight and then with the knee flexed. A walking–jogging progression on a firm but forgiving surface can be initiated when the symptoms have resolved and ROM, strength, endurance, and flexibility have been normalized to the uninvolved extremity. The patient must be reminded that this progression is designed to improve the affected tendon's ability to tolerate stress in a controlled fashion and not to improve fitness level. Studies show that cardiovascular fitness can be maintained with biking and swimming.[23] Finally, it is important to educate the patient on the nature of the condition to set realistic expectations for a safe return without recurrence of the condition.

Criteria for Full Return

The patient may return to full activity when: (a) there has been full resolution of symptoms with ADL and minimal or no symptoms with sport-related activity; (b) ROM, strength, flexibility, and endurance are equal to the opposite uninvolved extremity; and (c) all contributing biomechanical faults have been corrected during walking and running gait analysis with proper footwear and/or custom foot orthotics.

Achilles Tendon Rupture

Pathomechanics

The Achilles tendon is the largest tendon in the human body. It serves to transmit force from the gastrocnemius and soleus musculature to the calcaneus. Tension through the Achilles tendon at the end of stance phase is estimated at 250% of body weight.[63] Rupture of the Achilles tendon usually occurs in an area 2 to 6 cm proximal to the calcaneal insertion, which has been implicated as an avascular site prone to degenerative changes.[17,34,39] The injury presents after a sudden plantarflexion of the ankle, as in jumping or accelerating with a sprint. The patient will often feel or hear a pop and note a sensation of being kicked in the back of the leg. Plantarflexion of the ankle will be painful and limited but still possible with the assistance of the tibialis posterior and the peroneals. A palpable defect will be noted along the length of the tendon, and the Thompson test will be positive. The patient will require the use of crutches to continue ambulation without an obvious limp.

Injury Mechanism

Achilles tendon rupture is usually caused by a sudden forceful plantarflexion of the ankle. It has been theorized that the area of rupture has undergone degenerative changes and is more prone to rupture when placed under higher levels of tensile loading.[34,49,62,63] The degenerative changes may be a result of excessive compensatory pronation at the subtalar joint to accommodate for structural deviations of the forefoot, rear-foot, and lower leg during walking and running. This pronation can place an increased tensile stress on the medial aspect of the Achilles tendon. Also, a chronically inflexible gastrocnemius–soleus complex will reduce the available amount of dorsiflexion at the ankle joint, and excessive subtalar joint pronation will assist in accommodating this loss. The above mechanisms may result in tendinitis symptoms that precede the tendon rupture, but this is not always the case. Fatigue of the deconditioned patient or weekend warrior may also contribute to tendon rupture, as well as improper warm-up prior to ballistic activities such as basketball or racquet sports.[33]

Rehabilitation Concerns

After an Achilles tendon rupture, the question of surgical repair vs cast immobilization will arise. Cetti et al report that surgical repair of the tendon is recommended to allow the patient to return to previous levels of activity.[17] Surgical repair of the Achilles tendon may require a period of immobilization for 6 to 8 weeks to allow for proper tendon healing.[15,34,43] The deleterious effects of this lengthy immobilization include muscle atrophy, joint stiffness including intra-articular adhesions and capsular stiffness of the involved joints, disorganization of the ligament substance, and possible disuse osteoporosis of the bone.[15] Isokinetic strength deficits for the ankle plantarflexors, especially at lower speeds, have been documented with periods of cast immobilization for 6 weeks.[41] Steele et al noted significant deficits isokinetically of ankle plantarflexor strength after 8 weeks of immobilization.[68] Some feel that the primary limiting factor that influences functional outcome might be the duration of postsurgical immobilization.[72] Several studies have been done using early controlled ankle motion and progressive weight bearing without immobilization.[3,15,34,43,63,69,71,81] It is important not only to regain full ROM without harming the repair, but also to regain normal muscle function through controlled progressive strengthening. This can be performed through a variety of exercises, including isometrics, isotonics, and isokinetics (Figures 22-1 through 22-13). Open and closed kinetic chain activities can be incorporated into the progression to gradually increase weight-bearing stress on the tendon repair, as well as to improve proprioception (Figures 22-11, 22-14, 22-15, and 22-22 through 22-25). Cardiovascular endurance can be maintained with stationary biking and pool running with a flotation device. Gait normalization for walking and running can be performed using a treadmill.

Rehabilitation Progression

It is important for the athletic trainer to have an open line of communication with the physician in charge of the surgical repair. Decisions about length and type of immobilization, weight-bearing progression, allowable ROM, and progressive strengthening should be thoroughly discussed with the physician. Excellent results have been reported with early and controlled mobilization with the use of a splint that allows early plantarflexion ROM and that slowly increases ankle dorsiflexion to neutral and full dorsiflexion during a 6- to 8-week period.[15,34] More recent studies have noted excellent functional results with early weight bearing and ROM. Aoki et al reported a full return to sports activity in 13.1 weeks.[3] Controlled progressive weight bearing based on percentages of the patient's body weight can be done over 6 to 8 weeks postoperatively, with full weight bearing by the end of this time frame.

During the early stages of rehabilitation, ice, compression, and elevation are used to decrease swelling. A variety of ROM exercises are done to increase ankle ROM in all planes as well as initiate activation of the surrounding muscles (Figures 22-1 to 22-4, 22-9, 22-10, 22-14, 22-15, 22-18, and 22-20). By 4 to 6 weeks postoperatively, strengthening exercises with rubber tubing can be progressed to closed chain exercises using a percentage of the patient's body weight with heel raises on a Total Gym apparatus (Figures 22-5, 22-8, and 22-11). It is important to do more concentric than eccentric loading initially, so as not to place excessive stress on the repair. Gradual increases in eccentric loading can occur from 10 to 12 weeks postoperatively. Also at this time, isokinetic exercise can be introduced with submaximal high-speed exercise and be progressed to lower concentric speeds gradually over time (Figures 24-24 and 24-25). By 3 months, full weight-bearing heel raises can be performed (Figures 22-12 and 22-13). At the same time a walking/jogging program can be initiated. Isokinetic strength testing can be done between 3 and 4 months to determine if any deficits in ankle plantarflexor strength exist. The number of single-leg heel raises performed in a specified amount of time compared to the uninvolved extremity can also be used to determine functional plantarflexor strength and endurance. Sport-related functional activities can be initiated at 3 months along with a progressive jogging program. A

REHABILITATION PLAN

ACHILLES TENDINITIS

Injury situation: A 17-year-old male lacrosse player presents with pain in his right Achilles. He notes that the pain has been present for the past week, secondary to an increase in preseason conditioning that has included long runs on asphalt, hill running, and interval training on the track. He currently has morning stiffness and pain with walking, especially up hills and going down stairs. The patient is concerned that the pain will affect his conditioning for the lacrosse season, which will start in 3 weeks.

Signs and symptoms: The patient stands in moderate subtalar joint pronation with mild tibial varum. His single-leg stance balance is poor, with an increase in subtalar joint pronation and internal rotation of the entire lower extremity. Observation of the tendon reveals slight thickening. Palpation reveals mild crepitus with pain 4 cm proximal to the calcaneal insertion on the medial side of the tendon. ROM testing reveals tightness in both the gastrocnemius and soleus musculature vs the uninvolved side. A 6-inch lateral step-down demonstrates restricted closed kinetic chain ankle dorsiflexion that is painful, with compensation at the hip to get the opposite heel to touch the ground. The patient is able to perform 10 heel raises on the right with pain and 20 on the left without pain. Walking gait reveals increased pronation during the entire stance phase of gait. A 12-degree forefoot varus is noted on the right with the athlete in a prone subtalar joint neutral position.

Management plan: The goal is to decrease pain, address the issues of abnormal pronation, and provide a protected environment for the tendon to heal. Eventually address ROM and strength deficits that are preventing the athlete from functioning at his expected level.

PHASE ONE: Acute Inflammatory Stage

GOALS: Modulate pain, address abnormal pronation, and begin appropriate therapeutic exercise.

Estimated length of time (ELT): Day 1 to Day 4 Use ice and electrical stimulation to decrease pain. Nonsteroidal antiinflammatory drugs could help reduce inflammation. A foot orthotic could be fabricated to address the excessive pronation, which may be placing increased tensile stress on the medial aspect of the Achilles tendon. A heel lift could be built into the foot orthotic. It might be recommended that the patient wear a motion-control running shoe to address pronation and provide a heel lift. The patient could begin gentle, pain-free towel stretching for the gastrocnemius and soleus musculature several times per day. Conditioning could be done in a pool or on a bike.

PHASE TWO: Fibroblastic Repair Stage

GOALS: Increase gastrocnemius–soleus flexibility, gain strength, and improve single-leg stance (SLS) balance and SLS closed kinetic chain functional activity.

Estimated length of time (ELT): Days 5 to 14 As signs of inflammation decrease, the use of ultrasound could be introduced, first at a pulsed level and then at a continuous level. Stretching could be progressed to standing on a flat surface. Strengthening could be started with isometrics and progressed to open kinetic chain isotonics with rubber tubing. As the patient improves, standing double-leg heel raises can be introduced. SLS activity could be added, focusing on control of the lower extremity, especially foot pronation and lower-leg internal rotation. Conditioning at the end of this stage could be upgraded to weight-bearing activity, such as the elliptical trainer with the foot flat on the pedal, avoiding ankle plantarflexion.

PHASE THREE: Maturation Remodeling Stage

GOALS: Complete elimination of pain and full return to activity.

Estimated length of time (ELT): Week 3 to Full Return As ROM and strength improve, the athlete could be progressed to gastrocnemius–soleus stretching on a slant board and single-leg heel raises, with an increased focus on eccentric loading of the involved side. Dynamic muscle loading via double-leg hopping on a yielding surface such as jumping rope for short periods could be added. A running program on a flat, yielding surface such as grass or track could be initiated with good running shoes and the foot orthotic in place. The program should be sport specific and initially should be done every other day to allow the tendon to recover. A sport-specific functional program could also begin when straight running and sprinting are tolerated by the patient. Other forms of conditioning could also be continued to maintain fitness levels. Achilles taping may be of benefit when the athlete returns to training on a daily basis to reduce excess load to the tendon over the next several weeks.

Criteria for Returning to Competitive Lacrosse

1. No pain with walking, ADL, and running.
2. Gastrocnemius–soleus flexibility and strength are equal to the uninvolved extremity.
3. Improved SLS balance, closed kinetic chain function (step-down, squat, lunge).

DISCUSSION QUESTIONS

1. Why would an orthotic be helpful in this case?
2. Why would closed kinetic chain activities such as a SLS and reach and a step-down be painful and limited with this condition?
3. Explain what training errors may have caused this condition to arise with this patient.
4. Explain what intrinsic factors may have contributed to this condition occurring with this patient.
5. Explain why an Achilles tendon taping would benefit this patient during his sporting activity.

full return to unrestricted athletic activity can begin after 6 months, once the patient successfully meets all predetermined goals.

Criteria for Full Return

The patient can return to full activity after the following criteria have been met: (a) full AROM of the involved ankle compared to the uninvolved side; (b) isokinetic strength of the ankle plantarflexors at 90% to 95% of the uninvolved side; (c) 90% to 95% of the number of heel raises throughout the full ROM in a 30-second period compared to the uninvolved side; and (d) the ability to walk, jog, and run without an observable limp and successful completion of a sport-related functional progression without any Achilles tendon irritation.

Retrocalcaneal Bursitis

Pathomechanics

The retrocalcaneal bursae is a disc-shaped object that lies between the Achilles tendon and the superior tuberosity of the calcaneus.[12,63] The patient will report a gradual onset of pain that may be associated with Achilles tendinitis. Careful palpation anterior to the Achilles tendon will rule out involvement of the tendon. Pain is increased with AROM/ passive ROM ankle dorsiflexion and relieved with plantarflexion. Depending on the severity and swelling associated, it may be painful to walk, especially when attempting to attain full closed kinetic chain ankle dorsiflexion during the mid-stance phase of gait.

Injury Mechanism

Loading the foot and ankle in repeated dorsiflexion, as in uphill running, can be a cause of this condition. When the foot is dorsiflexed, the distance between the posterior/superior calcaneus and the Achilles tendon will be reduced, resulting in a repeated mechanical compression of the retrocalcaneal bursae. Also, structural abnormalities of the foot may lead to excessive compensatory movements at the subtalar joint, which may cause friction of the Achilles tendon on the bursae with running.

Rehabilitation Concerns

Because of the close proximity of other structures, it is important to rule out involvement of the calcaneus and Achilles tendon with careful palpation of the area. Rest and activity modification to reduce swelling and inflammation is necessary. If walking is painful, crutches with weight bearing as tolerated is recommended for a brief period. Gentle but progressive stretching and strengthening should be added as tolerated, with care being taken not to increase pain with gastrocnemius–soleus stretching (Figures 22-5, 22-12, 22-13, 22-18, and 22-19). If excessive compensatory pronation is noted during gait analysis, recommendations on proper footwear should be made, especially regarding the heel counter, and foot orthotics should be considered.

Rehabilitation Progression

The early management of this condition requires all measures to reduce pain and inflammation, including ice, rest from offending activity, proper footwear, and modified weight bearing with crutches if necessary. Cardiovascular fitness can be maintained with pool running with a flotation device. Gentle stretching of the gastrocnemius–soleus needs to be introduced slowly because this will tend to increase compression of the retrocalcaneal bursae. As pain resolves and ROM and walking gait are normalized, the patient may begin a progressive walking/jogging program. The patient can progress back to activity as the condition allows. Heel lifts in both shoes may be necessary in the early return to activity, with gradual weaning away from them as AROM/passive ROM dorsiflexion improves. The condition may allow full return in 10 days to 2 weeks, if treated early enough. If the condition persists, 6 to 8 weeks of rest, activity modification, and treatment may be needed before a successful result is attained with conservative care.

Criteria for Full Return

The following criteria need to be met before return to full activity: (a) no observable swelling and minimal to no pain with palpation of the area at rest or after daily activity; (b) full ankle dorsiflexion AROM and normal pain-free strength of the gastrocnemius and soleus musculature; and (c) normal and pain-free walking and running gait.

Summary

1. Although some injuries in the region of the lower leg are acute, most injuries seen in an athletic population result from overuse, most often from running.

2. Tibial fractures can create long-term problems for the patient if inappropriately managed. Fibular fractures generally require much shorter periods for immobilization. Treatment of these fractures involves immediate medical referral and most likely a period of immobilization and restricted weight bearing.

3. Stress fractures in the lower leg are usually the result of the bone's inability to adapt to the repetitive loading response during training and conditioning of the patient and are more likely to occur in the tibia.

4. CSS can occur from acute trauma or repetitive trauma of overuse. They can occur in any of the four compartments, but are most likely in the anterior compartment or deep posterior compartment.

5. Rehabilitation of MTSS must be comprehensive and address several factors, including musculoskeletal, training, and conditioning, as well as proper footwear and orthotics intervention.

6. Achilles tendinitis often presents with a gradual onset over time and may be resistant to a quick resolution secondary to the slower healing response of tendinous tissue.

7. Perhaps the greatest question after an Achilles tendon rupture is whether surgical repair or cast immobilization is the best method of treatment. Regardless of treatment method, the time required for rehabilitation is significant.

8. With retrocalcaneal bursitis the athlete will report a gradual onset of pain that may be associated with Achilles tendinitis. Treatment should include rest and activity modification to reduce swelling and inflammation.

References

1. Alfredson H, Pietila T, Jonsson P, et al. Heavy-load eccentric calf muscle training of the treatment of Achilles tendinosis. *Am J Sports Med*. 1998;26(3):360-366.

2. Andrish J, Work J. How I manage shin splints. *Phys Sportsmed*. 1990;18(12):113-114.

3. Aoki M, Ogiwara N, Ohta T, et al. Early active motion and weightbearing after cross stitch Achilles tendon repair. *Am J Sports Med*. 1998;26(6):794-800.

4. Batt M, Kemp S, Kerslake K. Delayed union stress fracture of the tibia: conservative management. *Br J Sports Med*. 2001;35:74-77.

5. Beck B, Osternig L. Medial tibial stress syndrome. *J Bone Joint Surg Am*. 1994;76(7):1057-1061.

6. Beckham S, Grana W, Buckley P, et al. A comparison of anterior compartment pressures in competitive runners and cyclists. *Am J Sports Med*. 1993;21(1):36-40.

7. Bennell K, Malcolm S, Thomas S, et al. The incidence and distribution of stress fractures in competitive track and field athletes: a twelve-month prospective study. *Am J Sports Med*. 1996;24(2):211-217.

8. Bennell K, Malcolm S, Thomas S, et al. Risk factors for stress fractures in track and field athletes: a twelve-month prospective study. *Am J Sports Med*. 1996;24(6):810-817.

9. Bennett J, Reinking M, Pleumer B, et al. Factors contributing to the development of medial tibial stress syndrome in high school runners. *J Orthop Sports Phys Ther*. 2001;31(9):504-511.

10. Bhatt R, Lauder I, Allen M, et al. Correlation of bone scintigraphy and histological findings in medial tibial stress syndrome. *Br J Sports Med*. 2000;34:49-53.

11. Blackburn T, Hirth C, Guskiewicz K. EMG comparison of lower leg musculature during functional activities with and without balance shoes. *J Athl Train*. 2002;38(3):198-203.

12. Bordelon R. The heel. In: DeLee J, Drez D, eds. *Orthopaedic and Sports Medicine: Principles and Practice*. Philadelphia, PA: WB Saunders; 1994.

13. Bullock-Saxton J. Local sensation changes and altered hip muscle function following severe ankle sprain. *Phys Ther*. 1994;74(1):17-31.

14. Bullock-Saxton J, Janda V, Bullock M. Reflex activation of gluteal muscles in walking. *Spine* (Philadelphia, PA 1976). 1993;21(6):704-708.

15. Carter T, Fowler P, Blokker C. Functional postoperative treatment of Achilles tendon repair. *Am J Sports Med*. 1992;20(4):459-462.

16. Case W. Relieving the pain of shin splints. *Phys Sportsmed*. 1994;22(4):31-32.

17. Cetti R, Christensen S, Ejsted R, et al. Operative versus nonoperative treatment of Achilles tendon rupture: a prospective randomized study and review of the literature. *Am J Sports Med*. 1993;21(6):791-799.

18. Chang P, Harris R. Intramedullary nailing for chronic tibial stress fractures: a review of five cases. *Am J Sports Med*. 1996;24(5):688-692.

19. Craig D. Medial tibial stress syndrome: evidence-based prevention. *J Athl Train*. 2008;43(3):316-318.

20. Dickson T, Kichline P. Functional management of stress fractures in female athletes using a pneumatic leg brace. *Am J Sports Med*. 1987;15(1):86-89.

21. Donatelli R. Normal anatomy and biomechanics. In: Donatelli R, Wolf S, eds. *The Biomechanics of the Foot and Ankle*. Philadelphia, PA: FA Davis; 1990.

22. Ekenman I, Tsai-Fellander L, Westblad P, et al. A study of intrinsic factors in patients with stress fractures of the tibia. *Foot Ankle*. 1996;17(8):477-482.

23. Eyestone E, Fellingham G, George J, Fisher G. Effect of water running and cycling on maximum oxygen consumption and 2-mile run performance. *Am J Sports Med*. 1993;21(1):41-44.

24. Fehlandt A, Micheli L. Acute exertional anterior compartment syndrome in an adolescent female. *Med Sci Sports Exerc*. 1995;27(1):3-7.

25. Feltner M, Macrae H, Macrae P, et al. Strength training effects on rearfoot motion in running. *Med Sci Sports Exerc*. 1994;26(8):102-107.

26. Fick D, Albright J, Murray B. Relieving painful shin splints. *Phys Sportsmed*. 1992;20(12):105-113.

27. Fredericson M, Bergman A, Hoffman K, Dillingham M. Tibial stress reaction in runners: A correlation of clinical symptoms and scintigraphy with a new magnetic resonance imaging grading system. *Am J Sports Med*. 1995;23(4):472-481.

28. Garrick J, Couzens G. Tennis leg: how I manage gastrocnemius strains. *Phys Sportsmed*. 1992;20(5):203-207.

29. Giladi M, Milgrom C, Simkin A, et al. Stress fractures: identifiable risk factors. *Am J Sports Med.* 1991;19(6):647-652.

30. Goldberg B, Pecora C. Stress fractures: a risk of increased training in freshmen. *Phys Sportsmed.* 1994;22(3):68-78.

31. Gross M. Lower quarter screening for skeletal malalignment: suggestions for orthotics and shoeware. *J Orthop Sports Phys Ther.* 1995;21(6):389-405.

32. Gross M. Chronic tendinitis: pathomechanics of injury factors affecting the healing response and treatment. *J Orthop Sports Phys Ther.* 1992;16(6):248-261.

33. Hamel R. Achilles tendon ruptures: making the diagnosis. *Phys Sportsmed.* 1992;20(9):189-200.

34. Heinrichs K, Haney C. Rehabilitation of the surgically repaired Achilles tendon using a dorsal functional orthosis: a preliminary report. *J Sport Rehabil.* 1994;3:292-303.

35. Hirth C. *Rehabilitation Strategies in the Management of Foot and Ankle Dysfunction: Research and Practical Applications.* Paper presented at the National Athletic Trainers Association 52nd Annual Meeting and Clinical Symposium, Los Angeles, CA, 19-23 June 2001.

36. Howard J, Mohtadi N, Wiley J. Evaluation of outcomes in patients following surgical treatment of chronic exertional compartment syndrome in the leg. *Clin J Sport Med.* 2000;10(3):176-184.

37. Janda V, VaVrova M. Sensory motor stimulation [video]. Brisbane, Australia: Body Control Systems; 1990.

38. Kaper B, Carr C, Shirreffs T. Compartment syndrome after arthroscopic surgery of knee: a report of two cases managed nonoperatively. *Am J Sports Med.* 1997;25(1):123-125.

39. Karjalainen P, Aronen H, Pihlajamaki H, et al. Magnetic resonance imaging during healing of surgically repaired Achilles tendon ruptures. *Am J Sports Med.* 1997;25(2):164-171.

40. Kohn H. Shin pain and compartment syndromes in running. In: Guten G, ed. *Running Injuries.* Philadelphia, PA: WB Saunders; 1997.

41. Leppilahti J, Siira P, Vanharanta H, et al. Isokinetic evaluation of calf muscle performance after Achilles rupture repair. *Int J Sports Med.* 1996;17(8):619-623.

42. Magnusson H, Westlin N, Nyqvist F, et al. Abnormally decreased regional bone density in athletes with medial tibial stress syndrome. *Am J Sports Med.* 2001;29(6):712-715.

43. Mandelbaum B, Myerson M, Forster R. Achilles tendon ruptures: a new method of repair, early range of motion, and functional rehabilitation. *Am J Sports Med.* 1995;23(4):392-395.

44. 44. Masse' Genova J, Gross M. Effect of foot orthotics in calcaneal eversion during standing and treadmill walking for subjects with abnormal pronation. *J Orthop Sports Phys Ther.* 2000;30(11):664-675.

45. Matheson G, Clement B, McKenzie C, et al. Stress fractures in athletes: a study of 320 cases. *Am J Sports Med.* 1987;15(1):46-58.

46. Micheli L, Solomon K, Solomon R, et al. Surgical treatment for chronic lower leg compartment syndrome in young female athletes. *Am J Sports Med.* 1999;27:197-201.

47. Michell T, Guskiewicz K, Hirth C, et al. *Effects of Training in Exercise Sandals on 2-D Rearfoot Motion and Postural Sway in Abnormal Pronators* [undergraduate honors thesis]. Chapel Hill: University of North Carolina; 2000.

48. Myers R, Padua D, Prentice W, et al. *Electromyographic Analysis of the Gluteal Musculature During Closed Kinetic Chain Exercises* [master's thesis]. Chapel Hill: University of North Carolina; 2002.

49. Myerson M, McGarvey W. Instructional course lectures, The American Academy of Orthopaedic Surgeons: disorders of the insertion of the Achilles tendon and Achilles tendinitis. *J Bone Joint Surg.* 1998;80:1814-1824.

50. National Academy of Sports Medicine. *Performance Enhancement Specialist Online Manual.* Callabassus, CA: Author; 2002.

51. Pedowitz R, Hargens A, Mubarek S, et al. Modified criteria for the objective diagnosis of chronic compartment syndrome of the leg. *Am J Sports Med.* 1990;18(1):35-40.

52. Petersen W, Welp R, Rosenbaum D. Chronic Achilles tendinopathy: a prospective randomized study comparing the therapeutic effect of eccentric training, the Air Heel Brace and a combination of both. *Am J Sports Med.* 2007;35:1659-1667.

53. Puddu G, Cerullo G, Selvanetti A, DePaulis F. Stress fractures. In: Harries M, Williams C, Stanish W, Micheli L, eds. *Oxford Textbook of Sports Medicine.* New York, NY: Oxford University Press; 1994.

54. Reber L, Perry J, Pink M. Muscular control of the ankle in running. *Am J Sports Med.* 1993;21(6):805-810.

55. Reeder M, Dick B, Atkins J, et al. Stress fractures: current concepts of diagnosis and treatment. *Sports Med.* 1996;22(3):198-212.

56. Rettig A, Shelbourne K, McCarrol J, et al. The natural history and treatment of delayed union stress fractures of the anterior cortex of the tibia. *Am J Sports Med.* 1988;16(3):250-255.

57. Rettig A, McCarroll J, Hahn R. Chronic compartment syndrome: surgical intervention in 12 cases. *Phys Sportsmed.* 1991;19(4):63-70.

58. Romani W. Mechanisms and management of stress fractures in physically active persons. *J Athl Train.* 2002;37(3):306-314.

59. Roos E, Engstrom M, Lagerquist A, et al. Clinical improvement after 6 weeks of eccentric exercise in patients with mid-portion Achilles tendinopathy: a randomized trial with 1 year follow-up. *Scand J Med Sci Sports.* 2004;14:286-295.

60. Sallade J, Koch S. Training errors in long distance runners. *J Athl Train.* 1992;27(1):50-53.

61. Schepsis A, Martini D, Corbett M. Surgical management of exertional compartment syndrome of the lower leg: longterm followup. *Am J Sports Med.* 1993;21(6):811-817.

62. Schepsis A, Wagner C, Leach R. Surgical management of Achilles tendon overuse injuries: a long-term follow-up study. *Am J Sports Med.* 1994;22(5):611-619.

63. Schepsis A, Jones H, Haas H. Achilles tendon disorders in athletes. *Am J Sports Med.* 2002;30(2):287-305.

64. Schon L, Baxter D, Clanton T. Chronic exercise-induced leg pain in active people: more than just shin splints. *Phys Sportsmed.* 1992;20(1):100-114.

65. Shaffer S, Uhl T. Preventing and treating lower extremity stress reactions and fractures in adults. *J Athl Train.* 2006;41(4):466-469.

66. Shwayhat A, Linenger J, Hofher L, et al. Profiles of exercise history and overuse injuries among United States Navy Sea, Air, and Land (SEAL) recruits. *Am J Sports Med.* 1994;22(6):835-840.

67. Simon R. The tibial and fibular shaft. In: Simon R, Koenigshnecht S, eds. *Emergency Orthopedics: The Extremities.* 3rd ed. Norwalk, CT: Appleton-Lange; 1995.

68. Slimmon D, Bennell K, Bruker P, et al. Long-term outcome of fasciotomy with partial fasciectomy for chronic exertional compartment syndrome of the lower leg. *Am J Sports Med.* 2002;30:581-588.

69. Solveborn S, Moberg A. Immediate free ankle motion after surgical repair of acute Achilles tendon ruptures. *Am J Sports Med.* 1994;22(5):607-610.

70. Sommer H, Vallentyne S. Effect of foot posture on the incidence of medial tibial stress syndrome. *Med Sci Sports Exerc.* 1995;27(6):800-804.

71. Speck M, Klaue K. Early full weightbearing and functional treatment after surgical repair of acute Achilles tendon rupture. *Am J Sports Med.* 1998;26:789-793.

72. Steele G, Harter R, Ting A. Comparison of functional ability following percutaneous and open surgical repairs of acutely ruptured tendons. *J Sport Rehabil.* 1993;2:115-127.

73. Strudwick W, Stuart G. Proximal fibular stress fracture in an aerobic dancer: a case report. *Am J Sports Med.* 1992;20(4):481-482.

74. Stuart M, Karaharju T. Acute compartment syndrome: recognizing the progressive signs and symptoms. *Phys Sportsmed.* 1994;22(3):91-95.

75. Styf J, Nakhostine M, Gershuni D. Functional knee braces increase intramuscular pressures in the anterior compartment of the leg. *Am J Sports Med.* 1992;20(1):46-49.

76. Swenson E, DeHaven K, Sebastianelli J, et al. The effect of a pneumatic leg brace on return to play in athletes with tibial stress fractures. *Am J Sports Med.* 1997;25(3):322-338.

77. Taube R, Wadsworth L. Managing tibial stress fractures. *Phys Sportsmed.* 1993;21(4):123-130.

78. Tiberio D. Pathomechanics of structural foot deformities. *Phys Ther.* 1988;68(12):1840-1849.

79. Tiberio D. The effect of excessive subtalar joint pronation on patellofemoral mechanics: a theoretical model. *J Orthop Sports Phys Ther.* 1987;9(4):160-165.

80. Thacker S, Gilchrist J, Stroup D, et al. The prevention of shin splints in sports: a systematic review of literature. *Med Sci Sports Exerc.* 2002;34(1):32-40.

81. Twaddle B, Poon P. Early motion for Achilles tendon ruptures: is surgery important. *Am J Sports Med.* 2007;35:2033-2038.

82. Vincent N. Compartment syndromes. In: Harries M, Williams C, Stanish W, Micheli L, eds. *Oxford Textbook of Sports Medicine.* New York, NY: Oxford University Press; 1994.

83. Vincenzino B, Griffiths S, Griffiths L, et al. Effect of antipronation tape and temporary orthotics on vertical navicular height before and after exercise. *J Orthop Sports Phys Ther.* 2000;30(6):333-339.

84. Wilder R, Brennan D, Schotte D. A standard measure for exercise prescription for aqua running. *Am J Sports Med.* 1993;21(1):45-48.

85. Wiley J, Clement D, Doyle D, et al. A primary care perspective of chronic compartment syndrome of the leg. *Phys Sportsmed.* 1987;15(3):111-120.

86. Willy C, Becker B, Evers H. Unusual development of acute exertional compartment syndrome due to delayed diagnosis: a case report. *Int J Sports Med.* 1996;17(6):458-461.

87. Whitelaw G, Wetzler M, Levy A, et al. A pneumatic leg brace for the treatment of tibial stress fractures. *Clin Orthop.* 1991;270:301-305.

88. Yasuda T, Miyazaki K, Tada K, et al. Stress fracture of the right distal femur following bilateral fractures of the proximal fibulas: a case report. *Am J Sports Med.* 1992;20(6):771-774.

SOLUTIONS TO CLINICAL DECISION-MAKING EXERCISES

22-1   AROM exercises for the foot and ankle in a warm whirlpool would assist in addressing ROM deficits and muscle activation issues of the lower leg. Specific joint mobilization exercises for the foot and ankle would also be indicated. Stretching of the gastrocnemius–soleus complex would also work on ankle ROM and flexibility issues. Addressing weakness of the proximal hip and thigh musculature via quadriceps and gluteal setting, along with four direction straight leg raises (SLR), would assist in dealing with lower-extremity disuse atrophy. Gait training emphasizing normal lower-extremity mechanics with assisted weight bearing and the use of crutches would be recommended. Most of these activities could be performed by the patient several times per day on his own.

22-2 The athletic trainer should refer the patient to a physician to rule out a stress fracture. Depending on the severity, an assistive device such as crutches may be warranted. Application of a pneumatic splint may assist in pain reduction and healing. Ice and electrical stimulation would be helpful for pain reduction. Training modifications including swimming, deep-water running, and cycling would be beneficial. Proper running shoes that meet the needs of the patient's foot type would be helpful not only for running but for ADLs. The patient should be encouraged to train on a more yielding surface than concrete. Lastly, educating the patient and coach regarding bone remodeling relative to increases in training volume would be helpful in devising a return-to-activity plan.

22-3 Clinically, the athletic trainer should address the potential causes of excessive compensatory pronation. This can include gastrocnemius–soleus stretching, fabrication of a foot orthosis, and use of motion- control running shoes. Addressing any myofascial restrictions via soft-tissue mobilization may provide some help. Conditioning on the bike and in the pool, along with non-impact activity on a Stairmaster or elliptical machine, would be appropriate. The patient needs to be counseled about the nature of the condition and what types of fitness training, training intensity, and training surface may affect the condition. Conditioning on a flat, yielding surface would reduce stress to the anterior compartment musculature. Also, conditioning that is more sport specific (eg, shorter runs vs long-distance running) may also benefit.

22-4 Once the initial pain and inflammation have subsided, the patient could begin AROM ankle dorsiflexion with the knee straight, stressing the involved muscle. Seated towel stretching of the gastrocnemius is next and could be progressed to standing calf stretching with the knee extended. Lastly, performing the same stretch on a slant board would place the most tensile stress on the medial head of the gastrocnemius muscle. Strengthening can begin with submaximal, pain-free isometric plantarflexion, progressing to maximal isometric strengthening. Isotonics can be introduced with manual resistance and progressed to concentric and eccentric isotonics with rubber tubing. The patient can then be progressed to weight-bearing, double-leg heel raises (concentric and eccentric) and then single-leg heel raises (concentric and eccentric). Single-leg eccentric lowering with body weight will place the greatest tensile load on the muscle. Dynamic muscle loading can be initiated with jumping rope. Multidirectional double-leg hopping can be progressed to multidirectional single-leg hopping on the involved side. The patient can be progressed to plyometrics with two legs and then to the involved leg at various heights.

22-5 The patient appears to have medial tibial stress syndrome. The increase in her training volume, along with running on non-yielding surfaces, may be the primary cause of the problem. She should be counseled to reduce her training volume and frequency to allow for soft-tissue healing. Non-impact cross-training would help her maintain her fitness level during this time. New running shoes along with a stretching program would be beneficial. When the symptoms have decreased, the patient should be educated to return to 50% of her training volume and increase by about 10% to 15% per week initially to not provoke the condition. Running on softer surfaces than concrete would also help reduce impact loading. A regimented stretching program of the gastrocnemius-soleus musculature would also be helpful.

22-6 Several structural alignment issues could be implicated in excessive pronation. In standing, the athletic trainer could look for a leg length discrepancy. The longer leg will attempt to shorten and equal out the pelvic heights, which can increase pronatory forces in the lower extremity. Femoral anteversion can be observed if the patella appears to be facing inward and can be confirmed with the patient prone on the table. Tibial varum and external tibial torsion can also be observed and measured in standing and sitting, respectively. The foot will most likely compensate with excessive pronation if these structural variations are present. Assessing rear-foot and fore-foot position in a prone position will usually reveal a rear-foot varus or valgus and most likely a forefoot varus when the subtalar joint is placed in a neutral position.

Please see videos on the accompanying website at

www.healio.com/books/sportsmedvideos

CHAPTER 23

Rehabilitation of Ankle and Foot Injuries

William E. Prentice, PhD, PT, ATC, FNATA
Stuart L. (Skip) Hunter, PT, ATC
Steven M. Zinder, PhD, ATC

After completion of this chapter, the athletic training student should be able to do the following:

- Review the biomechanics and functional anatomy of the foot and ankle.

- Identify the various injuries that occur at the ankle joint.

- Recognize the various treatment options for rehabilitating an ankle sprain.

- Analyze the effect of forefoot varus, forefoot valgus, and rear-foot varus on the foot and lower extremity.

- Explain the biomechanical examination of the foot.

- Demonstrate techniques for orthotic fabrication.

- Break down problems associated with the foot and the treatment options for each.

FUNCTIONAL ANATOMY AND BIOMECHANICS

The Talocrural Joint

The ankle joint, or talocrural joint, is a hinge joint that is formed by an articular facet on the distal extremity of the tibia, which articulates with the superior articular surface (trochlea) of the talus; the medial malleolus, which articulates with the medial surface of the trochlea of the talus; and the lateral malleolus, which articulates with the lateral surface of the trochlea. The axis of motion of the talocrural joint passes transversely through the body of the talus. This bony arrangement forms what is referred to as the ankle mortise.[72]

The talus provides a link between the lower leg and the tarsus. The talus, the second largest tarsal and the main weight-bearing bone

Prentice WE, ed.
Rehabilitation Techniques for Sports Medicine and Athletic Training (pp 749-799).
© 2015 SLACK Incorporated.

of the articulation, rests on the calcaneus and articulates with the lateral and medial malleoli. The relatively square shape of the talus allows the talocrural joint only two movements: dorsiflexion and plantarflexion. Because the talus is wider anteriorly than posteriorly, the most stable position of the ankle is with the foot in dorsiflexion. In this position the wider anterior aspect of the talus comes in contact with the narrower portion of the tibia lying between the malleoli, gripping it tightly. By contrast, as the ankle moves into plantarflexion, the wider portion of the tibia is brought in contact with the narrower posterior aspect of the talus, creating a less stable position than in dorsiflexion.[72]

The lateral malleolus of the fibula extends further distally so that the bony stability of the lateral aspect of the ankle is more stable than the medial. Motion at the talocrural joint ranges from 20 degrees of dorsiflexion to 50 degrees of plantarflexion depending on the patient. A normal foot requires 20 degrees of plantarflexion and 10 degrees of dorsiflexion with the knee extended for a normal gait.

Talocrural Joint Ligaments

The ligamentous support of the ankle consists of the articular capsule, three lateral ligaments, two ligaments that connect the tibia and fibula, and the medial or deltoid ligament (Figure 23-1). The three lateral ligaments are the anterior talofibular, the posterior talofibular, and the calcaneofibular. The distal anterior and posterior tibiofibular ligaments hold the tibia and fibula and form the distal portion of the interosseus membrane. The thick deltoid ligament provides primary resistance to foot eversion. A thin articular capsule encases the ankle joint.

Talocrural Joint Muscles

The muscles passing posterior to the lateral malleolus will produce ankle plantarflexion along with toe flexion. Anterior muscles serve to dorsiflex the ankle and to produce toe extension. The anterior muscles include the extensor hallucis longus, the extensor digitorum longus, the peroneus tertius, and the tibialis anterior. The posterior muscle group falls into three layers: at the superficial layer is the gastrocnemius; the middle layer includes the soleus and the plantaris; and the deep layer contains the

tibialis posterior, the flexor digitorum longus, and the flexor hallucis longus.[72]

The Subtalar Joint

The subtalar joint consists of the articulation between the talus and the calcaneus[80] (Figure 23-2). Supination and pronation are normal movements that occur at the subtalar joint. These movements are triplanar movements, that is, movements that occur in all three planes simultaneously.[24,63,69] In weight bearing, the subtalar joint acts as a torque convertor to translate the pronation/supination into leg rotation.[89,101] The movements of the talus during pronation and supination have profound effects on the lower extremity both proximally and distally. When weight bearing, in supination the talus abducts and dorsiflexes on the calcaneus while the calcaneus inverts on the talus. The foot moves into adduction, plantarflexion, and inversion. Conversely, when weight bearing in pronation, the talus adducts and plantarflexes while the calcaneus everts on the talus. The foot moves into abduction, dorsiflexion, and eversion.[24,60]

The Midtarsal Joint

The midtarsal joint consists of two distinct joints: the calcaneocuboid and the talonavicular joint. The midtarsal joint depends mainly on ligamentous and muscular tension to maintain position and integrity. Midtarsal joint stability is directly related to the position of the subtalar joint. If the subtalar joint is pronated, the talonavicular and calcaneocuboid joints become hypermobile. If the subtalar joint is supinated, the midtarsal joint becomes hypomobile. As the midtarsal joint becomes more or less mobile, it affects the distal portion of the foot because of the articulations at the tarsometatarsal joint.[63]

Effects of Midtarsal Joint Position During Pronation

During pronation, the talus adducts and plantarflexes and makes the joint articulations of the midtarsal joint more congruous. The long axes of the talonavicular and calcaneocuboid joints are more parallel and thus allow more motion. The resulting foot is often referred to as a "loose bag of bones."[24,80] As more motion

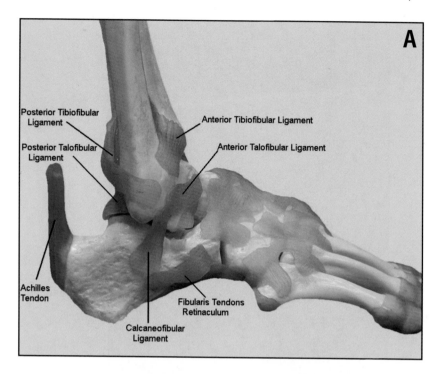

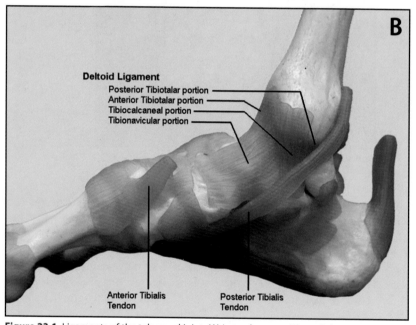

Figure 23-1. Ligaments of the talocrural joint. (A) Lateral aspect; (B) medial aspect.

occurs at the midtarsal joint, the lesser tarsal bones, particularly the first metatarsal and first cuneiform, become more mobile. These bones comprise a functional unit known as the first ray. With pronation of the midtarsal joint, the first ray is more mobile because of its articulations with that joint.[64] The first ray is also stabilized by the attachment of the long peroneal tendon, which attaches to the base of the first metatarsal. The long peroneal tendon passes posteriorly around the base of the lateral malleolus and then through a notch in the

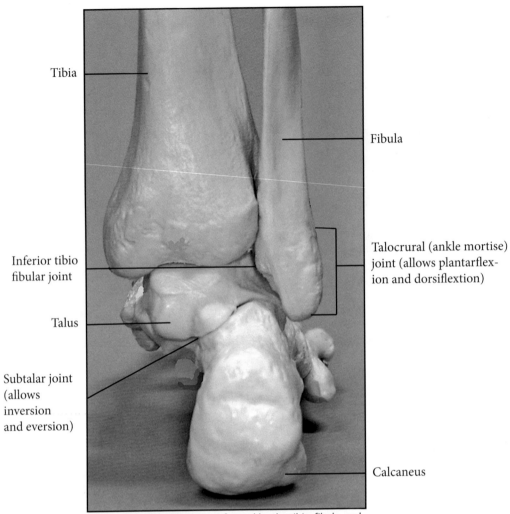

Figure 23-2. The ankle joint is formed by the tibia, fibula, and talus. The subtalar joint is formed by the talus and calcaneus.

cuboid to cross the foot to the first metatarsal. The cuboid functions as a pulley to increase the mechanical advantage of the peroneal tendon. Stability of the cuboid is essential in this process. In the pronated position, the cuboid loses much of its mechanical advantage as a pulley; therefore, the peroneal tendon no longer stabilizes the first ray effectively. This condition creates hypermobility of the first ray and increased pressure on the other metatarsals (Figure 23-3).

Effects of Midtarsal Joint Position During Supination

During supination, the talus abducts and dorsiflexes, which raises the level of the talonavicular joint superior to that of the calcaneocuboid joint and allows lesser surface areas of both joint articulations to become congruous.[79] Also the long axes of the joints become more oblique. Both allow less motion to occur at this joint, making the foot very rigid and tight. Since less movement occurs at the calcaneocuboid joint, the cuboid becomes hypomobile. The long peroneal tendon has a greater amount of tension since the cuboid has less mobility and thus will not allow hypermobility of the first ray. In this case the majority of the weight is borne by the first and fifth metatarsals (Figure 23-4).

The Tarsometatarsal Joint

The tarsometatarsal joint is composed of the cuboid; first, second, and third cuneiforms; and

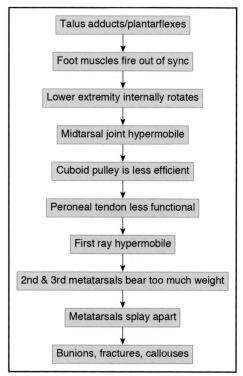

Figure 23-3. The effects of a forefoot varus.

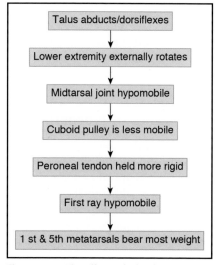

Figure 23-4. The effects of a forefoot valgus.

the bases of the metatarsal bones. These bones allow for rotational forces when engaged in weight-bearing activities. They move as a unit, depending on the position of the midtarsal and subtalar joints. Also known as the Lisfrancs' joint, the tarsometatarsal joint provides a locking device that enhances foot stability.

The Metatarsal Joints

Together with subtalar, talonavicular, and tarsometatarsal interrelationships, foot stabilization depends on the function of the metatarsal joints. The first metatarsal bone contact of the foot is on the lateral aspect of the calcaneus with the subtalar joint in supination.[4] At initial contact, the subtalar joint is supinated. Associated with this supination of the subtalar joint is an obligatory external rotation of the tibia. As the foot is loaded, the subtalar joint moves into a pronated position until the forefoot is in contact with the running surface. The change in subtalar motion occurs between initial heel strike and 20% into the support phase of running. As pronation occurs at the subtalar joint, there is obligatory internal rotation of

the tibia. Transverse plane rotation occurs at the knee joint because of this tibial rotation.[4] Pronation of the foot unlocks the midtarsal joint and allows the foot to assist in shock absorption and to adapt to uneven surfaces. It is important during initial impact to reduce the ground reaction forces and to distribute the load evenly on many different anatomical structures throughout the foot and leg. Pronation is normal and allows for this distribution of forces on as many structures as possible to avoid excessive loading on just a few structures. The subtalar joint remains in a pronated position until 55% to 85% of the support phase with maximum pronation is concurrent with the body's center of gravity passing over the base of support.[72] The foot begins to resupinate and will approach the neutral subtalar position at 70% to 90% of the support phase. In supination the midtarsal joints are locked and the foot becomes stable and rigid to prepare for push-off. This rigid position allows the foot to exert a great amount of force from the lower extremity to the running surface,[45] and along with the first cuneiform bone, forms the first ray. The first ray moves independently from the other metatarsal bones. As a main weight bearer, the first ray is concerned with body propulsion. Stabilization depends on the peroneus longus muscle that attaches on the medial aspect of the first ray. As with the other segments of the foot, stability of the first metatarsal bone depends on the relative position of the subtalar and talonavicular joints. The fifth metatarsal bone, like the first metatarsal bone, moves independently. In plantarflexion it moves into adduction and inversion; conversely, in dorsiflexion it moves the foot into abduction and eversion.[40]

Biomechanics of Normal Gait

The action of the lower extremity during a complete stride in running can be divided into two phases. The first is the stance, or support, phase that starts with initial contact at heel strike and ends at toe-off. The second is the swing or recovery phase. This represents the time immediately after toe-off in which the leg is moved from behind the body to a position in front of the body in preparation for heel strike.

The foot's function during the support phase of running is twofold. At heel strike, the foot acts as a shock absorber to the impact forces and then adapts to the uneven surfaces. At push-off, the foot functions as a rigid lever to transmit the explosive force from the lower extremity to the running surface. In a heel-strike running gait, initial contact of the foot is on the lateral aspect of the calcaneus with the subtalar joint in supination.[4]

At initial contact, the subtalar joint is supinated. Associated with this supination of the subtalar joint is an obligatory external rotation of the tibia. As the foot is loaded, the subtalar joint moves into a pronated position until the forefoot is in contact with the running surface. The change in subtalar motion occurs between initial heel strike and 20% into the support phase of running. As pronation occurs at the subtalar joint, there is obligatory internal rotation of the tibia. Transverse plane rotation occurs at the knee joint because of this tibial rotation.[4] Pronation of the foot unlocks the midtarsal joint and allows the foot to assist in shock absorption and to adapt to uneven surfaces. It is important during initial impact to reduce the ground reaction forces and to distribute the load evenly on many different anatomical structures throughout the foot and leg. Pronation is normal and allows for this distribution of forces on as many structures as possible to avoid excessive loading on just a few structures. The subtalar joint remains in a pronated position until 55% to 85% of the support phase with maximum pronation is concurrent with the body's center of gravity passing over the base of support.[72]

The foot begins to resupinate and will approach the neutral subtalar position at 70% to 90% of the support phase. In supination the midtarsal joints are locked and the foot becomes stable and rigid to prepare for push-off. This rigid position allows the foot to exert a great amount of force from the lower extremity to the running surface.[45]

REHABILITATION TECHNIQUES FOR SPECIFIC INJURIES

Ankle Sprains

Pathomechanics and Injury Mechanism

Ankle sprains are among the more common injuries seen in sports medicine.[8,21,103] Injuries to the ligaments of the ankle may be classified according to either their location or the mechanism of injury.

Inversion Sprains

An inversion ankle sprain that results in injury to the lateral ligaments is by far the most common. The anterior talofibular ligament is the weakest of the three lateral ligaments. Its major function is to stop forward subluxation of the talus. It is injured in an inverted, plantarflexed, and internally rotated position.[48,94] The calcaneofibular and posterior talofibular ligaments are also likely to be injured in inversion sprains as the force of inversion is increased. Increased inversion force is needed to tear the calcaneofibular ligament. Because the posterior talofibular ligament prevents posterior subluxation of the talus, its injuries are severe, such as is the case in complete dislocations.[9]

Eversion Sprains

The eversion ankle sprain is less common than the inversion ankle sprain, largely because of the bony and ligamentous anatomy. As mentioned previously, the fibular malleolus extends

REHABILITATION TECHNIQUES

Stretching Exercises

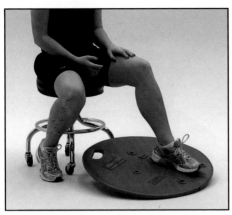

Figure 23-5. Seated BAPS board exercises are an AROM exercise that are useful in regaining normal ankle motion.

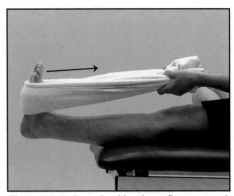

Figure 23-6. Seated ankle plantarflexors stretch using a towel.

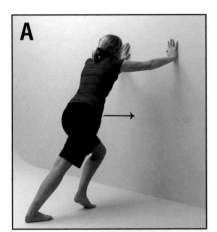

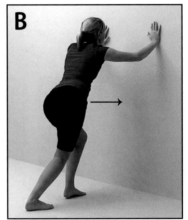

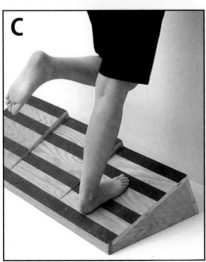

Figure 23-7. Standing ankle plantarflexors stretch. (A) Gastrocnemius; (B) soleus; (C) stretching may also be done using a slant board.

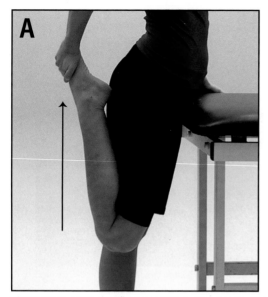

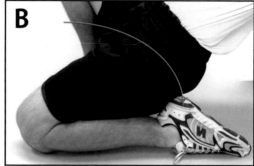

Figure 23-8. Ankle dorsiflexors stretch for the anterior tibialis. (A) Standing; (B) kneeling.

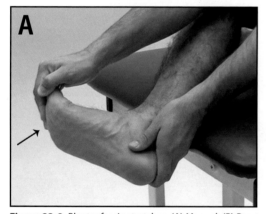

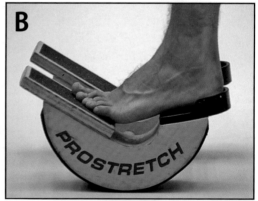

Figure 23-9. Plantar fascia stretches. (A) Manual. (B) Prostretch.

Isometric Strengthening Exercises

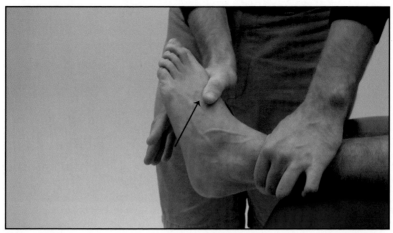

Figure 23-10. Isometric inversion against a stable resistance, used to strengthen the posterior tibialis, flexor digitorum longus, and flexor hallucis longus.

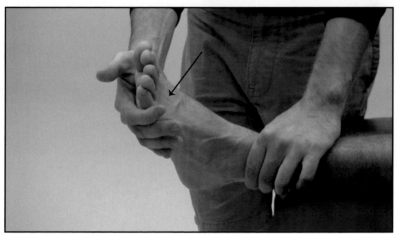

Figure 23-11. Isometric eversion against a stable resistance. Used to strengthen the peroneus longus, brevis, tertius, and extensor digitorum longus.

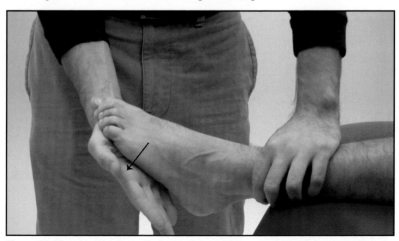

Figure 23-12. Isometric plantarflexion against a stable resistance. Used to strengthen the gastrocnemius, soleus, posterior tibialis, flexor digitorum longus, flexor hallucis longus, and plantaris.

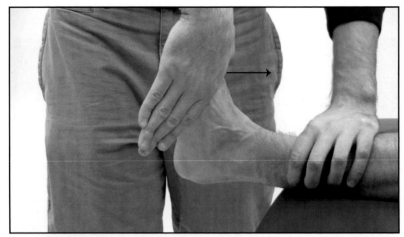

Figure 23-13. Isometric dorsiflexion against a stable resistance. Used to strengthen the anterior tibialis and peroneus tertius.

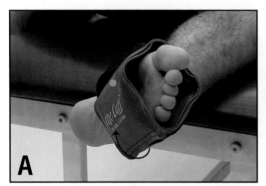

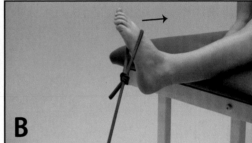

Figure 23-14. Inversion exercise. (A) Using a weight cuff; (B) using resistive tubing. Used to strengthen the posterior tibialis, flexor digitorum longus, and flexor hallucis longus.

Isotonic Strengthening Exercises

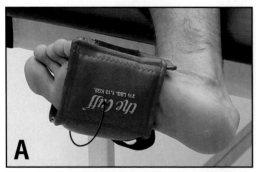

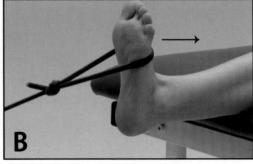

Figure 23-15. Eversion exercise. (A) Using a weight cuff; (B) using resistive tubing. Used to strengthen the peroneus longus, brevis, tertius, and extensor digitorum longus.

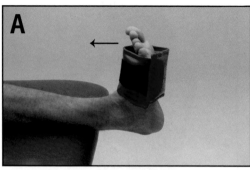

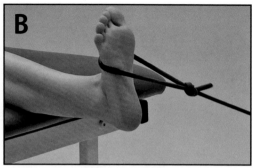

Figure 23-16. Dorsiflexion exercise. (A) Using a weight cuff; (B) using resistive tubing. Used to strengthen the anterior tibialis and peroneus tertius.

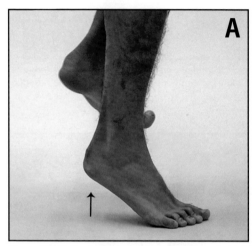

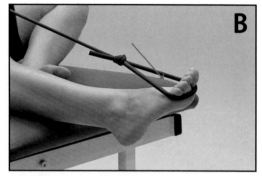

Figure 23-17. Plantarflexion exercise using surgical tubing. Used to strengthen the gastrocnemius, soleus, posterior tibialis, flexor digitorum longus, flexor hallucis longus, and plantaris. (A) Body weight resisted; (B) using surgical tubing.

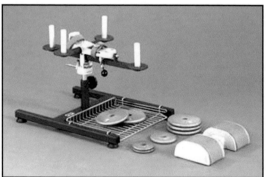

Figure 23-18. Multidirectional Elgin ankle exerciser. (Reprinted with permission from Elgin.)

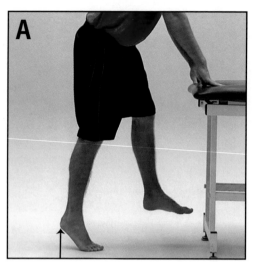
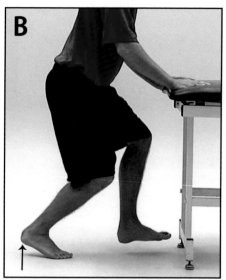

Figure 23-19. Toe raises. Used to strengthen the gastrocnemius, soleus, posterior tibialis, flexor digitorum longus, flexor hallucis longus, and plantaris. (A) Extended knee strengthens the gastrocnemius; (B) flexed knee strengthens the soleus.

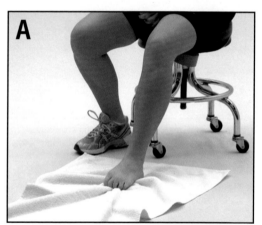
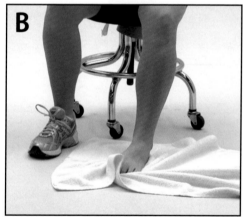

Figure 23-20. Towel-gathering exercise. (A) Toe flexion. Used to strengthen the flexor digitorum longus and brevis, lumbricales, and flexor hallucis longus. (B) Inversion/eversion exercises. Used to strengthen the posterior tibialis, flexor digitorum longus, flexor hallucis longus, peroneus longus, brevis, tertius, and extensor digitorum longus.

Closed Kinetic Chain Strengthening Exercises

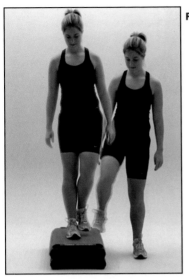

Figure 23-21. Lateral step-ups.

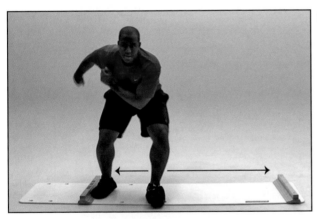

Figure 23-22. Slide board exercises.

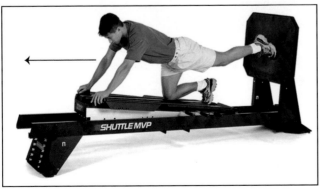

Figure 23-23. Shuttle MVP exercise machine.

Isokinetic Strengthening Exercises

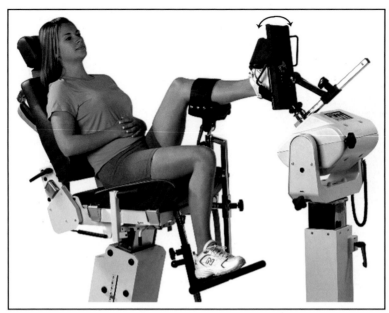

Figure 23-24. Isokinetic inversion/eversion exercise. Used to improve the strength and endurance of the ankle inverters and everters in an open chain. Also can provide an objective measurement of muscular torque production. (Reprinted with permission from Biodex Medical Systems.)

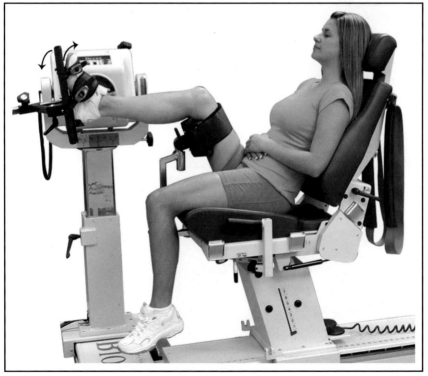

Figure 23-25. Isokinetic plantarflexion/dorsiflexion exercise. Used to improve the strength and endurance of the ankle dorsiflexors and plantarflexors in an open chain. Also can provide an objective measurement of torque production. (Reprinted with permission from Biodex Medical Systems.)

Proprioceptive Neuromuscular Facilitation Strengthening Exercises

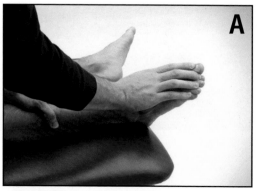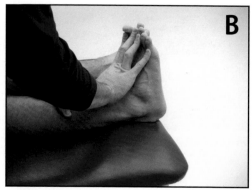

Figure 23-26. D1 pattern moving into flexion. (A), Starting position, ankle plantarflexed, foot everted, toes flexed. B) Terminal position, ankle dorsiflexed, foot inverted, toes extended.

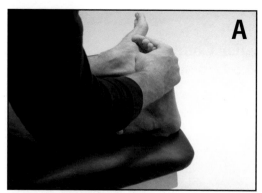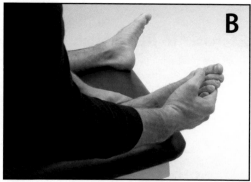

Figure 23-27. D1 pattern moving into extension. (A) Starting position, ankle dorsiflexed, foot inverted, toes extended. (B) Terminal position, ankle plantarflexed, foot everted, toes flexed.

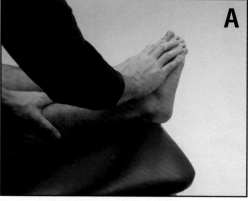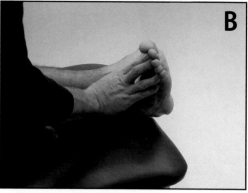

Figure 23-28. D2 pattern moving into flexion. (A) Starting position, ankle plantarflexed, foot inverted, toes flexed. (B) Terminal position, ankle dorsiflexed, foot everted, toes extended.

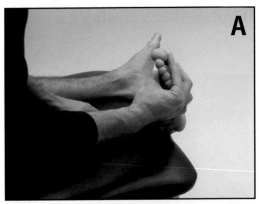
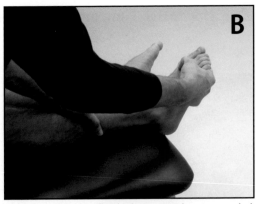

Figure 23-29. D2 pattern moving into extension. (A) Starting position, ankle dorsiflexed, foot everted, toes extended. (B) Terminal position, ankle plantarflexed, foot inverted, toes flexed.

Exercises to Reestablish Neuromuscular Control

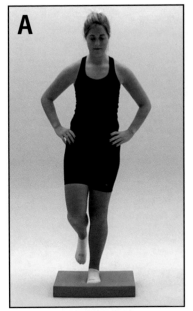
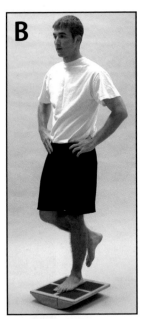
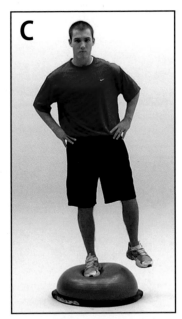

Figure 23-30. Standing single-leg balance activity. Used to activate the lower-leg musculature and improve balance and proprioception of the involved extremity. (A) Foam surface; (B) Rocker board; (C) Bosu balance trainer.

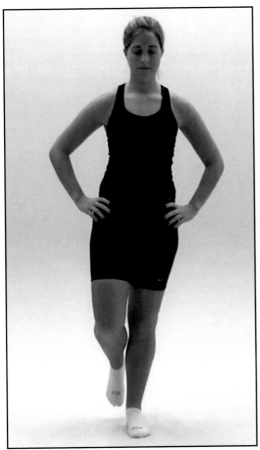

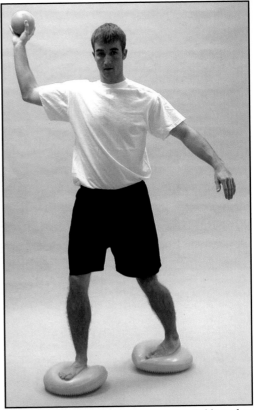

Figure 23-32. Single-leg stance on an unstable surface while performing functional activities.

Figure 23-31. Static single-leg standing balance progression. Used to improve balance and proprioception of the lower extremity. This activity can be made more difficult with the following progression: (A) single-leg stand, eyes open; (B) single-leg stand, eyes closed; (C) single-leg stand, eyes open, toes extended so only the heel and metatarsal heads are in contact with the ground; (D) single-leg stand, eyes closed, toes extended.

Figure 23-33. Single-leg standing rubber-tubing kicks. Using kicks resisted by surgical tubing of the uninvolved side while weight bearing on the involved side may encourage neuromuscular control.

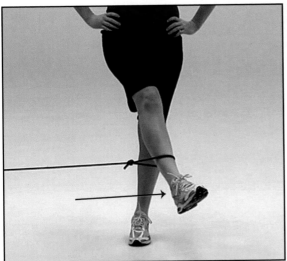

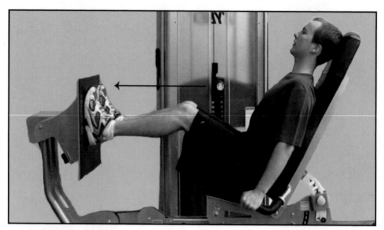

Figure 23-34. Leg press.

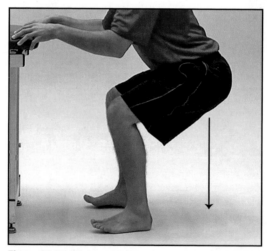

Figure 23-35. Mini-squats.

Exercises to Improve Cardiorespiratory Endurance

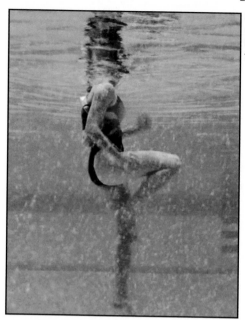

Figure 23-36. Pool running with flotation device. Used to reduce impact weight-bearing forces on the lower extremity while maintaining cardiovascular fitness level and running form.

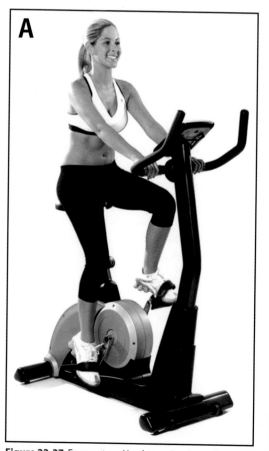

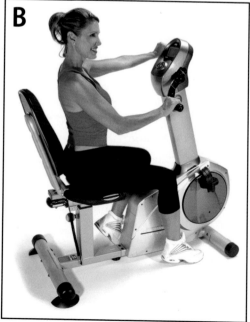

Figure 23-37. Ergometers. Used to maintain cardiovascular fitness when use of a lower-extremity ergometer is contraindicated or too difficult to use. (A) Upright stationary exercise ergometer; (B) upper body ergometer.

further inferiorly than does the tibial malleolus. This, combined with the strength of the thick deltoid ligament, prevents excessive eversion. More often eversion injuries may involve an avulsion fracture of the tibia before the deltoid ligament tears.[14] The deltoid ligament may also be contused in inversion sprains due to impingement between the fibular malleolus and the calcaneus. Despite the fact that eversion sprains are less common, the severity is such that these sprains may take longer to heal than inversion sprains.[66]

Syndesmotic Sprains

Isolated injuries to the distal tibiofemoral joint are referred to as syndesmotic sprains. The anterior and posterior tibiofibular ligaments are found between the distal tibia and fibula and extend up the lower leg as the interosseous ligament or syndesmotic ligament. Sprains of the syndesmotic ligaments are more common than has been realized in the past. These ligaments are torn with increased external rotational or forced dorsiflexion and are often injured in conjunction with a severe sprain of the medial and lateral ligament complexes.[92] Initial rupture of the ligaments occurs distally at the tibiofibular ligament above the ankle mortise. As the force of disruption is increased, the interosseous ligament is torn more proximally. Sprains of the syndesmotic ligaments are extremely difficult to treat and often require months to heal. Treatments for this problem are essentially the same as for medial or lateral sprains, with the difference being an extended period of immobilization. Functional activities and return to sport may be delayed for a longer period than for inversion or eversion sprains.

Severity of the Sprain

In a grade 1 sprain, there is some stretching or perhaps tearing of the ligamentous fibers with little or no joint instability. Mild pain, little swelling, and joint stiffness may be apparent. With a grade 2 sprain, there is some tearing and separation of the ligamentous fibers and moderate instability of the joint. Moderate to severe pain, swelling, and joint stiffness should be expected. Grade 3 sprains involve total rupture of the ligament, manifested primarily by gross instability of the joint. Severe pain may be present initially, followed by little or no pain

due to total disruption of nerve fibers. Swelling may be profuse, and thus the joint tends to become very stiff some hours after the injury. A grade 3 sprain with marked instability usually requires some form of immobilization lasting several weeks. Frequently the force producing the ligament injury is so great that other ligaments or structures surrounding the joint may also be injured. With cases in which there is injury to multiple ligaments, surgical repair or reconstruction may be necessary to correct instability.

Rehabilitation Concerns

During the initial phase of ankle rehabilitation, the major goals are reduction of post-injury swelling, bleeding, and pain and protection of the already healing ligament. As is the case in all acute musculoskeletal injuries, initial treatment efforts should be directed toward limiting the amount of swelling.[71] This is perhaps more true in the case of ankle sprains than with any other injury. Controlling initial swelling is the single most important treatment measure that can be taken during the entire rehabilitation process. Mawdsley, Hoy, and Erwin found the figure-of-eight method of measuring ankle edema to be reliable and valid.[55] There is no question that limiting the amount of acute swelling can significantly reduce the time required for rehabilitation. Initial management includes compression, ice, elevation, rest, and protection.

Compression

Immediately following injury and evaluation, a compression wrap should be applied to the sprained ankle. An elastic bandage should be firmly and evenly applied, wrapping distal to proximal. It is also recommended that the elastic bandage be wet to facilitate the passage of cold. To add more compression, a horseshoe-shaped felt pad may be inserted under the wrap over the area of maximum swelling.

Following initial treatment, open Gibney taping may be applied under an elastic wrap to provide additional compression and support. Care should be taken not to compartmentalize this treatment by placing tape across the top and bottom of the open area of the open Gibney (Figure 23-38). Uneven pressure or uncovered

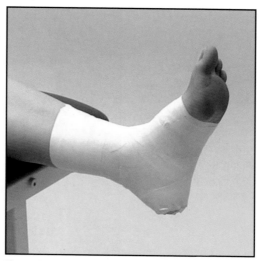

Figure 23-38. Closed basketweave tape.

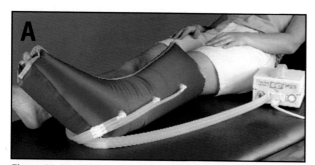
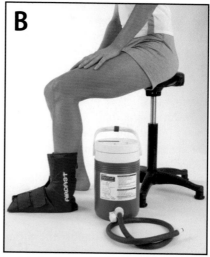

Figure 23-39. (A) Intermittent air compression device. (B) Cryo-cuff. (Reprinted with permission from of DonJoy.)

areas over any part of the extremity may allow the swelling to accumulate.

Other devices are available that apply external compression to the ankle to control or reduce swelling. These can be used both initially and throughout the rehabilitative process. Most of these use either air or cold water within an enclosed bag to provide pressure to reduce swelling. Among these are intermittent compression devices such as a Josbt Pump or a Cryo-cuff (Figure 23-39).

Ice

The use of ice on acute injuries has been well documented in the literature. Ice must initially be used with compression, because ice used alone is not as effective as ice used in conjunction with compression.[86] The initial use of ice has its basis in constricting superficial blood flow to prevent hemorrhage, as well as in reducing the hypoxic response to injury by decreasing cellular metabolism. Long-term benefits may be from reduction of pain and guarding.[72] Garrick suggests the use of ice for a minimum of 20 minutes once every 4 waking hours.[31] Ice should not be used longer than 30 minutes, especially over superficial nerves such as the peroneal and ulnar nerves; prolonged use of ice in such areas can produce transient nerve palsy.[25]

Current literature suggests that ice can be used during all phases of rehabilitation,[51] but is most effective if used immediately after injury.[73] Ice can certainly do no harm if used properly, but heat, if applied too soon after injury, may lead to increased inflammation. Often the switch from ice to heat cannot be made for weeks or months. The switch to heat should be made based on symptomatology rather than a strict time schedule.

Elevation

Elevation is an essential part of edema control. Pressure in any vessel below the level of the heart is increased, which may lead to increased edema.[15] Elevation allows gravity to work with the lymphatic system rather than against it and decreases hydrostatic pressure to decrease fluid loss and also assists venous and lymphatic return through gravity.[73] Patients with ankle sprains should be encouraged to maintain an elevated position as often as possible, particularly during the first 24 to 48 hours following injury. An attempt should be made to treat in the elevated position rather than the gravity-dependent position. Any treatment done in the dependent position will allow edema to increase.[73,84]

Rest

It is important to allow the inflammatory process a chance to accomplish what it is supposed to during the first 24 to 48 hours before incorporating aggressive exercise techniques. However, rest does not mean that the injured patient does nothing. Contralateral exercises may be performed to obtain cross-transfer effects on the muscles of the injured side. Isometric exercises may be performed very early in dorsiflexion, plantarflexion, inversion, and eversion (Figures 23-10 through 23-13). These types of exercises may be performed to prevent atrophy without fear of further injury to the ligament. Active plantarflexion and dorsiflexion may be initiated early because they also do not endanger the healing ligament as long as they are done in a pain-free range.

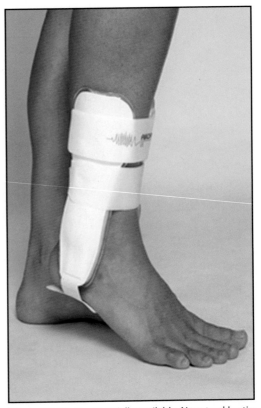

Figure 23-40. Commercially available Aircast ankle stirrup. (Reprinted with permission from DonJoy.)

These active plantarflexion and dorsiflexion exercises can be done while the patient is iced and elevated. Inversion and eversion are to be avoided, because they might initiate bleeding and further traumatize ligaments.

Protection

Several appliances are available to accomplish this early protected motion. Quillen recommends the ankle stirrup, which allows motion in the sagittal plane while limiting movement of the frontal plane and thus avoids stressing the ligaments through inversion and eversion[74] (Figure 23-40). Glascoe et al found that weight-bearing immobilization combined with an early exercise program was effective treatment for grade 2 ankle sprains.[34] Several commercially available braces accomplish this goal and also apply cushioned pressure to help with edema.[88] When a commercially available product is not feasible, a similar protective device may be fashioned from thermoplastic materials such as hexalite or orthoplast (Figure 23-41).

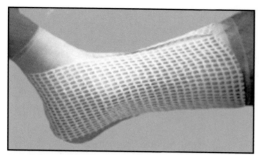

Figure 23-41. Molded hexalite ankle stirrup.

Gross, Lapp, and Davis compared the effectiveness of a number of commercial ankle orthoses and taping in restricting eversion and inversion. All of these support systems significantly reduced inversion and eversion immediately after initial application and after exercise when compared to preapplication measures. Of the orthoses tested, taping provided the least support after exercise.[37] Early application of these devices allows early ambulation.

Functional Ankle Instability

Most minor ankle sprains completely resolve with conservative treatment, while others persist with pain, weakness, and other symptoms of chronic instability. The rate of repeated lateral ankle sprain has been shown to be as high as 80%.[38,63,104] The most common sequelae following lateral ankle sprain are mechanical and functional instability.[81] Mechanical instability (MI) refers to a range of motion (ROM) beyond the normal physiological limits of a joint.[16] *Functional ankle instability* (FAI), a term first proposed by Freeman,[26] describes proprioceptive deficits that occur following a lateral ankle sprain and is commonly described as the sensation of the ankle "giving way." FAI is often considered the most viable reason for the high recurrence rate of lateral ankle sprain.[38]

The relationship between MI and FAI remains unclear. While it is somewhat rare to find individuals who suffer from MI who do not develop some semblance of FAI,[38] the reverse is not always true. Tropp et al[96] found that only 42% of patients with FAI showed any signs of ligamentous laxity, and Birmingham et al[6] found no differences in passive inversion ROM in 30 patients with unilateral FAI. Many of the differences obtained across studies may stem from the lack of a unified definition of

FAI. While MI is a purely objective measure of joint displacement, the measure of FAI is somewhat more subjective in nature. Many functional assessment tools exist in the literature in an attempt to quantify FAI.[23]

Rehabilitation Progression

In the early phase of rehabilitation, vigorous exercise is discouraged. The injured ligament must be maintained in a stable position so healing can occur. Thus, during the period of maximum protection following injury, the patient should be either non-weight-bearing or perhaps partial-weight-bearing on crutches. Partial weight bearing with crutches will help control several complications to healing. Muscle atrophy, proprioceptive loss, and circulatory stasis are all reduced when even limited weight bearing is allowed. Weight bearing also inhibits contracture of the tendons, which can lead to tendinitis. For these reasons, early ambulation, even if only touchdown weight bearing, is essential.[54] Aquatic therapy may be beneficial, in that it allows light to moderate weight bearing in a gravity-reduced environment.[34] It has been clearly demonstrated that a healing ligament needs a certain amount of stress to heal properly. The literature suggests that early limited stress following the initial period of inflammation might promote faster and stronger healing.[9,68] These studies found that protected motion facilitated proper collagen reorientation and thus increased the strength of the healing ligament.

As swelling is controlled and pain decreases, indicating that ligaments have reached that point in the healing process at which they are not in danger from minimal stress, rehabilitation can become more aggressive.

Range of Motion

In the early stages of the rehabilitation, inversion and eversion should be minimized. Light joint mobilization concentrating on dorsiflexion and plantarflexion should be started initially.[53] It can be accomplished by manual joint mobilization techniques (see Figures 13-63 through 13-66) or through exercises such as towel stretching for the plantarflexors (Figure 23-6) and standing or kneeling stretches for the dorsiflexors (Figure 23-8). Patients

REHABILITATION PLAN

ANKLE SPRAINS

Injury situation: A 30-year-old female recreational indoor soccer player attempted to cut on her right ankle when she experienced a grade 1 ankle sprain. The injury occurred 1 hour prior to her arrival in the athletic training clinic. Her local physician diagnosed a grade 1 ankle sprain. X-rays were negative.

Signs and symptoms: Physical findings include (1) mild swelling and tenderness to palpation over the anterior talofibular ligament; (2) negative anterior drawer test; (3) negative talar tilt test; (4) AROM: dorsiflexion=0 degrees, plantar flexion=50 degrees, inversion=0 degrees, eversion=20 degrees.

Management plan: The overall goal is to reduce inflammation initially, proceed through a ROM and strengthening program, address proprioceptive and neuromuscular control, and implement a return-to-sport program.

PHASE ONE: Acute Inflammatory Stage

GOALS: Control pain, limit swelling, regain ROM.

Estimated length of time (ELT): Days 1 to 5 Use PRICE (protection, rest, ice, compression, and elevation) to address the symptoms of the acute inflammatory stage. The use of tape/bracing allows early weight bearing while protecting the healing ligament from further motion. Exercises may be begun, stressing plantar flexion and dorsiflexion. Inversion–eversion exercises should be avoided during this stage to protect the healing ligament. Alternative forms of conditioning may be needed to maintain cardiovascular status during the entire rehabilitation. This may include swimming, cycling, pool running, and upper body ergometer work.

PHASE TWO: Fibroblastic Repair Stage

GOALS: Increase ROM in all planes, restore neuromuscular control, and restore proprioception.

Estimated length of time (ELT): Days 5 to 14 PRICE may be continued to control swelling and pain. ROM exercises should be performed in all planes. Strengthening exercises should address not only the musculature surrounding the ankle but also the intrinsic musculature of the foot. Full weight bearing should be encouraged as quickly as possible. Proprioceptive exercises should be begun as early as tolerated. These exercises may be started as non-weight-bearing exercises and progress to exercises as strenuous as standing BAPS board exercises with perturbations.

PHASE THREE: Maturation Remodeling Stage

GOALS: Elimination of swelling and pain, full ROM, full strength, and restoration of proprioception. These criteria are followed by a carefully instituted return-to-sport program.

Estimated length of time (ELT): Days 14 to 21 The patient continues to perform all the strengthening, ROM, and proprioceptive exercises. A gradual progression of walking to running and protection in the form of bracing, taping, and high-top shoes may be needed to allow these steps to be taken. Once cutting and sprinting have been performed without an antalgic gait, the athlete may be returned gradually to sports.

DISCUSSION QUESTIONS

1. How might the rehabilitation progression change if the patient had sustained a medial ankle sprain of the same degree?
2. Describe a proprioceptive exercise progression for this patient.
3. What steps can be taken to reduce the chance of reinjury for ankle sprains?
4. How might this patient's recovery time change if the injury had been to the tibiofibular ligament and the interosseus membrane?

are encouraged to do these exercises slowly, without pain, and to use high repetitions (two sets of 40).

As tenderness over the ligament decreases, inversion–eversion exercises may be initiated in conjunction with plantarflexion and dorsiflexion exercises. Early exercises include pulling a towel from one side to the other by alternately inverting and everting the foot (Figure 23-20B) and alphabet drawing in an ice bath, which should be done in capital letters to ensure that full range is used.

Exercises performed on a foam surface, Rocker board, or Bosu (Figure 23-30) may be beneficial for ROM, as well as a beginning exercise for regaining neuromuscular control.[95] These exercises should at first be done seated, progressing to standing (Figure 23-5). Initially the patient should start in the seated position with a wedge board in the plantarflexion-dorsiflexion direction. As pain decreases and ligament healing progresses, the board may be turned in the inversion–eversion direction. As the patient performs these movements easily, a seated BAPS board may be used for full ROM exercises (Figure 23-5). When seated exercises are performed with ease, standing balance exercises should be initiated. They may be started on one leg standing without a board. The patient then supports weight with the hands and maintains balance on a wedge board in either plantarflexion–dorsiflexion or inversion–eversion. Next, hand support may be eliminated while the patient balances on the wedge board. The same sequence is then used on the BAPS board. The BAPS board is initially used with assistance from the hands. Then balance is practiced on the BAPS board unassisted.

Vigorous heel cord stretching should be initiated as soon as possible (Figure 23-7). McCluskey, Blackburn, and Lewis[57] found that the heel cord acts as a bowstring when tight and may increase the chance of ankle sprains.

Strengthening

Isometrics may be done in the major ankle motion planes, frontal and sagittal (Figures 23-10 through 23-14). They may be accompanied early in the rehabilitative phase by plantarflexion and dorsiflexion isotonic exercises, which do not endanger the ligaments (Figures 23-16 and 23-17). As the ligaments heal further and ROM increases, strengthening exercises may be begun in all planes of motion (Figures 23-14 and 23-15). Care must be taken when exercising the ankle in inversion and eversion to avoid tibial rotation as a substitute movement. Pain should be the basic guideline for deciding when to start inversion–eversion isotonic exercises. Light resistance with high repetitions has fewer detrimental effects on the ligaments (2 to 4 sets of 10 repetitions). Resistive tubing exercises, ankle weights around the foot, or a multidirectional Elgin ankle exerciser (Figure 23-18) are excellent methods of strengthening inversion and eversion. Tubing has advantages in that it may be used both eccentrically and concentrically. Isokinetics have advantages in that more functional speeds may be obtained and they provide accommodating resistance (Figures 23-23 and 23-25). Proprioceptive neuromuscular facilitation (PNF) strengthening exercises that isolate the desired motions at the talocrural joint can also be used (Figures 23-26 through 23-29).

Proximal Stability

It is essential that when managing a patient with foot and ankle pathology or pathomechanics, that proximal stability is addressed, specifically that of the knee, hip, and trunk musculature.[12] As already discussed, ROM, strength, flexibility, and neuromuscular control are all key components. More detailed information is available in several previous chapters, including those on the core, hip, and knee.

To further expand on strengthening exercises, when a patient has weight-bearing restrictions, initiating exercises for proximal trunk and hip stability early in the rehabilitation process are recommended. For example, exercises for gluteus medius, hip lateral rotators, trunk extensors, and gluteus maximus can be initiated against gravity, against resistance or using an exercise ball. Once weight bearing is progressed to full and pain-free, then a more functional program can be implemented.[50]

Finally, it is important when managing a patient with a proximal movement-related dysfunction or diagnosis, to examine the foot and ankle. It is well accepted that when the foot comes into contact with the ground, there is a biomechanical influence up the kinetic chain.[12] Thus, the assumption can be made that overuse injuries involving knees, hips, or back could be related to foot or ankle pathomechanics.[12]

Proprioception and Neuromuscular Control

The role of proprioception in repeated ankle trauma has been questioned.[13,27,29,31] The literature suggests that proprioception is certainly a factor in recurrent ankle sprains. Rebman reported that 83% of his patients experienced a reduction in chronic ankle sprains after a program of proprioceptive exercises.[75] Glencross and Thornton found that the greater the ligamentous disruption, the greater the proprioceptive loss.[35] Early weight bearing has previously been mentioned as a method of reducing proprioceptive loss. During the rehabilitation phase, standing on both feet with closed eyes with progression to standing on one leg is an exercise to recoup proprioception (Figure 23-31). This exercise may be followed by standing and balancing on a BAPS board (Figure 22-23), a Dynadisc, a Bosu Balance Trainer, or an Extreme Balance Board (see Chapter 7), which should be done initially with support from the hands. As a final-stage exercise, the patient can progress to free standing and controlling the board through all ranges (Figure 23-30). A recent systematic review[58] assessing the effectiveness of balance training on the risk of incurring an ankle sprain found that prophylactic balance training significantly reduced the risk of sustaining future ankle sprains. The greatest effect was found in those patients with a history of previous sprain.[58]

Other closed kinetic chain exercises may be beneficial. Leg presses (Figure 23-34) and minisquats (Figure 23-35) on the involved leg will encourage weight bearing and increase proprioceptive return. Single-leg standing kicks using abduction, adduction, extension, and flexion of the uninvolved side while weight bearing on the affected side will increase both strength and proprioception. This may be accomplished either free-standing (Figure 23-33) or on a machine.

Clinical Decision-Making Exercise 23-1

A 21-year-old recreational basketball player suffered a grade 2 lateral ankle sprain last night. It is the third episode of the same injury in 3 years. His initial symptoms are limited swelling, pain, and loss of ROM. Talar tilt and anterior drawer testing are within normal limits. The patient states that previous rehabilitation included strengthening and ROM exercises. What type of additional rehabilitative exercises can the athletic trainer suggest that might reduce the likelihood of this injury recurring?

Cardiorespiratory Endurance

Cardiorespiratory conditioning should be maintained during the entire rehabilitation process. Pedaling a stationary bike (Figure 23-37B) or an upper-extremity ergometer (Figure 23-37B) with the hands provides excellent cardiovascular exercise without placing stress on the ankle. Pool running using a float vest and swimming are also good cardiovascular exercises (Figure 23-36).

Functional Progressions

Functional progressions may be as complex or simple as needed. The more severe the injury, the greater the need for a detailed functional progression. The typical progression begins early in the rehabilitation process as the patient becomes partially weight bearing. Full weight bearing should be started when ambulation is performed without a limp. Running may be begun as soon as ambulation is pain-free. Pain-free hopping on the affected side may also be a guideline to determine when running is appropriate. Exercising in a pool allows for early running. The patient is placed in the pool in a swim vest that supports the body in water. The patient then runs in place without touching the bottom of the pool. Proper running form should be stressed. Eventually the patient is moved into shallow water so that more weight is placed on the ankle. Progression is then made to running on a smooth, flat surface, ideally a track. Initially the patient should jog the straights and walk the curves and then progress to jogging the entire track. Speed may be increased to a sprint in a straight line. The cutting sequence should begin with circles of diminishing diameter. Cones may be set up for the patient to run figure eights as the next cutting progression. The crossover or sidestep is next.[1]

The patient sprints to a predesignated spot and cuts or sidesteps abruptly. When this progression is accomplished, the cut should be done without warning on the command of another person. Jumping and hopping exercises should be started on both legs simultaneously and gradually reduced to only the injured side.

The patient may perform at different levels for each of these functional sequences. One functional sequence may be done at half speed while another is done at full speed. An example of this is the patient who is running full speed on straights of the track while doing figure eights at only half speed. Once the upper levels of all the sequences are reached, the patient may return to limited practice, which may include early teaching and fundamental drills.

Criteria for Full Return

Estimates are that 30% to 40% of all inversion injuries result in reinjury.[27,43,44,56,82] In the past, patients were simply returned to sports once the pain was low enough to tolerate the activity. Cross, Worrell, Leslie, et al found that self-reported measures of impairment correlated well with clinical measures of limitation in predicting the number of days to return to sport.[20] Returning to full activity should include a gradual progression of functional activities that slowly increase the stress on the ligament.[49] The specific demands of each individual sport dictate the individual drills of this progression.

It is most desirable to have the patient return to sport without the aid of ankle support. However, it is common practice that some type of ankle support be worn initially. It appears that ankle taping does have a stabilizing effect on unstable ankles[30,97] without interfering with motor performance.[28,57] Nishikawa found that application of an ankle brace increased the excitability of the peroneus longus motoneuron.[67] This increase was attributed to a number of mechanoreceptors, one of which was cutaneous. McCluskey and others[57] suggest taping the ankle and also taping the shoe onto the foot to make the shoe and ankle function as one unit. High-topped footwear may further stabilize the

ankle.[39] Ricardo, Schulthies, and Soret found that high-top shoes reduced the rate of inversion.[76] If cleated shoes are worn, cleats should be outset along the periphery of the shoe to provide stability.[57] An aircast or some other supportive ankle brace can also be worn for support as a substitute for taping (Figure 23-40).

The patient should have complete ROM and at least 80% to 90% of preinjury strength before considering a return to sport.[83] Finally, if full practice is tolerated without insult to the injured part, the patient may return to competition.

Clinical Decision-Making Exercise 23-2

A 19-year-old volleyball player sprained her right ankle as she attempted to spike a ball at the net. The injury mechanism was external rotation and forced dorsiflexion. Initial pain was between the tibia and fibula above the ankle mortise, extending between the tibia and fibula superiorly halfway to the knee. What are the implications of these symptoms for the athletic trainer in assessing the likelihood that the patient will be ready for the conference championship in 2 weeks?

Ankle Fractures and Dislocation

Pathomechanics and Injury Mechanism

When dealing with injuries to the ankle joint, the athletic trainer must always be cautious about suspecting an ankle sprain when a fracture might actually exist. A fracture of the malleoli will generally result in immediate swelling. Ankle fractures can occur from several mechanisms that are similar to those for ankle sprains. In an inversion injury, medial malleolar fractures are often accompanied by a sprain of the lateral ligaments of the ankle. A fracture of the lateral malleolus is often more likely to occur than a sprain if an eversion force is applied to the ankle. This is due to the fact that the lateral malleolus extends as far as the distal aspect of the talus. With a fracture of the lateral malleolus, however, there may also be a sprain of the deltoid ligament. Fractures result from either avulsion or compression forces. With avulsion injuries, it is often the injured ligaments that prolong the rehabilitation period.[36]

Osteochondral fractures are sometimes seen in the talus. These fractures may also be referred to as dome fractures of the talus. Generally they will be either undisplaced fractures or compression fractures.[36]

While sprains and fractures are very common, dislocations in the ankle and foot are rare. They most often occur in conjunction with fractures and require open reduction and internal fixation.[83]

Rehabilitation Concerns

Generally, undisplaced ankle fractures should be managed with rest and protection until the fracture has healed, whereas displaced fractures are treated with open reduction and internal fixation. Undisplaced fractures are treated by casting in a short-leg walking cast for 6 weeks with early weight bearing. The course of rehabilitation following this period of immobilization is generally the same as for ankle sprains.

Following surgery for displaced or unstable fractures, the patient may be placed in a removable walking cast. However, it is essential to closely monitor the rehabilitative process to make certain that the patient is compliant.[36] If an osteochondral fracture is displaced and there is a fragment, surgery is required to remove the fragment. In other cases, if the fragment has not healed within a year, surgery may be considered to remove the fragment.[36]

Rehabilitation Progression

Following open reduction and internal fixation, a posterior splint with the ankle in neutral should be applied, and the patient should be non-weight-bearing for about 2 weeks. During this period efforts should be directed at controlling swelling and wound management.

At 2 to 3 weeks, the patient may be placed in a short-leg walking brace (Figure 23-42), which allows for partial weight bearing that should continue for 6 weeks. Active ROM plantarflexion and dorsiflexion exercises can begin and should be done 2 to 3 times a day, along with general strengthening exercises for the rest of the lower extremity.

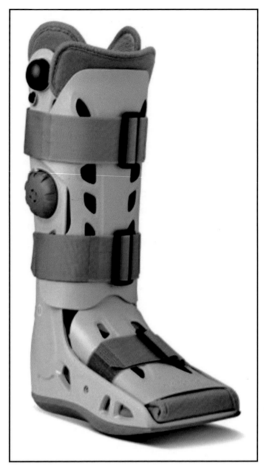

Figure 23-42. Short-leg walking brace.

At 6 weeks, the patient can be weight bearing in the walking brace, and this should continue for 2 to 4 weeks more. Isometric exercises (Figures 23-10 through 23-13) can be performed initially without the brace, progressing to isotonic strengthening exercises (Figures 23-14 through 23-17) that concentrate on eccentrics. Stretching exercises can also be incorporated (Figures 23-5 through 23-9). Joint mobilization exercises should be used to reduce capsular tightness (see Figures 14-63 through 14-68). Exercises to regain proprioception and neuromuscular control can progress from sitting to standing as tolerated (Figures 23-30 through 23-35). As strength and neuromuscular control continue to increase, more functional closed kinetic chain strengthening activities can begin (Figures 23-21 through 23-23).

Criteria for Full Return

Once near-normal levels of strength, flexibility, and neuromuscular control have been regained and the injured patient has progressed through an appropriate functional progression, full activity may be resumed.

Subluxation and Dislocation of the Peroneal Tendons

Pathomechanics

The peroneus brevis and longus tendons pass posterior to the fibula in the peroneal groove under the superior peroneal retinaculum. Peroneal tendon dislocation may occur because of rupture of the superior retinaculum or because the retinaculum strips the periosteum away from the lateral malleolus, creating laxity in the retinaculum. It appears that there is no anatomic correlation between peroneal groove size or shape and instability of the peroneal tendons.[47] An avulsion fracture of the lateral ridge of the distal fibula may also occur with a subluxation or dislocation of the peroneal tendons.

Injury Mechanism

Subluxation of peroneal tendons can occur from any mechanism causing sudden and forceful contraction of the peroneal muscles that involves dorsiflexion and eversion of the foot.[47] This forces the tendons anteriorly, rupturing the retinaculum and potentially causing an avulsion fracture of the lateral malleolus. The patient will often hear or feel a "pop." And, differentiating peroneal subluxation from a lateral ligament sprain or tear, there will be tenderness over the peroneal tendons and swelling and ecchymosis in the retromalleolar area. During active eversion the foot subluxation of the peroneal tendons may be observed and palpated. This is easier to observe when acute symptoms have subsided. The patient will typically complain of chronic "giving way" or popping. If the tendon is dislocated on initial evaluation, it should be reduced using gentle inversion and plantarflexion with pressure on the peroneal tendon.[47]

Rehabilitation Concerns and Progression

Following reduction, the patient should be initially placed in a compression dressing with a felt pad cut in the shape of a keyhole strapped over the lateral malleolus, placing gentle pressure on the peroneal tendons. Once the acute symptoms abate, the patient should be placed in a short-leg cast in slight plantarflexion and non-weight bearing for 5 to 6 weeks (Figure 23-42). Aggressive ankle rehabilitation, as previously described, is initiated after cast removal. In the case of an avulsion injury or when this becomes a chronic problem, conservative treatment is unlikely to be successful and surgery is needed to prevent the problem from recurring. A number of surgical procedures have been recommended, including repair or reconstruction of the superior peroneal retinaculum, deepening of the peroneal groove, or rerouting the tendon. Following surgery, the patient should be placed in a non-weight-bearing short-leg cast for about 4 weeks. The course of rehabilitation is similar to that described for ankle fractures with increased emphasis on strengthening of the peroneal tendons in eversion.[47]

Criteria for Full Return

The patient may return to full activity at about 10 to 12 weeks as tolerated, when normal strength, ROM, and neuromuscular control in the ankle joint are demonstrated.

Clinical Decision-Making Exercise 23-3

Following a recent grade 2 lateral ankle sprain, a patient has begun to complain that he feels a "popping" sensation accompanied by "giving way" of the ankle. X-rays are negative. Examination reveals full ROM, but there is palpable tenderness and slight swelling over the posterior aspect of the lateral malleolus, particularly in the retromalleolar area. What is the probable cause of this "popping" and "giving way"?

Tendinopathies

Pathomechanics and Injury Mechanism

Inflammation of the tendons surrounding the ankle joint is a common problem in patients. The tendons most often involved are the posterior tibialis tendon behind the medial malleolus, the anterior tibialis under the extensor retinaculum on the dorsal surface of the ankle, and the peroneal tendons both behind the lateral malleolus and at the base of the fifth metatarsal.[92]

Tendinopathies in these tendons may result from one specific cause or from a collection of mechanisms including faulty foot mechanics, which will be discussed later in this chapter; inappropriate or poor footwear that can create faulty foot mechanics; acute trauma to the tendon; tightness in the heel chord complex; or training errors. Training errors would include training at intensities that are too high or too frequent, changing training surfaces, or changes in activities within the training program.[92]

Patients who develop tendinopathies are likely to complain of pain with both active movement and passive stretching, swelling around the area of the tendon due to inflammation of the tendon and the tendon sheath, crepitus on movement, and stiffness and pain following periods of inactivity but particularly in the morning.

Rehabilitation Concerns and Progression

In the early stages of rehabilitation, exercises are used to increase circulation. The increased lymphatic flow facilitates removal of fluid and the by-products of the inflammatory process, and increases nutrition to the healing tendon. Exercise should also be used to limit atrophy, which can occur with disuse, and to minimize loss of strength, proprioception, and neuromuscular control. As is the case with the majority of tendinopathies, eccentric exercise has been the recommended treatment of choice for many years. However recent studies have questioned whether this is the only approach that should be used with tendinopathies in general and additional studies looking at different protocols should be conducted.[83]

Rehabilitation should incorporate techniques that reduce or eliminate inflammation. These include rest, therapeutic modalities (ice, ultrasound, diathermy), and anti-inflammatory medications.

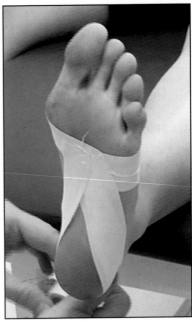

Figure 23-43. Low-dye taping for arch support.

If faulty foot mechanics are a cause of tendinopathy, it may be helpful to construct an appropriate orthotic device to correct the biomechanics. Taping of the foot may also help reduce stress on the tendons (Figure 23-43).

In many instances, if the mechanism that is causing the irritation and inflammation of the tendon is removed, and the inflammatory process is allowed to accomplish what it is supposed to, the tendinitis will often resolve within 10 days to 2 weeks. This is particularly true if rest and treatment are begun as soon as the symptoms begin. Unfortunately, if treatment does not begin until the symptoms have been present for several weeks or even months, as is most often the case, the tendinopathy will take much longer to resolve. Long-standing inflammation causes the tendon to thicken and significantly increases the period required for that tendon to remodel.

Criteria for Full Return

In our experience, it is better to allow the patient sufficient rest so that tendon healing can take place. The rehabilitation philosophy in sports medicine is usually aggressive, but with tendinopathy an aggressive approach that does not allow the tendon to minimize the inflammatory response and then to begin tissue realignment and remodeling will not allow the tendon to heal and can exacerbate the existing inflammation. The rehabilitation progression must be slow and controlled, with full return only when the patient seems to be free of pain.

Excessive Pronation and Supination

Pathomechanics and Injury Mechanism

Often, when we hear the terms pronation or supination, we automatically think of some pathological condition related to gait. It must be reemphasized that pronation and supination of the foot and subtalar joint are normal movements that occur during the support phase of gait. However, if pronation or supination is excessive or prolonged, overuse injuries may develop. Excessive or prolonged supination or pronation at the subtalar joint is likely to result from some structural or functional deformity in the foot or leg. The structural deformity forces the subtalar joint to compensate in a manner that will allow the weight-bearing surfaces of the foot to make stable contact with the ground and get into a weight-bearing position. Thus, excessive pronation or supination is a compensation for an existing structural deformity. Three of the most common structural deformities of the foot are a forefoot varus (Figure 23-44), a forefoot valgus (Figure 23-45), and a rear-foot varus (Figure 23-46).

Structural forefoot varus and structural rear-foot varus deformities are usually associated with excessive pronation. A structural forefoot valgus causes excessive supination. The deformities usually exist in one plane, but the subtalar joint will interfere with the normal functions of the foot and make it more difficult for it to act as a shock absorber, adapt to uneven surfaces, and act as a rigid lever for push-off. The compensation, rather than the deformity itself, usually causes overuse injuries.

Excessive or prolonged pronation of the subtalar joint during the support phase of running is one of the major causes of stress injuries.[5] Overload of specific structures results when excessive pronation is produced in the support phase or when pronation is prolonged into the propulsive phase of running. Excessive pronation during the support phase will cause compensatory subtalar joint motion such that the midtarsal joint remains unlocked, resulting in an excessively loose foot. There is also an increase in tibial rotation, which forces the knee joint to absorb more transverse rotation motion. Prolonged pronation of the subtalar joint will not allow the foot to resupinate in time to provide a rigid lever for push-off, resulting in a less powerful and less efficient force. Thus various foot and leg problems occur with excessive or prolonged pronation during the support phase. These include callus formation under the second metatarsal, stress fractures of the second metatarsal, bunions due to hypermobility of the first ray, plantar fasciitis, posterior tibial tendinitis, Achilles tendinitis, tibial stress syndrome, and medial knee pain.[5]

Several extrinsic keys may be observed that indicate pronation.[80] Excessive eversion of the calcaneus during the stance phase indicates pronation (Figure 23-47). Excessive or prolonged internal rotation of the tibia is another sign of pronation. This internal rotation can cause increased symptoms in the shin or knee, especially in repetitive sports such as running. A lowering of the medial arch accompanies pronation. It may be measured as the navicular differential,[55] the difference between the height of the navicular tuberosity from the floor in a non-weight-bearing position and its height in a weight-bearing position (Figure 23-48). Pronatory foot type as measured by a navicular drop test has been identified as an accurate predictor for the development of tibial stress syndrome.[42] As previously discussed, the talus plantarflexes and adducts with pronation. It may be seen as a medial bulging of the talar head (Figure 23-49). This same talar adduction causes increased concavity below the lateral malleolus in a posterior view while the calcaneus everts[60] (Figure 23-50).

At heel strike in prolonged or excessive supination, compensatory movement at the subtalar joint will not allow the midtarsal joint to unlock, causing the foot to remain excessively rigid. The foot cannot absorb the ground reaction forces as efficiently. Excessive supination limits tibial internal rotation. Injuries typically associated with excessive supination include

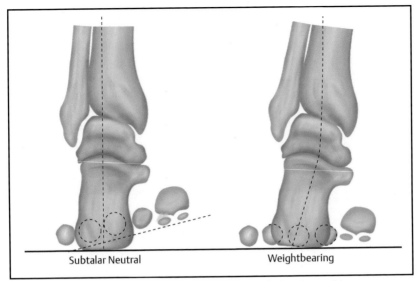

Figure 23-44. Forefoot varus. Comparing neutral and weight-bearing positions.

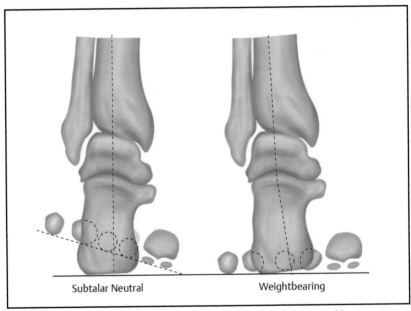

Figure 23-45. Forefoot valgus. Comparing neutral and weight-bearing positions.

inversion ankle sprains, tibial stress syndrome, peroneal tendinitis, iliotibial band friction syndrome, and trochanteric bursitis.

Structural deformities originating outside the foot also require compensation by the foot for a proper weight-bearing position to be attained. Tibial varum is the common bowleg deformity.[60] The distal tibia is medial to the proximal tibia[24] (Figure 23-51). This measurement is taken weight-bearing with the foot in neutral position.[41] The angle of deviation of the distal tibia from a perpendicular line from the calcaneal midline is considered tibial varum.[32] Tibial varum increases pronation to allow proper foot function.[10] At heel strike the calcaneus must evert to attain a perpendicular position.[89]

Ankle joint equinus is another extrinsic deformity that may require abnormal compensation. It may be considered an extrinsic or intrinsic problem.

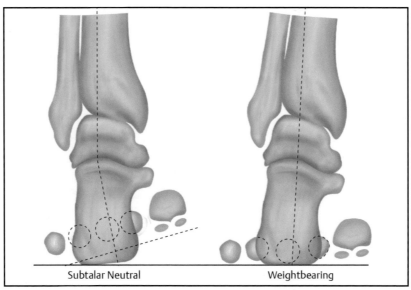

Figure 23-46. Rear-foot varus. Comparing neutral and weight-bearing positions.

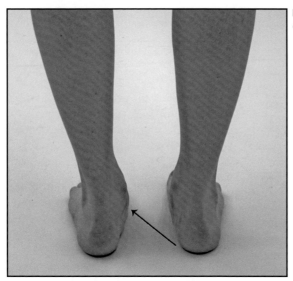

Figure 23-47. Eversion of the calcaneus on the left foot indicating pronation.

During normal gait, the tibia must move anterior to the talar dome.[60] About 10 degrees of dorsiflexion are required for this movement[60] (Figure 23-52).

Lack of dorsiflexion may cause compensatory pronation of the foot with resultant foot and lower-extremity pain. Often this lack of dorsiflexion results from tightness of the posterior leg muscles. Other causes include forefoot equinus, in which the plane of the forefoot is below the plane of the rear-foot.[60] It occurs in many high-arched feet. This deformity requires more ankle dorsiflexion. When enough dorsiflexion is not available at the ankle, the additional movement is required at other sites, such as dorsiflexion of the midtarsal joint and rotation of the leg.

Rehabilitation Concerns

In individuals who excessively pronate or supinate, the goal of treatment is quite simply to correct the faulty biomechanics that occur due to the existing structural deformity. An accurate biomechanical analysis of the foot and lower extremity should identify those deformities that require abnormal compensatory

Figure 23-48. Measurement of the navicular differential.

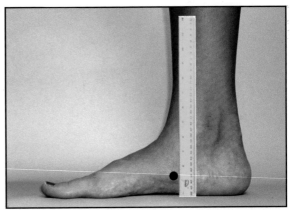

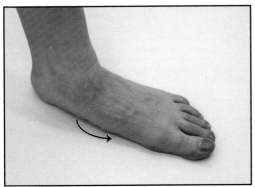

Figure 23-49. Medial bulge of the talar head indicating pronation.

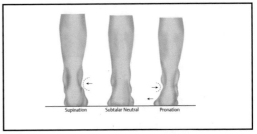

Figure 23-50. Concavity below the lateral malleolus indicating pronation.

movements. In the majority of cases, faulty biomechanics can be corrected by constructing an appropriate orthotic device.

Despite arguments in the literature, some have found orthotic therapy to be of tremendous value in the treatment of many lower extremity problems. This view is supported in the literature by several clinical studies. Donatelli et al[24] found that 96% of their patients reported pain relief from orthotics and that 52% would not leave home without the devices in their shoes. McPoil, Adrian, and Pidcoe found that orthotics were an important treatment for valgus forefoot deformities only.[59] Riegler reported that 80% of his patients experienced at least a 50% improvement with orthotics.[78] This same study reported improvements in sport performance with orthotics. Hunt reported decreased muscular activity with orthotics.[41] Oschendorff and Mattacola found that molded orthotics reduced postural sway in fatigued ankles.[70]

The process for evaluating the foot biomechanically, for constructing an orthotic device, and for selecting the appropriate footwear is detailed below.

Examination

The first step in the evaluation process is to establish a position of subtalar neutral. The patient should be prone with the distal third of the leg hanging off the end of the table (Figure 23-53). A line should be drawn bisecting the leg from the start of the musculotendinous junction of the gastrocnemius to the distal portion of the calcaneus[93] (Figure 23-54). With the patient still prone, the athletic trainer palpates the talus while the forefoot is inverted and everted. One finger should palpate the talus at the anterior aspect of the fibula and another finger at the anterior portion of the medial malleolus (Figure 23-55). The position at which the talus is equally prominent on both sides is considered neutral subtalar position.[46] Root, Orien, and Weed[80] describe this as the position of the subtalar joint where it is neither pronated nor supinated. It is the standard position in

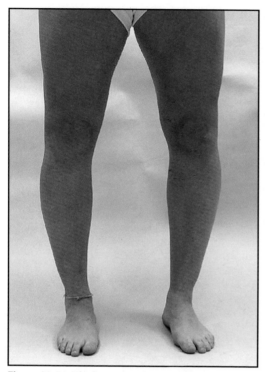

Figure 23-51. Tibial varum, or bowleg deformity.

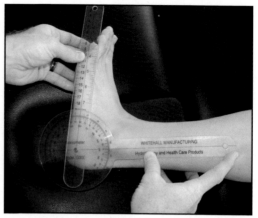

Figure 23-52. Ten degrees of dorsiflexion is necessary for normal gait.

which the foot should be placed to examine deformities.[69] In this position, the lines on the lower leg and calcaneus should form a straight line. Any variance is considered to be a rear-foot valgus or varus deformity. The most common deformity of the foot is a rear-foot varus deformity.[61] A deviation of 2 to 3 degrees is normal.[99]

Another method of determining subtalar neutral position involves the lines that were drawn previously on the leg and back of the heel. With the patient prone, the heel is swung into full eversion and inversion, with measurements taken at each position. Angles of the two lines are taken at each extreme. Neutral position is considered two-thirds away from maximum inversion or one-third away from maximum eversion. The normal foot pronates 6 to 8 degrees from neutral.[80] For example, from neutral position a foot inverts 27 degrees and everts 3 degrees. The position at which this foot is neither pronated nor supinated is that point at which the calcaneus is inverted 7 degrees.

Once the subtalar joint is placed in a neutral position, mild dorsiflexion should be applied while observing the metatarsal heads in relation to the plantar surface of the calcaneus. Forefoot varus is an osseous deformity in which the medial metatarsal heads are inverted in relation to the plane of the calcaneus (Figure 23-44). Forefoot varus is the most common cause of excessive pronation, according to Subotnick.[90] Forefoot valgus is a position in which the lateral metatarsals are everted in relation to the rear-foot (Figure 23-45). These forefoot deformities are benign in a non-weight-bearing position, but in stance the foot or metatarsal heads must somehow get to the floor to bear weight. This movement is accomplished by the talus rolling down and in and the calcaneus everting for a forefoot varus. For the forefoot valgus, the calcaneus inverts and the talus abducts and dorsiflexes. McPoil, Knecht, and Schmit[61] report that forefoot valgus is the most common forefoot deformity in their sample group.

In a rear-foot varus deformity, when the foot is in subtalar neutral position non-weight-bearing, the medial metatarsal heads are inverted as in a forefoot varus, and the calcaneus is also in an inverted position. To get to foot flat in weight bearing, the subtalar joint must pronate (Figure 23-46). Minimal osseous deformities of the forefoot have little effect on the function of the foot. When either forefoot varus or valgus is too large, the foot compensates through abnormal movements to bear weight.

Constructing Orthotics

Almost any problem of the lower extremity appears at one time to have been treated

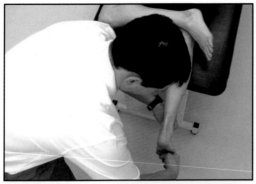

Figure 23-53. Examination position for neutral position.

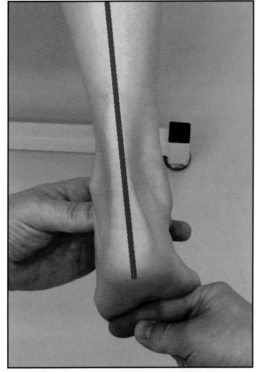

Figure 23-54. Line bisecting the gastrocnemius and posterior calcaneus.

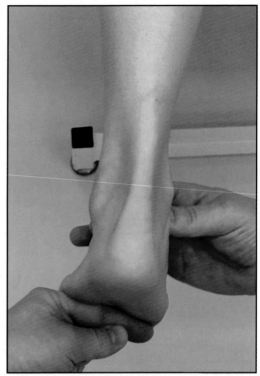

Figure 23-55. Palpation of the talus to determine neutral position.

an orthotic should help prevent compensatory problems. For problems that have already occurred, the orthotic provides a platform of support so that soft tissues can heal properly without undue stress.

Basically there are three types of orthotics:[42,51,89]

1. Pads and soft flexible felt supports (Figure 23-56). These soft inserts are readily fabricated and are advocated for mild overuse syndromes. Pads are particularly useful in shoes, such as spikes and ski boots, that are too narrow to hold orthotics.

2. Semirigid orthotics made of flexible thermoplastics, rubber, or leather (Figure 23-57). These orthotics are prescribed for patients who have increased symptoms. These orthotics are molded from a neutral cast. They are well tolerated by patients whose sports require speed or jumping.

3. Functional or rigid orthotics are made from hard plastic and also require neutral casting (Figure 23-58). These orthotics allow control for most overuse symptoms.

by orthotic therapy. The use of orthotics in control of foot deformities has been argued for many years.[3,17,19,33,46,79,89,90,101] The normal foot functions most efficiently when no deformities are present that predispose it to injury or exacerbate existing injuries. Orthotics are used to control abnormal compensatory movements of the foot by "bringing the floor to the foot."[42]

The foot functions most efficiently in neutral position. By providing support so that the foot does not have to move abnormally,

Many athletic trainers make a neutral mold, put it in a box, mail it to an orthotic laboratory, and several weeks later receive an orthotic back in the mail. Others like to complete the entire orthotic from start to finish (Figure 23-69A), which requires a much more skilled technician than the mail-in method, as well as about $1,000 in equipment and supplies. The obvious advantage is cost if many orthotics are to be made.

When the orthotics are received, time must be allowed for proper break-in. The patient should wear the orthotic for 3 to 4 hours the first day, 6 to 8 hours the next day, and then all day on the third day. Sports activities should be started with the orthotic only after it has been worn all day for several days.[42]

Shoe Selection

The shoe is one of the biggest considerations in treating a foot problem.[91] Even a properly made orthotic is less effective if placed in a poorly constructed shoe.

As noted, pronation is a problem of hypermobility. Pronated feet need stability and firmness to reduce this excess movement. Research indicates that shoe compression may actually increase pronation, compared to barefoot.[2] The ideal shoe for a pronated foot is less flexible and has good rear-foot control.

Conversely, supinated feet are usually very rigid. Increased cushion and flexibility benefit this type of foot. Several construction factors may influence the firmness and stability of a shoe. The basic form upon which a shoe is built is called the last.[2] The upper is fitted onto a last in several ways. Each method has its own flexibility and control characteristics. A slip-lasted shoe is sewn together like a moccasin (Figure 23-60A) and is very flexible. Board lasting provides a piece of fiberboard upon which the upper is attached (Figure 23-60B), which provides a very firm, inflexible base for the shoe. A combination-lasted shoe is boarded in the back half of the shoe and slip-lasted in the front (Figure 23-60C), which provides rear-foot stability with forefoot mobility. The shape of the last may also be used in shoe selection. Most patients with excessive pronation perform better in a straight-lasted shoe,[2] that is, a shoe in which the forefoot does not curve inward in relation to the rear-foot (Figure 23-61). Midsole

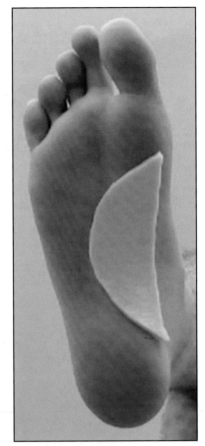

Figure 23-56. Felt pads.

design also affects the stability of a shoe. The midsole separates the upper from the outsole.[10] Ethylene vinyl acetate (EVA) is one of the most commonly used materials in the midsole.[65] Often denser EVA, which is colored differently to show that it is denser, is placed under the medial aspect of the foot to control pronation (Figure 23-62).

In an effort to control rear-foot movement, many shoe manufacturers have reinforced the heel counter both internally and externally, often in the form of extra plastic along the outside of the heel counter[61] (Figure 23-63). Other factors that may affect the performance of a shoe are the outsole contour and composition, lacing systems, and forefoot wedges.

Shoe Wear Patterns

Patients with excessive pronation often wear out the front of the running shoe under the second metatarsal (Figure 23-64). Shoe wear patterns are commonly misinterpreted by patients

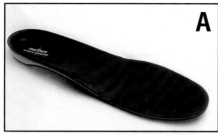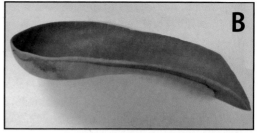

Figure 23-57. Semirigid orthotics. (A) Thermomoldable commercial orthotic blank; (B) custom made orthotic from thermoplastic materials.

Figure 23-58. Rigid orthotic. (Reprinted with permission from It K Orthotics Cedar Falls, IA.)

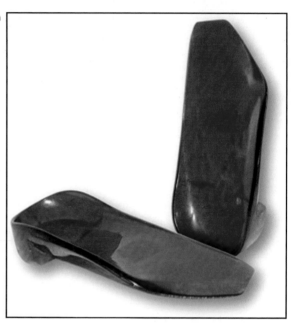

who think they must be pronators because they wear out the back outside edges of their heels. Actually, most people wear out the back outside edges of their shoes. Just before heel strike, the anterior tibial muscle fires to prevent the foot from slapping forward. The anterior tibial muscle not only dorsiflexes the foot but also slightly inverts it, hence the wear pattern on

---

Clinical Decision-Making Exercise 23-4

A 14-year-old cross-country runner has been diagnosed with a second-metatarsal stress fracture. After 8 weeks she is ready to return to running. Biomechanical examination of her foot shows a moderate forefoot varus deformity. With weight bearing there is a marked navicular differential and moderate calcaneal eversion. What shoe characteristics might be desirable for this individual as she returns to sport?

---

the back edge of the shoe. The key to inspection of wear patterns on shoes is observation of the heel counter and the forefoot.

Stress Fractures in the Foot

Pathomechanics and Injury Mechanism

The most common stress fractures in the foot involve the navicular, the second metatarsal (March fracture), and the diaphysis of the fifth metatarsal (Jones fracture). Navicular and second metatarsal stress fractures are likely to occur with excessive foot pronation, while fifth metatarsal stress fractures tend to occur in a more rigid pes cavus foot.

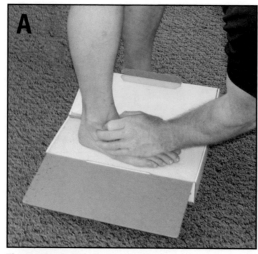
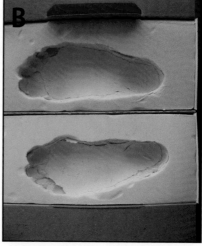

Figure 23-59. Making a mold. (A) The patient steps into a piece of foam to make an impression of the foot with the subtalar joint in a neutral position. (B) The mold is placed in a box and sent to a manufacturer to create an orthotic.

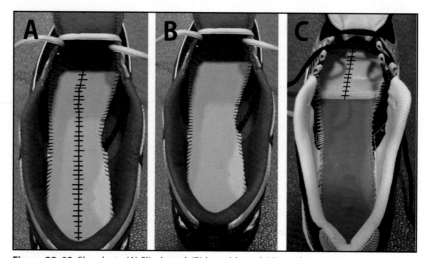

Figure 23-60. Shoe lasts. (A) Slip-lasted; (B) board-lasted; (C) combination-lasted.

Navicular Stress Fractures

Individuals who excessively pronate during running gait are likely to develop a stress fracture of the navicular. Of the tarsal bones it is the most likely to have a stress fracture.

Second Metatarsal Fractures

Second metatarsal stress fractures occur most often in running and jumping sports. As is the case with other injuries in the foot associated with overuse, the most common causes include rear-foot varus and forefoot varus structural deformities in the foot that result in excessive pronation, training errors, changes in training surfaces, and wearing inappropriate shoes. The base of the second metatarsal extends proximally into the distal row of tarsal bones and is held rigid and stable by the bony architecture and ligament support. The second metatarsal is particularly subjected to increased stress with excessive pronation, which causes a hypermobile foot. In addition, if the second metatarsal is longer than the first, as seen with a Morton's toe, it is theoretically subjected to greater bone stress during running. A bone scan, rather than a standard radiograph, is frequently necessary for diagnosis.

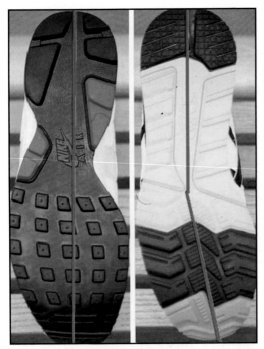

Figure 23-61. The last of the shoe may be either straight or curved.

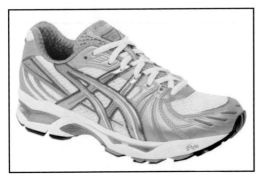

Figure 23-62. EVA in a midsole.

Fifth Metatarsal Stress Fractures

Fifth metatarsal stress fractures can occur from overuse, acute inversion, or high-velocity rotational forces. A Jones fracture occurs at the diaphysis of the fifth metatarsal most often as a sequela of a stress fracture.[83] The patient will complain of a sharp pain on the lateral border of the foot and will usually report hearing a "pop." Because of a history of poor blood supply and delayed healing, a Jones fracture may result in nonunion requiring an extended period of rehabilitation.

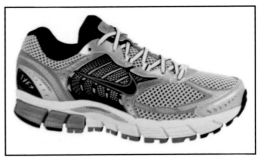

Figure 23-63. External heel counter.

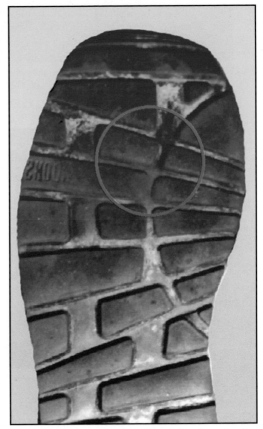

Figure 23-64. Front forefoot of a running shoe showing the typical wear pattern of a pronator.

Rehabilitation Concerns

Rehabilitation efforts for stress fractures should focus on determining and alleviating the precipitating cause or causes. Second metatarsal stress fractures tend to do well with modified rest and non-weight-bearing exercises such as pool running (Figure 23-36), upper-body ergometer (Figure 23-37B), or stationary bike (Figure 23-37A) to maintain the patient's cardiorespiratory fitness for 2 to 4 weeks. This is followed by a progressive return to running and jumping sports over a 2- or 3-week period using appropriately constructed orthotics and appropriate shoes. Stress fractures of both the navicular of the proximal shaft of the fifth metatarsal usually require more aggressive treatment, requiring non-weight-bearing short leg casts for 6 to 8 weeks for nondisplaced fractures. With cases of delayed union, nonunion, or especially displaced fractures, both the Jones and navicular fractures require internal fixation, with or without bone grafting. In the highly competitive patient, immediate internal fixation should be recommended.

Plantar Fasciitis/Fasciosis

Pathomechanics

Heel pain is a very common problem in the athletic and nonathletic population. This phenomenon has been attributed to several etiologies, including heel spurs, plantar fascia irritation, and bursitis. Plantar fasciitis is a catchall term that is commonly used to denote pain in the proximal arch and heel.

The plantar fascia (plantar aponeurosis) runs the length of the sole of the foot. It is a broad band of dense connective tissue that is attached proximally to the medial surface of the calcaneus. It fans out distally, with fibers and their various small branches attaching to the metatarsophalangeal articulations and merging into the capsular ligaments. Other fibers, arising from well within the aponeurosis, pass between the intrinsic muscles of the foot and the long flexor tendons of the sole and attach themselves to the deep fascia below the bones. The function of the plantar aponeurosis is to assist in maintaining the stability of the foot and in securing or bracing the longitudinal arch.[91]

Tension develops in the plantar fascia both during extension of the toes and during depression of the longitudinal arch as the result of weight bearing. When the weight is principally on the heel, as in ordinary standing, the tension exerted on the fascia is negligible. However, when the weight is shifted to the ball of the foot (on the heads of the metatarsals), fascial tension is increased. In running, because the push-off phase involves both a forceful extension of the toes and a powerful thrust by the ball of the foot (on the heads of the metatarsals), fascial tension is increased to about twice the body weight.

Patients who have a mild pes cavus are particularly prone to fascial strain. Modern street shoes, by the nature of their design, take on the characteristics of splints and tend to restrict foot action to such an extent that the arch may become somewhat rigid because of shortening of the ligaments and other mild abnormalities. The patient, when changing from such footwear into a flexible gymnastic slipper or soft track shoe, often experiences trauma when the foot is subjected to stress.[100] Trauma may also result from running, either from poor technique or because of lordosis, a condition in which the increased forward tilt of the pelvis produces an unfavorable angle of foot-strike when there is considerable force exerted on the ball of the foot.

Injury Mechanism

A number of anatomical and biomechanical conditions have been studied as possible causes of plantar fasciitis. They include leg length discrepancy, excessive pronation of the subtalar joint, inflexibility of the longitudinal arch, and tightness of the gastrocnemius–soleus unit. Wearing shoes without sufficient arch support, a lengthened stride during running, and running on soft surfaces are also potential causes of plantar fasciitis.

The patient complains of pain in the anterior medial heel, usually at the attachment of the plantar fascia to the calcaneus that eventually moves more centrally into the central portion of the plantar fascia. This pain is particularly troublesome upon arising in the morning or upon bearing weight after sitting for a long time. However, the pain lessens after a few steps. Pain also will be intensified when the toes and forefoot are forcibly dorsiflexed.

Rehabilitation Concerns

Orthotic therapy is very useful in the treatment of this problem. The authors have found that soft orthotics in combination with exercises can significantly reduce the pain level of these patients. A soft orthotic works better

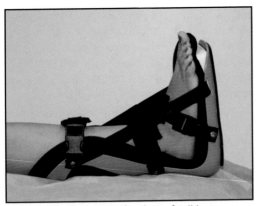

Figure 23-65. Night splint for plantar fasciitis.

than a hard orthotic. An extra-deep heel cup should be built into the orthotic. The orthotic should be worn at all times, especially upon arising from bed in the morning. Always have the patient step into the orthotic rather than ambulating barefoot.[10]

Use of a heel cup compresses the fat pad under the calcaneus, providing a cushion under the area of irritation. When soft orthotics are not feasible, taping may reduce the symptoms. A simple arch taping or alternative taping often allows pain-free ambulation.[105]

The use of a night splint to maintain a position of static stretch has also been recommended (Figure 23-65). In some cases it may be necessary to use a short-leg walking cast for 4 to 6 weeks.

Vigorous heel cord stretching should be used, along with an exercise to stretch the plantar fascia in the arch.

Exercises that increase dorsiflexion of the great toe also may be of benefit to this problem (Figure 23-19). Stretching should be done at least three times a day.

Anti-inflammatory medications are recommended. Steroidal injection may be warranted at some point if symptoms fail to resolve.

Criteria for Full Return

Management of plantar fasciitis will generally require an extended period of treatment. It is not uncommon for symptoms to persist for as long as 8 to 12 weeks. The patient's persistence in doing the recommended stretching exercises is critical. In some cases, particularly during a competitive season, the patient may continue to

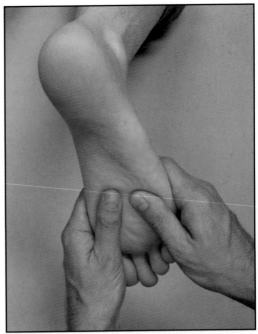

Figure 23-66. A cuboid manipulation is done with the patient prone. The lateral plantar aspect of the forefoot is grasped by the thumbs, with the fingers supporting the dorsum of the foot. The thumbs should be over the cuboid. The manipulation should be a thrust downward to move the cuboid into its more dorsal position. Often, a pop is felt as the cuboid moves back into place.

train and compete if symptoms and associated pain are not prohibitive.

Clinical Decision-Making Exercise 23-5

A 30-year-old tennis coach has complained of morning heel pain for several weeks. The pain began after changing to a very flexible shoe during training. His pain is intense upon arising in the morning. Forcible dorsiflexion of the toes and forefoot increases this heel pain. A local physician has diagnosed plantar fasciitis. X-rays were unremarkable. What treatment options might the athletic trainer consider for this patient?

Cuboid Subluxation

Pathomechanics

A condition that often mimics plantar fasciitis is cuboid subluxation. Pronation and trauma have been reported to be prominent causes of this syndrome.[102] This displacement of the cuboid causes pain along the fourth and fifth metatarsals, as well as over the cuboid. The primary reason for pain is the stress placed on the long peroneal muscle when the foot is in pronation. In this position, the long peroneal muscle allows the cuboid bone to move downward medially. This problem often refers pain to the heel area as well. Many times this pain is increased upon rising after a prolonged non-weight-bearing period.

Rehabilitation Considerations

Dramatic treatment results may be obtained by manipulating to restore the cuboid to its natural position. The manipulation is done with the patient prone (Figure 23-66). The plantar aspect of the forefoot is grasped by the thumbs with the fingers supporting the dorsum of the foot. The thumbs should be over the cuboid. The manipulation should be a thrust downward to move the cuboid into its more dorsal position. Often a pop is felt as the cuboid moves back into place. Once the cuboid is manipulated, an orthotic often helps to support it in its proper position.

Criteria for Full Return

If manipulation is successful, quite often the patient can return to play immediately with little or no pain. It should be recommended that the patient wear an appropriately constructed orthotic when practicing or competing to reduce the chances of recurrence.

Hallux Valgus Deformity (Bunions)

Pathomechanics and Injury Mechanism

A bunion is a deformity of the head of the first metatarsal in which the large toe assumes a valgus position[1] (Figure 23-67).

Commonly it is associated with a structural forefoot varus in which the first ray tends to splay outward, putting pressure on the first metatarsal head. The bursa over the first metatarsophalangeal joint becomes inflamed and eventually thickens. The joint becomes enlarged and the great toe becomes malaligned, moving laterally toward the second toe, sometimes to such an extent that it eventually overlaps the second toe. This type of bunion may

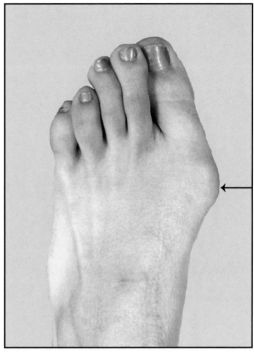

Figure 23-67. Hallux valgus deformity with a bunion.

also be associated with a depressed or flattened transverse arch. Often the bunion occurs from wearing shoes that are pointed, too narrow, too short, or have high heels. A bunion is one of the most frequent painful deformities of the great toe. As the bunion is developing there is tenderness, swelling, and enlargement with calcification of the head of the first metatarsal. Poorly fitting shoes increase the irritation and pain.

Rehabilitation Concerns

If the condition progresses, a special orthotic device may help normalize foot mechanics. Often an orthotic designed to correct a structural forefoot varus that can help increase stability of the first ray significantly reduces the symptoms and progression of a bunion. Shoe selection may also play an important role in the treatment of bunions. Shoes of the proper width cause less irritation to the bunion. Local therapy, including moist heat, soaks, and ultrasound, may alleviate some of the acute symptoms of a bunion. Protective devices such as wedges, pads, and tape can also be used. Surgery to correct the hallux valgus deformity is very common during the later stages of this condition.

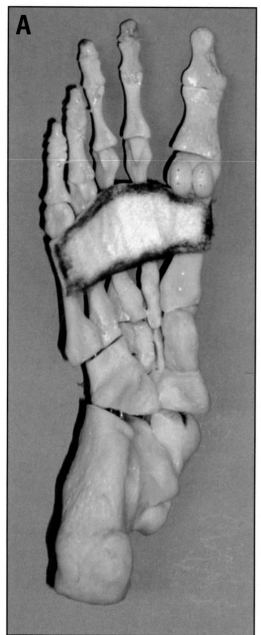

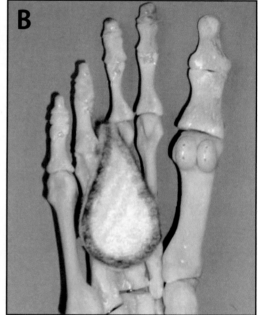

Figure 23-68. Metatarsal support pads. (A) Metatarsal bar; (B) teardrop pad.

Criteria for Full Return

It is likely that a patient with this condition can continue to compete while wearing an appropriately constructed orthotic, shoes with a wide toe box, and some type of donut pad over the bunion to disperse pressure.

Morton's Neuroma

Pathomechanics

A neuroma is a mass occurring about the nerve sheath of the common plantar nerve where it divides into the two digital branches to adjacent toes. It occurs most commonly between the metatarsal heads and is the most common nerve problem of the lower extremity.

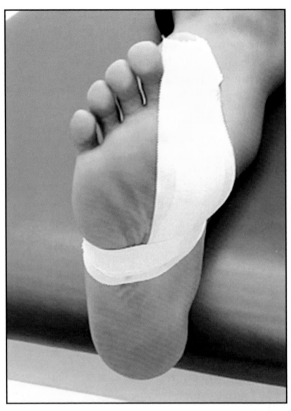

Figure 23-69. Turf toe tapping to prevent dorsiflexion.

A Morton's neuroma is located between the third and fourth metatarsal heads where the nerve is the thickest, receiving both branches from the medial and lateral plantar nerves. The patient complains of severe intermittent pain radiating from the distal metatarsal heads to the tips of the toes and is often relieved when non-weight-bearing. Irritation increases with the collapse of the transverse arch of the foot, putting the transverse metatarsal ligaments under stress and thus compressing the common digital nerve and vessels. Excessive foot pronation can also be a predisposing factor, with more metatarsal shearing forces occurring with the prolonged forefoot abduction.

The patient complains of a burning paresthesia in the forefoot that is often localized to the third web space and radiating to the toes.[89] Hyperextension of the toes on weight bearing, as in squatting, stair climbing, or running, can increase the symptoms. Wearing shoes with a narrow toe box or high heels can increase the symptoms. If there is prolonged nerve irritation, the pain can become constant. A bone scan is often necessary to rule out a metatarsal stress fracture.

Rehabilitation Concerns

Orthotic therapy is essential to reduce the shearing movements of the metatarsal heads. To increase this effect, either a metatarsal bar is placed just proximal to the metatarsal heads or a teardrop-shaped pad is placed between the heads of the third and fourth metatarsals in an attempt to have these splay apart with weight bearing (Figure 23-68). It may decrease pressure on the affected area.

Therapeutic modalities can be used to help reduce inflammation. The author has used phonophoresis with hydrocortisone with some success in symptom reduction.

Shoe selection also plays an important role in treatment of neuromas. Narrow shoes, particularly women's shoes that are pointed in the toe area and certain men's boots, may squeeze the metatarsal heads together and exacerbate the problem. A shoe that is wide in the toe box area should be selected. A straight-laced shoe often provides increased space in the toe box.[85]

On a rare occasion surgical excision may be required.

Criteria for Full Return

Appropriate soft orthotic padding often will markedly reduce pain and allow the patient to continue to play despite this condition.

Turf Toe

Pathomechanics and Injury Mechanism

Turf toe is a hyperextension injury resulting in a sprain of the metatarsophalangeal joint of the great toe, from either repetitive overuse or trauma.[98] Typically these injuries occur on unyielding synthetic turf, although they can occur on grass. Many of these injuries occur because many artificial turf shoes are more flexible and allow more dorsiflexion of the great toe.

Rehabilitation Concerns

Some shoe companies have addressed this problem by adding steel or other materials to the forefoot of their turf shoes to stiffen them. Flat insoles that have thin sheets of steel under the forefoot are also available. When commercially-made products are not available, a thin, flat piece of Orthoplast may be placed under the shoe insole or may be molded to the foot.[98] Taping the toe to prevent dorsiflexion may be done separately or with one of the shoe-stiffening suggestions (Figure 23-69). Modalities of choice include ice and ultrasound. One of the major ingredients in any treatment for turf toe is rest. The patient should be discouraged from returning to activity until the toe is pain-free.

Criteria for Full Return

The patient with turf toe can return to activity when the swelling in the metatarsophalangeal joint has resolved and full pain-free ROM from 0 to 90 degrees has been regained. In less severe cases, the patient can continue to play with the addition of a rigid insole. With more severe sprains, 3 to 4 weeks may be required for pain to reduce to the point where the patient can push off on the great toe.

Clinical Decision-Making Exercise 23-6

A 25-year-old professional football player has sustained a hyperextension injury to the metatarsophalangeal joint of the right great toe in the previous week's game. X-rays were negative, and a diagnosis of acute turf toe was given by the team physician. Following treatments with ultrasound and ice, the patient has regained full ROM with only slight residual soreness. What shoe modifications might the athletic trainer suggest to lessen the chance of reinjury in the following week's game?

Tarsal Tunnel Syndrome

Pathomechanics and Injury Mechanism

The tarsal tunnel is a loosely defined area about the medial malleolus that is bordered by the retinaculum, which binds the tibial nerve.[33] Pronation, overuse problems such as tendinitis, and trauma may cause neurovascular problems in the ankle and foot. Symptoms may vary, with pain, numbness, and paresthesia reported along the medial ankle and into the sole of the foot.[7] Tenderness may be present over the tibial nerve area behind the medial malleolus.

Rehabilitation Concerns

Neutral foot control may alleviate symptoms in less involved cases. Surgery is often performed if symptoms do not respond to conservative treatment or if weakness occurs in the flexors of the toes.[7]

Summary

1. The movements that take place at the talocrural joint are ankle plantarflexion and dorsiflexion. Inversion and eversion occur at the subtalar joint.

2. The position of the subtalar joint determines whether the midtarsal joints will be hypermobile or hypomobile. Dysfunction at either joint can profoundly affect the foot and lower extremity.

3. Ankle sprains are very common. Inversion sprains usually involve the lateral ligaments of the ankle, and eversion sprains

frequently involve the medial ligaments of the ankle. Rotational injuries often involve the tibiofibular and syndesmodic ligaments and can be very severe.

4. The early phase of treatment uses compression, ice, elevation, rest, and protection, all of which are critical components in preventing swelling.

5. Early weight bearing following ankle sprain is beneficial to the healing process. Rehabilitation may become more aggressive following the acute inflammatory response phase of healing.

6. Undisplaced ankle fractures should be managed with rest and protection until the fracture has healed. Displaced fractures are treated with open reduction and internal fixation.

7. Neutral casting is essential for the production of an orthotic, whether it is to be produced in-house or by someone else.

8. Subluxation of peroneal tendons can occur from any mechanism causing sudden and forceful contraction of the peroneal muscles that involves dorsiflexion and eversion of the foot. In the case of an avulsion injury or when this becomes a chronic problem, conservative treatment is unlikely to be successful and surgery is needed to prevent the problem from recurring.

9. Tendinitis in the posterior tibialis, anterior tibialis, and the peroneal tendons can result from one specific cause or from a collection of mechanisms. Rehabilitation should incorporate techniques that reduce or eliminate inflammation, including rest, therapeutic modalities (ice, ultrasound, diathermy), and anti-inflammatory medications.

10. Excessive or prolonged supination or pronation at the subtalar joint is likely to result from some structural or functional deformity, including forefoot varus, a forefoot valgus, or a rear-foot varus, which forces the subtalar joint to compensate in a manner that will allow the weight-bearing surfaces of the foot to make stable contact with the ground and get into a weight-bearing position.

11. Orthotics are used to control abnormal compensatory movements of the foot by "bringing the floor to the foot." By providing support so that the foot does not have to move abnormally, an orthotic should help prevent compensatory problems.

12. Shoe selection is an important parameter in the treatment of foot problems. The type of foot will dictate specific shoe features.

13. The most common stress fractures in the foot involve the navicular, the second metatarsal (March fracture), and the diaphysis of the fifth metatarsal (Jones fracture). Navicular and second metatarsal stress fractures are likely to occur with excessive foot pronation. Fifth metatarsal stress fractures tend to occur in a more rigid pes cavus foot.

14. A number of anatomical and biomechanical conditions have been studied as possible causes of plantar fasciitis. There is pain in the anterior medial heel, usually at the attachment of the plantar fascia to the calcaneus. Orthotics in combination with stretching exercises can significantly reduce pain.

15. Subluxation of the cuboid will create symptoms similar to those of plantar fasciitis and can be corrected with manipulation.

16. A bunion is a deformity of the head of the first metatarsal in which the large toe assumes a valgus position that is commonly associated with a structural forefoot varus in which the first ray tends to splay outward, putting pressure on the first metatarsal head.

17. In treating a Morton's neuroma, a metatarsal bar is placed just proximal to the metatarsal heads or a teardrop-shaped pad is placed between the heads of

the third and fourth metatarsals in an attempt to have these splay apart with weight bearing.

18. Turf toe is a hyperextension injury resulting in a sprain of the metatarsophalangeal joint of the great toe.

References

1. Andrews, J. R., W. McClod, and T. Ward, et al. 1977. The cutting mechanism. *American Journal of Sports Medicine* 5:111–121.

2. Baer, T. 1984. Designing for the long run. *Mechanical Engineering* (Sept.):67–75.

3. Bates, B. T., L. Osternig, and B. Mason, et al. 1979. Foot orthotic devices to modify selected aspects of lower extremity mechanics. *American Journal of Sports Medicine;* 7:338.

4. Baxter, D. 1995. *The foot and ankle in sport.* St. Louis: Mosby.

5. Bennett, J., M. Reinking, and B. Plaemer. 2001. Factors contributing to MTSS in high school runners. *Journal of Orthopedic and Sports Physical Therapy;* 31(9):504–510.

6. Birmingham, T. B., B. M. Chsworth, H. D. Hartsell, A. L. Stevenson, G. L. Lapenskie, and A. A. Vandervoort. 1997. Peak passive resistive torque at maximum inversion range of motion in subjects with recurrent ankle inversion sprains. *Journal of Orthopedic Sports Physical Therapy;* 25:342–348.

7. Birnham, J. S. 1986. *The musculoskeletal manual.* Orlando: Grune & Stratton.

8. Bosien, W. R., O. S. Staples, and R.W. Russell. 1955. Residual disability following acute ankle sprains. *Journal of Bone and Joint Surgery;* 37[A]:1237.

9. Bostrum, L. 1966. Treatment and prognosis in recent ligament ruptures. *Acta Chiropodist Scandanavia;* 132:537–550.

10. Brotzman, B., and J. Brasel. 1996. Foot and ankle rehabilitation. In *Clinical orthopaedic rehabilitation,* edited by B. Brotzman. St. Louis: Mosby.

11. Brody, D. M. 1982. Techniques in the evaluation and treatment of the injured runner. *Orthopedic Clinics of North America* 13:541.

12. Brown, C., Padua, D. 2011. Hip kinematics during a stop-jump task in patients with chronic ankle instability. *Journal of Athletic Training* 46(5):461-467.

13. Burgess, P. R., and J. Wei. 1982. Signalling of kinesthetic information by peripheral sensory receptors. *Annual Review of Neuroscience* 5:171–187.

14. Calliet, R. 1968. *Foot and ankle pain.* Philadelphia: F. A. Davis.

15. Canoy, W. F. 1975. *Review of medical physiology,* 7th ed., Los Altos, CA: Lange Medical.

16. Caulfield, B. 2000. Functional instability of the ankle joint: Features and underlying causes. *Physiotherapy;* 86(8): 401–411.

17. Cavanaugh, P. R. 1978. *An evaluation of the effects of orthotics force distribution and rearfoot movement during running.* Paper presented at the meeting of the American Orthopedic Society for Sports Medicine, Lake Placid, NY.

18. Choi, J. 1978. Acute conditions: Incidence and associated disability. *Vital Health Statistics; 120:*10.

19. Collona, P. 1989. Fabrication of a custom molded orthotic using an intrinsic posting technique for a forefoot varus deformity. *Physical Therapy Forum;* 8(5): 3.

20. Cross, K., T. Worrell, and J. Leslie. 2002. The relationship between self-reported and clinical measures and the number of days to return to sport following acute lateral ankle sprains. *Journal of Orthopedic and Sports Physical Therapy;* 32(1):16–23.

21. Cutler, J. M. 1984. Lateral ligamentous injuries of the ankle. In *Lateral ligamentous injuries of the ankle,* edited by Hamilton, W. C. New York: Springer-Verlag.

22. Delacerda, F. G. 1980. A study of anatomical factors involved in shin splints. *Journal of Orthopaedic and Sports Physical Therapy;* 2:55–59.

23. Donahue, M, Simon, J. 2011. Critical review of self-reported functional ankle instability measures, *Foot and Ankle International;* 32:1149-1146.

24. Donatelli, R. 1985. Normal biomechanics of the foot and ankle. *Journal of Orthopaedic and Sports Physical Therapy;* 7:91–95.

25. Drez, D., D. Faust, and P. Evans. 1981. Cryotherapy and nerve palsy. *American Journal of Sports Medicine;* 9:256–257.

26. Freeman, M. 1965. Instability of the foot after injuries to the lateral ligament of the ankle. *Journal of Bone and Joint Surgery;* 47-B: 669–677.

27. Freeman, M., M. Dean, and I. Hanhan. 1965. The etiology and prevention of functional instability at the foot. *Journal of Bone and Joint Surgery;* 47[Br]: 678–85.

28. Fumich, R. M., A. Ellison, and G. Guerin, et al. 1981. The measured effect of taping on combined foot and ankle motion before and after exercise. *American Journal of Sports Medicine;* 9:165–169.

29. Garn, S. N., and R. A. Newton. 1988. Kinesthetic awareness in subjects with multiple ankle sprains. *Journal of the American Physical Therapy Association;* 68:1667–1671.

30. Garrick, J. G., and R. K. Requa. 1977. Role of external supports in the prevention of ankle sprains. *Medicine and Science in Sports and Exercise;* 5:200.

31. Garrick, J. G. 1981. When can I . . .? A practical approach to rehabilitation illustrated by treatment of an ankle injury. *American Journal of Sports Medicine;* 9:67–68.

32. Giallonardo, L. M. 1988. Clinical evaluation of foot and ankle dysfunction. *Physical Therapy;* 68:1850–1856.

33. Gill, E. 1985. Orthotics. *Runners World,* February, pp. 55–57.

34. Glascoe, W., M. Allen, and B. Autrey. 1999. Weight bearing, immobilization, and early exercise treatment following a grade II ankle sprain. *Journal of Orthopedic and Sports Physical Therapy*; 29(7): 395–399.

35. Glencross, D., and E. Thornton. 1981. Position sense following joint injury. *Journal of Sports Medicine and Physical Fitness*; 21:23–27.

36. Glick, J., and T. Sampson. 1996. Ankle and foot fractures in athletics. In *The lower extremity and spine in sports medicine*, edited by Nicholas, J. and E. Hershman. St. Louis: Mosby.

37. Gross, M., A. Lapp, and M. Davis. 1991. Comparison of Swed-O-Universal ankle support and Aircast Sport Stirrup orthoses and ankle tape in restricting eversion-inversion before and after exercise. *Journal of Orthopaedic and Sports Physical Therapy*; 13(1): 11–19.

38. Hertel, J. 2000. Functional instability following lateral ankle sprain. *Sports Medicine*; 29(5): 361–371.

39. Hirata, I. 1974. Proper playing conditions. *Journal of Sports Medicine*; 4:228–234.

40. Hoppenfield, S. 1976. *Physical examination of the spine and extremities*. New York: Appleton-Century-Crofts.

41. Hunt, G. 1985. Examination of lower extremity dysfunction. In *Orthopedic and sports physical therapy*, vol. 2, edited by Gould, J. and G. Davies. St Louis: Mosby.

42. Hunter, S., M. Dolan, and M. Davis. 1996. *Foot orthotics in therapy and sport*. Champaign, IL: Human Kinetics.

43. Isakov, E., J. Mizrahi, P. Solzi, et al. 1986. Response of the peroneal muscles to sudden inversion of the ankle during standing. *International Journal of Sport Biomechanics*; 2:100–109.

44. Itay, S. 1982. Clinical and functional status following lateral ankle sprains: Follow-up of 90 young adults treated conservatively. *Orthopedic Review*; 11:73–76.

45. James, S. L., B. T. Bates, and L. R. Osternig. 1978. Injuries to runners. *American Journal of Sports Medicine*; 6:43.

46. James, S. L. 1979. Chondromalacia of the patella in the adolescent. In *The injured adolescent*, edited by Kennedy, S. C. Baltimore: Williams & Wilkins.

47. Jones, D., and K. Singer. 1996. Soft-tissue conditions of the foot and ankle. In *The lower extremity and spine in sports medicine*, edited by Nicholas, J. and E. Hershman. St. Louis: Mosby.

48. Kelikian, H., and A. S. Kelikian. 1985. *Disorders of the ankle*. Philadelphia: W. B. Saunders.

49. Kergerris, S. 1983. The construction and implementation of functional progressions as a component of athletic rehabilitation. *Journal of Orthopaedic and Sports Physical Therapy*; 5:14–19.

50. Kivlan, B., and Martin, R. 2012. Functional performance testing of the hip in athletes: A systematic review for reliability and validity. *International Journal of Sports Physical Therapy*; 7(4):402–412.

51. Kowal, M. A. 1983. Review of physiologic effects of cryotherapy. *Journal of Orthopaedic and Sports Physical Therapy*; 5:66–73.

52. Lockard, M. A. 1988. Foot orthoses. *Physical Therapy*; 68:1866–1873.

53. Loudin, J., and S. Bel. 1996. The foot and ankle: An overview of arthrokinematics and selected joint techniques. *Journal of Athletic Training*; 31(2): 173–178.

54. Mandelbaum, B. R., G. Finerman, and T. Grant, et al. 1987. Collegiate football players with recurrent ankle sprains. *Physician and Sports Medicine*; 15(11): 57–61.

55. Mawdsley, R., D. Hoy, and P. Erwin. 2000. Criterion-related validity of the figure-of-eight method of measuring ankle edema. *Journal of Orthopedic and Sports Physical Therapy*; 30(3): 149–153.

56. Mayhew, J. L., and W. F. Riner. 1974. Effects of ankle wrapping on motor performance. *Athletic Training* 3:128–130.

57. McCluskey, G. M., T. A. Blackburn, and T. Lewis. 1976. Prevention of ankle sprains. *American Journal of Sports Medicine*; 4:151–157.

58. McKeon, P. O., and J. Hertel. 2008. Systematic review of postural control and lateral ankle instability, Part II: Is balance training clinically effective? *Journal of Athletic Training*; 43(3): 305–315.

59. McPoil, T. G., M. Adrian, and P. Pidcoe. 1989. Effects of foot orthoses on center of pressure patterns in women. *Physical Therapy*; 69:149–154.

60. McPoil, T. G., and R. S. Brocato. 1985. The foot and ankle: Biomechanical evaluation and treatment. In *Orthopedic and sports physical therapy*, edited by Gould, J. and G. Davies. St. Louis: Mosby.

61. McPoil, T. G., H. G. Knecht, and D. Schmit. 1988. A survey of foot types in normal females between the ages of 18 and 30 years. *Journal of Orthopaedic and Sports Physical Therapy*; 9:406–409.

62. McPoil, T. G. 1988. Footwear. *Physical Therapy*; 68:1857–1865.

63. Monteleone, B, Ronsky, J. 2014. Ankle kinematics and muscle activity in functional ankle instability. *Clinical Journal of Sports Medicine*; 24(1):62-68.

64. Morton, D. J. 1937. Foot disorders in general practice. *Journal of the American Medical Association*; 109:1112–1119.

65. Nawoczenski, D. A., M. Owen, and M. Ecker, et al. 1985. Objective evaluation of peroneal response to sudden inversion stress. *Journal of Orthopaedic and Sports Physical Therapy*; 7:107–119.

66. Nicholas, J. A., and E. B. Hershman. 1990. *The lower extremity and spine in sports medicine*. St. Louis: Mosby.

67. Nishikawa, T., and M. Grabiner. 1999. Peroneal motorneuron excitability increases immediately following application of a semirigid ankle brace. *Journal of Orthopedic and Sports Physical Therapy*; 29(3): 168–173.

68. Noyes, F. R. 1977. Functional properties of knee ligaments and alterations induced by immobilization: A correlative biomechanical and histological study in primates. *Clinical Orthopedics*; 123:210–243.

69. Oatis, C. A. 1998. Biomechanics of the foot and ankle under static conditions. *Physical Therapy*; 68:1815–1821.

70. Oschendorff, D., and C. Mattacola. 2000. Effect of orthoticas on postural sway after fatigue of plantar flexors and dorsiflexors. *Journal of Athletic Training*; 35(1): 26–30.

71. Pagliano, J. N. 1988. Athletic footwear. *Sports Medicine Digest*; 10:1–2.

72. Prentice, W. 2014. *Principles of athletic training*. New York: McGraw-Hill.

73. Prentice, W. 2011. *Therapeutic modalities in Rehabilitation*. New York: McGraw-Hill.

74. Quillen, S. 1980. Alternative management protocol for lateral ankle sprains. *Journal of Orthopaedic and Sports Physical Therapy*; 12:187–190.

75. Rebman, L. W. 1986. Ankle injuries: Clinical observations. *Journal of Orthopaedic and Sports Physical Therapy*; 8:153–156.

76. Ricardo, M., S. Schulthies, and J. Saret. 2000. Effects of high top and low top shoes on ankle inversion. *Journal of Athletic Training*; 35(1): 38–43.

77. Ricardo, M., S. Sherwood, and S. Schultheis. 2000. Effects of type of exercise on dynamic ankle inversion. *Journal of Athletic Training*; 35(1): 31–37.

78. Riegler, H. F. 1987. Orthotic devices for the foot. *Orthopedic Reviews*; 16:293–303.

79. Rogers, M. M., and B. F. LeVeau. 1982. Effectiveness of foot orthotic devices used to modify pronation in runners. *Journal of Orthopaedic and Sports Physical Therapy*; 4:86–90.

80. Root, M. L., W. P. Orien, and J. H. Weed. 1977. *Normal and abnormal functions of the foot*. Los Angeles: Clinical Biomechanics.

81. Rose, A., R. J. Lee, R. M. Williams, L. C. Thomson, and A. Forsyth. 2000. Functional instability in non-contact ankle ligament injuries. *British Journal of Sports Medicine*; 34: 332–358.

82. Sammarco, J. G. 1975. Biomechanics of foot and ankle injuries. *Athletic Training*; 10:96.

83. Silbernagel, K. 2014. Does one size fit all when it comes to exercise treatment for Achilles tendinopathy? *Journal of Orthopaedic and Sports Physical Therapy*; 44(2):42–44.

84. Sims, D. 1986. Effects of positioning on ankle edema. *Journal of Orthopaedic and Sports Physical Therapy*; 8:30–33.

85. Sims, D. S., P. R. Cavanaugh, and J. S. Ulbrecht. 1988. Risk factors in the diabetic foot. Physical Therapy 68:1887–1901.

86. Sloan, J. P., P. Guddings, and R. Hain. 1988. Effects of cold and compression on edema. *Physician and Sports Medicine*; 16:116–120.

87. Smith, R. 1986. Treatment of ankle sprains in young athletes. *American Journal of Sports Medicine*; 14:465–471.

88. Stover, C. N., and J. M. York. 1980. Air stirrup management of ankle injuries in the patient. *American Journal of Sports Medicine*; 8:360–365.

89. Subotnick, S. I., and S. G. Newell. 1975. *Podiatric sports medicine*. Mt. Kisko, NY: Futura.

90. Subotnick, S. I. 1981. The flat foot. *Physician and Sports Medicine*; 9:85–91.

91. Subotnick, S. I. 1977. *The running foot doctor*. Mt. Vias, CA: World.

92. Taunton, J., C. Smith, and D. Magee. 1996. Leg, foot, and ankle injuries. In *Athletic injuries and rehabilitation*, edited by Zachazewski, J. D. Magee, and W. Quillen. Philadelphia: W. B. Saunders.

93. Tiberio, D. 1988. Pathomechanics of structural foot deformities. *Physical Therapy*; 68:1840–1849.

94. Tippett, S. R. 1982. A case study: The need for evaluation and reevaluation of acute ankle sprains. *Journal of Orthopaedic and Sports Physical Therapy*; 4:44.

95. Tropp, H., C. Askling, and J. Gillquist. 1985. Prevention of ankle sprains. *American Journal of Sports Medicine*; 13:259–266.

96. Tropp, H., P. Odenrick, and J. Gillquist. 1985. Stabilometry recordings in functional and mechanical instability of the ankle joint. *International Journal of Sports Medicine*; 6:180–182.

97. Vaes, P., H. DeBoeck, and F. Handleberg, et al. 1985. Comparative radiologic study of the influence of ankle joint bandages on ankle stability. *American Journal of Sports Medicine*; 13:46–49.

98. Visnich, A. L. 1987. A playing orthoses for "turf toe." *Athletic Training*; 22:215.

99. Vogelbach, W. D., and L. C. Combs. 1987. A biomechanical approach to the management of chronic lower extremity pathologies as they relate to excessive pronation. *Athletic Training*; 22:6–16.

100. Wilk, K., K. Fisher, and W. Gutierrez. 2000. Defective running shoes as a contributing factor in plantar fasciitis in a triathlete. *Journal of Orthopedic and Sports Physical Therapy*; 30(1): 21–31.

101. Williams, J. G. P. 1980. The foot and chondromalacia: A case of biomechanical uncertainty. *Journal of Orthopaedic and Sports Physical Therapy*; 2:50–51.

102. Woods, A., and W. Smith. 1983. Cuboid syndrome and the techniques used for treatment. *Athletic Training*; 18:64–65.

103. Yablon, I. G., D. Segal, and R. E. Leach. 1983. *Ankle injuries*. New York: Churchill Livingstone.

104. Yeung, M. S., K. Chan, C. H. So, 1994. An epidemiological survey on ankle sprain. *British Journal of Sports Medicine*; 28:112–116.

105. Zylks, D. R. 1987. Alternative taping for plantar fasciitis. *Athletic Training*; 22:317.

SOLUTIONS TO CLINICAL DECISION-MAKING EXERCISES

23-1 Regaining strength and ROM are certainly important components of a rehabilitation following ankle injury. Key elements that are frequently omitted in rehabilitation of the ankle are balance, proprioception, and neuromuscular control. These are very important components of ankle rehabilitation for recurrent ankle sprains.

23-2 Sprains of the syndesmosis and interosseus are very hard to treat and often take months to heal. It is not likely that this patient will be ready in 2 weeks following symptoms of this severity.

23-3 Peroneal tendon subluxation is a frequent cause of "popping" and "giving way" in ankle injuries. Peroneal subluxation will cause tenderness and ecchymosis in the retromalleolar space behind the lateral malleolus.

23-4 This patient's foot exam suggests moderate pronation. This condition often creates hypermobility of the first ray, increasing pressure on the other metatarsals. The most desirable shoe characteristic for a pronated foot is a shoe that is firm and gives good support. Straight, board-lasted shoes with dual density midsoles will provide the best pronation control.

23-5 Orthotic fabrication is very useful for this condition. Use of these orthotics is critical during the first few steps in the morning. Vigorous heel cord stretching should be performed several times daily. The use of a dorsiflexion night splint has also been recommended.

23-6 Some type of material should be added to the forefoot of the shoe to stiffen the shoe. Some shoe companies address this problem by placing steel in the forefoot of their shoes. Taping of the toe to prevent hyperextension is one alternative method of preventing reinjury.

Please see videos on the accompanying website at

www.healio.com/books/sportsmedvideos

CHAPTER 24

Rehabilitation of Injuries to the Spine

Daniel N. Hooker, PhD, PT, ATC
William E. Prentice, PhD, PT, ATC, FNATA

After completing this chapter, the athletic training student should be able to do the following:

- Discuss the functional anatomy and biomechanics of the spine.

- Describe the difference between spinal segmental stabilization and core stabilization.

- Explain the rationale for using the different positioning exercises for treating pain in the spine.

- Conduct a thorough evaluation of the back before developing a rehabilitation plan.

- Compare and contrast the importance of using either joint mobilization or core stabilization exercises for treating spine patients.

- Differentiate between the acute vs reinjury vs chronic stage models for treating low back pain.

- Explain the eclectic approach for rehabilitation of back pain in the athletic population.

- Describe basic- and advanced-level training in the reinjury stage of treatment.

- Discuss the rehabilitation approach to conditions of the thoracic spine.

- Incorporate the rehabilitation approach to specific conditions affecting the low back.

- Discuss the rehabilitation approach to conditions of the cervical spine.

Prentice WE, ed.
Rehabilitation Techniques for Sports Medicine and Athletic Training (pp 801-854).
© 2015 SLACK Incorporated.

FUNCTIONAL ANATOMY AND BIOMECHANICS

From a biomechanical perspective, the spine is one of the most complex regions of the body with numerous bones, joints, ligaments, and muscles, all of which are collectively involved in spinal movement. The proximity to and relationship of the spinal cord, the nerve roots, and the peripheral nerves to the vertebral column adds to the complexity of this region. Injury to the cervical spine has potentially life-threatening implications, and low back pain is one of the most common ailments known to humans.

The 33 vertebrae of the spine are divided into five regions: cervical, thoracic, lumbar, sacral, and coccygeal. Between each of the cervical, thoracic, and lumbar vertebrae lie fibrocartilaginous intervertebral disks that act as important shock absorbers for the spine.

The design of the spine allows a high degree of flexibility forward and laterally and limited mobility backward. The movements of the vertebral column are flexion and extension, right and left lateral flexion, and rotation to the left and right. The degree of movement differs in the various regions of the vertebral column. The cervical and lumbar regions allow extension, flexion, and rotation around a central axis. Although the thoracic vertebrae have minimal movement, their combined movement between the first and twelfth thoracic vertebrae can account for 20 to 30 degrees of flexion and extension.

As the spinal vertebrae progress downward from the cervical region, they grow increasingly larger to accommodate the upright posture of the body, as well as to contribute to weight bearing. The shape of the vertebrae is irregular, but the vertebrae possess certain characteristics that are common to all. Each vertebra consists of a neural arch through which the spinal cord passes, and several projecting processes that serve as attachments for muscles and ligaments. Each neural arch has two pedicles and two laminae. The pedicles are bony processes that project backward from the body of the vertebrae and connect with the laminae. The laminae are flat bony processes occurring on either side of the neural arch that project backward and

inward from the pedicles. With the exception of the first and second cervical vertebrae, each vertebra has a spinous and transverse process for muscular and ligamentous attachments, and all vertebrae have multiple articular processes.

Intervertebral articulations are between vertebral bodies and vertebral arches. Articulation between the bodies is of the symphysial type. Besides motion at articulations between the bodies of the vertebrae, movement takes place at four articular processes that derive from the pedicles and laminae. The direction of movement of each vertebra is somewhat dependent on the direction in which the articular facets face. The sacrum articulates with the ilium to form the sacroiliac joint, which has a synovium and is lubricated by synovial fluid.

Ligaments

The major ligaments that join the various vertebral parts are the anterior longitudinal, the posterior longitudinal, and the supraspinous. The anterior longitudinal ligament is a wide, strong band that extends the full length of the anterior surface of the vertebral bodies. The posterior longitudinal ligament is contained within the vertebral canal and extends the full length of the posterior aspect of the bodies of the vertebrae. Ligaments connect one lamina to another. The interspinous, supraspinous, and intertransverse ligaments stabilize the transverse and spinous processes, extending between adjacent vertebrae. The sacroiliac joint is maintained by the extremely strong dorsal sacral ligaments. The sacrotuberous and the sacrospinous ligaments attach the sacrum to the ischium.

Muscle Actions

The muscles that extend the spine and rotate the vertebral column can be classified as either superficial or deep. The superficial muscles extend from the vertebrae to ribs. The erector spinae is a group of superficial paired muscles that is made up of three columns or bands, the longissimus group, the iliocostalis group, and the spinalis group. Each of these groups is further divided into regions, the cervicis region in the neck, the thoracis region in the middle back, and the lumborum region in the

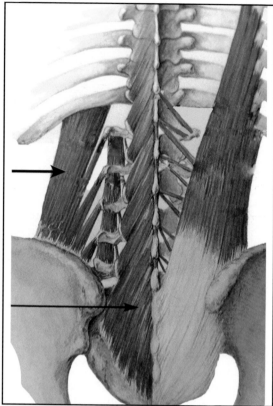

Quadratus lumborum

Multifidus lumborum

Figure 24-1. Muscles of the low back. The multifidus and the quadratus lumborum muscles.

low back. Generally the erector spinae muscles extend the spine. The deep muscles attach one vertebra to another and function to extend and rotate the spine. The deep muscles include the interspinales, multifidus, rotators, thoracis, and the semispinalis cervicis.

Flexion of the cervical region is produced primarily by the sternocleidomastoid muscles and the scalene muscle group on the anterior aspect of the neck. The scalenes flex the head and stabilize the cervical spine as the sterno-cleidomastoids flex the neck. The upper trapezius, semispinalis capitis, splenius capitus, and splenius cervicis muscles extend the neck. Lateral flexion of the neck is accomplished by all of the muscles on one side of the vertebral column contracting unilaterally. Rotation is produced when the sternocleidomastoid, the scalenes, the semispinalis cervicis, and the upper trapezius on the side opposite to the direction of rotation contract in addition to a contraction of the splenius capitus, splenius

cervicis, and longissimus capitus on the same side of the direction of rotation.

Flexion of the trunk primarily involves lengthening of the deep and superficial back muscles and contraction of the abdominal muscles (rectus abdominus, internal oblique, external oblique) and hip flexors (rectus femoris, iliopsoas, tensor faciae lata, sartorius). Seventy-five percent of flexion occurs at the lumbosacral junction (L5-S1), whereas 15% to 70% occurs between L4 and L5. The rest of the lumbar vertebrae execute 5% to 10% of flexion.[13] Extension involves lengthening of the abdominal muscles and contraction of the erector spinae and the gluteus maximus, which extends the hip. Trunk rotation is produced by the external obliques and the internal obliques. Lateral flexion is produced primarily by the quadratus lumborum muscle, along with the obliques, latissimus dorsi, iliopsoas, and the rectus abdominus on the side of the direction of movement.

Transversus abdominis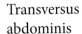

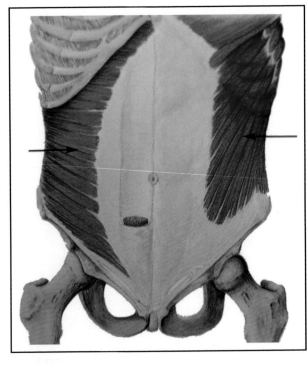

External oblique

Spinal segment stability is produced by the deep muscles of the spine (multifidi, medial quadratus lumborum, iliocostalis lumborum, interspinales, intertransversarii) working in concert with the transversus abdominis and internal abdominal oblique (Figure 24-1). Their location is close to the center of rotation of the spinal segment and their short muscle lengths are ideal for controlling each spinal segment. The transversus abdominis, because of its pull on the thoracolumbar fascia, and its ability to create increased intra-abdominal pressure as it narrows the abdominal cavity, is a major partner in spinal segment stability (Figure 24-2). This combination creates a rigid cylinder and in concert with the deep spinal muscles provides significant segmental stability to the lumbar spine and pelvis.[22,40-42,59-61,63,67-69]

Spinal Cord

The spinal cord is that portion of the central nervous system that is contained within the vertebral canal of the spinal column. Thirty-one pairs of spinal nerves extend from the sides of the spinal cord, coursing downward and outward through the intervertebral foramen passing near the articular facets of the vertebrae.

Any abnormal movement of these facets, such as in a dislocation or a fracture, may expose the spinal nerves to injury. Injuries that occur below the third lumbar vertebra usually result in nerve root damage but do not cause spinal cord damage.

The spinal nerve roots combine to form a network of nerves, or a plexus. There are five nerve plexuses: cervical, brachial, lumbar, sacral, and coccygeal.

THE IMPORTANCE OF EVALUATION IN TREATING BACK PAIN

In many instances after referral for medical evaluation, the patient returns to the athletic trainer with a diagnosis of low back pain. Even though this is a correct diagnosis, it does not offer the specificity needed to help direct the treatment planning. The athletic trainer planning the treatment would be better served with a more specific diagnosis such as spondylolysis, disk herniation, quadratus lumborum strain, piriformis syndrome, or sacroiliac ligament sprain.

Regardless of the diagnosis or the specificity of the diagnosis, the importance of a thorough evaluation of the patient's back pain is critical to good care. The athletic trainer should become an expert on this individual patient's back. Taking the time to perform a comprehensive evaluation will pay great rewards in the success of treatment and rehabilitation. The evaluation has six major purposes:

1. To clearly locate areas and tissues that might be part of the problem. The athletic trainer should use this information to direct treatments and exercises.[36,41,56]

2. To establish the baseline measurements used to assess progress and guide the treatment progression and help the athletic trainer make specific judgments on the progression of or changes in specific exercises. The improvement in these measurements also guides the return-to-activity decision and provides one measure of the success of the rehabilitation plan.[44,52,70]

3. To provide some provocative guidance to help the patient probe the limits of his or her condition, help him or her better understand his or her problem, present limitations, and understand the management of his or her injury problem.[44,52,70]

4. To establish confidence in the athletic trainer. This increases the placebo effect of the athletic trainer–patient interaction.[88,89]

5. To decrease the anxiety of the patient. This increases the patient's comfort, which will increase his or her compliance with the rehabilitation plan; a more positive environment is created, and the athletic trainer and patient avoid the "no one knows what is wrong with me" trap.[19]

6. To provide information for making judgments on pads, braces, and corsets.

Table 24-1 provides a detailed scheme for evaluation of back pain.

REHABILITATION TECHNIQUES FOR THE LOW BACK

Positioning and Pain-Relieving Exercises

Most patients with back pain have some fluctuation of their symptoms in response to certain postures and activities. The athletic trainer logically treats this patient by reinforcing pain-reducing postures and motions and by starting specific exercises aimed at specific muscle groups or specific ranges of motion (ROM). A general rule to follow in making these decisions is as follows: Any movement that causes the back pain to radiate or spread over a larger area should not be included during this early phase of treatment. Movements that centralize or diminish the pain are correct movements to include at this time.[56] Including some exercise during initial pain management generally has a positive effect on the patient. The exercise encourages him or her to be active in the rehabilitation plan and helps him or her to regain lumbar movement.[31,89]

When a patient relieves pain through exercise and attention to proper postural control, he or she is much more likely to adopt these procedures into a daily routine. A patient whose pain is relieved via some other passive procedure, and then is taught exercises, will not be able to readily see the connection between relief and exercise.[22,43,60,69]

The types of exercises that may be included in initial pain management include the following:

- Spinal segment control, transverse abdominis, and multifidus coactivation;

- Lateral shift corrections;

Table 24-1 Lumbar and Sacroiliac Joint Objective Examination

1. Standing position

   a. Posture–alignment

   b. Gait

       i. Patient's trunk frequently bent laterally or hips shifted to one side

       ii. Walks with difficulty or limps

   c. Alignment and symmetry

       iii. Trochanteric levels

       iv. PSIS and ASIS levels

       v. Levels of iliac crests

   Recent studies have raised the concern that these clinical assessments of alignment are not valid because of the small movements available at the sacroiliac joints. These tests should be used as a small part of the overall evaluation and not as stand-alone tests. In sacroiliac dysfunction, the ASIS, PSIS, and iliac crests may not appear to be in the same horizontal plane.

   d. Lumbar spine active movements

       i. With sacroiliac dysfunction, the patient will experience exacerbation of pain with side bending toward the painful side

       ii. Often a lumbar lesion is present along with a sacroiliac dysfunction

   e. Single-leg standing backward bending is a provocation test and can provoke pain in cases of spondylolysis or spondylolisthesis

2. Sitting position

   a. Lumbar spine rotation ROM

   b. Passive hip internal rotation and external rotation ROM

       i. Piriformis muscle irritation would be provoked by internal rotation and could be present from sacroiliac joint dysfunctions or myofascial pain from overuse of this muscle

       ii. Limited ROM of the hip can be a red flag for hip problems

   c. Sitting knee extension produces some stretch to the long neutral structures

   d. Slump sit is used to evaluate lumbar flexibility and neutral tension

3. Supine position

   a. Hip external rotation in a resting position may indicate piriformis muscle tightness

   b. Palpation of the transversus abdominis, as the patient is directed to contract, can help in the assessment of spinal segment control. Can the patient isolate this contraction from the other abdominal muscles?

   c. Palpation of the symphysis pubis for tenderness. Some sacroiliac problems create pain and tenderness in this area. Sometimes the presenting subjective symptoms mimic adductor or groin strain but the objective evaluation does not show pain or weakness on muscle contraction or muscle tenderness that would support this assessment

   d. Straight-leg raise (passive)

       I. Interpretation of straight-leg raise: pain provoked before

   - 30 degrees—hip problem or very inflamed nerve
   - 30 to 60 degrees—sciatic nerve involvement
   - 70 to 90 degrees—sacroiliac joint involvement
   - Neck flexion—exacerbates symptoms—disk or root irritation

(continued)

Table 24-1 Lumbar and Sacroiliac Joint Objective Examination (*continued*)

- Ankle dorsiflexion or Lasegue's sign—exacerbated symptoms usually indicate sciatic nerve or root irritation

e. Sacroiliac loading test (compression, distraction, posterior shear or P4 Test, Gasenslen's Scissor Stretch)—pain provoked by physical stress through the sacroiliac joints can be helpful in assessing for sacroiliac joint dysfunction

f. FABER (flexion, abduction, external rotation), also known as Patrick's test—at end range assesses irritability of the sacroiliac joint; hip muscle tightness can also be assessed using this test

g. FADIR (flexion, adduction, internal rotation) produces some stretch on the iliolumbar ligament

h. Bilateral knees to chest—will usually exacerbate lumbar spine symptoms as the sacroiliac joints move with the sacrum in this maneuver

i. Single knee to arm pit can provoke pain from a variety of sources from sacroiliac joint to lumbar spine muscles and ligaments; make patients be specific about their pain location and quality

4. Side-lying position

a. Iliotibial band length—sacroiliac joint problems sometimes create tightness of the iliotibial band and stress to the IT band will provoke pain in the SI joint area

b. Quadratus lumborum stretch and palpation

c. Hip abduction and piriformis muscle test. Pain provocation in muscular locations with either of these tests indicates primary myofascial pain problems or secondary tightness, weakness, and pain from muscle guarding associated with different pathologies. Pain provocation in the SI joint area would help confirm an SI joint dysfunction

5 Prone position

a. Palpation

i. Well-localized tenderness medial to or around the PSIS indicates sacroiliac dysfunction

ii. Tenderness lateral and superior to the PSIS indicates gluteus medius irritation or myofascial trigger point

iii. Gluteus maximus area—sacrotuberous and sacrospinous ligaments are in this area, as well as piriformis muscle and sciatic nerve. Changes in tension and tenderness can help make the evaluation more specific

iv. Tenderness around spinous processes or postural alignment faults from S-1 to T-10 could implicate some lumbar problems

b. Anterior—posterior or rotational provocational stresses can be applied to the spinous processes

c. Sacral provocation stress test—pain from anterior–posterior pressure at the center of the sacral base and/or on each side of the sacrum just medial to the PSIS may be indicative of sacroiliac joint dysfunction

d. Hip extension—knee flexion stretch will provoke the L3 nerve root and create a nerve quality pain down the anterolateral thigh

e. Anterior rotation stress to the sacroiliac joint can be delivered by using passive hip extension and PSIS pressure; pain in the SI joint area on either side would be indicative of sacroiliac dysfunction

6. Manual muscle test

If the lumbar spine or posterior hip musculature is strained, active movement against gravity and/or resistance should provoke a pain complaint similar to patient's subjective description of the problem

a. Hip extension

b. Hip internal rotation

e. Hip adduction

f. Trunk extension—arm and shoulder extension

g. Trunk extension—arm, shoulder, and neck extension

h. Trunk extension—resisted

i. Multifidus activation and control

j. Spinal segment coactivation of transversus abdominis and multifidi[29,44,52,69,70]

- Extension exercises—stretching and mobilization
- Flexion exercises—stretching and mobilization
- Postural traction positions
- Gentle rhythmic movements in flexion, extension, rotation, and side-bending
- Spinal manipulation

SPINAL SEGMENT CONTROL EXERCISE

In devising exercise plans to address the different clinical problems of the lumbo-pelvic-hip complex, the use of core-stabilizing exercises is a must for every problem for recovery, maintenance, and prevention of reinjury. Clinically, the core stabilization rehabilitation exercise sequence begins with relearning the muscle activation patterns necessary for segmental spinal stabilization. This beginning exercise plan is based on the work of Richardson, Jull, Hodges, and Hides.[40-43,61,68,69]

The first step in segmental spinal stabilization is to reestablish separate control of the transversus abdominis and the lumbar multifidii (Figures 24-1 and 24-2). The control and activation of these deep muscles should be separated from the control and activation of the global or superficial muscles of the core. Once the patients have mastered the behavior of coactivation of the transversus abdominis and multifidii to create and maintain a corset-like control and stabilization of the spinal segments, they may then progress to using the global muscles in the core stabilization sequence and more functional activities. Segmental spinal stabilization is the basic building block of core stabilization exercises and should be an automatic behavior to be used in every subsequent exercise and activity.[40,41,43,59,60]

The basic exercise that the patient must master is coactivation of the transversus abdominis and multifidii, isolating them from the global trunk muscles. This contraction should be of sufficient magnitude to create a small increase in the intra-abdominal pressure. This is a simple concept, but these muscle contractions are normally under subconscious automatic control; and in patients with low back pain, the subconscious control of timing and firing patterns become disturbed and the patient loses spinal segmental control.[41] To regain this vital skill and return the subconscious timing and firing patterns of these muscles, the patient will need individual instruction and testing to prove that he or she has mastered the conscious control of each muscle individually and in a coactivation pattern. The next step is to incorporate this coactivation pattern into functional exercise and other activities. The success of this exercise is dependent upon this muscular coactivation becoming a habitual postural control movement under both conscious and subconscious control.

A muscle contraction of 10% to 15% of the maximum voluntary contraction of the multifidus and the transversus abdominis is all that is necessary to create segmental spinal stability. Contraction levels greater than 20% of maximum voluntary contraction will cause overflow of activity to the more global muscles and negate the exercise's intent of isolating control of the transversus abdominis and multifidii.[43] Precision of contraction and control is the intent of these exercises; the ultimate goal is a change in the patient's behavior. As this behavior is incorporated into more daily activities and exercise, the strength and endurance of these muscle groups will also improve and the core system will work more effectively and efficiently.[30,44,45,52,53]

Transversus Abdominis Behavior Exercise Plan

1. Test the patient's ability to consciously contract and control the transversus abdominis in isolation from the other abdominal muscles. The athletic trainer can assess the contraction through observation and palpation. The patient is positioned in a comfortable relaxed posture: stomach-lying, back-lying, side-lying, or hand-knee position. The best palpation location is medial to the anterior superior iliac spine (ASIS) about 1.5 inches (Figure 24-3). The internal abdominal oblique has more vertical fibers and is closest to the ASIS, whereas

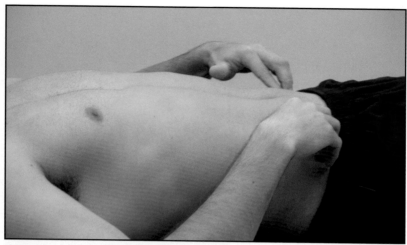

Figure 24-3. Palpation location to feel for isolated transversus abdominis contraction.

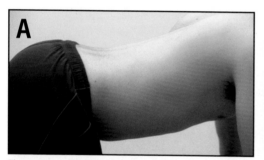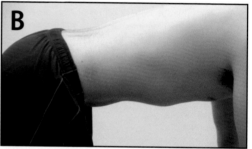

Figure 24-4. The quadruped position can be used to demonstrate and practice the isolated transversus abdominis contraction. The patient is instructed to (A) let his belly sag; then, (B) slowly and gently contract his pelvic floor muscles and practice holding this position for 10 seconds.

the transversus fibers run horizontal from ilia to ilia. The therapist monitors the muscle with light palpation and instructs the patient to contract the muscle, feeling for the transversus drawing together across the abdomen. As the contraction increases, the internal oblique fibers and external oblique fibers will start to fire. If the patients cannot separate the firing of the transversus from the other groups and/ or cannot maintain the separate contraction for 5 to 10 seconds, he or she will need individual instruction with various forms of feedback to regain control of this muscle behavior. In patients with low back pain, transversus contraction usually becomes more phasic and fires only in combination with the obliques or rectus.[43,69]

2. The patient is positioned in a comfortable pain-free position and instructed to breathe in and out gently, stop the breathing, and slowly, gently contract and hold the contraction of his or her transversus—and then resume normal light breathing while trying to maintain the contraction. Changes in body position (positions of choice are prone, side-lying, supine, or quadruped), verbal cues, and visual and tactile feedback will speed and enhance the learning process (Figures 24-4A and B). The use of imaging ultrasound as visual biofeedback to visualize the contractions of these muscles provides visualization of the tendon movement and can help in isolating and bringing these muscle contractions under cognitive control.[43,69]

3. The lumbar multifidii contractions are taut with tactile pressure over the muscle bellies next to the spinous processes (Figure 24-5). The patient is asked to contract the muscle so that the muscle swells up directly under the finger pressure. The feeling should be a

Figure 24-5. Palpation location to feel for isolated lumbar multifidii contractions.

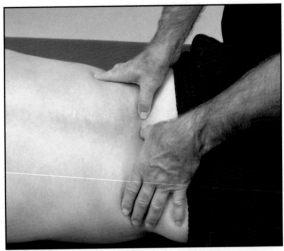

Figure 24-6. Palpation location to feel contractions, to give the patient feedback on his ability to perform a coactivation segmental spinal stabilization contraction.

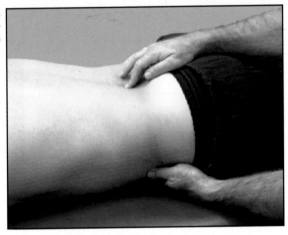

deep tension. A rapid superficial contraction or a contraction that brings in the global muscles is not acceptable, and continued trial and error with feedback is used until the desired contraction and control are achieved.[43,69]

4. As soon as cognitive control of the transversus and multifidii is achieved, more functional positions and exercises aimed at coactivation of both muscles are begun. The therapist should attempt to have the patient use the transversus and multifidii coactivation in a comfortable neutral lumbopelvic position with restoration of a normal lordotic curve so that the muscle coactivation strategies can start to be incorporated into the patient's daily life (Figure 24-6). Repetition improves the effectiveness of this contraction, and as it is used

more, the cognitive control becomes less and the subconscious pattern of segmental spinal stabilization returns to normal.[43,69]

5. Incorporating the coactivation contraction back into activities is the next step and is accomplished by graduating the exercises to include increases in stress and control. Supine-lying with simple leg and arm movements is a good starting point. Using a pressure biofeedback unit for this phase will help patients measure their ability to use the coactivation contraction effectively during increased exercise. The Stabilizer pressure biofeedback unit is inflated to a pressure of about 40 mm Hg. As the patient coactivates the transversus abdominis and multifidi, the pressure reading should stay the same or decrease slightly and remain at that level throughout the increased

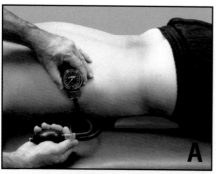
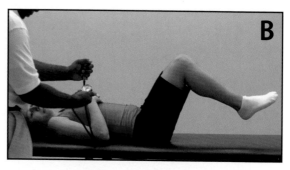

Figure 24-7. The Stabilizer pressure biofeedback unit can be used as an indirect method of measuring correct activation of the spinal segment stabilization coactivation contraction. The stabilizer is inflated to 40 mm Hg pressure and placed under the patient's (A) abdomen, or (B) back. The patient should be instructed to contract the transversus in a way that does not make the pressure in the cuff start to rise or fall.

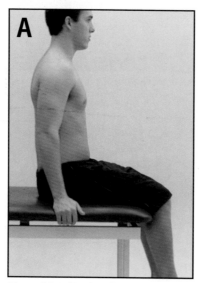
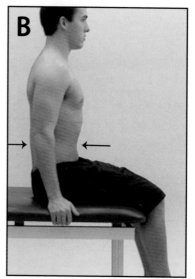

Figure 24-8. Trunk inclination exercise. The patient finds a comfortable neutral spine position and coactivates their transversus abdominis and lumbar multifidii to provide the segmental spinal stabilization.

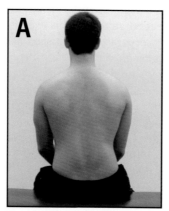
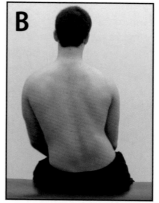

Figure 24-9. The patient challenges his or her spinal segment control by leaning away from the vertical position while holding the neutral spine position for 10 seconds.

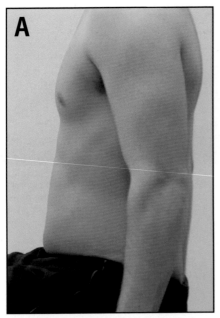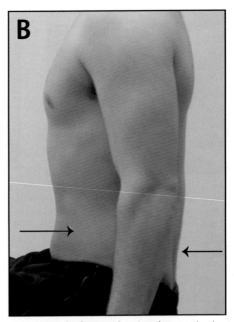

Figure 24-10. The patient is instructed to become posture savvy by frequently using the coactivation contraction throughout his day. The coactivation thereby becomes a subconscious movement pattern the patient incorporates into all they do.

movement exercises (Figures 24-7A and B). This is an indirect measure of the spinal segment stabilization, but gives the patients an outside feedback source to keep them more focused on the exercise.[43,69]

6. This can be followed with trunk inclination exercises in which patients maintain a neutral lumbo-pelvic position and incline their trunk in different positions away from the vertical alignment and hold in positions of forward-lean to side-lean for specific time periods (Figures 24-8A and B and 24-9A and B). This is first done in the sitting position. As control, strength, and endurance increase, the positions can become more exaggerated and the holding times longer.

7. Return the patient to a structured progressive resistive core exercise program (see Chapter 5). The incorporation of the segmental spinal stabilization coactivation contraction as the precursor to each exercise is the goal at this point in returning the patient back to functional activity.

8. The athletic trainer should teach this technique both as an exercise and as a behavior. The exercises should be taught and

monitored in an individual session with opportunity for feedback and correction. Patients must also use this skill in the functional things they do every day. The patients are asked to trigger this spinal segment control skill in response to daily tasks, postures, pains, and certain movements (Figures 24-10A and B). As their pain is controlled, the coactivation contraction should be incorporated into activities of daily living.

Segmental spinal stabilization is complementary for all forms of treatment and different pathologies. This exercise program can be incorporated and started at the same time as other therapies. The different forms of therapy summate, and the patient improves more quickly and maintains the gains in range and strength achieved with other therapies. Spinal segment control may also decrease pain and give the patient a measure of control to use in minimizing painful stress through the injured tissues.

Lateral Shift Corrections

Lateral shift corrections and extension exercises probably should be discussed together

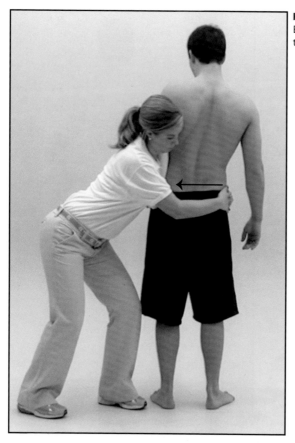

Figure 24-11. Lateral shift correction exercise. Emphasis is on pulling the hips, not on pushing the ribs.

because the indications for use are similar, and extension exercises will immediately follow the lateral shift corrections.

The indications for the use of lateral shift corrections are as follows:

- Subjectively, the patient complains of unilateral pain reference in the lumbar or hip area.

- The typical posture is scoliotic with a hip shift and reduced lumbar lordosis.

- Walking and movements are very guarded and robotic.

- Forward bending is extremely limited and increases the pain.

- Backward bending is limited.

- Side bending toward the painful side is minimal to impossible.

- Side bending away from the painful side is usually reasonable to normal.

- A test correction of the hip shift either reduces the pain or causes the pain to centralize.

- The neurological examination may or may not elicit the following positive findings:

  1. Straight-leg raising may be limited and painful, or it could be unaffected.

  2. Sensation may be dull, anesthetic, or unaffected.

  3. Manual muscle test may indicate unilateral weakness of specific movements, or the movements may be strong and painless.

  4. Reflexes may be diminished or unaffected.[56]

The patient will be assisted by the athletic trainer with the initial lateral shift correction. The patient is then instructed in the techniques of self-correction. The lateral shift correction is designed to guide the patient back to a more symmetrical posture. The athletic trainer's pressure should be firm and steady and more guiding than forcing. The use of a mirror to provide visual feedback is recommended for both the athletic trainer-assisted and self-corrected maneuvers. The specific technique guide for athletic trainer-assisted lateral shift correction is as follows (Figure 24-11):

1. Prepare the patient by explaining the correction maneuver and the roles of the patient and the athletic trainer.

   a. The patient is to keep the shoulders level and avoid the urge to side bend.

   b. The patient should allow the hips to move under the trunk and should not resist the pressure from the athletic trainer but allow the hips to shift with the pressure.

   c. The patient should keep the athletic trainer informed about the behavior of the back pain.

   d. The patient should keep the feet stationary and not move after the hip shift correction until the standing extension part of the correction is completed.

   e. The patient should practice the standing extension exercise as part of this initial explanation.

2. The athletic trainer should stand on the patient's side that is opposite his or her hip shift. The patient's feet should be a comfortable distance apart, and the athletic trainer should have a comfortable stride stance aligned slightly behind the patient.

3. Padding should be placed around the patient's elbow, on the side next to the athletic trainer to provide comfortable contact between the patient and the athletic trainer.

4. The athletic trainer should contact the patient's elbow with the shoulder and chest, with the head aligned along the patient's back. The athletic trainer's arms should reach around the patient's waist and apply pressure between the iliac crest and the greater trochanter (Figure 24-11).

5. The athletic trainer should gradually guide the patient's hips toward him or her. If the pain increases, the athletic trainer should

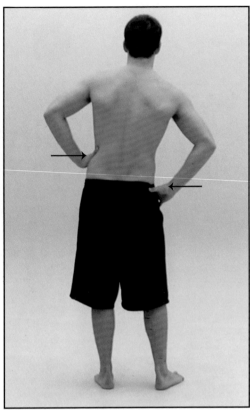

Figure 24-12. Hip shift self-correction. The patient can use a mirror for visual feedback as he applies the gentle guiding force to correct their hip shift posture. The patient uses one hand to stabilize himself at the rib level and uses the other hand to guide the hips across to correct their alignment. This position is held for 30 to 45 seconds, and then the patient is instructed to go into the standing extension position for 5 to 6 repetitions, holding the position for 20 to 30 seconds.

ease the pressure and maintain a more comfortable posture for 10 to 20 seconds, and then again pull gently. If the pain increases again, the athletic trainer should again lessen the pull and allow comfort, then instruct the patient to actively extend gently, pushing the back into and matching the resistance supplied by the athletic trainer. The goal for this maneuver is an overcorrection of the scoliosis, reversing its direction.

6. Once the corrected or overcorrected posture is achieved, the athletic trainer should maintain this posture for 1 to 2 minutes. This procedure may take 2 to 3 minutes to complete, and the first attempt may be less than a total success. Repeated efforts 3 to

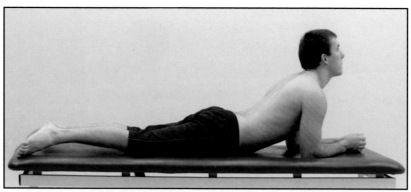

Figure 24-13. Prone extension on elbows.

4 minutes apart should be attempted during the first treatment effort before the athletic trainer stops the treatment for that episode.

7. The athletic trainer gradually releases pressure on the hip while the patient does a standing extension movement (Figure 24-16). The patient should complete about 6 repetitions of the standing extension movement, holding each for 15 to 20 seconds.

8. Once the patient moves the feet and walks even a short distance, the lateral hip shift usually will recur, but to a lesser degree. The patient then should be taught the self-correction maneuver (Figure 24-12). The patient should stand in front of a mirror and place one hand on the hip where the athletic trainer's hands were and the other hand on the lower ribs where the athletic trainer's shoulder was.

9. The patient then guides the hip under the trunk, watching the mirror to keep the shoulders level and trying to achieve a corrected or overcorrected posture. He or she should hold this posture for 30 to 45 seconds and then follow with several standing extension movements as described in step 7 (Figure 24-16).[56]

Extension Exercises

The indications for the use of extension exercise are as follows:

- Subjectively, back pain is diminished with lying down and is increased with sitting. The location of the pain may be unilateral, bilateral, or central, and there may or may not be pain radiating into either or both legs.

- Forward bending is extremely limited and increases the pain, or the pain reference location enlarges as the patient bends forward.

- Backward bending can be limited, but the movement centralizes or diminishes the pain.

- The neurological examination is the same as outlined for lateral shift correction.[56,57]

The efficacy of extension exercise is theorized to be from one or a combination of the following effects:

- A reduction in the neural tension.

- A reduction of the load on the disk, which in turn decreases disk pressure.

- Increases in the strength and endurance of the extensor muscles.

- Proprioceptive interference with pain perception as the exercises allow self-mobilization of the spinal joints.

Hip shift posture has previously been theoretically correlated to the anatomical location of the disk bulge or nucleus pulposus herniation. Creating a centralizing movement of the nucleus pulposus has been the theoretical emphasis of hip shift correction and extension exercise. This theory has good logic, but research on this phenomenon has not been supportive.[64] However, in explaining the exercises to the patient, the use of this theory may help increase the patient's motivation and compliance with the exercise plan.

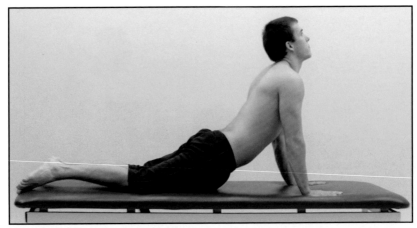

Figure 24-14. Prone extension on hands.

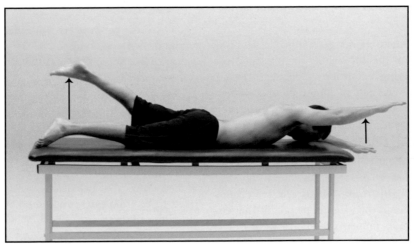

Figure 24-15. Alternate arm and leg extension.

End-range hyperextension exercise should be used cautiously when the patient has facet joint degeneration or impingement of the vertebral foramen borders on neural structures. Also, spondylolysis and spondylolisthesis problems should be approached cautiously with any end-range movement exercise using either flexion or hyperextension.

Figures 24-13 through 24-20 are examples of extension exercises. These examples are not exhaustive but are representative of most of the exercises used clinically.

The order in which exercises are presented is not significant. Instead, each athletic trainer should base the starting exercises on the evaluative findings. Jackson, in a review of back exercise, stated, "No support was found for the use of a preprogrammed flexion regimen that

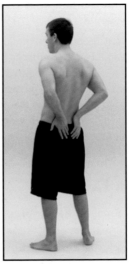

Figure 24-16. Standing extension.

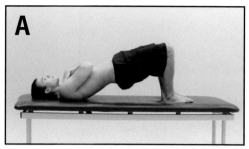
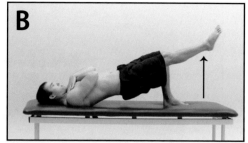

Figure 24-17. Supine hip extension—butt lift or bridge. (A) Double-leg support; (B) single-leg support.

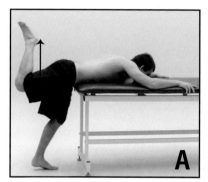
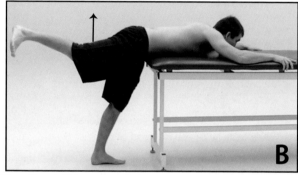

Figure 24-18. Prone single-leg hip extension. (A) Knee flexed; (B) knee extended.

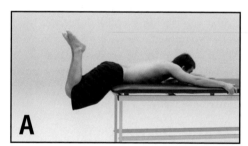
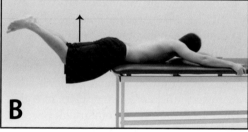

Figure 24-19. Prone double-leg hip extension. (A) Knees flexed; (B) knees extended.

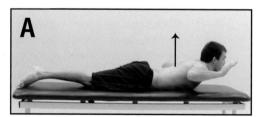
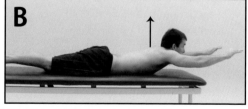

Figure 24-20. Trunk extension—prone. (A) Hands near head; (B) arms extended—superman position.

includes exercises of little value or potential harm and is not specific to the current needs of the patient, as determined by a thorough back evaluation." The review also included a report of Kendall and Jenkin's study, which stated that one-third of the patients for whom hyperextension exercises had been prescribed worsened.[36]

Flexion Exercises

The indications for the use of flexion exercises are as follows:

- Subjectively, back pain is diminished with sitting and is increased with lying down

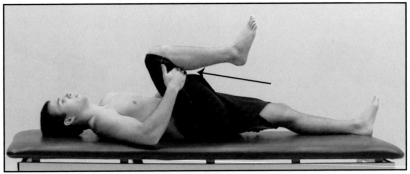

Figure 24-21. Single knee to chest. Stretch holding 15 to 20 seconds. Alternate legs.

or standing. Pain is also increased with walking.

- Repeated or sustained forward bending eases the pain.
- The patient's lordotic curve does not reverse as he or she forward bends.
- The end range of sustained backward bending is painful or increases the pain.
- Abdominal tone and strength are poor.

In his approach, Saal elaborates on the thought that "No one should continue with one particular type of exercise regimen during the entire treatment program."[74] We concur with this and feel that starting with one type of exercise should not preclude rapidly adding other exercises as the patient's pain resolves and other movements become more comfortable.

The efficacy of flexion exercise is theorized to derive from one or a combination of the following effects:

- A reduction in the articular stresses on the facet joints;
- Stretching to the thoraco-lumbar fascia and musculature;
- Opening of the intervertebral foramen;
- Relief of the stenosis of the spinal canal;
- Improvement of the stabilizing effect of the abdominal musculature;
- Increasing the intra-abdominal pressure because of increased abdominal muscle strength and tone;
- Proprioceptive interference with pain perception as the exercises allow self-mobilization of the spinal joints.[46]

Flexion exercises should be used cautiously or avoided in most cases of acute disk prolapse and when a laterally shifted posture is present. In patients recovering from disk-related back pain, flexion exercise should not be commenced immediately after a flat-lying rest interval longer than 30 minutes. The disk can become more hydrated in this amount of time, and the patient would be more susceptible to pain with postures that increase disk pressures. Other, less stressful exercises should be initiated first and flexion exercise done later in the exercise program.[56]

Figures 24-21 to 24-31 show examples of flexion exercises. Again, these examples are not exhaustive but are representative of the exercises used clinically.

Joint Mobilizations

The indications for the use of joint mobilizations are as follows:

- Subjectively, the patient's pain is centered around a specific joint area and increases with activity and decreases with rest.
- The accessory motion available at individual spinal segments is diminished.
- Passive ROM is diminished.
- Active ROM is diminished.
- There may be muscular tightness or increased fascial tension in the area of the pain.
- Back movements are asymmetrical when comparing right and left rotation or side bending.

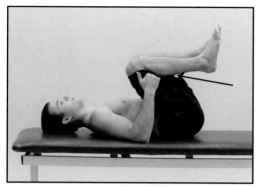

Figure 24-22. Double knee to chest. (A) Stretching—holding posture 15 to 20 seconds. Mobilization can be done using a rhythmic rocking motion within a pain-free ROM.

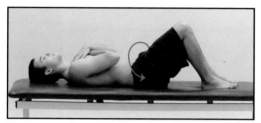

Figure 24-23. Posterior pelvic tilt.

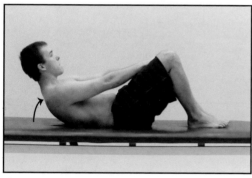

Figure 24-24. Partial sit-up.

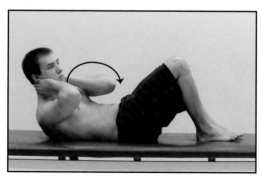

Figure 24-25. Rotation partial sit-up.

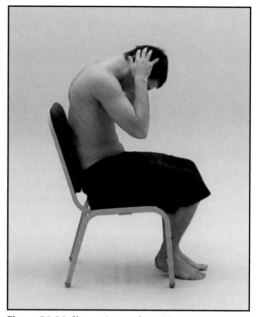

Figure 24-26. Slump sit stretch position.

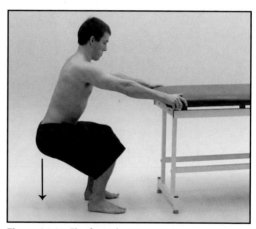

Figure 24-27. Flat-footed squat stretch.

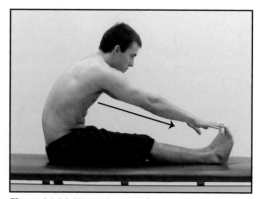

Figure 24-28. Hamstring stretch.

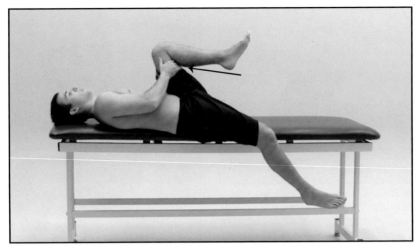

Figure 24-29. Hip flexor stretch.

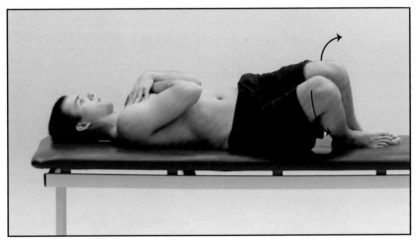

Figure 24-30. Knee rocking side to side.

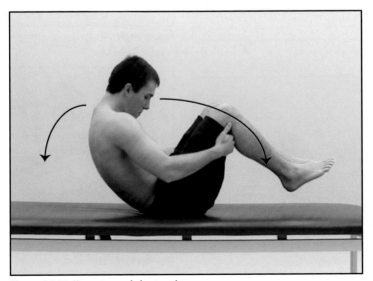

Figure 24-31. Knees toward chest rock.

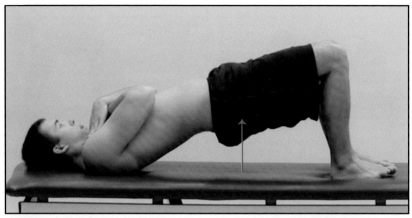

Figure 24-32. Supine hip lift-bridge-rock.

- Forward and backward bending may steer away from the midline.

The efficacy of mobilization is theorized to be from one or a combination of the following effects:

- Tight structures can be stretched to increase the ROM.

- The joint involved is stimulated by the movement to more normal mechanics, and irritation is reduced because of better nutrient–waste exchange.

- Proprioceptive interference occurs with pain perception as the joint movement stimulates normal neural firing whose perception supersedes nocioceptive perception.

Mobilization techniques are multidimensional and are easily adapted to any back pain problem. The mobilizations can be active or passive or assisted by the athletic trainer. All ranges (flexion, extension, side bending, rotation, and accessory) can be incorporated within the exercise plan. The mobilizations can be carried out according to Maitland's grades of oscillation as discussed in Chapter 13. The magnitude of the forces applied can range from grade 1 to grade 4, depending on levels of pain. The theory, technique, and application of the athletic trainer-assisted mobilizations and manipulation are best gained through guided study with an expert practitioner.[52]

Figures 24-30 to 24-39 show the various self-mobilization exercises.

Figures 13-35 to 13-45 show joint mobilizations that can be used by the athletic trainer.

Spinal Joint Manipulation

The research from the mid-1990s through 2000 is clarifying the role of spinal mobilization and manipulation in the overall scheme of back and neck rehabilitation. Treatment algorithms have evolved and the role of mobilization and manipulation techniques are better understood and are taking their rightful place in rehabilitation plans. The literature supports manipulation for the short-term benefits of pain relief and quicker return to functional activities. Long-term results show no detriment to this approach compared to other specific treatment plans. The reverse, however, is true. When manipulation is not included in a population that would benefit, the pain and loss-of-function symptoms last longer and can worsen.[11] This makes the case for including greater use of spinal manipulation in rehabilitation plans than might have previously been used by athletic trainers.[11,15,24,26]

The techniques used are shared among osteopathic, physical therapy, chiropractic, and athletic training disciplines with theoretical rationales for use, and matching certain techniques to certain evaluative findings varying between groups. The basic technique is simple and can be learned and used by any athletic trainer from the undergraduate student to the most experienced practitioner. Figures 24-39, 24-58, and 24-59 show the basic positioning for the athletic trainer and the patient. Once the

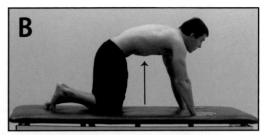

Figure 24-33. Pelvic tilt or pelvic rock. (A) Swayback horse; (B) scared cat.

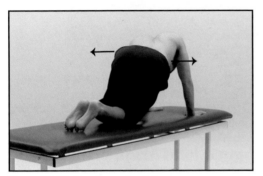

Figure 24-34. Kneeling—dog-tail wags.

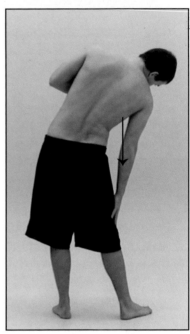

Figure 24-36. Sitting or standing side bending.

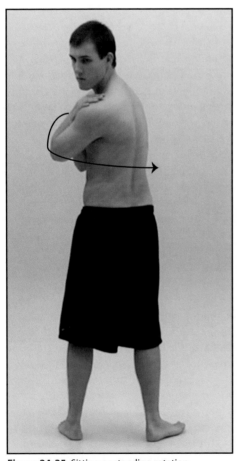

Figure 24-35. Sitting or standing rotation.

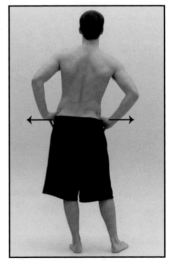

Figure 24-37. Standing hip-shift side to side.

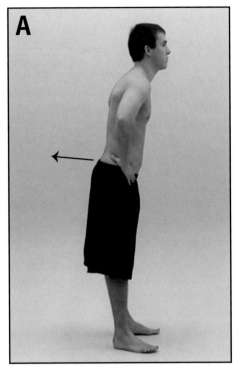 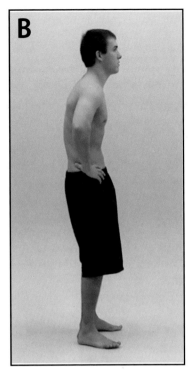

Figure 24-38. Standing pelvic rock. (A) Butt out; (B) tail tuck.

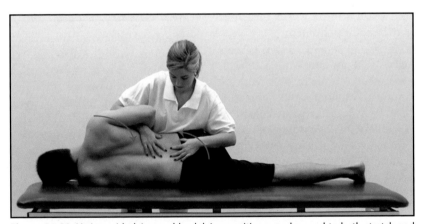

Figure 24-39. Various side-lying and back-lying positions can be used to both stretch and mobilize specific joints in the lumbar area.

positioning is set, the athletic trainer delivers a high velocity, low amplitude thrust mobilization to the lumbar spine or innominate that creates a sudden perturbation of the general lumbar and sacroiliac region. Although there is often an associated popping sound attributed to a cavitation of one or more of the facet joints, the success of the treatment and pain relief mechanisms are not attributed to this sound. The pain relief effect of the manipulation is poorly understood but the action mechanism will likely be multimodal and will include the afferent input to the central nervous system (CNS) and its effect on the endogenous pain control systems.[4,5,16,17,27,47,66,72]

The increased use of a technique adds to increased skill in performance, and security with that particular technique.

The indications for joint manipulation in the lumbar spine and pelvis are as follows:

- Subjectively, the patient's pain is limited to the low back and hip area and does not radiate below the knee.

- The symptoms have a recent onset, less than 16 days since onset.

- One lumbar segment is thought to be hypomobile.

- One hip has limited internal rotation.

- The patient will score low on a fear and avoidance to physical activity and work questionnaire.[89]

The athletic population should have a high proportion of low back pain patients that meets this clinical prediction rule. Manipulation should definitely be included in their rehabilitation plan.

Athletic trainers are usually entry-level care givers for patients with low back pain and are well positioned to use manipulation in the first treatments aimed at reducing back pain and increasing function.[15,23,24,25] If the patient has only three of the above findings, the treatment results might not be as good, but including manipulation would still be worth the effort and would not be contraindicated.

The side effects and potential adverse events are frequently used as contraindication to lumbar spinal manipulation but, in fact, are unproven and in most studies the complaints are musculoskeletal in nature and consist of mild pain, stiffness, and guarding of movements. These changes are usually self-limiting and do not affect the long-term outcome of the patient. The risk for serious complications (disk herniation, cauda equina syndrome) is very low.[8,10,25,73]

REHABILITATION TECHNIQUES FOR LOW BACK PAIN

Low Back Pain

Pathomechanics

In most cases, low back pain does not have serious or long-lasting pathology. It is generally accepted that the soft tissues (ligament, fascia, and muscle) can be the initial pain source.

The patient's response to the injury and to the provocative stresses of evaluation is usually proportional to the time since the injury and the magnitude of the physical trauma of the injury. The soft tissues of the lumbar region should react according to the biological process of healing, and the timelines for healing should be like those for other body parts. There is little substantiation that injury to the low back should cause a pain syndrome that lasts longer than 6 to 8 weeks. Pain avoidance and fear mechanisms are issues that also play a big role in return to activity and require some inclusion in the rehabilitation plan.[19,74,70]

Injury Mechanism

Back pain can result from one or a combination of the following problems: muscle strain, piriformis muscle or quadratus lumborum myofascial pain or strain, myofascial trigger points, lumbar facet joint sprains, hypermobility syndromes, disk-related back problems, or sacroiliac joint dysfunction.

Rehabilitation Concerns

Acute vs Chronic Low Back Pain

The low back pain that most often occurs is an acute, painful experience rarely lasting longer than 3 weeks. As with many injuries, athletic trainers often go through exercise or treatment fads in trying to rehabilitate the patient with low back pain. The latest fad might involve flexion exercise, extension exercise, joint mobilization, dynamic muscular stabilization, abdominal bracing, myofascial release, electrical stimulation protocols, and so on. To keep perspective, as athletic trainers select exercises and modalities, they should keep in mind that 90% of people with back pain get resolution of the symptoms in 6 weeks, regardless of the care administered.[74,89]

There are patients who have pain persisting beyond 6 weeks. This group of patients will generally have a history of reinjury or exacerbation of previous injury. They describe a low back pain that is similar to their previous back pain experience.

These patients are experiencing an exacerbation or reinjury of previously injured tissues by continuing to apply stresses that may have created their original injury. This group of patients needs a more specific and formal treatment and rehabilitation program.[19,74]

There are also people who have chronic low back pain. This is a very small percentage of the population that suffers from low back pain. The difference between the patient with an acute injury or reinjury and a person with chronic pain has been defined by Waddell. He states, "Chronic pain becomes a completely different clinical syndrome from acute pain."[89] Acute and chronic pain not only are different in time scale but are fundamentally different in kind. Acute and experimental pains bear a relatively straightforward relationship to peripheral stimulus, nociception, and tissue damage.

There may be some understandable anxiety about the meaning and consequences of the pain, but acute pain, disability, and illness behavior are generally proportionate to the physical findings. Pharmacological, physical, and even surgical treatments directed to the underlying physical disorder are generally highly effective in relieving acute pain. Chronic pain, disability, and illness behavior, in contrast, become increasingly dissociated from their original physical basis, and there may be little objective evidence of any remaining nociceptive stimulus. Instead, chronic pain and disability become increasingly associated with emotional distress, depression, failed treatment, and adoption of a sick role. Chronic pain progressively becomes a self-sustaining condition that is resistant to traditional medical management. Physical treatment directed to a supposed but unidentified and possibly nonexistent nociceptive source is not only understandably unsuccessful but may also cause additional physical damage. Failed treatment may both reinforce and aggravate pain, distress, disability, and illness behavior.[89]

Rehabilitation Progression

A discussion of the rehabilitation progression for the patient with low back pain can be much more specific and meaningful if treatment plans are grouped into two stages. Stage I (acute stage) treatment consists mainly of the modality treatment and pain-relieving exercises. Stage II treatment involves treating patients with a reinjury or exacerbation of a previous problem. The treatment plan in stage II goes beyond pain relief, strengthening, stretching, and mobilization to include trunk stabilization and movement training sequences and to provide a specific, guided program to return the patient to functional activity.[74,75]

Stage I (Acute Stage) Treatment

Modulating pain should be the initial focus of the athletic trainer. Progressing rapidly from pain management to specific rehabilitation should be a primary goal of the acute stage of the rehabilitation plan. The most common treatment for pain relief in the acute stage is to use ice for analgesia. Rest, but not total bed rest, is used to allow the injured tissues to begin the healing process without the stresses that created the injury. If the patient fits the clinical prediction rules for spinal manipulation, this should be initiated as soon as the patient can tolerate the positioning.[25]

Along with rest, during the initial treatment stage, the patient should be taught to increase comfort by using the appropriate body positioning techniques described previously, which may involve (1) lateral shift corrections (Figure 24-11); (2) extension exercises (Figures 24-13 to 24-20); (3) flexion exercises (Figures 24-21 to 24-31); (4) self-mobilization exercises (see Figures 13-46 and 13-47); or (5) spinal manipulation (Figures 24-39 and Figure 24-58). Segmental spinal stabilization exercise should be initiated concurrently with these other exercises. Outside support, in the form of corsets and the use of props or pillows to enhance comfortable positions, also needs to be included in the initial pain-management phase of treatment.[74,89] The patient should also be taught to avoid positions and movements that increase any sharp, painful episodes. The limits of these movements and positions that provide comfort should be the initial focus of any exercises.

The patient should be encouraged to move through this stage quickly and return to activity as soon as range, strength, and comfort will allow. The addition of a supportive corset during this stage should be based mostly on patient comfort. We suggest using an eclectic approach to the selection of the exercises, mixing the various protocols described according to the findings of the patient's evaluation. Rarely will a patient present with classic signs and symptoms that will dictate using one variety of exercise.

Stage II (Reinjury Stage) Treatment

In the reinjury or chronic stage of back rehabilitation, the goals of the treatment and training should again be based on a thorough evaluation of the patient. Identifying the causes of the patient's back problem and recurrences is very important in the management of his or her rehabilitation and prevention of reinjury. A goal for this stage of care is to make the patient responsible for the management of his or her back problem. The athletic trainer should identify specific problems and corrections that will help the patient better understand the mechanisms and management of the problem.[74]

Specific goals and exercises should be identified about the following:

- Which structures to stretch.

- Which structures to strengthen.

- Incorporating segmental spinal stabilization and abdominal bracing into the patient's daily life and exercise routine.

- Progression of core stabilization exercises.

- Which movements need a motor learning approach to control faulty mechanics.[74]

Stretching

The therapist and the patient need to plan specific exercises to stretch restricted groups, maintain flexibility in normal muscle groups, and identify hypermobility that may be a part of the problem. In planning, instructing, and monitoring each exercise, adequate thought and good instruction must be used to ensure that the intended structures are stretched and areas of hypermobility are protected from overstretching.[37] Inadequate stabilization will lead to exercise movements that are so general that the exercise will encourage hyperflexibility at already hypermobile areas. Lack of proper stabilization during stretching may help perpetuate a structural problem that will continue to add to the patient's back pain.

In the athletic trainer's evaluation of the patient with back pain, the following muscle groups should be assessed for flexibility[44]:

- Hip flexors;

- Hamstrings;

- Low back extensors;

- Lumbar rotators;

- Lumbar lateral flexors;

- Hip adductors;

- Hip abductors;

- Hip rotators.

Strengthening

There are numerous techniques for strengthening the muscles of the trunk and hip. Muscles are perhaps best strengthened by using techniques of progressive overload to achieve specific adaptation to imposed demands (the SAID principle). The overload can take the form of increased weight load, increased holding time, increased repetition load, or increased stretch load to accomplish physiologic changes in muscle strength, muscle endurance, or flexibility of a body part.[21]

The treatment plan should call for an exercise that the patient can easily accomplish successfully. Rapidly but gradually, the overload should push the patient to challenge the muscle group needing strengthening. The athletic trainer and the patient should monitor continuously for increases in the patient's pain or recurrences of previous symptoms. If those changes occur, the exercises should be modified, delayed, or eliminated from the rehabilitation plan.[46,74]

Core Stabilization

Core stabilization training, dynamic abdominal bracing, and finding the neutral position all describe a technique used to increase the stability of the trunk (see Chapter 5). This increased stability will enable the patient to maintain the spine and pelvis in the most comfortable and acceptable mechanical position that will control the forces of repetitive microtrauma and protect the structures of the back from further damage. Core muscular control is one key to giving patients the ability to stabilize their trunk and control their posture. Abdominal strengthening routines are rigorous, and the patient must complete them with vigor. However, in their functional activities, the patients need to take advantage of their abdominal strength to stabilize the trunk and protect the back.[36,53,76]

Richardson et al focus attention on motor control of the transversus abdominis and

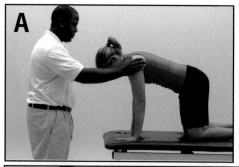

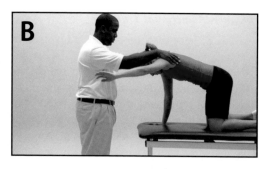

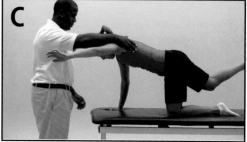

Figure 24-40. Weight shifting and stabilization exercises should progress from (A) quadruped, to (B) triped, to (C) biped.

lumbar multifidii in various positions.[41,74] Once this control is established, different positions and movements are added. As the vigor of the exercise is progressively increased, the patient will incorporate the more global muscles in stabilizing his or her core (see Chapter 5). Then the patient moves into the functional exercise progression with the spinal segment stabilization as the base movement in core stabilization, which is needed to perform functionally.[74] The concept of increasing trunk stability with muscle contractions that support and limit the extremes of spinal movement is important.

Basic Functional Training

Patients must be constantly committed to improving body mechanics and trunk control in all postures in their activities of daily living. The athletic trainer needs to evaluate the patients' daily patterns and give them instruction, practice, and monitoring on the best and least stressful body mechanics in as many activities as possible.

The basic program follows the developmental sequence of posture control, starting with supine and prone extremity movement while actively stabilizing the trunk. The patient is then progressed to all fours, kneeling, and standing (Figure 24-40).

Emphasis on trunk control and stability is maintained as the patient works through this exercise sequence.[36,55,74]

The most critical aspect for developing motor control is repetition of exercise. However, variability in positioning, speed of movement, and changes in movement patterns must also be incorporated. The variability of the exercise will allow patients to generalize their newly learned trunk control to the constant changes necessary in their movements. The basic exercise, transversus abdominis and lumbar multifidii coactivation, is the key. Incorporating this stabilization contraction into various activities helps reinforce trunk stabilization and returns trunk control to a subconscious automatic response.

The use of augmented feedback (EMG, palpation, ultrasound imagery, pressure gauges) of the transversus abdominus and lumbar multifidii contractions may be needed early in the exercise plan to help maximize the results of each exercise session supervised by the athletic trainer. The athletic trainer should have the patient internalize this feedback as quickly as possible to make the patient apparatus-free and more functional. With augmented feedback, it is recommended that the patient be rapidly and progressively weaned from dependency on external feedback.

Advanced Functional Training

Each activity that the patient is involved in becomes part of the advanced exercise rehabilitation plan. The usual place to start is with the patient's strength and conditioning program. Each step of the program is monitored, and emphasis is placed on spinal segmental stabilization for even the simple task of putting the weights on a bar or getting on and off exercise equipment. Each exercise in their strength and conditioning program should be retaught, and patients are made aware of their best mechanical position and the proper stabilizing muscular contraction. The strength program is patient-specific, attempting to strengthen weak areas and improve strength in muscle groups needed for better function.[74]

The patients should be taught to start their stabilizing contractions before starting any movement. This presets their posture and stabilization awareness before their movement takes place. As the movement occurs, they will become less aware of the stabilization contraction as they attempt to complete an exercise.

They might revert to old postures and habits, so feedback is important.

Each patient is different, not only with the individual back problem but also with the abilities to gain motor skill and to overcome the fear and avoidance associated with chronic back pain.[89] Patients differ in degree of control and in the speed at which they acquire these new skills of core stabilization.

Reducing stress to the back by using braces, orthotics, shoes, or comfortable supportive furniture (beds, desks, or chairs) is essential to help patients minimize chronic or overload stresses to their back. The stabilization exercise should also be incorporated into their activities of daily living.[60] Use of a low back corset or brace may also make the patient more comfortable (Figure 24-56).

Criteria for Return

For most low back problems the stage I treatment and exercise programs will get patients back into their activities quickly. If the pain or dysfunction is pronounced or the problem becomes recurrent, an in-depth evaluation and treatment using stage I and stage II exercise protocols will be necessary. The team approach, with patient, doctor, and athletic trainer working together, will provide the comprehensive approach needed to manage the patient's back problem. Close attention to and emphasis on the patient's progress will provide both the patient and the athletic trainer with the encouragement to continue this program.

Muscular Strains

Injury Mechanism

Evaluative findings include a history of sudden or chronic stress that initiates pain in a muscular area during the workout. There are three points on the physical examination that must be positive to indicate the muscle as the primary problem. There will be tenderness to palpation in the muscular area; the muscular pain will be provoked with contraction and with stretch of the involved muscle.

Rehabilitation Progression

The treatment should include the standard protection, ice, and compression. Ice may be applied in the form of ice massage or ice bags, depending on the area involved. An elastic wrap or corset would protect and compress the back musculature. Additional modalities would include pulsed ultrasound for a biostimulative effect and electrical stimulation for pain relief and muscle reeducation. The exercises used in rehabilitation should make the involved muscle contract and stretch, starting with very mild exercise and progressively increasing the intensity and repetition loads. In general this would include active extension exercises such as hip lifts (Figures 24-17 to 24-19), alternate arm and leg, hip extension (Figure 24-15), trunk extension (Figure 24-20), and quadratus hip hike exercises (Figures 24-41 to 24-43). A good series of abdominal spinal segmental stabilization and core stabilization exercises would also be helpful (Figures 24-23 and 24-24). Stretching exercises might include the following: knee to chest (Figures 24-21 and 24-22), side-lying leg hang to stretch the hip flexors (Figure 24-29), slump sitting (Figure 24-26), and knee rocking side to side (Figure 24-30).

Criteria for Return

Initially, patients may wish to continue to use a brace or corset, but they should be

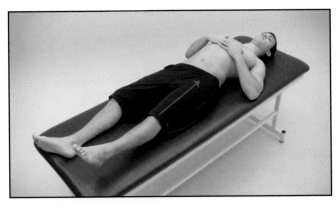

Figure 24-41. Back-lying—hip-hike shifting.

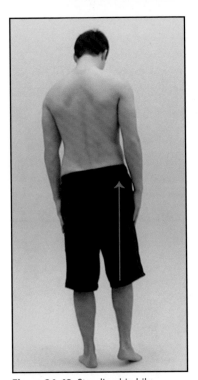

Figure 24-42. Standing hip hike.

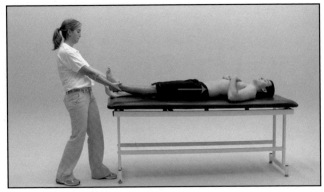

Figure 24-43. Back-lying—hip-hike resisted.

encouraged to do away with the corset as their back strengthens and their performance returns to normal.[21,46]

Piriformis Muscle Strain

Pathomechanics

Piriformis syndrome was discussed in detail in Chapter 20. The piriformis muscle refers pain to the posterior sacroiliac region, to the buttocks, and sometimes down the posterior or postero-lateral thigh. The pain is usually described as a deep ache that can get more intense with exercise and with sitting with the hips flexed, adducted, and medially rotated. The pain gets sharper and more intense with activities that require decelerating medial hip and leg rotation during weight bearing.[7]

Tenderness to palpation has a characteristic pattern, with tenderness medial and proximal to the greater trochanter and just lateral to the posterior superior iliac spine (PSIS). Isometric abduction in the sitting position produces pain in the posterior hip buttock area, and the movement will be weak or hesitant. Passive hip internal rotation in the sitting position will also bring on posterior hip and buttock pain.[62]

Rehabilitation Progression

Rehabilitation exercises should include both strengthening and stretching.[7,62] Strengthening exercises should include prone lying hip internal rotation with elastic resistance (Figure 24-44), hip-lift bridges (Figure 24-45), hand-knee position fire hydrant exercise (Figure 24-46), side-lying hip abduction straight leg raises (Figure 24-47), and prone hip extension exercise (Figure 24-48).

Figure 24-44. Prone-lying hip internal rotation with elastic resistance.

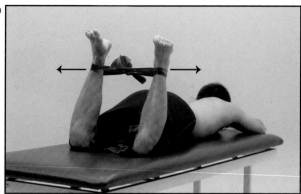

Figure 24-45. Hip-lift bridges.

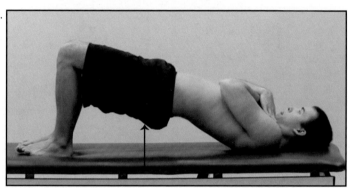

Figure 24-46. Hand-knee position—fire hydrant exercise.

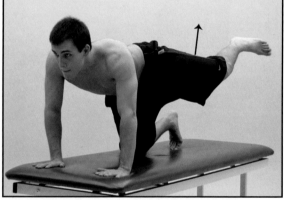

Stretching exercises for the piriformis include back-lying legs-crossed hip adduction stretch (Figure 24-49); back-lying with the involved leg crossed over the uninvolved leg, ankle to knee position, pulling the uninvolved knee toward the chest to create the stretch (Figure 24-50); and contract-relax-stretch with elbow pressure to the muscle insertion during the relaxation phase (Figures 24-51A and B).[48,80,83] This can also be done in the sitting position with the same mechanics, but the patient leans over at the waist and brings the chest toward the knee.

Quadratus Lumborum Strain

Pathomechanics

Pain from the quadratus lumborum muscle is described as an aching, sharp pain located in the flank, in the lateral back area, and near the posterior sacroiliac region and upper buttocks. The patient usually describes pain on moving from sitting to standing, standing for long periods, coughing, sneezing, and walking. Activities requiring trunk rotation or side

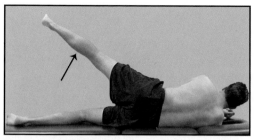

Figure 24-47. Side-lying hip abduction straight-leg raises.

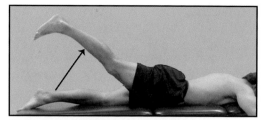

Figure 24-48. Prone hip extension exercise.

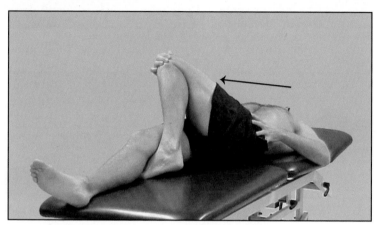

Figure 24-49. Back-lying legs-crossed hip adduction stretch.

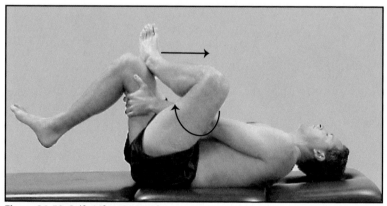

Figure 24-50. Self piriformis stretch.

bending aggravate the pain. The muscle is tender to palpation near the origin along the lower ribs and along the insertion on the iliac crest. Pain will be aggravated on side bending, and the pain will usually be localized to one side. For example, with a right quadratus problem, side bending right and left would provoke only right-side pain. Supine hip-hiking movements would also provoke the pain.

Rehabilitation Progression

Rehabilitation strengthening exercise should include back-lying hip-hike shifting (Figure 24-54), standing with one leg on elevated surface and the other free to move below that level, hip-hike on the free side (Figure 24-55), and back-lying hip-hike resisted by pulling on the involved leg (Figure 24-43).

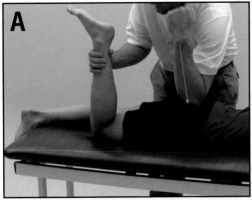
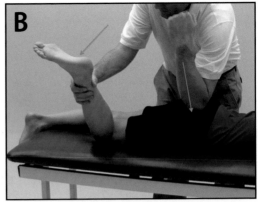

Figure 24-51. Piriformis stretch using elbow pressure. (A) Start-contract; (B) relaxation-stretch.

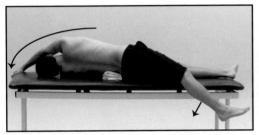

Figure 24-52. Side-lying stretch over pillow roll.

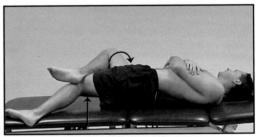

Figure 24-53. Supine self-stretch—legs crossed.

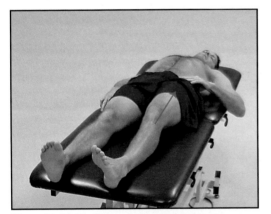

Figure 24-54. Hip-hike exercise with hand pressure.

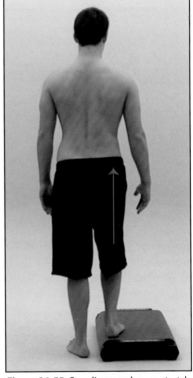

Figure 24-55. Standing one-leg-up stretch.

Stretching exercises should include side-lying over a pillow roll leg-hand stretch (Figure 24-52), supine self-stretch with legs crossed (Figure 24-53), hip-hike exercise with hand pressure to increase stretch (Figure 24-54), and standing one leg on a small book stretch (Figure 24-55).[90]

Myofascial Pain and Trigger Points

Pathomechanics and Injury Mechanism

The previous examples of muscle-oriented back pain in both the piriformis and quadratus lumborum could also have a myofascial origin. The major component in successfully changing myofascial pain is stretching the muscle back to a normal resting length. The muscle irritation and congestion that create the trigger points are relieved and normal blood flow resumes, further reducing the irritants in the area. Stretching through a painful trigger point is difficult.

A variety of comfort and counterirritant modalities can be used preliminary to, during, and after the stretching to enhance the effect of the exercise. Some of the methods used successfully are dry needling, local anesthetic injection, ice massage, friction massage, acupressure massage, ultrasound electrical stimulation, extracorporeal shock wave therapy, and cold sprays.[45]

The indications for treating low back pain with myofascial stretching and treatment techniques are as follows[45]:

1. Subjectively, muscle soreness and fatigue from repetitive motions are common antecedent mechanisms. Patients are also susceptible as fatigue and stress overload specific muscle groups. There may be a history of sudden onset during or shortly after an acute overload stress, or there may be a gradual onset with repetitive or postural overload of the affected muscle. The pain may be an incapacitating event in the case of acute onset, but it may also be a nagging, aggravating type of pain with an intensity that varies from an awareness of discomfort to a severe unrelenting type of pain. The pain location is usually a referred pain area remote from the actual myofascial trigger point. These trigger points can be present but quiescent until they are activated by overload, fatigue, trauma, or chilling. These points are called latent trigger points. This deep, aching pain can be specifically localized, but the patient is not sensitive to palpation in these areas. This pain can often be reproduced by maintaining pressure on a hypersensitive myofascial trigger point.

2. Passive or active stretching of the affected myofascial structure increases pain.

3. The stretch range of muscle is restricted.

4. The pain is increased when the muscle is contracted against a fixed resistance or the muscle is allowed to contract into an extremely shortened range. The pain in this case is described as a muscle cramping pain.

5. The muscle may be slightly weak.

6. Trigger points may be located within a taut band of the muscle. If taut bands are found during palpation, explore them for local hypersensitive areas.

7. Pressure on the hypersensitive area will often cause a "jump sign"; as the athletic trainer strums the sensitive area, the patient's muscle involuntarily jumps in response.

8. The primary muscle groups that create low back pain in patients are the quadratus lumborum and the piriformis muscles.[48,80,81,83]

Simons and Travell have devoted two volumes to the causes and treatment of various myofascial pains.[80,81] They have done a very thorough job of describing the symptoms and signs of each area of the body, and they give very specific guidance on exercises and positioning in their treatment protocols.

Rehabilitation Technique

Myofascial trigger points may be treated using the following steps:

1. Position the patient comfortably but in a position that will lead him or her to stretching the involved muscle group.

2. Caution the patient to use mild progressive stretches rather than sudden, sharp, hard stretches.

3. Hot pack the area for 10 minutes, and follow with an ultrasound and electrical stimulation treatment over the affected muscle.

4. Use an ice cup, and use two to three slow strokes starting at the trigger point and moving in one direction toward the pain reference area and over the full length of the muscle.

5. Begin stretching well within the patient's comfort. A stretch should be maintained for a minimum of 15 seconds. The stretch should be released until the patient is comfortable again. The next stretch repetition should then be progressively more intense if tolerated, and the position of the stretch should also be varied slightly. Repeat the stretch 4 to 6 times.

6. Hot pack the area, and have the patient go through some active stretches of the muscle.

7. Refer to Simons and Travell's manual for specific references on other muscle groups.[48,80,81]

8. Soft tissue mobilization and positional release techniques are used to treat and resolve trigger points (see Chapter 8). Therapeutic eccentric active massage has shown some clinical success. In this technique, the muscle for fascia associated with the identified trigger point is actively contracted to its shortest possible length. Using a small amount of lubricant, the active trigger point is compressed with a firm steady pressure. The athletic trainer provides resistance to the shortened muscle, and the patient is instructed to continue to resist but also allow the eccentric lengthening of the muscle to occur in a smooth, controlled manner. As the muscle lengthens under the compressive massage, the trigger point is compressed and the irritants in the area are dispersed over a greater area. This helps the pain decrease, and the muscle begins to function more normally.

The first repetition is usually uncomfortable for the patient. Subsequent repetitions are more comfortable and the patient can control the contraction better. Six to eight repetitions are used for each trigger point treated. This technique is empirically based, and research studies are needed to establish their validity.

> **Clinical Decision-Making Exercise 24-1**
>
> A basketball player has been having tightness in the low back and right hip region. After a regular workout without any known trauma, the patient started to have an intense ache in the right buttock area. The next day, pain is radiating laterally across the buttock and down the posterior thigh. There are two distinct tender areas lateral to the sacrum that reproduce the patient's pain. What strategies can the athletic trainer use to reduce the patient's discomfort? Should the patient continue to train?

Lumbar Facet Joint Sprains

Pathomechanics and Injury Mechanism

Sprains may occur in any of the ligaments in the lumbar spine. However, the most common sprain involves lumbar facet joints. Facet joint sprain typically occurs when bending forward and twisting while lifting or moving some object. The patients will report a sudden acute episode that caused the problem, or they will give a history of a chronic repetitive stress that caused the gradual onset of a pain that got progressively worse with continuing activity. The pain is local to the structure that has been injured, and the patient can clearly localize the area. The pain is described as a sore pain that gets sharper in response to certain movements or postures. The pain is located centrally or just lateral to the spinous process areas and is deep.

Local symptoms will occur in response to movements, and the patient will usually limit the movement in those ranges that are painful. When the vertebra is moved passively with a posterior–anterior or rotational pressure through the spinous process, the pain may be provoked.

Rehabilitation Progression

The treatment should include the standard protection, ice, and compression as mentioned previously. Both pulsed ultrasound and electrical stimulation could also be used similarly to the treatment of muscle strains but localized to the specific joint area.

Joint mobilization using posterior–anterior glides (see Figure 13-36) and rotational glides (see Figures 13-38 and 13-39) should help reduce pain and increase joint nutrition. The patient should be instructed in segmental spinal stabilization exercises using transversus abdominis and lumbar multifidii coactivation and good postural control (Figures 24-3 through 24-10). Strengthening exercises for abdominals (Figures 24-23 through 24-25) and back extensors (Figures 24-17 through 24-20) should initially be limited to a pain-free range. Stretching in all ranges should start well within a comfort range and gradually increase until trunk movements reach normal ranges. Patients should be supported with a corset or range-limiting brace, which should be used only temporarily until normal strength, muscle control, and pain-free range are achieved.[21,51,52,85,86] It is important to guard against the development of postural changes that might occur in response to pain.

Hypermobility Syndromes (Spondylolysis/Spondylolisthesis)

Pathomechanics

Hypermobility of the low back may be attributed to spondylolysis or spondylolisthesis. Spondylolysis involves a degeneration of the vertebrae and, more commonly, a defect in the pars interarticularis of the articular processes of the vertebrae.[58] This condition is often attributed to a congenital weakness, with the defect occurring as a stress fracture. Spondylolysis may produce no symptoms unless a disk herniation occurs or there is sudden trauma such as hyperextension. Commonly spondylolysis begins unilaterally. However, if it extends bilaterally, there may be some slipping of one vertebra on the one below it. A spondylolisthesis is considered to be a complication of spondylolysis often resulting in hypermobility of a vertebral segment.[23] Spondylolisthesis has the highest incidence with L5 slipping on S1.[58]

Injury Mechanism

Movements that characteristically hyperextend the spine are most likely to cause this condition.[58]

Rehabilitation Concerns

Patients usually have a relatively long history of feeling "something go" in their back. They complain of a low back pain described as a persistent ache across the back (belt type). This pain does not usually interfere with their workout performance but is usually worse when fatigued or after sitting in a slumped posture for an extended time. Patients may also complain of a tired feeling in the low back. They describe the need to move frequently and get temporary relief of pain through self-manipulation. They often describe self-manipulative behavior more than 10 times a day. Their pain is relieved by rest, and they do not usually feel the pain during exercise. On physical examination, patients usually will have full and painless trunk movements, but there may be a wiggle or hesitation in forward bending at the midrange. On backward bending, movement may appear to hinge at one spinal segment. When extremes of range are maintained for 15 to 30 seconds, patient feel a lumbo-sacral ache. On return from forward bending, patients will use thigh climbing to regain the neutral position. On palpation there may be tenderness localized to one spinal segment.[58,65]

Rehabilitation Progression

Patients with this problem will fall into the reinjury stage of back pain and may require extensive treatment to regain stability of the trunk. The patient's pain should be treated symptomatically. Initially, bracing and occasionally bed rest for 1 to 3 days will help reduce pain. The major focus in rehabilitation should be on segmental spinal stabilization exercises that control or stabilize the hypermobile segment (Figures 24-3 through 24-10). Progressive trunk-strengthening exercises, especially through the midrange, should be incorporated. Core stabilization exercises that concentrate on transversus abdominis behavior and endurance should also be used (see Chapter 5).[40,41,43,54,61,63,67-69] The patient should avoid manipulation and self-manipulation, as well as stretching and flexibility exercises. Corsets and braces are beneficial if the patient uses them only for support during higher-level activities

Figure 24-56. A lower-lumbar corset or brace.

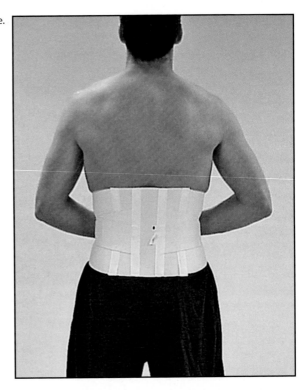

and for short (1 to 2 hour) periods to help with pain relief and fatigue (Figure 24-56).[36,74] Hypermobility of a lumbar vertebrae may make the patient more susceptible to lumbar muscle strains and ligament sprains. Thus it may be necessary for the patient to avoid vigorous activity. The use of a low back corset or brace may also make the patient more comfortable (Figure 24-56).[39]

Clinical Decision-Making Exercise 24-2

A female gymnast arrives at your school with a previously diagnosed spondylolysis at L5-S1. The patient has had periodic problems with back pain and has not been on a formal program to rehabilitate her back. What program should the athletic trainer recommend for this patient?

Disk-Related Back Pain

Pathomechanics

The lumbar disks are subject to constant abnormal stresses stemming from faulty body mechanics, trauma, or both, which, over time, can cause degeneration, tears, and cracks in the annulus fibrosus.[14] The disk most often injured lies between the L4 and L5 vertebrae. The L5-S1 disk is the second most commonly affected.[82]

Injury Mechanism

The mechanism of a disk injury is the same as that for the lumbosacral sprain–forward bending and twisting that places abnormal strain on the lumbar region. The movement that produces herniation or bulging of the nucleus pulposus may be minimal, and associated pain may be significant. Besides injuring soft tissues, such a stress may herniate an already degenerated disk by causing the nucleus pulposus to protrude into or through the annulus fibrosis. As the disk progressively degenerates, a prolapsed disk may develop in which the nucleus moves completely through the annulus.

REHABILITATION PLAN

TREATMENT OF DISK-RELATED BACK PAIN

Injury situation: A 31-year-old mother was attempting to put her 2-year-old daughter in the child restraint seat of her minivan. After picking up the child, she bent forward and twisted to get the child into the seat and felt immediate intense pain in her low back and down the back of her right leg. Her right leg gave way, and she collapsed to the floor with back and right-leg pain. She was referred to an athletic trainer for evaluation and treatment by a family practice physician.

Functionally she was very guarded and stiff-looking. On forward bending, she was very guarded and used compensating movement patterns to move from sit to stand or standing to lying down. Lumbar spine forward bending and right straight-leg raising provoked central back pain that radiated into her right posterior thigh. Backward bending provoked central pain and was restricted at 50% of normal range. Sitting knee extension movement with the right leg provoked central pain and posterior thigh pain when the knee flexion angle reached 60 degrees. Dorsiflexion at the ankle and chin to chest movement increased this pain. Posterior–anterior mobilizations to the sacrum and the L5 spinous process increased central back pain and caused some shooting pain down the right leg. On manual muscle test, trunk extension was strong and painless. Left hip extension and left hip internal rotation and external rotation were strong but provoked right posterior leg pain. A sensory check demonstrated normal feeling over both lower extremities. On palpation, she was non-tender over all major structures.

PHASE ONE: Acute Phase

GOALS: Decrease pain, encourage rest, maintain spinal segment stability, and create safe, pain-free movement behaviors that minimize the stress on the disk complex.

Estimated length of time (ELT) Days 1 to 3 The patient was treated with 3 days of relative bed rest. She was encouraged to work on spinal segment stability exercises, knees toward chest, and knee-rocking mobilizations while in a flat-lying position (supine, side-lying, or prone). Multiple bouts of the 90/90 position and prone-on-elbows position were used for their positional traction benefit. Activities of daily living were kept to a necessary level—remain at home, avoid sitting posture. Standing and walking for brief periods (less than 10 minutes) were allowed. The physician prescribed analgesic and anti-inflammatory medications.

PHASE TWO: Intermediate Phase

GOALS: Decrease pain, encourage motion. Encourage rest positions that enhance centralization of the disk nucleus and provide optimum nourishment for the disk complex.

Estimated length of time (ELT): Day 4 to week 4 After 3 days, the patient was encouraged to come to the physical therapy clinic for treatment, once a day. The above activities were preceded with the comfort modalities of hot packs and electrical stimulation. Spinal segment stabilization was reassessed, and the patient started on the beginning-level core stability exercises. The patient was instructed to be flat-lying for 20 to 30 minutes four times daily and to continue to minimize time spent in sitting postures. At 1 week, the patient was encouraged to walk for conditioning and movement purposes, starting with 10 minutes and working up to 30 minutes. The walking was followed by flat-lying and positional traction periods of 20 to 30 minutes. The core stability exercises were gradually progressed to continue to challenge strength and endurance as the pain became more manageable. At 3 weeks, more functional exercises were included. Squats, balance activities, and light weight lifting (no axial loading) were begun. Flat-lying postures, 4 times daily, were encouraged. At 4 weeks, the patient was instructed to gradually increase sitting times, guided by comfort.

PHASE THREE: Advanced Phase

GOALS: Maximize core stability strength and endurance, retrain functional movement patterns to include spinal segment and core stability, return normal flexibility and strength to lower extremities, and encourage good mechanics in activities of daily living.

Estimated length of time (ELT): Week 5 to 6 months The patient was reevaluated, and specific flexibility and strengthening problems were identified. Tight muscle groups were stretched 3 or 4 times a day, weak muscle groups were isolated and progressively strengthened. Spinal segment stability and core stability were stressed with more challenging exercises. Normal strength and conditioning exercises were encouraged, but technique was monitored closely, and the patient was encouraged to use spinal segment stability coactivation patterns in every exercise. Functional activities of daily living drills were begun, with the patient being encouraged to incorporate spinal segment co-activation patterns into her motor planning for each drill.

Criteria for Return to Function

1. The patient demonstrates good spinal segment control in the physical therapy clinic.
2. The patient has normal flexibility and strength in her lower extremities.
3. Functional performance test scores are at least 90% of previous baseline scores.
4. The patient tolerates 1 to 1.5 hours of exercise with no system.
5. The patient demonstrates in exercises that she can perform the activities of daily living with no noticeable compensatory movement patterns.

If the nucleus moves into the spinal canal and comes in contact with a nerve root, this is referred to as an extruded disk. This protrusion of the nucleus pulposus may place pressure on the spinal cord or spinal nerves, causing radiating pains similar to those of sciatica, as occurs in piriformis syndrome. If the material of the nucleus separates from the disk and begins to migrate, a sequestrated disk exists.[82]

Rehabilitation Concerns

Patients will report a centrally located pain that radiates unilaterally or spreads across the back. They may describe a sudden or gradual onset that becomes particularly severe after they have rested and then tried to resume their activities. They may complain of tingling or numb feelings in a dermatomal pattern or sciatic radiation. Forward bending and sitting postures increase their pain. The patient's symptoms are usually worse in the morning on first arising and get better through the day. Coughing and sneezing may increase their pain.[82]

On physical examination, the patient will have a hip-shifted, forward-bent posture. On active movements, side bending toward the hip shift is painful and limited. Side bending away from the shift is more mobile and does not provoke the pain. Forward bending is very limited and painful, and guarding is very apparent. On palpation, there may be tenderness around the painful area. Posterior–anterior pressure over the involved segment increases the pain. Passive straight-leg raising will increase the back or leg pain during the first 30 degrees of hip flexion. Bilateral knee-to-chest movement will increase the back pain. Neurological testing (strength, sensory reflex) may be positive for differences between right and left.[82]

Rehabilitation Progression

The patient should be treated initially with pain-reducing modalities (ice, electrical stimulation, rest). The athletic trainer should then use the lateral shift correction (Figure 24-11), followed by a gentle extension exercise (Figure 24-16). The patient is then sent home with the following rest and home-exercise program.

The patient must commit to resting in a flat-lying position three to four times a day for 20 to 30 minutes. During that time, the patient can use some prone press-up extension exercises, holding the stretched position for 15 to 20 seconds for each repetition (Figures 24-13 and 24-14). Another recommended pain-relieving position is the 90/90 position—90 degrees of hip flexion and 90 degrees of knee

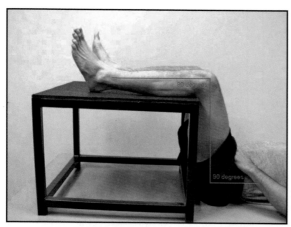

Figure 24-57. The 90-90 position. The patient is positioned back-lying with hips flexed to 90 degrees and knees supported at 90 degrees by stool or pillows.

flexion (Figure 24-57). Both of these exercises provide very mild traction to the lumbar spine that enhances the centralization and nourishment effect of the flat-lying position on the disk, which in turn leads to decreased pain and increased function. Segmental spinal stabilization exercises can also be incorporated into the rest positions and may be used concurrently with other modalities (Figures 24-3 through 24-10).[87]

The goal is to reduce the disk protrusion and restore normal posture. When posture, pain, and segmental spinal control return to normal, the core stabilization exercises should be emphasized and progressed. The patient may recover easily from the first episode, but if repeated episodes occur, the patient should start on the reinjury stage of back rehabilitation.

When the patient changes positions—sit to stand or lying to stand— he or she should do a lateral shift self-correction (Figures 24-12 and

24-16), followed by a segmental spinal coactivation contraction (Figures 24-8 through 24-10). Some gentle flexion exercises, low back corsets, and heat wraps may make the patient more comfortable.

If the disk is extruded or sequestrated, about the only thing that can be done is to modulate pain with electrical stimulation. Flexion exercises and lying supine in a flexed position may help with comfort. The use of a low back corset or brace may also make the patient more comfortable (Figure 24-56). Sometimes the symptoms will resolve with time. But if there are signs of nerve damage, surgery may be necessary.[87]

Clinical Decision-Making Exercise 24-4

A wrestler has recently recovered from disk-related back pain and is entering the strength and functional recovery part of the rehabilitation process. What are the important factors to consider to prevent a recurrence of his problem?

Sacroiliac Joint Dysfunction

Pathomechanics and Injury Mechanism

A sprain of the sacroiliac joint may result from twisting with both feet on the ground, stumbling forward, falling backward, stepping too far down and landing heavily on one leg, or forward bending with the knees locked during lifting.[51] Activities involving unilateral forceful movements are the usual activities associated

---

Clinical Decision-Making Exercise 24-3

A crew rower has been having central low back pain since the third week of the season. There are two weeks of the regular season and two weeks of championships left for this season. Recently she has experienced some parasthesia in the L5 and S1 dermatomes of her right leg. Neurological tests (reflex, strength, sensory) are all equal to her other leg. An MRI shows a disk herniation at L5 that is not compromising the nerve root. Her major findings are central lumbar spine discomfort, some stiffness on forward bending, and tingling sensations in the right leg. Should this patient continue to participate for the remainder of the season?

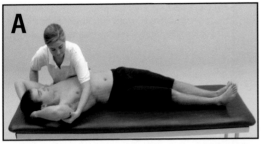 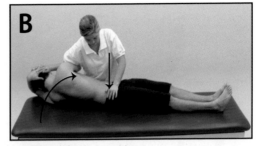

Figure 24-58. Posterior innominate rotation. (A) Starting position; (B) mobilization position.

with the onset of pain. Any of these mechanisms can produce stretching and irritation of the sacroiliac, sacrotuberous, or sacrospinous ligaments.[54]

Rehabilitation Concerns

The patient will report a dull, achy back pain near or medial to the PSIS, with some associated muscle guarding. The pain may radiate into the buttocks or posterior lateral thigh. The patient may describe a heaviness, dullness, or deadness in the leg or referred pain to the groin, adductor, or hamstring on the same side. The pain may be more noticeable during the stance phase of walking, on stair climbing, and rolling in bed.[91]

Side bending toward the painful side will increase the pain. Straight-leg raising will increase pain in the sacroiliac joint area after 45 degrees of hip motion. On palpation, there may be tenderness over the PSIS, medial to the PSIS, in the muscles of the buttocks, and anteriorly over the pubic symphysis. The back musculature will have increased tone on one side.[29,44,70]

If a sacroiliac joint is stressed and reaches an end-range position in rotation, the joint can become dysfunctional as pain, mechanical form-closure locking, and/or muscle guarding create hypomobility at the joint. This hypomobility is usually temporary, and often spontaneous repositioning will occur. This allows the pain to go away and muscle guarding to disappear. With the joint back to normal alignment, function returns to normal.[44,70]

When normal alignment does not spontaneously return, treatment efforts should initially mobilize or manipulate the joints and then work on spinal segment stabilization to maintain and improve sacroiliac joint stability. These exercises, along with core stability training are the key to preventing recurrences. The athletic trainer should consider sacroiliac dysfunction as a problem with pelvic stability rather than mobility.[44,68]

Rehabilitation Progression

Recent studies of sacroiliac joint testing cast severe doubt on our ability to recognize the postural asymmetries that have been associated with directionally specific techniques.[29,44,70] The treatment of sacroiliac dysfunction has been grounded in the empiricism of performing techniques that reduce pain. Postural asymmetries have given the athletic trainer a starting point for directionally specific techniques, but the instruction in deciding on appropriate technique is to try one and, if the outcome is not satisfactory, move on to the next technique, which may be biomechanically opposite to the first technique.[21,54] Empirically, these mobilizations have been used for many years and have demonstrated a good effect on sacroiliac dysfunctions with an asymmetry of the pelvis and pain. Each technique will have about the same effect on the pelvis and sacroiliac joints because the joints are part of an arch, and forces at any point in the arch can be translated throughout the structure to the affected part of the arch. These stretches should be used only at the beginning stage of treatment to free the joint from the initial hypomobility.[91]

A posterior innominate rotation may be used to treat sacroiliac dysfunction (Figure 24-58). The patient is positioned with legs and trunk moved toward the side of the low ASIS. This locks the lumbar spine so that the mobilization effect will be primarily at the sacroiliac joint. The athletic trainer stands on the side away from the low ASIS and rotates the patient's trunk toward the athletic trainer. The patient is

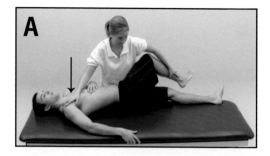

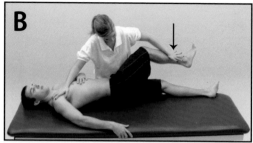

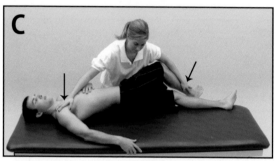

Figure 24-59. Sacroiliac stretch, position 1. (A) Starting position; (B) position for isometric resistance; (C) stretch position.

instructed to breathe and relax as the athletic trainer overpressures the rotation to take up the slack. The lower hand contacts the low ASIS and mobilizes or manipulates the innominate into posterior rotation.[65]

The athletic trainer should also mobilize the sacroiliac joint using stretching positions 1 and 2 or the anterior–posterior sacroiliac joint rotation stretch to correct the postural asymmetry (Figures 24-59 and 24-60).[12–14,35,90]

The stretch exercise should be done two or three times a day, three or four repetitions each time, holding the stretch position for 20 to 30 seconds. Spinal segment stability exercises are used after each stretching bout (Figures 24-4 through 24-10).[68] These stretches should not be continued longer than 2 or 3 days. The spinal segmental stabilization exercises are continued to try to create the behaviors that stabilize the sacroiliac joints and strengthen the muscles that support the joint. The exercises should be progressed to include more core

Clinical Decision-Making Exercise 24-5

A physician sends a patient to the athletic training clinic with a diagnosis of low back strain. The patient has pain around the PSIS area and some restriction of range. What rehabilitation exercise plan should the athletic trainer use to help this patient?

stabilization and functional training, leading to return to sports. Corsets and pelvic stabilizing belts are also helpful during higher-level activities and/or if the patient is having problems with recurrences (Figure 24-56).[65]

Sacroiliac stretch positions 1 and 2 will help realign the patient's pelvis when he or she is having sacroiliac dysfunction. Position 1 (Figure 24-59) and position 2 (Figure 24-60) stretches can be done in both right side-lying and left side-lying positions. The starting position of the position 1 stretch is side-lying with the upper hip flexed 70 to 80 degrees and the knee flexed about 90 degrees (Figure 24-59). The patient's trunk is then rotated toward the upper side as far as is comfortable. The patient is instructed to lift the top leg into hip abduction and internal rotation, and resist the athletic trainer for 5 seconds. The patient is instructed to breathe and exhale as the athletic trainer gently overpressures the trunk rotation. The patient is then instructed to relax the hip and leg and allow the leg to drop toward the floor. As the patient relaxes, the athletic trainer applies a gentle overpressure to the foot and takes up the slack as the patient allows the hip and leg to drop further to the floor.

In the position 2 stretch (Figure 24-60), the patient is positioned on either the right or left side. The patient is side-lying with the trunk

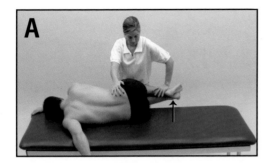

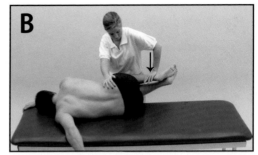

Figure 24-60. Sacroiliac stretch, position 2. (A) Starting position; (B) position for isometric resistance; (C) stretch position.

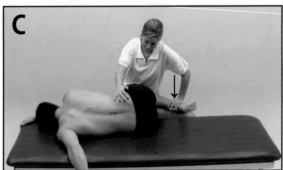

rotated so that the lower arm is behind the hip and the upper arm is able to reach off the table toward the floor. Both knees and hips are flexed to about 90 degrees. The patient's knees are supported on the athletic trainer's thigh. The athletic trainer also supports the feet in this stage of the stretch.

Before beginning the stretch component of the position 2 stretches, the athletic trainer provides isometric resistance to lifting both legs toward the ceiling, holding the contraction for 5 seconds. The patient is instructed to exhale while relaxing the legs and allowing them to drop toward the floor. The athletic trainer adds a light pressure to the feet and shoulder blade area to guide the stretch and take up slack. The athletic trainer holds the patient in a comfortable maximum stretch for 20 to 30 seconds.

REHABILITATION TECHNIQUES FOR THORACIC SPINE CONDITIONS

Injuries to the thoracic region of the spine have a much lower rate of incidence than do injuries to the cervical, lumbar, and sacral regions. This lower rate of acute injury is due primarily to the articulation of the thoracic vertebrae with the ribs, which acts to stabilize and limit motion of the vertebrae. However, there are two conditions that affect the thoracic region of the spine and thus posture that should be discussed: Scheuermann's kyphosis, and scoliosis.

Scheuermann's Kyphosis

Kyphosis refers to the natural sagittal plane curve of the thoracic spine, which normally has a forward curve of 20 to 40 degrees. If the thoracic curve is more than 40 to 50 degrees, it is considered excessive. This is an abnormal spinal deformity. There are many possible causes of excessive kyphosis, including posture, healed vertebral fractures, osteoporosis, rheumatoid arthritis, or Scheuermann's disease.[32]

Pathomechanics

Scheuermann's disease occurs during growth in the adolescent.[92] In lay terms this deformity has been described as "hunchback" posture. In this condition, the thoracic curve is usually 45 to 75 degrees. This is due to vertebral wedging of greater than 5 degrees of three or more adjacent vertebrae. In patients with Scheuermann's disease, the anterior longitudinal ligament is thickened. Tightness of this ligament may affect the growth of the vertebrae during childhood, leading to too much growth in the posterior portion of the vertebrae and too little anteriorly, which produces wedged vertebrae. Problems with the mechanics of the spine, muscle imbalances, and avascular necrosis may also play a role in the development of kyphosis. Wedging of the vertebrae in this triangular shape causes an excessive curve in the spine. In addition, Schmorl's nodes can also develop, where the disc between the affected vertebrae herniates through the bone at the bottom and/ or the top of that vertebrae's endplate.[92] Males are twice as likely to develop this type of kyphosis as females, and there also seems to be a high genetic predisposition to this disease.[32,33]

Rehabilitation Concerns

Symptoms of Scheuermann's disease generally develop around puberty, between the ages of 10 and 15 years. When the problem actually begins is hard to determine because X-rays will not show the changes until the patient is about 10 or 11 years. The disease is often discovered when parents notice the onset of poor posture, or slouching, in their child. Alternatively, the adolescent might experience fatigue and some pain in the mid back. The pain is rarely disabling or severe at this point, unless the deformity is severe. The onset of excessive kyphosis is generally slow. With Scheuermann's disease, there is generally a rigid deformity or curvature. It worsens with flexion and partially corrects with extension. Pain typically increases with time and length of the deformity. About one-third of patients with Scheuermann's kyphosis will also have scoliosis. As the patient ages, arthritic changes may appear on the X-rays.

If the kyphosis is less than 75 degrees, the deformity will usually be treated without surgery. The usual option is casting, or bracing.[34] The brace will be successful in straightening the spine only in patients who are still growing. The brace is designed to hold the spine in a straighter, upright posture. The goal of bracing is to try to "guide" the growth of the vertebrae to straighten the spine. This is thought to work by taking pressure off the anterior portion of the vertebrae, and allowing the anterior bone growth to catch up with the posterior growth. In older patients, a brace may be used to support the spine and relieve pain, but it will not actually change the curve. Though many braces are available, the Milwaukee brace is the most commonly used. The brace will include lateral pads to keep the shoulders pulled back and a chin extension. The brace is usually effective in adolescents with curves of less than 75 degrees. If the patient wears the brace 16 hours each day, there is often correction of the deformity with 2 years of treatment.[38]

Surgery for the correction of Scheuermann's kyphosis typically consists of a fusion of the abnormal vertebrae. The operation has two phases—one operation is done on the front of the spine and another on the back of the spine. A posterior-only fusion is rare because of the rigidity of the curves. In the operation, the spine is fused anteriorly and posteriorly with surgical implants.[32,38]

Rehabilitation Progression

In nonoperative cases, exercises are used in combination with a brace. Extension exercises for the upper back (Figures 24-13 through 24-20) can improve posture and prevent the spine from slouching forward. Hamstring stretches (Figure 24-28) and pelvic tilt exercises (Figure 24-33) improve posture by preventing extra lordosis in the low back. Pain should also be addressed by applying heat, cold, ultrasound, and massage treatments. Adults who have had kyphosis for many years (and the resulting low back pain from too much lordosis) benefit from postural exercises to reduce the lumbar curve, followed by core stabilization exercises to help them keep better posture.

Rehabilitation after surgery is more complex. In-hospital treatment sessions should help patients learn to move and do routine activities of daily living without putting extra strain on the back. Patients should wear a back brace or support belt. They should be cautious about overdoing activities in the first few weeks after surgery. Many patients wait up to 3 months before beginning a rehabilitation program after fusion surgery for Scheuermann's disease. Exercises should include both flexion and extension activities and should particularly concentrate on core stabilization. Treatment should last for 8 to 12 weeks. Full recovery may take up to 8 months.[34]

Scoliosis

Pathomechanics

A scoliosis is an abnormal curve that occurs in the coronal or frontal plane in the thoracic spine or in the lumbar spine, or in both regions simultaneously. The curves can range from as minor as 10 degrees to severe cases of more than 100 degrees. The most common type of scoliosis, called idiopathic adolescent scoliosis, is first observed and treated in childhood or adolescence at the growth spurt of puberty.[71] Idiopathic adolescent scoliosis is generally treated with a brace, or in severe cases, surgery at the end of the teenager's growth spurt.[18]

A condition called adult scoliosis develops after puberty.[9] Adult scoliosis can be the result of untreated or unrecognized childhood scoliosis, or it can actually arise during adulthood. Sometimes adult scoliosis is the result of changes in the spine due to aging and degeneration of the spine. The causes of scoliosis that begins in adulthood are usually very different from the childhood types.

The cause of scoliosis can be either functional or structural. Functional scoliosis results from extra-spinous factors such as leg length discrepancy or pelvic obliquity. This type of scoliosis corrects itself once the underlying problem is eliminated. Structural scoliosis is a fixed deformity that results from paralytic, congenital, or, most often, idiopathic conditions.[37]

Rehabilitation Concerns

Initially, the majority of cases of scoliosis are painless. Patients with scoliosis seek medical attention when they note a problem with how the back looks or some asymmetrical abnormalities including one shoulder or hip that is higher than the other and sticks out farther; a "rib hump" appears when scoliosis causes the chest to twist, causing a hump on one side of the back as the ribs stick out farther when bending forward; or, one arm hanging longer than the other because of a tilt in the upper body. As the condition progresses, back pain can develop. The deformity may cause pressure on nerves leading to weakness, numbness, loss of coordination, and pain in the lower extremities. If the chest is deformed due to the scoliosis, the lungs and heart may be affected leading to breathing problems and fatigue. Bracing is usually considered with curves between 25 and 40 degrees, particularly if the patient is still growing and the curve is likely to get bigger.[71]

Adult scoliosis has a variety of treatment options. Whenever possible, the first choice of treatment for adult scoliosis is always going to be conservative. Spinal surgery will always be the last choice of treatment because of the risks involved. Conservative treatment that is commonly recommended includes medications, exercise, and certain types of braces to support the spine. The use of a spinal brace may provide some pain relief. However, in adults, it will not cause the spine to straighten. Usually, curves of less than 40 degrees will be treated nonsurgically whereas curves over 40 degrees might be recommended for surgery.[9]

The most common reason for surgery is pain relief. Surgery will nearly always be recommended for curves above 60 degrees, as the twisting of the torso can lead to more serious lung and heart conditions. Generally, the only cases where surgery is considered are severe cases that lead to continual physical pain, difficulty in breathing, significant disfigurement, or continued progression of the curve. The goal is to first straighten the spine and then fuse the vertebrae together. Nearly all surgeries will use some type of fixation, or rods to help straighten the spine and hold the vertebrae in place while the fusion heals and becomes solid.[9,37]

Curves above 100 degrees are rare, but they can be life-threatening if the spine twists the body so much that the heart and lungs do not function properly.

Rehabilitation Progression

A well-designed exercise program can provide pain relief in many patients. Initially, the best treatment for patients having spinal fusion surgery will be walking as much as possible to regain strength and facilitate healing. The goal will be to increase walking distance each day. It is not advisable for patients to begin physical therapy sooner than 6 weeks after surgery as excessive and premature exercise may impede healing. After about 6 weeks, the patient can begin general conditioning, extremity strengthening and stretching, and learning correct body mechanics to maintain erect posture that counteracts the effects of the scoliosis. Patients are usually able to return to activities of daily living within 3 months following spinal fusion surgery. Rehabilitation after spinal fusion surgery should usually continue for about 6 months. Even after full recovery and rehabilitation from spinal fusion surgery for scoliosis, patients should avoid high-contact sports. They may pursue other activities such as tennis, hiking, and swimming.[9,38]

REHABILITATION TECHNIQUES FOR THE CERVICAL SPINE

Acute Facet Joint Lock

Pathomechanics

Acute cervical joint lock is a very common condition, more frequently called wryneck or stiff neck. The patient usually complains of pain on one side of the neck following a sudden backward bending, side bending, and/or rotation of the neck. Pain can also occur after holding the head in an unusual position over time, as when awakening from sleep. This problem can also occasionally follow exposure to a cold draft of air. There is no report of other acute trauma that could have produced the pain. This usually occurs when a small piece of synovial membrane lining the joint capsule or a meniscoid body is impinged or trapped within a facet joint in the cervical vertebrae. During inspection, there is palpable point tenderness and marked muscle guarding. The patient will report that the neck is "locked." Side bending and rotation are painful when moving in the direction opposite to the side on which there is locking. Other movements are relatively painless.[79]

Rehabilitation Progression

Various therapeutic modalities may be used to modulate pain in an attempt to break a pain-spasm-pain cycle. Joint mobilizations involving gentle traction (Figure 24-61), rotation (see Figure 16-24), and lateral bending (see Figure 16-33), first in the pain-free direction and then in the direction of pain, can help reduce the guarding. Occasionally pain will be relieved almost immediately following mobilization. If not, it may be helpful to wear a soft cervical collar to provide for comfort (Figure 24-62). This muscle guarding will generally last for 2 or 3 days as the patient progressively regains motion.

Cervical Sprain

Pathomechanics and Injury Mechanism

A cervical sprain usually results from a moderate to severe trauma. More commonly the head snaps suddenly, while unprepared. Frequently muscle strains occur with ligament sprains. A sprain of the neck can produce tears in the major supporting tissue of the anterior or posterior longitudinal ligaments, the interspinous ligament, and the supraspinous ligament. There may be palpable tenderness over the transverse and spinous processes that serve as sites of attachment for the ligaments.[93]

The sprain displays all the signs of the facet joint lock, but the movement restriction is much greater and can potentially involve more than one vertebral segment. The main difference between the two is that acute joint lock can usually be dealt with in a very short time, but a sprain will require a significantly longer period for rehabilitation. Pain may not be significant initially but always appears the day after the trauma. Pain stems from the inflammation of injured tissue and a protective muscle guarding that restricts motion.[93]

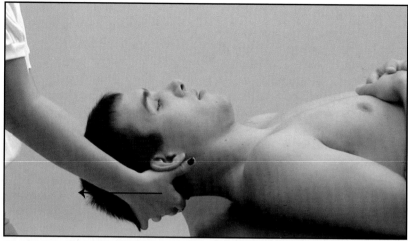

Figure 24-61. Cervical traction. With a severe injury, the physician may prescribe 2 to 3.

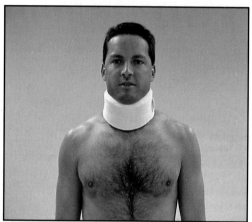

Figure 24-62. The use of a soft or hard collar can increase comfort.

Rehabilitation Progression

As soon as possible, the patient should have a physician evaluation to rule out the possibility of fracture, dislocation, disk injury, or injury to the spinal cord or nerve root. A soft cervical collar may be applied to reduce muscle guarding (Figure 24-62). Ice and electrical stimulation are used for 48 to 72 hours, while the injury is in the acute stage of healing. Days of bed rest, along with analgesics and anti-inflammatory medication should be helpful. ROM exercises through a pain-free range should begin as soon as possible, including flexion (Figure 24-63), extension (Figure 24-64), rotation (Figure 24-65), and side bending (Figure 24-66). It has been demonstrated that using early ROM exercises, instead of long periods of

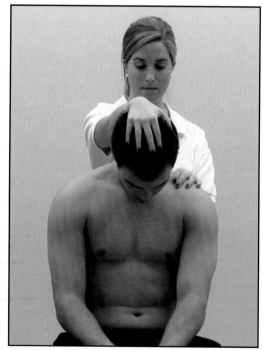

Figure 24-63. Manually assisted flexion stretching exercise.

immobility, tends to reduce the likelihood of neck hypomobility when the healing process is complete.[93] It is important to regain motion as soon as possible.

REHABILITATION PLAN

TREATMENT PROTOCOL TO CORRECT SACROILIAC DYSFUNCTION

Injury situation: 47-year-old male was crossing an intersection when he stepped off the curb onto his left foot and misjudged the height. He felt immediate sharp pain in his low back. He was referred to physical therapy for evaluation and treatment. The patient complained of mild pain and a stiff-tight feeling in his left groin area, with hip flexion and adduction increasing his discomfort. His previous medical history was unremarkable for hip, sacroiliac, or muscle problems, and he was in excellent physical condition with no other injuries at this time.

Functionally, the patient walked with a reduced stride length on the left, which produced a mild limp. Walking produced some mild left groin pain, and stair climbing increased this pain in his left groin. ROM was assessed. Lumbar spine range was full in all ranges, but side-bending left and backward bending created pain in the left sacroiliac region. Holding the backward bent position created some left groin pain similar in nature to the pain that occurred initially. Passive hip ROM was full in all ranges, with mild groin pain provoked on the end range of flexion, abduction, and internal rotation. On manual muscle test, hip flexion and abduction were strong but produced pain in the left groin similar in nature to the presenting pain. Right and left straight-leg raise tests were positive for left groin pain. Bilateral knees-to-chest test was full-range and painless, as were the stress test of iliac approximation, iliac rotation, and posterior–anterior spring test. On palpation, there was mild tenderness along the left sacroiliac joint and over the left gluteus medius just lateral to the PSIS. The hip abductors, hip flexors, and hamstring muscles were non-tender but had increased tone.

PHASE ONE: Acute Phase

GOALS: Modulate the pain, stretch, and strengthen the sacroiliac joint to return them to a more symmetric position.

Estimated length of time (ELT): Days 1 to 3 The patient was treated with stretching to bring his sacroiliac joints into symmetric positions. Spinal segment stabilization was initiated along with beginning core stabilization exercises (hip-lift bridges, isometric hip adduction ball squeezes). The left groin and sacroiliac area were treated with ice. The patient was instructed to repeat stretching and the strengthening exercises three times a day. He was also given analgesic medication to make him more comfortable.

On day 2, stretching was continued, and the stretching exercise load was increased by adding repetitions. A stretching program was begun for the hip abductors, hip internal rotators, hip flexors, and hamstrings. His usual weight-lifting session was modified to a non-weight-bearing program. His conditioning workout was done on the exercise bike and in the pool. Hot packs were applied to the adductor area preliminary to the exercise and stretching programs. The sacroiliac area was treated with ice and electrical stimulation at a moderate sensory intensity.

On day 3, stretching was discontinued. Strengthening was increased with the addition of elastic resistance to hip abduction and adduction. Functional exercises were initiated, including line walking, mini-squats, and side shuffle with tubing resistance. Modalities remained the same.

PHASE TWO: Intermediate Phase

GOALS: Increase spinal segment awareness, core stabilization strength, return to functional exercises, and return to practice and play status.

Estimated length of time (ELT): Day 4 to 7 Pain modalities were continued. Stretching exercises to the left hip abductors, flexors, and internal rotators were continued. Strengthening exercises continued with increased repetitions, resistance, and difficulty. Hot packs and electrical stimulation were continued, as were the spinal segment and core stabilization exercises.

PHASE THREE Advanced Phase

GOALS: Maintain spinal segment strength, increase core strength, and return to normal exercise routines.

Estimated Length of Time (ELT): Day 8 to 6 weeks Post Injury Pain modalities should be used if needed. Tight muscle groups should continue to be stretched two or three times a day. Strengthening routines should become more challenging but not more time-consuming.

Criteria for Return to Function

The patient demonstrates that he can perform functional activities and activities of daily living with no noticeable compensatory movements.

However, it is critical to understand that a sprain, particularly one that involves a complete ligament tear, causes hypermobility. Thus strengthening exercises (Figures 24-67 to 24-70) along with stabilization exercises (Figures 24-71 and 24-72) should also be incorporated into the rehabilitation program.[93] Mechanical traction may also be prescribed to relieve pain and muscle guarding (Figures 24-71 and 24-72).

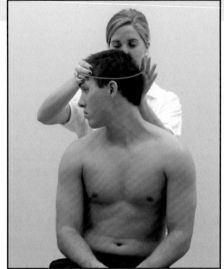

Figure 24-65. Manually assisted rotation stretching exercise.

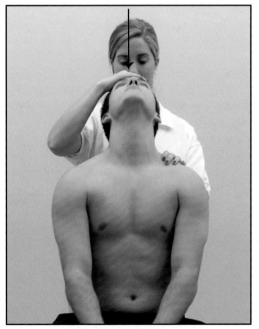

Figure 24-64. Manually assisted extension stretching exercise.

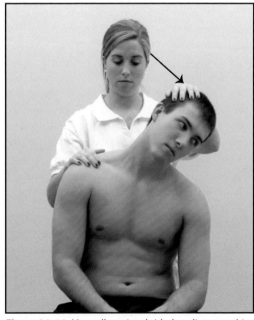

Figure 24-66. Manually assisted side-bending stretching exercise.

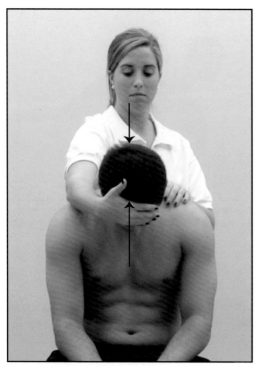

Figure 24-67. Manually resisted flexion strengthening exercise.

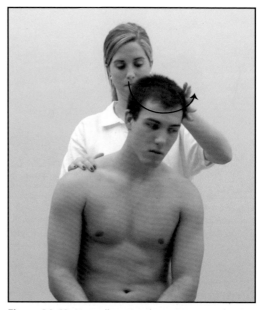

Figure 24-69. Manually resisted rotation strengthening exercise.

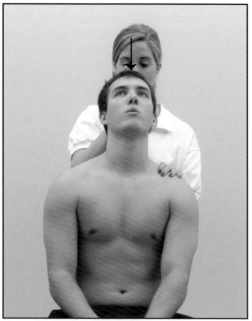

Figure 24-68. Manually resisted extension strengthening exercise.

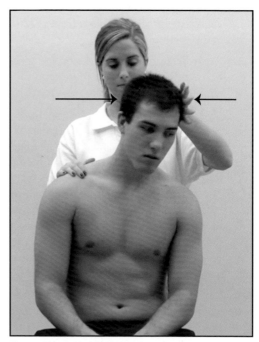

Figure 24-70. Manually resisted side-bending strengthening exercise.

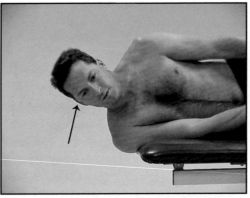

Figure 24-71. Gravity-resisted cervical stabilization exercise done on a treatment table with the head maintaining a static position. May be done side-lying (right and left), prone, and supine.

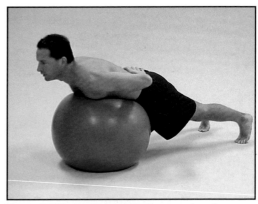

Figure 24-72. Cervical stabilization exercises done on a Swiss ball.

Summary

1. The low back pain that patients most often experience is an acute, painful experience of relatively short duration that seldom causes significant time loss from practice or competition.

2. Regardless of the diagnosis or the specificity of the diagnosis, a thorough evaluation of the patient's back pain is critical to good care.

3. Back rehabilitation may be classified as a two-stage approach. Stage I (acute stage) treatment consists mainly of the modality treatment and pain-relieving exercises. Stage II treatment involves treating patients with a reinjury or exacerbation of a previous problem. In patients meeting the clinical prediction rule for being included in a manipulation treatment group, spinal manipulation should be initiated early in Stage I.

4. Segmental spinal stabilization and core exercise should be included in the exercise plan of every patient with back pain.

5. The types of exercises that may be included in the initial pain management phase include the following: lateral shift corrections, extension exercises, flexion exercises, mobilization exercises, and myofascial stretching exercises.

6. It is suggested that the athletic trainer use an eclectic approach to the selection of exercises, mixing the various protocols described according to the findings of the patient's evaluation.

7. Specific goals and exercises included in stage II should address which structures to stretch, which structures to strengthen, incorporating segmental spinal stabilization into the patient's daily life and exercise routine, and which movements need a motor learning approach to control faulty mechanics.

8. The rehabilitation program should include functional training that may be divided into basic and advanced phases.

9. Back pain can result from one or a combination of the following problems: muscle strain, piriformis muscle or quadratus lumborum myofascial pain or strain, myofascial trigger points, lumbar facet joint sprains, hypermobility syndromes, disk-related back problems, or sacroiliac joint dysfunction.

10. Cervical pain can result from muscle strains, acute cervical joint lock, ligament sprains, and various other problems.

References

1. Adams, M.A., S. May, B.J.C. Freeman, H.P. Morrison, and P. Dolan. 2000. Effects of backward bending on lumbar intervertebral discs. *Spine; 25*(4):431–437.

2. Barr, K.P., M. Griggs, and T. Cadby. 2005. Lumbar stabilization. *Am J Phys Med Rehabil; 84*(6):473–80.

3. Beattie, P. 1992. The use of an electric approach for the treatment of low back pain: A case study. *Phys Ther; 72*(12):923–928.

4. Beffa, R., and R. Mathews. 2004. Does the adjustment cavitate the targeted joint? An investigation into the location of cavitation sounds. *J of Manipulative and Physiological Therapeutics; 27*(2):1–5.

5. Bialosky, J.E., S.Z. George, and M.D. Bishop. 2008. How spinal manipulative therapy works: Why ask why? *J Orthop Sports Phys Ther; 38*(6) 293–295.

6. Binkley, J., E. Finch, and J. Hall, et al. 1993. Diagnostic classification of patients with low back pain: Report on a survey of physical therapy experts. *Phys Ther; 73*(3):138–155.

7. Broadhurst, N. 2004. Piriformis syndrome: Correlation of muscle morphology with symptoms and signs. *Arch Phys Med Rehabil; 85*(12):2036–2039.

8. Cagnie, B., E. Vinck, A. Beerneart, and D. Cambier. 2004. How common are side effects of spinal manipulation and can these side effects be predicted? *Manual Ther; 9*:151–156.

9. Childs, J.D., T.W. Flynn, and J.M. Fritz. 2006. A perspective for considering the risks and benefits of spinal manipulation in patients with low back pain. *Manual Ther; 11*:316–320.

10. Childs, J.D., J.M. Fritz, and T.W. Flynn, et al. 2004. A clinical prediction rule to identify patients with low back pain most likely to benefit from spinal manipulation: A validation study. *Annals of Internal Med; 141*(12):920–928.

11. Cibulka, M. 1992. The treatment of the sacroiliac joint component to low back pain: A case report. *Phys Ther; 72*(12):917–922.

12. Cibulka, M., A. Delitto, and R. Koldehoff. 1988. Changes in innominate tilt after manipulation of the sacroiliac joint in patients with low back pain: An experimental study. *Phys Ther; 68*(9):1359–1370.

13. Cibulka, M., S. Rose, and A. Delitto, et al. 1986. Hamstring muscle strain treated by mobilizing the sacroiliac joint. *Phys Ther; 66*(8):1220–1223.

14. Cleland, J.A., J.M. Fritz, J.M. Whitman, J.D. Childs, and J.A. Palmer. 2006. The use of a lumbar spine manipulation technique by a physical therapist in patients who satisfy a clinical prediction rule: A case series. *J Orthop Sports Phys Ther; 36*(4)209–214.

15. Colloca, C.J., T.S. Keller, and R. Gunzburg. 2003. Neuromechanical characterization of in vivo lumbar spinal manipulation. Part II neurophysiologic response. *J of Manipulative and Physiological Therapeutics; 26*(9): 579–591.

16. Colloca, C.J., T.S. Keller, and R. Gunzberg. 2004. Biomechanical and neurophysiological responses to spinal manipulation in patients with lumbar radiculopathy. *J Manipulative & Physiological Therapeutics; 27*(1):1–15.

17. DeRosa, C., and J. Porterfield. 1992. A physical therapy model for the treatment of low back pain. *Phys Ther; 72*(4):261–272.

18. Deyo, R., A. Diehl, and M. Rosenthal. 1986. How many days of bed rest for acute low back pain? A randomized clinical trial. *N Engl J Med; 315*:1064–1070.

19. Donley, P. 1977. Rehabilitation of low back pain in patients: The 1976 Schering symposium on low back problems. *Athlet Train; 12*(2):65–69.

20. Ebenbichler, G.R., L.I. Oddsson, J. Kollmitzer, and Z. Erim. 2001. Sensory-motor control of the lower back: Implications for rehabilitation. *Med Sci Sport Exerc; 33*(11):1889–1898.

21. Erhard, R., and R. Bowling. 1979. The recognition and management of the pelvic component of low back and sciatic pain. *Am Phys Ther Assoc; 2*(3):4–13.

22. Erhard, R.E., A. Delitto, and M.T. Chibulka. 1994. Relative effectiveness of an extension program and a combined program of manipulation and flexion and extension exercise in patients with acute low back pain. *Phys Ther; 74*(12):1093–1100.

23. Flynn, T.W. 2002. Move it and move on [Editorial]. *J Orthop Sports Phys Ther; 32*(5):193.

24. Flynn, T.W. 2006. There's more than one way to manipulate a spine [Editorial]. *J Orthop Sports Phys Ther; 36*(4):199.

25. Flynn, T.W., J.D. Childs, and J.M. Fritz. 2006. The audible pop from high-velocity manipulation and outcome in individuals with low back pain. *J Manipulative & Physiological Therapeutics; 29*(1): 40–45.

26. Flynn, T., J. Fritz, and J. Whitman, et al. 2002. A clinical predication rule for classifying patients with low back pain who demonstrate short-term improvement with spinal manipulation. *Spine; 27*(24):2835–2843.

27. Freburger, J.K., and D.L. Riddle. 2001. Using published evidence to guide the examination of the sacroiliac joint region. *Phys Ther; 81*(5):1135–1143.

28. Friberg, O. 1983. Clinical symptoms and biomechanics of lumbar spine and hip joint in leg length inequality. *Spine; 8*(6):643–650.

29. Frymoyer, J. 1988. Back pain and sciatica: Medical progress. *N Engl J Med; 318*(5):291–300.

30. Grieve, G. 1976. The sacroiliac joint. *Physiotherapy; 62*:384–400.

31. Grieve, G. 1982. Lumbar instability: Congress lecture. *Physiotherapy; 68*(1):2–9.

32. Herman, M. 2003. Spondylolysis and spondylolisthesis in the child and adolescent patient. *Orthop Clin N Am; 34*(3): 461–467.

33. Hides, J.A., C.A. Richardson, and G.A. Jull. 1996. Multifidus muscle recovery is not automatic after resolution of acute, first-episode low back pain. *Spine; 21(23):2763–2769.*

34. Hodges, P.W., and C.A. Richardson. 1996. Inefficient muscular stabilization of the lumber spine associated with low back pain. *Spine; 21(22):2640–2650.*

35. Hodges, P.W., and C.A. Richardson. 1997. Contraction of the abdominal muscles associated with movement of the lower limb. *Phys Ther; 77(2):132–144.*

36. Hodges, P.W. 2002. *Science of stability: clinical application to assessment and treatment of segmental spinal stabilization for low back pain.* Course Handbook and Course Notes, September 27, Northeast Seminars, Durham, N.C.

37. Hooker, D.N. 2001. *Evaluation of the lumbar spine and sacroiliac joint: What, why, and how?* Paper presented at the N.A.T.A. National Convention, Los Angeles.

38. Huguenin, L. 2004. Myofascial trigger points: The current evidence. *Phys Ther Sport; 5(1):2–12.*

39. Jackson, C., and M. Brown. 1983. Analysis of current approaches and a practical guide to prescription of exercise. *Clin Orthop Rel Res; 179:46–54.*

40. Jull, G., and A. Moore. 2002. Are manipulative therapy approaches the same? Editorial. *Manual Ther; 7(2):63.*

41. Lederman, E. 2010. The fall of the postural-structural-biomechanical model in manual and physical therapies: Exemplified by lower back pain. *CPDO Online Journal;* 1–14. http://www.cpdo.net

42. Lewit, K., and D. Simons. 1984. Myofascial pain: Relief by postisometric relaxation. *Arch Phys Med Rehabil; 65(8):452–456.*

43. Lindstrom, I., C. Ohlund, and C. Eek, et al. 1992. The effect of graded activity on patients with subacute low back pain: A randomized prospective clinical study with an operant-conditioning behavioral approach. *Phys Ther; 72(4):279–290.*

44. MacDonald, D.A., G.L. Moseley, and P.W. Hodges. 2006. The lumbar multifidus: Does the evidence support clinical beliefs? *Manual Ther; 11:254–263.*

45. Maigne, R. 1980. Low back pain of thoracolumbar origin. *Arch Phys Med Rehabil; 61(9):391–395.*

46. Maitland, G, Hengeveld, E. 2014. Maitland's vertebral manipulation, 8th ed. London, Churchill Livingstone.

47. Mapa, B. 1980. An Australian programme for management of low back problems. *Physiotherapy; 66(4):108–111.*

48. McGrath, M. 2004. Clinical considerations of sacroiliac joint anatomy: A review of function, motion and pain. *J Osteopath Med; 7(1):16–24.*

49. McGraw, M. 1966. *The Neuro-muscular maturation of the human infant.* New York: Hafner.

50. McKenzie, R. 1972. Manual correction of sciatic scoliosis. *N Z Med J; 76(484):194–199.*

51. McKenzie, R. 2003. *The lumbar spine: Mechanical diagnosis and therapy.* New Zealand: Lower Hutt.

52. McNeely, M. 2003. A systematic review of physiotherapy for spondylolysis and spondylolisthesis. *Man Ther; 8(2):80–91.*

53. Moseley, G.L., M.K. Nicholas, and P.W. Hodges. 2004. A randomized controlled trial of intensive neurophysiology education in chronic low back pain. *The Clinical Journal of Pain; 20(5):324-330.*

54. Moseley, G.L. 2005. Is successful rehabilitation of complex regional pain syndrome due to sustained attention to the affected limb? A randomized clinical trial. *Pain; 114:54-61.*

55. Moseley, G.L., and H. Flor. 2012. Targeting Cortical Representations in the Treatment of Chronic Pain: A Review. *Neurorehabilitation and Neural Repair; 26(6):646-652.*

56. Moseley, L. 2003. Unraveling the Barriers to Reconceptualization of the Problem in Chronic Pain: The Actual and Perceived Ability of Patients and Health Professionals to Understand the Neurophysiology. *The Journal of Pain; 4(4):184-189.*

57. Moseley, G.L. 2005. Widespread brain activity during an abdominal task markedly reduced after pain physiology education: fMRI evaluation of a single patient with chronic low back pain. *Australian Journal of Physiotherapy; 51(1):49-52.*

58. Norris, C.M. 1995. Spinal stabilization. *Physiotherapy; 81(2):61–79.*

59. Norris, C.M. 1995. Spinal stabilization. *Physiotherapy; 81(3):127-146.*

60. O'Sullivan, P.B., L.T. Twomey, and G.T. Allison. 1997. Evaluation of specific stabilizing exercise in the treatment of chronic low back pain with radiologic diagnosis of spondylolysis or spondylolisthesis. *Spine; 22(24):2959-2967.*

61. Papadopoulos, E. 2004. Piriformis syndrome. *Orthopedics; 27(8):797-799.*

62. Pizzutillo, P.D., and C.D. Hummer. 1994. Nonoperative treatment for painful adolescent spondylolysis or spondylolisthesis. *J Pediatr Orthop; 9(5):538–540.*

63. Porter, R., and C. Miller. 1986. Back pain and trunk list. *Spine; 11(6): 596–600.*

64. Prather, H. 2003. Sacroiliac joint pain: Practical management. *Clin J Sport Med; 13(4):252–255.*

65. Price, D.D., L.S. Milling, I. Kirsch, A. Duff, G.H. Montgomery, and S.S. Nicholls. 1999. An analysis of factors that contribute to the magnitude of placebo analgesia in an experimental paradigm. *Pain; 83:147–156.*

66. Puentedura, E.J. and A. Louw. 2012. A neuroscience approach to managing athletes with low back pain. *Physical Therapy in Sport; (13):123-133.*

67. Rantanen, J., M. Hurme, and B. Falck, et al. 1993. The lumbar multifidus muscle five years after surgery for a lumbar intervertebral disc herniation. *Spine; 18(5):568–574.*

68. Richardson, C.A., C.J. Snijders, J.A. Hides, L. Damen, M.S. Pas, and J. Storm. 2002. The relationship between the transversus abdominis muscles, sacroiliac joint mechanics, and low back pain. *Spine; 27(4):399–405.*

69. Richardson, C., P. Hodges. 2004. *Therapeutic exercise for Lumbopelvic Stabilization: A Motor Control Approach for the Treatment and Prevention of Low Back Pain.* Sydney: Churchill Livingstone.

70. Riddle, D., and J. Freburger. 2002. Evaluation of presence of sacroiliac joint region dysfunction using a combination of tests: A multicenter intertester reliability study. *Phys Ther; 82(8):*772–781.

71. Ross, J.K., D.E. Bereznick, and S.M. McGill. 2004. Determining cavitation location during lumbar and thoracic spinal manipulation: is spinal manipulation accurate and specific? *Spine; 29(13):*1452–1457.

72. Rubinstein, S.M. 2008. Adverse events following chiropractic care for subjects with neck or low back pain: Do the benefits outweigh the risks? *J Manipulative & Physiological Therapeutics; 31(6):*461–464.

73. Saal, J. 1988. Rehabilitation of football players with lumbar spine injury. *Physician Sports Med; 16(9):*61–68.

74. Saal, J. 1988. Rehabilitation of football players with lumbar spine injury. *Physician Sports Med; 16(10):*117–125.

75. Saal, J. 1990. Dynamic muscular stabilization in the nonoperative treatment of lumbar pain syndromes. *Orthop Rev; 19(8):*691–700.

76. Saal, J.A., J.S. Saal. 1989. Nonoperative treatment of herniated lumbar intervertebral disk with radiculopathy: An outcome study. *Spine; 14(4):*431–437.

77. Santilli, V., E. Beghi, S. Finucci. 2006. Chiropractic manipulation in the treatment of acute back pain and sciatica with disc protrusion: A randomized double-blind clinical trial of active and simulated spinal manipulations. *The Spine Journal; 6:*131–137.

78. Simons, D., and J. Travell. 1998. *Myofascial pain and dysfunction: The lower extremities.* Baltimore: Lippincott Williams & Wilkins.

79. Simons, D., and J. Travell. 2005. *Myofascial pain and dysfunction: The trigger point manual.* Baltimore, Lippincott Williams & Wilkins.

80. Solomon, J. 2004. Discogenic low back pain. *Crit Rev Phys Rehabil Med; 16(3):*177–210.

81. Steiner, C., C. Staubs, and M. Ganon, et al. 1987. Piriformis syndrome: Pathogenesis, diagnosis, and treatment. *J Am Orthop Acad; 87(4):*318–323.

82. Tenhula, J., S. Rose, and A. Delitto. 1990. Association between direction of lateral lumbar shift, movement tests, and side of symptoms in patients with low back pain syndrome. *Phys Ther; 70(8):*480–486.

83. Threlkeld, A. 1992. The effects of manual therapy on connective tissue. *Phys Ther; 72(12):*893–902.

84. Twomey, L. 1992. A rationale for treatment of back pain and joint pain by manual therapy. *Phys Ther; 72(12):*885–892.

85. Verrills, P. 2004. Interventions in chronic low back pain. *Aust Fam Physician; 33(6):*421–426 and 447–448.

86. Waddell, G. 1987. Clinical assessment of lumbar impairment. *Clin Orthop Relat Res; 221:*110–120.

87. Waddell, G. 1987. A new clinical model for the treatment of low-back pain. *Spine; 12(7):*632–644.

88. Walker, J. 1992. The sacroiliac joint: A critical review. *Phys Ther; 72(12):*903–916,

89. Warren, P. 2003. Management of a patient with sacroiliac joint dysfunction: A correlation of hip range of motion asymmetry with sitting and standing postural habits. *J Man Manipulative Ther; 11(3):*153–159.

90. Walker, J. 1992. The sacroiliac joint: A critical review. *Phys Ther; 72(12):*903–916,

91. Warren, P. 2003. Management of a patient with sacroiliac joint dysfunction: A correlation of hip range of motion asymmetry with sitting and standing postural habits. *J Man Manipulative Ther; 11(3):*153–159.

92. Wood, K. 2002. Spinal deformity in the adolescent patient. *Clin Sports Medicine; 21(1):*77–92.

93. Zmurko, M. 2003. Cervical sprains, disc herniations, minor fractures, and other cervical injuries in the patient. *Clin Sports Med; 22(3):*513–521.

SOLUTIONS TO CLINICAL DECISION-MAKING EXERCISES

24-1 The patient most likely has myofascial trigger points in his piriformis. The muscle's hyper-irritability could be helped with exercise and stretch, ischemic pressure and stretch, and modalities to decrease pain and increase circulation in conjunction with exercise. The sciatic nerve should also be considered as a possible source of the discomfort. The play-and-practice decision is complex. The trigger point does not inherently compromise function. The patient's reaction to the pain and use of compensatory behaviors will dictate the activity modifications necessary to balance the patient's recovery against his need to perform in his sport.

24-2 The patient needs to be fully evaluated, and problems with flexibility and weakness should be specifically identified. Spondylolysis is considered a hypermobility problem and could be a reason the patient might experience some pain with increased activity. With good spinal segment stabilization and core strength and endurance, this patient should be capable of participation in all athletic activities without provoking this pain. If the patient does develop back pain, she should be monitored for continued problems from this spondylolysis, such as a slip of L5 on Sl creating a spondylolisthesis.

24-3   Each patient's situation should be evaluated on an individual basis. The patient, athletic trainer, physician, parents, and coach should confer on the risks associated with continued participation in crew. Potential treatments and possible surgical interventions should be discussed, focusing on how continued participation might affect the eventual recovery and long-term health of the patient. If the risks are negligible, and the primary problem is the patient's pain, the patient herself should be able to decide whether to continue for the rest of the season.

24-4   The patient should be continuing forever on a program of spinal segmental stabilization and core stabilization. Strength-training exercises should be structured so that axial loads are minimized until the disk has healed. Doing knee extension and flexion, and leg-press exercises instead of squats and lunges with weight on the shoulders, would provide a strengthening load for the legs while keeping the axial load reduced. To promote the centralization of the disk nucleus in the disk space, the patient should routinely lie flat or inverted after workouts.

24-5   The diagnosis from the physician is non-specific. The athletic trainer should first evaluate the patient to identify the specific muscle groups that are weak and painful. Appropriate exercise plans can then be established. Muscle strain diagnoses are overused in cases of low back pain. To confirm a diagnosis of muscle strain, the evaluation should demonstrate pain and tenderness over a muscle area. The pain should be reproduced by stretching the muscle and contracting the muscle.

Please see videos on the accompanying website at

www.healio.com/books/sportsmedvideos

GLOSSARY

A

abduction: The movement of a body part away from the midline of the body.

accessory motion: The movement of one articulating joint surface relative to another, involving spin, roll, glide.

active range of motion: That portion of the total range of motion through which a joint can be moved by an active muscle contraction.

acute injury: An injury with a sudden onset and short duration.

adduction: The movement of a body part toward the midline of the body.

adherence: A term used in a behavior modification setting/program for what is usually a long-term commitment to a rehabilitation program.

aerobic activity: An activity in which the intensity of the activity is low enough that a sufficient amount of oxygen can be delivered to continue activity for an indefinite period.

agonist muscle: The muscle that contracts to produce a movement.

anaerobic activity: An activity in which the intensity is so great that the demand for oxygen is greater than the body's ability to deliver oxygen.

analgesia: A loss of sensitivity to pain.

anemia: An iron deficiency.

antagonist muscle: The muscle being stretched in response to contraction of the agonist muscle.

anteversion: Tipping forward of a part as a whole, without bending.

antiemetics: Drugs used to treat nausea and vomiting arising from any of a variety of causes.

antipyretic: An agent that relieves or reduces fever.

antitussives: Drugs that suppress coughing.

aponeurosis: A thin, sheet-like tendon made of dense connective tissue.

apophysis: Bony outgrowth to which muscles attach.

arthokinematics: The physiology of joint movement. The manner in which two articulated joint surfaces move relative to one another.

arthroscopic: Technique, using an arthroscope, which uses a small camera lens, to view the inside of a body part, such as a joint.

arthrosis: A degenerative process involving destruction of cartilage, remodeling of bone, and possible secondary inflammation.

atrophy: A decrease in muscle size due to inactivity.

attenuation: A decrease in energy intensity as the ultrasound wave is transmitted through various tissues; caused by scattering and dispersion.

avulsion: Forcible tearing away of a part or a structure of a tissue from its normal attachment.

B

Bad Ragaz technique: An aquatic therapy technique where buoyancy is used for flotation purposes only.

ballistic stretching: A stretching technique in which repetitive contractions of the agonist muscle are used to produce quick stretches of the antagonist muscle.

basal metabolic rate: The rate at which calories are used for carrying on the body's vital functions and maintenance activities when the body is at rest.

biomechanics: The mechanics of biological movement, regarding forces that arise either from within or outside of the body.

buffers: Techniques that allay the symptoms of stress but do not address the problem that initially caused the stressor.

buoyant force: A force that assists motion toward the water's surface and resists submersive motion.

bursitis: Inflammation of a bursa, especially of a bursa located around a joint.

C

calisthenic exercises: Exercises that use body weight as resistance.

capacitor electrodes: Air space plates or pad electrodes that create a stronger electrical field than a magnetic field.

cardiac output: The volume of blood the heart is capable of pumping in exactly 1 minute.

cardiorespiratory endurance: The ability to persist in a physical activity requiring oxygen for physical exertion without experiencing undue fatigue.

cavitation: The formation of gas-filled bubbles that expand and compress because of ultrasonically induced pressure changes in tissue fluids.

chronic injury: A injury with long onset and long duration.

circuit training: A series of exercise stations typically consisting of various combinations of weight training, flexibility, calisthenics, and brief aerobic exercises.

closed fracture: A fracture that involves little or no displacement of bones and thus little or no soft-tissue disruption.

closed kinetic chain: A position in which at least one foot or one hand are in a weight-bearing position.

collagen: The main organic constituent of connective tissue.

compliance: A term used in the rehabilitation setting to describe a patient's attitude toward the caregiver's instructions. The patient is obedient to the physician or health caregiver's directions, the caregiver is in an authoritative position, and the treatment is short-term and usually has been prescribed.

concentric contraction: A contraction in which the muscle shortens.

continuous training: A technique that uses exercises performed at the same level of intensity for long periods.

contractile tissue: Tissue capable of contraction (ie, muscles).

coping rehearsal: A technique in which an individual visually rehearses a problem they feel may be an obstacle to reaching a goal, such as a return to competition, and envisions being successful.

core stability: The ability to transfer the vertical projection of the center of gravity around a stationary supporting base.

crepitation: A crackling sound heard and felt during the movement of broken bones or in a case of soft tissue inflammation.

cryotherapy: Cold therapy.

cubital tunnel syndrome: Entrapment of the ulnar nerve in the cubital tunnel.

cyanosis: Slightly bluish, grayish, slatelike, or dark purple discoloration of the skin caused by a lack of sufficient oxygen.

D

degeneration: Deterioration of tissue.

diapedesis: A passage of blood cells via ameboid action through the intact capillary wall.

disassociation: A technique that can be used in rehabilitation for temporary pain modulation. The individual thinks about something other than the pain, such as a sunny day at the beach or the game-winning shot at the buzzer.

distal: Farthest from center, from the midline, or from the trunk.

dorsiflexion: Bending toward the dorsum or rear of the foot; opposite of plantarflexion.

E

eccentric contraction: A contraction in which the muscle lengthens while contracting.

edema: Swelling as a result of a collection of fluid in connective tissue.

energy: Biologically, the ability to do work that is produced as body cells break down the chemical units of glucose, fats, or amino acids.

epiphysis: A cartilaginous growth region of a bone.

etiology: The science of dealing with causes of disease or trauma; or the chain of conditions that give rise to a disease or trauma.

eversion: Turning the foot outward.

exudate: An accumulation of fluid in an area.

F

fartlek: A type of workout that involves jogging at varying speeds over varying terrain.

fascia: A fibrous membrane that covers, supports, and separates muscles.

fasciotomy: An incision into the fascia to release pressure within the compartment.

fast-twitch muscle fibers: A type of muscle fiber responsible for speed or power activities such as sprinting or weight lifting.

fibrinogen: A blood plasma protein that is converted into a fibrin clot.

fibroblast: Any cell component from which fibers are developed.

fibrocartilage: A type of cartilage (eg, intervertebral disks) in which the matrix contains thick bundles of collaginous fibers.

fibroplasia: The period of scar formation that occurs during the fibroblastic-repair phase.

flexibility: The ability to move the arms, legs and trunk freely throughout a full, nonrestricted, pain-free range of motion.

foot pronation: Combined foot movement of eversion and abduction.

foot supination: Combined foot movement of inversion and abduction.

force: A push or a pull produced by the action of one object or another; measured in pounds or newtons.

force couple: Action of two forces in opposing direction about some axis of rotation.

force-velocity relationship: The faster a muscle is loaded or lengthened eccentrically, the greater the resultant force output.

frequency: With therapeutic modalities, the number of cycles per seconds that a specific exercise is performed during a training cycle.

functional progression: A series of gradual progressive activities designed to prepare an individual for return to a specific sport.

G

genu recurvatum: Hyperextension at the knee joint.

genu valgum: Knock-knee.

genu varum: Bowleg.

Golgi tendon organ (GTO): A mechanoreceptor sensitive to changes in tension of the musculotendinous unit.

H

hemorrhage: A discharge or loss of blood.

herniation: A bulging or enlargement of soft tissue.

hip pointer: A subcutaneus contusion that can cause, in most cases, a separation or tearing of the origins or insertions of the muscles. The injury is usually caused by a direct blow to the iliac crest or anterosuperior iliac spine.

hyperextension: Extreme stretching of a body part.

hypermobile: Extreme mobility of a joint.

hypertonic: Having a higher osmotic pressure than a compared solution.

hypertrophy: An increase in muscle size in response to training.

hyperventilation: Abnormally deep breathing that is prolonged, resulting in too much oxygen intake and too little carbon dioxide outtake.

hypoxia: Oxygen deficiency.

I

idiopathic: Cause of a condition is unknown.

imagery: A technique in which the athlete vividly imagines a sensory experience to practice or prepare for a situation.

infrared: The portion of the electromagnetic spectrum associated with thermal changes. Infrared wavelengths, located adjacent to the red portion of the visible light spectrum.

interosseous membrane: Connective tissue membrane between bones.

interval training: Alternating periods of relatively intense work followed by active recovery.

inversion: Turning the foot inward.

iontophoresis: A therapeutic technique that involves introducing ions into the body tissue by means of a continuous direct electrical current.

ischemia: Local anemia.

isokinetic exercise: An exercise in which the speed of movement is constant regardless of the strength of a contraction.

isometric exercise: An exercise in which the muscle contracts against resistance but does not change in length.

isotonic exercise: An exercise in which the muscle contracts against resistance and changes in length.

J

joint capsule: A saclike structure that encloses the ends of bones in a diarthrodial joint.

K

kinesthesia, kinesthesis: Sensation or feeling of movement; the awareness one has of the spatial orientation of his or her body and the relationships among its parts.

M

macrotears: Tears usually caused by acute trauma, involving significant destruction of soft tissue and resulting in clinical symptoms and function alteration.

margination: An accumulation of leukocytes on blood vessel walls at the site of an injury during early stages of inflammation.

maximal aerobic capacity: The maximal amount of oxygen an individual can use during exercise.

microstreaming: The unidirectional movement of fluids along the boundaries of cell membranes, resulting from the mechanical pressure wave in an ultrasonic field.

microtears: Soft-tissue tears that involve only minor damage and most often are associated with overuse.

muscle guarding: A protective response in muscle that occurs because of pain or fear of movement.

muscle spindle: Mechanoreceptors within skeletal muscle sensitive to changes in length and rate of length changes in muscle.

muscular endurance: The ability to perform repetitive muscular contractions against some resistance for an extended period.

muscular strength: The ability of a muscle to generate force against some resistance.

myofilaments: Small protein structures that are the contractile elements in a muscle fiber.

myositis: Inflammation or soreness of muscle tissue.

N

negative reinforcement: A punishment (verbal or a stimulus) to elicit a certain behavior or inhibit a specific behavior.

nerve entrapment: Compression of a nerve between bone or soft tissue.

neuroma: A tumor consisting mostly of nerve cells and nerve fibers.

neuromuscular control: The interaction of the nervous and muscular systems to create coordinated movement.

O

open fracture: A fracture that involves enough displacement of the fracture ends that the bone actually disrupts the cutaneous layers and breaks through the skin.

open kinetic chain: The foot and hand are not in contact with the floor or any other surfaces.

orthosis: An appliance or apparatus used in sports to support, align, prevent, or correct deformities or to improve function of a movable body part.

orthotics: Devices used to control abnormal compensatory movement of the foot.

osteochondritis dissecans: Trauma in which fragments of cartilage and underlying bone are detached from the articular surface.

osteokinematic motion: A physiological movement that results from either concentric or eccentric active muscle contraction that moves a bone or joint.

osteoporosis: A decrease in bone density.

overload: Exercising at a higher level than normal.

P

pain threshold: The amount of noxious stimulus required before pain is perceived.

painful arc: Pain that occurs at some point in the midrange but disappears as the limb passes this point in either direction.

par cours: A technique for improving cardiorespiratory endurance that basically combines continuous training and circuit training.

passive range of motion: That portion of the total range of motion through which a joint may be moved passively with no muscle contraction.

pathology: Science of the structural and functional manifestation of disease; the manifestations of disease.

pathomechanics: Mechanical forces applied to a living organism that adversely change the body's structure and function.

periosteum: A highly vascularized and innervated membrane lining the surface of bone.

phagocytosis: Destruction of injurious cells or particles by phagocytes (white blood cells).

phalanges: Bones of the fingers and toes.

phalanx: Any one of the bones of the fingers or toes.

phonophoresis: A technique in which ultrasound is used to drive a topical application of a selected medication into the tissue.

plyometric exercise: A technique of exercise that involves a rapid eccentric (lengthening) stretch of a muscle, followed immediately by a rapid concentric contraction of that muscle for the purpose of producing a forceful explosive movement.

positive reinforcement: A reward (verbal or a stimulus) that elicits a desired behavior.

posterior interosseus nerve compression: Compression of the posterior interosseus nerve within the radial tunnel, producing motor weakness with no pain.

power: The ability to generate great amounts of force against a certain resistance in a short period.

progression: Gradually increases in the level and intensity of exercise.

progressive resistance exercise: A technique that progressively strengthens muscles through a muscle contraction that overcomes some fixed resistance.

prone: To be positioned, lying down, on one's ventral surface.

proprioception: The ability to determine the position of a joint in space.

proprioceptive neuromuscular facilitation (PNF): A group of manually resisted strengthening and stretching techniques.

prothrombin: A substance that interacts with calcium to produce thrombin.

proximal: Nearest to the point of reference.

R

radial tunnel syndrome: Entrapment of the radial nerve within the radial tunnel, which produces pain with no motor weakness.

rating of perceived exertion (RPE): A technique used to subjectively rate exercise intensity on a numerical scale.

regeneration: The repair, regrowth, or restoration of a part of a tissue.

retroversion: Tilting or turning backward of a part.

S

SAID principle: When the body is subjected to stresses and overloads of varying intensities, it will gradually adapt, over time, to overcome whatever demands are placed on it.

scapulohumeral rhythm: The movement of the scapula relative to the movement of the humerus throughout a full range of abduction.

scoliosis: Lateral rotary curve of the spine.

slow-twitch muscle fibers: Muscle fibers that are resistant to fatigue and more useful in long-term, endurance activities.

somatosensation: Specialized variation of the sensory modality of touch that encompasses the sensation of joint movement (kinesthesia) and joint position (joint position sense).

speed: The ability to perform a particular movement very rapidly. It is a function of distance and time.

spondylolysis: Degeneration of the vertebrae: most commonly it is a defect in the pars interarticularis of the articular processes of the vertebrae.

sprains: Damage to a ligament that provides support to a joint.

static balance: The ability to maintain a center of gravity over a fixed base of support (unilateral or bilateral) while standing on a stable surface.

static stretching: Passively stretching a given antagonist muscle by placing it in a maximal position of stretch and holding it there for an extended time.

steadiness: The ability to keep the body as motionless as possible; this is a measurement of postural sway.

strain: The extent of deformation of tissue under loading.

stress: A positive or negative force that can disrupt the body's equilibrium.

stressor: Anything that affects the body's physiological or psychological condition, upsetting the homeostatic balance.

stroke volume: The volume of blood being pumped out of the heart with each beat.

subluxation: A partial or incomplete dislocation of an articulation.

supine: To be positioned, lying down, on one's dorsal surface.

symmetry: The ability to distribute weight evenly between both feet in an upright stance.

T

target heart rate: A specific heart rate to be achieved and maintained during exercise.

tendinitis: Inflammation of a tendon.

tenosynovitis: Inflammation of a tendon synovial sheath.

thermotherapy: Heat therapy.

torque: The moment of force applied during rotational motion (measured in foot-pounds or Newton-meters).

traction: A tension applied to a body segment which separates joint surfaces.

translation: Equality of body parts on one side of the body when compared to the opposite side.

traumatic: Pertaining to an injury or wound.

trigger point: Localized deep tenderness in a palpable firm band of muscle. When stretched, palpating finger can snap the band like a taut string, which produces local pain, a local twitch of that portion of muscle, and a jump by the patient. Sustained pressure on a trigger point reproduces the pattern of referred pain for that site.

V

valgus: Position of a body part that is bent outward.

varus: Position of a body part that is bent inward.

vasoconstriction: A decrease in the diameter of a blood vessel.

vasodilation: An increase in the diameter of a blood vessel.

volar: Referring to the palm or the sole.

volume: Regarding exercise, the total amount of work that is performed in a single workout session.

W

Wolff's law: A law that states that bone remodels itself and provides increased strength along the lines of the mechanical forces placed on it.

FINANCIAL DISCLOSURES

Ms. Jolene L. Bennett has not disclosed any relevant financial relationships.

Dr. Troy Blackburn has not disclosed any relevant financial relationships.

Dr. Michelle C. Boling has not disclosed any relevant financial relationships.

Mr. Michael Clark has not disclosed any relevant financial relationships.

Dr. Bernard DePalma has not disclosed any relevant financial relationships.

Dr. Joe Gieck has not disclosed any relevant financial relationships.

Dr. Kevin M. Guskiewicz has not disclosed any relevant financial relationships.

Mr. Doug Halverson has no financial or proprietary interest in the materials presented herein.

Dr. Elizabeth G. Hedgpeth has not disclosed any relevant financial relationships.

Mr. Christopher J. Hirth has not disclosed any relevant financial relationships.

Dr. Barbara J. Hoogenboom has not disclosed any relevant financial relationships.

Dr. Daniel N. Hooker has not disclosed any relevant financial relationships.

Mr. Stuart L. (Skip) Hunter has not disclosed any relevant financial relationships.

Dr. Scott Lephart has not disclosed any relevant financial relationships.

Ms. Nancy E. Lomax has not disclosed any relevant financial relationships.

Dr. Michael McGee has not disclosed any relevant financial relationships.

Dr. Joseph B. Myers has no financial or proprietary interest in the materials presented herein.

Dr. Darin A. Padua has not disclosed any relevant financial relationships.

Dr. William E. Prentice has not disclosed any relevant financial relationships.

Ms. Terri Jo Rucinski has not disclosed any relevant financial relationships.

Ms. Anne Marie Schneider has not disclosed any relevant financial relationships.

Mr. Rob Schneider has not disclosed any relevant financial relationships.

Mr. Patrick Sells has not disclosed any relevant financial relationships.

Dr. Steven R. Tippet has not disclosed any relevant financial relationships.

Dr. C. Buz Swanik has not disclosed any relevant financial relationships.

Mr. Michael L. Voight has not disclosed any relevant financial relationships.

Dr. Steven M. Zinder has not disclosed any relevant financial relationships.

Mr. Pete Zulia has not disclosed any relevant financial relationships.

INDEX